Field Manual for Small Animal Medicine

# Field Manual for Small Animal Medicine

*Edited by*

*Katherine Polak*

Four Paws International

*Ann Therese Kommedal*

AniCura Dyresykehus Stavanger,
AWAKE International Veterinary Outreach,
WSAVA Animal Welfare and Wellness Committee,
International Companion Animal Management Coalition

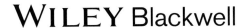

*Registered Office*
John Wiley & Sons, Inc., 111 River Street, Hoboken, NJ 07030, USA

*Editorial Office*
111 River Street, Hoboken, NJ 07030, USA

For details of our global editorial offices, customer services, and more information about Wiley products visit us at www.wiley.com.

Wiley also publishes its books in a variety of electronic formats and by print-on-demand. Some content that appears in standard print versions of this book may not be available in other formats.

*Library of Congress Cataloging-in-Publication Data*

Names: Polak, Katherine, 1984- editor. | Kommedal, Ann Therese, 1977- editor.
Title: Field manual for small animal medicine / edited by Katherine Polak,
    Ann Therese Kommedal.
Description: Hoboken, NJ : Wiley, 2018. | Includes bibliographical references
    and index. |
Identifiers: LCCN 2018000474 (print) | LCCN 2018001335 (ebook) | ISBN
    9781119243182 (pdf) | ISBN 9781119243199 (epub) | ISBN 9781119243274
    (paper)
Subjects: | MESH: Dog Diseases | Cat Diseases | Poverty Areas | Veterinary
    Medicine–methods | Sterilization, Reproductive–veterinary
Classification: LCC SF991 (ebook) | LCC SF991 .F54 2018 (print) | NLM SF 991
    | DDC 636.7/0896–dc23
LC record available at https://lccn.loc.gov/2018000474

Cover Design: Wiley
Cover Images: (Left and right images) Courtesy of Raymond Gerritsen, Soi Dog Foundation;
(Middle image) Courtesy of Katherine Polak

Set in 10/12 pt WarnockPro-Regular by Thomson Digital, Noida, India
Printed and bound in Singapore by Markono Print Media Pte Ltd

10  9  8  7  6  5  4  3  2  1

*This textbook is dedicated to the dogs and cats around the world that we share our lives with, who provide us with companionship, protection, and service; and to the veterinarians, volunteers, and caretakers who dedicate their lives to keep them safe and healthy, no matter the circumstance.*

# Table of Contents

# List of Contributors

**Valerie A.W. Benka, MS, MPP**
Alliance for Contraception in Cats & Dogs
11145 NW Old Cornelius Pass Rd., Portland
OR 97231, USA

**Lori Bierbrier, DVM**
American Society for the Prevention
of Cruelty to Animals
424 East 92nd Street, New York, NY 10128, USA

**Jennifer Bolser, DVM**
International Veterinary Consultant
Qijiayuan Diplomatic Compound
9 Jianwai Dajie, Chaoyang District
Beijing 100600
China

**Amie Burling, DVM, MPH, DACVPM, DABVP
(Shelter Medicine Practice)**
University of Missouri
College of Veterinary Medicine
900 E. Campus Dr., Columbia, MO 65211, USA

**Hillary Causanschi, VMD**
Bucks County Society for the Prevention
of Cruelty to Animals
60 Reservoir Road, Quakertown, PA 18951, USA

**Cynthia Delany, DVM**
Koret Shelter Medicine Program
University of California Davis
1 Shields Avenue, CCAH, Davis, CA 95616, USA

and

California Animal Shelter Friends
34511 State Highway 16, Woodland, CA 95695, USA

**Brian A. DiGangi, DVM, MS, DABVP
(Canine & Feline Practice, Shelter Medicine Practice)**
ASPCA
PO Box 142275, Gainesville, FL 32614, USA

**Joshua S. Eaton, VMD, DACVO**
School of Veterinary Medicine, Ocular Services
on Demand (OSOD), LLC
University of California
Davis, CA 95616, USA

**Consie von Gontard**
Florida State Animal Response Coalition
235 Apollo Beach Boulevard, Suite #311, Apollo
Beach, FL 33572, USA

**Elly Hiby, BSc, PhD**
International Companion Animal Management
(ICAM) Coalition, Chaired by IFAW
International Headquarters
290 Summer Street, Yarmouth Port, MA 02675
USA

**Lawrence Hill, DVM, DABVP**
College of Veterinary Medicine, Clinical Sciences
The Ohio State University
232 Veterinary Medical Center, 601 Vernon Tharp
St., Columbus, OH 43210, USA

**Mark R. Johnson, DVM**
Dog Capture and Care Resources
Greenbank, WA 98253
USA

**Tamara Kartal, MS**
Humane Society International
2100 L St., NW Washington, DC 20037, USA

**Patrick J. Kenny, BVSc, DipACVIM (Neurology)
DipECVN, FHEA, MRCVS**
Small Animal Specialist Hospital
Level 1, 1 Richardson Place, North Ryde
Sydney, NSW 2113, Australia

**Ann Therese Kommedal, DVM**
AniCura Dyresykehus Stavanger
AWAKE International Veterinary Outreach, Nedre
Stokkavei 12, 4023 Stavanger, Norway

**Rachael Kreisler, VMD, MSCE**
Midwestern University
5715 W. Utopia Rd., Glendale, AZ 85308, USA

**Kate Kuzminski, DVM**
Humane Society Veterinary Medical Association –
Rural Area Veterinary Services (HSVMA-RAVS)
PO Box 1589, Felton, CA 95018, USA

**Jennifer Landis, DVM**
Animal Welfare Consultant
PO Box 74621, Phoenix, AZ 85087, USA

**Natasha Lee, DVM, MSc**
Asia Animal Happiness
Jalan Kerja Ayer Lama, Ampang Jaya
Ampang, Selangor 68000, Malaysia

**I. Kati Loeffler, DVM, PhD, MRCVS**
Community Animals Program
International Fund for Animal Welfare
290 Summer Street, Yarmouth Port, MA 02675
USA

**Carolyn McKune, DVM, DACVAA**
Affiliated Veterinary Specialists
Orange Park Specialty Center
Orange Park, FL 32073, USA

**Laurie M. Millward, DVM, MS, DACVP**
Department of Veterinary Clinical Sciences
College of Veterinary Medicine
601 Vernon L. Tharp Street, Columbus, OH 43210,
USA

**Susan Monger, DVM**
International Veterinary Consultants
Austin, TX 78757, USA

**Tatiana Motta, DVM, MS**
College of Veterinary Medicine, Clinical Sciences
The Ohio State University
601 Vernon Tharp St., Columbus, OH 43210, USA

**Adam Parascandola**
Humane Society International
(Global Headquarters)
1255 23rd Street, NW, Suite 450, Washington, DC
20037, USA

**Katherine Polak, DVM, MPH, MS, DACVPM, DABVP
(Shelter Medicine Practice)**
Four Paws International
11th Floor B, Gypsum Metropolitan Tower, 539/2
Sri Ayudhaya Road, Thanon Phaya Thai
Ratchathewi, Bangkok, 10400 Thailand

**J.F. Reece, BSc, BVSc, MRCVS**
Help in Suffering
Maharani Farm
Durgapura, Jaipur 302018, Rajasthan, India

**Sheilah Robertson, BVMS (Hons), PhD, DACVAA,
DECVAA, DACAW, DECAWBM (WSEL), CVA, MRCVS**
Lap of Love Hospice
17804 N US Highway 41, Lutz, FL 33549, USA

**Andrew N. Rowan, PhD**
Humane Society International
2100 L St., NW Washington, DC 20037, USA

**Amanda Shelby, CVT, VTS (Anesthesia and Analgesia)**
Jurox Animal Health
Avon, IN 46123, USA

**Ahne Simonsen, DVM**
Humane Society Veterinary Medical Association –
Rural Area Veterinary Services (HSVMA-RAVS)
PO Box 1589, Felton, CA 95018, USA

**Emily Walters, DVM, MS, DACVP**
Antech Diagnostics
17672 Cowan
Irvine, CA 92614, USA

# Acknowledgments

This manual was born out of a passion for animal welfare, veterinary outreach, and field medicine, and it truly took a village to make it happen. Providing a resource for those working in the field was only made possible by the generous contribution of knowledge and experience from numerous authors and contributors who set aside time between clinic jobs, international travel, teaching, and otherwise hectic schedules to contribute to this text.

While publications on veterinary outreach and field medicine exist, the information has remained scattered and we want to recognize Wiley Publishing for their support in the creation of a text designed to provide a comprehensive resource to those that need it most. We also want to thank the authors for helping us gather valuable material that included both peer-reviewed information and recommendations, and anecdotes based on practical experience, particularly when published literature was lacking.

We want to acknowledge the people working tirelessly to help animals and people living in limited-resourced areas who dedicate their lives, spare time, knowledge, care, and money to help improve animal welfare, veterinary training, and contribute to One Health initiatives in communities all over the world. You inspire us every day and your work, stories, questions, and compassion was what kept us going when motivation was running low after countless hours spent in front of the computer screen at home.

A special thank you to the Koret Shelter Medicine Program at the University of California Davis and Maddie's Shelter Medicine Program at the University of Florida and our mentors who helped guide us through our shelter medicine residencies when shelter medicine was neither considered popular or trendy, and who have continued to support and encourage our quests to make the world a better place for homeless and free-roaming animals. We also appreciate the support of international animal welfare charities including Humane Society International and International Fund for Animal Welfare who encouraged us to pursue this lofty endeavor back when it was merely an idea.

While editing this book, Katherine would like to personally acknowledge the many animal welfare charities throughout Southeast Asia working under extremely challenging conditions who provided daily inspiration and ongoing advice as to what materials would be most practical to include. She'd also like to thank her family who supported her international career and for their understanding when she couldn't always make it home for Christmas. A special thanks to her mother for spending countless hours assisting with editing, and undoubtedly learning a lot about field medicine along the way. Special thanks also to her colleagues and friends for their understanding of occasional tardiness and missed deadlines resulting from the preparation of this text. To her faithful dog and cat, Mangosteen Queen (มังคุด) and Grace for getting her away from the computer and onto the beautiful beaches of Thailand. To Drs. Julie Levy, Cynda Crawford, and Brenda Griffin for setting the bar so very high and supporting their resident down a unique career path. And last but certainly not least, to Dr. Claudia Baldwin, a mentor, friend, and inspiration to her and so many others.

Tess would like to thank Kate Hurley for making her think it is realistic to try and make a difference and save the world, Pixie the rottie for walking her over fields, along beaches and atop mountains, to her amazingly supportive family, friends, and colleagues for making her laugh, love, and share a lot of great memories and bubbles (may there be many more!). To Katherine for being the perfect partner in editing even across oceans. Special thanks to shelter medicine for making her heart sing, and for bringing adventure, friends, pets, and an extended family all over the world into her life.

# 1

# Introduction to Working in the Field

*Katherine Polak[1] and Ann Therese Kommedal[2]*

[1]*Four Paws International, 11th Floor B, Gypsum Metropolitan Tower, 539/2 Sri Ayudhaya Road, Thanon Phaya Thai, Ratchathewi, Bangkok, 10400 Thailand*
[2]*AniCura Dyresykehus Stavanger, AWAKE International Veterinary Outreach, Nedre Stokkavei 12, 4023 Stavanger, Norway*

## 1.1 Overview

Veterinary outreach and field medicine projects are expanding across international boundaries at a rapid pace. Projects span from small, local initiatives to robust country-wide programs operated by international animal welfare charities. Both small- and large-scale disaster relief efforts involving animals are also becoming increasingly common. Although the majority of larger animal welfare organizations have operating manuals, guidance documents, and participant guidelines to follow, smaller groups often have few to no protocols or resources to use, other than a passion to help make a difference for the animals in a community. A Field Manual for Small Animal Medicine was born out of the editors' passion for providing a resource for those working in this exciting and challenging field.

This manual is intended to assist veterinarians, veterinary technicians, veterinary students, and those involved in animal welfare projects with improving the health and welfare of animals in remote, rural, and international contexts. The contributing authors recognize the challenges faced when executing field surgical clinics, disaster response, and treatment of free-roaming dogs and cats in the face of limited resources. Like many other textbooks, some gold-standard recommendations are provided; however, this manual strives to also provide practical and cost–effective recommendations where the ideal solution may not be available. Readers will encounter highlighted tips and tricks that suggest innovative ways to best allocate resources to provide the best animal care possible.

Practicing veterinary medicine in limited-resourced environments requires a multitude of skills and training in a variety of subjects ranging from soft tissue surgery to emergency medicine. The topics chosen for inclusion in this manual were those deemed most critical for small animal practitioners, spay/neuter surgeons, shelter administrators and program managers. On an individual animal level, treatment protocols for commonly observed canine and feline diseases, euthanasia considerations, emergency medicine, and diagnostic techniques are discussed. As fieldwork often consists of high-volume spay/neuter activities, information pertaining to humane handling and capture techniques for free-roaming animals, surgical asepsis, high-volume surgical techniques, and cost-effective anesthetic and pain management is included.

On a programmatic level, the editors also felt that it was necessary to include material on dog population management, methods of measuring programmatic success, and community engagement. Those working in limited-resourced shelters might find information on sanitation, wellness and preventive care, and emergency sheltering useful to their operations.

Although much has been published on these topics in the past decade in various journals, textbooks, and organizational manuals, the information remains scattered. The editors attempted to centralize such

*Field Manual for Small Animal Medicine*, First Edition. Edited by Katherine Polak and Ann Therese Kommedal.
© 2018 John Wiley & Sons, Inc. Published 2018 by John Wiley & Sons, Inc.

information in a readily accessible format. Although the majority of material included is derived from peer-reviewed sources, readers should be aware that some recommendations may be anecdotal and based on practical experience, particularly when published literature is lacking. Easy-to-read tables, charts, tips, and practical advice are included that can be quickly referenced in a field environment.

A total of 32 authors from around the world with extensive in-the-field experience contributed to the manual under the editorial guidance of Drs. Katherine Polak and Tess Kommedal. It is the editors' hope that it will ultimately improve the lives of animals worldwide by serving as a resource for practicing medicine in the face of limited resources. Readers should be compelled to not only take up the challenge of working in the field but also contribute to advancing and improving traditional medical and surgical standards and practices. It is likely that field veterinary medicine will continue to evolve into its own veterinary specialty one day.

## 1.2 Scope of This Manual

Although the editors appreciate that practical resources are needed for all animals, the focus of this manual is on dogs and cats. Large animals, pocket pets, and exotic animals are outside of the scope of this text. Readers may note a bias toward dogs in several of the chapters pertaining to humane animal capture and population management. In the editors' experience, most international projects tend to focus on dogs more so than cats due to the public health threat of rabies attributable to free-roaming dog populations.

## 1.3 What Constitutes "in the Field"?

Poverty and geographic isolation often make routine veterinary care inaccessible or unavailable due to a lack of resources; limitations may include medications, surgical supplies, staffing, local infrastructure, and even expertise. The expansion of veterinary medicine into rural and international settings has given rise to complex dilemmas on how to provide adequate medical care with minimal resource investment. Veterinarians may find themselves deciding

how to best utilize limited resources to improve the health and welfare of as many animals as possible. When faced with such limitations, staff must be creative and adaptive.

For the purpose of this book, the term "in the field" will refer to any under-resourced environment that challenges the ability of workers to meet the standards of care that would otherwise be achieved in a traditional clinical or shelter setting. As veterinary professionals are increasingly involved in a variety of such settings, this manual is widely applicable to different environments including service-learning international projects, rabies control programs, spay/neuter clinics in low-income communities, rural and remote areas with limited veterinary resources, and disaster and emergency settings.

## 1.4 Who Is This Manual Written for?

Field-based projects tend to attract and recruit staff with a variety of skill sets and professional backgrounds. Therefore, although veterinarians and veterinary technicians are the primary intended audience, this manual is useful to a variety of readers:

- Veterinarians
- Veterinary students
- Veterinary technicians
- Emergency responders
- Animal care staff
- Animal welfare program directors
- Lay persons/volunteers participating in veterinary service projects

## 1.5 Benefits, Opportunities, and Challenges of Working in the Field

The opportunity to make an immediate and meaningful difference in the lives of animals in need is what draws most people to field medicine. Animals living in underserved communities often suffer from a lack of preventive health care, treatment, and spay/neuter services. For some, the motivating factor is the degree of animal suffering in some communities. For others, motivation may not stem from first-hand experience but rather indirectly, through exposure to the increasing media attention of international companion animal welfare issues. Most recently, these have included the inhumane culling of dogs following a rabies outbreak in Penang, Malaysia, annual Yulin Dog Meat Festival in China, and the systematic slaughter of dogs in Sochi, Russia, before the 2014 Winter Olympic Games, to name a few [1–3].

International and rural veterinary outreach programs help bring medical services to animals that would otherwise likely never receive it. Such programs may focus on providing care to the individual animal, or work on a population-level through mass spay/neuter and vaccination activities. Fieldwork can undoubtedly also have direct effects on human health. One Health initiatives are becoming more widely advocated for by the public health and medical communities to control zoonotic diseases and promote both human and animal health. Canine rabies is a perfect example of a disease in which One Health initiatives have been successful in eradication efforts. Around the world, mass dog vaccination programs underpin the success of rabies eradication programs. In light of the fact that up to 99% of human rabies cases worldwide are the result of dog bites, in theory rabies should be an easily preventable disease through vaccination programs and education [4]. Unfortunately, as the World Health Organizations (WHO) explains, the cost of rabies post-exposure prophylaxis can be catastrophically expensive for those living in developing nations, costing approximately $40 in Africa and $49 in Asia per person [5]. There are therefore few opportunities in veterinary medicine that have a greater impact on both animal welfare and public health.

Many field-based programs focus on the spaying and neutering of free-roaming animals in an effort to reduce overpopulation. When the number of free-roaming animals is larger than a community can care for, animals frequently suffer from infectious disease, malnutrition, vehicular trauma, and inhumane culling. Although many factors contribute to animal welfare in a community, evidence suggests that targeted and sustainable spay/neuter programs are one of the more effective and humane methods for managing free-roaming dog and cat populations. In addition to improving the health of the individual animal, spay/neuter programs can also promote responsible pet ownership and community acceptance of sterilized and vaccinated free-roaming animals. As a result, the number of spay/neuter-based programs is increasing and such programs are receiving increasing attention within the veterinary community. Spay/neuter clinics are often fast-paced, challenging, and bring together diverse groups of people from around the world.

In addition to helping animals in need, those working in the field enjoy the change of pace of working in an environment other than their daily clinical practice. Scrubbing in to perform a castration under a tent in Latin America may appeal to the small animal practitioner in Kansas. Many veterinarians will use their vacation time to donate their spay/neuter services. Veterinary students may participate in service-based projects during their holiday breaks. Others may determine that such work fulfills their personal and professional goals and dedicate their careers to such pursuits.

Working in non-traditional field settings also allows veterinarians the opportunity to manage a diverse and robust caseload of medical conditions not commonly seen in private practice. Transmissible venereal tumors, canine brucellosis, canine distemper virus, and tick-borne disease are just a few conditions commonly seen in free-roaming dogs in many under-served communities.

Although field medicine offers many exciting opportunities, it also has its fair share of challenges and disadvantages. Field clinics often have limited diagnostic and therapeutic modalities and are frequently understaffed. Due to their temporary nature, such clinics rarely have a traditional clinic building to work out of; many must make do with a tent or municipal building. Staff must get creative in their approach to maximize limited resources to provide care for as many animals as possible. This requires both a special professional and personal skill set. Field clinics can be mentally as well as physically challenging. The work is hard and the hours are often long. Clinic staff must be able to work well together, quickly adjust to change, and exercise sound judgment. Clinics may be in remote areas with limited basic amenities such as running water and electricity. Potential participants of field projects should ask themselves if they could live for prolonged periods without the comfort of a fan or air-conditioning, eat an unfamiliar diet, and tolerate extreme weather and insects.

Fieldwork can also be emotionally tolling, particularly during disaster relief. The severity of animal suffering can be great, and it is not uncommon for responders to have strong emotional reactions. Even in non-emergency situations, dogs and cats in rural and international environments frequently lack basic veterinary services leading to malnutrition and untreated chronic conditions. When working in a field environment, animals commonly present as victims of poisoning, vehicular trauma, abuse, and neglect or starvation. Responders may also be confronted with animal hoarding, which frequently results in neglect, illness and death.

There is also an increased public health risk for those involved in field projects as dogs and cats can serve as competent vectors of zoonotic diseases. Depending on the location, many animals in field environments will be unvaccinated and have a high parasite burden. Rabies is an important consideration as well when working in the field, and all staff in contact with animals should be up-to-date on their rabies vaccinations. Traditional methods of handling animals are also often more challenging than in private practice settings. Patients are often fractious and difficult to handle due to limited socialization or prior mistreatment by humans. Furthermore, many veterinarians in local communities have little experience with handling free-roaming dogs. All staff should receive adequate training and wear appropriate personal protective equipment. Safe and humane handling and capture techniques as described in this book are crucial for ensuring animal and human safety.

Finally, a major drawback of this type of work is that it typically pays significantly less than a traditional veterinary position in a clinic. Most people working in the field full-time work for non-profit organizations. These organizations historically offer lower salaries than jobs in the private, corporate, or government sector. Therefore, one must consider a lower pay grade than what would be considered normal back in their home country when deciding whether or not to get involved. Even U.S.-registered, non-profit organizations often compensate international staff using local salary scales in the project country.

## 1.6 A Closer Look at the Book's Content

Although veterinary professionals perform a wide range of activities from medical treatment to surgery, the editors attempted to limit the scope of the book to topics most relevant to field-based work. Therefore, only the most practical of information was included to manage the challenges met in the field. A compilation of forms, checklists, and other helpful material that can be used and adapted by the reader are included as appendices.

### 1.6.1 Stray Dog Population Management

Free-roaming dogs may suffer from a wide range of welfare issues including disease, injury, malnutrition, and abusive treatment. Misguided attempts to control free-roaming animal populations often involve cruel methods of handling, inhumane methods of killing, and poor animal shelter management. Although most field service projects focus on providing spay/neuter services to reduce the population size over time, there is no single intervention that will work for all situations. The most effective strategies are multifactorial involving public education, legislative initiatives, waste management, and spay/neuter services. This chapter provides case studies to reflect on what we are learning about global dog populations and opportunities for humane dog management programs.

### 1.6.2 Community Engagement

Community engagement is crucial for ensuring long-term sustainable solutions for animal welfare issues. Dog and cat welfare issues are complex and intertwined with community beliefs and practices. This chapter discusses methods of engagement and empowerment of community members and provides case studies of effective community engagement.

### 1.6.3 Humane Canine Handling, Capture, and Transportation

The capture, handling, and transportation of free-roaming dogs is typically required for providing medical and surgical services in the field. The World Organization for Animal Health mandates that handling, capture, and transport be conducted humanely and safely [6]. This chapter discusses effective capture techniques and transportation considerations. It also includes descriptions of how to use catching equipment and photographs for quick reference.

### 1.6.4 Operating a Spay/Neuter Clinic

Spay/neuter programs have received increased attention over the last decade in the effort to improve animal welfare by curbing the overpopulation of free-roaming cats and dogs. This chapter provides guidance on all aspects of running a spay/neuter clinic in the field from clinic setup to patient discharge. It outlines the basic standard of care that should be upheld in any field clinic, with special attention to animal identification techniques, record keeping, and clinic animal flow-through. It provides practical tips on how to increase clinic efficiency and effectiveness on a limited budget.

### 1.6.5 General Anesthesia and Analgesia

The field environment presents unique challenges when implementing safe and balanced anesthetic protocols. Animals typically present with unknown medical histories, drug availability and staffing may be limited, patients may be fractious, and field clinics often involve large numbers of animals requiring anesthesia. No matter the setting, however, a balanced anesthetic and analgesic protocol is a must. This chapter discusses effective and economical anesthetic and pain management protocols that have proved successful in the field.

### 1.6.6 Regional Anesthesia and Local Blocks

Local anesthesia can be used to reduce pain and distress during and after a surgical procedure. Techniques involving local and regional anesthesia are used quite extensively in large animals for a variety of minor and major surgical procedures, but much less so in small animal medicine. For many of our small animal patients, a combination of general and local anesthesia techniques will provide the optimal level of anesthesia during the procedure as well as improve post-operative analgesia. In this chapter, easy-to-use local and regional anesthesia techniques are described.

### 1.6.7 Non-surgical Fertility Control

Over the last decade, there has been tremendous growth in the field of non-surgical fertility control as an alternative to traditional spay/neuter surgical procedures. Many communities lack the resources

necessary to provide surgical spay/neuter services, while some may resist surgical spay/neuter practices due to cultural aversion. Non-surgical fertility control methods have the potential of being easier, faster, and less expensive than surgery. This chapter provides an overview of non-surgical techniques and case studies of how they are being used in free-roaming dog population management programs around the world.

### 1.6.8 Surgical Techniques: Spay/Neuter

Although there are many surgical techniques for performing spay/neuter procedures described in the literature, this chapter shares tried and tested techniques used by the authors. The information presented is not designed to be an all-inclusive surgery course, and it is expected that veterinarians will already have basic knowledge of surgical anatomy and technique. This chapter provides recommendations regarding instrument and suture selection, surgical knots, and time-saving techniques. Special attention is devoted to the flank approach for ovariohysterectomies. Common surgical mistakes and ways to avoid them are also discussed.

### 1.6.9 Surgical Techniques: Ancillary Procedures

Veterinarians working in the field are frequently confronted with free-roaming dogs and cats requiring amputations and enucleations due to trauma. This chapter is designed to provide practitioners with easy-to-follow descriptions of forelimb, hindlimb, and digit amputations, as well as enucleations.

### 1.6.10 Sanitation and Surgical Asepsis

Infectious disease control is challenging in most hospital settings and even more so in field clinics. Many of the patients served are unvaccinated, arrive in poor health, may be malnourished, and are highly stressed. Some will be shedding harmful pathogens, with or without any clinical signs of disease. This necessitates a plan to guard against infections and disease spread. Aseptic technique, sterile surgical instruments, and prevention of postoperative infections also need to be addressed. This chapter discusses commonly used disinfectants, how to set up a practical sanitation protocol for a facility, animal handling equipment, and surgical instruments.

### 1.6.11 Treatment Protocols

Many charitable organizations attempt to provide medical care to free-roaming dogs and cats, often with limited medical knowledge and resources. Free-roaming animals can serve as competent reservoir hosts of several zoonotic pathogens and a multitude of infectious diseases due to a lack of preventive veterinary care. Gastrointestinal parasites, dermatopathies, ectoparasites, tick-borne diseases, heartworm disease, and transmissible venereal disease (TVT) are some of the more commonly observed conditions in field patients. Effective treatment protocols for field patients must take into account the need for a condensed treatment timeline, ease of drug administration, and cost. Such protocols are especially important when rescue groups engage in international adoptions. This chapter provides practical treatment protocols and strategies for managing commonly observed diseases in free-roaming animals, while recognizing that the gold-standard treatment is often unavailable.

### 1.6.12 Diagnostic Techniques

Diagnostic testing is often underutilized in the field because of limited availability and expense. This chapter is divided into three sections, each chosen due to their clinical application in the field: point-of-care testing, microscopy, and neurological examination.

#### 1.6.12.1 Point-of-care Testing
Point-of-care tests are designed to diagnose diseases or patient immunity "bench-side" or "patient-side" with a limited investment of resources. This allows the user to save both money, time, and animal lives by rapidly identifying an infectious disease or medical condition. The focus of this section is on inexpensive and practical methods for diagnosing commonly seen diseases such as canine parvovirus and fecal parasites.

#### 1.6.12.2 Microscopy
With the assistance of a microscope, those working in the field with limited resources can practice high-quality medicine by making the best use of diagnostic specimens. This chapter outlines practical techniques for diagnostic testing in the field, focusing on the analysis of cytological samples to derive accurate diagnostic and prognostic information. Practical interpretation of skin cytology, ear cytology, blood smears, dry-mount fecal cytology, and vaginal cytology will be described to diagnose various pathological processes in dogs and cats.

#### 1.6.12.3 Neurological Examination
In the field, veterinarians tend to struggle with performing a good neurological examination, and interpreting its findings. As it is a part of the overall patient examination, it is the most portable and cost-effective diagnostic techniques we have – one that can be performed almost anywhere. A neurological examination should not be considered a "specialist procedure" but rather one that can be performed by any veterinarian as described in this section.

### 1.6.13 Emergency Medicine

Managing emergency situations in the field will tax a clinician's knowledge, experience, and judgment. Although most field clinics are designed to provide spay/neuter services, it is very likely that emergency cases will also be seen. This chapter provides an overview on how to evaluate, resuscitate, and stabilize the critical patient, as well as instructions on how to perform various lifesaving procedures including thoracocentesis, CPR, and blood transfusions.

### 1.6.14 Wellness and Preventive Care

The prevention of animal physical and emotional disease is an efficient, cost-effective, and humane approach to animal care. Wellness and preventive care should be integrated into all field spay/neuter clinics, rabies control programs, and animal shelters. For many animals, the treatment provided during field clinics may be the only veterinary care they ever receive. In this chapter, proper husbandry, vaccination, parasite prevention, nutrition, and elective sterilization are discussed.

### 1.6.15 Prevention Considerations for Common Zoonotic Diseases

A range of pathogens including viruses, bacteria, fungi, and parasites can cause zoonotic diseases. Around 60% of all human infections and 75% of all emerging infectious diseases are reported to be zoonoses [7]. For personnel handling and treating dogs and cats with unknown vaccination histories and health statuses, the risk of contracting a zoonotic disease is increased. Therefore, it is important to know how to recognize suspect animals and how to be prepared and protected should the suspicion arise. This chapter discusses some of the more common and potentially dangerous zoonotic diseases that should be considered when working in the field, with an emphasis on prevention.

### 1.6.16 Euthanasia

When working in the field, every practitioner will be faced at some point with making the difficult decision of how to handle suffering animals. When suffering cannot be appropriately addressed or when an animal presents a significant risk to human health or the safety of other animals, ending the life in a humane manner may be required. This chapter discusses euthanasia considerations in the field, provides an algorithm for guiding euthanasia decisions, and discusses recommended and unacceptable euthanasia methods.

### 1.6.17 Emergency Sheltering

Responding to large-scale cruelty cases or natural disasters often requires the sheltering of hundreds of animals with little to no notice. The many components of a temporary animal shelter are discussed including design, setup, staffing, daily operations, and demobilization. Photographs and a schematic of a temporary shelter are included.

### 1.6.18 Program Monitoring and Evaluation

Programmatic monitoring requires systematic and routine data collection. This chapter provides valid, practical, and reliable ways of assessing the impact of population management interventions both on the population and individual animal. Evaluation then uses the data collected through monitoring to answer the fundamental question, "Is this program making a difference?" The use of cost-effective measurable indicators is discussed to improve program planning and performance.

### 1.6.19 Formulary

An alphabetical formulary is included for quick-reference. A brief description of commonly used drugs, dosages, side effects, and considerations important for the clinician are included. The information included here is compiled from both the clinical experience of the editors, authors, and other textbooks as referenced in the chapter. Handy reference charts and compounding recipes are included.

## 1.7 Veterinary Oath

International veterinary oaths vary by geographic region and country. Depending on where a veterinarian graduates, many take an oath to practice veterinary medicine ethically and conscientiously for the benefit of both animals and humans. Furthermore, veterinarians swear to maintain professional standards, promote animal and public health, and relieve animal suffering. In 2010, the American Veterinary Medical Association revised the Veterinarian's Oath to emphasize the importance of animal welfare [8]. Veterinarians have a responsibility to not only protect animal health but also welfare; to not only relieve animal suffering but also prevent it.

The veterinary oath should be central to everything we do as medical professionals, guiding our decisions, and ensuring that we act in the best interests of our patients at all times. Yet many countries do not have an oath or other professional affirmation of their role in the community. In some countries with an oath, most fail to recognize the concept of animal welfare, focusing purely on the importance of relieving suffering. In 2014, the World Small Animal Veterinary Association's (WSAVA) animal welfare and wellness committee developed an international oath to highlight the importance of animal welfare and that is relevant to all veterinary practitioners:

> "As a global veterinarian, I will use my knowledge and skills for the benefit of our society through the protection of animal welfare and health, the prevention and relief of animal suffering, and the promotion of One Health.[1] I will practice my profession with dignity in a

---

1 One Health is a worldwide approach to obtain optimum human, animal, and environmental health though interdisciplinary collaboration and communication between physicians, veterinarians, and other scientific-health-related personnel.

correct and ethical manner, which includes lifelong learning to improve my professional competence" [9].

At a minimum, veterinarians must "do no harm." The best interest of the individual patient should be the first consideration in any decision on care. The health of animals, people, and the environment are inextricably connected.

In the field, dogs and cats are more likely to be free-roaming and semi-owned by multiple members of a community rather than owned by a single person. While ownership patterns may vary from that in more traditional settings, we should always strive to provide the highest level of individual animal care possible, just as if the animal was a pet living in a home.

## 1.8 Minimally Acceptable Standards of Care

Before engaging in any veterinary activity, one must have an understanding of ideal or "gold-standard" practices as well as minimum requirements. This applies to everything from equipment, facilities, staffing, medication selection, and surgical procedures. Although we can often find alternative and compromised methods to continue working in challenging situations, it is essential to know what the minimum requirements are. This will help those involved to recognize when to stop, preventing unacceptable situations for the animals and people involved.

Any attempts to provide medical care or perform surgical operations in remote areas require special attention to minimally acceptable standards to safely operate. If a program cannot maintain minimal requirements for each patient, we must re-evaluate the approach.

This manual is not meant to define the exact minimum standards of care but rather provide resources for achieving better standards of care. There are currently no universally accepted, international standards of veterinary care but we have several guiding documents that can be applied. These include the Association of Shelter Veterinarians Veterinary Medical Care Guidelines for Spay–Neuter Programs [10] and International Spay–Neuter Clinic Guidelines published by the Humane Society

Veterinary Medical Association-Rural Area Veterinary Services [11]. This manual provides guidelines based on published evidence and expert opinion that can be adapted to varying circumstances. Throughout the text practices deemed unacceptable by guidance documents are also noted.

## 1.9 Ways to Get Involved

Opportunities abound for veterinarians, veterinary technicians, students, and animal welfare enthusiasts to work in the field, effectively combining travel and veterinary service projects. For veterinary students, many veterinary colleges offer structured international externships. Several colleges such as the Ohio State University have formal institutional arrangements with foreign veterinary colleges to facilitate student externships. Student certificate programs in International Veterinary Medicine are offered by a handful of colleges, such as the University of Georgia, in an effort to familiarize students with issues and opportunities in this field. Most students, however, can find opportunities through their college's student chapter of the International Veterinary Student Association (IVSA).

For veterinarians, there are short- and long-term volunteer projects, as well as paid permanent positions. Unfortunately, there is no single centralized database for advertising international work and most projects are posted on various organizational websites. The American Veterinary Medical Association (AVMA) website offers some information on jobs, externships, and exchange opportunities at www.avma.org.

Although most involved in fieldwork tend to participate in short-term or temporary projects involving spay/neuter activities, some may decide that fieldwork is better suited to their career aspirations and choose to pursue such work on a full-time basis. For those interested in permanent work, there are positions available ranging in degree of responsibility, expertise, and job duty. Some prefer hands-on clinical work abroad or in low-income environments locally, whereas others may choose to impact the strategic direction of a nongovernmental organization at a managerial level. International positions for veterinarians, however, may be difficult to find as the U.S. lags behind other countries in the advertising of such opportunities.

Potential applicants of both volunteer and paid positions should be warned of the frequent requirement for prior international experience. This can be frustrating particularly for new graduates eager to gain experience. The reason for this requirement is usually to weed out applicants that may not adapt well to the challenges of working in the field.

For those who are not able to provide on-the-ground support, organizations are frequently in need of donations. Money, medical supplies, and expertise are always appreciated and can go a long way in limited-resourced environments. Project V.E. T.S., based out of Boulder, Colorado, accepts donated veterinary equipment and supplies and redistributes them to charities in need around the world.

## 1.10 Choosing a Project to Work with

Many get involved in fieldwork following a search of programs recruiting volunteers. Programs can vary from small, local initiatives to large-scale spay/neuter and rabies vaccination campaigns. Unfortunately, the quality of programs can vary dramatically and potential participants should research programs before committing. In the editors' opinion, the most effective programs collaborate with multiple local stakeholders including animal welfare groups, municipal agencies, non-governmental organizations, public health officials, and local veterinarians, rather than operate in a community independently. As dog and cat ecology is inextricably linked with human behavior, programs should not only focus on animals but also involve the public to have a long-lasting, positive impact on communities. Therefore, an integrated, comprehensive approach is ideal, rather than one focusing solely on the spaying and neutering of dogs and cats.

Successful programs should leave communities better equipped at dealing with their own animal populations than before. This can be achieved through collaboration with local veterinary schools, inviting local veterinarians to participate and train at the clinic site, and collaborating with local government. Such engagement helps enable communities to manage their own free-roaming animal population independently rather than relying on foreign intervention.

Participants should therefore be wary of programs focused solely on spaying and neutering animals with little engagement of the local community. Members of the local community are not only needed for long-term change but also for helping address practical, logistical issues during the clinic.

Word of mouth is often the most effective way to determine program quality. Program websites may provide a useful overview of the organizational mission and activities. Photos posted on program websites or social media can be good indicators of surgical quality and aseptic technique. Participants can also request clinic protocols ahead of time for review. Programs that are unable to provide protocols should likely be avoided. Table 1.1 lists reputable organizations that routinely invite volunteer veterinarians and technicians to participate in their international programs.

## 1.11 Cultural Considerations

There is growing recognition in the veterinary profession for improved cultural competency. Unfamiliar languages, cultural norms, and religions can challenge even the most seasoned of veterinarians. Working in the field typically involves rural and international settings that span across national, ethnic, and religious divides. Effective communication skills and cross-cultural sensitivity are essential for working in the field.

The most cited definition of cultural competency is, "a set of congruent behaviors, attitudes, and policies that come together in a system, agency, or among professionals that enables effective work in cross-cultural situations" [12]. In a nutshell, cultural competency involves understanding the culture and beliefs of the clients in the community that will be served. Developing cultural competency does not happen overnight and requires experience, exposure, and education. For those interested in learning more, Georgetown University offers the National Center for Culture Competency and the U.S. Department of Human Health Services' Office of Minority Health offers an online course in Cultural Competency Curriculum for Disaster Preparedness and Crisis Response [13].

It is imperative that those partaking in fieldwork be aware of cultural and religious differences, particularly as they pertain to animals. The human-animal bond and role cats and dogs play in the community can vary dramatically between cultures. Although in

**Table 1.1** Organizations routinely accepting volunteers for field companion animal projects.

| Organization | Description | Website |
| --- | --- | --- |
| Mission Rabies | Mission Rabies aims to eliminate rabies from the world by 2030 through the mass vaccination of dogs in rabies-endemic countries. Their primary working area is India. | www.missionrabies.com |
| Animal Balance | Animal Balance works on island nations around the world to gradually reduce the population of community dogs and cats through mass sterilization. | www.animalbalance.net |
| Worldwide Veterinary Service (WVS) | WVS veterinary teams work all over the world, providing a lifesaving resource to animal welfare charities and non-profit organizations. WVS also provides emergency response services and runs a veterinary training center in India. | www.wvs.org.uk |
| World Vets | World Vets develops, implements, and manages international veterinary and disaster relief programs. World Vets operates a veterinary field services program, disaster response program, training programs, civil–military humanitarian aid, and a veterinary supply donation program. | www.worldvets.org |
| International Veterinarians Dedicated to Animal Health (VIDAS) | VIDAS is a non-profit organization working in Mexico to combat dog and cat overpopulation through sterilization. | www.vidas.org |
| The Humane Society Veterinary Medical Association Rural Area Veterinary Services (HSVMA-RAVS) | HSVMA-RAVS combines high-quality, direct care veterinary field clinics with clinical training for future veterinary professionals to improve the health of animals in remote rural communities. With a service-learning approach, veterinary students work directly with experienced professional mentors to provide care to animals in need. | www.hsvama.org |
| The Esther Honey Foundation (EHF) | EHF established and continues to support the only veterinary clinic for the Cook Islands' thousands of companion animals. Volunteer veterinarians and technicians have traveled to the South Pacific islands to treat more than 3000 patients annually. | www.estherhoney.org |

most developed countries cats and dogs are viewed as pets and family members, in many countries these animals serve a very different purpose including guarding property, a status symbol for upper-income families, or even as food. According to some religions, dogs are ritually viewed as unclean and are often subject to culling.

In most developing countries, patterns of dog and cat ownership vary dramatically as well. Rather than having individual owners, most dogs and cats are allowed to roam outside of the house and are semi-owned by neighborhoods or groups of people. This collaborative ownership can lead to lapses in care

when no one person takes sole responsibility for the animal. This perceived lack of responsible pet ownership and human–animal bond is often met with suspicion from veterinarians accustomed to working in traditional private practices where cats and dogs are cherished companions. It is therefore important that all project participants are briefed on the role dogs and cats play in the community where they will be working.

Cultural differences may also exist regarding permissible veterinary practices. Euthanasia in some cultures is denounced, and procedures including limb amputations, ear notching, and the termination of pregnancy may be culturally inappropriate depending on the working area. Performing such procedures without appropriate consent may lead to animal abandonment or abuse.

---

**Textbox 1.1 Euthanasia in Thailand**

Most veterinarians generally accept euthanasia as a way to compassionately end an animal's life when the suffering is so great that it cannot be relieved or managed appropriately. Not all cultures share this view, however. In predominantly Buddhist countries such as Thailand, most veterinarians are compelled to allow death to take its natural course, rather than hasten it through euthanasia. Traditional Buddhist beliefs imply that dying with full awareness of the process contributes to spiritual progress in future lives. When euthanasia is not an option, veterinarians should be prepared to implement pain management protocols to alleviate animal suffering to the best of his or her abilities, if confronted with such a situation.

---

## 1.12   Stay Positive

At the end of the day, even the most excellent technical skills will be wasted if a person is perceived as rude, condescending, or disrespectful. A positive attitude is perhaps the most important determining factor for success when working in the field. As discussed earlier, fieldwork often requires working within cultures foreign to the participant. This requires open and adaptive attitudes toward change and new environments.

At a minimum, volunteer veterinarians and staff must show respect for the people in the community in which they are working. They should remember that they are guests and behave accordingly. Also, as fieldwork is rarely performed individually, participants should have a "team-player" attitude and communicate effectively with others.

## 1.13   Before you Go

When it comes to having a successful trip, good travel is the result of good planning. Included is a checklist that can be used to prepare for a safe and effective trip. Although much of this information is designed for those traveling internationally, several suggestions are applicable to domestic travel as well.

Textbox 1.3 includes a packing list written by veterinarians and veterinary technicians experienced in packing for field service projects. Of course no two travelers are the same and every destination has unique packing needs; this list is designed to be a starting point when considering what to pack for a trip.

In general, it is recommended that belongings be packed in a traveler's backpack rather than a suitcase, as smaller flights may have stricter baggage restrictions than others. The suggested packing list is designed for a 2-week trip and travelers should customize it to their needs.

## Disclaimer

Throughout the manual, authors attempted to cover a wide range of topics by assimilating materials from a variety of sources to provide readers with a practical and robust resource. Although the editors believe the material to be up-to-date and accurate, veterinary medicine is constantly evolving and clinicians should determine and verify all treatments and surgical procedures before performing them.

The material presented here is not intended to be a substitute for formal training and education. Veterinarians and technicians should only perform medical procedures within their comfort zone and in accordance to their level of training. In regards to the surgical procedures described in this manual, the methods presented are not intended to serve as the only way to perform a specific procedure but rather are suggested methods or approaches.

As we recognize that those working with limited resources must be innovative and devise compromised treatment strategies, the authors have attempted to include a variety of treatment options for varying medical conditions dependent on the resources available. One should always attempt to provide the highest level of care given the situation. Although certain products such as animal-handling equipment are mentioned in the book, the authors, editors, and publisher do not endorse specific products.

---

**Textbox 1.2 Traveler's checklist and tips to make travel easier**

☐ *If you have an American passport, visit the U.S. Department of State website for information on visa requirements and travel warnings.* Travelers should enroll in the Smart Traveler Enrollment Program (STEP), which facilitates communication between the embassy or consulate and the traveler in the event of an emergency. There is an official State Department Smart Traveler iPhone app available for mobile access to up-to-date information.

☐ *Make sure that your passport is up to date.* Many countries require your passport to be valid for at least 3 months beyond the period of travel. The U.S. Department of State website has up-to-date passport information and assistance in finding your nearest passport facility. Some countries require that passports be valid for at least 3 or 12 months after your ticketed date of return. This means that even if your passport does not expire for a few months, you will still be denied entry into a country.

☐ *Check the visa requirements for your destination.* Arranging visas can be costly and time-consuming. Some countries participating in a visa waiver program do not require citizens of reciprocating countries to pre-arrange a visa, but others may require a visa stamp in the traveler's passport beforehand.

☐ *Purchase travel insurance.* Most health insurance providers will not cover you while you are traveling abroad. Depending on your destination, you should consider purchasing a short-term policy including evacuation coverage in the unlikely event that something should happen. Frequently, travel insurance is intended to cover not only medical expenses but also trip cancellation, lost luggage, and other losses that might be incurred while traveling.

☐ *Determine driving requirements.* If you think you will be driving during your trip, you may need to obtain an International Driving Permit (IDP), which can be obtained through the American Automobile Association, Inc (AAA) or National Auto Club in the USA. Check with the embassy or consulate of the destination country to find out driver's license and insurance requirements. You should also check to see what side of the road drivers use in the destination country.

☐ *Call your cell phone company to discuss international calling plans.* Different rates may be available for calling or texting. Pre-paid calling cards can also come in handy. Be sure to also determine the access code for the country you will be visiting beforehand.

☐ *Notify your bank to let them know where and when you will be traveling.* If companies see foreign charges without receiving prior notice, they may temporarily freeze the account.

☐ *Determine the electrical standards of the country you will be visiting.* Different countries have different size electrical plugs and voltage requiring a converter or plug adapter. Items that heat up such as hair dryers may not work correctly even with a converter.

☐ *Look up the international monetary exchange rate by searching online currency converters.* Be familiar with what the foreign currency equates to in your home currency.

☐ *Be prepared to always have local currency.* Many countries do not accept credit or debit cards. Most international airport have currency exchange kiosks.

☐ *Visit the Centers for Disease Control (CDC) and WHO travelers' health pages for travel health advisories and immunization recommendations.* Immunizations against certain diseases may be required to enter some countries. Countries might also require travelers to carry an International Certificate of Vaccination (ICV), also known as a Carte Jaune or Yellow Card.

☐ *Copy key documents such as your passport and travel itinerary.* In the unfortunate event that such documents are lost are stolen, it is always a good idea to have copies of important documents that are stored separately from the originals. Such documents might include the passport photo page, visa, flight itinerary, hotel bookings, driver's license, credit cards, and health insurance information.

---

**Textbox 1.3 Sample 2-week packing list**

*Clothing*

Pack clothing that is easy to wash and fast drying. As a general rule, bring modest clothing that respects local culture.

- Two pairs lightweight capris or long pants
- Two long-sleeved shirts
- Two short-sleeved shirts
- Two tank tops or sleeveless shirts
- Five pairs of underwear
- Three pairs of socks
- One windbreaker or waterproof jacket
- One bandana
- One hat

*Shoes*

- One pair of athletic or hiking shoes
- One pair of flip flops or easily removable sandals

*Personal Items*

Unless you are packing a prescription product, most toiletries can be purchased at the destination. Remember to consider Transportation Security Administration (TSA) restrictions if you want to bring liquids and gels in a carry-on bag.

- Shampoo
- Soap
- Toothbrush
- Deodorant
- Razor
- Contact lenses and solution
- Necessary medications including motion sickness tablets, anti-diarrheals, and pain medication
- Hairbrush or comb
- Hair ties/headband
- Band aids
- Mosquito repellent
- Sunblock
- Anti-malaria drugs (if recommended by a doctor)

*Technical Gear*

- Power converters and adapters
- Camera with extra battery and memory card
- Laptop or tablet

*Other necessary items*

- Passport and necessary visa
- Copies of important documents
- Sunglasses
- Quick-drying towel
- Necessary maps, guidebooks, language guide
- Headlamp
- Notebook
- Headlamp
- Luggage lock
- Water bottle. Depending on the destination, travelers may also consider bringing a portable water purifier such as a SteriPEN® or LifeStraw®
- Wet wipes
- Backpack
- Sleeping bag (if needed)
- Ear plugs
- Fishing line. Extremely durable and can be used as a clothesline, etc.
- Inflatable travel pillow
- Eating utensils
- All-purpose tool such as Swiss Army® knife or Leatherman® (Remember to not store in a carry-on bag)

*If There Is Still Room*

- *Gifts for children.* Curious local children will inevitably visit almost every mobile clinic site. Small gifts such as pencils or treats can help engage the local community.

*Remember: Never put valuables in checked luggage and empty your wallet of unnecessary items such as credit cards that you will not be using on the trip.*

With respect to the formulary, dosages are derived from a number of professional sources. Although authors attempted to utilize the most up-to-date information available, readers should refer to the approved labeling of drugs for further guidance.

## References

1 Mok, O. (2015). Penang firm on stray dogs cull despite public outrage. Malay Mail [online]. www.themalaymailonline.com (accessed 18 February 2016).

2 Quin, A. (2015). Chinese city defends dog meat festival, despite scorn. The New York Times [online]. www.nytimes.com (accessed 16 February 2016).

3 Herszenhorn, D. (2014). Racing to save the stray dogs of Sochi. The New York Times [online]. http://www.nytimes.com (accessed 10 February 2016).

4 WHO (2013). WHO expert consultation on rabies: second report. World Health Organization [online]. http://apps.who.int./iris/handle/10665/85346 (accessed 2 February 2016).

5 WHO (2016). Rabies. World Health Organization [online]. http://www.who.int./mediacentre/factsheets/fs099/en/ (accessed 5 March 2016).

6 WHO (2010). Terrestrial animal health code 2010. World Organization for Animal Health [online]. http://web.oie.int./eng/normes/mcode/a_summry.htm (accessed 5 March 2016).

7 Taylor, L., Latham, S., and Woolhouse, M. (2001). Risk factors for human disease emergence. *Philosophical Transactions of the Royal Society, B: Biological Sciences* **356**: 983–989.

8 Nolen, S. (2010) Veterinarian's oath revised to emphasize animal welfare commitment. The American Veterinary Medical Association [online]. http://www.avma.org (accessed 07 December 2017).

9 The World Small Available Veterinary Association (2014). WSAVA veterinary oath. www.wsava.org/sites/default/files/WSAVA%20Veterinary%20Oath.pdf (accessed 5 January 2016).

10 Looney, A.L., Bohling, M.W., Bushby, P.A. et al. (2008). The Association of Shelter Veterinarians veterinary medical care guidelines for spay-neuter programs. *Journal of the American Veterinary Medical Association* **233**: 74–86.

11 Fundamentals and Standards of Small Animal Field Clinic Surgery (2011). Humane society veterinary medical association-rural area veterinary services. www.ruralareavet.org (accessed 1 February 2016).

12 Cross, T., Bazron, B., Dennis, K., and Isaacs, M. (1989). Towards a Culturally Competent System of Care, vol. I. Washington, DC: CASSP Technical Assistance Center, Georgetown University Child Development Center.

13 U.S. Department of Health and Human Services (HHS). (2000). Office of minority health. Assuring cultural competency in health care: recommendations for national standards and an outcomes-focused research agenda [online]. www.omhrc.gov (accessed 15 February 2016).

**2**

# Stray Dog Population Management

*Tamara Kartal and Andrew N. Rowan*

*Humane Society International, 2100 L St., NW Washington, DC 20037, USA*

## 2.1 Introduction

There are a number of terms such as "stray" and "owner" that are used relatively loosely when referring to dogs in developing countries. Municipal authorities commonly talk of the unregulated breeding, increasing numbers, and worsening nuisance problem caused by "stray" dogs. However, it is not at all clear how many dogs are truly "strays" nor whether or not dog populations are changing substantially. An important paper reporting on this issue was published in 2014 and indicated that over 90% of the community dogs in four communities in Bali and South Africa were "owned" [1]. Clearly, these dogs are not "owned" in the same way as a confined pet in Europe or North America will be, but treating all street dogs as unowned "strays" is problematic. In general, we recommend that such terminology not be used without better clarification and that simply referring to dogs as street dogs or "controlled/uncontrolled" dogs is preferable to use of the terms "stray" or "unowned."

This chapter does not spend much time on issues such as the above but, in the following sections, will raise a number of issues dealing with street dog management and, in some cases, suggests ways forward as animal advocates attempt to encourage a more humane approach to human–dog interactions globally.

## 2.2 Dog Population Numbers

There are several estimates of the total global dog population ranging from around 400 million to 1 billion [2] but we estimate (using a range of external sources and our own survey data) that there are 700 million dogs across the globe, an average of roughly 10 dogs for every 100 people, of which around 300 million are "street" dogs [3]. However, even a cursory examination of dog population estimates indicates that the rate of dog ownership varies over a wide range across the globe (Table 2.1). It is fairly obvious that, in a population of controlled pet dogs, the size of the dog population will depend to a very significant extent on human choices and behavior. However, it is not as obvious that the size of uncontrolled street dog populations is also very dependent on human choices and behaviors [1]. Municipal authorities commonly talk of growing dog populations and the increased problems associated with that growth when the actual relative number of dogs (in terms of dogs per 100 humans) is probably not changing substantially from year to year.

The range of street dog populations in different communities around the world is very large (variances of 500 or more). We suspect that much of the variance can most plausibly be attributed to differences in human behavior rather than variations in canine reproduction potential. Among countries with prevalent street dog populations, their magnitudes can be very different; India is estimated to have a street dog population of around 30–40 million dogs (or 3 per 100 people), whereas Sri Lanka is estimated to have around 1–2 million street dogs (5–10 per 100 people) and Bhutan has about 75,000 street dogs (10 per 100 people) [15]. By contrast, South America is estimated to have 20+ street dogs per 100 people dependent on the region (Table 2.1). Other countries

*Field Manual for Small Animal Medicine*, First Edition. Edited by Katherine Polak and Ann Therese Kommedal.
© 2018 John Wiley & Sons, Inc. Published 2018 by John Wiley & Sons, Inc.

Table 2.1 Dog populations around the globe.

| Region | Number of dogs per 100 people | Source |
|---|---|---|
| Central/Eastern Tanzania | 7.1 | Knobel et al. [4] |
| Mauritius | 20 | HSI [5] |
| Malawi – Lilongwe district | 4.7 | HSI [6] |
| Ireland | 8.5 | Euromonitor [7] |
| Italy | | |
| – owned dogs | 11.3 | Euromonitor [7] |
| – free-roaming dogs | 1.4 | Di Nardo et al. [8] |
| Sweden | 7.2 | Euromonitor [7] |
| United Kingdom | | |
| – owned dogs | 13.8 | Euromonitor [7] |
| – free-roaming dogs | 0.2 | Dogs Trust [9] |
| USA | 22.4 | AVMA [10] |
| Canada | 14.3 | Euromonitor [7] |
| Mexico – Yucatan | 29.4 urban 58.8 rural | Bolio-Gonzalez et al. [11] |
| Bolivia – Santa Cruz de la Sierra | 21.7 | Suzuki et al. [12] |
| Brazil – Sao Paulo | 25 | Goi Porto Alves et al. [13] |
| Bahamas – Marsh Harbor, Abaco | 33–36 | HSI [14] |

like the United States (22.4 dogs per 100 people) or Sweden (7.2 dogs per 100 people) have almost no street dog populations.

Dog densities are commonly reported as dogs per square kilometer, but we would argue that this is an inappropriate measure. Dogs are almost always clustered around human habitation and reporting density in terms of dogs per 100 humans (or per household) is a far better density measure and more relevant to the challenges of managing dogs in communities. We have, through numerous surveys of dog populations in India and elsewhere, observed an inverse relationship between human density (humans/km$^2$) and dogs per 100 humans.

This inverse relationship holds so far for dog populations in India (Mumbai, Haryana, Jamshedpur, and Ahmedabad), in Bangladesh (Dhaka), in the USA (looking at dog populations by state), and in Mauritius. The highest numbers of dogs per 100 humans are found in rural communities. As human density increases, the number of dogs per 100 humans tends to fall. In Haryana State, India, we designed and conducted a dog population survey in 1-km$^2$ blocks of different human densities across the state and preliminary results demonstrate this inverse relationship (Figure 2.1) [16]. Additional analyses will provide further insights into how human density and settlement type may influence dog densities and if total dog population sizes respond to a multivariate combination of both factors or if one of them is predominant.

This inverse relationship can be observed across a large range of scales of human density (40 humans/km$^2$ to 40,000 humans/km$^2$). However, in a recent study from Chile, the authors reported that dog numbers per person increased in urban areas, which is contrary to our findings [17].

## 2.3 Understanding the Evolution of Dog Management

Differentiating between dog populations can be difficult and challenging as dogs form a variety of relationships with humans. Street dogs have usually been assumed to be un-owned strays or community dogs. However, recent research shows that the percentage of street dogs being claimed by people as "owned" could be much higher than traditionally assumed. Morters et al. in 2014 reports that more than 90% of the street dogs in two villages in Bali and two townships in South Africa were "owned" – somebody in the community claimed they "owned" a particular dog or dogs [1]. This finding is very important when considering management options for street dogs in developing countries.

We are just now beginning to understand the demographics of the overall dog population globally as points on a continuum, which is the key first step to effectively plan strategic humane management programs [16].

Although the human–dog relationship differs from developed to developing countries, it appears that there is an evolution over time of human behavior from letting dogs roam freely to developing more and more control over dogs and eventually keeping them

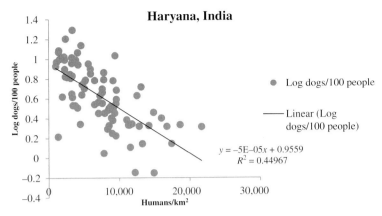

**Figure 2.1** Semi-log graph of dogs per 100 people as a function of humans/km$^2$.

almost exclusively controlled in the home or on a leash. For example, there are almost no street dogs in most of the United States today but, in the 1960s, about 25% of dogs were estimated to be street dogs and millions of unwanted dogs and cats were killed in U.S. shelters every year [18]. In a 1973 survey of shelters nationwide, The Humane Society of the United States (HSUS) estimated that 13.5 million dogs and cats (equal to 65 dogs and cats per 1,000 people) were euthanized in shelters. This was around 20% of the owned dog and cat populations at the time [19]. In the early 1970s, a flurry of articles brought together major stakeholders to address the issue of stray and unwanted companion animals in the United States [19]. Phyllis Wright developed an approach designated as LES (Legislation, Education and Sterilization), pet owners were urged to control their animals at all times, and a countrywide pet sterilization movement was launched [20]. According to data available on the Petpoint website (http://www .petpoint.com/), stray dogs now constitute about 50% of the dogs taken in by shelters, whereas shelter euthanasia rates have fallen dramatically from 65 dogs and cats euthanized per 1,000 people to less than 10 dogs and cats euthanized per 1,000 people today. It is estimated that about 2.7 million cats and dogs were euthanized in shelters in 2014 (out of an estimated pet dog and cat population around 160 million) [21]. The significant decline in shelter intakes and euthanasia is, we speculate, largely attributable to a shift in veterinary attitudes and behavior toward sterilization and its subsequent influence on pet owners. In 1970, veterinarians basically discouraged sterilization of pets, but this changed rapidly in the following decade when some shelters opened low-cost spay/neuter operations. Today, private veterinary clinics sterilize an estimated five cats and dogs for every one sterilized through a shelter or subsidy program [22].

Responsible pet ownership may appear to be out of place in communities with large numbers of roaming street dogs, but these communities will probably engage in more responsible dog management as conditions and local assumptions change. The case study below describing changes in human–dog interaction in Costa Rica is an example of what is likely to happen in many countries across the globe. These changes toward greater control of dogs can be accelerated by appropriate animal NGO programs and educational efforts. Although such programs may involve the establishment of shelters to rescue and house dogs, typically we find that some form of sterilization and release/return program is the most effective initial strategy for communities with sizable street dog populations. Animal shelters are expensive to build and manage, especially in countries where euthanasia is actively discouraged or prohibited. It is usually much more effective to concentrate on nonboarding sterilization and veterinary care programs aimed at street dogs than it is to build and maintain significant shelter operations.

## 2.4 Street Animal Management Strategies

Street dog control measures usually consist either of some form of "capture-kill" or increasingly a humane dog management program. Lethal methods have historically been the dominant approach in attempts (usually fruitless) to reduce dog populations and address dog zoonotic threats – and even today continue to be the default approach to dog control in many countries. In the late 1980s, lethal approaches were challenged on both ethical and efficacy grounds by the World Health Organization (WHO) [23,24] and others [25,26].

### 2.4.1 Lethal Methods

Aside from animal welfare issues that arise with mass killing programs, these programs may increase the risk of human rabies by killing not only unvaccinated but also vaccinated dogs. The removed dogs will then be replaced by unvaccinated dogs, which results in higher rabies risk [27]. Mass removal of dogs may, therefore, be counterproductive and the WHO reported that it found no evidence that removal of dogs had ever had a significant effect on dog population densities or the spread of rabies [28]. Since at least 2001, the WHO has not considered capture and removal of dogs to be effective in rabies control and highlights vaccination and reproductive control instead as an integral part of an effective national rabies control and elimination program [29].

In 2007, following the OIE/WHO International Conference on Rabies Control in Eurasia, a questionnaire on dog population control was sent out to all 172 OIE member countries, with the goal of identifying the national approaches to street dog population issues. Dalla Villa et al. in 2010 analyzed the responses of the 81 OIE countries (47%) that responded [30]. There was a strong positive correlation between the stage of development of the countries and inhumane street dog management and a strong negative correlation between development level and the use of sterilization as a population control tool. In Figure 2.2, the commonly used euthanasia methods among the 81 countries are indicated. Injectable barbiturate or other injectable euthanasia agents were far more common among developed countries, whereas shooting, poisoned baits, and other lethal methods were significantly more common in developing countries.

### 2.4.2 Humane Nonlethal Methods

Humane dog management programs have recorded a good track record over the past two decades in efforts to control rabies. Long-term dog population management programs, whether they include sterilization/vaccination or vaccination-only programs have had notable success in Latin America and in certain Indian cities. Ad hoc and short-term attempts to create a solution to rabies and other zoonoses have not proven to be effective even if animal welfare concerns are not considered. Humans tend to look for immediate positive feedback, but solutions to

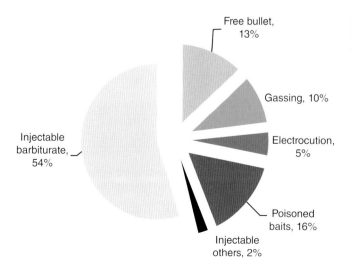

**Figure 2.2** Methods of euthanasia by dog control agencies among 81 Eurasian countries. Source: Dalla et al. [30]. Reproduced with permission of Elsevier.

Free bullet, 13%

Gassing, 10%

Electrocution, 5%

Injectable barbiturate, 54%

Poisoned baits, 16%

Injectable others, 2%

complex problems usually show their effectiveness over longer term time spans (at least 5–10 years), and this is certainly true of dog population management.

Data from programs that have been implemented for more than a decade have shown that high percentages of sterilized and vaccinated dogs alter a dog population dynamic (reducing overall street dog populations) while improving dog welfare and the public perception of dogs. Developed countries (e.g. United States) with their distinct pet culture show the positive effect of sterilization on overall dog population management and sterilization is likely to have a similar impact in developing countries. Additionally, well-controlled dog and cat populations usually provide new economic opportunities in the veterinary and pet care field.

Although some claim that there is not enough data to support the assumption that sterilization has a positive overall effect on street dogs' health and longevity, several projects anecdotally report improved canine welfare following sterilization. A study by Yoak et al. in 2014 reports that street dog sterilization improves overall dog welfare compared with similar cities that had not conducted sterilization programs [31]. In developed countries, it has been commonly assumed that sterilization produces better individual dog welfare as well, although several recent papers have begun to challenge that assumption.

Some argue that sterilization efforts are not an effective management tool for street dogs as street dogs have a low life expectancy and the high turnover of dogs will counteract sterilization efforts. Dog counts along index routes (counting dogs on the same routes at the same time of day) from the Pink City (Jaipur) between 1997 and 2013 (Figure 2.3) show that high levels of street dog sterilization are associated with a steady decline in street dog numbers. The figure looks at two trend lines for surveys carried out over two different periods of the year, from September to December (before puppies are born) and from January through April (when puppies are on the street). The two trend lines proceed virtually parallel to each other.

Reece et al. have also looked at the incidence of dog bites treated in hospitals in the Pink City [32]. They report that dog bites display a seasonal rise with the high point occurring when puppies are first born in December and January and then declining to July before the dog breeding season begins again. However, what is more interesting from the perspective of the impact of humane dog management programs is the large decline in the relative number of dog bites treated in medical facilities per 100,000 people from 1993 to 2010 (Figure 2.4).

In Ahmedabad, where a major street dog sterilization program was launched in 2006 with funding from the Municipal Corporation (45,000 street dogs out of an estimated 200,000 were sterilized in 10 months) but then came to a sudden halt because of local political infighting, the dog bites treated in municipal hospitals has risen steadily from 409 bites treated per 100,000 people in 2006 to 665 in 2011. In

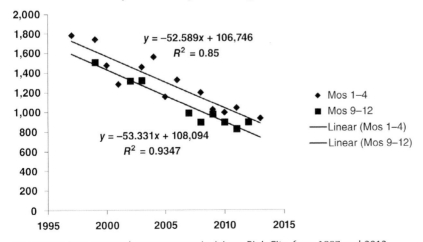

**Jaipur Pink City street dog counts**

$y = -52.589x + 106,746$
$R^2 = 0.85$

$y = -53.331x + 108,094$
$R^2 = 0.9347$

- ◆ Mos 1–4
- ■ Mos 9–12
- —— Linear (Mos 1–4)
- —— Linear (Mos 9–12)

**Figure 2.3** Dog counts along set routes in Jaipur, Pink City, from 1997 and 2013.

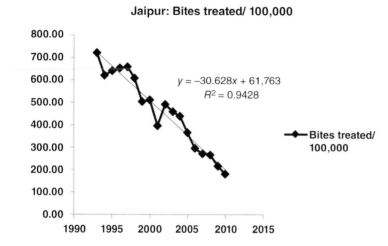

**Jaipur: Bites treated/ 100,000**

$$y = -30.628x + 61{,}763$$
$$R^2 = 0.9428$$

Bites treated/ 100,000

**Figure 2.4** Trends in dog bites treated in medical facilities in Jaipur's Pink City. Source: Courtesy of Jack Reece [32].

other words, a sustained sterilization program (Help in Suffering was sterilizing approximately 2,500 dogs a year) appears to have reduced the dog bite incidence in Jaipur, whereas the ending of the sterilization program in Ahmedabad led to an increased dog bite incidence. In India as a whole, it appears that there are somewhere between 700 and 1,000 dog bites treated by clinics and emergency rooms per 100,000 people annually. In developed countries, the rate of dog bites treated in emergency rooms per 100,000 people every year varies from around 40 to 100 (there are cases where it is much lower than this) [16].

## 2.5 The Catch–Neuter–Vaccinate– Return (CNVR) Program in Bhutan

In 2009, Humane Society International (HSI), India launched a CNVR pilot project in Thimphu, Bhutan, in an effort to help the Bhutanese government to address the nuisance concerns of street dogs including negative reactions by tourists to the presence of street dogs and virtually continuous barking at night. Bhutan is an excellent example where the stakeholders worked constructively together to implement a successful and sustainable CNVR program. In Bhutan, most dogs were free-roaming and uncontrolled, of which an estimated one-third to one-half were considered unowned street dogs.

Bhutan had tried several different approaches to address their street dog problem before partnering with HSI. An outbreak of rabies in dogs occurred in the eastern part of the country in 2005–2006, resulting in the death of one human and 106 dogs. High densities and movements of free-roaming dogs might have been responsible for the rapid spread and persistence of the infection for a longer period than expected in dogs [33]. The fear of rabies continued and, combined with the nuisance of excessive barking and litters of puppies roaming the streets, created something of a crisis. Not only did this adversely affect the local human population but it also started to hurt the country's tourism industry, an important part of Bhutan's economy. According to an unpublished report by K. Rinzin in 2012, "Efforts to control the stray dog population started in the 1970s by undertaking several measures. Dogs were once killed and poisoned but it was inhumane and strongly opposed. The impounding of dogs, which was undertaken in 2008, was a bitter experience and will not be pursued in future. The sterilization campaign which was initiated by the Department of Livestock (DOL) since 1991 was not successful to bring down the dog population to a manageable level due to poor coverage" [34].

Based on Bhutan's general attitude toward animals and the failure of traditional methods adequately to control rabies and the dog population, the Royal Government of Bhutan (RGoB) together with HSI created a CNVR pilot project in 2009 in Thimphu. Within 4 months, 2,846 dogs had been vaccinated and sterilized. In September 2009, a nationwide CNVR program was implemented and continued through June 2015. HSI's initial project goal was to sterilize around 50,000 dogs countrywide (an estimated 75% of the total dog population), covering 18 out of 20 districts. HSI and the RGoB shared the cost of the program equally. Veterinary teams rotated to designated communities that were chosen based on climate, population, and tourism statistics. In the first 9 months (the ramping up phase), 11,000 dogs were sterilized, 40% of which were "owned." By the end of the first year of the program, more than 14,000 dogs across seven districts had been sterilized and vaccinated [35].

The DOL in Bhutan created a program to build awareness and acceptance of the CNVR program in rural communities throughout the country [35]. In addition to holding meetings, local DOL staff went door-to-door to inform people before the veterinary teams arrived in a new location for their two- to three-month-long clinic. Although Norbu in 2012 notes some lack of cooperation from the public and interference with dog catching because of the Buddhist cultural views on sterilizing animals, generally the veterinary teams were accepted and even welcomed by locals [35,36]. The communities assisted by bringing dogs to a drop-off location for pickup or bringing their pet dogs to designated locations to have spay/neuter surgeries performed. Interviews showed wide acceptance of the program by residents and even thankfulness that HSI and the DOL were working together to offer a much-needed service for dogs that would help with dog safety around children.

Studies exploring public attitude, dog population estimates, and CNVR coverage were conducted throughout the program and provided valuable information to assess the value of CNVR programs and their effect on public health, animal welfare, livestock economics but also deficiencies that should be addressed in future CNVR projects. Rinzin in 2012 explored public attitudes toward the CNVR program as well as toward street dogs and found that in districts with CNVR programs, attitudes had become more positive toward street dogs because issues like biting, noise, and pollution were alleviated [34]. Fewer puppies and the overall better health of the remaining dogs was observed by Bhutanese and considered a positive outcome. Also, the notched ear of a dog indicated that it was vaccinated against rabies, resulting in less fear of street dogs. Rinzin also looked at public officials' opinions toward CNVR programs and found that it

was strongly positive especially praising the professional and efficient way HSI's CNVR programs were implemented [34].

Just 3 years after the implementation (in 2012), it was generally accepted that the project had been very successful. Rinzin reported the following public feedback on the program:

- Barking and noise caused by dogs during the night had been dramatically reduced.
- There are fewer nuisances during the breeding season.
- Most of the people know that notched dogs are neutered and vaccinated.
- There are relatively fewer puppies in the whelping seasons.
- There are lower numbers of lactating bitches.
- The CNVR program should be continued [34].

Some animal-based indicators such as body and skin conditions were also measured. Ear-notched dogs were found to be healthier than dogs that had not been involved in the CNVR program [37]. Other health problems observed included mange, pyometra, and venereal tumors [38].

By December 2011, 31,000 dogs had been sterilized, but the more accurate counts that were now possible using counts of the relative number of ear-notched versus un-notched dogs indicated that the actual dog population in the country was closer to 65,000 (or about 10 dogs per 100 people). HSI proposed that CNVR should be extended until 80% of the Bhutanese dog population was sterilized [36]. In June 2015, after sterilizing and vaccinating almost 65,000 dogs, HSI handed the CNVR program over to municipal authorities and a newly trained corps of veterinary personnel.

Overall, the sterilization rate of street dogs in Bhutan is now about 64% in urban and 44% in rural street dogs [15] and 50% overall [39]. The health of sterilized dogs in Bhutan appears to have improved. Based on an examination of 600 dogs, the body condition scores of sterilized dogs (thin = 16.1%, ideal = 68.3%, and overweight = 15.6%) was significantly higher than those of intact dogs (thin = 34.6%, ideal = 60.9%, and overweight = 4.5%) [39]. Control (keeping in homes) of dogs is slowly becoming more common and public support for humane CNVR programs continues to increase. Although 84% of survey participants in 2012 were in support of birth control programs, this number rose to 92% of respondents in 2015 [39].

Other data such as the number of human rabies cases (a slight downward trend, but there were only a few cases nationally – two to five a year) and bite incidence (which increased – possibly due to the public outreach about the importance of having bites treated) will continue to be monitored on a yearly basis. Rinzin found that treatment-seeking behaviors (e.g. visiting a hospital) following dog bites of people had increased from 84% in 2012 to 91% in 2015, and although many participants still consider street dogs a public health risk, more respondents (74%) took care of street dogs in 2015 (compared with 58% in 2012).

Since the implementation of the CNVR program, the number of human rabies deaths has declined and animal rabies cases in the main towns of the four southern Dzongkhags (where the greatest number of rabies cases occur) has declined since 2012. Rinzin in 2015 attributes this decline to the annual mass rabies vaccination campaign of both owned and stray dogs along the border towns as well as the regular CNVR campaigns implemented in these towns [39]. Additionally, a survey of dog bite victims found that people were significantly more aware of rabies and better informed about preventive measures (washing the bite wound with soap) in the Bhutan–India border areas than in the south–central areas [33].

In terms of overall population effect, in the beginning of 2011, there were 6.63 dogs per 100 people in Thimphu town. Three years later, the dog population had decreased by 10% (6.02 dogs per 100 people in September 2014).

The Bhutan project mostly involved net-catching of street dogs as necessary. However, the dogs quickly became familiar with the nets and with the catching vehicles and it became increasingly difficult to catch the dogs. In HSI's Jamshedpur (India) project (begun toward the end of the Bhutan project), we started out integrating a new technique of catching dogs via hand, exploiting the mostly friendly temperaments of the dogs in Jamshedpur (70% or so could be caught by hand). By putting community engagement and human behavior change at the center of what were usually animal-focused activities, challenges such as stress experienced during transport to and from sterilization clinics, catching techniques, limited knowledge of animal behavior science among the communities, as well as an apparent lack of compassion toward animals were successfully addressed [40]. Qualitatively, human–dog conflicts declined and the human–animal bond was strengthened [40].

## 2.6 Human Behavior Change – A Key Component

Communities appear to undergo significant changes in public attitude and public awareness concerning dog ownership after the implementation of a humane dog management program that includes high-volume sterilization. No systematic examination of this impact has yet been undertaken, but there are many anecdotal reports that it is real. In Marsh Harbor (Abaco, The Bahamas), residents reported that the street dogs were friendlier and healthier following a sterilization project [41]. On Koh Tao Island (Thailand), the proportion of residents who claimed that they owned dogs almost doubled after a sterilization project on the island was completed [42]. However, one of the most convincing datasets currently available on this topic is provided by data reported by a local shelter (AHPPA – Asociación Humanitaria para la Proteccion Animal de Costa Rica) in San Raphael (Costa Rica), a suburb of Heredia, and two surveys conducted by the World Society for the Protection of Animals (now World Animal Protection) in the region around San Jose, Costa Rica, in 2003 and 2011 [42].

### 2.6.1 Case Study: Costa Rica

The AHPPA was launched in 1991 when World Society for the Protection of Animals (WSPA) turned over a shelter with a few small cages, a leaky surgical room, and more than 100 cats and dogs to Ms. Lilian Schnog. At the time, Costa Rica's approach to animal overpopulation was to poison the animals in the streets. Dogs and cats "lucky" enough to have a home were seen as working animals. Some people believed that a hungry cat would catch more mice and a chained dog would be a better watchdog. Many of these animals were fed leftovers and if there were none, the animals remained hungry. When the animals were no longer useful or wanted by their owners, they would be left on the street. Unregulated breeding of these street animals created further problems.

Table 2.2 Animals handled/treated by AHPPA veterinarians and shelter staff.

| Year | Neutered area animals | Neutered outreach | Veterinary consultations | Animals received | Animals adopted | Animals euthanized |
|------|------|------|------|------|------|------|
| 2006 | 10,179 | 379 | 3,380 | 5,475 | 4,108 | 1,200 |
| 2007 | 10,815 | 287 | 2,878 | 5,201 | 3,758 | 1,440 |
| 2008 | 9,230 | 318 | 3,118 | 1,938 | 1,025 | 875 |
| 2009 | 7,975 | 984 | 4,733 | 2,035 | 1,798 | 227 |
| 2010 | 5,770 | 1,060 | 3,672 | 1,993 | 1,668 | 303 |
| 2011 | 4,023 | 2,301 | 4,902 | 2,322 | 1,899 | 423 |
| 2012 | 5,096 | 4,300 | 3,724 | 2,980 | 2,306 | 679 |
| 2013 | 5,517 | 5,873 | 5,013 | 2,477 | 2,325 | 152 |
| 2014 | 9,480 | 6,395 | 3,770 | 2,018 | 1,825 | 193 |
| 2015 | 10,310 | 4,701 | 11,807 | 2,405 | 2,380 | 25 |

For the first 10 years, the main challenge was simply to create an efficient and functional shelter and veterinary program. However, beginning in 2005, systematic record keeping began to document a change in how animals were being treated. One of us (ANR) first visited the shelter in 1999 and observed numerous street dogs in Heredia, the nearest major town. On a return at the beginning of 2014, no street dogs were observed. The only dogs in view were those behind fences. Table 2.2 documents changes that may have contributed to the disappearance of the street dogs.

The most dramatic trend in the above table is the decline in the number of animals euthanized by the shelter and the increase in adoptions. These trends are illustrated in Figure 2.5, and they would be a matter of considerable pride for a shelter in the United States.

The two WSPA surveys in the San Jose metro area (which includes Heredia) in 2003 and 2011 [42] complement the data reported by AHPPA (Table 2.3).

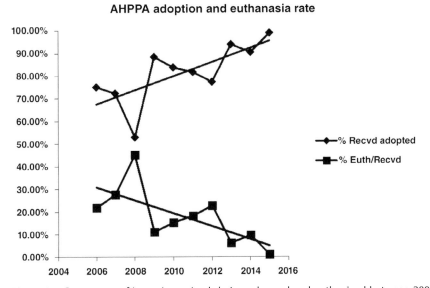

Figure 2.5 Percentage of incoming animals being rehomed and euthanized between 2006 and 2014.

Table 2.3 Results of survey question in Costa Rica.

| Question | 2003 (% respondents) | 2011 (% respondents) |
|---|---|---|
| Dogs aged 6 or higher | 17.5 | 27.6 |
| Households letting dog(s) sleep inside | 26.5 | 54.2 |
| Households permitting dogs on street without supervision | 34.0 | 17.0 |
| Households taking dog to veterinarian at least once a year | 61.0 | 80.0 |

On average, the WSPA surveys reported that around 50% of Costa Rican households "own" dogs and each owning household has an average of 1.67 dogs (for a total estimated dog population in 2011 in the metro area of 583,000). (There has been little change in the rate of dog ownership this century.) Costa Rica has approximately 20 dogs per 100 people (similar to the United States and Mexico).

The changes in human behavior in the 8 years between 2003 and 2011 reported by the WSPA surveys are large given the relatively short time involved. The changes are all in the direction of increasing control of and care for household dogs and indicate that it is possible to evolve from a culture of street dogs to a culture of controlled pets relatively quickly. Similar changes occurred in the United States in the 25 years following World War II.

## 2.7 Recommendations for Global Dog Management

There is a tendency to view dog management as a different challenge in different parts of the world. There are certainly big cultural and demographic differences that must be taken into account from one community or country to another, but there are also some constants. For example, no matter where in the world one is, there are people who love and care for dogs whether they are protected in homes or living in the streets. There are "dog mamas" in the slums of Mumbai (where people exist on less than a dollar or two a day), in Taiwan, and in Organization for Economic Co-operation and Development (OECD) member countries. Although dogs may be largely ignored in some communities, it is not difficult to elicit more caring behaviors with appropriate interventions. HSI is steadily documenting improved human–dog interactions and outcomes in communities and countries where we have initiated sterilization and vaccination campaigns. The International Fund for Animal Welfare reports similar positive changes in the communities where they have instituted community-wide humane dog management projects (K.N. Atema, personal communication). It may be that vaccination-only campaigns will achieve the same positive outcomes for dogs and humans, but vaccination-only programs may not deliver the same outcomes in terms of reduced dog turnover and reduced dog-bite incidence.

There are large gaps in our knowledge of typical human–dog interactions globally and in different communities. Improving our understanding of those interactions and the types of interventions that improve the situation for both dogs and people is an imperative need moving forward. Here are some data needs that should dispel the accepted dogma (pun intended) and unsubstantiated opinion that obscures and undermines effective public policy and dog management interventions.

A) Pre-program evaluations (including surveys – either of index routes or to estimate total dog population) should be conducted to tailor the intervention and to provide a benchmark against which progress can be evaluated. This is not an easy task. Even in developed countries, the dog population datasets available do not reliably estimate dog populations in different communities let alone produce reliable national estimates. In the United States, for example, the sources of the 9 million or so puppies annually required to maintain the national dog population has never been determined in any detail.

B) Continuous monitoring and evaluations should be used to track the development of the dog population size and demographics and inform the intervention. In the United States, a few individuals began to track the number of dogs entering shelters and being euthanized annually in the 1980s, but the first national data system to track trends in dog shelter demographics has only just been launched (see Shelteranimalscount.org).

Nonetheless, there is now sufficient data to demonstrate that there have been huge declines in the number of dogs abandoned and euthanized in shelters. In developing countries with large street dog populations and few shelters, tracking trends in dog management is even more challenging. The use of "index routes" to count dogs in Jaipur shows the type of effort that can produce useful results. It is also important to recognize that humane programs provide long-term solutions, but significant changes are usually only noticeable after several years of activity and then only if standardized data are collected. (Note: There are frequent claims that the population of street dogs in a particular community is increasing rapidly. These claims have never been supported by carefully collected data and we suspect that street dog populations are either relatively stable or in decline across the globe.)

C) High-volume sterilization programs such as CNVR, combined with educational outreach, not only affect the reproduction rate of the street animal population but also appear to enhance the human–animal relationship short and long term (e.g. dog bite rates and the number of human and canine rabies cases decline and "responsible" dog ownership leads to an increased demand for veterinary services).

D) Veterinary training and capacity building are vital components of successful and sustainable sterilization programs, but there are many unknown factors where data could help define the most effective, humane, and cost-efficient approaches. For example, it is widely assumed that the faster the surgery (up to a point), the better the outcomes for the dogs, but there is very limited data supporting this assumption. Reece et al. noted that surgical time increased as the length of incision increased, but even so, their average surgery time (11 min, 4 s) is apparently much quicker than the average reported for spays in developed countries [32]. It would be important to know a range of parameters for veterinarians involved in high-volume sterilization programs including the average surgery speed, the rate of adverse postoperative outcomes for each surgeon, as well as overall postoperative outcomes for the project as a whole. In addition, not all veterinary graduates will become skilled surgeons, and it will be important to know what metrics predict which veterinary trainees will make the best surgeons. Worldwide, the number of veterinarians being trained in high-volume sterilization surgery is increasing rapidly. For example, HSI has trained 132 veterinarians in the Philippines in high-volume sterilization and has trained many others in other parts of the world. Numerous other groups are also engaged in animal sterilization and veterinary training (e.g. Worldwide Veterinary Services in Ooty and other parts of India; the Soi Dog Foundation in Thailand; Animals Asia Foundation in China; IFAW in Africa, Latin America and Asia; Vier Pfoten in Eastern Europe; the Mayhew Home in Russia, Afghanistan and India, to pick out just a few). These training programs promise to have a long-term impact across the globe.

E) Although the prospect of sterilizing 100 million dogs (the number needed to sterilize 70% of the female street dogs globally assuming only females are sterilized) appears to be an impossible target, the resources available to tackle such a task are growing rapidly. We estimate that the funds currently being devoted to humane dog management by international animal groups is now somewhere in the range of $20–30 million (an increase from just a few million dollars at the turn of this century). This figure does not include funds devoted by local and national animal groups or by municipal and national authorities. If one considers that the global rabies burden is estimated to be $8.9 billion annually, and that approximately $2.5 billion are direct costs (postexposure treatment – $1.82 billion, dog vaccination – $155 million, and livestock losses – $550 million), it should not be difficult to persuade national and municipal authorities to increase the resources devoted to humane dog management [43]. At an average price of around $20–25 per sterilization, sterilizing 20 million dogs a year should produce significant savings in rabies costs and greatly reduce the nuisance impact of street dogs over the course of a decade.

## 2.8 Conclusion

High-volume and same-day release sterilization programs are a relatively new, cost-effective, humane (if carried out by skilled veterinary and catching staff and involving some form of post-release monitoring), and efficient way of managing street dog populations in developing countries. These programs are a successor to the sterilization programs launched in the United States in the 1970s (or the U.S. programs followed the advocacy of the Blue Cross of India in the 1960s to start sterilizing street dogs) that drove a dramatic decline in shelter euthanasia rates and to the stray/feral cat trap-neuter-return (TNR) programs in North America and Europe. This approach has the potential to change the lives of hundreds of millions of street dogs for the better over the next decades. Projects such as those described above (in Haryana, Jaipur, Costa Rica, and Bhutan) have shown that local communities can learn to catch street dogs humanely and local veterinary surgeons, if trained properly, become very skilled at sterilization because of the volume of the operations they perform. When implemented according to protocol, such surgery is minimally invasive and is accompanied by low mortality and infection rates. The rapid return of dogs to their capture sites means that dogs do not lose their community niche, they do not have to face the stress of a four-plus day stay in a shelter, and any disruption of street dog dynamics is kept to a minimum.

To deliver maximum impact, these programs must also be accompanied by a significant commitment from government bodies and assisting organizations, as well as uninterrupted and adequate financial support.

## Acknowledgment

The authors, in particular Andrew Rowan, would like to thank the entire HSI Street Animal Welfare team for its dedication and commitment to rigorously collect standardized data in programs across the world and their tireless efforts to improve the effect of HSI programs on street animal welfare and public policy. Special thanks to Companion Animal and Engagement Directors Kelly O'Meara and Rahul Sehgal and their program managers as well as the survey teams, which were led by Amit Chaudhari with advice and guidance from John D. Boone and Lex Hiby.

## References

1 Morters, M.K., McKinley, T.J., Restif, O. et al. (2014). The demography of free-roaming dog populations and applications to disease and population control. *Journal of Applied Ecology* **51** (4): 1096–1106.

2 Gompper, M.E. (2014). The dog–human–wildlife interface: assessing the scope of the problem. In: Free-Ranging Dogs and Wildlife Conservation (ed. M.E. Gompper). Oxford: Oxford University Press.

3 Rowan, A.N. (2010). Understanding the need: international panel. Fourth International Symposium on Non-Surgical Methods of Pet Population Control, Dallas, TX: Alliance for Contraception in Cats & Dogs. http://www.acc-d.org/resource-library/symposia/4th-symposium (accessed 20 October 2017).

4 Knobel, D.L., Laurenson, M.K., Kazwala, R.R. et al. (2008). A cross-sectional study of factors associated with dog ownership in Tanzania. *BMC Veterinary Research* **4**: 5.

5 Humane Society International (2013). Baseline Surveys in Mauritius for Street Dog Management. Unpublished report by Humane Society International, Washington, DC, USA.

6 Humane Society International (2013a). Baseline Survey for Street Dogs in Lilongwe, Malawi. Unpublished report by Humane Society International, Washington, DC, USA.

7 Euromonitor (2012). Pet care. http://www.euromonitor.com/pet-care.

8 Di Nardo, A., Candeloro, L., Budke, C.M., and Slater, M.R. (2007). Modelling the effect of sterilization rate on owned dog population size in Central Italy. *Preventive Veterinary Medicine* **82** (3–4): 308–313.

9 Dogs Trust (2014). Stray dogs survey 2014. https://www.dogstrust.org.uk/whats-happening/news/stray%20dogs%202014%20report.pdf (accessed 1 December 2016).

10 American Veterinary Medical Association (2012). Market Research Statistics: U.S. Pet Ownership & Demographics Sourcebook, 2007e. American Veterinary Medical Association http://www.avma.org/reference/marketstats/sourcebook.asp.

11 Bolio-Gonzalez, M.E., Rodriguez-Vivas, R.I., Sauri-Arceo, C.H. et al. (2007). Prevalence of the *Dirofilaria immitis* infection in dogs from Merida, Yucatan, Mexico. *Veterinary Parasitology* **148** (2): 166–169.

12 Suzuki, K., Pereira, J.A., Frías, L.A. et al. (2008). Rabies-vaccination coverage and profiles of the owned-dog population in Santa Cruz de la sierra, Bolivia. *Zoonoses and Public Health* **55** (4): 177–183.

13 Goi Porto Alves, M.C., Ruiz de Matos, M., Reichmann, M.L., and Harrison Dominguez, M. (2005). Estimation of the dog and cat population in the state of São Paulo. *Revista Saúde Pública* **39**: 891–897.

14 Humane Society International (2001). Case Study of an Incentive Program to Encourage Sterilization of Dogs (and Cats) and Greater Attention to Animal Welfare on Abaco Island in the Bahamas. Washington, DC: Humane Society International.

15 Hiby, L., Rinzin K., Verma, S., et al. (2015). Bhutan roaming dog survey May to June 2015. Unpublished report by Humane Society International, Washington, DC, USA.

16 Rowan and Kartal (unpublished). Humane Dog Management – A Global Perspective. *Manuscript in preparation.*

17 Astorga, F., Escobar, L.E., Poo-Muñoz, D.A., and Medina-Vogel, G. (2015). Dog ownership, abundance and potential for bat-borne rabies spillover in Chile. *Preventive Veterinary Medicine* **118** (4): 397–405.

18 Schneider, R. (1975). Observations on overpopulation of dogs and cats. *Journal of the American Veterinary Medicine Association* **167**: 281–284.

19 Rowan, A.N. and Williams, J. (1987). The success of companion animal management programs: a review. *Anthrozoös* **1** (2): 110–122.

20 Unti, B.O. (2004). Protecting All Animals. Washington, DC: Humane Society Press.

21 Clifton, M. (2015). Record low shelter killing raises both hopes & questions. http://www.animals24-7.org/2014/11/14/record-low-shelter-killing-raises-both-hopes-questions/ (accessed 12 November 2016).

22 Marsh, P. (2010). Replacing Myth with Math: Using Evidence-Based Programs to Eradicate Shelter Overpopulation. Town and Country Reprographics, Inc.

23 WHO/WSPA (1990). Guidelines for Dog Population Management. Geneva: World Health Organization (WHO/ZOON/90166).

24 WHO (2011). Rabies. Fact sheet No. 99. http://www.who.int/mediacentre/factsheets/fs099/en/ (accessed 8 October 2016).

25 Reece, J.F. (2005). Dogs and dog control in developing countries. In: The State of the Animals III: 2005 (ed. D.J. Salem and A.N. Rowan), 55–64. Washington, DC: Humane Society Press.

26 Jackman, J. and Rowan, A.N. (2007). Free-roaming dogs in developing countries: the benefits of capture, neuter, and return programs. In: The State of the Animals IV: 2007 (ed. D.J. Salem and A.N. Rowan), 55–64. Washington, DC: Humane Society Press.

27 Cleaveland, S., Kaare, M., Knobel, D., and Laurenson, M.K. (2006). Canine vaccination – providing broader benefits for disease control. *Veterinary Microbiology* **117** (1): 43–50.

28 World Health Organization (2005). Health situation and trends assessment: health situation in the South-East Asia region, 1998–2000. Trends in Health Status. http://www.searo.who.int/en/section1243/section1382/section1386/section1898_9262.htm (accessed 6 October 2016).

29 World Health Organization (2001). Strategies for the control and elimination of rabies in Asia: Report of a WHO Interregional Consultation. http://www.who.int/rabies/en/Strategies_for_the_control_and_elimination_of_rabies_in_Asia.pdf (accessed 6 October 2016).

30 Dalla Villa, P., Kahn, S., Stuardo, L. et al. (2010). Free-roaming dog control among OIE-member countries. *Preventive Veterinary Medicine* **97**: 58–63.

31 Yoak, A.J., Reece, J.F., Gehrt, S., and Hamilton, I.M. (2014). Disease control through fertility control: secondary benefits of animal birth control in Indian street dogs. *Preventive Veterinary Medicine* **113**: 152–156.

32 Reece, F., Nimesh, M.K., Wyllie, R.E. et al. (2012). Description and evaluation of a right flank, mini-laparotomy approach to canine ovariohysterectomy. *The Veterinary Record* **171**: 248–253.

**33** Tenzin, T., Dhand, N.K., Gyeltshen, T. et al. (2011). Dog bites in humans and estimating human rabies mortality in rabies endemic areas of Bhutan. *PLoS Neglected Tropical Diseases* **5** (11): e1391.

**34** Rinzin, K. (2012a). Community attitude assessment of Humane Society International's street dog sterilization & rabies vaccination program in Bhutan. Unpublished report by Humane Society International, Washington, DC, USA.

**35** Humane Society International (2011). Street dogs in Bhutan. http://www.hsi.org/issues/street_dog/ factsheets/street_dogs_bhutan.html (accessed 12 November 2016).

**36** Norbu, P. (2012). Bhutanese compassion prevents sterilization. Kuensel Online. http://www .kuenselonline.com/2011/?p=25830 (accessed 07 December 2017).

**37** Rinzin, K. (2012b). Evaluation of capture-neuter-vaccinate-release (CNVR) programme to control Rabies and Dog Population in Bhutan (A Report on monitoring of National Dog Population Management and Rabies Control Project). Unpublished report by Humane Society International, Washington, DC, USA.

**38** Rinzin, K. (2015). Population dynamics and health status of free-roaming dogs in Bhutan. Doctoral dissertation. Murdoch University.

**39** Rinzin, K. (2015). Monitoring and evaluation (M&E) of capture-neuter-vaccinate-release

(CNVR) programme in Bhutan. Unpublished report by Humane Society International, Washington, DC, USA.

**40** Lee, J. and Sehgal, R. (2015). Dog population management in Jamshedpur, India: a model for improving welfare and achieving impact through human behavior change. Second International Conference on Dog Population Management, Istanbul, Turkey. Available at: http://www.icam-coalition.org/downloads/ICAM_Abstract_book.pdf (accessed 10 October 2016).

**41** Humane Society International (2001). Case study of an incentive program to encourage the sterilization of dogs (and cats) and greater attention to animal welfare on Abaco Island in the Bahamas. http://www.hsi.org/assets/pdfs/eng_dogs_on_abaco.pdf (accessed 28 September 2016).

**42** World Society for the Protection of Animals (2012). Situación de la población en los hogares de la Gran Área Metropolitana, Costa Rica. Report by the World Society for the Protection of Animals, San Jose, Costa Rica. http://www.veterinarios.or.cr/ files/doc/Situacion-de-la-poblacion-canina-en-los-hogares-de-la-Gran-Area-Metropolitana-Costa-Rica-WSPA.pdf (accessed 28 October 2016).

**43** Hampson, K., Coudeville, L., Lembo, T. et al. (2015). Estimating the global burden of endemic canine rabies. *PLoS Neglected Tropical Diseases* **9**: e0003709.

# 3

# Community Engagement and Education

*Natasha Lee*

*Asia Animal Happiness, Jalan Kerja Ayer Lama, Ampang Jaya, Ampang, Selangor 68000, Malaysia*

## 3.1 Introduction

Community engagement and education are essential components of any animal welfare-related project, whether conducted by the government, nongovernmental organizations (NGOs), professional associations, or private practitioners. Projects designed to address animal welfare problems must target the root causes of the problem rather than solely the issue itself. Unfortunately, the root cause of much animal suffering is human behavior. Addressing animal welfare issues therefore almost always requires an element of human behavior change. For example, it may be tempting to focus solely on spay/neuter activities in an area with a stray dog overpopulation issue. Although that may be initially effective in reducing the canine reproductive rate, this approach fails to address the reason why the dogs are there in the first place. Change must come from within communities themselves. A frequent approach in many developing countries involves visiting veterinarians or NGOs operating spay/neuter projects in foreign communities to address stray animal overpopulation. Without involving the local community itself, however, such interventions are unlikely to have any type of long-term, sustainable impact following the departure of the group. Through engagement, community members are encouraged to participate in solving animal welfare issues in their own community. The long-term objective is to empower communities to take responsibility for enacting animal welfare change.

Community engagement and education should be purposefully incorporated into a project's design. Projects that effectively engage the community are far more likely to achieve long-term and sustainable outcomes.

### 3.1.1 Community Engagement

Community engagement is the process of working collaboratively with and through groups of people affiliated by geographic proximity, special interest, or similar situations to address issues affecting stakeholders in different stages of a project [1]. This includes policymaking, planning, implementation, monitoring, and evaluation. Engagement can be used to gather useful information, increase program acceptance and support, foster collaboration, and build local capacity. It is not always an easy process, but bringing together people from different backgrounds and with different beliefs allows for a more comprehensive understanding of issues at a local level, and allows for the development of a multifaceted solution to animal welfare issues.

There are various approaches to community engagement. When the community is involved in providing input during the planning stages of a project, it is referred to as a "bottom-up" approach. This tends to lead to more sustainable changes compared with a "top-down" approach, which occurs when members of upper management make decisions without much input from those actually working on the ground.

The goals of community engagement are:

1) *To inform and obtain feedback.* Requires minimal engagement with the community, involving only

*Field Manual for Small Animal Medicine*, First Edition. Edited by Katherine Polak and Ann Therese Kommedal.
© 2018 John Wiley & Sons, Inc. Published 2018 by John Wiley & Sons, Inc.

an exchange of information. Public involvement brings more information to particular decisions and knowledge about the context where projects are implemented. An example of this is conducting surveys to estimate the number of dog feeders in an area.

2) *To involve and collaborate.* Requires a medium level of engagement involving active participation from the individuals or groups within the community. The purpose of this approach is to include the community in decision making processes. An example of this is involving animal caretakers in identifying and catching free-roaming animals for vaccination.

3) *To build capacity and empower.* Requires high levels of engagement through training and assigning responsibilities to individuals within a community. This approach is designed to empower community members to take an active role in project implementation. An example of this is training animal health workers to catch and vaccinate free-roaming dogs so they can then conduct a program annually themselves.

### 3.1.2 Education

The goal of education in animal welfare projects or veterinary services is to change attitudes and behaviors through increasing specific knowledge or skills of the target audience. Education is typically considered either formal or informal. Formal education is usually conducted in schools using a defined curriculum, whereas informal education uses a less rigid structure, often taking place outside the classroom.

Learning can be an active or passive process. Passive learning typically consists of a one-way communication process through activities such as listening to lectures in a traditional classroom setting or watching a video. Active learning utilizes engaging methodologies to encourage the reflection of lessons. In other words, active learning occurs when students are guided in doing *and* thinking about the actions they are performing [2].

### 3.1.3 How Are Community Engagement and Education Related?

Community engagement is a *process*, whereas education is a *goal*. Therefore, community engagement can

be used to achieve educational objectives. The process of engaging in an educational activity makes it an active learning process, which facilitates the learning and retention of knowledge and skills. Engagement increases the likelihood that attitudes and behavior will change.

On the other hand, community engagement can be used to achieve educational objectives by collecting data and consulting with the community. Identifying lapses in education and the type of delivery methods appropriate for the target audience allows for the development of a sound implementation plan. For example, through discussions with local authorities and community leaders, researchers learned that most people in rural China listen to the radio compared with other forms of media. Therefore, radio announcements are probably the most effective way to educate the public about the importance of vaccinating dogs in that area.

## 3.2 The Value of Community Engagement and Education

Community engagement and education can bring about many benefits, several of which are discussed here further.

### 3.2.1 Informed Decisions

Integrating the community's aspirations, concerns, needs, and values into all levels of a project will allow for greater effectiveness and impact [3]. The local community has insight into the problems they face and are best positioned to develop practical solutions. A feedback loop whereby community members report back to project leaders on successes and failures will allow the community to assist in the continuous monitoring and evaluation of the project.

### 3.2.2 Increasing Acceptance and Participation

Perhaps the most important benefit of community engagement is the increased likelihood that projects or solutions will be widely accepted by the community. By engaging community members, their understanding of programmatic goals and how it benefits them and their community will be better understood. Even if a community member disagrees with a decision, through the engagement process he or she is exposed to other stakeholder opinions and reasons why that particular decision was made. Increased acceptance is crucial for community participation and program sustainability.

### 3.2.3 Changing Attitudes and Behaviors

Education can effectively increase public awareness about a certain issue; however, it may not be enough to motivate behavior change. Through community education, community members are invited to contribute to solving the problem at hand and reflect on their own attitudes and behaviors. This can create a path whereby individuals increasingly believe in the necessity for change, which then becomes the motivator to adopt the changes themselves. This level of buy-in can also increase the dissemination of information to other community members.

### 3.2.4 Sustainability

Through appropriate engagement, knowledge and skills can be developed and retained within a community, allowing the community itself to become more self-sufficient. Long-term behavior change can become the "new norm" that is continually practiced after a project has ended. This allows the community to become independent from the project.

### 3.2.5 Improving Veterinary Care and Knowledge

In many places throughout the developing world, there is a significant shortage of trained veterinarians and technicians. Topics such as shelter medicine, high-volume spay/neuter, dog population management, and infectious disease control are rarely taught in most veterinary curriculums. As a result, community engagement and education is often used to develop the local capacity both of medical professionals and lay persons to fill gaps in knowledge. Increased community engagement also helps improve public understanding of the importance of veterinary services and fosters trust in the veterinary profession.

In the developing field of participatory epidemiology, animal keepers, particularly those associated with livestock, are integrally involved in disease control programs from analysis of disease problems, to the design, implementation, and evaluation of the

program and policies [4]. In companion animal medicine, especially when access to veterinarians is limited, animal health workers can be trained to identify signs of rabies in dogs, obtain and send samples to the local laboratory for confirmation, and conduct annual vaccination campaigns.

Engagement and education of pet owners and animal caretakers can also increase treatment compliance and improve animal care. Spending time engaging clients allows practitioners to better understand barriers to treatment. In the long term, this engagement may increase the likelihood that pet owners will seek preventive health services such as annual rabies vaccinations for their pets in the future.

## 3.3 Important Principles of Community Engagement and Education

### 3.3.1 Theories on Learning

Learning can be accomplished using a variety of methods, and every individual has their own learning style. Learning styles are grouped into four categories: visual, auditory, kinesthetic, and reading/writing [5] (Table 3.1). Individuals typically have a mixture of these learning styles, with one or more styles dominating.

How much one learns can be influenced by the level of engagement during the learning process. The more participatory the learning, the more knowledge tends

Table 3.1 Description of learning styles.

| Learning style | Description | Activity examples |
| --- | --- | --- |
| Visual | Watching and imagining | Visualizing graphs, diagrams, pictures, videos, demonstrations |
| Auditory | Listening and talking | Listening to lectures, radio, podcasts, discussions, dialogues |
| Kinesthetic | Hands-on approach | Participating in demonstrations, simulations |
| Reading/writing | Text-based | Reviewing books, journals, brochures, writing essays |

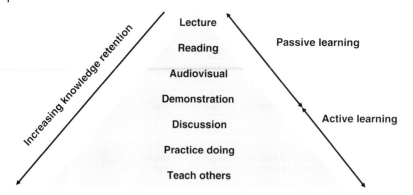

Figure 3.1 Learning pyramid. Source: Adapted from National Training Laboratories, Bethel, Maine.

to be retained. The learning pyramid in Figure 3.1 is often used as a visual representation of this theory.

A successful education program incorporates multiple learning styles, targets different senses, and has a participatory component. Confucius provided a nice assessment of how we learn, which should be considered when developing educational programs.

> "Tell me, and I will forget.
> Show me, and I may remember.
> Involve me, and I will understand."
> Confucius

### 3.3.2 Adult Learning

Pedagogy is the discipline that deals with the practice of education; in simpler terms, it refers to the best ways to teach. Pedagogy in elementary schools typically involves a curriculum, which is arranged by subject matter and is content-oriented. This approach is less effective in adult education, which is commonly referred to as andragogy. Andragogy must utilize a different approach as adults have specific learning requirements which are much different from children. Adults are assumed to be autonomous and must first be willing to learn before education can be effective. They have a wealth of experience that serves as the basis for learning, as opposed to children which respond more favorably to didactic approaches.

Adults are self-directed, so methods that allow them to discover knowledge and skills through guidance work well. They also learn best when the lesson content is relevant to them; problem-based approaches are often appropriate. Lessons that work well with adult learners have a participatory component including discussions, practical sessions, trial and error, and guided learning exercises.

These four principles outlined by Knowles [6] summarize adult learning:

1) *Involvement.* Adults need to be involved in the planning and evaluation of their lessons.
2) *Experience.* Actual experiences of adults, both successes and mistakes, should be leveraged as the basis for learning.
3) *Relevance.* Adults are most interested in learning subjects that are immediately relevant to their occupation or personal life.
4) *Problem-centered.* The content being taught should be centered around issues rather than a content-oriented approach.

### 3.3.3 Human Behavior Change

Most animal suffering is caused by humans doing, or not doing something. Although the typical approach to address animal welfare issues is to offer services that directly benefit the animals, this rarely influences the underlying reason of why people behave the way they do. In order to change human behavior, one must first understand the process of behavior change and the underlying motivations behind the change.

There are many theories of change in existence, and the five stages below describe the process of implementing a public health intervention. A similar process can be applied to animal-related projects where there is a desired human behavior change. It is important to note that awareness and education mainly influence the initial stages of change. Actual behavior change and maintenance of the behavior are influenced by many other factors, some of which are explored later in the chapter.

The stages of health behavior change described by Proschka [7] include:

1) *Precontemplation.* Not ready for change. They are yet to consider change, are in denial, or simply unaware of the need to change.
2) *Contemplation.* Beginning to recognize the need for change. They have started to think about the issues, are still ambivalent about change, and are weighing the pros and cons for change.
3) *Preparation.* Ready for change. They have intentions to take action, are gathering information, and are planning the change behaviors.
4) *Action.* Practicing new behavior. They are practicing new behaviors or have modified past behaviors.
5) *Maintenance.* Consolidating new behavior. They are working to sustain new behaviors and are actively preventing relapse.

## 3.4 How to Engage and Educate Your Community

### 3.4.1 Planning

The most vital component of program planning as it pertains to community engagement and education is defining clear goals and a mission that targets the root causes of the problem. A root cause is the primary factor in a chain of causal events that results in the main problem. For example, in the problem of free-roaming dog overpopulation, root causes can include irresponsible pet ownership, lack of reproductive control, and poor garbage management.

The more specific the goals, the more targeted the implementation activities. The target audience must be identified and understood, especially in terms of age groups, literacy levels, past experiences, and if possible, motivating factors. This enables the appropriate dissemination of messaging and selection of project activities.

Following identification of the target group and root causes, project logistics must be planned. This includes determining the program location, duration, programmatic activities, personnel involved, and what materials should be prepared. Although some community engagement activities may appear as being spontaneous, effective engagement requires significant preparation beforehand. Seemingly, simple tasks such as talking to community members require the development of clear and consistent messaging. Similarly, conducting informal interviews requires preparation of discussion points. Activities and communications should ideally be practiced first with friends or colleagues before going into the field.

Program planning also involves developing ways to evaluate project success. This is discussed briefly at the end of this chapter and in Chapter 19.

### 3.4.2 Community Engagement Methods

The overarching goal of engagement is to allow for two-way communication which imparts a project message while also listening to the community. Community engagement techniques are numerous. Rather than provide an exhaustive list, a few of the most commonly used methods in the animal welfare sector are included here as examples. The good news is that many engagement methods are not resource intensive, apart from time and manpower; how engagement occurs is only limited by the imagination.

#### 3.4.2.1 Surveys and Feedback

Surveys can serve two purposes, the first of which is to ascertain feedback from the survey taker; the second is to provide information to the survey taker. For example, in a survey used to collect data on sterilization rates among cat owners, questions can be written in a way that highlights the benefits of spay/neuter in an effort to raise awareness among owners. The sample survey below informs survey takers that a spay/neuter clinic is coming to their town, while also hinting at the health benefits of spay/neuter.

---

**Textbox 3.1 Sample survey**

Q: Is your cat sterilized?                          Yes   No

Q: Did you know that sterilizing can . . .

   a. Reduce the risk of mammary          Yes   No
      tumors in females?

   b. Reduce urine spraying in males?     Yes   No

   c. Keep your cat closer to home?       Yes   No

*A spay/neuter clinic is coming to your town next month. Call us to make an appointment to neuter your cat.*

---

Polls and online surveys can engage a large audience simultaneously, often requiring minimal effort. Some methods may be more time consuming such as focus groups or face-to-face interviews, but the data collected is detailed and potentially more useful. Conducting surveys and obtaining feedback constitute the lowest level of engagement.

Surveys can be performed quickly and simply, especially if the primary goal is to ascertain general views on particular issues. For example, a quick exit survey with clients at a veterinary clinic can help determine their level of satisfaction with the services provided. Such a survey can also serve a dual purpose of reminding them about the importance of follow-up vaccinations. Surveys can take a variety of forms including paper, electronic, or even physical forms such as voting using colored balls dropped into clear ballot boxes.

Before carrying out a survey, one must understand the target audience to allow for the tailoring of survey questions. Questions should be clear and precise, unbiased, and care must be taken to not lead the survey taker to give desirable answers. Surveys should be designed in such a way that the results can be analyzed to provide useful information for project planning, monitoring, and assessment.

Feedback can involve one- or two-way communication. Examples of one-way feedback include using suggestion boxes or "like" buttons on social media. Two-way feedback might include comments on social media, online discussion platforms, and open forums. Face-to-face feedback conversations are also two-way, allowing both parties to understand better what is being said. Less time-intensive than face-to-face interviews are focus groups, which use a cohort of the target audience. Focus groups enable a trained moderator to utilize the dynamics of a particular group to discuss animal welfare topics in depth. A focus group is not necessarily representative of all the target audience, but it can still provide useful information during project planning to understand the local culture and identify potential barriers. For example, a focus group of pet owners may give important insight into the human–animal bond in a particular community. In many cultures, cats and dogs are community-owned whereby a number of people in the community collectively feed the animals. Identifying how dogs are cared for can dramatically affect the design of an intervention intended to improve their welfare.

### 3.4.2.2 Participatory Planning

Participatory planning is a process a community takes to reach an animal welfare goal by consciously identifying its problems and developing a course of action to resolve them. Program planning often involves the following steps, all of which can involve stakeholders and community members.

- Performing a situational analysis
- Pin-pointing the problems
- Identifying the root causes of animal welfare issues
- Brainstorming solutions
- Agreeing on project objectives
- Delegating tasks for each objective
- Listing resources and budgetary needs
- Designing a system to monitor and evaluate the project.

Participatory planning workshops can help bring a group of people together to assess their knowledge, extract their opinions, and solve problems in a collaborative environment. Workshops can be particularly valuable when there is conflict between animal feeders or local animal welfare charities and the government regarding free-roaming animal management policies. Textbox 3.2 includes a sample schedule of a participatory planning workshop.

Planning sessions can vary in length from a few hours to several days. Sometimes two separate sessions are required, one for information gathering and situational analysis and the other for designing implementation plans. Sessions should be carried out using several different participatory activities to avoid monotony and keep participants engaged. Examples of different participatory activities can be found in Table 3.2.

Participants should be allowed to voice their individual opinions and concerns freely. They can take turns stating an opinion, allow anonymously written opinions, or use small group discussions, exchanging members when needed. Adequate time should be allocated for participants to reflect and provide feedback following each activity.

Participatory planning is not just limited to a particular project. Rather, it can be applied for achieving various objectives where multi-stakeholder involvement is crucial:

- Developing a euthanasia policy [8]
- Community disease surveillance [9]

---

**Textbox 3.2 Sample dog population management planning workshop schedule**

*Workshop focus.* Planning a dog population management and rabies control project in City X
*Participants.* Local animal welfare NGOs, animal welfare experts, rabies professionals, hospital representatives, municipality officials, central government officials (animal and human/public health departments), community leaders, religious leaders, members of the local and national veterinary associations, and private veterinary practitioners in City X.

| Day/Time | Topic | Details |
|---|---|---|
| **Day 1 Morning** | Workshop objectives, ice breaker Report of rabies situation in City X | Presentations by various stakeholders on their activities related to rabies and free-roaming dogs |
| **Afternoon** | Identification of problem and root causes of issues regarding free-roaming dogs | Groups carry out a cause-and-effect exercise to identify the root causes of the agreed-upon issues |
| **Day 2 Morning** | Defining project objectives to target root causes Brainstorming activities to achieve objectives | Group discussion to convert root causes into project objectives Groups list activities and tasks that can used to achieve set objectives |
| **Afternoon** | SWOT (strengths, weaknesses, opportunities, and threats of the project) analysis of the project Delegating tasks, budget, and resources | Groups perform a SWOT analysis to identify activities not yet included earlier Stakeholders are assigned to the project objectives; they then discuss the budget and resources needed. Proportional piling exercise can be used (see Table 3.2) |
| **Day 3 Morning** | Identifying ways to monitor progress Developing a systematic project plan | Groups identify possible indicators to measure Workshop results are put into an agreed upon project plan |
| **Afternoon** | Final discussions | Discuss any issues that arose during the workshop |

---

- Creating a collaborative community animal care plan
- Developing country-specific vaccination guidelines.

### 3.4.2.3   Project Implementation

Once a project starts community participation should be encouraged to foster project support, encourage long-lasting positive behavioral changes, disseminate project messages, and increase self-sustainability within the community.

During the initial implementation phase one tends to focus on the logistical aspects of carrying out the project while community engagement takes a back seat. However, the early stages of the project are the most vital to engage the community engagement to secure buy-in from community members from the very beginning. The following section provides specific examples of community engagement activities categorized by the underlying intent for engagement.

#### 3.4.2.3.1   *To Inform and Obtain Feedback*
Communication is the lowest level of engagement. Communication with the public often occurs during

**Table 3.2** Examples of participatory activities.

| Type | Activity | Description | Purpose | Example topic |
|---|---|---|---|---|
| Discussion | Structured discussion | Groups discuss a set of provided questions regarding an issue, taking turns providing answers | Providing feedback on a topic | Feasibility of implementing a mass vaccination campaign |
| | Open discussion | Groups discuss a general topic or set of open-ended questions; discussion is unguided | Providing feedback on a topic | Pros and cons of operating a no-kill shelter |
| | Debates | Groups argue for or against an idea or issue | Understanding various sides and complexity of an issue | Early age neutering in private practice, trap–neuter–return of cats in unmanaged colonies |
| | Role playing | Participants role play, taking the sides of various stakeholders | Understanding motivations of various stakeholders | Providing treatment for free-roaming animals lacking owners to pay for medical services |
| Analysis | SWOT | SWOT analysis | Identifying risks and opportunities | School education program on animal welfare, low-cost treatment clinic in urban areas |
| | PESTLE | PESTLE analysis (discuss the influence of politics, economy, social, technology, legal and environment on the project) | Understanding various programmatic aspects influencing factors | TNR project in a village, mobile clinics in refugee camps |
| Visual representation | Mind mapping | Create a diagram to visually organize information. Ideas are noted down around a central topic. Ideas can be grouped or linked in a diagram | Identifying the interconnectivity of ideas | Importance of education, ways to increase adoption rates |
| | Drawings | A topic is visually depicted using drawings | Enabling participants to think comprehensively about an issue, to visualize what an ideal/worst situation looks like, to report on something they have previously seen | Designing an ideal shelter for cats |
| | Timelines | List ideas or events against a timeline | Comparing between different times of the day/week/month/year, or effects of seasonality | Assessing the daily life of a free-roaming dog, seasonality of disease incidence |
| | Maps | Draw a map to visualize where programmatic activities or barriers are located (e.g. resources for food and shelter, potential dangers) | Understanding geographical effects, to identify strengths/barriers/places to focus on | Determining areas with free-roaming animals, finding suitable locations for setting cat traps |

**Table 3.2** (*Continued*)

| Type | Activity | Description | Purpose | Example topic |
|------|----------|-------------|---------|---------------|
| | Problem tree | With the main issue in the center, the causes of that issue are listed at the bottom while the effects of the issue are listed at the top. Several layers of causes or effects can be listed | Investigating the root causes and effects of an issue | Poor medical compliance of pet owners, absent free-roaming cat and dog animal management programs, poorly managed animal shelters |
| | Proportional piling | Respondents are asked to pile stones, beans, or pellets proportional in size to the relative number or importance of the items under discussion. Fixing the total number of beans makes the technique more reproducible | Understanding the perceived importance of each item | Impact of free-roaming dogs on various aspects of family life, resource distribution for different shelter activities |
| Matrix and scoring | Scoring/ rating | List and score each item, or rank the items by priority. This can be repeated at a later date to provide a comparison | Comparing and rating different components of a topic, to prioritize a list of components | Pain scores for medical conditions, animal welfare ratings, prioritizing actions items, rating the welfare of pets against the Five Freedoms |
| | Stakeholder analysis | Rank stakeholders by their ability to influence a program | Identifying and prioritizing project stakeholders | Identifying important stakeholders in a mass vaccination campaign |
| | Risk assessment | Rate each program risk by its possible impact and probability of occurence | Identifying potential risks to a project so mitigation plans can be put in place | Risks of offering free spay/ neuter, risks of a public rally against culling of free-roaming dogs |
| Small projects or group work | Presentation or lecture | Present or give a lecture to the class/group | Learning more about a specific topic | Feline neutering techniques |
| | Projects | Individual or groups collaborate to solve a problem. This activity can be hand written or delivered verbally | Building critical thinking, learning about various aspects of a topic | Designing a cattery to maximize welfare, creating a promotional video to promote vaccination |

activities that occur in the public eye including stray dog vaccination programs or trapping cats for neutering. Other examples of communication include the following:

- Explaining to community members about the project and its importance
- Handing out information leaflets on dog bite prevention
- Identifying local animal feeders

- Asking feeders where dogs normally hide during the day
- Informing pet owners of the benefits of spay/neuter and where to obtain services.

### 3.4.2.3.2 To Involve and Collaborate

The next level of engagement is community participation. The community can get involved and support animal welfare projects in many different ways. Some examples include:

**Textbox 3.3 Case study: Colombo, Sri Lanka**

Blue Paw Trust (BPT) is a nongovernmental organization based in Colombo, Sri Lanka. From 2007 to 2012, BPT managed the Colombo Project, which was designed to humanely manage free-roaming dogs in the capital city of Sri Lanka. The program was multifaceted, focusing on canine neutering and rabies vaccination, public education, and improving animal guardianship.

Project staff knew that community engagement would be critical to ensure buy-in from the community. A full-time Community Liaison Officer (CLO) was therefore hired for the sole purpose of increasing community participation. It was critical that this person was recruited from the very community that BPT was working in. Talking to community members in their own language and winning their trust was key.

A important responsibility of the CLO was to work with community leaders to educate them on the importance of BPT's neutering efforts. The CLO was also tasked with identifying community members to assist with the postoperative care of sterilized free-roaming dogs.

The CLO also organized community education events to improve rabies awareness and dog bite prevention. The sessions were held at times, often late at night, when members of the community were most likely to be able to participate and included videos and demonstrations on safe dog handling.

Over time, the acceptance of BPT's work grew within Colombo and human rabies and dog bite cases decreased significantly. There were also smaller victories, such as the increased ability to return surgical patients to their caretakers in the community on the same day as surgery. This allowed for increased clinic productivity as more animals could be sterilized and returned in a timely fashion. Furthermore, BPT became inundated with public requests for sterilization and vaccination.

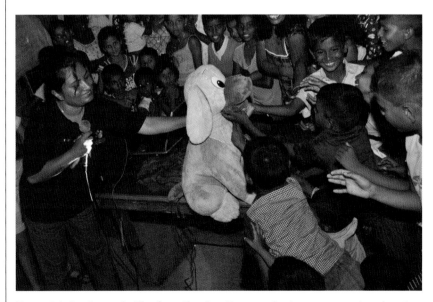

**Figure 3.2** Dr. Ganga de Silva from Blue Paw Trust conducting a community education session on safe dog handling, organized by the CLO. Using soft toys enables children and community members to participate, learn, and practice in a safe environment.

- Identify, locate, and restrain free-roaming animals for vaccination or collection for neutering
- Provide postoperative care and monitoring
- Identify adopters for unowned animals
- Establish feeding stations for responsible feeding of free-roaming cats and dogs
- Identify sick animals
- Disseminate project messages
- Petition the authorities to change policies
- Engage local businesses to determine their interest in financially supporting the project.

#### 3.4.2.3.3 To Build Capacity and Empower

The highest level of engagement is capacity building and delegating responsibility back to the community. This takes significant time and resources for preparation and implementation, but the benefits are enormous. The following individuals or groups can be trained to perform the following tasks:

- *Local animal caretakers.* Provide preventive animal care including vaccination and deworming
- *Local educators.* Conduct small group educational activities
- *Local animal welfare groups.* Establish and manage free-roaming cat colonies
- *Local veterinarians.* Perform high-volume, high-quality spay/neuter techniques.

The Colombo case study describes how dedicated staff successfully encouraged active community participation.

#### 3.4.2.4 Monitoring and Reporting

Monitoring and reporting are essential components of project management. Monitoring program performance allows for better evaluation of the project objectives and activities, and timely implementation of changes should they be required. Monitoring and reporting can also be used to keep the community, particularly the beneficiaries updated on program progress.

The community can be directly involved with monitoring their own community's progress or of the project itself. They can be trained to collect data and assess it on a regular basis; this might include counting the number of puppies or kittens born during a neutering project, measuring the improvement in welfare of the animals they care for, or

tracking the number of animal mortalities. Some community members can be trained to assess particular programmatic elements and data, and troubleshoot the project as needed. Table 3.2 lists activities that can be used as monitoring tools to help evaluate programmatic progress.

### 3.4.3 Teaching Methods

Similar to community engagement, there are countless ways to educate. The methodologies included here fall under two broad categories: passive and active learning. Passive learning is usually easier to conduct, less resource intensive, and can reach a wider audience. Active learning is more time consuming and requires advanced planning, but typically leads to increased knowledge retention and understanding.

#### 3.4.3.1 Information, Education, and Communication (IEC) Materials

Information, education, and communication, commonly referred to as IEC, is used to disseminate the intended project messages. IEC can be used to raise awareness, increase knowledge, change attitudes, or even change behaviors. Common IEC materials include posters, brochures, booklets, TV advertisements, radio broadcasts, social media posts, videos, talks, presentations, and lesson plans for schools.

IEC campaigns can be very successful in increasing awareness and knowledge if the materials are targeted and well planned [10,11]. This involves having a focused goal, specific target audience, clear issue to address, simple and consistent messaging, distribution plan, and a monitoring mechanism. IEC material must be suitable for the target audience and should be tested in a pilot project before launching it with a wider audience.

IEC can be made more engaging by incorporating a participatory component, such as surveys or feedback. Educational messaging can be incorporated into entertaining games that serve as an active learning opportunity. IEC campaigns alone are not always enough to achieve sustainable behavior change within the community [12]. Long-lasting change is better achieved by using an approach that also includes community engagement and/or social marketing.

#### 3.4.3.2 Traditional Classroom Setting

The traditional classroom is a teacher-focused environment where lessons are delivered through a series of lectures. In this setting, students learn through listening, watching, and reading, and knowledge is usually passively received. Formal examinations are then used to measure the acquisition of knowledge. A major benefit of the classroom setting is the fact that a structured curriculum can be standardized for a particular region or country and the same lessons can be used for different groups of students.

Standardized curriculums ensure that all students receive consistent messaging, and scripted curriculums minimize the harm that can be done by poor teachers. A major concern with standardized curriculums, however, is that they limit the opportunities for students to learn because of the one-size-fits all-course structure. Interestingly, animal welfare material can be skillfully incorporated into existing subjects found in standardized curricula such as reading and mathematics, rather than serve as a stand-alone topic. For example, educational materials on how to take care of a pet dog may be incorporated into an English language lesson. An assignment might be for students to write a short essay on how to properly feed and bath their dog. A mathematics assignment might be to add the number of free-roaming dogs on one street with the number of cats on another.

#### 3.4.3.3 Active Learning Methods

##### 3.4.3.3.1 "Flipped" Classrooms

The "flipped classroom" has gained popularity over the last decade since Bergmann and Sams adopted this strategy in teaching their class in Colorado. In a flipped classroom, the traditional delivery of the subject matter and homework are reversed [13]. Students are provided course materials to be reviewed outside of the classroom and the classroom sessions then focus on activities where students learn to apply their new knowledge or skills. The benefit of this system is that students can go through the material at their own pace using their preferred learning style. This enables the instructor to enhance the students' critical thinking skills by combining knowledge from different subjects to approach a problem [14], such as science and geography to learn about climate change. Examples of participatory activities that can be used

to facilitate learning in a flipped classroom are found in Table 3.2.

#### 3.4.3.4 Facilitated Community Education

Facilitated community education consists of workshops whereby community members are guided by a facilitator through a problem assessment. When dealing with free-roaming cats and dogs, the problem usually involves nuisance behaviors, animals perceived to be aggressive, and rabies. Through facilitated discussions, the participants discuss the issue at hand, share ideas, and brainstorm solutions. The goal of these workshops is to empower participants to collectively take ownership and responsibility for their own problems, rather than relying on foreign intervention. In international development, this approach is also known as participatory rural appraisal (PRA) or participatory learning and action (PLA). Table 3.2 includes examples of activities that can be used in workshops for facilitated community education. The case study from Cambodia describes the use of this approach to improve pony welfare.

### 3.4.4 Other Ways to Achieve Behavior Change

Awareness and education alone do not always lead to behavior change. Smoking is a perfect example of a behavior that is notoriously difficult to change; many smokers know about the health dangers of smoking but refuse to quit. Therefore, imparting awareness and knowledge are only the first steps in encouraging behavior change.

Besides campaigning for improved awareness and education, behavior change can be targeted through:

1) *Legislation.* Legislation and enforcement requires people to behave a certain way without necessarily understanding nor agreeing with it. For example, pet owners must comply with laws requiring the rabies vaccination of pet dogs and cats, regardless of their views on vaccination.

2) *Incentives.* Positive and negative incentives encourage behavior change. To be effective, incentives must be perceived more beneficial than the effort it takes to change the behavior. For example, the reduction in annual licensing fees should be significant enough to incentivize owners to sterilize their dogs. Alternatively, fines or penalties may be used as a negative incentive to encourage or deter certain behaviors. In some communities, pet

**Textbox 3.4 Case study: Phnom Penh, Cambodia**

Cambodia Pony Welfare Organization (CPWO) was founded in 2007 with the intent of improving the health and welfare of equines in Cambodia. In Cambodia, most equines are ponies used to transport equipment and goods. The livelihood of many local people depends on the performance of their ponies. Before CPWO, the welfare of most ponies was poor due to a lack of available veterinary services and limited owner knowledge and training. Many of the medical issues affecting the ponies were preventable, but without proper training, animals that might otherwise be productive and lead long, healthy lives suffered or died instead. Ponies were overworked, lacked regular hoof trimming, dental care, and endoparasite control.

To improve animal guardianship, CPWO launched a program that trained select pony owners to become community facilitators. These facilitators then went into the community and engaged other pony owners through interactive exercises on animal care. Each exercise was designed to help community members understand how their actions affect the welfare of their ponies. Facilitators then worked with community members to identify behaviors and cooperative activities that could improve pony welfare. Preventive health

practices including high-quality equine nutrition was emphasized. After initial local success, more facilitators were identified and employed in various communities throughout Cambodia.

Over time, CPWO became entrenched in their project communities. Pony owners better understood the relationship between pony health and increased productivity. Preventable diseases such as nutritional secondary hyperparathyroidism (due to an imbalance of Ca:P ratio in the diet) and wounds caused by inappropriate harness use decreased significantly. In some communities, pony owners worked together to design designated pony resting areas which provided much-needed shade and water. CPWO staff were able to monitor the program's progress through improved local understanding of pony welfare issues. This was demonstrated through interactive activities whereby pony owners would generate visual charts identifying potential pony health issues and obstacles.

Over the years, the program evolved to address more complex animal health issues including Surra (trypanosomiasis), grooming, skin diseases, and diarrhea. The success of this program was due entirely to an approach focused on community engagement and empowerment (Figure 3.3).

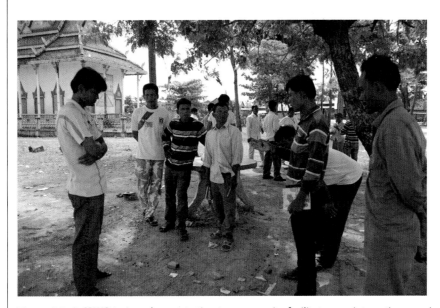

**Figure 3.3** A CPWO trainer demonstrating to community facilitators an interactive exercise known as, "Mapping of resources." Using dirt, sticks, and rocks, a simple map of the community is drawn on the ground and resources such as food, water, and shelter are marked. Beans or pebbles are used to represent the ponies within the communities. This exercise enables pony owners to identify common obstacles to animal health (e.g. damaged roads or inadequate shelter at rest stops) and develop strategies to overcome them.

owners are subject to fines for not registering their cat or dog.

3) *Convenience.* Behaviors that are convenient and easy to perform are far more likely to actually be carried out and sustained. For instance, the presence of a local low-cost spay/neuter clinic makes it easy for cat owners to have their cats sterilized.

4) *Social norms.* Human nature involves the tendency to follow behaviors set by peers. For example, owners may routinely vaccinate their pets if they believe it is common practice to do so.

5) *Influence.* The public is influenced by popular trends, celebrities, friends, etc. Many animal shelters have improved animal welfare awareness through the use of celebrities and media personalities.

### 3.4.4.1  Social Marketing

Social marketing is the integration of marketing principles with social science to sell ideas, attitudes, and behaviors to the community [15]. Social marketing examines what influences attitudes and behaviors, and develops ways of targeting them.

The main principles of social marketing can be summarized as the 4Ps: Product, Price, Placement and Promotion. Table 3.3 provides an example of each marketing principle as it relates to animal welfare.

## 3.5  Tips and Tricks

### 3.5.1  Facilitation Skills

Facilitation is one of the most important skills for conducting community engagement or education. A good facilitator is able to guide and solicit contributions from participants to achieve a collective solution or reach a decision. Those that are considered good lecturers and speakers however, may not be good facilitators. In the author's opinion, an effective facilitator should have the following key qualities:

- Able to maintain the role of the facilitator rather than a participant, leader, or teacher
- Stimulates the interaction and the free sharing of thoughts and ideas
- Creates a safe environment for the group to open up and become engaged
- Knows when to close a discussion, change topic, or encourage contribution
- Supports the well-being of participants
- Uses questions to stimulate new ways of thinking
- Effectively manages uncomfortable situations.

A good facilitator should seek to remain neutral throughout discussions, ensuring that the group feels that they have discovered new knowledge or that the outcome is based on their choices. This way, the end result is something that the community owns and feels invested in.

There are many courses available both online or through workshops to become an effective facilitator.

### 3.5.2  Local Staff

Trust and acceptance are vital to gain access into a community. Trust can be difficult to achieve but ultimately needs to come from within the community. Therefore, selecting someone from that community

**Table 3.3** Principles of social marketing.

| Marketing principles | Application to social science | Example |
|---|---|---|
| Product | What behavior or attitude needs to be fostered or changed? | Increase the number of owners neutering their cats |
| Price | How much will it cost? This can include money, time, or effort. The perceived benefits must outweigh the costs | Neutering is priced affordably and the benefit for pet owners is that cats are healthier and demonstrate less nuisance behaviors |
| Placement | Where can the product be sold or distributed? Is it convenient and easily accessible? | A mobile clinic that comes to the village once a month will reduce the need for pet owners to travel far for services |
| Promotion | How will this message be disseminated to the target audience? | Social media is used to effectively communicate the benefits of neutering cats |

itself as the key person to engage with community members is ideal. The more similarities this person has with the community, the better he or she can relate with its members. This person has to have confidence and leadership skills, but not be too authoritative otherwise the community will expect a more "top–down" approach, which could impede the sustainability of any behavior change. Once there is trust and acceptance, community members can be persuaded to participate in new approaches or adopt a better solution.

### 3.5.3 Negative Engagement

Community engagement can be both positive and negative. Negative engagement occurs when the project is perceived as detrimental to the community, and community members stop participating in the activity. Even worse, community members can work to actively sabotage the program. Negative engagement can also occur when a harmful attitude or behavior is permeated through the community.

Whenever a new approach, skill, or training occurs, adequate supervision and follow-up must take place to ensure that interventions do not have negative, unintended consequences. Well-intentioned and eager community members may want to apply their newly learned skills or knowledge immediately, without the proper guidance, supplies, or understanding on how they should be used. For example, the author has observed instances where surgical procedures were taught to veterinarians lacking basic veterinary skills and supplies. Without first teaching the basics of asepsis, wound healing, anesthesia, and pain management, staff can do more harm than good.

Other examples of negative engagement include the following:

1) A shelter advertising a no-kill policy indirectly promotes the abandonment of unwanted pets to the shelter.
2) A Highly Pathogenic Avian Influenza (HPAI) surveillance program relies on local reporting but simultaneously culls poultry flocks without compensating farmers. Community members, consisting of mostly small scale farmers, stop reporting and supporting the program [16].
3) A catch-and-kill policy for stray dogs reduces community participation in vaccination campaigns, due to reduced trust in the authorities.

4) An anti-dog-meat eating campaign launched in a particular country is perceived as shaming of the local culture, making the community feel more strongly opposed to the campaign to defend their cultural identity.
5) Humane dog capture training for local community members is carried out in an area that routinely removes and impounds stray dogs in overcrowded shelters. The training was conducted to facilitate the catching of dogs for surgery as part of a catch-vaccinate-neuter-return program. However, following departure of the trainers, community members preceded to remove and impound many more dogs than before as a result of their improved dog catching abilities.
6) A responsible pet ownership campaign stresses the importance of confining dogs to reduce public health issues and nuisance complaints. As a result of the campaign, dog owners begin using inhumane caging and tethering of dogs, creating additional animal welfare problems.

### 3.5.4 Keeping Everyone Motivated

A major challenge with community engagement is the seemingly slow progress, especially at the beginning of a program. As most engagement and educational goals involve long-term change, it can be difficult to appreciate immediate results. Project staff should always maintain focus on long-term objectives and find ways to keep motivated during the project's implementation phase. This can be accomplished by celebrating small achievements and sharing stories of how individual community members have directly benefited from the project. Once positive results of the program become evident, they can be used to further excite and motivate the team.

## 3.6 Monitoring and Evaluation

### 3.6.1 Short-, Medium-, and Long-term Educational Goals

Educational goals can be classified into three time-bound categories: short, medium, and long-term. Monitoring can be done against these three categories. In the short term, the goal is typically to increase the knowledge about a particular subject. Medium-term goals include improving knowledge retention, usually about 6–12 months posteducational event. A test or survey can be carried out to measure both short- and medium-term goals. Long-term goals aim to achieve sustained behavior change. This can be measured by calculating the percentage of people who performed the indicated behavior before and after the intervention. However, because of its long-term nature, the behavior changes can be difficult to attribute back to a specific activity.

### 3.6.2 Knowledge, Attitude, and Practice (KAP) Surveys

Knowledge, attitude, and practice (KAP) surveys are commonly performed as a means to guide interventions and measure program effectiveness. KAP surveys are focused evaluations that measure changes in human knowledge, attitudes, and practices in response to a specific intervention. They typically involve the use of a structured and standardized questionnaire [17]. KAP surveys are typically performed multiple times, often before and after a program, to assess changes or trends over time.

### 3.6.3 Quantitative versus Qualitative Evaluation

Measuring the impact of community engagement activities can be difficult, and will depend upon the specific goals of the program. Although quantitative measures are very useful for scientific evaluation qualitative data is equally valuable to understand what changes have occurred within the community. Numbers work well for analyzing statistics and progress, but they can't express motives, sentiments, and feelings about a particular program. Quantitative measures may include the number of community members participating in an activity, number of people demonstrating a change in behavior, and the number of communities participating in the project. Qualitative measures include stories from the community, feedback from the various stakeholders, and before and after photos.

## 3.7 Community Engagement Resources

A variety of resources are readily available for further discussion and self-study on this topic.

*Online*
*Participatory Epidemiology: A Toolkit for Trainers*
Manual edited by Stacie Dunkle and Jeffrey Mariner
https://cgspace.cgiar.org/handle/10568/35216
*A Handbook for Trainers on Participatory Local Development: The Panchayati Raj Model in India. Second Edition*
Food and Agricultural Organization of the United Nations
http://www.fao.org/docrep/007/ae536e/ae536e00.HTM
*Public Engagement in International Animal Welfare: Reflections and Cases*
Overseas Development Institute
Report written by Ajoy Datta
https://www.odi.org/sites/odi.org.uk/files/odi-assets/publications-opinion-files/7490.pdf
*Sharing the Load: Sustainable Community Action to Improve the Welfare of Working Animals in Developing Countries*
Report by Lisa van Dijk et al.
http://www.australiananimalwelfare.com.au/app/webroot/files/upload/files/Sharing the load.pdf

*Text*
*Questionnaire design, interviewing, and attitude measurement. Second edition*
Oppenheim, A.N. (2000). Bloomsbury Publishing.
*Fostering Sustainable Behavior: An Introduction to Community-Based Social Marketing. Third edition* McKenzie-Mohr, D. (2011) New Society Publishers.

# References

1 Centers for Disease Control and Prevention (1997). Principles of Community Engagement, 1ee. Atlanta: CDC/ATSDR Committee on Community Engagement.

2 Bonwell, C. and Eison, J. (1991). Active Learning: Creating Excitement in the Classroom. *AEHE-ERIC Higher Education Report No. 1.* George Washington University, Washington, DC.

3 Brisbane Declaration (2005). International Conference on Engaging Communities. Brisbane Declaration [online]. Available at: https://www.qld.gov.au/web/community-engagement/guides-factsheets/documents/brisbane_declaration.pdf (accessed 26 May 2016).

4 Catley, A., Alders, R.G., and Wood, J.L.N. (2012). Participatory epidemiology: approaches, methods, experiences. *The Veterinary Journal* **191**: 151–160.

5 Fleming, N.D. and Mills, C. (1992). Not another inventory, rather a catalyst for reflection. *To Improve the Academy* **11**: 137–155.

6 Knowles, M. (1984). Andragogy in Action. Applying Modern Principles of Adult Education. San Francisco, CA: Proquest Info & Learning.

7 Prochaska, J.O., DiClemente, C.C., and Norcross, J.C. (1992). In search of how people change. Applications to addictive behaviors. *American Psychologist* **47** (9): 1102–1114.

8 The Welfare Basis for Euthanasia of Dogs and Cats and Policy Development (2011). International Companion Animal Management Coalition. The welfare basis for euthanasia of dogs and cats and policy development [online]. Available at: http://www.icam-coalition.org/downloads/ICAM-Euthanasia%20Guide-ebook.pdf (accessed 08 December 2017).

9 Jost, C.C., Mariner, J.C., Roeder, P.L. et al. (2007). Participatory epidemiology in disease surveillance and research. *Revue Scientifique Et Technique* **26** (3): 537–549.

10 Noar, S.M. (2006). A 10-year retrospective of research in health mass media campaigns: where do we go from here? *Journal of Health Communication* **11** (1): 21–42.

11 World Health Organization (2001). Information, education and communication: lessons from the past; Perspectives for the future. Occasional Paper. Available at: http://apps.who.int/iris/bitstream/10665/67127/1/WHO_RHR_01.22.pdf (accessed 08 December 2017).

12 Cofie, P., De Allegri, M., Kouyate, B., and Sauerborn, R. (2013). Effects of information, education, and communication campaign on a community-based health insurance scheme in Burkina Faso. *Global Health Action* **6**: 20791.

13 Bergmann, J. and Sams, A. (2012). Flip Your Classroom: Reach Every Student in Every Class Every Day, 1ee. International Society for Technology in Education.

14 Lage, M.J., Platt, G.J., and Treglia, M. (2000). Inverting the classroom: a gateway to creating an inclusive learning environment. *The Journal of Economic Education* **31** (1): 30–43.

15 Lee, N.R. and Kotler, P. (2015). Social Marketing: Changing Behaviors for Good, 5ee. Sage Publications.

16 Azhar, M., Lubis, A.S., Siregar, E.S. et al. (2010). Participatory disease surveillance and response in Indonesia: strengthening veterinary services and empowering communities to prevent and control highly pathogenic avian influenza. *Avian Diseases* **54**: 761–765.

17 World Health Organization (2008). Advocacy, Communication and Social Mobilization for TB Control: A Guide to Developing Knowledge, Attitude and Practice Surveys. Switzerland: WHO Press.

# 4

# Humane Canine Handling, Capture, and Transportation

*Mark R. Johnson,[1] Katherine Polak,[2] and Consie von Gontard[3]*

[1]*Dog Capture and Care Resources, Greenbank, WA 98253, USA*
[2]*Four Paws International, 11th Floor B, Gypsum Metropolitan Tower, 539/2 Sri Ayudhaya Road, Thanon Phaya Thai, Ratchathewi, Bangkok, 10400 Thailand*
[3]*Florida State Animal Response Coalition, 235 Apollo Beach Boulevard, Suite #311, Apollo Beach, FL 33572, USA*

## 4.1 Introduction

Humane animal handling underpins every veterinary field operation intent on improving animal welfare. The objective of most field programs is to humanely reduce stray animal populations and improve community acceptance and attitudes toward animals. In fact, the success of catch–vaccinate–neuter–return (CVNR) and rabies control programs often depends on the capture of at least 70–80% of a given animal population [1,2]. This may require the physical handling of tens of thousands of animals depending on the given location. In order to accomplish such ambitious goals, careful attention should be paid to choosing the most effective and humane techniques. While numerous capture and handling methods exist, the most appropriate technique will depend on staffing, available supplies, working environment, animal population, and cost. Irrespective of the method employed, sound handling skills are essential to protect both handler and animal.

While animal capture is primarily seen as a way of collecting animals for spay/neuter clinics or rabies vaccination, it should also be viewed as an opportunity for community engagement and promotion of humane animal care and treatment. The long-term success of most stray animal population management programs is contingent upon changes in community attitudes toward animals. Free-roaming animals may be perceived as having very little value in a community, subject to frequent abuse and neglect. Treating animals with respect during capture programs demonstrates compassion and can set a precedent for humane animal treatment. This chapter is designed to provide an overview of the most common handling and capture techniques used in the field. While the chapter emphasizes techniques used primarily for free-roaming dogs, special mention is given when particular methods apply to both cats and dogs.

## 4.2 Humane Handling

Humane handling methods improve working conditions for staff by reducing their chances of being bitten or scratched. Handlers must be appropriately trained in such methods to prevent both human injury and unnecessary animal suffering. While this chapter provides a brief overview of some of the most commonly used techniques in the field, hands-on training is necessary to ensure handler and animal safety. Advice and training may be available through international animal welfare organizations including Humane Society International (HSI), International Fund for Animal Welfare (IFAW), and the Royal Society of Prevention of Cruelty to Animals (RSPCA). Another valuable training resource is Dog Capture and Care Resources (www.dogcaptureandcare.com), which provides detailed descriptions of techniques and equipment for capturing free-roaming dogs. Local animal shelters and humane organizations may also offer training courses in dog handling.

In addition to being adequately trained, animal handlers must also be appropriately rabies vaccinated, have the necessary equipment, and understand their role and responsibilities. Depending on the project, handlers may choose to work in pairs or small groups rather than individually, which is typically safer and more effective.

The safest and most humane method of capture will depend on the particular animal and working environment. As a general rule, the least invasive method of handling and restraint should be employed first.

### 4.2.1 Approaching a Free-Roaming Dog in the Field

There are a few general considerations that can increase both capture success and handler safety in the field. Firstly, free-roaming dogs are frequently unfamiliar with handling by humans and are therefore often more fearful of people than traditionally owned dogs. Furthermore, since free-roaming animals may be less likely to receive routine veterinary care and are more likely to be victims of vehicular trauma, these dogs may exhibit signs of aggression due to underlying painful medical conditions. Therefore, these animals should be approached slowly and handled with caution.

When approaching any unfamiliar dog, one should consider approaching from the dog's side rather than head on, avoiding direct eye contact which could trigger a flight response. While approaching, the handler should watch closely for signs of fear or aggression. Appendix 4.A includes a description of canine body language signals.

Upon getting closer to the dog, many handlers will attempt to make their bodies "smaller" by crouching down perpendicularly to the dog. At this point, the

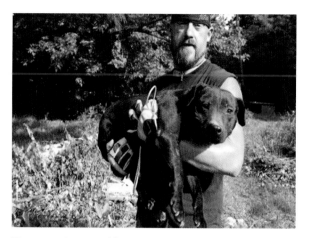

**Figure 4.1** Humane lifting and handling of a dog in the field. Source: Courtesy of The HSUS.

animal can sometimes be lured toward to the handler using food held in the palm of an open hand or a second member of a capture team can approach the animal from behind if necessary.

### 4.2.2 Lifting and Carrying

Proper lifting and carrying techniques are essential to protect both the animal and handler. Both ends of the animal must be supported at all times. When lifting and carrying dogs, dogs should not be scruffed (grasping tightly behind the neck). This is particularly pertinent to brachycephalic breeds (those that have a domed head, flat nose, and protruding eyes).

It is unacceptable to carry any animal by the scruff, loose skin, legs, or tail. Both the head/chest area and the abdominal/hip area must be supported as demonstrated in Figure 4.1. A muzzle wrap consisting of a lead wrapped several times around the muzzle with a towel over the head can help control the head/mouth to facilitate handling. With larger dogs,

---

**Textbox 4.1 Tips for approaching unfamiliar dogs in the field**

- Prior to approaching, assess the area for any hazards that the animal could run into if scared, such as trafficked roads. Be on the lookout for safe areas that the animal can be driven towards.
- Remain calm and approach slowly. Avoid making quick movements.

- Keep catching equipment hidden from the dog being caught. Certain equipment such as collapsible nets and leads can be hidden behind the back of the handler.
- Consider using a tasty treat as a lure.
- Assuming a crouched position may appear less threatening to the dog.

handlers should work together as a team to safely and gently transport the animal.

### 4.2.3 The Y Pole

The Y pole is a humane tool for handling fearful dogs that was recently introduced to the animal welfare community by the author, Dr. Mark Johnson of Dog Capture and Care Resources [3]. The Y pole is simply a Y-shaped metal pole with a long handle that facilitates the handling of dogs that are already caught or cornered, or are unsafe for catching with a lead alone. The Y pole is particularly useful when working with fearful dogs in kennels. In shelters, the Y pole can significantly replace most uses of the catch pole for more compassionate handling.

Companies that sell the Y pole incorrectly describe it as a tool for pinning a dog to a wall or fence. Rather it is used as a safe and compassionate extension of the handler's arm to invite the animal to comply with whatever action is desired. The Y pole is carefully placed on the dog's neck without using excessive pressure (Figure 4.2). Such force is unnecessary because the Y pole is intended to be used *in cooperation* with the dog, allowing for the placement of a lead around the neck or head cover, a physical exam, administration of injections, or use of a syringe pole. It is imperative that the handler works in a calm and kind manner when using a Y pole.

#### 4.2.3.1 How to Use the Y Pole

The handler should first walk slowly towards the cornered animal and stop when or if the dog appears tense. If this happens, the handler should remain calm, let the dog settle, then slowly approach the dog again. The Y pole should be held in both hands so that the upper tine is slightly below the dog's eye level. As the handler continues to approach the dog calmly, the Y pole should be moved toward the corner of the dog's mouth. The dog should be allowed to bite the Y pole if necessary, and the handler should remain calm, and not pull back if he bites the pole. Most dogs will soon look away, offering their neck and allowing the Y pole to be softly placed over the neck. Following acceptance of the Y pole, a lead can then be placed around his neck for additional restraint and/or a towel placed over his head for stress reduction.

If the dog refuses to comply and repeatedly bites the Y pole, it can be used as a pin stick to hold the animal against a wall or ground as a last resort. If the handler wishes to anesthetize the dog, this is a good time to use a Y pole in conjunction with a syringe pole to administer appropriate sedatives.

#### 4.2.3.2 Other Uses for the Y Pole

The Y pole can be used after a dog is netted to reduce struggling in the net. After netting the dog, the net is quickly twisted to secure the dog and a second person can then place the Y pole over the twisted portion of the net. This will facilitate securing the net and controlling the dog while administering intramuscular injections such as rabies vaccines. A towel placed over the dog will also help reduce struggling. Some find the Y pole of particular use in shelter environments to humanely work with kenneled dogs, particularly those that might be aggressive.

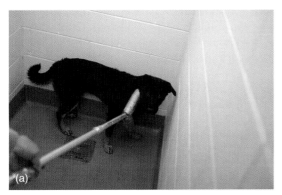 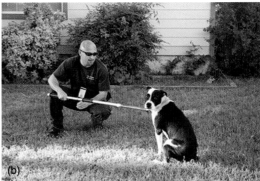

**Figure 4.2** (a) Approaching a dog with a Y pole. Source: Courtesy of Mark R. Johnson DVM, Dog Capture and Care Resources. (b) Calmly restraining a dog using a catch pole. Source: Courtesy of The HSUS.

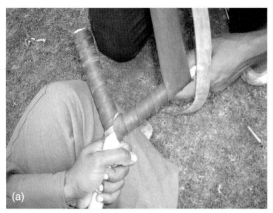
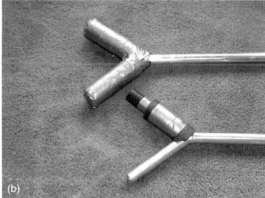

**Figure 4.3** Finishing the construction of a Y pole. (a) Y pole is wrapped with bicycle inner tubing. (b) A demo Y pole showing each layer (bottom) and a finished Y pole (top). Source: Courtesy of Mark R. Johnson DVM, Dog Capture and Care Resources.

### 4.2.3.3 Constructing a Y Pole

To build a Y pole, one should find a welder who is familiar with working with aluminum. Aluminum ensures that the Y pole will be both light and strong. The handle is typically about 4.5 ft (1.37 m) long. The welder should weld 6 in. (15 cm) tines to the handle in the shape of a "Y" so the tines form a 70–80° angle as shown in Figure 4.3. This size is effective when handling most dogs. Y poles can be made in different lengths and shapes to fit a variety of animal sizes and situations.

The first layer should be wrapped over each tine and consist of a rugged material to prevent the dog's teeth from contacting the metal. Such material may include PVC tubing, automotive heater hose, or several layers of bicycle inner tubing. This first layer should be reinforced with duct tape and a second layer consisting of closed-cell foam added. Such foam is used because it does not absorb water. The easiest foam to work with is long, tube-shaped pipe insulation. Multiple layers of duct tape are then applied as tightly as possible ensuring that the ends of each tine are thoroughly covered. This helps prevent dogs from fracturing their teeth should they bite on the pole.

### 4.2.4 Catch Pole

The catch pole, also known as a control pole or rabies pole, is a rigid metal pole with an adjustable plastic-coated cable loop at one end designed to maneuver an animal. They are primarily used in the field to guide a dog onto a transport vehicle or into a cage. The catch pole may be one of the most commonly used tools for catching and controlling dogs, particularly in North America; yet they should be considered the last tool in the authors' opinion. Catch poles are easily misused and often result in serious injury to the animal if used incorrectly. However, when used properly with care and concern for the animal, the catch pole can be a versatile and effective tool in certain situations. The poles come in varying lengths and with different options for adjusting and releasing the cable from around the animal's neck. When purchasing a catch pole, one should ensure that it has an instant release mechanism and a swivel.

---

**Textbox 4.2 Online Y pole training resources**

The Y Pole Page
Y pole history, construction, and techniques along with training videos.
Dog Capture and Care Resources
www.dogcaptureandcare.com

One Cool Tool – article on the Y pole in Animal Sheltering Magazine
www.wildliferesources.com/wp-content/uploads/2010/04/One-Cool-Tool.pdf

---

**Textbox 4.3 How to correctly use a catch pole:**

Step 1. Slowly approach the dog holding the catch pole directly behind you or at your side. Never approach a dog with the catch pole facing the dog.

Step 2. Using both hands, slip the noose (cable) over the dog's head until fully encompassing the neck. Pull the release cord with one hand to tighten the cable until the loop fits snugly. Never over-tighten the cable lead around the animal's neck.

Step 3. While keeping your hands spaced on the pole, stand beside the dog and guide him ahead, in the desired direction. Most dogs will begin to walk, but if not, adjust your location to be slightly behind the dog.

Step 4. Once in the desired location, loosen the cord to free the dog.

*Helpful hint #1. Wrap the end of the catch pole with multiple layers of vet wrap or place a large Kong®-type toy around the end of the pole. This will prevent injury if the dogs bite the pole.*

*Helpful hint #2. Those who have acquired the skill working with a Y pole recommend using the catch pole as if it is a Y pole.*

---

Catch poles should *never* be used to do the following:

- Catch or restrain a cat
- Lift an animal off the ground
- Drag, yank, or pull an animal.

Appendix 4.B further describes how to use a catch pole. In addition to using them correctly, catch poles must also be properly maintained to ensure their functionality. Catch poles should be stored on their side, on a flat surface, or using clips rather than hanging them by the loop which causes the loop to become deformed. The loop should maintain a tear shape. The standard "spring-loaded" cable release may also jam and become unusable if the cable is frayed, bent, or has been chewed on. This can create a dangerous situation for both the animal and handler. Cables should generally be replaced every 18–24 months.

### 4.2.5 Jhali

Another humane tool for handling fearful dogs in kennels is a modified version of a pig board known as a *jhali*, which means "mesh" or "screen" in Hindi. This method is commonly used in CVNR programs in India [2]. The *jhali* is made of an angle iron frame roughly 1 square yard (1 m) covered with 1 in. (2.54 cm) welded wire or mesh. This provides a physical barrier between the dog and handler, allowing the handler to safely work with the dog in a confined kennel space. Attaching handles on the handler side of the *jhali* improves safety and ease

of handling. With a soft gentle pressure against the dog, the handler can move the animal toward a corner or against the wall to observe wounds, apply topical treatments, and administer injections (Figure 4.4). In some situations, two *jhalis* can be used to contain a dog.

## 4.3 Capture Techniques

Preferred capture methods reduce animal stress, minimize the risk of animal and human injury, and protect the public. All handling and capture techniques rely on the animal handler first having a general understanding of how to safely approach an animal in the

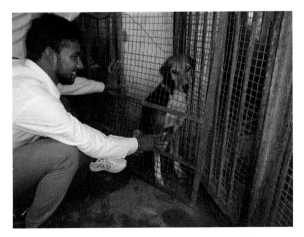

**Figure 4.4** Use of a *jhali* for humane restraint in a kennel in India. Source: Courtesy of Help in Suffering, Jaipur, India.

field. As mentioned earlier, catching is typically the safest and most efficient when catchers work in pairs or small teams. Multiple catch teams should be used in programs requiring the capture of many animals spread out over a large geographical area.

### 4.3.1 Hand Capture

Hand capture refers to using a lead placed around the dog's neck and walking him to a transport vehicle or cage, or physically lifting and carrying the animal. This method works best in areas where dogs are accustomed to people and can be safely handled. Feeders and those who have a relationship with the particular animal can be used to help pick animals up and place them into a transport vehicle or box trap.

Hand capture requires minimal equipment but significant training and experience in dog handling. This method can result in serious bite wounds to handlers if attempted with improper technique on fearful or aggressive dogs. Table 4.1 lists some of the advantages and disadvantages of this method.

The technique for hand capturing a dog in principle is quite simple. A skilled handler entices a dog with food or treats, waiting for him or her to approach. Once close enough to touch, the handler places one arm under the belly or around the rump of the animal with the other arm around the neck as close to the head as possible. Handlers should be wearing protective gloves as hands and arms are close to the animal's mouth. The dog should then be gently lifted and placed into either a truck or transport cage. A

temporary wrap around the dog's muzzle with the lead can help protect the handler from accidental bites. Adding a towel to cover the head minimizes animal stress and increases human safety, particularly while carrying.

### 4.3.2 Slip Leads

Slip leads are useful for catching friendly, socialized dogs particularly in areas where there is a large number of owned animals. They are relatively easy to use; the large loop is first placed around the dog's head and the handle pulled. The loop gets tighter as the animal pulls away. The most functional leads used in fieldwork are slip leads, rather than trigger-clip leads that attach to a dog's collar. The majority of free-roaming dogs are not wearing reliable collars suitable for restraint.

To control a fractious or difficult-to-handle dog, the handler may consider placing two slip leads around the dog's head and positioning a handler on both sides of the animal. One should ensure that there is adequate slack in at least one of the leads. This technique of using two leads allows better control of the dog without creating excessive tension on the neck and also prevents the dog from thrashing and rolling. A third person can also place a towel or sheet over the animal's head for stress reduction. Alternatively, if the dog has a long enough muzzle, a two-handed scruff can be used to temporarily control the head while another handler wraps a lead a few turns around the dog's muzzle.

Slip leads should never be placed around the neck of a cat. A safer alternative for feline restraint is to wrap them up tightly in a towel, minimizing the potential for scratching and escape.

There are a variety of canine slip leads to choose from and only the most commonly used types are described here (Figure 4.5).

#### 4.3.2.1 Flat Slip Lead

Flat slip leads are made of an inexpensive nylon or cotton ribbon style lead with a "D" ring on one end and a loop handle on the other end. This style of slip lead is inexpensive and can also be fashioned into a muzzle or harness if needed. The drawback to this lead is that dogs can easily and quickly chew through the material and escape.

Table 4.1 Advantages and disadvantages of hand capture.

| Advantages | Disadvantages |
| --- | --- |
| Reduces the risk of injury to the animal. | Animal responses can be unpredictable as many free-roaming animals are unfamiliar with restraint and handling. |
| Can be more visually pleasing to the public than other capture methods. | |
| Can be one of the most humane capture methods when performed correctly. | Requires considerable skill and comfort with animal handling. |

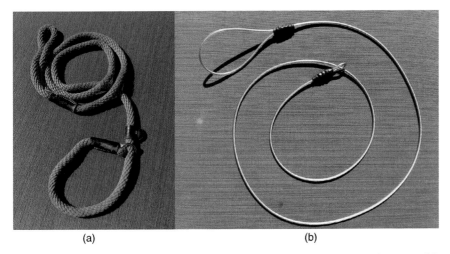

(a)         (b)

**Figure 4.5** (a) British-style slip lead and (b) plastic-coated cable lead. Source: Courtesy of Consie Von Gontard.

#### 4.3.2.2 British-Style Slip Lead

British-style slip leads are made of rope with a sliding leather tab that can be positioned to prevent the lead from loosening after it is placed around the dog's neck. The British-style slip lead is much more durable than the flat/ribbon style slip lead and can also be fashioned into a muzzle or harness. Due to the thickness of the rope, it is also more difficult for the animal to chew through and escape. This style lead is more expensive than the flat slip lead, but in the authors' opinion it is worth the extra cost due to its sturdiness and functionality.

#### 4.3.2.3 Plastic-Coated Cable Lead

Plastic-coated cable leads are also known as an ACO's Friend Lead and consist of a plastic-coated braided cable, which is virtually "bite proof." They are typically 5–7 ft (1.5–2.1 m) in length. This style lead should be used as a last resort as the cable can be difficult to loosen when an animal struggles. Due to the size of the cable and the inability to loosen it, there is a possibility of damage to the trachea and even asphyxiation. One advantage of this lead is that the stiffness of the coated cable allows the handler to carefully slide the lead over a dog's head as it is leaning against a wall. If one is not an advanced animal handler and familiar with using this lead, it is recommended that a British-style or flat slip lead be used instead. Uncoated wire cable leads should never be used under any circumstances.

### 4.3.3 Netting

Nets are the most commonly used catching tool in the field worldwide because they can be used to catch large numbers of moving animals quickly. Netting is particularly useful for programs that require quick capture and release, such as during rabies vaccination campaigns. Table 4.2 describes the various advantages and disadvantages of netting.

There are multiple types of nets used in the field including pole nets, throw nets, and hoop nets, which are all described here. Nets vary in cost depending on the materials and quality. The type of net used will depend on the animal to be captured and the working conditions and environment. Nets can be effective for catching both dogs and cats. If used to catch cats however, the diameter of the holes in the net must be small enough to prevent the cat's legs from becoming entangled. The preferred mesh hole size in nets for cats is no larger than 0.5 in. (1.27 cm). Nets should consist of a material that can be easily cleaned and disinfected to prevent disease transmission, such as polypropylene or polyethylene. For both cats and dogs, nets are to be placed over the animal rather than trying to "scoop" them from beneath.

#### 4.3.3.1 Pole Nets

Pole nets are commonly used to capture unsocialized dogs, and the hoop diameter should be quite large. In the United States, salmon nets have an ideal hoop

**Table 4.2** Advantages and disadvantages of net capture.

| Advantages | Disadvantages |
| --- | --- |
| Cost of obtaining or fabricating nets is often significantly less than other types of capture tools (i.e. box traps). Nets can be easily made using an aluminum frame and fishing net. | Mesh netting may require frequent replacement. |
| Technically easier than chemical capture or trapping. | Requires extensive practice, experience, and a degree of physical fitness to use. May also require a team effort. |
| During rabies vaccination campaigns, dogs can be easily vaccinated through the net and released. | May be visually displeasing to the public. |

diameter of $32 \times 41$ in. ($81 \times 104$ cm). The net itself must be deep enough for the handler to twist the net multiple times, safely securing the dog. Most nets are between 4 and 5 ft (1.2–1.5 m) deep. Twisting the dog in the net is important to prevent escape and minimize struggling. Some nets have a feature that allows the pole to be removed, enabling two people to carry the netted dog away using the hoop frame. Other types have drawstring closures to quickly secure and release the animal. After a dog is caught in a net, a Y pole can be placed over the twisted part of the net and the animal covered with a towel for stress reduction, as demonstrated in Figure 4.6.

#### 4.3.3.2 Throw Nets

Throw nets, also known as cast nets, typically consist of a simple design of a $25.8\,\text{ft}^2$ ($2.4\,\text{m}^2$) mesh with a weighted rim. These are cast over an animal, often when they are lying down [2]. The net typically takes the animal by surprise and works by entangling them within the net. Note that animals entangled in these nets are still capable of moving and possibly running away; the nets may simply just slow them down.

#### 4.3.3.3 Hoop Nets

Hoop nets are large circular nets designed for casting over the top of the target animal. They typically consist of a 39–50 in. (100–150 cm) lightweight aluminum hoop with an attached net.

### 4.3.4 Sack Method (Do Bora)

Every spay/neuter or municipal program should have as many humane tools as possible for catching dogs. While nets are fast and reliable, the sack method, also

known as *do bora*, meaning "two sacks" in Hindi, is another valuable catching tool. These are easy to make, inexpensive, and can catch dogs in locations where traditional nets cannot [2].

The *do bora* is made from two burlap sacks. To make one, one side seam on each sack should be opened and sewed together into one large sack. Eight metal rings are then be sewn evenly spaced along the top edge. A long rope of approximately 6 ft (1.8 m) is threaded through the rings and finally tied to the last ring, which acts as a draw string. The free end of the rope should have a loop to place around the handler's wrist. The sack is thrown over the dog and the rope is quickly pulled, tightening the sack and securing the dog. Figure 4.7 depicts the capture process using a *do bora*.

In difficult-to-maneuver places such as narrow streets, traditional nets are too large and difficult to hide. With the sack method, the handler can easily tuck it under his arm and approach a dog casually, without scaring him away. Dogs are experts at reading body language and as such, handlers should be as casual and calm as possible when approaching dogs. Handlers should not think only about catching the dog when approaching. If they do, their body language is usually tense, and the handler will look like a predator. Instead, handlers are encouraged to be cognizant of how they look, stay relaxed, and hide their intentions.

When using the *do bora*, two handlers typically work as a team. One staff member distracts the dog with food, while the other throws the sack over the dog and pulls the rope tight, trapping the dog inside. The sack is later lifted into the transport

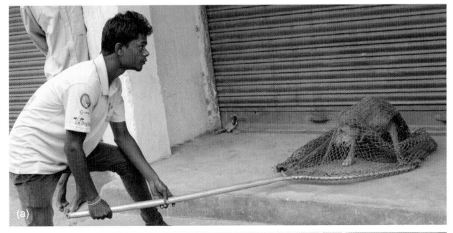

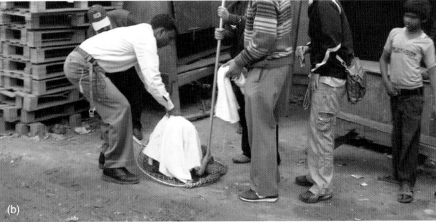

Figure 4.6 (a) Handler using a handmade pole net to capture a free-roaming dog in India. The net is locally made, using a frame constructed of an aluminum rod measuring 4 ft and a hoop frame of approximately 2 × 2 ft. Fishing net is attached to the frame using a strong fishing line. Source: Courtesy of Praveen Ohal, Mission Rabies, World Veterinary Services. (b) Dog captured with a net and Y pole. A towel is placed over the dog's head for immediate stress reduction. Source: Courtesy of Mark R. Johnson DVM, Dog Capture and Care Resources.

vehicle and the rope is loosened, which releases the dog. With use, sacks will become soiled and require frequent washing.

### 4.3.5 Trapping

Humane live trapping can be the safest and least stressful means of capturing difficult-to-catch dogs and cats when performed correctly. Trapping refers to the use of a box-style trap to safely and humanely capture an animal; it does not refer to the use of traps that capture the animal by the leg or snaring. These are referred to as leg hold or snare traps, which should never be used in the field.

Because trapping can require a significant amount of time per animal, it is best suited for CVNR programs where the animals require transport to a clinic site for surgery rather than for mass-vaccination programs, which require quick capture and release. Table 4.3 describes the advantages and disadvantages of using traps in the field for catching free-roaming cats and dogs.

#### 4.3.5.1 Choosing a Live Capture Trap

There are a wide variety of traps to choose from. For smaller animals such as cats, traps should be constructed of lightweight materials. A basic cat trap is constructed from 1 × 1 in. 14-gauge galvanized steel

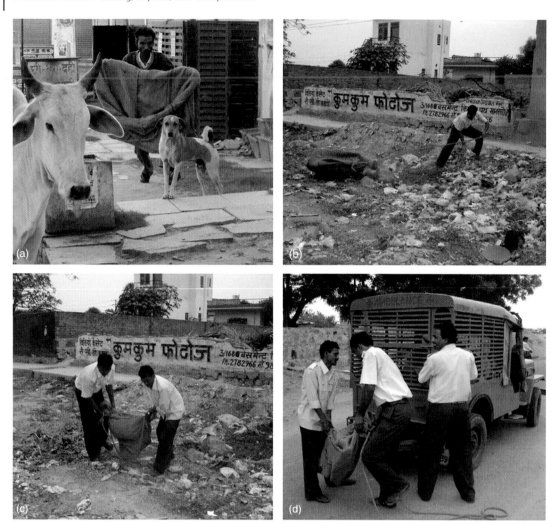

**Figure 4.7** Catching a dog using the sack (*do bora*) method. Source: (a) Courtesy of Danny Chambers MRCVS (b,c,d) Courtesy of Jack Reece, Help in Suffering.

**Table 4.3** Advantages and disadvantages of trapping.

| Advantages | Disadvantages |
| --- | --- |
| While trap closure may cause initial panic, animals typically calm down quickly. | Traps can be expensive and cumbersome to transport, store, and maintain. |
| Allows for the capture of many animals over a short period of time given an adequate number of traps. | May take hours or days to trap a single animal. |
| Poses minimal risk of human injury. | Forgotten set traps can be deadly. |
| | Can be easily stolen if not secured while in use. |
| Ideal for CVNR and TNR clinics to safely transport animals to a clinic for surgery. | |

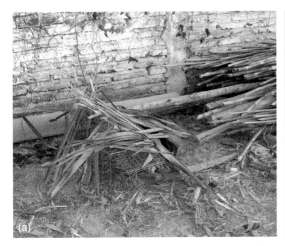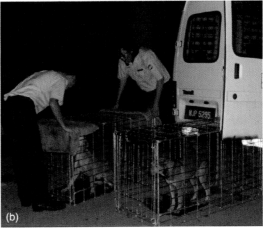

**Figure 4.8** (a) Disguised cat trap. Source: Courtesy of Consie von Gontard (b) Dogs trapped using box traps in Malaysia. Source: Courtesy of Adrian Johnson Lim, Aurum Paradisa Sdn Bhd, Malaysia.

mesh wire grid measuring $26 \times 9 \times 9$ in. ($66 \times 23 \times 23$ cm). For animals weighing more than 20 pounds (9 kg), traps must be durable and well-constructed, with a sturdy trip plate. A high-quality trap is well worth the money spent. A major disadvantage of larger "dog-sized" traps is their size, making them cumbersome to store and transport. For this reason, it is advisable to purchase folding traps. Medium-sized dogs trapped in box traps are illustrated in Figure 4.8b.

As opposed to traditional box traps, live capture drop traps for cats can be purchased or constructed inexpensively. A wooden frame, covered by netting or mesh is propped up on one side. Food is placed in the back under the trap. The trapper, who stands at a distance, pulls on a string attached to a prop-stick when the cat is inside, allowing the trap to drop,

capturing the cat. Animals captured in the drop trap can then enter a transport cage through a small trap door on the side of the drop trap. The disadvantage of these traps is that they must be constantly monitored and manually triggered when the animal enters the trap.

### 4.3.5.2 Creating a Trapping Plan

Successful trapping for CVNR and TNR programs requires planning, surveying, adequate staffing and equipment, and monitoring of the animal population over time. Success also depends on the cooperation of multiple stakeholders including local animal shelters, TNR groups, and community members. Chapter 3 describes effective methods of community engagement.

Running a successful trapping campaign requires organization and accountability. Working within an

---

**Textbox 4.4 Capture considerations**

- Why is a capture program necessary?
- What are the safety concerns?
- What are the legalities of trapping free-roaming owned animals in the working area?
- What species will be trapped? Cats, dogs, or both?
- What is the target number per day to trap? How many total animals require trapping?
- How many traps are available? What type of sizes will be used?
- Who is responsible for record-keeping?
- Who will return the animals to the field and when?
- Who will provide transport/vehicles?
- Where will trapped animals be housed?

established organizational structure prevents duplication of effort and streamlines operations and communications.

### 4.3.5.3 Legal Issues

Certain locations may have legal restrictions on both the trapping and feeding of free-roaming animals. It is important to first identify pertinent legislation prior to performing any actual field work to ensure program activities are legally permissible. Plans should also be in place for the accidental capture of an obviously owned, roaming animal. A concerted effort should be made to identify the owner of any animal with physically affixed identification (collars, tags) or microchip. When trapping owned animals for spay/neuter surgery, owners should always be encouraged to sign waivers, permitting such activity.

### 4.3.5.4 Community Consideration

Animal capture programs must respect the local customs, religious beliefs, and the role animals play in the community. In advance of any trapping taking place, community members must be informed that free-roaming animals will be collected, on what dates, and that this could affect roaming owned pets as well. Effective communication media include radio, television, newspapers, posters, and going door-to-door.

Preparations for the clinic should include communication with members of the community in regards to where animal populations reside. Children are often a wealth of information as to the movements and locations of the community animals, particularly those in whelping dens.

### 4.3.5.5 Feeding Stations

Setting up feeding stations in target trapping areas can "train" animals to congregate in specific areas facilitating capture. Feeding stations should be established in areas that are safe for the animals and can minimize potential negative interactions with humans or other animals. Feeding stations or trapping areas located on private property rather than public grounds are preferred, which provide a more controlled, safe environment for both animals and handlers.

Ideally, the area selected for such stations should be large enough to create several feeding stations with a significant distance between them. This will ensure all animals have safe access to food. Feeding stations should be set up ideally 2 weeks prior to the onset of trapping. Feeding should be done at the same time each day, preferably around dusk or dawn. When feeding, the authors recommend the use of white- or light-colored plates/bowls to feed with. The white color can be easily seen at night from a distance, facilitating recognition of the station. If birds steal the food, bowls can be placed over it for protection, as dogs and cats will generally still be able to locate it. Consistent feeding of animals at a feeding station might also help identify animals that have medical issues requiring attention during the clinic.

Once the animals are accustomed to being fed in a certain location they should be fed in unset traps. This should ideally be done for a minimum of a week prior to the clinic start date. The trap doors can be wired open to ensure that they do not close once the animal enters the trap. This allows the animals to acclimate to the traps and facilitate capture once the clinic starts. This works particularly well for trap-shy animals. The evening before the clinic, the wires keeping the trap doors open can be removed to set the traps. Note that traps that are wired open must be visited at least once daily to prevent accidental captures.

### 4.3.5.6 Getting Organized

Before going into the field, capture teams should be briefed on the overall goal of the trapping program, a plan for the working period, the boundaries of the working areas, all paperwork procedures including trap records and intake/release paperwork, staff and animal safety issues, and a communication plan.

Trapping supplies should also be inventoried and ready to go. Recommended supplies include the following:

- Traps and trap covers
- Food trays, can openers, spoons/forks
- Baits
- Personal supplies such as first-aid kits, water, snacks
- Heavy duty gloves
- Headlamps
- Notebook and pen
- Trapping records.

### 4.3.5.7 Trap Preparations

All traps must be cleaned and disinfected prior to use to prevent the spread of disease between animals. This is particularly important when working with

---

**Textbox 4.5 Potential trapping safety issues**

*Inclement weather.* Animals are vulnerable in traps, and extremes in temperature and rain can be life-threatening. Avoid trapping in the rain or heat of the day without appropriate weatherproofing and/or shade.

*Vehicular traffic.* Traps should not be positioned in such a way that the animal has to cross a busy street to get to them.

*Human interference.* Ideally, position traps well away from pedestrian walkways or public areas.

*Theft.* Traps are sometimes stolen for metal recycling or repurposed as fish and crab traps. In certain areas, chains or cables and sturdy padlocks should be used to secure traps.

---

different colonies of animals. Traps should be inspected well in advance of the trapping, as well as prior to each use, to ensure that they are functioning properly.

Traps should be individually numbered and equipped with permanent signage indicating the name and contact information for the organization trapping. Additional trap signage may include a "Spay/neuter program in progress" sign. Members of the public may damage a trap trying to "rescue" a trapped animal that he or she believes is stuck in the trap. Traps can also be color-coded if multiple teams are catching animals from distinct colonies or areas.

Whenever possible, traps should be prepared away from the trapping location. The activity and commotion associated with preparing traps may scare animals away. Traps should be set just before normal feeding time and as quietly as possible. If headlamps or flashlights are required, one may consider using red- or green-colored lights to avoid scaring off other animals in the area.

All set traps must be recorded and mapped. Each team should maintain trap records for every trap they set along with a map of the exact location the trap was set. The most catastrophic trapping scenario is a trap that is set and forgotten. Records should also contain the trap number and color codes, date, exact location, time set, bait used, capture time, and animal details including species, sex, color and markings, and return time and date.

A holding area should be prepared to place trapped animals before and after the clinic. A garage or other protected area free from temperature extremes with newspapers or tarps lining the floor is ideal. If possible, animals being trapped for spay/neuter should be trapped overnight to minimize the amount of pre-surgical time spent in the trap.

#### 4.3.5.8 Trap Placement

There are many considerations for determining trap placement. In general, capture staff should consider the following:

- Find flat and high ground. Animals are far less likely to enter traps that are unstable or on an incline. Traps should never be placed on sloping ground or where water may collect or run off.
- Choose areas that minimize potential harassment of trapped animals by other animals. Dogs may attack cats in a trap.
- Choose an area that can be easily checked by the trapper, either physically or using binoculars from a distance.
- Determine animal movement and place traps in an area frequently visited by the particular animal. If animals are traveling along roads, consider using scent lures and feeding stations to draw them to a safer location.
- If trapping in a public area, choose areas farthest from pedestrian traffic.
- Remember to map all set traps in an area! Label and record every trap set; trappers must account for each trap before leaving the area.

All five senses should be used to improve trapping success. Animals rely heavily on their senses, particularly sight, sound, and smell. Trappers can use this to their advantage to improve trapping odds.

#### 4.3.5.8.1 Sight

Traps should be disguised so that they are integrated into the environment and are inviting to the animal. One should closely examine the surroundings and use readily available materials to camouflage the traps. Traps can be disguised by placing them against foliage and/or leaning branches on the top of the traps (see Figure 4.8a). In urban areas where there may be little "nature" to disguise traps, traps can be placed against a wall, behind a trash can, or any object that is found consistently in the trapping environment.

#### 4.3.5.8.2 Sound

Trappers should be aware of the natural sounds in the trapping area and use common sense. If a nearby house is having a large party, trapping should not occur on that night. Similarly, the sound of tarps or plastic liners used to waterproof traps might scare animals away on a windy night. As a general rule, noise levels should be kept to a minimum at the trapping site. One exception to this is the noise of kittens or puppies, which can be used to attract the mother.

#### 4.3.5.8.3 Smell

Scents can be used to lure animals to a trap. Using urine from a female dog in heat can serve as an attractant for male dogs. Likewise, trapping a queen in heat can be an alluring scent for tomcats in the area. Conversely, a territorial tomcat/male dog that sprays on a trap or marks the area may repel other animals.

When baiting traps with food, those that are oily or packed in oil, such as tuna or mackerel, tend to maintain their scent longer. "Scent lures" can be created by soaking a paper towel in the urine of a female dog in heat. These can be hung from a tree, downwind from the target animals. A liquid scent lure can also be created using a mixture of water and oily food. Conversely, human scent can potentially repel animals.

#### 4.3.5.8.4 Touch

Animals often react negatively to the wire bottom of traps as it is a foreign substrate to walk on. Trap bottoms should be covered with materials from the surrounding environment including dirt, gravel, or leaves that will create a familiar surface for animals to walk on. A piece of cardboard can be used to line the bottom of the trap. Any materials used to disguise the trap bottom should not interfere with the functionality of the trip plate or trap door.

#### 4.3.5.8.5 Taste

Small amounts of "lure" foods can be placed outside the trap to entice animals to enter the trap. These should be small amounts of food that reward the animal for coming close to the trap and putting their head inside the door. A "mother lode" of food should be placed at the far back of the trap or possibly underneath the trap wires so the animal must spend time working to get the food. This increases the probability that the animal will actually step on the trip plate. Note that metal food cans should never be left inside the trap to prevent inadvertent trauma to the animal.

#### 4.3.5.9 Saturation Trapping

Saturation trapping involves catching as many animals in one area in the shortest time possible. A good rule of thumb is to use 50% more traps than the estimated number of animals. For example, in a colony of 20 cats, one should consider setting 30 traps. Saturation trapping helps prevent animals from becoming trap-savvy, whereby animals learn to avoid traps after observing other animals being trapped.

#### 4.3.5.10 Monitoring the Traps

Ideally, set traps should never be left in an unprotected area and should be monitored from a distance. Traps can be monitored from a parked vehicle using binoculars. If physically close enough, trappers may be able to hear the traps close. If monitoring the traps from a distance is not possible, traps should be physically checked every 1–2 h.

Once an animal is trapped, the trap should be transported to a quiet area to check if he or she was previously sterilized, juvenile or adult, or lactating. The traps should be covered by a towel whenever possible to reduce animal stress.

As a general rule, trapped animals should be removed from the trapping site immediately to prevent them from scaring off other animals. Special considerations include the following:

- *Lactating females*. One must carefully inspect all trapped females for lactation to determine if there might be kittens or puppies dependent on her for nutrition nearby. If part of an ongoing project, releasing the lactating female may result in catching her and her offspring at another time. If the clinic is the only chance to perform surgery however, one must weigh the risk of the offspring not having access to the mother for up to 8–12 h with not sterilizing her at all. If surgery is pursued, the time from pickup to release should be minimized, releasing her as soon as she is recovered from anesthesia.
- *Kittens/puppies*. Whenever juvenile animals are observed or trapped, efforts should be made to locate the mother and any litter-mates. One may

consider using kittens or puppies to attract other siblings and the mother by placing the trapped kitten or puppy in another trap or transfer cage adjacent to an empty set trap. The access to the trap containing the puppies or kittens should be blocked in such a way that the only way for the mother to get close to the juvenile is to enter the adjacent trap.

- *Wildlife.* All wildlife should be released quietly.
- *Already sterilized animals.* Sterilized animals (those with obvious ear tips/notches) should be released unless they require booster vaccines, examination, etc.

Trappers may consider setting another trap in the same spot where a trapped animal was removed if it is a "hot spot" for catching. Note that any animals trapped overnight should be the priority for the next day's surgery schedule.

Nothing is more frustrating than animals either avoiding traps altogether or eating food out of the trap without actually setting off the trap. Textbox 4.6 includes some simple tips for trapping trap-savvy animals.

#### 4.3.5.11 Returning Trapped Animals

Following surgery, animals must be returned to the *exact* location where they were trapped. This is critical to the animal's survival. Working closely with the veterinarians at the clinic will ensure that it is safe for the animals to be returned. Animals must be fully ambulatory prior to return. If possible, it is preferred that animals are monitored overnight in their traps and released the following morning. The exception to this are lactating females, which should be returned as soon as possible. If there is any doubt regarding the safety of return, return should be delayed or reassessed. When returning animals, the area of release should be free from danger, including busy streets. During release, traps should be pointed away from streets or potential danger as animals will typically bolt out. Release dates, times, and locations should be logged for each animal.

## 4.4 Chemical Capture

Chemical capture refers to the use of anesthetic drugs to immobilize an animal for capture. It is a veterinary procedure that requires specialized drugs, equipment, and knowledge of caring for the drugged animal including monitoring temperature, pulse, and respiration. Drugs are typically administered using some type of drug delivery system such as a blowpipe, dart gun, or pole syringe. Many programs require handlers to have specific training before they can chemically capture dogs. Although there are entire reference manuals detailing chemical capture, the handler is encouraged to receive professional training rather than train himself or herself prior to undertaking this potentially dangerous activity.

Chemical capture should typically be reserved as a last resort for capture due to its inherent complexities and danger to both humans and animals. Training provides information on how to address these complexities and human and animal risks, an understanding of the legal aspects of using immobilizing drugs, and will inform the handler which immobilizing

---

**Textbox 4.6 Tips for trapping trap-savvy animals**

1) *Acclimatize animals to enter the trap for food ahead of time.* Several days prior to the clinic, wire the traps open so that the animals can enter without triggering the trap. Visit traps every day to provide fresh food and confirm no animals were accidentally caught.

2) *Withhold food for 24 h prior to trapping.* Hungry animals are more likely to enter a trap. Also notify others who may feed animals in the area to not leave food out.

3) *Extend the length of the trip plate.* If the trip plate is too short, clever animals may walk into the trap, have a snack, and walk out without actually setting off the trap. Alternatively, hang a piece of deboned chicken above the trip plate to ensure the animal has to actually step on it to eat.

4) *Use a larger trap.* Some animals refuse to enter traps that are small relative to their body size.

5) *Eliminate unnatural smells.* If using trap covers, store them outside so that they lose their "human" or "unnatural" scent.

6) *Position the trap in a more secluded location.*

**Table 4.4** Advantages and disadvantages of chemical capture.

| Advantages | Disadvantages |
|---|---|
| Can facilitate catching animals from a distance. | Requires extensive training and skill. |
| Reduces both handler and animal stress when working with fractious animals as it requires minimal physical restraint. | Can be a serious hazard to operators, bystanders, and animals. Requires a knowledge of addressing animal health such as monitoring temperature, pulse, and respiration. |
| May facilitate the capture and transport of injured animals for treatment. | Can be expensive, depending on the drugs and equipment used. |
| | May require special permits or be illegal depending on the area. |
| | Only for use in particular environments where there is minimal potential danger to the animal. Not for use in areas with traffic and/or near bodies of water. |
| | Should never be used for dogs weighing less than 5 kg or domestic cats. |

drugs are available, safe, and effective for use in their region. Dart guns/pistols, for instance, may require a special permit to own. Darting and chemical capture should only be performed under veterinary supervision. Before electing to use chemical capture, one should carefully consider the advantages and disadvantages of this technique (Table 4.4).

### 4.4.1 Equipment

Equipment for chemical capture and darting is very specialized and requires expertise and practice to use safely. At a minimum, the following equipment is required:

- A drug delivery system such as a dart gun rifle or pistol (also called projectors), blowpipe, or pole syringe.
- Immobilizing drugs from a veterinarian kept under lock and key.
- Basic handling equipment for animal care including a head cover, thermometer, and stethoscope.
- Items to cool or warm the animal and a crash kit with basic veterinary supplies to address emergencies. See Chapter 15 for information on handling medical emergencies.

Following chemical capture, staff must also have the ability to safely and humanely transport the anesthetized animal to a veterinary facility.

An essential tool for chemical capture is a towel or head cover. If a dog is drugged in a crate or trap, the trap should be covered with a sheet or towel. Covering the head/trap/crate will reduce animal fear and stress,

increase human safety, and demonstrate professionalism and humane animal care. Covering the trap or crate may also increase the effectiveness of the drugs by shortening the induction time and minimizing the need to redose.

#### 4.4.1.1 Pole Syringe

Pole syringes are syringes (with needle attached) mounted on a long pole of typically 3–6 ft (1–2 m) used to inject animals from a distance or through a trap/net. They are essentially an extension of the handler's arm and can only be used over short distances as determined by the length of the pole. Homemade pole syringes can be easily and cheaply made; however, none seem to work as well as commercially available models. Some commercial pole syringes are reusable and require only a new needle with each use. Other commercial pole syringes provide a long handle and plunger and the handler replaces both a new syringe and new needle with each use. Using a Y pole on the dog first may increase the chances of successful injection with the pole syringe.

#### 4.4.1.2 Blowpipe

Blowpipes are used for delivering small volumes of drugs at short distances of typically less than 20 ft (6.1 m). They propel a dart containing drugs through a pipe or tube by rapid expulsion of breath. They are quiet and typically cause little injury to the animal. Blowpipes require considerable skill but can be cheap, effective, and made with local materials such as small-diameter PVC pipes.

### 4.4.1.3 Dart Guns (Projectors)

The most accurate and reliable drug delivery systems that are also safest for the animals have a pressure gauge and use $CO_2$ cartridges to propel the darts. These are available as either $CO_2$ rifles or pistols. The major companies producing these humane projectors are Pneu-Dart (http://www.pneudart.com), Dan-Inject (http://dan-inject.com), and TeleDart (http://teledart.com/en). Cartridge-fired rifles or pistols using blank 0.22 charges should not be used on dogs.

### 4.4.1.4 Darts and Needles

Darts are essentially flying syringes delivered by the $CO_2$ rifle or pistol. They consist of a needle, body, plunger, and tailpiece [3]. Because darts typically expel their contents in 0.001 s, large-bore needles are required. Pneudart darts are disposable and are the easiest to use. DanInject and TeleDart darts are reusable but require cleaning and maintenance after each use. They may also cause less tissue damage than Pneudart. Regardless of the system used, darts must always be recovered if they bounce off or fall out of the animal to avoid a potential public health accident. Anyone darting animals must practice often, order darts with collared needles, and always put a slight arc in the flight of the dart to prevent excessive impact. Pneudart, DanInject, and TeleDart darts are pictured in Figure 4.9.

### 4.4.2 Recommended Drugs

The following information on pharmaceuticals is intended for veterinarians only. Handlers wishing

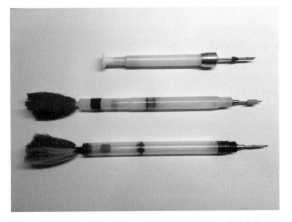

**Figure 4.9** Darts from Pneudart, DanInject, and TeleDart (top to bottom). Source: Courtesy of Mark R. Johnson DVM, Dog Capture and Care Resources.

to chemically capture dogs must first receive appropriate training and work under veterinary supervision. Descriptions of the most commonly used drug combinations are included here. The drugs selected for chemical capture often depend upon local product availability and cost. However, cost should be the least important factor. If a budget for the purchasing of appropriate drugs is lacking, chemical capture should not be used.

Immobilizing drugs are always administered intramuscularly (IM), and capture staff should aim for the large muscles in the hind limb. Most drug combinations do not work instantaneously and doses listed here are only recommendations. Doses should also be adjusted depending on the dog. Young and excited animals may require more drug per unit body weight, whereas a sick or injured animal may require less.

### 4.4.2.1 Ketamine/Xylazine

Ketamine is the most commonly used anesthetic agent for chemical capture. When used alone, ketamine can produce excessive muscle tension, tremors, seizures, and other complications; therefore, ketamine should always be used in combination with a sedative or tranquilizer such as xylazine or medetomidine. There is no antagonist for ketamine.

Ketamine is frequently paired with xylazine due to its relatively low cost and wide availability. Unfortunately, this drug combination can be inconsistent in its quality and effectiveness however with unpredictable knockdowns, sudden wake-ups, and long rough recoveries. Adding butorphanol (0.2 mg/kg), a weak opioid, to either a ketamine/xylazine or ketamine/medetomidine cocktail is recommended to produce a more consistent, effective, and smooth anesthetic experience. Recommended doses for such cocktails in feral dogs includes ketamine 10 mg/kg, xylazine 2 mg/kg, and butorphanol 0.2 mg/kg. Xylazine is reversed with yohimbine 0.25 mg/kg IM, tolazoline 4 mg/kg, or atipamezole at 1 mg for every 10 mg of xylazine administered. Antagonists should not be given until at least 30 min after the last dose of ketamine is administered [4]. Butorphanol does not require reversal.

### 4.4.2.2 Ketamine/Medetomidine

This combination is very similar to ketamine/xylazine, but medetomidine is much stronger and more effective than xylazine. Therefore, less ketamine is required and reversal is quicker and more effective [5].

A recommended ketamine/medetomidine/butor-phanol cocktail for feral dogs includes the following: ketamine 4 mg/kg, medetomidine 0.8 mg/kg, and butorphanol 0.2 mg/kg. Medetomidine is reversed with an equal volume of atipamezole at least 30 min after the last ketamine administration [4].

### 4.4.2.3 Telazol® (Zoletil®)

Telazol is a combination of two drugs: tiletamine (an anesthetic) and zolazepam (a tranquilizer). Tiletamine is five times stronger than ketamine, so this combination can produce a faster knockdown, which is valuable when free-roaming dogs have places to run and hide, but the duration of anesthesia can last much longer. Even though Telazol is labeled for use as a sole agent in dogs, the authors recommend using it in combination with another drug. A suggested Telazol cocktail is Telazol 10 mg/kg and xylazine 2 mg/kg. Both Zoletil and xylazine are manufactured in various concentrations, so it is important to check product labels prior to use.

### 4.4.2.4 Oral Drugging

While the oral administration of various drugs such as acepromazine or diazepam is sometimes attempted, this tends to be unreliable and largely ineffective as a routine capture tool.

### 4.4.3 Predarting Considerations

Before attempting chemical capture, it is imperative to consider every possible scenario for what could go wrong. For example, the dart itself can cause significant muscle or nerve trauma, if inappropriately placed. Therefore, one must pay special attention to the dart's placement and force in which the dart will impact the animal.

After darting, animals often attempt to flee and can stumble into traffic or a body of water as the drug takes effect. This can lead to a potentially dangerous situation for both the animal and catching team. In an urban environment, darted animals can be difficult to track with many obstructions to a handler's line of sight including vehicles and pedestrian traffic. Packs of free-roaming dogs also require special consideration. Rarely, a pack of dogs may attack a darted dog as it becomes disoriented and displays ataxia. In such a situation, capture team members must move quickly to diffuse the situation and protect that animal from being harmed or killed.

Capture staff should always note the time the dart hits the dog. It typically takes between 5 and 20 min for the drugs to take effect, depending on the animal and sedatives used. When watching the dog and waiting for the drug to take effect, the following should be assessed:

- Was the dog actually darted?
- What muscle group did the dart hit?
- Was the weight estimate and drug dose accurate?
- Did the dart malfunction?

Re-darting a dog may be considered with the same initial dose *only* after 20 min have passed and the dog is not adequately immobilized.

### 4.4.4 Postdarting Care

Darted dogs should be followed visually from a distance and approached when almost or fully unresponsive. Chasing or approaching the dog prematurely before the drugs have taken full effect will increase the dog's epinephrine response, reduce drug effectiveness, and potentially create an emergency situation should the dog take off running.

Dogs under chemical restraint should be transported to the clinic site or attended to as quickly as possible. Drugged animals may be unable to properly thermoregulate, swallow, or blink. Therefore, capture staff must assume the responsibility for caring for an anesthetized animal during the transportation process, which includes covering the head with a towel, immediately monitoring temperature, pulse, and respiration (TPR), and addressing any capture-related emergencies. Ideally, a TPR measurement should be taken as soon as the dog is in hand, the dog's body temperature should be normalized if needed, and breathing ensured before placing the dog in a transport vehicle.

Hyper- or hypothermia, respiratory distress, and circulatory failure are the most common emergencies associated with chemical capture. The risk of hyperthermia can be reduced by not darting on hot days, not chasing the animal for prolonged periods prior to darting, monitoring the body temperature, and cooling the animal when needed. The risk of hypothermia can best be minimized by quickly monitoring body

**Textbox 4.7 Additional chemical capture resources**

Silvy, N.J. (2012) *The Wildlife Techniques Manual,* 7th edition.

Kreeger, T. & Arnemo, J. (2012). *Handbook of wildlife chemical immobilization* 4th edition.

West, G., Heard, D. & Caulkett, N. (2014) *Zoo Animal and Wildlife Immobilization and Anesthesia,* 2nd edition.

Brothers, B. (2010) *Operational Guide for Animal Care and Control Agencies: Chemical Capture.* Available at: http://www.americanhumane.org/.

undertaken without having additional capture and handling equipment on-hand. This includes nets, cages, slip leads, handling gloves, and cage covers.

## 4.5 Transportation

Whenever animals are transported, care must be taken to protect them from injury, stress, or unnecessary suffering. Dogs and cats should be healthy enough for the intended journey, and injured and sick animals should only be transported for veterinary care [4]. Distressed dogs should ideally be allowed to calm down prior to travel. Using a dark, enclosed kennel can help facilitate this.

### 4.5.1 Cages

Dogs and cats should be comfortably confined during transport. If an animal is transported in a transportation cage or crate, he should be able to stand, sit upright, lie in a natural position, and turn around normally while standing. If dogs are transported together with other dogs, such as in the back of a caged truck, there should be sufficient space for all dogs to turn around and lie down without touching

temperature and using blankets if necessary to keep the dog warm. A normal canine body temperature is 100–103 °F (37.8–39.5 °C). The handler is responsible for keeping the dog's body temperature within this normal range.

Dogs should be recovered from anesthesia in a timely manner to minimize self-trauma during the recovery process. Because chemical capture can be unpredictable, no darting program should be

**Textbox 4.8 Transportation suggestions**

1) Transportation practices must comply with relevant legislation.
2) Transportation vehicles must safeguard animal health and welfare.
3) Captured animals should be transported as soon as possible following capture to the holding facility or clinic for unloading, minimizing the amount of time spent in the vehicle. If the journey is long or the dog's health is compromised, breaks should be taken to provide water and rest.
4) Whenever possible, animals displaying obvious signs of illness (discharge from the nose or eyes, excessive drooling) should be isolated from other animals during transport to minimize the potential for disease transmission.
5) Cats should not be transported in the cargo area of a vehicle when dogs are also onboard.
6) Care should be taken when loading and securing animals in a vehicle. If transport cages and crates require stacking, they must be safely secured.
7) Temperature extremes in the vehicles must be avoided. Vehicles should be designed to moderate temperatures and driver practices should maximize animal care.
8) Transport containers and cargo holds should be made of materials that can be thoroughly cleaned and disinfected after each transfer of animals to a facility.
9) The use of sedatives during transport is generally discouraged unless the animals can be continuously monitored, which is rare in the field.

each other. The authors recognize that this may or may not be possible during emergency situations.

## 4.5.2  Vehicles

A suitable vehicle must be available for transporting animals. Animals should never be left unattended for prolonged periods in any transport vehicle. To help minimize transport times, times of traffic congestion and adverse weather should be avoided. A well-designed vehicle for transporting animals should provide or include the following:

- Low ground clearance to facilitate animal loading and unloading. If this is not possible, a ramp can be used to gain access to the animal holding area.
- Adequate natural air flow or fitted with an appropriate ventilation system. In Southeast Asia, pickup trucks are often fitted with cages enclosing the flatbed (see Figure 4.10).

- A full bulkhead or dividing wall should isolate the personnel in the cabin from animals in the cargo. Ideally, a window allows for the viewing of the animals from the cabin.
- Individual transport crates that can be easily removed. This allows the crate to be brought to the dog rather than the dog brought to the vehicle.

Animals should never be transported in the closed cargo area of a box truck due to a lack of ventilation and climate control. Furthermore, unconfined or tethered animals should never be transported in the back of an open pickup truck [5]. Regardless of the type of vehicle used, transport vehicles can serve as a reservoir for disease if not thoroughly disinfected. See Chapter 11 for cleaning suggestions.

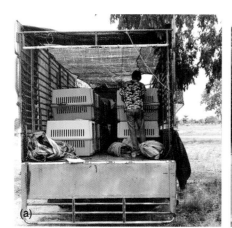 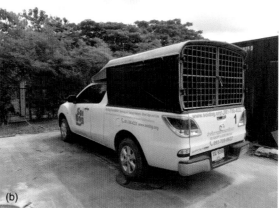

Figure 4.10  (a) The transport of dogs across central Thailand. Crates are stacked two high and secured using cable ties. Source: Courtesy of Cristy Baker. (b) Animal transport vehicle in Thailand used for transporting free-roaming dogs for spay/neuter surgery. Tarps on each side of the vehicle are rolled down, effectively shielding transported animals from rain during the monsoon season. Source: Courtesy of Katherine Polak, Soi Dog Foundation.

# Appendix

## 4.A   Identifying Fearful Body Language in Dogs

## Identifying fearful body language in dogs

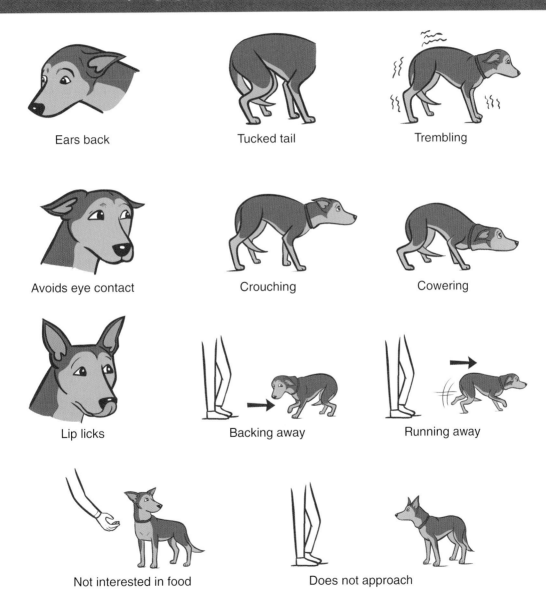

**These body language signals indicate that a dog may be fearful.**

Ears back

Tucked tail

Trembling

Avoids eye contact

Crouching

Cowering

Lip licks

Backing away

Running away

Not interested in food

Does not approach

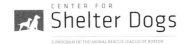

© 2013 Center for Shelter Dogs, Animal Rescue League of Boston
Illustrated by Lili Chin www.doggiedrawings.net

Source: Center for Shelter Dogs, Animal Rescue League of Boston.

## 4.B   How to Use a Control Pole

# How to Use a Control Pole

> *Most animal control officers consider the control pole one of the most valuable tools of the trade. But like a carpenter's hammer or drill, a control pole is only as effective as the person holding it in his or her hands.*

The next time a call comes in, whether it's for a stray dog or a raccoon, remember that the control pole ("catch pole," "come-along," or "rabies pole" as it's sometimes called) is designed to gently coax animals to safety. Its use as a weapon is inappropriate, and could easily endanger the animal and the animal control officer. Remember that control poles should not be used on cats. The use of a net is the most humane and effective way of capturing a cat, and it will be detailed in the next issue of *Animal Sheltering*.

Lastly, before you hop out of the truck, it's important to quickly examine the control pole, making sure that cable and release mechanisms are operating smoothly. Be sure the loop retains a rounded shape rather than a tear shape by storing the pole on a flat surface or using broom clips. Replace cables every 18-24 months as a part of regular maintenance.

### 1: Easy Does It.

Approach the dog slowly, holding the control pole directly behind you or at your side, with the cable loop hanging loosely. *Never* approach a dog with a control pole held high, like a weapon, as this will set the tone for the entire encounter.

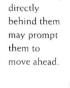

### 3: Lead By Following.

Keep both hands a slight distance apart on the pole. Once the loop is secured about the animal's neck, stand beside the dog and slowly guide the animal ahead. Most dogs will readily walk forward if you remain in their field of vision, but in some cases walking directly behind them may prompt them to move ahead.

### 2: It's All In The Wrist.

Using both hands, slip the noose smoothly over the dog's head until the loop is around the animal's neck. Use one hand to pull the release cord to tighten the cable until the loop fits snugly, but not too tight. The pole is designed to maneuver the animal, so it is important *never* to use the control pole to choke the animal or force him into submission.

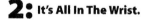

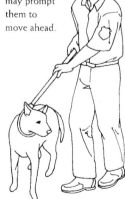

Illustrations by Susie Duckworth

*Continued on reverse side*

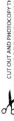

## 4.B    How to Use a Control Pole (*Continued*)

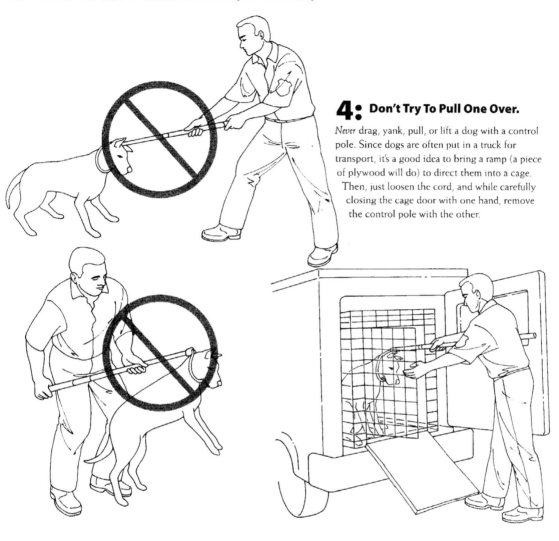

**4:** **Don't Try To Pull One Over.**

*Never* drag, yank, pull, or lift a dog with a control pole. Since dogs are often put in a truck for transport, it's a good idea to bring a ramp (a piece of plywood will do) to direct them into a cage. Then, just loosen the cord, and while carefully closing the cage door with one hand, remove the control pole with the other.

**Wild Ones.**

It may be necessary to temporarily restrain some wild animals (such as raccoons) using the control pole. These animals should *never* be looped solely around the neck or chest. Instead, the cable should be looped "bandolier-style" around the neck and under one of the front legs, and the animal should be guided in the manner described previously.

Source: The HSUS.

# References

1 Davlin, S.L. and Vonville, H.M. (2012). Canine rabies vaccination and domestic dog population characteristics in the developing world: a systematic review. *Vaccine* **30** (24): 3492–3502.

2 WHO (2010). Rabies vaccines: WHO position paper-recommendations. *Vaccine* **23** (44): 7140–7142.

3 Johnson, M. (2017). The Y-pole. Global Wildlife Resources, Inc. http://wildliferesources.com/the-y-pole/ (accessed 11 December 2016).

4 National Dog Warden Association (2012). Guidance for handling dogs. http://www.ndwa.co.uk/media/guidance-for-handling-dogs.pdf (accessed 10 December 2016).

5 Newbury, S., Blinn, M.K., Bushby, P.K. et al. (2010). Guidelines for Standards of Care in Animal Shelters. Association of Shelter Veterinarians: Corning, NY.

# 5

## Operating a Field Spay/Neuter Clinic

*Susan Monger*

*International Veterinary Consultants, Austin, TX 78757, USA*

## 5.1 Introduction

Spay/neuter clinics require tremendous planning irrespective of the setting. Field clinics in particular face numerous unique challenges including limited supply availability, lack of reliable electricity and running water, and compromised patient health. Regardless of these conditions, clinics must uphold a minimal standard of care to ensure the safety and well-being of both staff and animals alike. Such standards affect not only patient outcomes but also the relationship with the community.

Improving animal welfare requires more than just spay/neuter. A long-term change in community behaviors and attitudes is also required. As such, cultural, professional, and diplomatic sensitivity is imperative to building community trust and operating a successful clinic. The crafting of effective protocols requires a multidisciplinary approach that is best achieved by a veterinary team that understands the community's goals, limitations, and opportunities and is sympathetic to the local situation. If a clinic cannot establish and/or maintain an acceptable level of care, then one must reassess the approach and strategy.

In the literature and among those practicing in limited-resourced environments, there is a wide range of what are considered "minimally acceptable" practices and standards [1]. The recommendations presented in this chapter are based on published best practices, hundreds of national and international spay/neuter clinics that have been organized by the author, lessons learned from failures and successes, as well as ongoing evaluation of the changing field of high-quality, high-volume spay neuter and shelter medicine.

This chapter provides guidelines and suggestions to plan a field clinic and establish an acceptable standard of practice based on the availability of equipment, supplies, trained staff, and volunteers. Readers will note an emphasis on international field clinics (those conducted outside the organizer's home country). For detailed descriptions of anesthetic and spay/neuter surgical procedures, the reader is encouraged to refer to the relevant chapters within this book. A list of relevant websites and guidance documents is also available at the end of the chapter.

---

**Textbox 5.1 Practical tips for success**

Tip #1. Determine the standards of practice and level of care that is achievable given the specific working environment. Every effort should be made to provide the highest level of care possible through proper planning, prioritization of resources, use of volunteers, and creative decision-making.

Tip #2. Learn to say no. If animal welfare is compromised, reassess the clinic's goals and capacity. Capacity is often determined by the type of clinic, project budget, and staffing.

Tip #3. Be flexible. The best-laid plans can sometimes go awry.

Tip #4. Be culturally aware. Every attempt should be made prior to the clinic to gain knowledge and insight into the country and area where the field clinic will be held.

---

*Field Manual for Small Animal Medicine*, First Edition. Edited by Katherine Polak and Ann Therese Kommedal.
© 2018 John Wiley & Sons, Inc. Published 2018 by John Wiley & Sons, Inc.

Tip #5. Hire translators, if needed. If the language spoken locally differs from that of the staff, consider staffing medically trained translators to ensure appropriate communication.

Tip #6. Recruit volunteers with field experience. Field clinic limitations and the conditions of the animals can be shocking to inexperienced volunteers.

## 5.2 Planning

Field clinics require extensive planning. Even with careful attention to detail, unforeseen circumstances can undermine the best-laid plans. Potential obstacles, particularly those that could completely halt clinic operations, should be identified well in advance.

In general, clinics held for the first time require more time to plan compared with subsequent clinics. A reconnaissance trip to the community where the clinic will take place can help with planning, logistics, and establishing a relationship with local residents and animal welfare organizations. During the planning phase, common logistical challenges that require particular attention including finding an appropriate clinic site, locating accomodations for a large professional/support team, and sourcing medications to perform the large number of surgeries required.

### 5.2.1 Determine the Type of Clinic

- Stationary clinics take place at a "fixed" site (permanent structure or building) and may be equipped with many of the same supplies and equipment found in a traditional hospital.
- MASH-type clinics, short for Mobile Army Surgical Hospital, can occur in a variety of locations including under a tent in the jungle or in a gymnasium (Figure 5.1). These clinics can operate for a single or multiple days. As a general rule, MASH-type clinics are very labor intensive. They relocate frequently, which requires time to set-up and tear down the clinic. Such excessive movement can also cause wear and tear on equipment and supplies.
- Mobile clinics usually involve a vehicle where surgeries are performed. Vehicles can move from community to community, permitting access to

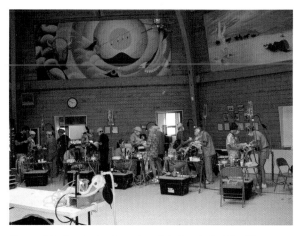

**Figure 5.1** Surgical setup at a clinic located at the Pine Ridge Indian Reservation Cultural Center in Kyle, South Dakota.

areas where animal transport might be challenging. Drawbacks of this type of clinic include a significant initial overhead and maintenance costs. Weather and roads may also compromise the ability to travel to certain locations. Depending on the vehicle, mobile clinics may lack enough cages to house patients for multiple days following surgery.

### 5.2.2 Create a Timeline and "To-do" Checklist

Planning should typically begin at least 6–8 months prior to the clinic start date to ensure adequate time for the procurement of supplies, acquisition of permits, and staff/volunteer travel arrangements. A suggested timeline for clinic planning is included in Appendix 5.A.

### 5.2.3 Investigate In-Country Communications

A local, on-site person should be identified to handle logistics and communication. Clinic success depends on having a reliable staff member or volunteer to coordinate activities, organize personnel, and engage with the public in the local language. Staffing local people also demonstrates respect to the community which facilitates trust.

Depending on the location, one should consider the likely possibility of limited Internet and phone availability which can compromise communication.

Meetings with local government authorities should be held to facilitate immediate and/or future

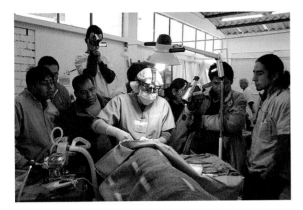

**Figure 5.2** Enucleation demonstration to local veterinarians in La Paz, Bolivia. Note the blankets used to keep the patient warm due to freezing temperatures and lack of supplemental heat.

assistance with planning, monetary, in-kind or personnel support, advertising, and community awareness of the clinic. These meetings can be challenging for multiple reasons. (1) Animal welfare is often not a priority of government agencies (2) Municipalities may have limited financial resources for spay neuter efforts, and (3) There is often a lack of knowledge, even among the locals about who is the appropriate person or government department to communicate with.

Local veterinarians in communities where field clinics are held may perceive clinics as a threat to their livelihood. There may also be feelings of embarrassment due to differing levels of knowledge, skill, and professional standing. In order to address these concerns, it is highly recommended that clinic organizers involve local veterinarians during the planning process. Through effective communication and collaboration, field clinics can serve to not only sterilize animals, but also be an opportunity for training and information exchange. It is often the engagement component of field clinics that ultimately elevates the overall level of veterinary care in a community (Figure 5.2).

### 5.2.4 Acquire Permits

Acquiring permits can be one of the most difficult, time-consuming, frustrating, and, sometimes expensive aspects of the clinic. Countries have the right to hold or confiscate equipment and supplies upon arrival at customs. Furthermore, export and import regulations vary from country to country. It pays to research specific requirements well in advance.

If equipment and pharmaceuticals are to be imported, import permits are often required. Import permit applications can vary with some requiring detailed information including a specific equipment and medication list provided by the importee, lists of lot numbers, manufacturers and expiration dates of medications and vaccines, letters of invitation from the local organization sponsoring the clinic, and proof of professional licensure. The author recommends traveling with multiple copies of permits and documented communications.

#### 5.2.4.1 How to Acquire Permits

- Permits always require a local person capable of communicating with authorities.
- Asking other animal welfare groups working in-country for advice can shed light on the permitting process. One might consider reaching out to human medical or dental groups working in that country as well.
- It may take several attempts and perseverance to identify the proper government agency to contact.
- Authorities may not respond to or acknowledge permit requests. If this is the case, it is advisable to document attempts to communicate with the local authorities. These communications may suffice when attempting to enter a country or receive proper authorization to export or import equipment and supplies.
- Almost all official permits are in the recognized language of the destination country. Some official government organizations may require official translation into their respective languages. For example, the United States Drug Enforcement Agency (DEA) requires permits received from the destination country be translated into English.
- Official customs brokers can facilitate the import process but at a cost and without guarantee. One must ensure brokers are legitimate and credentialed.
- *Know the laws.* Just because one animal welfare group provided medical services without permits does not mean their import process was legal.

#### 5.2.4.2 Consider Controlled Substances

Bringing controlled drugs into a country often requires separate permits from both the origin and destination country. When transporting controlled drugs, the transporter must hold a valid DEA (or equivalent) and veterinary license, and carry copies of both. One must keep in mind that drugs that are not considered controlled in one country may be a designated controlled substance in another. For example, acepromazine is a recognized controlled substance in El Salvador but not in the United States.

---

**Textbox 5.2  Controlled drugs considerations**

- Information from the DEA import/export department in the United States can be found at: http://www.deadiversion.usdoj.gov/imp_exp/
- The DEA in the United States maintains contact information for the recognized Competent Authority (host country equivalent of the DEA), which is the recognized point of contact by the DEA for the respective host country.
- For countries other than the United States, it is recommended to contact the government agency responsible for granting exportation permission for controlled substances.
- Consider the possibility of leftover controlled drugs and how to address a potential surplus.

---

Even with appropriate paperwork, supplies may still be confiscated, held in customs, and/or taxed for import. Unexpected "fees" may therefore need to be paid. The confiscation of supplies can cause a trip to be cancelled and/or severely compromise clinic operations.

### 5.2.5  Determine Local and National Holidays

Local and national holidays can greatly affect the success or failure of a clinic. Many countries shut down local operations in order to celebrate a specific religious event or holiday.

It is therefore advisable to check local calendars for holidays and events before setting clinic dates. Note that holidays can often vary from region to region, even within the same country.

Unforeseen celebrations and rites of passage such as a funeral or wedding sometimes occur during planned clinic dates. These cannot be avoided and must be respected.

### 5.2.6  Obtain Medical Evacuation Coverage

Medical evacuation insurance is relatively inexpensive and strongly recommended for all team members.

The lead organizer should create a list of all team members and their respective contacts and evacuation policy information, in case of an emergency.

Suggested sources for evacuation insurance include:

- *MedExAssist.* https://www.medexassist.com
- *International SOS.* https://www.internationalsos.com

### 5.2.7  Plan Airline Travel

While traveling, staff should have personal identification and flight information both inside and outside of all pieces of luggage. Identification should include a contact name and address at the destination.

Baggage should be planned well in advance. Baggage fees can be costly, especially if exceeding designated weight allowances. It may be worth dividing up supplies among traveling team members so if one or two bags are lost, the entire trip isn't compromised. Dividing supplies among team members also helps reduce excess baggage fees. Airlines should be contacted prior to the date of travel to confirm baggage arrangements.

---

**Textbox 5.3  Know your embargos**

- *Weight embargos.* Airlines may have specific times of the year that they limit the amount and weight of checked baggage.
- *Box embargo.* Certain airlines occasionally have a "box" embargo. American Airlines has been known to reject "boxes" such as Rubbermaid® Action Packers at particular times throughout the year.

---

### 5.2.8  Investigate Professional Licensure Restrictions

License requirements of veterinary professionals providing services in foreign countries vary dramatically country to country. The United States has strict requirements regarding the licensure of foreign veterinarians practicing in the United States, yet other countries have few or no such requirements. One should also note that the cost of services provided may affect licensure restrictions. Some countries do not require licensure if the services are provided free of charge, whereas charging for services may affect the need to acquire and/or demonstrate licensure. It is the responsibility of the person in charge of organizing the clinic to investigate specific licensure requirements. All veterinarians should be of good standing and licensed to practice in their respective countries. Veterinarians should also carry copies of their respective country's licensure and controlled drug permit if indicated.

### 5.2.9 Create a Supply List

It is essential to identify critical supplies for clinic operations. Supply lists can vary widely from clinic to clinic and are dictated by the clinic's protocols. Team members should be aware of the potential for limited in-country drug and supply availability. Limited clinic resources may not allow for the purchasing of ideal anesthetics, supplies, and monitoring equipment. However, clinics can still provide quality care with minimal supplies and inexpensive medications.

#### 5.2.9.1 Create a Supply Manifest

A manifest or checklist of required equipment and supplies (with approximate amounts) is needed prior to the start of every clinic. The manifest can be divided into various clinic categories such as anesthesia, recovery, and surgery to ensure the appropriate supplies are available for each area of the clinic. At first, one should make the list detailed and comprehensive, and later pare down depending on the specifics of the clinic and ability to transport supplies. A sample supply list is included as Appendix 5.B.

#### 5.2.9.2 Acquire Supplies In-Country

One should investigate the cost and ease of supply acquisition in the host country versus the cost in the country of origin. This includes both the purchase cost as well as the logistical cost of time and effort of exporting medications (i.e. controlled drugs) and permits to import supplies into the country. Often, an increased cost in the host country is worth it if it minimizes the incurred cost of transport and avoids customs and permits.

If working in a foreign country, it may be difficult or impossible to acquire specific medications or equipment. This is especially true with regard to opiates and analgesics that are readily available and affordable in developed countries. Medical volunteers should note that there can be a marked difference in *quality* of medications acquired in-

country. It has been described that a "routine" dose of certain anesthetics acquired in certain countries will not achieve surgical planes of anesthesia. For example, ketamine acquired in one country required almost twice the recommended dose to attain a surgical plane of anesthesia than in another. Several patients have also demonstrated seizure-like activity such as tremors or convulsions while under ketamine-induced anesthesia.

There should be a plan in place for the safe storage of leftover supplies. Donating them to local veterinary professionals is recommended.

### 5.2.10 Arrange Food, Lodging, and Transportation

Food, lodging, and transportation arrangements will vary depending on the clinic site and team size. The safety of all team members is paramount, and they should be comfortably accommodated, given the circumstances. Arrangements should be made well before the start of the clinic.

#### 5.2.10.1 Food and Water

Every effort should be made to address the dietary considerations of team members, relative to local diet and customs. It is recommended to research and prepare the team ahead of time to ensure the local culture is respected. If a team member has specific dietary restrictions that fall outside the cultural or physical capabilities of the host site, he or she should be responsible for bringing their own snacks to supplement their diet.

Food and water to be provided throughout the working days should be addressed by the local organizer. Clarifying who will be responsible for providing food and water will ensure supplies are always adequate. Local restaurants and community members can also be organized to support the clinic by providing food and meals. Team members should be encouraged to bring supplemental food and water in case either becomes difficult to obtain. When food and lodging is provided by local people, team members should be sure to thank whoever is responsible.

#### 5.2.10.2 Lodging

Safe and secure lodging should be identified for the appropriate number of team members prior to arrival. In some locations, certain amenities like showers, beds, and blankets may or may not be available, and participants need to be informed so that they can prepare accordingly. Local hotels and community members are often willing to support the clinic by hosting team members.

### 5.2.10.3 Transportation

Transportation for team members should be arranged both to and from the clinic site and airport (if arriving from another country). If daily local transportation is needed for team members from lodging to the clinic, this requires arranging in advance. MASH-style clinics require additional advanced planning to ensure seamless transportation of equipment and supplies.

Four-wheel drive vehicles may be required for transportation to some locales. This requires discussion with the in-country coordinator prior to arrival as four-wheel drive vehicles may require time to reserve and be expensive.

### 5.2.10.4 Communications and Advertising

If the clinic intends to admit owned animals, advertising is needed to inform community members accordingly (Figure 5.3).

Advertising is also a means to educate the community on the benefits of the clinic. If the intent of the clinic is to trap, neuter, and return free-roaming cats and dogs, the community needs to be informed as many stray dogs and cats are "owned" yet roam free. Some owners or caregivers may object to sterilization without consent. If more than one language is spoken,

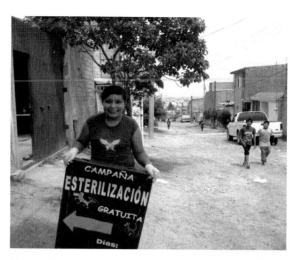

**Figure 5.3** A volunteer advertising a spay/neuter clinic in Bucerias, Mexico.

ensure that there are enough people for translation when required.

### 5.2.10.5 Organizational Meeting and Chain of Command

An initial organizational meeting prior to the start of the clinic is essential for team building, identifying key personnel, and reviewing clinic protocols and procedures. Attendance to this meeting is mandatory for all participants, even if a team member has participated in many clinics before. If team members or volunteers arrive late and are unable to make the initial meeting, brief them individually, as soon as they arrive.

Clinics can quickly become chaotic once they begin. A chain of command should be created to streamline both in-clinic and public communication. Identifying key personnel who can address specific aspects of the clinic will maximize efficiency and minimize complications.

The meeting should address the following:

1) Identification of team leaders and team members
   - Team leader(s)
     - If there is only one team leader, this should be a veterinarian to address medical issues that may arise. Note that this may be a shared position (i.e. local coordinator and lead veterinarian)
   - Professional staff
     - Veterinarians
     - Technicians
     - Experienced volunteers

---

**Textbox 5.4 Clinic advertisement mediums**

- Radio
- Schools
- Churches
- Local markets
- Social media
- Flyers
- Mobile public announcing[a] (this consists of loud speakers in the back of a truck or on top of a car driving through the community announcing clinic details)
- Local government officials such as mayors and public health officials.

*a* One of the most commonly used methods in most of the world.

- Volunteers
  - Volunteer coordinator
  - Identification of clinic areas requiring help
  - Identification of experienced and inexperienced volunteers.
2) Chain of command
  - Identify who is in charge of specific clinic areas
  - Determine how and who will make specific decisions regarding clinic issues
  - Identify who is responsible for making final decisions regarding patient care and treatment.

#### 5.2.10.6 Rounds
A debriefing meeting should be planned for the end of each clinic day to discuss any issues and improve operations. This can be challenging as many clinic days are long and tiring. At a minimum, key team members should meet and discuss logistics and/or veterinary issues daily.

### 5.2.11 Assessing Local Needs and Patient Selection

During the clinic planning process, assessment of animal welfare issues in the community should be performed to target the intervention. Clinics designed to address a specific population such as free-roaming animals may be overwhelmed by requests by another segment of the population (community members wanting the same services for their pets). This creates a potential logistical as well as public relations issue. The goal of the clinic should be established and communicated prior to the start of the clinic.

#### 5.2.11.1 Caseload Selection
The clinic organizers will decide how patients will be admitted. Whatever the approach, appointments, first-come, first-serve, or capture, the intake criteria should be well-defined. The clinic should also have a protocol in place to address emergency cases that might present, such as pyometra or dystocia.

#### 5.2.11.2 Determining Daily Caseload
The number of surgeries that can be performed safely and humanely will vary greatly depending on staffing, anesthesia, surgical skill, supply availability, and logistics. The animal holding capacity (number of cages) at the clinic and transport can limit the caseload even when staffing and medical supplies are adequate. Sufficient numbers of experienced veterinarians, technicians, clinic assistants, and volunteers are necessary to ensure an adequate standard of care and safety for all patients and team members. Overly ambitious plans regarding the number of surgeries can easily compromise the humane care and life of individual animals. The caseload should be estimated conservatively keeping the following considerations in mind:

- The daily caseload is usually determined by the lead veterinarian in conjunction with the local coordinator.
- The projected daily caseload must be acknowledged and understood by all team members.
- The caseload may be increased or decreased by the lead veterinarian based on logistical or technical issues.
- Patients often present in less than ideal health. As a result, surgical candidacy is determined by veterinary staff. It is important to remember that most sterilization surgeries are elective procedures; sometimes, postponing or canceling surgery is in the best interest of the animal. If the clinic happens to be the only opportunity to sterilize a patient, one must weigh the risk of surgery against the benefit to the animal.

---

**Textbox 5.5 Caseload considerations**

- Will the caseload rely on the public bringing animals on a first-come, first-serve basis as a result of local advertising?
- Will it be by appointment?
  - If so, identify how and who will be responsible for making and confirming appointments.
  - In many cultures, "no-shows" are common despite having appointments. This can affect the overall numbers of surgeries each day.
- Will clinic admission rely on the trapping of free-roaming animals?
- Will there be a fee for service?

### 5.2.12 Working with the Local Veterinary Community

The in-country or on-site clinic organizer should determine if any small animal veterinarians provide medical services in the general vicinity of the proposed clinic site. An attempt should be made to meet with any local veterinarians to discuss the clinic and extend an invitation for their involvement. It is likely that the local veterinarian(s) will address any postoperative complications should they arise, and therefore should be well informed of the clinic. In the author's experience, many veterinarians welcome the opportunity to work with foreign veterinary professionals when offered. This cooperation establishes a professional relationship conducive to a mutually beneficial clinic.

### 5.2.13 Bite Incidence

An animal bite policy should be created prior to the start of a clinic. Many clinics are located in remote locations with limited access to medical services. One should research the incidence of rabies in the working area prior to the trip, and determine the nearest medical facility to the clinic site. Bite policies should specify where clinic participants should go for medical attention if they get bitten as animal bites can easily become infected with potential long-lasting sequelas. All team members must acknowledge the bite policy, and a protocol must be in place should a team member decline medical care.

Despite extensive rabies control programs in many countries, the vaccination status of individual animals is often unknown, particularly those that are free roaming. Following a bite, quarantining animals for the recommended 10 days is often difficult or impossible to do in a field setting. The team organizers must integrate quarantine procedures as part of the bite policy prior to the clinic.

Examples of bite policies are available online, which can be adapted to particular clinics depending on resources and logistics. Clinic supervisors should know which team members have been rabies vaccinated or have adequate protective antibody titers. Prior rabies vaccination should be a requirement for all staff and volunteers handling animals.

## 5.3 Site Consideration

Field clinics can be held in almost any location. They can be MASH-type, mobile, or stationary, and many are held outdoors, on soccer fields, in garages or community centers, with or without access to water or electricity. When choosing a clinic site, consider the ability to transport equipment, supplies, and team members to the site, water and electricity availability, the ability to adequately clean and disinfect the site prior to and throughout the clinic, the ability to safely handle and confine animals, protection from rain and wind, and overall ability to conduct humane surgery.

### 5.3.1 Clinic Type

The first step in clinic planning is to determine the type of clinic: stationary, MASH-type, or mobile. Once the clinic type has been determined, additional considerations such as access to electricity and water can be taken into account.

### 5.3.2 Accessibility

Site accessibility affects the cost and success of the clinic. Important considerations include the distance, ease of access, and cost for team members to arrive safely to the clinic site. Other considerations include:

- Ease and cost of travel for team members to the country or region
- Ease of access and travel time to the local clinic site
- Safety of local transport
- Food and lodging accessibility.

The site should be reasonably accessible to members of the community, keeping in mind that many may not have access to cars. It is not uncommon to see owners walking, carrying, riding a bicycle, motorcycle, or horseback ride long distances to bring their animals to a clinic. One should investigate whether or not there are local taxis or similar transportation such as tuk-tuks that can service owners with dogs or cats.

Consider transportation of postoperative patients. In many situations, caregivers may not recognize the invasiveness and seriousness of the surgical procedure and will attempt to walk the patient home following surgery. Patients released on the same day of surgery may still be groggy or have impaired neurologic status due to anesthesia. Walking home after a surgical procedure may contribute to increased postoperative complications. The mode of transportation should be identified, and if inappropriate, pet owners educated and encouraged to use alternative transport, if possible.

Cats warrant special mention as many caregivers carry their cats to the clinic loose, without appropriate carriers. The same owners expect to carry the animals home in the same manner following surgery. Many anesthetic protocols employed in field surgery cause delayed recoveries in cats. There is also an increased potential for a cat to escape or inadvertently hurt its caregiver if one attempts to carry the cat home without appropriate containment.

### 5.3.3  Weather Patterns and Altitude

Weather and altitude can affect both clinic and team members. Annual weather patterns should be investigated to determine if there is a rain, monsoon, hurricane, or other natural weather event that may compromise the transport of staff, ability to conduct a clinic safely, and/or ability of local community members to reach the clinic.

Similarly, seasonal weather patterns such as hot or cold seasons in the working area may affect the ability to perform surgery and recover animals safely. Cold and rainy weather can compromise patient thermoregulation. Conversely, hot and humid weather can compromise some team member's ability to perform. Altitude may also affect some individuals and possibly anesthesia.

### 5.3.4  Water

Access to clean water is essential to the clinic, but may be challenging in some places due to scarcity and cost. This may take some team members by surprise who are accustomed to regular, unrestricted access to water in their respective work places.

If running water is unavailable at a clinic site, a plan must be devised for accessing clean water throughout the clinic. Sufficient quantities of water are needed for animals to drink, patient and surgeon preparations, and cleaning of kennels and animal care products. Buckets, tubs, clean dish pans, and hoses stretching to a remote water source can help supply clean water during a clinic. While hot water is preferred, it is not absolutely necessary to conduct a clinic. The use of hot water also increases the community's cost of hosting the clinic. Over-the-counter hand sanitizer strategically located throughout the clinic can reduce the amount of water required.

### 5.3.5  Material to Dry Hands, Instruments, and Clinic Supplies

Supplies to dry hands, instruments, or other supplies should be on hand. Hospitals in the United States throw away a large number of huck towels (blue surgery towels) every day. Many hospitals are willing to save and donate these unwanted towels. Old sheets and towels from local hotels are another good source of material for cleaning and bedding. This also reduces the amount of paper towels consumed over the course of a clinic. The ability to do laundry in a timely manner to maintain adequate numbers of towels and rags during the clinic must be investigated.

### 5.3.6  Electricity

Electricity is very expensive in many places in the world. In some places, access is restricted during certain parts of the day to conserve resources. Frequent power outages may also be common. Even if electricity is available, one should plan for occasional disruption in service.

> **Textbox 5.6 Strategies for operating with limited or no electricity**
>
> - Keep adequate numbers of headlamps, flashlights, and batteries on hand.
> - Consider keeping a portable generator on-site for use in the event of a power outage.
> - Invest in inverters that attach to a car battery or a solar generator with a 12 V output. This will convert 12 V battery power to 110 V.
> - Maintain a stock of batteries for battery-powered devices.

The number of functioning outlets at the clinic site should be noted. One should plug an electrical device into an outlet to determine if it is functioning rather than relying on the fact that "there are a lot of outlets present." An adequate number of extension cords and power strips should also be kept on hand. Clinic staff

**Textbox 5.7 110 versus 220 V**

- If working in a country with different voltage than your home country, it is imperative to have adequate numbers of adapters. Everyone on the team must be aware of differences in electrical voltage. Electrical equipment can be damaged from being plugged into an inappropriate voltage source.
- Adapters are readily available online from Amazon.com or in home goods and recreational sporting goods stores.
- Note the difference between an adapter, converter, and transformer:
  - An adapter adapts the local electricity to the electricity required by the electrical device.
  - A converter actually converts electricity from one voltage to another. Converters should be used with products with mechanical motors or heating devices. Converters are designed for short periods of use (1–2 h).
  - Transformers step up or down the voltage but are significantly more expensive. Transformers can be operated continuously.

should exercise caution when plugging in multiple devices as fuse boxes in many places are unable to handle a heavy electrical demand.

### 5.3.7 Lighting

Lighting can be one of the most challenging aspects of a clinic; however, most clinic areas do not require high-wattage lighting. There are many simple and easily adapted lighting sources for these areas including floodlights and lamps. Surgical areas however require sufficient light to adequately visualize inside the body cavity. Surgical lighting can be augmented with lights on the end of the table, headlamps worn by surgeons and assistants, and, if necessary, flashlights held by volunteers.

### 5.3.8 Disinfection and Cleaning

Adequate sanitation and disinfection protocols are necessary to prevent in-clinic disease transmission. Additional information is described in Chapter 11.

### 5.3.9 Laundry and Newspapers

Clean, soft, and absorbent material such as towels and sheets are needed to address patient care throughout the clinic, from admission to recovery. Newspaper, albeit less ideal, can also be used in place of towels. Donations of such items may come from local community members and businesses; old sheets and towels may be donated from local hotels.

Newspaper or cardboard can facilitate patient thermoregulation and has the advantage of being disposed of after a single use. When additional thermoregulation is needed such as during a lengthy procedure, blankets, towels or sheets should be used instead. These require laundering however in between patients and laundry facilities may or may not be available depending on the location.

Laundry facilities can include a laundromat or a local volunteer with access to a washing machine. One must be aware of the degree of contamination (fecal material, blood) of the laundry and take appropriate measures to address cleaning. Blood and fecal material may be culturally offensive to some local volunteers.

**Textbox 5.9 Laundry tip**

Blood contamination can be cleaned using a large container with hydrogen peroxide mixed with water in equal amounts and placed in strategic locations, such as next to the surgical tables. Hydrogen peroxide assists in breaking down the red blood cells and permits more thorough cleaning.

**Textbox 5.8 Sanitation tips and tricks**

- Place squirt bottles of disinfectant in multiple places throughout the clinic.
- Potassium peroxymonosulfate (Trifectant®, Virkon®) is a broad-spectrum disinfectant that comes in easy-to-transport tablets. Dilute as per instructions. Note that the tablets absorb moisture and crumble in high humidity over time and should therefore be stored in the low-humidity environment or in a refrigerator.
- Bleach is usually readily available. A diluted bleach solution can be used as a general disinfectant, provided that all organic material has been removed first.
- Hand sanitizer placed in strategic locations helps reduce the reliance on water and decreases the spread of disease.

### 5.3.10 Proper Disposal of Sharps Materials and Biological Wastes

The required disposal method of trash and sharps can vary from location to location and country to country. It is the responsibility of the team leader to dispose of sharps in accordance to the rules and regulations of the community to minimize the possibility of injury to humans and animals. Proper disposal of sharps is particularly important in some communities as members of the public may walk barefoot. Dogs, chickens, pigs, horses, and other animals are also often free roaming and may be injured in any number of ways by the inappropriate disposal of sharps materials. Although local disposal may consist of rather simple or primitive methods including burying the sharps container in the ground, filling the containers with concrete, or burning the containers in a fire, every effort must be made to minimize injury and contamination. Local health departments, clinics, and hospitals can advise on proper disposal methods and may supply appropriate sharps containers.

Some countries have strict laws regarding the proper disposal of biological waste while other countries have few requirements at all. Local cultural beliefs may dictate if or how body tissues are handled and disposed of. The clinic organizer is responsible for investigating local rules, regulations, and cultural practices regarding the proper disposal of biological waste.

### 5.3.11 Bathroom Facilities

Bathroom facilities vary greatly from country to country. Team members should be aware of possible differences prior to the clinic to avoid surprise while on-site. In many international settings, septic systems are nonexistent or unable to handle toilet paper and personal hygiene products. Such products should be disposed of in a wastebasket, not in the toilet.

## 5.4 Staffing and Volunteers

The "ideal" number of team members and volunteers is dependent on many variables. A clinic must have the appropriate number of staff and volunteers to ensure that every animal is cared for in a safe and humane manner from capture or admission to recovery. It is the lead veterinarian's responsibility to determine how many surgeries can be performed safely and humanely, given the clinic's staffing.

Every effort should be made in advance to inform the team members of conditions where they will be working. That being said, oftentimes the reality of the clinic and the conditions of the animals can be shocking to some team members.

On-site, the clinic manager needs to be able to effectively address situations that may arise. This can include having uncomfortable discussions such as asking team members to assist in other areas more suitable to their skill set or asking team members or volunteers to leave. The cohesiveness of the working team is paramount to demonstrate to both staff and local community the team's desire and ability to provide medical services, which will ultimately improve animal welfare.

Veterinarians, technicians, and volunteers lacking field experience should be paired up with more experienced team members. Anesthesia warrants particular attention as anesthesia drugs and protocols may be very different from those used in their usual place of work. Ideally, one veterinarian has at least one staff member to monitor anesthesia and another to attend to additional surgical supplies as needed; field clinics often lack this "ideal" number however.

---

**Textbox 5.10 Waste disposal suggestions**

- Official sharps containers and biological bags, both usually red, are often available from the local health department.
- Biological waste (body parts and tissue) may require special trash bags (usually red and heavy duty) and a specific manner of disposal.
- Many containers suffice as sharps containers including plastic milk cartons and soda bottles. Once filled, the containers should be closed with a proper lid or taped shut with heavy tape such as duct tape.
- Place a trash bag on each surgery table as well other strategic locations throughout clinic to facilitate garbage collection.
- Trash should be collected and disposed of in a secure manner that minimizes the risk of stray animals ripping into bags, disseminating garbage in the community.

**Textbox 5.11 Field clinic case study**

A passionate local charity working in a rural village in Mexico wants to host a 5-day spay/neuter clinic to sterilize and rabies-vaccinate 250 dogs. The majority of dogs are owned, but allowed to free-roam. The charity lacks any trained medical staff, and as a result, foreign veterinarians and nurses are invited to assist. During the planning process, the following challenges are immediately flagged and strategies devised to move forward with the clinic.

| | Challenges identified | Proposed remedies |
| --- | --- | --- |
| *Clinic site* | The proposed clinic site is located on a soccer field. The source of electricity is a single house with two outlets on the edge of the field. There is no running water | A. Move the clinic site closer to the house/power source<br>B. Run an extension cord across the field<br>C. Order a potable-water truck or haul in water from an outside source<br>D. Use waterless products including Avagard™ and hand sanitizer |
| *Staffing* | The local charity is only able to provide a total of 5 nonmedically trained volunteers to help with the clinic | A. Recruit 3 veterinarians, 4 nurses, and 3 nonmedically trained volunteers (at a minimum) to support clinic operations |
| *Instruments* | There are only 5 surgical instrument packs available. A small pressure cooker is available for instrument sterilization, but only has the capacity to sterilize up to 5 packs at a time and the sterilization cycle is 1 h | A. Bring extra surgical packs to the clinic<br>B. Have cold sterilization on hand<br>C. Investigate purchasing a pressure cooker locally with a larger capacity |
| *Medications* | NSAID and opioid availability is largely unknown | A. Determine the feasibility of importing pain medications if they cannot be sourced locally |
| *Animal capture* | In the community, free-roaming dogs are typically captured using chemical capture (blow darting) | A. Determine if nets can be sourced/made locally<br>B. Train staff to use nets or other hand capture techniques<br>C. Encourage community members to bring friendly dogs to the clinic<br>D. Devise anesthesia protocols to account for dogs presenting to the clinic following chemical capture |
| *Travel* | The road to the clinic site is frequently compromised by flooding | A. Ensure access to a vehicle with 4-wheel drive |

Recruiting suitable team members and volunteers can be challenging. Many are passionate and dedicated to animal welfare and want to share their passion in places less fortunate than their own, yet are unfamiliar with the sometimes striking cultural and professional differences in field settings. Many volunteers also lack experience in animal handling, restraint, and postoperative monitoring.

There are many avenues of recruitment, but determining the degree of experience and skill of potential volunteers can be challenging. Skills required in field clinics can be very different than skills required in traditional clinic settings. Field clinics often lack diagnostic and monitoring equipment and even the most experienced veterinarian or technician from a high-quality hospital can be challenged by having to determine how many drops per second of an intravenous fluid to deliver, how to administer the correct amount of injectable anesthesia to maintain a surgical plane of anesthesia, or how to use a pressure cooker for instrument sterilization.

## 5.4.1 In-country or On-site Coordinator

An in-country or on-site coordinator is critical to the success of the clinic. This person is responsible for various aspects of the clinic from community education and advertising the clinic to assuring the specifics of food, lodging, transportation, and clinic essentials are ready when the team arrives. The coordinator is the ambassador of the team. Local language skills are essential and they must be familiar and respectful of the culture.

If a person other than the on-site coordinator is addressing logistical details from outside the clinic or country, the on-site coordinator must have the ability to communicate and liaise with that person.

## 5.4.2 Lead Veterinarian

The designated lead veterinarian is responsible for all medical and animal care protocols. These protocols may be developed collaboratively, involving other members of the team, and discussed before the clinic. Some protocols may require amending during the clinic. Decisions regarding specific animals and medical cases can be difficult to make in field clinics, but ultimately the lead veterinarian is responsible for final decisions.

In the case of owned animals, the owner wishes and requests must be respected. It takes skill and diplomacy to explain difficult cases and options to an owner and community. The lead veterinarian oversees these communications and ensures that every aspect of the patient or case is addressed as best as possible. He or she is also responsible for communication of these difficult decisions to the team. Free-roaming patients pose a particular challenge as aftercare is often minimal or questionable. The lead veterinarian takes responsibility for decisions made regarding the appropriate release of such patients.

## 5.4.3 Recruitment Methods

Several methods and venues for recruiting volunteers and staff for a field clinic include:

- Personal recommendations
- Word of mouth
- Posting on recognized listservs such as High-Quality, High-Volume, Spay/Neuter (HQHVSN) and The Association of Shelter Veterinarians (ASV). Membership is required to post.
- Recruitment via a non-profit animal welfare organization's Web page and application process
- Local advertising
  - Local volunteers and community members
  - Expatriates living in the area
- *Social media*. Facebook is used widely by many organizations and campaigns. It is recommended to have a person affiliated with the field clinic or campaign to address and filter Facebook inquiries and applications.

## 5.4.4 Areas Requiring Professional Staff and Volunteers

The number of designated "stations" of a clinic will vary depending on the specifics of the clinic. A mobile clinic, due to limited space, will have fewer stations compared to a stationary, high-volume campaign. A clinic targeting free-roaming animals will require staff experienced in animal capture and transport. Required staffing in each area will vary greatly depending on the type of clinic, the goals of the clinic, and the number of experienced team members.

---

**Textbox 5.13 Clinic positions requiring staff**

- *Animal trapping/capture.* If catching feral or free-roaming animals
- *Animal transport.* If planning an animal capture-based campaign or if providing animal transport services for owners
- Check-in and admission
- Patient assessment. Can be performed at admission
- Patient preparation
- Anesthesia
- Surgery
- Recovery
- Instrument care
- Logistics
- Cleaning crew
- Intensive care unit (ICU) (if needed)
- Volunteer coordinator
- Discharge

---

### 5.4.5 Professional Team Members

#### 5.4.5.1 Licensure

In the author's experience, many countries do not require acquisition of licensure to provide temporary veterinary services; however, requirements vary from country to country. Some may only require proof of current licensure in the veterinary professional's home country. If a fee for service is implemented, this may affect licensure requirements. It is the responsibility of the lead veterinarian to investigate licensure and professional insurance requirements.

All licensed veterinary professionals (veterinarians and technicians) must be current on licensure and in good standing in their respective country and/or state, and all licensed professionals should carry a copy of their current license.

#### 5.4.5.2 Qualifications and Skill Sets

Licensed veterinarians and technicians, as well as unlicensed technicians, should provide references if requested. If volunteers are unfamiliar or lack experience in field clinics, it is advisable for them to first work with experienced staff.

Veterinarians and technicians should work in areas in which they have experience. If they desire to work in an unfamiliar area, they should work under the guidance of a recognized, experienced team member. Team members must acknowledge if they are placed in an area or on a case that exceeds their capabilities and skill set, and ask for assistance or reassignment if needed.

#### 5.4.5.3 Veterinarians

Spay and neuter surgical experience is critical. Conditions in field clinics can be austere and patients are often physically compromised; common medical conditions include upper respiratory tract infection, transmissible venereal tumors, *Ehrlichia* infection, pregnancy, and being in heat. Veterinarians whose surgical skills are not sufficient to perform safe surgery in the field can provide invaluable assistance at other stations in the clinic including patient assessment, recovery, and anesthesia.

#### 5.4.5.4 Technicians

Participating technicians must be experienced in patient preparation, patient monitoring, anesthesia, and recovery. If they are inexperienced or feel that the caseload or patient requirements are beyond their capability, they should be reassigned or partnered with a more experienced staff member.

#### 5.4.5.5 Ratio of Veterinarians to Technicians

An ideal ratio for a surgical spay/neuter clinic is one veterinarian to one experienced technician per surgery, and one assistant to address preparation and other needs during the procedure. Field clinics are often not an "ideal" clinic setting, however, and staffing adjustments may be necessary. If staffing one technician and one assistant per veterinarian is not possible, one experienced team member should be dedicated to the anesthesia area to address anesthetic events and emergencies.

Adequate staffing is particularly important for patient monitoring during preparation, surgery, and recovery. If sufficient numbers of skilled, experienced staff are lacking, the lead veterinarian must determine the number of anesthetized and recovering patients that can be safely monitored simultaneously.

#### 5.4.5.6 Support Staff and Volunteers

Volunteers and support staff can be immensely helpful in overseeing patient care and providing logistical support. The number of support staff and volunteers needed will vary depending on the type of clinic (MASH-type, mobile, or stationary) and proposed number of surgeries.

One must appreciate that volunteers often lack experience in many aspects of clinic work and animal care. Time and care should be taken at the beginning of the clinic to identify volunteer strengths and weaknesses, although this may be difficult in a large clinic setting. For this reason, a volunteer coordinator is essential. If the clinic is large or occurs over many days, more than one coordinator may be required. This helps streamline services and communication between the various clinic stations, identifying where the particular volunteers' skills may best be utilized. Good communication skills are essential.

Once skills are identified, team members should be identified using nametags and staffed at their respective stations.

```
Textbox 5.14  Ways to utilize support staff

• Handle and transport animals from station to station
• Check-in and admit patients
• Clip and scrub patients prior to surgery
• Monitor patients during recovery
• Clean surgical instruments
• Provide food and water for team members
• Provide transport
    – Animals
    – Team members.
```

### 5.4.6 Animal Handling

Animal handling is often challenging in a field clinic due to the following:

• The clinic environment can be novel and frightening for the animal.
• Many free-roaming or feral animals are unaccustomed to restraint and confinement.
• Dogs and cats often wait together in the same area during check-in.
• Cats often arrive to the clinic without any form of confinement or restraint.

Experienced animal handlers are essential to minimize patient stress as well as protect animal handlers and others working with the animal. Competent handlers should be staffed in admission, presurgery exam, premedication/anesthesia, and recovery stations. All animal bites must be reported to the team leader and treated appropriately.

There are many techniques for minimizing animal stress and potential for escape, while also protecting the handler (Figure 5.4).

```
Textbox 5.15  Tips for handling fearful animals

• Move slowly with nonthreatening body language.
• Talk softly.
• Placing towels or blankets over the animal's head
  creates a "safe" environment for the animal and
  adds an extra layer of protection for the handler.
• Have a net and Y pole available, and train staff in
  using them. Nets are practical for loose cats or
  those that need immediate restraint upon arrival.
• Use slip leashes in place of loose collars on dogs.
• Consider using "figure-eight" leashes on cats.
  Leashes applied in this manner do not tighten
  around the throat should a cat become fractious
  during handling.
• Have muzzles[a] on hand

a   A muzzle should only be placed on an animal to examine a
patient or to sedate/anesthetize the animal. Muzzles must
always be immediately removed after the task at hand is
completed.
```

In the author's experience, catch poles are rarely needed and are often used inappropriately. If an animal is extremely difficult to handle, the lead veterinarian should determine if it is worth the stress to the animal and safety of the handler to proceed. Having a pole syringe available to administer sedatives and anesthetics safely in aggressive or feral animals can be helpful. A pole syringe can also be constructed using 4-feet PVC pipe. The thumb piece off the plunger of a 3cc syringe is cut off and forced into the end of the pipe. The D-ring on a nylon leash can then be slipped over the top of the syringe to make it inject or administer medication orally (D. Fakkema, personal communication).

## 5.5 Medical, Surgical, and Clinic Supplies

Clinic supplies will vary greatly depending on number of projected animals, clinic duration, ability to transport supplies to the site, and budget. A supply manifest is essential to ensure that the necessary items are

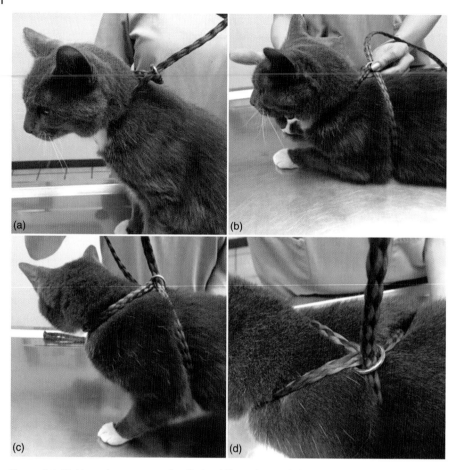

**Figure 5.4** Making a harness out of a slip lead (from the top left to bottom left, read clockwise). First, pass the lead around the neck and through the metal loop. Then pass the lead behind the front legs and back through the metal loop. Be sure to go around the neck first, then behind the legs, which reduces tension on the neck should the cat struggle to get away.

available to conduct a safe and humane clinic. It is best to start with a very detailed, comprehensive manifest to help minimize possible oversight of critical items. Critical supplies should be highlighted.

Acquiring and transporting the proper amount of supplies to address clinic needs can be difficult. Some team members may have easy and inexpensive access to supplies in their home working environments. The team should understand the efforts and cost involved to transport supplies and account for the potential scarcity of simple items such as gauze and paper towels at the clinic site.

The quantity of required supplies such as suture material and anesthetics can vary greatly depending on the quality of medications and material, surgical skill, surgical caseload, and budget. Every effort should be made to ensure an adequate inventory of supplies

deemed most critical. The author recommends having more critical supplies than one thinks will be needed. It is also advisable to determine if there are local places to acquire more critical supplies if need be. If the clinic does not have appropriate numbers of critical supplies due to a variety of reasons, the surgical caseload should be addressed accordingly.

Medical and surgical supplies warrant special mention. The lead veterinarian should be aware of what medications and supplies will be available for use and should develop protocols accordingly. This may involve importing medications and supplies and investigating the ability of acquiring them locally. It is advisable to inform team members of the medications and supplies that will be available so they are aware of the possible difference in approach to analgesia, anesthesia, and surgery.

---

**Textbox 5.16 Tips for planning medical, surgical, and clinic supplies**

1) Highlight critical supplies on the manifest.
2) The lead veterinarian should be aware of what medications and supplies are available.
3) Understand that there can be a marked difference in quality of locally acquired medications and supplies.
4) Investigate the ability to obtain oxygen locally and its cost.
5) Verify that regulators will fit on respective oxygen tanks.
6) Be prepared to adapt to and use injectable anesthesia if there are issues with inhalant anesthesia.
7) Have a backup plan for sterilizing instruments in case of equipment failure. Cold disinfectant may need to be employed if other options are unavailable, but should be a last resort. Dry ovens are usually not an acceptable method of instrument and equipment sterilization unless proper materials are available.

---

### 5.5.1 Supplies

#### 5.5.1.1 Acquisition
One of the first decisions when planning a field clinic is whether to procure supplies locally, import them, or both. (See notes on permit acquisition if importing re: permits and encountering excess baggage fees and/or embargos.) The cost of the same or similar materials can vary greatly between the host country and country of origin. This may dictate the origin of supplies if there are budgetary concerns. However, there can be a marked difference in quality of suture material and medications, especially analgesics and anesthetics. This can affect the amounts required to adequately address patient care, anesthesia, and surgery.

#### 5.5.1.2 Sourcing Oxygen
If oxygen is to be used in the clinic, one should investigate the ability to acquire and deliver to clinic site and verify the cost, as oxygen can be very expensive in some countries. If sourcing it locally, it is important to verify the specifics of oxygen tanks and regulators as regulator threads from one country may not be compatible with threads on the oxygen tank in the host country. Always be prepared to use injectable anesthesia if oxygen is not available or there are issues with the tank or regulator.

#### 5.5.1.3 Surgical Drapes
The number of surgical drapes required should account for possible contaminations and a higher surgical caseload than initially expected. In the author's experience, one should bring at least 20% more drapes than the forecasted number of procedures, to ensure an adequate supply.

#### 5.5.1.4 Surgical Instruments
While surgical instruments used for routine spay/neuter procedures can vary from veterinarian to veterinarian, most high-volume surgeons only use five or six instruments per surgery.

Sterile instruments should be readily available in the event of contamination or complications. Instruments can be sterilized in appropriate autoclave material such as pack wraps or drape material, or in self-sealing sterilization pouches. Such pouches are readily available for purchase online.

Surgery team members should be familiar with the instruments they will have available to them. Additional instruments should be available and ready.

---

**Textbox 5.17 Surgical instrument tips**

- Surgical instruments are usually limited. Use staff effectively to continuously clean and sterilize instruments throughout the day.
- It is advised to have cold disinfectants readily available to sterilize instruments should an autoclave or pressure cooker be unavailable.
- Local human hospitals and clinics may have an autoclave that can be used after their normal operating hours to sterilize packs, if needed.

---

### 5.5.2 Sterilization of Equipment Before and During Clinic

The number of instrument packs available for use throughout the clinic may be limited. Establishing how many packs are available and the manner in which they will be resterilized or chemically disinfected throughout the day and clinic should be done well in advance. The number of available instrument packs must be sufficient to support the caseload and pace of the clinic.

To maximize efficiency, a separate station and team member(s) should be dedicated to instrument cleaning and sterilizing. This ensures proper cleaning and care and minimizes the possibility of lack of sterile instruments when a patient is on the surgery table awaiting surgery. Surgeon time is precious and should not be wasted by waiting for instruments.

If chemical disinfection is to be used, sufficient time must be allotted per pack to ensure adequate disinfection. If an autoclave or pressure cooker is to be used, sufficient time is needed to run a complete cycle.

Dry ovens warrant special mention as they are frequently used in most of the world due to their affordability and relative ease of use. Most materials will not tolerate dry ovens; cloth and paper will catch fire for example. Dry ovens also use a relatively long cycle time and many materials will not attain time and temperatures sufficient for adequate sterilization. Metal containers, aluminum foil, and self-sealing sterilization pouches can be used in dry ovens to contain instruments and gauze during sterilization. If metal containers and/or self-sealing sterilization pouches are not available, dry ovens should not be used for the sterilization of surgical supplies (drapes, instruments, gauze).

In some areas, a local human hospital may allow access to their autoclave during off-hours.

## 5.6 Medical Records

Every animal admitted to or treated by the clinic must have a medical record. This includes free-roaming, aggressive, and feral/trapped animals. The medical record is a written log of owner or responsible party information and signed consent, patient information, physical exam findings, and all medications administered to the patient. Additionally, it serves as an anesthesia, surgery, and recovery log. All team members should be familiar with the medical record. Medical records can be color-coded (blue for males, pink for females) to facilitate patient identification.

---

> **Textbox 5.18  Medical record requirements**
>
> - Every animal admitted to the clinic must have a medical record.
> - Perform a brief physical exam on all patients prior to anesthesia, unless feral or too aggressive, and record the results in the medical record.
> - Document all medications, doses, routes of administration, and the time administered to a patient in the medical record.
> - Monitor quantities of medications and supplies on-hand throughout the clinic.

---

Medical records also provide valuable patient information should an animal have a postoperative complication or require additional care. This information can be critical for any veterinarian or responsible party providing follow-up care.

Medical histories of most patients will be unknown, particularly if they are feral or free-roaming. In such cases, the medical record should require only information deemed absolutely necessary such as caregiver contact information and a signed consent by the responsible party. A sample patient medical record is included in Appendix 5.C.

### 5.6.1  Storage of Medical Records

Medical records should be stored in a place where the person responsible for post-clinic communications and care has access to them. The length of time records should be stored post-clinic will depend on the local legal regulations and/or clinic organizer's need for access. Most records are stored for a minimum of 3 years.

### 5.6.2  Medication and Drug Logs

The local or national requirements regarding the logging of specific medications used during the clinic must be determined. This can be challenging information to obtain as it can vary from country to country and location to location. Some countries require a log of every medication, including antibiotics used during the clinic. This can create logistical difficulties, yet every effort should be made to comply with the local and national law.

A log should be maintained for both non-controlled and controlled drugs. The definition of a controlled substance is drug or chemical whose manufacture, possession, or use is regulated by a government. The designation of a "controlled" drug, however, varies from country to country. What is considered a controlled drug in one country may not be so in another country. A sample controlled drug log is included in Appendix 5.D.

### 5.6.3 Inventory Log

All supplies and medications should be carefully inventoried prior to the start of a clinic. A specific person should be designated to monitor quantities on hand throughout the clinic. Sudden changes in caseload or situations requiring a larger amount of certain medications can quickly deplete drug stocks. This is particularly important for anesthetics and analgesics.

### 5.6.4 Catching Manifest

If trapping cats and dogs, a manifest is required to document information including the number of animals captured and their locations. See Chapter 4 for additional information on trapping.

## 5.7 Preoperative Considerations

Many factors affect the decision of whether or not to perform surgery on an individual animal. All animals presenting for surgery must be assessed for anesthesia and surgical candidacy. If the clinic is trapping animals, plans should be in place to minimize patient stress during the assessment of surgical candidacy (physical examination). The decision to proceed with surgery is determined by the veterinary team, and the lead veterinarian makes all final decisions.

Zoonotic diseases always warrant attention, particularly rabies. It helps to know the rabies incidence in the working area so that a bite policy can be implemented prior to the start of the clinic. In most places, quarantining animals for rabies can be difficult to impossible. The clinic organizer should maintain a list of which team members are vaccinated for rabies.

The decision to proceed with surgery can be difficult. Field clinics frequently lack comprehensive postoperative care capacity, aside from what is required for a routine spay/neuter surgery. One should consider the following:

- Will the animal benefit from surgery today versus postponing or cancelling surgery?
- Is the veterinary team ready and capable of addressing possible intraoperative or postoperative complications should they arise?
- Will the mobile team, local clinic, or caregiver have the capacity to provide postoperative care for the amount of time required for the patient to heal?

### 5.7.1 Patient Selection

Preoperative examinations are essential in determining whether or not animals qualify for surgery. Written protocols developed prior to the clinic and amended during the clinic if necessary will make this process more efficient.

Common considerations regarding surgical candidacy include the following:

- *Age and weight limits.* To be determined based on the veterinary skill of team members and logistics of the field clinic. General recommended age and weight guidelines include:
  - Minimum 8 weeks and 1 kg in healthy patients with appropriate anesthesia
  - Minimum 12 weeks and 1.5 kg in areas where dogs and cats are nutritionally and medically challenged
  - Maximum age of 7 years
- *Pregnant animals.* Most field clinics spay pregnant females. Anesthesia and surgical risk must be determined by physical examination and addressed accordingly.
- *Pediatric animals.* Generally defined as 8–16 weeks of age
- *Medical issues*
  - Upper respiratory tract infection
  - Anemia
  - Mange
  - Late-stage pregnancy
  - Pyometra
  - Postwhelping or queening
  - Transmissible venereal tumor
- *Free-roaming animals/trapped animals.* Must determine if postoperative care be provided, if needed.

### 5.7.2 Common Diseases

The clinic organizer and lead veterinarian should be aware of canine and feline disease prevalence in the working area as routine diagnostic testing is usually unavailable. *Ehrlichia* spp. and other tick borne diseases that affect coagulation are endemic in many parts of the world. Any clinical signs (i.e. petechia, ecchymosis, prolonged bleeding after an injection) found on physical exam related to tick-borne disease should be brought to the attention of the lead veterinarian or designated section head. Clinical signs of a coagulopathy may not be noted until intraoperatively, so mechanisms should be implemented to address such issues prior to the start of the clinic.

### 5.7.3 Food and Water Recommendations

It is generally recommended to withhold food the morning of surgery, with the exception of pediatric patients, which can rapidly become hypoglycemic. Pediatric surgeries should be performed early in the day and patients fed as soon as they have recovered sufficiently to eat. If the surgical wait time is more than 4 h, offer a small amount of food to pediatric patients and note the time and amount in the medical record. Honey or Karo syrup rubbed on the gums also helps prevent hypoglycemia.

Patients should be allowed to drink water until arrival at the clinic. Many surgical candidates suffer from mild to moderate dehydration as they may wait the entire day without water before surgery. The conditions at a field clinic can be hot, humid, and stressful. Therefore, it is recommended to permit water consumption prior to arrival. If an animal is expected to wait more than 4 h and the physical exam or the climate suggests that water is needed, a small bowl should be offered.

### 5.7.4 Thermoregulation

Thermoregulation intra- and postoperatively is essential for patient care and recovery. Thermo-regulation is one of the most neglected aspects of patient care. It is much easier to maintain normal temperatures during surgery and recovery than to address hypo- or hyperthermia.

Many field clinic sites are in hot climates or in areas with little to no ventilation. Animals sitting all day in such conditions without access to water can have elevated temperatures preoperatively. Conversely, field clinics in colder climates or higher altitudes will need to address thermoregulation and risk of hypothermia intra- and postoperatively.

Hypothermia is one of the most common post-operative complications and contributes to slow recoveries and delayed wound healing. Anesthesia, wet body surfaces, prolonged surgical times, and large incisions all contribute to lowering the core body temperature. Be aware that intravenous or sub-cutaneous administration of fluids can contribute to hypothermia as room temperature of the fluids is colder than the core temperature of the patient.

Methods to address thermoregulation should be determined before the clinic starts. Certain items can be kept on-hand to maintain a preoperative and recovery area conducive to minimizing adverse conditions. Table 5.1 details specific measures to minimize patient hypo- and hyperthermia.

---

**Textbox 5.19 Tools for thermoregulation**

- Thermometers and lubrication
  - Insulating material for use intra- and postoperative
  - Towels
  - Blankets
  - Newspapers
  - Yoga mats, foam mats, straw mats
  - Mylar or space blankets
- Microwave for heating rice socks or water bottles
- Heat sources[a]
  - Socks filled with uncooked rice (rice socks) to heat in microwave
  - Recycled water bottles
  - Heating pads
- Warm water baths for Lactated Ringers or similar fluids
  - Do not administer warm solutions subcutaneously without veterinary oversight
- Fans
- Frozen ice packs, water bottles.

*a* NEVER put a heat source directly against the patient's skin.

Table 5.1 Methods to facilitate thermoregulation.

| Minimizing hypothermia | Minimizing hyperthermia |
|---|---|
| • Minimize excess water/prep solutions during patient preparation. Wet animals get cold faster<br>• Limit the use of alcohol in preparations. Alcohol rapidly reduces body temperature<br>• Change out the material used for surgery table insulation or in recovery if wet<br>• Place appropriately protected heat sources alongside patient intra or postoperatively<br>• Place socks or plastic wrap over paws<br>• Place patient on insulating material intra- or postoperatively<br>   – Yoga mats covered in plastic trash bags on the surgery table are great sources of insulation and easy to clean between patients<br>   – Towels<br>   – Newspapers<br>• Cover patients with blankets or towels in recovery<br>• Administer warm subcutaneous fluids[a] | • Place the patient directly on surgery table or recovery floor without insulation<br>• Administer intravenous or subcutaneous fluids at room temperature<br>• Use fans<br>• Apply ice packs in the axillary and inguinal areas, if needed<br>• Use gauze soaked alcohol on paws, if needed |

a) Only to be done under the guidance of an experienced veterinarian.

### 5.7.5 Perioperative Medications

#### 5.7.5.1 Vaccinations

Ideally, vaccines would be given well in advance of the day of surgery to allow for the production of protective antibodies and to minimize potential adverse reactions. If there is an adverse reaction, it may be difficult to recognize and treat during anesthesia and surgery. For example, if an animal postoperatively becomes lethargic with pale mucous membranes, it may be difficult to differentiate between an adverse vaccine reaction and potential bleeding or hypotensive event. However, vaccinations administered at the time of the surgery in field clinics may be the only opportunity to vaccinate the animal. Therefore, the benefits typically far outweigh the risks. It is wise to establish a consistent time for vaccination, i.e. all vaccines are given during recovery. Giving vaccines during or before anesthesia is not recommended due to the difficulty in differentiating between intraoperative problems due to anesthesia versus vaccine reaction.

#### 5.7.5.2 Deworming

Similar to vaccination, deworming during field surgery/campaigns may be the only time the animal receives this medication. Oral dewormers are routinely administered during recovery. If given prior to surgery, there is a good chance that they might vomit the medication, depending on the premedication used.

#### 5.7.5.3 Antibiotics

The routine administration of antibiotics perioperatively in field clinics is controversial. The routine administration of antibiotics in surgical patients, in the presence of aseptic technique, has been shown to increase the prevalence of antibiotic-resistant bacteria and is not recommended [2].

#### 5.7.5.4 Analgesics

All surgical patients should receive at least one analgesic perioperatively.

#### 5.7.5.5 Dosing Charts

The use of dosing charts ($\times$ ml/kg of medications) in a clinic will help minimize dosing errors and increase the efficiency in determining medication dosages for individual patients. Dosing charts are especially useful for emergency drugs and anesthesia cocktails.

## 5.8 Clinic Areas and Flow

Clinic efficiency is dependent on the clinic layout. Although field clinics vary greatly, every effort should be made to facilitate patient movement from check-in through recovery, with an emphasis on minimizing patient stress. Patient movement from clinic station to station is also referred to as clinic flow.

Clinic flow is usually fairly simple in mobile clinics due to limited space. Stationary and MASH-type clinic flow will be determined by the available space, access to water and electricity, and, possibly, the elements such as sunlight and ventilation.

A major barrier to clinic flow occurs when a patient presents with a medical condition that requires a surgical procedure other than spay/neuter. The clinic

---

**Textbox 5.20 Tips and tricks to maintain a safe and efficient clinic**

- The medical record stays with the patient at all times throughout the clinic.
- Know the surgical limit. Learn to say "no" and stop admissions when indicated.
- Have a supply checklist for each clinic station.
- Mark the oxygen tank psi level at the beginning and end of each day to monitor for excessive use and/or leaks.
- Monitor patients until they can be safely returned to a kennel or discharged to their owner.
- Postoperative instructions must be provided to every caregiver/owner (Appendix 5.E).

---

should determine well ahead of time if surgeons will perform ancillary procedures such as wound repairs,

amputations, or administer treatment for transmissible venereal tumors. If these will not be performed on-site, a local veterinary clinic should be identified to provide such services.

While clinic setups can vary, the most commonly used clinic stations are described here (Figure 5.5).

### 5.8.1 Check-in

Patient check-in is often the most chaotic area of the clinic. Public turnout can be overwhelming, and more animals may present to the clinic than the clinic can accommodate. Pet owners may begin to line up extremely early in the morning (Figure 5.6).

Every animal admitted or treated at the clinic must have a medical record that is completed at the clinic. *It is imperative the medical record stay with the animal at all times, from check-in until discharge. This includes feral and free-roaming animals.*

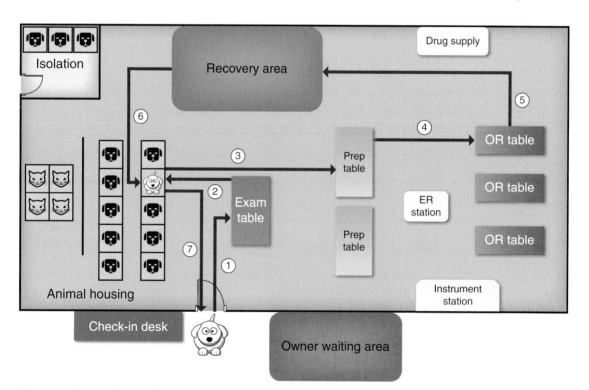

**Figure 5.5** Suggested route for surgical patients in a field clinic. 1. After a patient is checked in, an intake examination is performed. A weight is typically obtained at this time. The patient may be premedicated for surgery here, or later following placement in a housing unit. 2. The patient is moved to an individual cage or group-housing area, depending on the patient housing available. 3. Once sedated, the patient is moved to a preparation table where anesthesia is induced and the patient is prepared for surgery. 4. The patient is moved to an operating table where the surgical procedure is performed. 5. The patient is moved into the recovery area to receive any additional medications and monitoring. 6. Following recovery, the patient is moved back into his or her original housing unit. 7. The patient is discharged following an examination confirming adequate recovery from anesthesia and surgery.

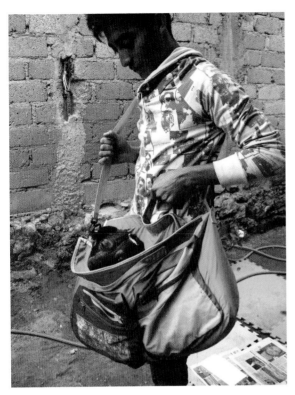

**Figure 5.6** Patient arriving to the clinic for check-in.

### 5.8.2 Monitoring the Number of Admitted Patients

Each clinic day should have a predetermined number of surgeries. If the clinic is to be a first-come, first-serve basis, there must be a method in place to monitor the number of animals accepted for surgery. A recommended practice is to have a sign in sheet and numbers assigned as the animals arrive. *Numbers are to be assigned per individual animal.* Some people may arrive with more than one animal and each should receive a unique number. One person can be designated to assign numbers on entry and to avoid errors in numbering. If the clinic is by appointment, the lead veterinarian should predetermine the number of appointments. The person in charge of monitoring the caseload must check the list frequently and stop admission once the predetermined number is achieved.

The lead veterinarian should have the ability to increase or decrease the predetermined number based on equipment, supplies, anesthesia, surgical skill, and staffing to safely address patient care.

Care must be taken to admit only the number of animals that can be safely and humanely addressed for the day.

One practical option is to have a dry erase board or similar method to track patients. A dry erase board can be used to identify the surgeries that have special requirements such as those that may need to be done earlier in the day or provide notes regarding a specific patient such as "aggressive". Dry erase boards also allow tracking of completed procedures by volunteers.

A list of required items is helpful to ensure all supplies are on hand prior to the start of the clinic.

---

**Textbox 5.21 Patient check-in supply list**

- Sign in sheet, pens, sharpies, or other permanent markers
- Medical records (suggestion: pink for females, blue for males)
- Clipboards for medical records
- Nametags for volunteers (suggestion: write both name and clinic position)
- Stapler
- Materials for patient identification and numbering:
  - Masking tape on the top of the head with a number.
  - Preprinted numbers on adhesive paper to number animals and charts.
  - Self-adhering neckbands. Note that neckbands must be removed at the time of discharge to avoid injury to the patient.
- Leashes
- Kennels (clean and ready-to-use)
- Supplies to attach medical records to the patient and kennel
  - If the owner is waiting with the animal, the owner keeps the medical record with them until the animal is moved to a kennel or surgery.
  - If an animal is placed in a kennel, attach the medical record to the kennel.
    Clothes pins: color coded, blue = male, pink = female
    Clipboards with the medical record placed in front of cage or carabiners to attach onto kennel doors
    Tape for securing the medical record
- Consent forms
  - Free-roaming animals and pets should have a responsible person provide consent.

---

### 5.8.3 Pick-up Times

If same-day release is planned, owners need to be informed of an approximate pick-up time. Anesthesia protocols will determine the necessary recovery time, and a patient must be fully conscious to be released. Owners should be prepared to wait until their animal is cleared for release by an experienced team member. In general, surgeries are performed in the order that patients were admitted. Exceptions to this include pediatric patients, pregnant animals, or metabolically compromised patients.

### 5.8.4 Preoperative Area

Preoperative areas involve any areas where animals are waiting for surgery, either with their owners or in kennels. Ideally, this area should be far away from patient preparation, surgery, and recovery areas as dogs awaiting surgery tend to bark, which can arouse other clinic patients. Having slip leashes and kennels available in this area to assist owners with animal handling and restraint if necessary is also recommended.

Every patient must have a brief physical exam prior to anesthesia to determine if he or she is a surgical candidate. The only exceptions to this rule are extremely aggressive or feral animals, which may require sedation or anesthesia prior to examination.

An experienced veterinarian can usually perform a physical exam in 2–3 min. If abnormalities are found that may affect surgical candidacy, additional time may be required. A brief physical exam includes the following:

- Heart rate, rhythm, and character
- Respiratory rate and character
- Mucous membrane color
- Capillary refill time
- A brief whole body palpation
- Temperature. Taking an animal's temperature can be very stressful. If too stressful for the animal or unsafe for the handler, this can be postponed until the animal is under sedation or anesthesia.
  - Non-contact thermometers such as the Rycon Portable Non-Contact Infrared Thermometer have proved to be very useful for stressed, anxious, or aggressive animals. The thermometer should be pointed at an area with little hair such as the axillary region or medial thigh.

- Weight. Every effort should be made to obtain an accurate weight of each animal. A digital scale is ideal but often unavailable. A bathroom scale can be used whereby a volunteer or owner lifts the dog and weighs both the dog and himself, then subtracts the weight of the person. Baby scales are an excellent way to obtain an accurate weight of small animals.

To facilitate examinations, reference ranges for normal vital sign values should be posted and readily visible for staff to use (see Chapter 20).

### 5.8.5 Patient Housing

Ensuring adequate pre- and postoperative patient housing can be a challenging aspect of the clinic. Many organizations lack sufficient, safe housing for the number of surgeries planned. The clinic space and the number of kennels/cages available may limit the number of surgeries possible.

Animals awaiting surgery or discharge require housing in individual, species appropriate cages to prevent fighting and possible injury. This is especially true during recovery as anesthesia can affect patient behavior. Cats accustomed to living together in a household will often become temporarily aggressive while recovering from anesthesia if placed in a cage together. Dogs that were too aggressive or fractious to safely handle preoperatively will require a cage immediately upon completion of surgery to recover in a safe manner (Figure 5.7).

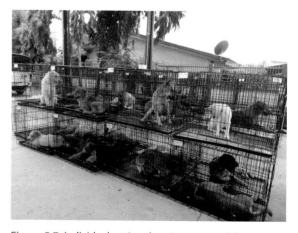

**Figure 5.7** Individual patient housing at a mobile spay/neuter clinic in Thailand. Photo credit: Katherine Polak, Soi Dog Foundation.

Clinics using an appointment or first-come, first-serve system may allow owners to wait with their pets until housing becomes available. Exceptions to this include aggressive or fractious animals, which will require immediate housing for safety reasons. Ideally patients are discharged on a rotational basis, freeing up cage space as the clinic proceeds through the day. Trap–neuter–return (TNR) programs will have animals already in traps, and patients will be returned to their respective traps for recovery.

Clinic organizers must know the number of appropriate patient housing units available for the clinic and reconcile this number with the projected number of surgeries. If there is an insufficient quantity of appropriate housing units, plans must be made as to how patients will be housed appropriately pre- and postoperatively. In some clinic situations, dogs are housed collectively in pens. This practice is less ideal due to the potential for fighting and infectious disease transmission.

### 5.8.6 Patient Preparation

Patients are usually prepared for surgery in a separate, designated area. In the field, this may not be an option due to limited space or tables and patients are prepared on the surgical table. If this is the case, care must be taken to prepare the patient in a manner that minimizes contamination of the surgical area. A portable, small vacuum or lint brush will greatly reduce contamination. If a separate area is available, the area for patient preparation should be adjacent to the surgery area, minimizing the distance needed to carry an anesthetized patient from the preparation area to the surgical table. During patient transport, care must be taken to not contaminate the prepared surgical site (Figure 5.8).

The patient preparation protocol including endotracheal intubation and placement of an intravenous catheter, if needed, should be written prior to the start of the clinic. If gas anesthesia is to be used, endotracheal (ET) tubes of various sizes are required. The lead veterinarian determines the specific protocol for the clinic based on the budget and supplies available. ET intubation and the placement of intravenous catheters will increase preparation time yet may increase patient safety. If ET tubes and intravenous catheters are not routinely placed, they need to be easily accessible in the preparation area for emergencies.

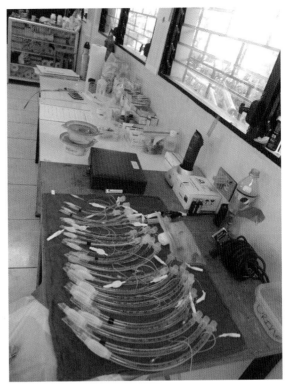

**Figure 5.8** Anesthesia station at a spay/neuter clinic in San Salvador, El Salvador.

---

**Textbox 5.22 Preparation area supply list**

- Preparation solution and scrub
- Gauze
- Eye lubrication. A drop of corn or vegetable oil can replace commercial eye lubricants such as Paralube
- Clippers
  - Keep straight razors as a backup in case of electricity failure or broken clippers
- Vacuum or lint brushes to remove hair from the clipped surgical site
- ET tubes of various sizes and materials to hold them in place
  - Tube gauze, recycled IV lines, rubber bands
- Miscellaneous items
  - Intravenous catheters and injection caps
  - 1 in. white adhesive tape or similar tape
  - ET tubes of various sizes (if not routinely used)
  - A bag valve mask ("Ambu bag") for respiratory assistance
  - Intravenous or subcutaneous fluids
  - Extra 1 and 3 ml syringes.

### 5.8.7 Anesthesia

Most field clinics have a dedicated area for the storage and use of anesthetic drugs. Certain medications should also be made accessible to the necessary clinic stations including patient preparation, induction, and recovery.

A veterinarian or veterinary technician experienced in field clinics should be in charge of anesthesia to minimize dosing errors and miscommunications. Anesthesia personnel must communicate with the surgeon so that the surgeon is ready and waiting for the patient when the patient arrives at the table. Irrespective of the protocol, everything necessary for anesthesia should be ready and in place prior to premedicating and inducing the first animal. The veterinary professional in charge should walk through the clinic prior to the first procedure to ensure the proper equipment and supplies are ready.

---

**Textbox 5.23 Anesthesia supply considerations**

- Designate a place for storing emergency medications and equipment.
  - All experienced veterinarians and technicians must know where emergency medications and supplies are. Red is the recognized color for emergencies. Use red containers to house emergency equipment and supplies.
- Ensure basic supplies are kept on hand:
  - 1, 3, and 6 ml syringes (a few 12, 20, or 35 ml syringes available if needed)
  - 18, 20, 22, and 25 gauge needles
  - Analgesics
  - Anesthetics
  - Intravenous catheters, injection ports, and appropriate tapes
  - Catheter flush solution
  - Supply of permanent markers to label syringes
  - Stethoscope
  - Thermometer
- Provide access to monitoring equipment, if available.
- Designate an area in surgery (a table in a central location or a carryall per surgery table) with additional anesthesia supplies.
  - Additional anesthetics
  - Extra syringes

---

  - Intravenous flush solution (if using IV catheters)
  - Needles
  - Permanent markers
- If using gas anesthesia, check levels of inhalant anesthetic in the vaporizer frequently. Pressure check gas machines at the beginning of each day.
- Check oxygen tanks to ensure sufficient oxygen for the day or clinic. Put a piece of duct tape on the tank and record the psi at the beginning of the day. This helps ascertain if there are leaks.

---

### 5.8.8 Surgeon Preparation

For proper surgeon preparation, access to water is essential. This may be in a bathroom, a sink, or bucket with fresh water. The use of "waterless" hand antiseptic products such as Avagard will decrease the reliance on running water for surgeon preparation but may be cost prohibitive.

Ideally, the area of surgeon preparation should be closest to the surgery table; however, this may be dictated by the location of accessible water for scrubbing hands. Surgeons will need to scrub and dry their hands in a satisfactory manner and be able to don sterile surgery gloves in an area that will permit them to maintain sterility until they reach the surgery table. This should be in a relatively traffic-free area, without wind, and close to the surgery table. See Chapter 12 for further information on surgeon preparation.

### 5.8.9 Surgery

The surgery area will be adjacent to patient preparation, or, in some cases, the same as patient preparation. Establish an area for surgical supplies adjacent to this area. This should include equipment and supplies most commonly used during surgery such as suture, surgical blades, instruments, drapes, sterile gauze, tissue glue, tattoo ink, and extra sterile instruments.

Surgeons or volunteers should gather necessary supplies and place them on the instrument table (or the end of the surgery table if no instrument table is available) prior to the surgeon's arrival at the table. The surgeon should be at the table and ready to perform surgery by the time the patient arrives at the table. Valuable anesthesia time is lost if an anesthetized patient is waiting for a surgeon and/or

**Table 5.2** Recommended supplies to have on hand at the surgery station.

| Required supplies | Recommended ancillary supplies |
|---|---|
| • Sterile, single-use surgery gloves<br>• Surgical caps and masks, if available<br>• Surgical blades<br>• Suture material<br>• Sterile drape<br>• Sterile gauze<br>• Sterile surgical instruments | • Extra sterile gauze and sterile laparotomy pads<br>• Extra sterile instruments<br>  – Hemostats of all sizes<br>  – Scissors<br>  – Needle drivers<br>  – Tissue forceps<br>  – Retractors<br>• Extra sterile drapes<br>• Auto transfusion kit<br>• Sterile surgical gowns, if available |

surgical equipment to arrive. Table 5.2 includes a list of required and recommended surgical supplies for spay/neuter procedures.

### 5.8.10 Surgical Schedule

It is easiest to perform surgeries in the order that the patients are admitted; however, there will be surgeries that will need to be performed as early as possible to allow adequate recovery time. As mentioned earlier, a white board can be used to identify special cases that may need to be done earlier in the day. This includes patients that are:

• Pediatric
• Pregnant
• Metabolically compromised
• Feral or free-roaming
• Large, obese female dogs

### 5.8.11 Tables

An ideal surgery table should be portable, adjustable, and made of a material that is easy to clean and disinfect. Stainless steel is ideal as it is durable and disinfectable. Plastic, light, portable adjustable tables of varying lengths are affordable and available at many home improvement-type stores. Some field clinics with limited-resources may need to adapt whatever table or furniture is readily available. Spacing between tables should be sufficient for team members to transport patients on and off surgical tables.

Tables vary in height. If adjustable tables are unavailable, placing concrete blocks under the legs of the tables can be used to raise them. Conversely, surgeons can stand on an item such as a book while performing surgery. When selecting surgery tables, identify the following:

• What is the available space for tables?
• Do they need to be portable?
• What is the expected average weight and size of the patients?

Patient positioners (V trays) may or may not be available. If unavailable, IV fluid bags, sand bags, or rice socks can be placed along the sides of the patient to assist with positioning. Crossing the front legs of the patient when tied to the table can also assist with the positioning of large or deep-chested dogs.

### 5.8.12 Recovery, Postoperative Care and Monitoring

Postoperative care and monitoring of patients recovering from anesthesia and surgery is critical to ensure patient health and safety. The sooner an anesthetic complication such as pale mucous membranes, weak pulses, or a low temperature is identified and addressed, the better the patient outcome. Patients in recovery should be monitored until an acceptable level of recovery is achieved to allow the patient to be returned to a kennel or discharged to the owner. *If an animal is intubated, a team member MUST stay with the patient constantly until extubated.*

The recovery area should be near the surgery area, within sight of veterinarians. This minimizes the distance an anesthetized animal needs to be carried for possible emergency care. Traffic and noise in the

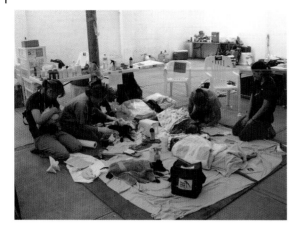

Figure 5.9 Postoperative recovery area.

medications allow easy transport from animal to animal. Carryalls should be restocked at the beginning of each day.

**Textbox 5.24 Recommended recovery area supplies**

- Reference chart with normal canine and feline vital sign parameter ranges
- Thermometer and lubrication
- Stethoscope
- Towels, blankets, newspapers
- Foam mats or other insulating materials to place the patient on
- Honey or corn syrup (to apply to the gums of pediatrics or small animals in the case of hypoglycemia)
- Medications to be administered postoperatively and dosing charts
  - Flea and tick medications
  - Deworming
- Vaccines (stored at an appropriate temperature in a cooler or refrigerator)
- Non-sterile syringes to administer topical/oral medications
- Materials to address thermoregulation
- Cleaning and disinfecting solutions and supplies
- Tape or vet wrap to apply bandages if intravenous catheters were placed and removed
- Bandage scissors
- Toe nail trimmers and Kwik Stop (styptic powder)
- Flea combs
- Tweezers
- Q-tips or cotton balls
- Ear cleaner
- Jar of isopropyl alcohol to collect ticks after removal
- Bandages for abdominal wraps, if needed.

recovery area should be minimized, to avoid overstimulating recovering patients. A slip lead should be kept around a dog's neck or leash wrapped around a cat in a figure-eight fashion, not around the neck, in the event of a sudden recovery and attempt to flee. An experienced team member must be appointed to oversee recovery at all times. All communications should go through the lead recovery person except in the case of an acute animal emergency. These should be directly referred to an experienced veterinarian or veterinary technician (Figure 5.9).

This station is also an area where patients receive additional care including vaccinations, flea and tick preventative, deworming, toe nail trimming, and ear cleaning. Team members should be reminded to exercise caution as some of these practices can overstimulate a recovering patient, resulting in an acute and/or aggressive response that may injure both animal and handler. Injections should be administered by a team member with experience in performing injections. Many volunteers want to assist in recovery yet lack experience in working with animals recovering from anesthesia or monitoring vital parameters. It is one of the most common areas where bites occur so experienced recovery leaders should help train volunteers to ensure staff and patient safety.

Entry to the recovery area should be restricted to designated volunteers. Children should be prohibited from this area. A central location where medications and materials that will be routinely used in recovery should be readily accessible for recovery staff. Portable carryalls with frequently used equipment and

### 5.8.13 Discharge: Postoperative Care and Instructions

Spay/neuter surgeries require postoperative care in order to minimize complications and ensure the patient the best possible care and recovery. Postoperative care instructions must be provided to all owners and patient caregivers.

Many owners fail to appreciate the invasiveness of spay/neuter surgery. Feline and canine spays are major abdominal procedures and need to be treated as such. Castrations, although not as invasive as spays, are painful, and severe complications can occur without proper postoperative care. Owners may be deceived as most patients appear "normal" upon release.

---

**Textbox 5.25 Recommendations for postoperative care**

- Instructions must be written clearly, simply, and in a language the owner/caregiver can understand.
- Designated person(s) must explain and discuss the following with the owner/caregiver:
  - Feeding instructions
  - Activity restriction
  - Housing for the immediate postoperative period
  - Explanation of incision and suture absorption
  - Any abnormalities noted on physical exam
  - Explanation of any additional medications dispensed to the patient
  - Contact information of a person who can address postoperative questions or complications
- Have a protocol in place for communication between caregiver and veterinary care provider in the event of questions or complications.
- Ensure all intravenous catheters and band aids are removed prior to release.
- An experienced team member must inspect the incision and observe the patient's mentation and ambulation prior to release.

---

### 5.8.13.1 Same Day Release or Postoperative Housing and Confinement

All postoperative patients benefit from confinement, activity restriction, and a warm, dry place to recover. Patients returning to homes and caregivers will hopefully have such needs addressed, although that can never be ensured, even in the best of households. For this reason, some field clinics choose to house patients for 1–5 days following surgery to ensure proper healing and recovery, even though most patients in a field clinic are sufficiently recovered from anesthesia to permit same–day release. Programs working primarily with free-roaming dogs in communities that offer little care may consider keeping patients several days postoperatively to ensure proper recovery. This

practice must be weighed against the stress of confinement on the patient, the number of cages available, and the potential for infectious disease transmission, particularly if animals are co- or group-housed. Table 5.3 lists the advantages and disadvantages of same-day release versus housing dogs and cats for an extended period of time.

The veterinary team must be ready to address any indication that a patient requires overnight or additional care. The team should be prepared to care for the patient on-site, at their site of lodging, or refer the

Table 5.3 Same-day release vs. hospitalization.

|  | Same-day release | Housing animals postoperatively for 1–5 days |
|---|---|---|
| Advantages | Reduced patient stress as patients are able to return home sooner | Confinement and activity restriction is ensured |
|  | Reduced staffing is needed to care for in-patients | Improved ability to monitor incisional healing and recovery |
|  | Reduced clinic cost | Patient access to food, water, and warmth is ensured |
|  | Reduced clinic supplies required (bowls, secure kennels, food, cleaning supplies) | Easier to keep incisions clean and dry |
|  | Waste disposal minimized |  |
|  | Higher owner reclamation rate |  |
| Disadvantages | Inability to monitor the patient and incisional healing following discharge | Potential for infectious disease transmission, increased stress, and compromised welfare |
|  | Loss to follow-up | Capacity to perform additional surgeries may be reduced |
|  | Access to food, water, and shelter cannot be ensured | Owner reclamation may be affected |

patient to a local veterinary professional for monitoring and care.

### 5.8.13.2 Surgeries Requiring Extended Care and Special Instructions

Surgeries that require additional instructions and care necessitate a trained and experienced team member to discuss the specific postoperative care and instructions in a language and wording the caregiver can understand. The importance of ensuring appropriate postoperative care cannot be overemphasized.

- All instructions must be written down.
- Allow enough time to discuss the case and patient with the caregiver and answer questions.
- A designated staff member should be available for questions after the patient is released, or be able to refer the client to a local veterinary professional.

For patients requiring a more complicated surgery, clinic veterinarians often have the surgical skills to perform the procedure, but aftercare may be questionable. In such cases, the veterinary team should discuss the case and determine the best possible approach. This can be difficult for team members or volunteers, especially if euthanasia is the most humane option, or if the caregiver decides on a course of treatment that differs from that recommended by the veterinary team.

### 5.8.13.3 Free-roaming and TNR Patients

Free-roaming animals collected for spay/neuter and those undergoing a TNR-type program are often released on the same day of, or morning after surgery. Occasional exceptions include stationary clinics equipped with facilities and staff to properly house and care for patients longer. The majority of these patients will not receive any aftercare in their communities, although some of the patients may live in locations where local people will observe their activity and note possible complications. These patients need as much time as possible in recovery on the day of surgery to allow adequate time to recover from anesthesia and surgery so that they are as fit as possible for release.

### 5.8.14 Instrument and Equipment Care Station

Instruments are expensive and should be maintained in good working condition. To do so, clean water must be readily available. The author recommends designating a specific area and team members for instrument cleaning and prep throughout the clinic. This ensures proper care and cleaning and that the instruments are ready when needed for surgery. Having designated team members for autoclave or pressure cooker use will also increase efficiency and decrease potential equipment misuse.

The method of instrument sterilization should be determined prior to the clinic, and adequate supplies to facilitate cleaning and care should be kept on hand. Readers can refer to Chapter 11 for additional information.

---

**Textbox 5.26 Recommended equipment for surgical equipment care**

- Water (distilled for autoclaves)
- Buckets or tubs
- Liquid dish washing detergent
- Toothbrushes or similar brush for cleaning instrument teeth and hinges
- Syringe to inflate cuff of ET tubes for cleaning
- Pipe cleaning brush to clean inside ET tubes (available at cigar and pipe smoking stores)
- Towels or rags to dry instruments
- Chemical disinfectant (if using for surgical instruments)
- Autoclave or pressure cooker (if using for surgical instruments)
- Autoclave tape +/− sterilization monitor strips such as OK strips placed inside a pack to indicate sterility after autoclaving.

---

### 5.8.15 Intensive Care Unit (ICU)

If space allows, a designated area for animals requiring intensive care is recommended. If space is limited, an area separate from high-activity areas can be created to increase isolation and minimize noise and activity. An experienced team member can be designated to oversee patient monitoring and treatment. Every patient in the ICU requires a treatment sheet to minimize miscommunications and allow for a rapid assessment of patient status.

### 5.8.16 Isolation

Many field clinics work in areas with a high prevalence of infectious disease due to a lack of preventive health services, husbandry, and proper nutrition. Animals may therefore present to the clinic with clinical signs consistent with diseases such as distemper and parvovirus. Staff must be trained to recognize clinical signs suggestive of a possible contagious disease and isolate sick animals to the best of their ability. In an ideal scenario, sick patients should be transferred off-site to a local clinic, if one is available.

Having an isolation area as far as possible from the other animals, especially if puppies and kittens are present, is strongly recommended. If separate rooms are unavailable, curtains and tarps can be hung to create temporary isolation areas. The number of people with access to the isolation area should be minimized, and specific team members dedicated to patient care. Appropriate gloves, gowns, or scrubs tops are needed for handling isolated animals, as well easy access to disinfectants.

---

**Textbox 5.27 Isolation supply list**

- Treatment care sheets
- Disinfectant and sprayer
- Exam gloves +/− gowns
- Towels, rags, newspapers
- Separate trash containers
- Kennels
- Thermometer and lube
- IV catheters
- Fluids
- Needles and syringes
- Antibiotics/antiemetics.

---

## 5.9 Conclusion

Field clinics are conducted in a variety of settings all over the world. Planning clinics in one's home community can be difficult; planning clinics in a remote part of the world is exponentially more difficult, requiring careful planning, discussion, patience, and more patience. Field clinics demand the ability to adapt to adverse conditions and unforeseen circumstances, while working with a patient caseload that can be challenging as well as heartbreaking. Careful planning allows veterinary professionals, team members, volunteers, and community members to provide humane care for patients and educate by example, thereby enhancing animal welfare and decreasing animal suffering around the world. This can occur even in communities where the clinic team does not even share a common language with local people.

It is recognized that a minimal standard of care will vary based on the logistics of the clinic. Lack of an adherence to a defined and acknowledged approach to humane patient care for each clinic can adversely affect the patient's outcome and community perception of the clinic, and undermine community trust. Adhering to high-quality practices and maximizing upon limited resources helps develop an important relationship with the community. This can have a long-lasting, positive impact on the provision of care to pets, free-roaming animals, trust in the veterinary profession, and also in the lives of the countless volunteers who devote their time and skills to selflessly deliver animal care.

## 5.10 Suggested Websites

International Veterinary Consultants: http://internationalveterinaryconsultants.org
ASPCA Spay/Neuter Alliance: www.aspca.org/humane-alliance
The Association of Shelter Veterinarians: http://www.sheltervet.org
The World Small Animal Veterinary Association: www.wsava.org
The Humane Society Veterinary Medical Association–Rural Area Veterinary Services Volunteer Training Manual: www.ruralareavet.org/
Sterile instrument pouches: www.sterilizerusa.com
Pole Syringe: www.animal-care.com/product/aces-pole-syringe/

# Appendix

## 5.A  Sample Clinic Timeline

### 5.A.1  Suggested Timeline for Arranging an International Spay/Neuter Clinic

**12 Months Pre-clinic**

☐ Investigate which national government officials/departments need to be contacted
☐ Perform a reconnaissance trip:
  ○ Identify potential logistical/travel issues
  ○ Meet with local people responsible for organizing the clinic
  ○ Assess community receptiveness for the clinic
  ○ Identify a local lead veterinarian
  ○ Meet with relevant government officials/departments, if possible

**8–12 Months Pre-clinic**

☐ Determine clinic dates
☐ Confirm a local lead veterinarian
☐ Create a supply manifest
☐ Determine what supplies will be imported versus acquired in-country
☐ Write clinic protocols
☐ Obtain invitation letters from local officials or sponsors of the clinic to facilitate permit acquisition and entry into the country

**6–8 Months Pre-clinic**

☐ Determine staffing requirements
☐ Establish if/what professional licensure is required and begin to address the requirements
☐ Start recruiting volunteers

**6 Months Pre-clinic**

☐ Begin permit acquisition to import equipment and medicines into the clinic country, if required[1]
☐ Begin permit acquisition to export controlled drugs, if required
☐ Plan travel to the country of the proposed clinic
☐ Determine transport of equipment and supplies to the country:
  ○ With volunteers
  ○ Commercial shipping
  ○ Local acquisition
☐ Delegate specific tasks to volunteers

**4 Months Pre-clinic**

☐ Meet with local officials to reconfirm clinic dates
☐ Determine the specific clinic location
☐ Confirm team members and support staff
☐ Begin to confirm volunteer travel arrangements to the country

---

1  This varies by country. Some countries will not accept permit applications or submissions more than 1 month in advance of the clinic. Others require months of communication to receive a response. Permit acquisition will be ongoing until permits are actually received. Be prepared for this to take months.

## 5.A    Sample Clinic Timeline (*Continued*)

**3 Months Pre-clinic**

☐ Secure team accommodation
☐ Meet with local government officials/departments who may be assisting with specific aspects of the clinic
  o Tourism
  o Health department
  o Education
☐ Begin collecting supplies locally

**2 Months Pre-clinic**

☐ Reconfirm clinic dates
☐ Reconfirm clinic location
☐ Begin planning on-site meals
☐ If the clinic will involve trapping, begin scouting locations for trapping and planning animal transport
☐ Purchase any supplies that will be imported and have them delivered to the respective team members who will be transporting supplies in their luggage[2]
☐ Begin cutting, folding, and sterilizing surgical drapes (if not buying prefolded and sterilized drapes)
☐ Begin sterilizing gauze packets

**1 Month Pre-clinic**

☐ Meet with team leaders and local participants to delegate specific tasks
☐ Define tasks and assign responsibilities
☐ Reconfirm participation of team members and volunteers
☐ Reconfirm on-site meals
☐ Reconfirm clinic location
☐ Confirm local acquisition of supplies such as tables, chairs, and lights
☐ Reconfirm team accommodation
☐ If a TNR clinic, confirm local assistance with animal transport and identifying trapping sites
☐ Plan transportation details
  o Airport pickup
  o Transportation required during the clinic
    ▪ Volunteers
    ▪ Animals
    ▪ Supplies
☐ Begin publicizing the clinic
  o Radio
  o Schools
  o Churches
  o Community meetings
  o Mobile loudspeaker
  o Social media
☐ Confirm access to and delivery of oxygen (if using for anesthesia)

---

2  This may be done as early as 6 months in advance if needed for permit acquisition. This will vary from country-to-country and trip-to-trip.

## 5.A   Sample Clinic Timeline (*Continued*)

**2 Weeks Pre-clinic**

- ☐ Have local supplies ready and accounted for
- ☐ Reconfirm all transportation details
- ☐ Perform a publicity blitz
- ☐ Conduct a volunteer meeting and training
  - ○ Determine the volunteer leader
  - ○ Discuss training and clinic details
  - ○ Assign tasks
  - ○ Assign positions and shifts
    - ▪ Transportation of team members to and from clinic
    - ▪ Check-in
    - ▪ Surgery prep
    - ▪ Surgical assistants
    - ▪ Recovery
    - ▪ Discharge
    - ▪ Instruments
    - ▪ Food/water
    - ▪ Animal handling
    - ▪ Animal transport
    - ▪ Kennel cleaning
- ☐ Arrange laundry facilities

**1 Week Pre-clinic**

- ☐ Confirm airport pick-ups
- ☐ Confirm on-site meals
- ☐ Reconfirm location and access (is a key needed? security guard?)
- ☐ Perform another publicity blitz
- ☐ Finalize the volunteer schedule
- ☐ Prepare adequate copies of all necessary forms
  - ○ Sign-in sheets
  - ○ Numbering system
  - ○ Medical records
  - ○ Discharge instructions
- ☐ If sterilizing surgical instrument packs locally, have packs wrapped and sterilized

**1 Day Pre-clinic**

- ☐ Team meeting
  - ○ Organizational discussion
  - ○ Identification of leaders
  - ○ Acknowledgement of protocols
- ☐ *Clinic set-up.* Clinic should be ready to admit the first patient, examine him, anesthetize him, recover him, and discharge him!

**CLINIC DAY**

## 5.B   Sample Clinic Supply Manifest

MANIFEST

Location of Clinic_____Date_____

| √ | Category | Item | Need | Have | Comments |
|---|----------|------|------|------|----------|
| | Anesthesia drugs, emergency drugs, and reversals | Acepromazine | | | |
| | | Atipamezole | | | |
| | | Atropine | | | |
| | | Buprenorphine | | | |
| | | Dexamethasone | | | |
| | | Dexmedetomidine | | | |
| | | Diazepam | | | |
| | | Diphenhydramine | | | |
| | | Epinephrine | | | |
| | | Isoflurane | | | |
| | | Ketamine | | | |
| | | Morphine | | | |
| | | Nalbuphine (or torbutrol) | | | |
| | | Naloxone | | | |
| | | PropoFlo 28 | | | |
| | | Sodium pentobarbital | | | |
| | | Sterile water for injection | | | |
| | | Tramadol injectable | | | |
| | | Telazol (Zolatil) | | | |
| | | Xylazine 100 mg/ml | | | |
| | | Xylazine 20 mg/ml | | | |
| | | Yohimbine | | | |
| | Anesthesia machine equipment and supplies | Anesthesia stand | | | |
| | | Isoflurane vaporizer | | | |
| | | Flow meter | | | |
| | | Absorber | | | |
| | | Adult breathing circuits | | | |
| | | Nonrebreathing system | | | |
| | | F air canisters | | | |
| | | Scavenger connectors | | | |
| | | Scavenger tubing | | | |
| | | Breathing bags 1 L | | | |
| | | Breathing bags 2 L | | | |

*(continued)*

## 5.B  Sample Clinic Supply Manifest (*Continued*)

| √ | Category | Item | Need | Have | Comments |
|---|----------|------|------|------|----------|
| | | Breathing bags 3 L | | | |
| | | Oxygen tank regulator E tank | | | |
| | | Oxygen tank regulator H tank | | | |
| | | Oxygen lines | | | |
| | | Soda lime | | | |
| | | Wrench small crescent | | | |
| | | Wrench large crescent | | | |
| | | Plumbers tape | | | |
| | | Extra tubing and connectors | | | |
| | Anesthesia equipment and supplies | Ambu bag | | | |
| | | Anesthesia mask large | | | |
| | | Anesthesia mask small | | | |
| | | Bandage scissors | | | |
| | | Blood pressure monitor | | | |
| | | Calculator | | | |
| | | Chlorhexidine solution | | | |
| | | Chlorhexidine scrub | | | |
| | | Clippers, electric (portable preferred) | | | |
| | | Clipper blade oil | | | |
| | | Clipper blade wash | | | |
| | | Cuff syringes | | | |
| | | Endotracheal tubes 3.0 | | | |
| | | Endotracheal tubes 3.5 | | | |
| | | Endotracheal tubes 4.0 | | | |
| | | Endotracheal tubes 4.5 | | | |
| | | Endotracheal tubes 5.0 | | | |
| | | Endotracheal tubes 5.5 | | | |
| | | Endotracheal tubes 6.0 | | | |
| | | Endotracheal tubes 6.5 | | | |
| | | Endotracheal tubes 7.0 | | | |
| | | Endotracheal tubes 7.5 | | | |
| | | Endotracheal tubes 8.0 | | | |
| | | Endotracheal tubes 8.5 | | | |
| | | Endotracheal tubes 9.0 | | | |
| | | Endotracheal tubes 9.5 | | | |
| | | Endotracheal tubes 10.0 | | | |

## 5.B  Sample Clinic Supply Manifest (*Continued*)

| √ | Category | Item | Need | Have | Comments |
|---|----------|------|------|------|----------|
| | | Endotracheal tube cleaning brushes | | | |
| | | Esophageal stethoscope 12 fr | | | |
| | | Esophageal stethoscope 18 fr | | | |
| | | Laryngoscope and blades | | | |
| | | Laryngoscope light bulbs, extra | | | |
| | | Non-sterile gauze | | | |
| | | Puralube eye ointment (or corn oil) | | | |
| | | Pulse oximeter | | | |
| | | Stethoscope | | | |
| | | Stylet | | | |
| | | Penlight or flashlight | | | |
| | | Prep table | | | |
| | | Tables for anesthesia supplies | | | |
| | | Thermometer | | | |
| | | Tube gauze | | | |
| | | Tupperware containers for prep solution and scrub | | | |
| | | Vacuum or lint brushes | | | |
| | Analgesics | Tramadol oral | | | |
| | | Carprofen, meloxicam, or ketoprofen injectable | | | |
| | | Carprofen or meloxicam oral (or other NSAID) | | | |
| | | Lidocaine | | | |
| | Surgery supplies | Sterile surgery blades, # 10 or #15 | | | |
| | | Sterile, single-use surgery gloves 6.0 | | | |
| | | Sterile, single-use surgery gloves 6.5 | | | |
| | | Sterile, single-use surgery gloves 7.0 | | | |
| | | Sterile, single-use surgery gloves 7.5 | | | |
| | | Sterile, single-use surgery gloves 8.0 | | | |
| | | Sterile, single-use surgery gloves 8.5 | | | |
| | | Suture material, monofilament absorbable 3-0, swaged on 3/8 circle cutting or reverse cutting needle | | | |
| | | Suture material, monofilament absorbable 2-0, swaged on 3/8 or 1/2 circle, cutting or reverse cutting needle | | | |
| | | Suture material, monofilament absorbable 0, swaged 1/2 circle cutting or reverse cutting needle | | | |
| | | Misc. size monofilament, absorbable suture material (4-0, 1) w/swaged on needle | | | |

(*continued*)

## 5.B   Sample Clinic Supply Manifest (*Continued*)

| √ | Category | Item | Need | Have | Comments |
|---|----------|------|------|------|----------|
| | | Suture material, cassette 3-0 monofilament | | | |
| | | Suture material, cassette 2-0 monofilament | | | |
| | | Suture material cassette 0 monofilament | | | |
| | | Cassette holder | | | |
| | | Suture material, cassette 1 monofilament | | | |
| | | Surgery needles, 3/8 circle cutting or reverse cutting, #12 | | | |
| | | Surgery needles, 3/8 circle cutting or reverse cutting, #16 | | | |
| | | Surgery needles 1/2 circle, cutting or reverse cutting, # 17 or 18 | | | |
| | | Surgical glue | | | |
| | | Sterile surgical drapes | | | |
| | | Instrument pack wraps | | | |
| | | Instrument stand and tray | | | |
| | | Surgery lights | | | |
| | | Surgery tables | | | |
| | | V trays small and large (thoracic positioner) | | | |
| | | Leg ties (slip leads work well) | | | |
| | | Sterile gauze | | | |
| | | Sterile lap pads | | | |
| | | Surgical caps | | | |
| | | Surgical masks | | | |
| | | Surgical gowns | | | |
| | | Tattoo ink or paste | | | |
| | | Clipper blades #40 | | | |
| | | Clipper blades #10 | | | |
| | | Straight razor | | | |
| | | Gel foam | | | |
| | | Scrub brushes for surgeon prep | | | |
| | | Avagard (waterless prep) | | | |
| | | Yoga mat (covered in plastic) for surgery table insulation | | | |
| | | Headlamps (participants to bring) | | | |
| | | Yunnan Baiyao | | | |
| | | Tables, for surgical supplies | | | |
| | Surgery instruments | Towel clamps | | | |
| | | Halsted Mosquito curved hemostats 5″ | | | |
| | | Halsted Mosquito straight hemostats, 5″ | | | |
| | | Kelly or Crile curved hemostats | | | |

## 5.B    Sample Clinic Supply Manifest (*Continued*)

| √ | Category | Item | Need | Have | Comments |
|---|----------|------|------|------|----------|
| | | Kelly or Crile straight hemostats | | | |
| | | Carmalts, curved 6.25″ | | | |
| | | Carmalts, straight 6.25″ | | | |
| | | Metzenbaum scissors, straight or curved | | | |
| | | Mayo or similar scissors | | | |
| | | Needle holders (Olsen Heger preferred) | | | |
| | | Thumb forceps, Brown Adson | | | |
| | | Thumb forceps, rat tooth | | | |
| | | Spay hook, 8″ | | | |
| | | Allis tissue forceps | | | |
| | | Army Navy retractors | | | |
| | | Extra sterile instruments | | | |
| | | Extra, large hemostats (Rochester Peen, etc.) | | | |
| | Syringes and needles | Syringes, 1 cc insulin with 25 or 27 gauge needles | | | |
| | | Syringes, 1 cc TB with 25 gauge needles | | | |
| | | Syringes 3 cc with 22 gauge needles | | | |
| | | Syringes 5 or 6 cc | | | |
| | | Syringes 10 or 12 cc | | | |
| | | Syringes 20 or 35 cc | | | |
| | | Syringes 60 cc | | | |
| | | Needles 18 gauge | | | |
| | | Needles 20 gauge | | | |
| | | Needles 22 gauge | | | |
| | | Needles 25 gauge | | | |
| | Intravenous supplies | IV catheters 18 gauge | | | |
| | | IV catheters 20 gauge | | | |
| | | IV catheters 22 gauge | | | |
| | | IV catheters 24 gauge | | | |
| | | T-ports | | | |
| | | Injection ports luer lock | | | |
| | | Tape, 1″ white | | | |
| | | IV drips sets mini drips (60 drops/ml) | | | |
| | | IV drips sets, maxi drips (10, 15 or 20 drops/ml) | | | |
| | | IV extensions | | | |

(*continued*)

## 5.B   Sample Clinic Supply Manifest (*Continued*)

| √ | Category | Item | Need | Have | Comments |
|---|---|---|---|---|---|
| | | Sterile saline 0.9% | | | |
| | | Heparin | | | |
| | | Lactated Ringers or similar fluid | | | |
| | | Hetastarch | | | |
| | | IV pole | | | |
| | | Bandage scissors | | | |
| | Antibiotics injectable/vitamins | Baytril 22.7 mg/ml | | | |
| | | Cefazolin 1 g | | | |
| | | Procaine Pen G 250 ml bottle | | | |
| | | Vitamin K1 injectable | | | |
| | Antibiotics oral and topical medications | Amoxicillin 500 mg | | | |
| | | Cephalexin 250 mg (or Cefpodoxime 100 mg) | | | |
| | | Cephalexin 500 mg | | | |
| | | Clavamox drops 62.5 mg/ml | | | |
| | | Clavamox 125 mg | | | |
| | | Doxycycline 100 mg (or minocycline 100 mg) | | | |
| | | Metronidazole 250 mg | | | |
| | | Triple antibiotic ophthalmic ointment (or similar eye ointment) | | | |
| | | Antibiotic plus hydrocortisone ophthalmic ointment | | | |
| | | Antibiotic ointment, topical | | | |
| | Vaccines | Rabies | | | |
| | | DHPP/DHLPP | | | |
| | | FVRCP | | | |
| | | Cooler and ice packs or small refrigerator | | | |
| | | Rabies certificates/tags | | | |
| | Dewormers | Pyrantel pamoate | | | |
| | | Ivermectin injectable 1% (for oral use) | | | |
| | | Fenbendazole | | | |
| | Instrument and endotracheal tube cleaning | Autoclave or pressure cooker | | | |
| | | Autoclave tape | | | |
| | | Distilled water (for autoclave only) | | | |
| | | Indicator strips (OK strips) | | | |

## 5.B  Sample Clinic Supply Manifest (*Continued*)

| √ | Category | Item | Need | Have | Comments |
|---|---------|------|------|------|----------|
| | | Detergent (liquid) or instrument enzyme cleaner | | | |
| | | Instrument milk | | | |
| | | Toothbrushes or similar brush to clean instruments | | | |
| | | Tubs for instrument washing and rinsing | | | |
| | | Spray bottle or Tupperware container for instrument milk | | | |
| | | Towels to dry instruments | | | |
| | | Instrument pack wraps | | | |
| | | Tupperware containers for chemical disinfectant (in place of autoclave) | | | |
| | | Benz-All or similar glutaraldehyde chemical disinfectant concentrate | | | |
| | | Syringe, non-sterile, to inflate cuffs on ET tubes for cleaning | | | |
| | | Pipe cleaners or similar brushes to clean inside endotracheal tubes | | | |
| | Office supplies/check-in | Table(s) | | | |
| | | Medical records | | | |
| | | Clip boards | | | |
| | | Clothes pins, carabiners, or other manner to attach record to kennel | | | |
| | | Weight scale | | | |
| | | Baby scale | | | |
| | | Leashes | | | |
| | | Muzzles | | | |
| | | Permanent markers | | | |
| | | Pens | | | |
| | | Dry erase markers | | | |
| | | Dry erase white board | | | |
| | | ID bands | | | |
| | | Masking tape | | | |
| | | Ziploc quart size | | | |
| | | Ziploc gallon | | | |
| | | Stapler | | | |
| | | Paper clips | | | |
| | | Restraint gloves | | | |
| | | Catch pole | | | |
| | | Disinfectant in spray bottle | | | |

(*continued*)

## 5.B Sample Clinic Supply Manifest (*Continued*)

| √ | Category | Item | Need | Have | Comments |
|---|----------|------|------|------|----------|
| | | Note pads or scrap paper | | | |
| | | Post-its | | | |
| | Recovery | Foam mats, straw mats, or similar insulating material for patients | | | |
| | | Carryalls (tackle box) for recovery items | | | |
| | | Stethoscope | | | |
| | | Thermometer | | | |
| | | Vaseline | | | |
| | | Bandage scissors | | | |
| | | Tape, 1″ white tape | | | |
| | | Vet wrap | | | |
| | | Microwave | | | |
| | | Rice, uncooked | | | |
| | | Socks for rice or recycled water bottles | | | |
| | | Heating pad | | | |
| | | Mylar space blankets | | | |
| | | Cotton balls | | | |
| | | Hydrogen peroxide | | | |
| | | Tick jar | | | |
| | | Tweezers | | | |
| | | Nail trimmer | | | |
| | | Cotton tip applicators | | | |
| | | Towels | | | |
| | | Blankets | | | |
| | | Newspaper | | | |
| | | Disinfectant spray bottle | | | |
| | | Paper towels | | | |
| | | Fans | | | |
| | | Ice packs | | | |
| | | Ace bandages | | | |
| | | Quik Stop (styptic powder) | | | |
| | | Hemostat for ear tipping cats | | | |
| | | Honey or Karo syrup | | | |
| | | Dog or puppy food dry (in sealed containers to minimize ants and other bugs) | | | |
| | | Cat of kitten food, dry (in sealed containers to minimize ants and other bugs) | | | |

## 5.B    Sample Clinic Supply Manifest (*Continued*)

| √ | Category | Item | Need | Have | Comments |
|---|---------|------|------|------|----------|
| | | Cat food, canned | | | |
| | | Dog food, canned | | | |
| | | Food bowls | | | |
| | | Water bowls | | | |
| | | Toilet paper | | | |
| | Miscellaneous | Alcohol | | | |
| | | Chairs | | | |
| | | Trash bags small | | | |
| | | Trash bags large | | | |
| | | Duct tape | | | |
| | | Extension cords | | | |
| | | Exam gloves, S, M, and L | | | |
| | | Power strips | | | |
| | | Voltage converter | | | |
| | | Tupperware containers small (for needles in anesthesia and recovery, etc.) | | | |
| | | Tupperware containers medium (syringes) | | | |
| | | Tupperware containers large (for cleaning and storage) | | | |
| | | Blue surgery towels (Huck towels) | | | |
| | | Bucket | | | |
| | | Mop | | | |
| | | Sharps containers | | | |
| | | Dish detergent | | | |
| | | Spray bottles | | | |
| | | Zip ties | | | |
| | | Kennels small | | | |
| | | Kennels medium | | | |
| | | Kennels large | | | |
| | | Net | | | |
| | | Cat litter | | | |
| | | Cooler | | | |
| | | Broom | | | |
| | | Dustpan | | | |
| | | Bleach | | | |
| | | Scrub brushes for cleaning kennels | | | |
| | | Batteries AAA | | | |

(*continued*)

## 5.B Sample Clinic Supply Manifest (*Continued*)

| √ | Category | Item | Need | Have | Comments |
|---|---|---|---|---|---|
| | | Batteries AA | | | |
| | | Batteries C | | | |
| | | Clock | | | |
| | | Suture removal scissors | | | |
| | | Flashlight, battery or rechargeable | | | |
| | | Hand sanitizer | | | |
| | | Laundry basket | | | |
| | | Laundry detergent | | | |
| | | First aid kit | | | |
| | | Paper towels | | | |
| | | Prescription labels | | | |
| | | Veterinary formulary | | | |
| | | Chairs | | | |
| | | Tables | | | |
| | | Sterile lube | | | |
| | | Cling 3″ | | | |
| | | Cast padding | | | |
| | | Telfa nonadhering bandages | | | |
| | | Vet wrap, 2″, 3″, or 4″ or Elastikon | | | |
| | | ICU sheets | | | |
| | | Basic care treatment sheets | | | |
| | Optional | Stretcher | | | |
| | | Cat traps | | | |
| | | Dog traps | | | |
| | | E Collars | | | |
| | | Cat carriers, cardboard | | | |
| | | Hemo-Nate blood filters | | | |

## 5.C  Patient Medical Record (Pages 1 and 2)

**ANIMAL BALANCE** SOLUTIONS WITHOUT SUFFERING

| Clinic Location: | Date: | MASH # | Patient Weight *(lbs)*: |
|---|---|---|---|

**①** **Patient Information** | **Presurgical Examination**

| Patient Information | Presurgical Examination | WNL | Abnormal |
|---|---|---|---|
| Name: _____ Dog  Cat | General Appearance | | |
| Breed/Looks Like: _____ . Sex:_____ | Mucous Membranes | | |
| Coat Color: _____ Age: | Hydration | | |

**②** **Caretaker Information**

| Caretaker Information | | | |
|---|---|---|---|
| Name: _____ | Cardiovascular | | |
| Phone Number: _____ | Urogenital | | |
| Address: | Other | | |
| | **Cage-Side Exam Performed:** *(Fractious Patient)* | | |

**③** **Colony Information**

| Colony Information | **Additional Notes:** |
|---|---|
| Colony Location: | |
| 1 of _____ cats | |

**④** **Patient Medical History**

| Patient Medical History | Yes | No |
|---|---|---|
| Eating/Drinking Normally in past 48 hours? | | |
| On any medications? (including mange, flea and tick treatment in last 30 days) If yes, please describe: | | |

I confirm that I have examined this patient and it appears healthy enough for spay/neuter surgery.

| Current Medical Conditions including coughing, sneezing, vomiting, diarrhea? If yes, please describe: | Vomiting | | |
|---|---|---|---|
| | Diarrhea | | |
| | Coughing | | |
| | Sneezing | | |
| Has patient ever had a vaccine reaction? | | | |
| Has patient recently had a litter? *If yes, how long ago?* | | | |
| Does the patient spend most of their time indoors or outdoors? | | | |

**Patient Prep**

| Patient Prep | mL | Time |
|---|---|---|
| TTDex: | | |
| Meloxicam: | | |
| TVT:    None    1    2    3    4    5 | | |
| Circle One: | Flank | Midline |
| Isoflurane: | Yes | No |
| Ear Tip: | Yes | No |
| Notes: | | |
| Technician's Initials: | | |

**Treatments and Services**

| Treatments and Services | Yes | No |
|---|---|---|
| Ear Tip | | |
| FVRCP / DHLPP Vaccine | | |
| Microchip | | |
| Parasite Treatment | | |

**⑤** **Surgical Release**

**Patient Release * (required)**

I hereby give permission to Animal Balance (AB) to sterilize my pet. If my pet has medical problems, I understand that Animal Balance will treat with medications that are available in the clinic. I understand there are risks with the procedure and a very small percentage of patients die. I agree to hold harmless AB, its officers, managers, veterinarians, technicians, volunteers and agents for any of my pet's problems arising as a result of surgery. I will provide treatment and care at home for my pet as directed. Furthermore, I give permission to Animal Balane to sterilize my pet and permanently identify him/her as sterilized via a tip or tattoo. I also agree to return for this pet and will not abandon the pet at the Animal Balance clinic.

**Caretaker Signature**

Signature:_____    Date:_____

## 5.C Patient Medical Record (Pages 1 and 2) (*Continued*)

| Date: | MASH # | Patient Weight *(lb*s): |
|---|---|---|

### Surgery

| Procedures Performed (*Check All that Apply*) | | | | Additional Notes | | |
|---|---|---|---|---|---|---|
| Castration | | Ovariohysterectomy | | | | |
| Zeuter | | Ovariectomy | | | | |
| Cryptorchid: | | Pregnant:  Early<br>Middle  Late | | | | |
| Inguinal | L / R | Postpartum | | | | |
| Abdominal | L / R | Pyometra / Hydrometra | | | | |
| | | Estrus | | Tattoo: | | |
| Surgeon: | | | | Time: | | |

### Recovery

| Time In Recovery : | | Recovery Technician Initials: | | |
|---|---|---|---|---|

| Vaccines and Treatments | | | Fluids | | | |
|---|---|---|---|---|---|---|
| FVRCP<br>DHPP | | | Saline | SQ / IV | mL: | |
| Flea<br>Treatment | | | LRS | SQ / IV | mL: | |
| Ivermectin | | mL: | Reversal : | Yes / No | mL: | Time: |
| Pyrantel | | mL: | Notes | | | |
| Microchip | | ID # | | | | |
| Toe Nail<br>Trim: | | Matts: Y / N | | | | |

### Patient Discharge

| Take Home Medication? | | Additional Post-Operative Instructions | |
|---|---|---|---|
| Staying Overnight? | Yes / No | | |
| Post-Op Instructions<br>Given to Caretaker? | Yes / No | | |
| Veterinarian's Signature for Release: | | | Time: |

Source: Courtesy of Meredith Hippert & Emma Clifford, Animal Balance.

## 5.D   Controlled Drug Log Template

UNOPENED CONTROLLED DRUG LOG

Name of medication_____ Strength_____

| DATE | LOT NUMBER | BOTTLE NUMBER | EXPIRATION DATE | QUANTITY | DATE RECEIVED | DATE DISPENSED TO USE | LOCATION DISPENED FOR USE | INITIALS |
|------|-----------|---------------|-----------------|----------|---------------|------------------------|---------------------------|----------|
|      |           |               |                 |          |               |                        |                           |          |
|      |           |               |                 |          |               |                        |                           |          |
|      |           |               |                 |          |               |                        |                           |          |
|      |           |               |                 |          |               |                        |                           |          |
|      |           |               |                 |          |               |                        |                           |          |
|      |           |               |                 |          |               |                        |                           |          |
|      |           |               |                 |          |               |                        |                           |          |
|      |           |               |                 |          |               |                        |                           |          |
|      |           |               |                 |          |               |                        |                           |          |
|      |           |               |                 |          |               |                        |                           |          |
|      |           |               |                 |          |               |                        |                           |          |
|      |           |               |                 |          |               |                        |                           |          |
|      |           |               |                 |          |               |                        |                           |          |
|      |           |               |                 |          |               |                        |                           |          |
|      |           |               |                 |          |               |                        |                           |          |
|      |           |               |                 |          |               |                        |                           |          |
|      |           |               |                 |          |               |                        |                           |          |
|      |           |               |                 |          |               |                        |                           |          |
|      |           |               |                 |          |               |                        |                           |          |
|      |           |               |                 |          |               |                        |                           |          |
|      |           |               |                 |          |               |                        |                           |          |
|      |           |               |                 |          |               |                        |                           |          |
|      |           |               |                 |          |               |                        |                           |          |
|      |           |               |                 |          |               |                        |                           |          |
|      |           |               |                 |          |               |                        |                           |          |
|      |           |               |                 |          |               |                        |                           |          |
|      |           |               |                 |          |               |                        |                           |          |
|      |           |               |                 |          |               |                        |                           |          |
|      |           |               |                 |          |               |                        |                           |          |
|      |           |               |                 |          |               |                        |                           |          |
|      |           |               |                 |          |               |                        |                           |          |
|      |           |               |                 |          |               |                        |                           |          |
|      |           |               |                 |          |               |                        |                           |          |
|      |           |               |                 |          |               |                        |                           |          |
|      |           |               |                 |          |               |                        |                           |          |
|      |           |               |                 |          |               |                        |                           |          |
|      |           |               |                 |          |               |                        |                           |          |
|      |           |               |                 |          |               |                        |                           |          |
|      |           |               |                 |          |               |                        |                           |          |
|      |           |               |                 |          |               |                        |                           |          |
|      |           |               |                 |          |               |                        |                           |          |
|      |           |               |                 |          |               |                        |                           |          |
|      |           |               |                 |          |               |                        |                           |          |
|      |           |               |                 |          |               |                        |                           |          |
|      |           |               |                 |          |               |                        |                           |          |

## 5.E   Postoperative Instructions for Clients

## POST-OPERATIVE INSTRUCTIONS

PATIENT NAME: _____

PROCEDURE: _____          DATE OF SURGERY: _____

**FOOD AND WATER**: Offer approximately one-half of the animal's normal amount of food this afternoon or evening.   Your pet can drink water in small amounts every 2 -3 hours until bedtime. Do not allow them to eat or drink excessive amounts at one time as they may vomit. Offer water and their normal amount of food tomorrow morning.

**ELIMINATIONS:** It is possible your pet may not urinate or defecate for the 12 hours following the surgery. This can be normal as they have not had much to eat or drink.

**INCISION:** The incision was closed with absorbable sutures underneath the skin. You do not need to return for suture removal. They will dissolve in the next few months.  Male cats do not have any sutures. A small amount of ink may have been placed in or near the incision to indicate your pet has been sterilized. Do not place any topical medications on the incision. Monitor the incision twice daily. There should be no swelling, opening or drainage.

**MONITOR**: If your pet has any of the following symptoms or problems, please contact the number below.
- No eating or drinking for more than 24 hours
- Lethargy or depression
- Problems with the incision, (inflamed, swollen, discharge, open)
- Vomiting
- Appears painful
- Difficulty breathing
- Any other questions

**ACTIVITY AND BATHING RESTRICTIONS:**  Upon return to your home, keep the animal in a quiet, warm and dry place so he or she may fully recover from anesthesia and surgery. Minimize animal activity for the next 7-10 days in order to minimize post-operative complications. Dogs should only be leash walked, if possible. Do not bathe your pet for 7-10 days.

**MEDICATIONS:**  Your pet received injections for pain before and after the procedure.  Please call us if you see signs of pain.

**SPECIAL INSTRUCTIONS:**

_____
_____
_____
_____

If you have any questions or problems, please call or text _____

Thank you for letting us take care of your pet.


Sincerely,

# References

1 Griffin, B., Bushby, P.A., McCobb, E. et al. (2016). The Association of Shelter Veterinarians' 2016 veterinary medical care guidelines for spay-neuter programs. *Journal of the American Veterinary Medical Association* **249**(2): 165–188.

2 Treparie, L.A. (2013). Rational Use of Presurgical Antibiotics. Auckland, New Zealand: World Small Animal Veterinary Association World Congress http://www.vin.com/apputil/content/defaultadv1.aspx?pId=11372&meta=Generic&id=5709855&print=1(accessed 10 September 2016).

# 6

# General Anesthesia and Analgesia

*Carolyn McKune[1] and Sheilah Robertson[2]*

[1]*Affiliated Veterinary Specialists, Orange Park Specialty Center, Orange Park, FL 32073, USA*
[2]*Lap of Love Hospice, 17804 N US Highway 41, Lutz, FL 33549, USA*

## 6.1 Introduction: Developed versus Developing Countries

> *"The future of pain management and anesthesia in my country . . . is beautiful."*
> – Emmanuella A. O Sogebi,
> Nigerian Veterinarian

The first task of this chapter is to dispel any assumptions that people might make about the state of veterinary medicine in a location where they have not practiced. This is especially important if an individual comes from a developed country and will participate in remote area medicine in a developing country. Many false assumptions may be made, which collectively create unrealistic expectations about resources that will be at their disposal. These assumptions may include the following:

1) Structure and organized veterinary medicine is the typical model in an underdeveloped country.
2) Widespread awareness of animal welfare in some basic form exists.
3) Because animal welfare is considered, veterinary medicine is a respected profession.
4) There is trust by authority figures in their countries' veterinarians, allowing them to extend certain privileges (i.e. use of controlled substances).
5) A drug licensed for use implies *availability* of the drug to veterinary professionals.
6) Veterinarians in that country understand that balanced anesthesia is necessary for a surgical procedure.

7) Veterinarians in that country view pain management as part of the perioperative plan.

In fact, many, if not all, of these assumptions are the exception but not the norm in some developing nations struggling with organization at a local and national level. The ability to obtain controlled drugs is in the hands of those with power and authority (e.g. government officials and police officers), and colleagues from other countries often require express permission in native languages to bring in necessary uncontrolled substances (i.e. tranquilizers). Often the question is not "what drugs are licensed for use in this country?" but rather "to what extent can I provide a service?" and "what do I currently have in my possession that might aid this animal?" Although the author will list drugs that are currently available in some (not all) countries, it is important to remember it may mean relatively few choices in some environments. *The most invaluable tool for someone who practices remote area veterinary anesthesia is a local contact who can provide most of what is necessary.*

Based on these challenges, the Association of Shelter Veterinarians (ASV) charged a task force with creating guidelines for spay/neuter programs. The initial guidelines, published in 2008, were recently updated in 2016 [1] and are available for free download online (http://avmajournals.avma.org/doi/pdf/10.2460/javma.249.2.165) and (www.sheltervet.org). The intent of these guidelines is to provide principles applicable and achievable for any veterinary group providing sterilization services. The authors refer to these recommendations throughout this chapter, but encourage the reader to review these guidelines for themselves.

The World Small Animal Veterinary Association (WSAVA) charged their Global Pain Council with developing guidelines for recognition, assessment, and treatment of pain (http://www.wsava.org/sites/default/files/jsap_0.pdf). Detailed protocols for commonly performed surgeries are provided for use in countries with controlled drug availability, without controlled drug availability and in scenarios with limited availability of analgesic drugs.

## 6.2 Preparation for Field Anesthesia

Performing anesthesia requires good planning and preparation. The correct equipment, drugs, and knowledge must be available for the job. When developing a plan for anesthesia, the authors find it helpful to consider the concerns related to the patient, anesthesia, and the procedure itself.

---

**Textbox 6.1 Important questions to formulate an anesthetic plan**

*Patient Specific Concerns the Following Information*

- What is the patient's age?
- What is the patient's breed?
- What is the patient's presenting complaint and the duration of that complaint?
- What, if any, diagnostic information is present?
- What does physical exam reveal?
- What other comorbidities are present?
- Has the patient been fasted?

*Anesthesia Concerns the Following*

- Hypotension
- Hypoventilation
- Hypothermia

*Procedural Concerns the Following*

- What procedure(s) will be performed?
- How invasive is the procedure?
- Is significant hemorrhage possible?

---

For example, an adult dog with an unknown history but unremarkable physical exam, presenting for an ovariohysterectomy would have a problem or "concern" list that includes

- Unknown comorbidities
- Estimated age
- Hypotension
- Hypoventilation
- Hypothermia
- Noxious stimuli/pain from the procedure
- Potential hemorrhage.

The problem list includes factors we would ideally monitor for and manage. The following supplies allow the veterinarian to achieve a good outcome:

- Mask and portable oxygen
- Endotracheal tubes or supraglottic airway devices
- Blood pressure monitors
- Capnograph or apnea alarm (see Figure 6.3)
- Thermometer
- Catheters and fluids.

With the presence of two "unknowns" (concurrent disease and age), the veterinarian prepares for unexpected complications, such as those resulting from subclinical respiratory disease or profound effects from a "traditional" dose of anesthetic drugs if the dog is geriatric. One of the most important attributes of an anesthetist/veterinarian in the field is to know *your* limitations. Having the foresight to suggest a potential patient is *not* a suitable candidate allows the veterinarian to one of two things: do no harm or have a crucial conversation with the "owner" and staff, confirming that we are electing to proceed despite some risks, including death. It is demoralizing

---

**Textbox 6.2 Characteristics of a patient and procedure suitable for a field procedure**

A patient that can be restrained (i.e. does not possess an imminent threat of harm to the staff).
ASA Category 1 or 2.
Age > 4 months to nongeriatric adults.
Elective procedure.
No outward abnormalities on physical exam that would interfere with the surgery.
Patient fasted for minimum of 4 h.
Risk of hemorrhage is low.
Predicted pain level is considered low to moderate.
Duration of procedure is 60 min or less.

to the team and to the community to have an animal die under anesthesia. While the veterinarian may understand that is always a risk, assuming that the rest of the community and the staff understand this may result in loss of trust. Some limitations may be cultural in nature, for example, in predominantly Buddhist communities, euthanasia is not an option. Therefore, the patient may experience significant suffering if an attempt is not made to operate, even if surgical intervention risks the demise of the patient. See Section 6.2.1.

Relying on memory alone has resulted in avoidable morbidity and mortality in numerous medical settings, and the use of a checklist reduces human error. A checklist is a living document; that is, when initially created, it is not possible to know everything which will become important. It is a document that starts with core building blocks and then evolves as the team works together and debriefs following an adverse event. The World Health Organization (WHO)'s website provides an example of a well-studied, basic checklist: www.who.int/patientsafety/safesurgery/tools_resources/SSSL_Checklist_final Jun08.pdf?ua=1.

The checklist should be short, ideally limited to a single page. Brevity ensures the checklist is not intentionally skipped over due to time constraints. There is also a difference between a standard operating procedure (SOP) and a presurgical checklist. An SOP is intentionally comprehensive to ensure a novice or new employee has all the details to familiarize themselves with the correct execution of a procedure. A checklist assumes the user is already familiar with a procedure and, therefore, covers only the critical points that are often overlooked. It is advisable to create both; however, only the checklist is performed before every procedure. A group can begin with the WHO checklist and then remove things that are not applicable for their situation and add applicable things (e.g. a section for cats) (Figure 6.1).

## 6.2.1 Patient and Procedure Selection

Anesthesia has been described as "careful controlled and reversible poisoning," and this is not a wholly untruthful description. There are very few drugs available that do not have profound physiologic consequences; however, because the use of anesthetics is "routine," veterinarians often underestimate the risks.

Underlying a safe anesthetic event, however, is the critical defining point: a safe anesthetist. The first job of the anesthetist, therefore, is to select the appropriate patient for a field setting. Body size may or may not be a limiting factor, based on available equipment. Age is controversial. It is the recommendation of the ASV that animals are 4 months or older; however, neutering at a younger age can be acceptable if the animal is otherwise healthy. When working with free-roaming animals, recapturing an animal when it has reached the ideal age is often impossible; practitioners thus often elect to perform the procedure on animals as young as 8 weeks of age if they are of good health and BCS, as it may be the only opportunity to sterilize these animals. Another consideration is that neutering an animal prior to adoption may improve the chances of a successful placement. Early neutering has the benefit of preventing unintended litters and pyometra, as well as reducing the risk of mammary neoplasia. A few studies have suggested that some orthopedic and neoplastic conditions are increased in certain breeds if they are neutered at a young age, but the advantages of early neutering outweigh this risk when managing free-roaming dogs and homeless pets [2].

Ideally, adult patients have food withheld for approximately 4 h prior to surgery, while younger ones may receive a soft food meal within 2 h of the procedure. Water is not withheld. Exceptions for feral patients, where a feeding history is not available, may be necessary.

The American Society of Anesthesiologists (ASA) scoring system helps to create a rubric for patient classification purposes [3] (Table 6.1). A full physical examination is performed when possible. In feral animals, the best guess as to ASA status (and usually weight) is made. Patients appropriate for field procedures will fall into an ASA 1–2 category. Occasionally, a field veterinarian will be asked to perform a procedure for an ASA 3–5 patient. In the words of Steve Haskins, an outstanding anesthesiologist-turned criticalist, "If death is the alternative, *anything* is a good option." The author wishes to modify that statement to "If death is the alternative, *anything* is a good option . . . after a crucial conversation with the caregiver and the team that death may very well be the outcome." In some cases, for example, subclinical infectious diseases or pre-existing medical conditions that increase anesthetic risk, this trade-off may be acceptable.

**AVS**
AFFILIATED
VETERINARY
SPECIALISTS
Centers for **Advanced** Medical Care

**Anesthetic Checklist**

Age: _____ Weight: **0.0** kg **0.0** lb
Species: **Canine** Sex: **Select**

**Prior to induction**

- [ ] Has the owner been called?
- [ ] Bloodwork approved by a doctor
- [ ] Confirm patient information
  - [ ] Identity
  - [ ] Age
  - [ ] Surgical site
  - [ ] Procedure
  - [ ] Consent
  - [ ] CPR status
  - [ ] 1 ASA status
- [ ] Is hemorrhage possible (>60mL/kg for cats and >90mL/kg for dogs)?
  - [ ] Crossmatch (MANDATORY if feline) or Universal Donor?
  - [ ] Blood available?
  - [ ] Second IV catheter placed?
- [ ] Anesthetic equipment check
  - [ ] Propofol less than 3mL drawn in 1mL syringes?
  - [ ] Appropriate breathing system and bag?
  - ***Feline only***
- [ ] Lidocaine for airway?
- [ ] Clear endotracheal tube cut to size?
- [ ] Cuff minimally inflated?
- [ ] Fluid rate set to 2-3 mL/kg/hr?

**Anesthesia Notes**

0

**After induction and before clipping:**

- [ ] To what measurement is the endotracheal tube placed?
- [ ] Surgeon confirms surgical site
- [ ] Bladder expressed?
- [ ] Epidural successful?

**Prior to incision**

- [ ] Surgeon confirms:
  - [ ] Patient
  - [ ] Procedure
  - [ ] Introduce all team members and their role
- [ ] Are there any critical or non routine steps:
  - [ ] Anesthesia? _____ If yes, what?
  - [ ] Surgery? _____ If yes, what?
- [ ] Duration of surgery?
- [ ] Anticipated blood loss?
- [ ] Any current patient specific concerns? _____ If yes, what?
- [ ] Has sterility been maintained?
- [ ] Sponge count complete? _____ Count?
- [ ] Equipment issues/concerns? _____ If yes, what?
- [ ] Have antibiotics been given in the last 60 minutes? _____ Time:
- [ ] Essential imaging displayed?

**Prior to leaving the operating room**

- [ ] Name of the procedure?
- [ ] Sponge and needle count complete?
- [ ] Specimen(s) labeled?
- [ ] Equipment problems to be addressed? _____ If yes, what?
- [ ] Key concerns for recovery _____ If yes, what?
- [ ] Bladder expressed (if epidural was successful)?
- [ ] Radiographs to be taken?

**Figure 6.1** Sample anesthetic checklist.

Procedural selection is equally important for a successful outcome in a field setting. In addition to the general characteristics listed, soft tissue procedures make up the vast majority of surgeries performed. Many orthopedic procedures require an implant, which could serve as a source of infection if sterility is compromised. It is important to perform a daily evaluation of the program's schedule, to avoid overtaxing the team. Examples of ideal field procedures include minor mass removal, sterilization, and

**Table 6.1** ASA scoring schematic with examples.

| ASA score | Definition | Example |
|-----------|------------|---------|
| 1 | A normal healthy patient | A healthy dog for an ovariohysterectomy |
| 2 | A patient with mild-to-moderate disease | A brachycephalic cat for an ovariohysterectomy |
| 3 | A patient with severe systemic disease | A cat with hypertrophic cardiomyopathy for mass removal |
| 4 | A patient with severe systemic disease that is a constant threat to life | A dog with a splenic tumor |
| 5 | A moribund patient who is unlikely to survive without an intervention | An animal with septic shock from GI perforation |

enucleation. The experience of the primary surgeon will dictate expansion of this list; for example, an experienced surgeon may choose to perform more extensive soft tissue procedures such as an amputation (limb, tail), whereas a less experienced one may not.

## 6.2.2 Components of General Anesthesia

General anesthesia for a procedure requires provision of what were once four but now five essential components [4]. These five components are unconsciousness, amnesia, muscle relaxation, lack of purposeful movement in response to surgical stimulation, and analgesia. Amnesia is difficult to assess in animals, so we rely on information from humans and assume it applies to our patients. The inclusion of a benzodiazepine, such as midazolam, provides amnesia [5]. Analgesia is a property of certain drugs (traditionally opioids, $\alpha_2$-adrenergic agonists, ketamine, local anesthetics, and nonsteroidal anti-inflammatory drugs (NSAIDs)). Volatile inhalant anesthetics are thought to provide the necessary elements of unconsciousness, muscle relaxation, and lack of purposeful moment in response to surgical stimulation, although they do not produce amnesia [6] or analgesia (the exception being methoxyflurane) [7]. However, it is possible to provide these three components of general anesthesia without inhalant anesthetics by using appropriate injectable techniques. Table 6.2 lists injectable agents with these properties. The reason why an $\alpha_2$-adrenergic agonist

**Table 6.2** Drugs and their families providing characteristics of general anesthesia.

| Characteristic | Drug families | Example |
|----------------|---------------|---------|
| Unconsciousness [8] | Barbiturates, nonbarbiturate anesthetics, NDMA antagonists | Thiopental, etomidate, alfaxalone, propofol, ketamine, tiletamine and zolazepam, inhaled anesthetic agents |
| Amnesia [9] | Benzodiazepines, nonbarbiturate anesthetics (dose dependent), NMDA antagonists (dose dependent) | Midazolam, diazepam, zolazepam, propofol, ketamine |
| Muscle relaxation | $\alpha_2$-Adrenergic agonists, barbiturates, benzodiazepines, nonbarbiturate agonists, opioids | Dexmedetomidine, thiopental, midazolam, diazepam, etomidate, alfaxalone, propofol, zolazepam, butorphanol, hydromorphone, morphine, buprenorphine, nalbuphine, inhaled anesthetic agents |
| Lack of spontaneous movement in response to supramaximal noxious stimuli | Barbiturates, nonbarbiturate anesthetics | Thiopental, propofol, alfaxalone, etomidate |
| Analgesia | $\alpha_2$-agonists, NMDA antagonists, opioids | Dexmedetomidine, xylazine, ketamine, butorphanol, hydromorphone, morphine, buprenorphine, nalbuphine |

in conjunction with an NMDA antagonist (i.e. dexmedetomidine and ketamine) is so popular in the field is because this combination provides many of the important aspects of anesthesia. Currently, in many countries, ketamine is not scheduled and therefore does not require a special license for purchase or use. However, access to this essential drug has come under threat. In March of 2016, the United Nations Commission on Narcotic Drugs (CND) evaluated a petition to place ketamine under international scheduling. The CND agreed with The WHO's Expert Committee on Drug Dependence, which unequivocally recommends that ketamine *not* be placed under international control. Unfortunately, at least one country has vowed to continue to press for control at future conventions and meetings. While an ethical discussion on the importance of ketamine is beyond the scope of this chapter and perhaps this book, it is the strong recommendation of the authors that ketamine is an essential medicine in developing countries, without which countless animals, women, men, and children would suffer. Any reader with further interest in this subject is encouraged to visit the website of the WSAVA to learn the facts and how to help (http://www.wsava.org/educational/ketamine-campaign).

Routes of administration for maintenance will vary. Inhalational anesthesia in a field setting is traditionally limited by the requirements of specialized delivery devices and scavenging of waste anesthetic gases (WAG). While most field programs tend to rely on injectable-only anesthetic protocols, some have successfully incorporated the routine use of portable anesthesia machines. While such machines require

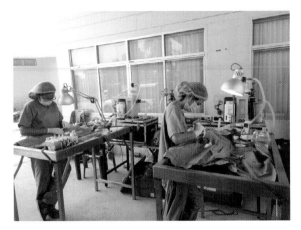

**Figure 6.2** Portable anesthetic machines in use during a field spay/neuter clinic. Note also the use of a pulse oximeter and apnea alert monitor for anesthetic monitoring. Source: Courtesy of Katherine Polak, Soi Dog Foundation.

an initial investment of up to 1500 USD, if well maintained they can be a long-lasting and valuable addition to mobile spay/neuter operations (Figure 6.2).

Many field procedures are performed with total intramuscular anesthesia (TIMA), with "top-up" doses given if needed to complete the procedure. Ideally, an intravenous catheter would be placed to allow for the administration of emergency drugs and for additional anesthetic drugs, either as a single bolus or as a constant rate infusion. Constant rate infusions (CRIs) are easier to set up than most people think (Textbox 6.3). While this example deals with a combination of analgesic drugs, it is also suitable to use CRIs for maintenance of anesthesia; see anesthesia maintenance below.

---

**Textbox 6.3  Preparing a constant rate infusion (CRI)**

For purposes of this example, the end goal is the creation of a hydromorphone, lidocaine, and ketamine mixture (HLK).

$ml = milliliter, \ kg = kilogram, \ mg = milligram, \ h = hour$

- Step 1. Select a convenient total volume in milliliters. This is often the volume of a bag of fluids, in the field (as syringe pumps are unlikely available).
  For this example, we will select a one-liter (L) bag.
  Total volume: 1000 ml LRS
- Step 2. Select a dosage in mg/kg/h.
  For this example, we'll use hydromorphone at 0.03 mg/kg/h, lidocaine at 2 mg/kg/h, and ketamine at 1.0 mg/kg/h intraoperatively.
  *Doses are based on current peer reviewed literature.*

- Step 3. Select a rate in ml/kg/h. Rate is selected based on user preference; for example, one could use fluid rate of 5 ml/kg/h for a dog.
- Step 4. Separate calculations are performed for each drug used using the following formula:
  Equation 6.1 – Calculating how many mgs of any drug to add for a constant rate infusion

$$\frac{\text{Dose (mg/kg/h)}}{\text{Rate (ml/kg/h)}} \times \text{Total volume(ml)} = \text{mg of drug to add}$$

The answers to the calculations are in milligrams; in the case of the above example, we would get the following results:
Equation 6.2 – Calculating how many mgs of hydromorphone, lidocaine, and ketamine to add for a constant rate infusion

$$\text{Hydromorphone}: \frac{0.03 \text{ mg/kg/h}}{5 \text{ ml/kg/h}} \times 1000 \text{ ml} = 6 \text{ mg of drug to add}$$

$$\text{Lidocaine}: \frac{2 \text{ mg/kg/h}}{5 \text{ ml/kg/h}} \times 1000 \text{ ml} = 400 \text{ mg of drug to add}$$

$$\text{Ketamine}: \frac{1 \text{ mg/kg/h}}{5 \text{ ml/kg/h}} \times 1000 \text{ ml} = 200 \text{ mg of drug to add}$$

The anesthetist divides by the concentration of the drugs used to determine the volume of each drug added to the bag of fluids.
Equation 6.3 – Calculating how many mls of hydromorphone, lidocaine, and ketamine to add for a constant rate infusion

$$\text{Hydromorphone}: 6 \text{ mg} \times \frac{\text{ml}}{2 \text{ mg}} = 3 \text{ ml}$$

$$\text{Lidocaine}: 400 \text{ mg} \times \frac{\text{ml}}{20 \text{ mg}} = 20 \text{ ml}$$

$$\text{Ketamine}: 200 \text{ mg} \times \frac{\text{ml}}{100 \text{ mg}} = 2 \text{ ml}$$

- Step 5. Creating: The total volume of the drugs to be added is removed from the bag of LRS first, and then the drugs are added.
- Loading doses of these drugs are administered. For this example, hydromorphone's loading dose is usually 0.1 mg/kg, lidocaine is 1.0 mg/kg, and ketamine is 0.5 mg/kg.
- Fluid drip rate calculations are used to determine drop/s for administration.

### 6.2.3 Risks of Anesthesia

There are various studies documenting the risk of sedation and general anesthesia. The largest studies done in veterinary medicine to date is work by Dave Brodbelt and colleagues [10] looking at just over 98 000 dogs and approximately 78 000 cats, and several other small companion animals. This data was collected from general practitioners, referral centers, and university hospitals in the United Kingdom. The study found that the risk of mortality under anesthesia was 0.17% in dogs overall and when stratified for ASA 1–2 dogs, about 0.05%. This translates into about 1 in 2000 dogs (classified as healthy) having an anesthetic-related mortality. While this number may outwardly appear satisfactory, risk in human medicine is as low as 0.82 in 100 000 [11]. In cats, sedation- and general anesthetic-related mortality overall is 0.24%, and 0.11% when only including

**Table 6.3** Normal basic vital parameters for the canine and feline patient.

| Species | HR (beats/min) | RR (breath/min) | Temp (F) | Temp (C) | CRT (s) | MMC |
|---------|----------------|-----------------|-----------|-----------|---------|-----|
| Canine | 80–160 | 16–40 | 99.5–102.0 | 37.5–38.9 | <2 | Pink or pigmented |
| Feline | 140–220 | 40–60 | 99.5–102.5 | 37.5–39.2 | <2 | Pink |

ASA 1–2 felines, which translates into 1 in 900 "healthy" cats dying due to anesthesia.

A review of over 7500 cats sterilized at a single feral cat clinic using TIMA reported an overall anesthetic mortality rate of 0.23% [12]. The outcome of two different total intravenous anesthesia (TIVA) techniques (ketamine/diazepam or propofol) following premedication with xylazine and butorphanol in free-ranging dogs have been reported. There were 50 dogs in each group; they were not intubated and breathed room air. There were no mortalities in either group, but recovery scores were better and $PaO_2$ higher in the propofol group [13].

However, it is important to note that the advanced safety in human anesthesia is not just a result of "better drugs and equipment," but of the strict adherence to checklists, following procedure and appropriate documentation of these events (i.e. accountability); this is something achievable for all areas where anesthesia is practiced. Additionally, according to Li et al., almost half of the anesthetic mortality in humans resulted from anesthetic overdose [11], which can likely be prevented in the veterinary world by accurately obtaining weights and careful calculations. Indeed, in many developing or underdeveloped countries, anesthesia is not always performed by a veterinarian or veterinary technician, underscoring the need for as much clarity as possible.

### 6.2.4 Monitoring and Management Under Anesthesia

The most important and critical monitor of anesthetic depth is a well-trained anesthetist. "Well-trained" in this context implies *experience* and formal education, and in settings where resources are limited, individuals without formal education and varying levels of experience may be performing anesthesia. This suggests that part of anesthetic planning

is teaching those who will monitor patients' vital signs (Table 6.3).

Textbox 6.4 describes the characteristics of light, moderate, and deep anesthesia. While it may seem basic, arousal or breakthrough pain is one of the most frequently encountered undesirable perianesthetic events requiring remedial intervention [14], and anesthetists must be prepared to deal with this.

---

**Textbox 6.4 Characteristics of light, moderate, and deep planes of anesthesia**

*Patients in a Light Anesthetic Plane*

- Palpebral reflex is present.
- Jaw tone is tight.
- Pupil position is central.
- Anal tone is present.

*Patients in a Moderate Anesthetic Plane*

- Palpebral reflex is absent.
- Jaw tone is loose.
- Pupil position is ventral and medial.
- Anal tone is minimally present.

*Patients in a Deep Anesthetic Plane*

- Palpebral reflex is absent.
- Jaw tone is absent.
- Pupil position is central.
- Anal tone is absent.

---

Several basic, small portable pieces of equipment can be used for monitoring – these should be considered an extension of the human senses, not a replacement for them. As mentioned previously, the three anticipated complications of anesthesia include hypotension, hypoventilation, and hypothermia; technology has made monitoring for these complications available in most settings. See Textbox 6.5 for a list of basic equipment that is useful in a field setting. Most of this equipment is battery powered, so a supply of suitable batteries, or a battery recharger, needs to be available. Follow the manufacturer's recommendations and practical experience to determine how long a set of batteries will last (Figure 6.3).

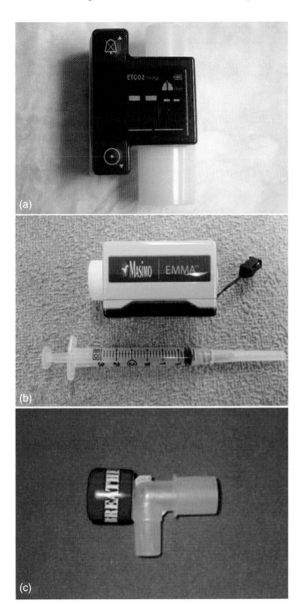

**Figure 6.3** Portable monitoring devices. (a) and (b) Portable capnographs. Allows for monitoring of respiration rate and end-tidal carbon dioxide and facilitates confirmation of ETT placement. (c) Breathe Safe Apnea Monitor. This relatively inexpensive device connects between the endotracheal tube and the anesthesia machine. The monitor beeps to indicate the patient has taken a breath. An alarm will sound if the patient fails to breathe for 30 s or more.

Hypotension (SBP < 90 mmHg, MAP < 60 mmHg) may or may not be present in the field setting, depending on the anesthetic protocol used and patient status. Hypotension is the result of a decrease in systemic vascular resistance and/or myocardial depression and is most commonly associated with the use of inhalant agents. If these agents are not used, for example in the case of TIMA, then hypotension may not occur. Should hypotension occur, strategies such as reducing or eliminating inhaled anesthesia (if it is used), fluid administration, and correcting a patient's heart rate to normal will restore adequate blood pressure in most cases. However, if hemorrhage has resulted in hypotension, controlling hemorrhage, fluid therapy, and possible transfusion may become necessary.

Guidelines from the ASV suggest that fluid therapy is not mandatory for all elective procedures, although it is recommended that all clinics have the ability to provide fluid therapy. Well-hydrated animals that undergo short procedures (<30 min), with minimal blood loss and with access to water after recovering from anesthesia, are unlikely to require intraoperative fluids. Cases that are greater than an ASA 3–5 warrant consideration for fluid therapy. Again, a veterinarian should make the final decision as to the necessity of intravenous fluid therapy and determine when the benefits to the patient outweigh the cost of providing fluid therapy. Subcutaneous fluids provide an alternative strategy if IV fluids are not used (e.g. any balanced crystalloid such as lactated Ringer's solution; daily requirements are 50–60 ml/kg).

End-tidal $CO_2$ is an indirect measure of $PaCO_2$ and alveolar ventilation and influenced by respiratory frequency, dead space, and tidal volume. Hypoventilation (elevated $EtCO_2$) is corrected by either increasing respiratory frequency, giving a more appropriate tidal volume, or a combination of these, which ideally requires a patient who is intubated. Patients can be ventilated using a face mask, but accumulation of gas in the stomach is likely, and this can impair diaphragmatic movement. The increase in respiratory frequency or tidal volume is typically accomplished by hand ventilating a patient with a respiratory rate of up to 25 breathes per minute (exceeding this may compromise expiratory time or giving a breath up to 20 cmH$_2$0 (as measured on the circuit manometer). The goal is to maintain an exhaled $CO_2$ between 35 and 50 mmHg (4.53–6.66 kPa).

Overventilation (PaCO$_2$ < 20 mmHg (2.66 kPa)) can result in vasoconstriction of cerebral blood vessels and compromised blood flow to the brain. Ventilation can also be performed with an Ambu bag.

Hypothermia occurs for a multitude of reasons, including but not limited to reduced metabolism, low environmental temperatures, inspiration of nonhumidified cold gases, and open body cavities. Simple things such as keeping animals in a dry, warm, and draft-free environment at all times help to combat heat loss; this is critical in sick or very young patients. Strategies such as prewarming a patient are not proved to help, but certainly cannot hurt [15]. Forced air warming is one of the most reliable methods to manage intraoperative hypothermia, but may not be available for all locations as it requires electrically operated specialized equipment [16]. Once a patient is induced, minimizing contact with cool surfaces, use of warmed scrub solution, preventing scrub solutions from wetting hair, maintaining an environmental temperature of 70 °F (21 °C) or warmer, and beginning surgery soon after patient preparation are common sense ways to maintain normothermia. Intraoperatively, reducing oxygen flow rates in circle systems will help a patient retain body heat. Even for large patients, flow rates as low as 0.5 l/min usually meet minimum oxygen requirements (5 ml/kg/min for the canine). Nonrebreathing circuits are used in smaller patients and require a high flow rates (200–300 ml/kg/min), which must be maintained to prevent rebreathing, so are often associated with

---

**Textbox 6.5 Basic equipment for a field setting**

- Airway access (laryngoscope or penlight and tongue depressor, laryngeal mask airway device, endotracheal tubes, lidocaine for feline arytenoids, ties to secure endotracheal tubes in place)
- Ambu bag
- Capnography
- Esophageal stethoscope
- Minimally invasive blood pressure unit (portable)
- Mylar blanket ("survival blanket")
- Portable oxygen tank (aluminum tanks are the lightest)
- Pulse oximeter
- Oxygen regulator and tubing for flow by oxygen
- Thermometer

---

hypothermia. Considering *healthy* patients as small as three kilograms can be safely placed on a rebreathing circle system, these (with pediatric hoses) are recommended when available. Additional thermal supports in the OR, including forced air warming and warm water blankets, are encouraged when available. Electrical heating blankets should never be used due to the risk of burns.

## 6.3 Equipment in the Field

### 6.3.1 Oxygen Sources

A portable oxygen source is critical in case of an emergency, and oxygen supplementation during anesthesia is good medical practice and it is becoming increasingly easier to bring oxygen to the field. Aluminum E tanks are light and portable, with enough compressed gas to deliver approximately 600 l of oxygen. Equation 6.4 demonstrates how many liters remain in an "E" tank. For those groups who do not wish to transport their own tanks, outside companies providing portable oxygen services exist (http://oxygentogo.com).

Equation 6.4 – Calculating how long an "E" tank will last:

$$PSI \times 0.3 = l \text{ remaining} \quad PSI = \text{Pounds per square in.}$$

Oxygen concentrators separate oxygen from air by chemical means. The maximum oxygen concentration produced is 95% and most commercial units can produce up to 10 l/min. Their limitation in a field situation is the need for an electrical source to operate them.

### 6.3.2 Airway Equipment

Endotracheal tubes (ETTs) or supraglottic airway devices (SGADs, see later in this section) are recommended even if patients breath room air because they secure the airway and prevent aspiration. Ambu bags can be attached and used for manual ventilation. Endotracheal intubation is suitable, especially if intravenous access is not utilized, as this is an alternative route for administration of emergency drugs such as epinephrine and atropine. ETTs are available in a variety of sizes and materials, although it is the recommendation of the authors to use "single-use"

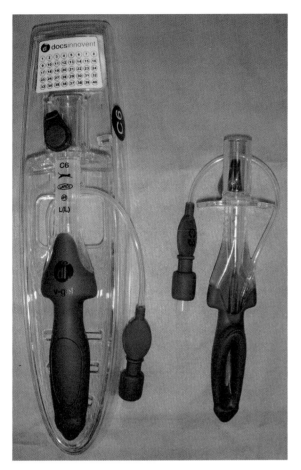

**Figure 6.4** Supraglottic airway device (SGAD) (feline specific).

human Polyvinyl chloride (PVC) ETTs. They can be cleaned and reused and represent a (minor) cost savings over silastic ETTs. An alternative is the use of a SGAD (Figure 6.4) for the feline patient. While these devices are significantly more expensive than ETTs, they are easy and quick to place, requiring minimal skill to do so. They can also be inserted at a lighter plane of anesthesia (i.e. less induction drug(s) are required). This is particularly important in cats, which are prone to laryngospasm and traumatic intubation, which could result in life-threatening postoperative airway obstruction. Cats may eat sooner with the use of these devices, which suggests that there is less laryngeal and pharyngeal irritation.

Additional airway equipment includes a facemask, a laryngoscope (bring extra batteries and light bulbs), and a simple means of securing the ETT (e.g. tie

gauze). If an anesthesia machine is used, a safety checklist should be completed daily to ensure it is in proper working order and appropriate maintenance of this machine is done annually (or more often, if used heavily). Carbon dioxide absorbent is checked daily and changed if required. While color change indicates the state of the $CO_2$ absorbent, things such as heat production (i.e. does the absorber still feel warm to the touch when in use as it should if chemical reactions are occurring?) and production of water (i.e. is there moisture beading on the wall of the canister?) also help to indicate the function of the absorbent. How quickly the $CO_2$ absorbent becomes exhausted depends on multiple factors, but most canisters used in veterinary anesthesia machines last less than 14 h of use; it is recommended to mark off on a piece of removable tape attached to the canister, each hour it is in use. In places where capnography is employed, an increase in inspired $CO_2$ (and therefore often an increase in end tidal $CO_2$) also indicates possible exhaustion of the carbon dioxide absorbent.

Charcoal canisters are excellent short-term scavengers of WAG, but require frequent changing in a high-volume setting (i.e. up to every 8 h, or more frequently as indicated by weight gain – a weight gain of 50 g indicates the need to change it).

An emergency ("crash") box should be available and contain the following: atropine, epinephrine (adrenaline), an emergency drug card (with weights and doses; available at: http://www.acvecc-recover.org), injection caps, ETTs (range of sizes), Ambu bag, catheters, fluid bags, and syringes.

Other items may include eye lubricant (corn oil can also be used for this purpose, which is easily and inexpensively purchased at most locations), an anesthetic record and pens for recording drug administration and any monitoring performed, IV flush (heparinized saline) for catheter placement, battery-powered clippers, scrub, alcohol, gauze squares, tape, and a container for used needles and syringes. Organizing for the field requires an awareness of what you would do each time you anesthetize a patient. It may be helpful here to acknowledge the limits of working memory and bring a worksheet or list of items to confirm all essential items are stocked and available. A small formulary, such as the one included in this book (Chapter 20), is helpful to have for important drug dosage information.

## 6.4 Drugs for Use in the Field

The perioperative period is often broken down into four parts: premedication, induction, maintenance, and recovery, and are described in these terms in the following sections. However, TIMA combines premedication and induction into one event and in some cases is sufficient for maintenance; this route is well suited to some field settings.

Record keeping must comply with local laws and regulations. At a minimum, drugs, route of administration, and time of administration should be recorded for each animal.

### 6.4.1 Premedication

The intention of premedication is to provide preemptive analgesia, decrease stress, render the animal easier to handle, and reduce the requirements for induction and maintenance drugs. The $\alpha_2$-adrenergic agonists are noncontrolled substances that meet these requirements. Drugs in this group include dexmedetomidine, medetomidine, and xylazine. Very few differences emerge between dexmedetomidine and medetomidine; for example, there is little difference in recovery time between the two drugs [17], especially when atipamezole is used. All $\alpha_2$-adrenergic agonists can cause vomiting, but this is especially true with xylazine. Vomiting may be distressing to the animal and increase the risk of aspiration. If not familiar with these drugs, one must be prepared for a profound level of sedation and biphasic cardiovascular effects. Initially, $\alpha_2$-adrenergic agonists result in profound vasoconstriction and a peripherally mediated bradycardia, and, secondarily, as vascular tone relaxes, a centrally mediated bradycardia results in a decrease in cardiac output. Because of this biphasic effect, it is inappropriate to coadminister $\alpha_2$-adrenergic agonists along with an anticholinergic drug, such as atropine. The initial bradycardia is anticipated as a normal consequence of vasoconstriction, and combining these two drugs will increase blood pressure and myocardial workload. As with any drug, it is important to assess whether the benefits of this drug outweigh the cardiovascular consequences.

$\alpha_2$-Adrenergic agonists result in some degree of hypoventilation [18], although the decrease in respiratory rate may be offset by an increase in tidal volume. Other side effects include hypothermia, increase in urinary output, and a transient hyperglycemia secondary to a decrease in insulin release. Atipamezole is intended for reversal of medetomidine and dexmedetomidine, although it works for all $\alpha_2$-adrenergic agonists. It is at the discretion of the anesthetist whether to routinely include reversal. In cats, if other analgesics are also present (such as an opioid), they are comfortable following reversal and recovery times are shortened [19].

Other sedative choices include acepromazine and midazolam. Acepromazine will provide mild-to-moderate sedation without reducing anxiety or providing analgesia. It is not reversible, but it has a fairly wide margin of safety [20]. Like dexmedetomidine, acepromazine ultimately results in a decrease in cardiac output and vasodilation, although this effect is minimized by ensuring the patient is euvolemic and using clinically appropriate doses. Midazolam, of all the sedatives, provides the most cardiovascular and respiratory stability. However, of the three sedatives, it is the only one that is internationally controlled. In young and very old or debilitated patients, the sedative effects are quite reliable and consistent; however, robust juvenile and adult dogs and cats will often become agitated and exited. In these patients, midazolam can be used as a coinduction agent with injectable induction drugs such as propofol or ketamine. Midazolam is one of the few drugs that reliably result in amnesia (an important component for anesthesia). When available, it is suitable for inclusion in many anesthetic plans, although this necessitates appropriate documentation and disposal as dictated by the regulatory bodies in the country where it is used.

It is appropriate to include an opioid as a component of premedication, both for the synergistic action of $\alpha_2$-adrenergic agonists and opioids [21, 22] and their preemptive analgesic effects. See additional information on nonsteroidal anti-inflammatories, which are also well suited as analgesic agents in these settings. The opioid chosen is often dictated by availability. The International Narcotics Control Board lists fentanyl (and its various derivatives), buprenorphine, hydromorphone, methadone, morphine, and oxymorphone as internationally controlled. This leaves butorphanol and tramadol as the only noncontrolled opioids available in some but not all regions (e.g. butorphanol and tramadol are scheduled drugs in the United States). Therefore, the most likely opioid for incorporation into an anesthetic plan is the one that is obtainable through a veterinarian with a license to access that country's controlled drugs. Preference for inclusion in a plan is given to full mu-opioid agonist opioids such as hydromorphone (which was comparable in its minimal cost to morphine in the United States at the time of writing). Morphine, oxymorphone, and methadone are also suitable. The reality is that butorphanol, a mu antagonist and kappa agonist, is the opioid most likely to be available. Butorphanol has a limited duration of action of about an hour in dogs, when administered at a dose of 0.4 mg/kg [23], although this may be longer in cats. A duration of almost 3 h was reported in cats; however, this study was not measuring clinical pain [24]. Clinically, it is appropriate to repeat the dose of butorphanol in dogs after an hour, if the procedure is not yet complete. The plan should include two administrations of this drug, unless one opts to use a constant rate infusion in the field; see Section 6.4.3. In combination with a local block (Chapter 5), a nonsteroidal anti-inflammatory, a skilled surgeon, and a procedure that evokes no more than moderate pain, this may be enough to provide adequate analgesia. Tramadol, a weak mu-agonist and serotonin/norepinephrine reuptake inhibitor, should not be considered a cornerstone drug for acute pain in dogs. Dogs produce very little of the key analgesic metabolite (O-desmethyltramadol [M1]) [25]. Cats, however, do produce O-desmethyltramadol and, therefore, are more likely to reap some benefits from this drug [26].

Buprenorphine is available in some countries, although it is internationally controlled. Buprenorphine is a longer acting partial mu agonist, meaning that although it occupies mu receptors, it only has about 80% of the efficacy of a full mu agonist (e.g. morphine) [27, 28]. Buprenorphine is probably best when combined with a nonsteroidal anti-inflammatory drug in dogs; the latter provides good analgesia of longer duration [29] as dogs often require rescue analgesia within the first 24 h after soft tissue surgery when buprenorphine is used alone [30, 31]. In cats, buprenorphine appears to provide quite satisfactory analgesia and has demonstrated a synergistic action when used with dexmedetomidine [22]. In multiple feline studies, buprenorphine was superior to butorphanol [32].

NSAIDs serve a vital role in pain management for field procedures. Their prolonged duration of action

(up to 24 h in many cases), lack of controlled substance designation, and applicability to a variety of painful stimuli make them an obvious choice in this setting. Additionally, many are available in an injectable formulation, which can be used perioperatively and in oral formulations for postoperative use. They are not true premedicants in the sense that they do not reduce the amount of drug necessary to provide analgesia or increase the handleability of a patient, although they do provide preemptive analgesia if administered prior to surgery. It is up to the veterinary personnel whether they are comfortable with routine use of NSAIDs preoperatively. NSAIDs vary in their disruption to normal homeostatic function. NSAIDs, which are considered preferential or selective (such as meloxicam, carprofen, deracoxib, robenacoxib), will inhibit cyclooxygenase (COX) enzymes traditionally increased after tissue injury (although there is some role for COX-2 enzymes is normal homeostatic processes, such as gastrointestinal healing). However, it is impossible to inhibit COX-2 without the potential for normal COX-1 homeostatic mechanisms (gastrointestinal protection, renal protection, and platelet function) becoming compromised. The extent of this disruption is correlated both to the selectivity of the NSAID (for example, ketoprofen does not select for COX-2) and to the severity of the disruption to COX-1-mediated functions. NSAIDs are used cautiously in cases where perioperative coagulopathy, hemorrhage, hypovolemia, hypotension, or preexisting renal disease is present. NSAIDs are contraindicated in patients who are receiving corticosteroids.

### 6.4.2 Induction and Maintenance of Anesthesia

#### 6.4.2.1 Intramuscular Administration

When revisiting the goals of premedication, including creating a manageable patient, there are certainly cases in the field where intramuscular injection of an induction agent (as opposed to IV injection) becomes an attractive option. No single agent can provide all five components of anesthesia, but TIMA is feasible if a combination of agents is used (Figure 6.5b). Ideally, these agents can be combined for single IM administration. Ketamine and alfaxalone are two induction drugs producing reliable results when given intramuscularly. TIMA is achieved when either of these drugs is used in combination with routine premedication (it is worth noting that amnesia is the only component of general anesthesia we may not achieve). Ketamine is a key component of many TIMA protocols and has been used for this purpose for almost 50 years. Ketamine is versatile in that it can be used IM or IV and has a high therapeutic index (TI) – the ratio between the desired effect and the toxic or lethal dose of a drug. Indeed, the author petitioned the United States government (through the Freedom of Information Act) for the TI as a reference source. The agency spent almost 2 years scouring records and could not retrieve a single study where the lethal dose could be found, due to the inability of ketamine to cause death in young laboratory species. This is not to say that ketamine cannot result in death of a patient, but rather confirms the drug's safety. Ketamine does not result in apnea, although an apneustic breathing pattern is often observed. Ketamine results in little cardiovascular depression because it is a sympathetic stimulant. However, ketamine is not without drawbacks. For example, ketamine used alone does not achieve all the components of general anesthesia (specifically, it will not inhibit spontaneous movement or produce muscle relaxation and its amnestic properties are unknown). Therefore, ketamine is combined with other drugs, such as $\alpha_2$-adernergic agonists, to achieve true TIMA. Ketamine, which is metabolized only to norketamine in cats, can result in suboptimal recoveries, and this is another reason that it is combined with other drugs. Some practitioners speculate that bladder expression (and thus removal of norketamine from the body via the emptying of urine) may improve recovery, a theory that has not been put to the test in an experimental study. A known advantage to expressing the bladder before recovery, however, is increased patient comfort and prevents urination and lying on a wet and cold surface. Additionally, ketamine is not controlled in many countries outside most North America and Europe, making it easily accessible for use in the field. Tiletamine/zolazepam (proprietary names Telazol or Zoletil), another *N*-Methyl-*D*-aspartate (NMDA) antagonist combined with a benzodiazepine, provides a good option if it is available. It is not internationally controlled in some countries, but may be in some regions, e.g. the United States. One of the advantages of tiletamine/zolazepam is the small volume required to produce deep sedation or a surgical plane of anesthesia.

The IM administration of alfaxalone in dogs and cats is the subject of several studies. When combined with an opioid and dexmedetomidine in cats, measured physiologic variables were well maintained [33]. Recovery from alfaxalone alone is not smooth, with animals exhibiting tremors and ataxia [34, 35], so it is the author's recommendation that if alfaxalone is used intramuscularly, it is coadministered with other drugs (see sample protocols for information on optimal dosing). Dogs do not appear to respond as favorably as cats to a combination of alfaxalone, $\alpha_2$-adrenergic agonists, and opioids [36], suggesting other intramuscular protocols are more suitable for dogs.

### 6.4.2.2 Intravascular Administration

Age, socialization, and disease status will dictate how easy an animal is to handle without chemical restraint. In dogs and cats that are easy to work with, it is possible to obtain venous access to induce anesthesia. This is advantageous because drugs can be titrated to effect, rather than committing to a "depot" (intramuscular) dose and hoping to get the desired effect without any adverse effects.

Several drugs are available for intravenous drug administration. Thiobarbiturates are available in some countries, but are not recommended for use in the field, as accidental perivascular administration, especially when IV catheters are not used, results in severe pain and ultimately necrosis of the skin at the site of extravasation [37]. Additionally, these drugs can cause ventricular bigeminy and respiratory depression and are controlled substances. Because redistribution rather than elimination results in recovery, additional "top-ups" (more than 1–2 times) are cumulative, resulting in prolonged and poor quality recoveries. However, in some countries (such as Thailand), pento- or thiobarbiturates are often selected due to cost and availability. If this is the case, it is highly recommended to ensure patency of IV access prior to administration and to use these drugs at conservative dosages, and minimizing repeat boluses. In ASA category 3–5 patients, it is advised to select alternative agents. Thiobarbiturates should not be used in sighthounds because in these breeds the recovery phase is prolonged and often violent.

Propofol, at the time of writing, was not a controlled substance and, therefore, was readily available for intravenous use in the field. Propofol is not an irritant if given perivascularly. However, the drug itself has a much lower therapeutic index than that of ketamine and, therefore, must be titrated to effect to prevent bradycardia, a decrease in systemic vascular resistance, hypoventilation, and apnea (probably the most common and serious side effect). Giving this drug slowly (over at least 60 s) appears to improve the margin of safety. Pain on injection has been reported [38]; however, propofol results in a smooth induction and recovery and is widely used. Because propofol can be given as a single bolus (dogs and cats), repeated injections (dogs) or as a CRI (dogs), without prolonging recovery, it is a versatile field anesthetic when the duration of a procedure is unpredictable. Multiple "top-ups" and CRIs of over 30 min result in prolonged recoveries in cats. Propofol with a preservative (benzyl alcohol) is available and has a shelf life of 28 days after the vial is breached, which reduces drug wastage. However, a sterile technique must be adhered to each time the drug is drawn up.

Alfaxalone causes minimal change in heart rate when administered slowly to effect, thus offering some advantages over propofol. Alfaxalone administration can result in apnea, but usually only at high dosages or if given quickly [39], although this is likely influenced by the choice and effect of premedicant agents. Similarly, cardiovascular depression was avoided when using clinically relevant dosages, but did occur at supraclinical dosages of 5 to 10 times the standard induction doses [40, 41]. This drug has a place in feline field anesthesia, because of cats' unique physiology. Cats have a variable ability to metabolize drugs heavily reliant on glucuronidation, resulting in unpredictable effects of those drugs. Alfaxalone is excreted virtually unchanged in the urine or undergoes oxidation and, therefore, has a very predictable profile in cats. Indeed, this likely accounts for the improved recovery with alfaxalone when used in combination with other premedications, as opposed to traditional induction drugs such as ketamine and diazepam [42]. It is worth noting that ketamine's dissociative properties likely result in some behavioral side effects, which is not the case for alfaxalone. Alfaxalone stands apart for its highly favorable profile in high-risk patients such as those underwent cesarean sections and with hyperthyroidism [43, 44] – although not common, these patients may be anesthetized in a field clinic. Some drawbacks of alfaxalone are linked to geographic locations; for example,

in the United States, alfaxalone is more expensive than propofol and is a scheduled drug.

Once a protocol is chosen, it is helpful to develop a dosing chart for premedication and induction agents. The ASV guidelines discourage the use of "one-size-fits-all" dosing (i.e. all cats get the same dose regardless of size), but does support the use of categorical dosing on common weight ranges. For example, dosages for cats that fall into 1–2 kg, 2–4 kg, 4–6 kg, etc. might help to reduce the possibility of errors that occur if calculations are done for each patient. On the other hand, many automated calculators are available for smart devices that may provide the best of both worlds. It is always appropriate to have a printed dosing chart, especially for emergency drugs (see Section 6.5) as a backup.

### 6.4.3 Maintenance

#### 6.4.3.1 Intravenous Drugs

Maintenance of anesthesia is often achieved with additional "top-ups" of injectable agents. In this regard, ketamine is safe and can be repeatedly redosed. Other injectable agents such as alfaxalone and propofol (as discussed earlier, the dose of propofol should be minimized in cats) are suitable for readministration, but should be given slowly and to effect to reduce the incidence of apnea. One study in which dogs were premedicated with medetomidine and maintained with IV ketamine or propofol "as needed" reported fewer side effects and better quality of recovery with propofol [45].

An alternative is the administration of a CRI to maintain anesthesia. A CRI maintains a constant plasma drug concentration so that repeated "top-ups" are not needed. A loading dose is given to achieve the target plasma concentration, followed by the CRI which maintains this. In the field setting, this can be accomplished with a catheter, a fluid administration set, and a bag of fluids. Equations 6.1–6.3 (see Textbox 6.3 for this information) assist in calculating and administering CRIs using fluid bags.

#### 6.4.3.2 Inhalant Anesthesia Agents

Portable anesthetic machines make the use of inhalant agents possible in some settings. The initial outlay for these machines may be relatively expensive but with proper upkeep will last many years. As described previously, oxygen cylinders and oxygen concentrators are also portable or may be available at the clinic location. By default, the use of inhalant agents provides oxygen supplementation. An advantage of inhalant techniques is that they can be used without IV access and provide continuous anesthesia and have the ability to change the plane of anesthesia quickly.

### 6.4.4 Recovery

The recovery phase includes extubation if applicable and at least the first 3 h after regaining consciousness because over 50% of canine and 60% of feline anesthetic mortalities occur during this time [10]. A patient is extubated when it is judged that they can maintain their own airway (e.g. strength to lift their head, swallowing). To facilitate a patent airway, the head is positioned in an extended position. The ET tube cuff is deflated after the patient swallows (unless otherwise indicated; for example, in the case of an animal who has regurgitated when it may be left wholly or partially inflated to prevent aspiration). During the recovery period, continuous observation and monitoring is recommended, with necessary support for common anesthetic comorbidities such as anxiety, dysphoria, pain, cardiopulmonary depression, vomiting or regurgitation, and hypothermia. Note, when littermates "huddle" for warmth, it is possible for inadvertent respiratory compromise to occur, so use commonsense when deciding whether it is appropriate to litters to recover together. It is also important to assess animals for pain at this time and provide additional analgesia if needed. Pain scoring tools are helpful in assessing the patient (see Appendices 6.A–6.C). The patient should recover in a quiet, warm, dry, clean environment on the floor (although not in direct contact with it), and elevated surfaces are not recommended due to the dangers of falling and injury. Young patients should have their blood glucose checked if possible; if not, application of corn syrup or dextrose to the gums is appropriate as the risk of hypoglycemia outweighs the risk of hyperglycemia. At a minimum, pulse rate and quality, respiratory rate, mucous membrane color, and body temperature are monitored during recovery.

Reversal of anesthetic drugs may be necessary in cases of emergency or prolonged recovery (see Reversal Agents). The benefits of reversal must be weighed against the possible detrimental effects including inadequate analgesia and a very abrupt recovery.

The timing of release from veterinary care will vary with each setting. Free-roaming animals that are to be released back to their environment must be fully recovered and if possible have eaten before release. This may require overnight holds in traps or cages.

Some dogs may be required to walk home with owners and should not be released until they can do so with no ataxia.

### 6.4.5 Sample Protocols

Figure 6.5 provides a tool to help those working in the field create their own balanced anesthetic protocol. The list of drugs is not meant to be all-inclusive or a gold standard, but rather to provide useful suggestions for field clinics. Selected doses are generally mid-range, with lower dosages suitable for geriatric or ill patients and higher dosages used for difficult-to-handle but otherwise healthy patients (i.e. fractious cats). The authors prefer to administer a nonsteroidal anti-inflammatory postoperatively, in case of unexpected intraoperative hypotension or bleeding. Appendix 6.D also lists some commonly used protocols from various animal welfare organizations working in international settings.

---

**Textbox 6.6 Additional tips from the field**

Take care to administer propofol SLOWLY, or severe respiratory or cardiovascular depression may result.

Editors of this book have used xylazine in place of dexmedetomidine in animals as a premedication, at a dose of 1.0–1.5 mg/kg. It is worth noting that xylazine comes in a concentration of 20 mg/ml, 100 mg/ml, and 200 mg/ml, so practitioners should verify concentration when creating these drug protocols.

Nalbuphine is a kappa agonist, mu antagonist opioid with properties similar to that of butorphanol. Its advantages include lower cost and it is not controlled. This allows nalbuphine to substitute for butorphanol in many protocols.

To create such dosing charts, it is imperative that we verify the concentration of the drugs for a given a geographic region prior to finalizing the chart. Stock concentration varies by country of drug origin in many cases. For example, ketamine may be available in 10, 50, or 100 mg/ml concentrations.

**Combined canine anesthesia**

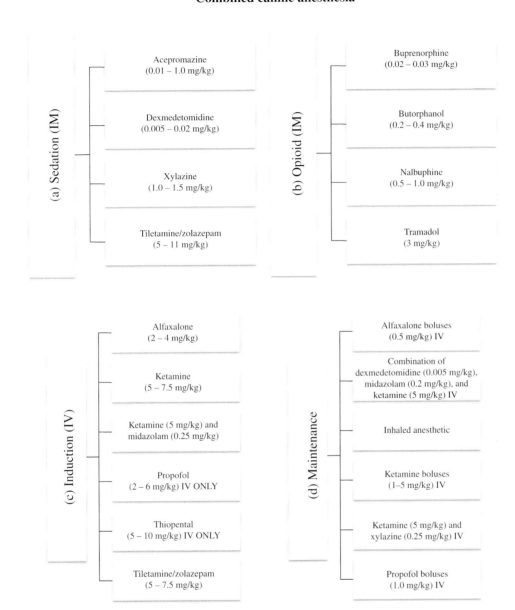

**Figure 6.5** Example protocols for field anesthesia and guide to their use.

Selections from (a) (sedation) and (b) (opioid) are always given together intramuscularly; (c) (induction) is administered together with (a) and (b) for total intramuscular anesthesia (TIMA), *or* (c) and (d) (maintenance) are administered via injection or inhalation if TIMA is not used. To use the figure below, select one choice each from (a)–(d). Traditionally, what one chooses in (a) and (b) will influence the selection from groups (c) and (d); that is, practicality would indicate continuation of drugs selected from (a) and (b) for (c) and (d) (unless inhalants are selected).

Keep in mind several things to make these protocols successful:

These protocols are intended as examples ONLY, and not as endorsements for best medical practice. See text; the best protocol is the one that meets the availability of drugs in one's area of practice and with which the practitioner is familiar.

The sample protocols listed above are for the anesthetic period *only*. Additional analgesia, such as NSAIDs and local blocks, should be included as appropriate.

Appropriate opioids targeted for the level of pain expected will provide the best anesthesia event possible. For example, butorphanol is unlikely to last more than 60–90 min in the canine patient.

**Combined feline anesthesia**

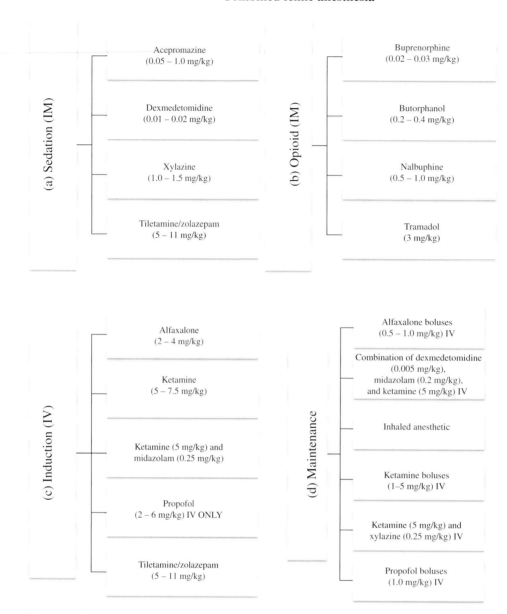

Figure 6.5 (*continued*)

## 6.5 Cardiopulmonary Resuscitation (CPR) in the Field

A key goal in anesthesia is *preventing* the occurrence of cardiopulmonary arrest (CPA). It is unwise, however, to assume that CPA does not occur in relatively healthy animals [10]. As with any event that occurs under anesthesia, cardiopulmonary resuscitation (CPR) is most successful when the team is prepared, the crisis is recognized early, and CPR is started immediately. Indeed, the most comprehensive veterinary CPR guidelines at the time of this writing

## Combined total intramuscular anesthesia (TIMA)

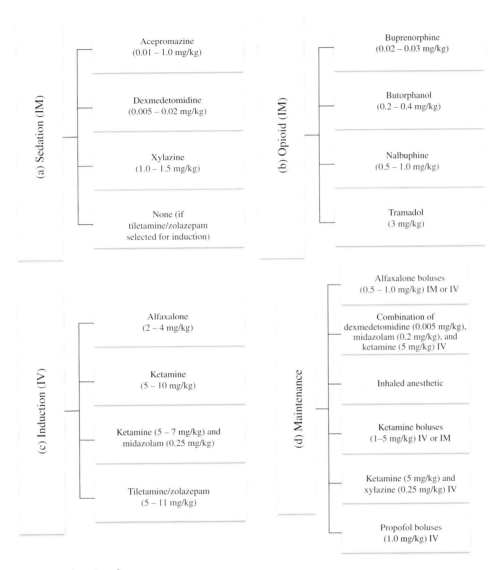

**(a) Sedation (IM)**

Acepromazine
(0.01 – 1.0 mg/kg)

Dexmedetomidine
(0.005 – 0.02 mg/kg)

Xylazine
(1.0 – 1.5 mg/kg)

None (if
tiletamine/zolazepam
selected for induction)

**(b) Opioid (IM)**

Buprenorphine
(0.02 – 0.03 mg/kg)

Butorphanol
(0.2 – 0.4 mg/kg)

Nalbuphine
(0.5 – 1.0 mg/kg)

Tramadol
(3 mg/kg)

**(c) Induction (IV)**

Alfaxalone
(2 – 4 mg/kg)

Ketamine
(5 – 10 mg/kg)

Ketamine (5 – 7 mg/kg) and
midazolam (0.25 mg/kg)

Tiletamine/zolazepam
(5 – 11 mg/kg)

**(d) Maintenance**

Alfaxalone boluses
(0.5 – 1.0 mg/kg) IM or IV

Combination of
dexmedetomidine (0.005 mg/kg),
midazolam (0.2 mg/kg), and
ketamine (5 mg/kg) IV

Inhaled anesthetic

Ketamine boluses
(1–5 mg/kg) IV or IM

Ketamine (5 mg/kg) and
xylazine (0.25 mg/kg) IV

Propofol boluses
(1.0 mg/kg) IV

**Figure 6.5** *(continued)*

strongly suggest beginning CPR immediately if there is a suspicion of CPA; see RECOVER guidelines for more information [46]. Animals that experience cardiac arrest under anesthesia have better survival rates than those that collapse in other settings. This is likely due to early recognition, established patent airway, oxygen delivery, and presence of an IV catheter (hence the recommendations to place these even in the field). There is strong evidence to support the use of a visual algorithm during CPR; see Figure 6.6 for an example from the RECOVER guideline itself.

1) The RECOVER and American Heart Association guidelines suggest bypassing palpating a pulse and beginning immediately with CPR if CPA is suspected. This is appropriate if the pulse

**Feline total intramuscular anesthesia (TIMA)**

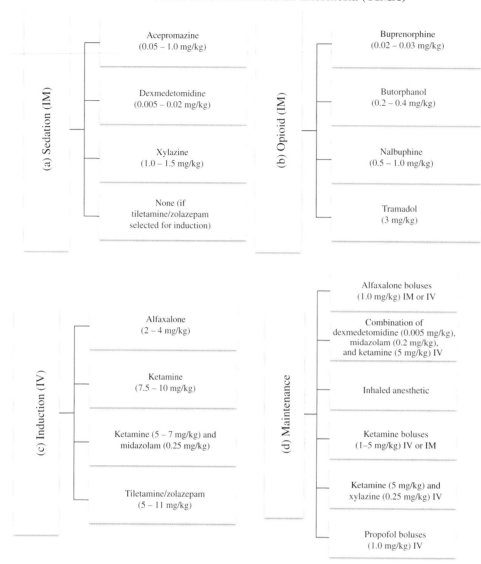

Figure 6.5 (*continued*)

is not being monitored during anesthesia. If a pulse is being continuously monitored (with monitoring equipment), it is sometimes the loss of that audio or visual signal that suggests CPA has occurred.

2) *Discontinue anesthesia* (turn off the vaporizer and flush the anesthetic circuit with oxygen, terminate CRIs of injectable agents and stop bolus administration).

3) *Begin basic life support with CAB.*

   *C = compressions.* Beginning compressions is the critical first step (even before securing an airway in a nonintubated patient); the importance of supporting circulating blood flow is more important than providing ventilation in the initial stages of resuscitation. The patient is placed in left lateral recumbency (although dorsal is acceptable for

# CPR algorithm

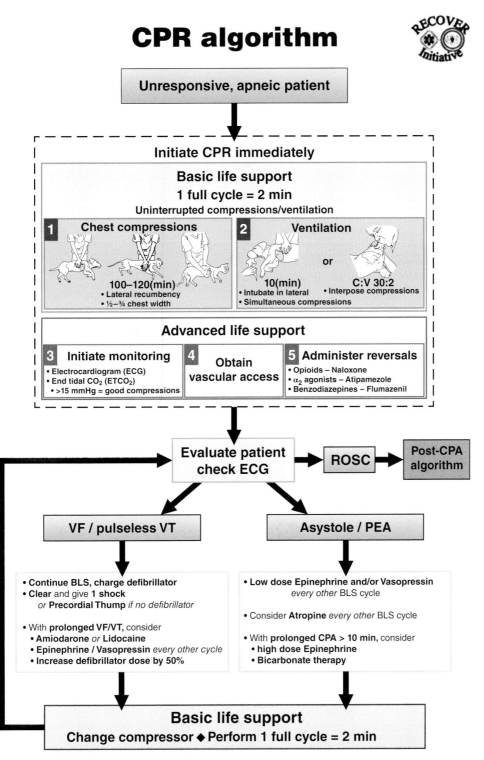

Figure 6.6 RECOVER visual aid during CPR. Source: Fletcher et al. 2012 [46]. Reproduced with permission of John Wiley & Sons.

"barrel-chested" dogs, e.g. bulldogs). Target rate of compressions is 100–120 bpm. Compressions are biphasic: initially, the compressor compresses downward, 1/3 of the width of the chest. Secondarily, and equally important, the compressor must allow full recoil of the chest before the next compression. Compressors are more effective and can reduce their fatigue by using appropriate posture. This posture includes leverage over the animal (using a stool if necessary), locked elbows, interlocked hands and bending at the waist to utilize the entire upper body to perform compressions. Interruption of chest compressions is minimized, as it is impossible to regain the same level of output each subsequent restart of CPR. It is appropriate to change the compressor every 2 min. Appropriate transition between compressors begins with communication regarding the hand off to the new compressor. Next, the new compressor will place their hands over the current compressor's hands, so transition is seamless.

$A = airway.$ A degree of ventilation is imparted through cardiac compressions. The most experienced person present should then attempt to intubate the patient (which will require an ETT, laryngoscope, and a secure tie, with oxygen support if available). While attempting intubation, compressions are not stopped unless absolutely necessary.

$B = breathing.$ Once intubated, deliver approximately 10 breaths per minute (with oxygen if available). If a manometer is available, the positive inspiratory pressure (PIP) is 10 cmH$_2$O per breath and tidal volume is 10 ml/kg; an Ambu bag is a suitable alternative to the anesthesia machine.

4) *Monitoring during CPR.* Place monitoring equipment. A capnograph is now considered standard of care for use during CPR (See Figure 6.3). This small, simple piece of equipment is usually easily placed and therefore one of the first monitors used. The target goal is 15 mmHg EtCO$_2$ or greater. If available, an ECG is placed on the patient for assessment of the rhythm during chest recoils.

5) *Drugs.* Administer drugs intravenously, if possible. If no catheter is present, initial epinephrine is delivered intratracheal (IT) and drugs are diluted with saline. In an ideal setting, the drug is delivered via a red rubber catheter inserted down the ET tube and of equal/longer length to the ET tube, and followed by a bolus of air to evacuate the drug from the red rubber catheter (consider this equipment for the emergency box). Attempts to secure an access site for drug administration is appropriate and may include placing an IV or intraosseous (IO) catheter. Compressions should not stop to facilitate this.

---

**Textbox 6.7 Emergency drugs for use in the field**

*Epinephrine, also known as adrenaline* (0.01 mg/kg IV/IO or 0.02–0.1 mg/kg diluted 1 : 1 with saline if given IT), is administered and repeated every 4 min.

*Vasopressin* (0.8 IU/kg IV/IO or 1.2 IU/kg IT) is an alternative to epinephrine, but is expensive and unlikely to be available in the field.

*Atropine* (0.04 mg/kg IV/IO or 0.08 mg/kg IT) is recommended by the author for use in the anesthetized patient, due to higher vagal tone; however, RECOVER guidelines suggest this is not mandatory for incorporation into routine CPR [46].

*Reversal Agents*
*Atipamezole.* Equal volume to dexmedetomidine administration for reversal of $\alpha_2$-adrenergic agonist in dogs and half the volume for use in cats.

*Flumazenil.* 0.04 mg/kg IV for benzodiazepine reversal.

*Naloxone.* 0.01 mg/kg IV for opioid reversal.

Fluids during CPR are used only if the patient is hypovolemic prior to arrest.

---

6) *Defibrillation.* In human CPR, ventricular fibrillation is the predominant arrest rhythm, and, thus, time to defibrillation is a major determinant of survival. However, asystole is more common in dogs and cats compared to ventricular fibrillation. It is unlikely that one would have a defibrillator in the field, but it is remiss not to mention this is the most appropriate intervention for animals with ventricular fibrillation.

Should return of spontaneous circulation occur, the next step is to begin postresuscitative care. The

RECOVER guidelines review this information in more depth [46].

## 6.6 Pain Management

*"There are no geographic limitations to the occurrence of pain, nor the ability to diagnosis it"* – Treatise on the recognition, assessment, and treatment of pain, WSAVA GVC.

The World Small Animal Veterinary Association Global Veterinary Community (WSAVA GVC) have guidelines for recognition, assessment, and treatment of pain applicable to all veterinary professionals worldwide [47]. This material is an excellent source for setting a program's pain management standards. This global network recognizes the challenges of pain management in different countries including the limited availability of drugs and has tailored these guidelines to enable good standards of care everywhere.

### 6.6.1 Acute versus Chronic Pain

The International Association for the Study of Pain defines pain and has recently proposed an updated definition of pain as follows: "Pain is a distressing experience associated with actual or potential tissue damage with sensory, emotional, cognitive and social components." [48] To help refine our treatment modalities, it is common to further classify pain, for example, acute versus chronic pain. However, the most helpful classification is to determine the underlying cause (e.g. inflammatory, neuropathic), which will guide the choice of drugs for treatment. The reader is referred to more comprehensive literature if they are interested in the physiology of pain management [49]. In general, acute pain is what we most commonly consider perioperatively; acute pain is thought of as the body's normal response to injury of less than an arbitrary duration (usually weeks to months). The pain an animal experiences from castration is an example of "acute pain." Chronic pain is pain of a longer duration than anticipated after apparent healing or with diseases such as osteoarthritis, and is expected to alter the processing of pain in the CNS. This is sometimes termed "maladaptive" pain and is of no benefit to the patient. In terms of treatments, this usually means that acute pain is managed in a comprehensive but straightforward manner. Chronic or maladaptive pain often requires a more extensive approach. In the field, preparing for acute pain is appropriate, as this will be the most common type of pain encountered. However, one must also be prepared for potential "acute-on-chronic" pain that may occur in some patients, for example, a dog with a chronic wound that undergoes surgical debridement or a dog with osteoarthritis that undergoes a surgical procedure.

### 6.6.2 Pain Assessment

It is impossible to overemphasize the importance of pain assessment in pain management. Just as there is no certain way to tell if a weight-loss diet is working without monitoring weight, it is impossible to tell if pain management strategies have achieved their goal without a structured assessment tool. Prerequisites of a successful tool include user friendliness, accuracy, reliability, sensitivity, and efficiency. Tools range from simple numeric rating scales or visual analogue scales to more complex composite scales. Although there are several pain assessment tools to choose from, many are not validated. Therefore, this section will focus predominantly on validated acute pain scales for the feline and canine patient. A validated and logical approach for assessing acute pain comes from combining a subjective assessment (for example, a behavior) with a numeric score (for example, from zero to two). This descriptor and score facilitates reproducibility and consistency of scoring, which is critical for successful pain management. It is important to note, however, that a pain assessment tool should not be used to *de*emphasize pain. In other words, and in accordance with WSAVA GCP Pain Treatise guidelines, if an animal has predictable pain (i.e. surgical pain), it is our moral and ethical obligation to manage for this, even if our pain scale values are low.

#### 6.6.2.1 Canine

In an acute pain setting, the Glasgow Composite Pain Scale Short Form (GCPS SF) is validated and these authors' personal preference for dogs [50, 51]. The assessment includes observation of the dog in its kennel, observation of the dog as it is taken out of its kennel, response to palpation, vocalization, and assessment of demeanor. Each of those broad categories is composed of parameters, for a total of 30 descriptors in 6 behavioral categories. See Appendix 6.A for an example of the GCPS. This tool is now available in multiple languages. (www.newmetric .com).

The maximum total for this scale is 24 (20 if mobility is excluded); values greater than 6 out of 24 suggests intervention is necessary (5 if mobility is excluded). The GCPS is validated for acute pain resulting from a variety of procedures. Pain scales are used to guide, not replace clinical judgment; therefore, should the score be less than the recommended intervention level, the observer should trust their instincts and not the score alone. After some experience, it generally takes less than a minute to complete this assessment, so the user is advised to familiarize themselves with this tool in their usual setting *prior* to using it in the field.

#### 6.6.2.2 Feline

Brondani and colleagues developed a pain scale for assessing acute postoperative pain in cats undergoing ovariohysterectomy [52]; the initial validation was in Brazilian Portuguese, but since then, this scale or it's translation has proved useful in a variety of languages (English, French, Spanish, and Italian) [53, 54]. This tool includes several behavioral and physiologic parameters for assessing pain. They fall broadly into four categories: psychomotor changes, protection of the wound area, a physiologic variable (blood pressure), and vocalization. Each parameter has descriptors with corresponding scales; see Appendix 6.B for the UNESP-Botucatu scale.

If all categories are included, the maximum value of the scale is 30, with 7 or greater considered pain that warrants intervention. Although more assessed categories enhance the power of the assessment, Brondani's pain scale is particularly user friendly albeit more time consuming, in that it retains value for pain assessment even if categories are excluded. For example, systolic blood pressure assessment or appetite are categories that, if removed, do not invalidate the scale.

The Glasgow Composite Measure Pain Scale -Feline was created by some of the same authors who provided the GCPS SF for dogs [55]. Like it's canine counterpart, there are several categories including observation of the cat in its cage, interaction with the cat, the cat's response to palpation, and assessment of the cat's well-being. Caricatures depicted underscore the importance of facial expression as a pain assessment tool. This scale has been validated in cats with a variety of causes of acute pain, not just ovariohysterectomy. See Appendix 6.C for an example of the Glasgow CMPS-Feline.

The maximum total for this scale is 20, and values greater than 5 of 20 suggest intervention is necessary. To reiterate, trust the animal and not the score alone, and ensure your familiarity with this tool in predictable setting before taking this tool into the field.

### 6.6.3 Multimodal Analgesia

Multimodal analgesia was described previously in this chapter, but its importance merits further discussion. The term *multimodal analgesia* implies combining analgesics, each with different methods of action, toward the goal of reducing or preventing nociceptive stimulation via multiple receptors and pathways. In theory, less of each drug is necessary to obtain adequate analgesia and a more robust protection against pain is achieved. There is mounting evidence of the importance of multimodal analgesia in veterinary studies and definitive evidence from human work suggesting a decrease in postoperative morbidity and mortality, improved quality of life, increased patient satisfaction, and reduced costs. One of the most profound ways to incorporate multimodal analgesia into a patient's plan is by including a local anesthetic block (see Chapter 7 for detailed local blocks suitable for field use).

As mentioned previously, opioids are the cornerstone of pain management in small-animal veterinary practice, owing to both a reduction in pain at the spinal cord and supraspinal level (i.e. where pain is processed and where it is perceived by the patient).

#### 6.6.3.1 Opioids and $\alpha_2$-Adrenergic Agonists

The mechanism of analgesia for $\alpha_2$-adrenergic agonists is twofold: these agents provide analgesia through a spinal and supraspinal mechanism, via the $\alpha_{2A}$ and/or $\alpha_{2C}$ receptor, and they also enhance opioid analgesia. Both buprenorphine and dexmedetomidine individually provide analgesia to cats. However, lower doses were effective (and duration was longer for analgesia) when dexmedetomidine was combined with buprenorphine [21] – a *synergistic* effect, in that the combination of buprenorphine and dexmedetomidine provided better sedation and analgesia than when either drug was used alone. However, it should be noted that the dose of dexmedetomidine required to produce sedation in cats is much lower than that needed for analgesia; therefore, dexmedetomidine should not be relied upon as the sole analgesic [56].

Studies support the synergistic effect of opioids and $\alpha_2$-adrenergic agonists in canine patients well. In a study by Valtolina and colleagues, when dexmedetomidine was given as a CRI, this drug was as effective an analgesic as morphine given as CRI. What is surprising is that both treatment groups required rescue analgesia (morphine) in approximately 50% of patients. Intriguingly, pain scores for dogs receiving dexmedetomidine CRIs and morphine rescue analgesia were *lower* than those dogs receiving morphine CRIs and given morphine rescue analgesia [21]. This suggests the combination of $\alpha_2$ adrenergic agonists and opioid was *more* effective than an opioid alone – supporting the importance of multimodal analgesia.

#### 6.6.3.2   Opioids and Nonsteroidal Anti-inflammatory Drugs (NSAIDs)

In veterinary species, a similar synergism is demonstrated between NSAIDs and opioids. Martins and his colleagues evaluated somatic pain of bone origin in the dog with a maxillectomy or mandibulectomy as a model. A significant degree of pain is the anticipated consequence with such procedures. This work is particularly pertinent to the field, in that it suggests that while opioids are essential parts of an analgesic plan, NSAIDs combined with weak opioid agonists may also provide adequate analgesia [57]. Both opioids used (codeine and tramadol) are weak opioids in dogs, with little demonstrable analgesia on their own [58]. Adding an NSAID allowed these weak opioids to be used as effective analgesics for these procedures. This is particularly important for fieldwork, where there are little other options than NSAIDs, with or without tramadol postoperatively.

The combination of an opioid and a NSAID in cats is also reported to be beneficial in cats. Two studies combined tramadol with an NSAID in cats undergoing ovariohysterectomy and suggested this combination provided better analgesia than either drug used alone [59, 60]. More recent work with robenacoxib suggests that this NSAID combined with buprenorphine does not offer a significant advantage over robenacoxib alone [61]. Robenacoxib showed superiority over meloxicam when only an NSAID was used for soft tissue surgeries in cats [62]. Robenacoxib may provide sufficient analgesia that it is difficult to see additional benefits when combining an opioid; however, it may be that our ability to assess pain in cats still requires improvement. In short, although information is limited, there appears to be no harm from including both an opioid and an NSAID, and one can harness the benefit of preemptive analgesia and a reduction in drug requirements conferred by the inclusion of an opioid.

*This chapter is dedicated to beautiful, bright stars, such as Dr. O Sogebi, who create hope by envisioning and fighting for a reality that does not yet exist.*

# Appendix

## 6.A   Glasgow Composite Pain Scale Short Form (Canine)

### 6.A.1   Glasgow Composite Measure Pain Score: CMPS – Short Form

#### 6.A.1.1   Guidance for Use

The short form composite measure pain score (CMPS-SF) can be applied quickly and reliably in a clinical setting and has been designed as a clinical decision-making tool developed for dogs in acute pain. It includes 30 descriptor options within 6 behavioral categories, including mobility. Within each category, the descriptors are ranked numerically according to their associated pain severity, and the person carrying out the assessment chooses the descriptor within each category which best fits the dog's behavior/condition. It is important to carry out the assessment procedure as described on the questionnaire, following the protocol closely. The pain score is the sum of the rank scores. The maximum score for the 6 categories is 24 or 20 if mobility is impossible to assess. The total CMPS-SF score has been shown to be a useful indicator of analgesic requirement, and the recommended analgesic intervention level is 6/24 or 5/20.

## 6.A   Glasgow Composite Pain Scale Short Form (Canine) (*Continued*)

### SHORT FORM OF THE GLASGOW COMPOSITE MEASURE PAIN SCALE

**Dog's name** _                       Date    /    /        Time

**Hospital Number** _____

**Procedure or Condition** _____

_____

*In the sections below please circle the appropriate score in each list and sum these to give the total score*

### A. Look at dog in Kennel
*Is the dog*

(i)
| | |
|---|---|
| Quiet | 0 |
| Crying or whimpering | 1 |
| Groaning | 2 |
| Screaming | 3 |

(ii)
| | |
|---|---|
| Ignoring any wound or painful area | 0 |
| Looking at wound or painful area | 1 |
| Licking wound or painful area | 2 |
| Rubbing wound or painful area | 3 |
| Chewing wound or painful area. | 4 |

In the case of spinal, pelvic or multiple limb fractures, or where assistance is required to aid locomotion do not carry out section **B** and proceed to **C**
*Please tick if this is the case* ☐ then proceed to C

### B. Put lead on dog and lead out of the kennel
*When the dog rises/walks is it?*

(iii)
| | |
|---|---|
| Normal | 0 |
| Lame | 1 |
| Slow or reluctant | 2 |
| Stiff | 3 |
| It refuses to move | 4 |

### C. If it has a wound or painful area including abdomen, apply gentle pressure 2 inches round the site
*Does it?*

(iv)
| | |
|---|---|
| Do nothing | 0 |
| Look round | 1 |
| Flinch | 2 |
| Growl or guard area | 3 |
| Snap | 4 |
| Cry | 5 |

### D. Overall
*Is the dog?*

(v)
| | |
|---|---|
| Happy and content or happy and bouncy | 0 |
| Quiet | 1 |
| Indifferent or non-responsive to surroundings | 2 |
| Nervous or anxious or fearful | 3 |
| Depressed or non-responsive to stimulation | 4 |

*Is the dog?*

(vi)
| | |
|---|---|
| Comfortable | 0 |
| Unsettled | 1 |
| Restless | 2 |
| Hunched or tense | 3 |
| Rigid | 4 |

### Total Score (i+ii+iii+iv+v+vi) = _____

Source: Courtesy of University of Glasgow.

## 6.B   UNESP-Botucatu Scale

UNESP-Botucatu Multidimensional Composite Pain Scale for assessing postoperative pain in cats.

| | **Subscale 1: PAIN EXPRESSION (0 – 12)** | |
|---|---|---|
| **Miscellaneous behaviors** | Observe and mark the presence of the behaviors listed below | |
| | **A** - The cat is laying down and quiet, but moving its tail | A |
| | **B** - The cat contracts and extends its pelvic limbs and/or contracts its abdominal muscles (flank) | B |
| | **C** - The cats eyes are partially closed (eyes half closed) | C |
| | **D** - The cat licks and/or bites the surgical wound | D |
| | • All above behaviors are absent | 0 |
| | • Presence of one of the above behaviors | 1 |
| | • Presence of two of the above behaviors | 2 |
| | • Presence of three or all of the above behaviors | 3 |
| **Reaction to palpation of the surgical wound** | • The cat does not react when the surgical wound is touched or pressed; or no change from pre-surgical response (if basal evaluation was made) | 0 |
| | • The cat does not react when the surgical wound is touched, but does react when it is pressed. It may vocalize and/or try to bite | 1 |
| | • The cat reacts when the surgical wound is touched and when pressed. It may vocalize and/or try to bite | 2 |
| | • The cat reacts when the observer approaches the surgical wound. It may vocalize and/or try to bite The cat does not allow palpation ofthe surgical wound | 3 |
| **Reaction to palpation ofthe abdomen/flank** | • The cat does not react when the abdomen/flank is touched or pressed; or no change from pre-surgical response (if basal evaluation was made). The abdomen/flank is not tense | 0 |
| | • The cat does not react when the abdomen/flank is touched, but does react when it is pressed. The abdomen/flank is tense | 1 |
| | • The cat reacts when the abdomen/flank is touched and when pressed. The abdomen/flank is tense | 2 |
| | • The cat reacts when the observer approaches the abdomen/flank. It may vocalize and/or try to bite The cat does not allow palpation of the abdomen/flank | 3 |
| **Vocalization** | • The cat is quiet, purring when stimulated, or miaows interacting with the observer, but does not growl, groan, or hiss | 0 |
| | • The cat purrs spontaneously (without being stimulated or handled by the observer) | 1 |
| | • The cat growls, howls, or hisses when handled by the observer (when its body position is changed by the observer) | 2 |
| | • The cat growls, howls, hisses spontaneously (without being stimulated or handled by the observer) | 3 |

## 6.B UNESP-Botucatu Scale (*Continued*)

| | | |
|---|---|---|
| | **Subscale 2: PSYCHOMOTOR CHANGE (0 – 12)** | |
| **Posture** | • The cat is in a natural posture with relaxed muscles (it moves normally) | 0 |
| | • The cat is in a natural posture but is tense (it moves little or is reluctant to move) | 1 |
| | • The cat is sitting or in sternal recumbency with its back arched and head down; or <br> The cat is in dorso-lateral recumbency with its pelvic limbs extended or contracted | 2 |
| | • The cat frequently alters its body position in an attempt to find a comfortable posture | 3 |
| **Comfort** | • The cat is comfortable, awake or asleep, and interacts when stimulated (it interacts with the observer and/or is interested in its surroundings) | 0 |
| | • The cat is quiet and slightly receptive when stimulated (it interacts little with the observer and/or is not very interested in its surroundings) | 1 |
| | • The cat is quiet and "dissociated from the environment" (even when stimulated it does not interact with the observer and/or has no interest in its surroundings) <br> The cat may be facing the back of the cage | 2 |
| | • The cat is uncomfortable, restless (frequently changes its body position), and slightly receptive when stimulated or "dissociated from the environment" <br> The cat may be facing the back of the cage | 3 |
| **Activity** | • The cat moves normally (it immediately moves when the cage is opened; outside the cage it moves spontaneously when stimulated or handled) | 0 |
| | • The cat moves more than normal (inside the cage it moves continuously from side to side) | 1 |
| | • The cat is quieter than normal (it may hesitate to leave the cage and if removed from the cage tends to return, outside the cage it moves a little after stimulation or handling) | 2 |
| | • The cat is reluctant to move (it may hesitate to leave the cage and if removed from the cage tends to return, outside the cage it does not move even when stimulated or handled) | 3 |
| **Attitude** | Observe and mark the presence of the mental states listed below | |
| | **A - Satisfied:** The cat is alert and interested in its surroundings (explores its surroundings), friendly and interactive with the observer (plays and/or responds to stimuli) <br> *The cat may initially interact with the observer through games to distract it from the pain. Carefully observe to distinguish between distraction and satisfaction games | A |
| | **B - Uninterested:** The cat does not interact with the observer (not interested by toys or plays a little; does not respond to calls or strokes from the observer) <br> *In cats which don't like to play, evaluate interaction with the observer by its response to calls and strokes | B |
| | **C - Indifferent:** The cat is not interested in its surroundings (it is not curious; it does not explore its surroundings) <br> *The cat can initially be afraid to explore its surroundings. The observer needs to handle the cat and encourage it to move itself (take it out of the cage and/or change its body position) | C |
| | **D - Anxious:** The cat is frightened (it tries to hide or escape) or nervous (demonstrating impatience and growling, howling, or hissing when stroked and/or handled) | D |
| | **E - Aggressive:** The cat is aggressive (tries to bite or scratch when stroked or handled) | E |
| | • Presence of the mental state A | 0 |
| | • Presence of one of the mental states B, C, D, or E | 1 |
| | • Presence of two of the mental states B, C, D, or E | 2 |
| | • Presence of three or all of the mental states B, C, D, or E | 3 |

## 6.B UNESP-Botucatu Scale (*Continued*)

| | | Subscale 3: PHYSIOLOGICAL VARIABLES (0 – 6) | |
|---|---|---|---|
| **Arterial blood pressure** | • 0% to 15% above pre-surgery value | | 0 |
| | • 16% to 29% above pre-surgery value | | 1 |
| | • 30% to 45% above pre-surgery value | | 2 |
| | • > 45% above pre-surgery value | | 3 |
| **Appetite** | • The cat is eating normally | | 0 |
| | • The cat is eating more than normal | | 1 |
| | • The cat is eating less than normal | | 2 |
| | • The cat is not interested in food | | 3 |

**TOTAL SCORE (0 – 30)**

### Directions for using the scale

Initially observe the cat's behavior without opening the cage. Observe whether it is resting or active; interested or uninterested in its surroundings; quiet or vocal. Check for the presence of specific behaviors (see "Miscellaneous behaviors"above).

Open the cage and observe whether the cat quickly moves out or hesitates to leave the cage. Approach the cat and evaluate its reaction: friendly, aggressive, frightened, indifferent, or vocal. Touch the cat and interact with it, check whether it is receptive (if it likes to be stroked and/or is interested in playing). If the cat hesitates to leave the cage, encourage it to move through stimuli (call it by name and stroke it) and handling (change its body position and/or take it out of the cage). Observe when outside the cage, if the cat moves spontaneously, in a reserved manner, or is reluctant to move. Offer it palatable food and observe its response.*

Finally, place the cat in lateral or sternal recumbency and measure its arterial blood pressure. Evaluate the cat's reaction when the abdomen/flank is initially touched (slide your fingers over the area) and in the sequence gently pressed (apply direct pressure over the area). Wait for a time, and do the same procedure to assess the cat's reaction to palpation of surgical wound.

*To evaluate appetite during the immediate postoperative period, initially offer a small quantity of palatable food immediately after recovery from anesthesia. At this moment most cats eat normally independent of the presence or absence of pain. Wait a short while, offer food again, and observe the cat's reaction.

Source: Brondani et al. [52], https://bmcvetres.biomedcentral.com/articles/10.1186/1746-6148-9-143.CC BY 2.0.

## 6.C Glasgow Composite Pain Scale (Feline)

### 6.C.1 Glasgow Composite Measure Pain Score: CMPS-Feline

#### 6.C.1.1 Guidance for Use

The Glasgow Feline Composite Measure Pain Scale (CMPS-Feline), which can be applied quickly and reliably in a clinical setting, has been designed as a clinical decision-making tool for use in cats in acute pain. It includes 28 descriptor options within 7 behavioral categories. Within each category, the descriptors are ranked numerically according to their associated pain severity, and the person carrying out the assessment chooses the descriptor within each category which best fits the cat's behavior/condition. It is important to carry out the assessment procedure as described on the questionnaire, following the protocol closely. The pain score is the sum of the rank scores. The maximum score for the 7 categories is 20. The total CMPS-Feline score has been shown to be a useful indicator of analgesic requirement and the recommended analgesic intervention level is 5/20.

## 6.C  Glasgow Composite Pain Scale (Feline) (*Continued*)

### Glasgow Feline Composite Measure Pain Scale: CMPS - Feline

Choose the most appropriate expression from each section and total the scores to calculate the pain score for the cat. If more than one expression applies choose the higher score

**LOOK AT THE CAT IN ITS CAGE:**

Is it?
**_Question 1_**

| | |
|---|---|
| Silent / purring / meowing | 0 |
| Crying/growling / groaning | 1 |

**_Question 2_**

| | |
|---|---|
| Relaxed | 0 |
| Licking lips | 1 |
| Restless/cowering at back of cage | 2 |
| Tense/crouched | 3 |
| Rigid/hunched | 4 |

**_Question 3_**

| | |
|---|---|
| Ignoring any wound or painful area | 0 |
| Attention to wound | 1 |

**_Question 4_**

    a) Look at the following caricatures. Circle the drawing which best depicts the cat's ear position?

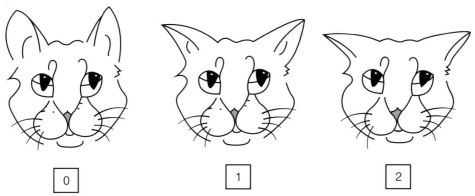

        0        1        2

    b) Look at the shape of the muzzle in the following caricatures. Circle the drawing which appears most like that of the cat?

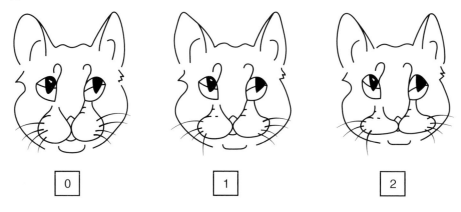

        0        1        2

## 6.C   Glasgow Composite Pain Scale (Feline) (*Continued*)

**APPROACH THE CAGE, CALL THE CAT BY NAME & STROKE ALONG ITS BACK FROM HEAD TO TAIL**

### *Question 5*
Does it?

|  |  |
|---|---|
| Respond to stroking | 0 |

Is it?

|  |  |
|---|---|
| Unresponsive | 1 |
| Aggressive | 2 |

**IF IT HAS A WOUND OR PAINFUL AREA, APPLY GENTLE PRESSURE 5 CM AROUND THE SITE. IN THE ABSENCE OF ANY PAINFUL AREA APPLY SIMILAR PRESSURE AROUND THE HIND LEG ABOVE THE KNEE**

### *Question 6*
Does it?

|  |  |
|---|---|
| Do nothing | 0 |
| Swish tail/flatten ears | 1 |
| Cry/hiss | 2 |
| Growl | 3 |
| Bite/lash out | 4 |

### *Question 7*
General impression

Is the cat?

|  |  |
|---|---|
| Happy and content | 0 |
| Disinterested/quiet | 1 |
| Anxious/fearful | 2 |
| Dull | 3 |
| Depressed/grumpy | 4 |

**Pain Score ... /20**

Source: Courtesy of University of Glasgow.

## 6.D   Sample Anesthetic Protocols

The following section includes anesthetic protocols compiled by the editors that are currently in use by various animal welfare organizations for spay/neuter procedures in the field. Most assume a lack of anesthetic gas, unless otherwise stated. Some protocols are comprehensive, inclusive of supplemental analgesia while others include anesthetic agents only. While these protocols are meant to serve as a reference for animal welfare organizations performing spay/neuter procedures, protocols should be tailored to the specific working environment and patient.

### 6.D.1   Feline-Specific Anesthetic Protocols

#### 6.D.1.1   Telazol/Butorphanol/Medetomidine (TTMed)

| Feline drug protocol | | | |
| --- | --- | --- | --- |
| Weight (lbs) | TT Med IM (cc) | Meloxicam SQ (cc) | Atipamezole IM (cc) |
| 1 | 0.01 | 0.01 | 0.01 |
| 1.5 | 0.02 | 0.01 | 0.02 |
| 2 | 0.03 | 0.02 | 0.02 |
| 2.5 | 0.03 | 0.02 | 0.03 |
| 3 | 0.04 | 0.03 | 0.04 |
| 3.5 | 0.05 | 0.03 | 0.05 |
| 4 | 0.05 | 0.04 | 0.06 |
| 4.5 | 0.06 | 0.04 | 0.06 |
| 5 | 0.07 | 0.05 | 0.07 |
| 6 | 0.08 | 0.05 | 0.07 |
| 7 | 0.10 | 0.06 | 0.08 |
| 8 | 0.11 | 0.07 | 0.09 |
| 9 | 0.12 | 0.08 | 0.10 |
| 10 | 0.12 | 0.09 | 0.11 |
| 11 | 0.13 | 0.10 | 0.12 |
| 12 | 0.13 | 0.11 | 0.14 |

| Drug | Concentration | Dosage | Route | Purpose |
| --- | --- | --- | --- | --- |
| TT Med | — | 0.03 ml/kg | IM | Induction |
| Meloxicam | 5 mg/ml | 0.1 mg/kg | SQ | NSAID |
| Atipamezole | 2 mg/ml | 0.1 mg/kg | IM | Reversal |

TTMed = One bottle of Telazol reconstituted with:
2.5 cc Butorphanol (10 mg/ml)
2.5 cc Medetomidine (1 mg/ml)
Source: Courtesy of Animal Balance.

#### 6.D.1.2   Telazol/Ketamine/Xylazine (TKX)

TKX = Telazol or Zoletil 100 (500 mg), ketamine (100 mg/ml), xylazine (100 mg/ml).

To mix, add 4.0 ml ketamine to 1 unconstituted bottle of Telazol, then add 0.8 ml xylazine (80 mg). This creates a total volume of 4.8 ml TKX cocktail.

| Weight (lbs) | Weight (kg) | Initial IM TKX Dose (ml) | TKX Redose (ml) | Buprenorphine (0.3 mg/ml) |
| --- | --- | --- | --- | --- |
| 3 | 1.4 | 0.07 | 0.02 | 0.05 |
| 4–5 | 1.8–2.3 | 0.10 | 0.03 | 0.10 |
| 5–6 | 2.3–2.7 | 0.12 | 0.04 | 0.10 |
| 6–9 | 2.7–4.1 | 0.15 | 0.05 | 0.15 |
| >10 | >4.5 | 0.20 | 0.05 | 0.15 |

Source: Data from Feral Cat Coalition.

## 6.D  Sample Anesthetic Protocols (*Continued*)

### Redose
If the cat is waking up prematurely, administer an additional dose of TKX (see column titled redose). Alternatively, for males undergoing a routine neuter and females that are close to the end of their procedure, inhalant anesthesia may substitute another dose of TKX.

### Reversal
Reversal (if needed) is achieved with yohimbine (2 mg/ml) 0.5 ml/cat IM or IV.

### Analgesia
Buprenorphine (0.3 mg/ml) 0.02–0.04 mg/kg IV, IM, SC, or TM.
   An NSAID may replace the buprenorphine when opioids are unavailable.

### 6.D.1.3  Injectable Anesthetic Protocols Commonly Used for Surgical Training in the Field
Feline protocol 1: Xylazine/tramadol/ketamine/diazepam.

|  | Medication | Route | Dose |
| --- | --- | --- | --- |
| Premedication | Xylazine | IM | 1 mg/kg (1.2–1.5 mg/kg if aggressive) |
|  | Tramadol | IM | 2.5 mg/kg |
| Induction | Ketamine | IV | 5 mg/kg |
|  | Diazepam | IV | 0.5 mg/kg (0.25 mg/kg if diazepam is limited) |
| Maintenance | Ketamine | IV | 5 mg/kg |
|  | Diazepam | IV | 0.25 mg/kg |
|  | Xylazine | IV | 0.25 mg/kg (can usually start with 1/3 to 1/2 of this dose) |

Feline protocol 2: Xylazine/tramadol/ketamine.

|  | Medication | Route | Dose |
| --- | --- | --- | --- |
| Premedication | Xylazine | IM | 1 mg/kg (1.2–1.5 mg/kg if aggressive) |
|  | Tramadol | IM | 2.5 mg/kg |
| Induction | Ketamine | IV | 5 mg/kg |
|  | OR |  |  |
|  | Ketamine | IM | 11 mg/kg |
| Maintenance | Ketamine | IV | 5 mg/kg |
|  | Xylazine | IV | 0.25 mg/kg |

Feline protocol 3: Xylazine/tramadol/Telazol.

|  | Medication | Route | Dose |
| --- | --- | --- | --- |
| Premedication | Xylazine | IM | 1 mg/kg (1.2–1.5 mg/kg if aggressive) |
|  | Tramadol | IM | 2.5 mg/kg |
| Induction | Telazol (Zoletil 100) | IV | 5 mg/kg |

*(continued)*

## 6.D Sample Anesthetic Protocols (*Continued*)

(*Continued*)

| | Medication | Route | Dose |
|---|---|---|---|
| | OR | | |
| | Telazol (Zoletil 100) | IM | 11 mg/kg |
| Maintenance | Telazol (Zoletil 100) | IV | 5 mg/kg |
| | Xylazine | IV | 0.25 mg/kg |

Source: Courtesy of International Veterinary Consultants.

### 6.D.2 Canine-specific anesthetic protocols

#### 6.D.2.1 Telazol/Butorphanol/Medetomidine (TTMed)

| Canine drug protocol | | | | |
|---|---|---|---|---|
| Weight (lbs) | TTMed IM (cc) | Meloxicam SQ (cc) | TTMed IV (cc) | Atipamezole IM (cc) |
| 1 | 0.01 | No NSAIDs | 0.01 | 0.01 |
| 2 | 0.03 | — | 0.01 | 0.02 |
| 3 | 0.04 | — | 0.02 | 0.02 |
| 4 | 0.05 | — | 0.03 | 0.03 |
| 5 | 0.07 | 0.09 | 0.03 | 0.04 |
| 6 | 0.08 | 0.11 | 0.04 | 0.05 |
| 8 | 0.11 | 0.15 | 0.05 | 0.06 |
| 10 | 0.14 | 0.18 | 0.07 | 0.08 |
| 12 | 0.16 | 0.22 | 0.08 | 0.10 |
| 14 | 0.19 | 0.25 | 0.10 | 0.11 |
| 16 | 0.22 | 0.29 | 0.11 | 0.13 |
| 18 | 0.25 | 0.33 | 0.12 | 0.14 |
| 20 | 0.27 | 0.36 | 0.14 | 0.16 |
| 25 | 0.34 | 0.45 | 0.17 | 0.20 |
| 30 | 0.41 | 0.55 | 0.20 | 0.24 |
| 35 | 0.41 | 0.64 | 0.20 | 0.28 |
| 40 | 0.45 | 0.73 | 0.23 | 0.32 |
| 45 | 0.51 | 0.82 | 0.26 | 0.36 |
| 50 | 0.57 | 0.91 | 0.28 | 0.40 |
| 60 | 0.68 | 1.09 | 0.34 | 0.48 |
| 70 | 0.80 | 1.27 | 0.40 | 0.56 |
| 80 | 0.91 | 1.45 | 0.45 | 0.64 |

## 6.D    Sample Anesthetic Protocols (*Continued*)

| Drug | Concentration | Route | Dosage | Purpose |
|------|---------------|-------|--------|---------|
| TTMed | — | IM | ≈0.03 ml/kg | Induction and maintenance of anesthesia |
| TTMed | — | IV | ≈0.015 ml/kg | |
| Meloxicam | 5 mg/ml | SQ | 0.20 mg/kg | NSAID |
| Atipamezole | 2 mg/ml | IM | 0.1 mg/kg | Reversal |

TTMed = One bottle of Telazol reconstituted with:
2.5 cc Butorphanol (10 mg/ml)
2.5 cc Medetomidine (1 mg/ml)
Source: Courtesy of Animal Balance.

- TTMed can be administered IV or IM. The IV dose is half the recommended IM dose.
- Listed doses are for a surgical plane of anesthesia lasting approximately 30 min. If surgery will last longer than 30 min and gas anesthesia is available, the patient should be placed on isoflurane or sevoflurane supplementation as needed. If gas anesthesia is unavailable, a second dose of TTMed (half the original volume) can be administered.
- The dexmedetomidine within the TTDex can be reversed with atipamezole (see dosing chart).

### 6.D.2.2    Injectable Anesthetic Protocols Commonly Used for Surgical Training in the Field

Canine protocol 1: Xylazine/tramadol/ketamine/diazepam.

| | Medication | Route | Dose |
|---|-----------|-------|------|
| Premedication | Xylazine | IM | 1.2 mg/kg (1.5–1.8 mg/kg if aggressive) |
| | Tramadol | IM | 3 mg/kg |
| Induction | Ketamine | IV | 5 mg/kg |
| | Diazepam | IV | 0.5 mg/kg (0.25 mg/kg if diazepam is limited) |
| Maintenance | Ketamine | IV | 5 mg/kg |
| | Diazepam | IV | 0.25 mg/kg |
| | Xylazine | IV | 0.25 mg/kg |

Canine protocol 2: Xylazine/tramadol/ketamine.

| | Medication | Route | Dose |
|---|-----------|-------|------|
| Premedication | Xylazine | IM | 1.2 mg/kg (1.5–1.8 mg/kg if aggressive) |
| | Tramadol | IM | 3 mg/kg |
| Induction | Ketamine | IV | 5 mg/kg |
| | OR | | |
| | Ketamine | IM | 11 mg/kg |
| Maintenance | Ketamine | IV | 5 mg/kg |
| | Xylazine | IV | 0.25 mg/kg |

## 6.D    Sample Anesthetic Protocols (*Continued*)

Canine protocol 3: Xylazine/tramadol/Telazol.

|  | Medication | Route | Dose |
|---|---|---|---|
| Premedication | Xylazine | IM | 1.2 mg/kg (1.5–1.8 mg/kg if aggressive) |
|  | Tramadol | IM | 3 mg/kg |
| Induction | Telazol (Zoletil 100) | IV | 5 mg/kg |
|  | OR |  |  |
|  | Telazol (Zoletil 100) | IM | 11 mg/kg |
| Maintenance | Telazol (Zoletil 100) | IV | 5 mg/kg |
|  | Xylazine | IV | 0.25 mg/kg |

Source: Courtesy of International Veterinary Consultants.

### 6.D.2.3    Anesthetic Protocols Used in Canine Catch-Vaccinate-Neuter-Return (CVNR) Programs

*Premedication*
Xylazine (20 mg/ml) 1–2 mg/kg IM (recommended maximum dose 2.0 ml)

- In young dogs (6–12 weeks of age), administer 0.5 mg/kg xylazine.
- Avoid if hypotension, hypovolemia, heart, or liver disease is present.

  OR
  Phenothiazine tranquilizer (i.e. triflupromazine, acepromazine) + (opiate analgesic or tramadol)

- Note that phenothiazines have no analgesic properties.
- Triflupromazine (Siquil) 2.2–4 mg/kg IM (use low end if combining with tramadol).

*Induction (to be given 10 min after administration of premedication)*
Ketamine (50 mg/ml) 2.5 mg/kg + diazepam (5 mg/ml) 0.25 mg/kg

- Mix equal parts in the same syringe.
- Give IV at a rate of 1.0 ml mixture per 10 kg, use top-up doses if required.
- Some clinics use two parts ketamine to one part diazepam in the mixture for top-up doses.
- When performing a high volume of surgeries, multiple 10 ml syringes of the mixture can be prepared at the start of the day.

  OR
  Xylazine (20 mg/ml) + ketamine (50 mg/ml)

- Mix in the same syringe one part xylazine to two parts ketamine (i.e. 3.0 ml xylazine to 6.0 ml ketamine).
- Give IV at a dose of 2.0 ml for 10 kg, 3.0 ml for 20 kg, 4.0 ml for 40 kg.
- Give top-up doses of 0.5 ml IV, if necessary.

  OR
  Thiopentone 2.5% IV

- A 2.5% solution is preferred to reduce the risk of severe perivascular reaction.
- Administer thiopentone (2.5% solution) at 4.0 ml/10 kg to a premedicated patient.
- Avoid use in cachexic, very lean, and geriatric patients.
- Avoid perivascular injection.

## 6.D  Sample Anesthetic Protocols (*Continued*)

- Administer small IV boluses if needed. Note that this will lead to prolonged anesthesia and longer recovery times.
- Less analgesic effect than ketamine (therefore premedication should include xylazine or opioids).

For all protocols: place an endotracheal tube immediate following induction to secure the airway and prevent inhalation of gastric contents should vomiting occur.

### Maintenance

- Ideally, inhalation anesthetic agents such as isoflurane should be used, in combination with medical oxygen.
- In the absence of inhalation agents, anesthesia can be maintained using incremental administration of induction agents.
- Ensure very careful placement of an IV catheter and tape securely to the limb. Monitor the depth of anesthesia closely to determine when top-up doses are needed.
- Intravenous fluids (preferably warmed to body temperature) are routinely administered intraoperatively.

### Recovery

- Provide an NSAID (i.e. meloxicam 0.2 mg/kg) following removal of the ET tube.

Source: Courtesy of Vets Beyond Borders.

### 6.D.3  Injectable Anesthetic Protocols Using Propofol

#### 6.D.3.1  Propofol Protocol 1 (Canine)

*Premedication*
Xylazine (20 mg/ml): 2 mg/kg (not more than 2.5 ml/dog) IM.
(If available, combine xylazine with butorphanol: 0.2 mg/kg IM)

*Induction*
Induction drugs are administered following the placement of an IV catheter:
Diazepam: 0.25 mg/kg IV.
Lidocaine: 1 mg/kg IV.
Propofol: 1 mg/kg IV slowly.

*Also given at the time of induction:*

Tramadol: 5–8 mg/kg IV.
Carprofen: 4 mg/kg IV.

*Maintenance*
Propofol 1 mg/kg IV as needed, based on depth of anesthesia (on average every 10 min).

IV fluids are administered throughout the procedure. A total of 3.0 ml of lidocaine (20 mg/ml) can be added to a 500 ml bag of normal saline or maintenance crystalloid fluids and administered at a routine anesthetic fluid rate throughout the procedure for additional analgesia. Using a fluid rate of 10 ml/kg/h will provide a constant rate infusion of 20 µg/kg/min. If needed, the dose can be doubled by increasing the fluid rate to 20 ml/kg/h. In the author's experience, using a lidocaine CRI intraoperatively can significant reduce the amount of propofol needed for maintenance of anesthesia.

Source: Courtesy of Dr. Maiju Tamminen.

## 6.D   Sample Anesthetic Protocols (*Continued*)

### 6.D.3.2   Propofol Protocol 2

*Premedication*
Xylazine (20 mg/ml): 1.0–2.0 mg/kg IM.

*Induction*
Propofol to effect: 3.0–5.0 mg/kg IV.
If diazepam is available, use at 0.25 mg/kg in conjunction with propofol:

- Protocol A – Give diazepam IV first, *flush catheter*, then administer propofol IV titrated to effect.
- Protocol B – Give 1/3 propofol IV, *flush catheter*, administer diazepam IV, *flush catheter*, then administer remainder of propofol titrated to effect.

*Maintenance*
Administer 0.2 mg/kg intermittent boluses of propofol in response to HR, RR, BP, and reflexes.
Start at 0.2 mg/kg and increase or decrease by 0.05 mg/kg increments based on monitoring parameters.

Source: Courtesy of International Veterinary Consultants

### 6.D.3.3   Propofol Protocol 3

*Premedication*
Same as propofol protocol 2.

*Induction*
Same as propofol protocol 2.

*Maintenance*
Administer propofol as a CRI – 0.05–0.1 mg/kg/min.

Source: Courtesy of International Veterinary Consultants.

### 6.D.4   Telazol–Torbugesic–Dexdomitor (TTDex) Dosing Chart for Cats and Dogs

TTDex = Combine 2.5 ml dexmedetomidine (500 mcg/ml) and 2.5 ml butorphanol (10 mg/ml) with 1 bottle (500 mg) of Telazol powder.

## 6.D    Sample Anesthetic Protocols (*Continued*)

| Weight (lbs) | Weight (kg) | Mild sedation (0.005 ml/kg IM) (ml) | Moderate sedation (0.01 ml/kg IM) (ml) | Profound sedation (0.02 ml/kg IM) (ml) | Surgical anesthesia (0.035 ml/kg IM) (ml) | Profound surgical anesthesia (0.04 ml/kg IM) (ml) |
|---|---|---|---|---|---|---|
| 2–4 | 1–2 | 0.005 | 0.01 | 0.02 | 0.035 | 0.04 |
| 4–7 | 2–3 | 0.013 | 0.025 | 0.05 | 0.09 | 0.12 |
| 7–9 | 3–4 | 0.018 | 0.035 | 0.07 | 0.12 | 0.15 |
| 9–11 | 4–5 | 0.023 | 0.045 | 0.09 | 0.16 | 0.19 |
| 11–22 | 5–10 | 0.038 | 0.075 | 0.15 | 0.26 | 0.37 |
| 22–29 | 10–13 | 0.06 | 0.12 | 0.24 | 0.40 | 0.48 |
| 29–33 | 13–15 | 0.07 | 0.14 | 0.28 | 0.49 | 0.58 |
| 33–44 | 15–20 | 0.09 | 0.18 | 0.36 | 0.61 | 0.78 |
| 44–55 | 20–25 | 0.12 | 0.23 | 0.46 | 0.79 | 0.98 |
| 55–66 | 25–30 | 0.14 | 0.28 | 0.56 | 0.96 | 1.25 |
| 66–73 | 30–33 | 0.16 | 0.32 | 0.64 | 1.10 | 1.30 |
| 73–81 | 33–37 | 0.18 | 0.35 | 0.70 | 1.20 | 1.45 |
| 81–99 | 37–45 | 0.21 | 0.41 | 0.82 | 1.44 | 1.70 |
| 99–110 | 45–50 | 0.24 | 0.48 | 0.96 | 1.66 | 1.95 |
| 110–121 | 50–55 | 0.26 | 0.53 | 1.10 | 1.84 | 2.20 |

*Considerations*

- If surgery will last longer than 30 min, the patient should be placed on isoflurane supplementation PRN (lower concentration at start (0.25%) and slowly increase isoflurane concentration to 1.5% by 45 min).
- The dexmedetomidine within the TTDex can be reversed with atipamezole (give half the volume of the TTDex dose IM).

Source: Ko and Berman 2010 [63]. Adapted with permission of Elsevier

### 6.D.5    Canine Anesthetic Dosing Chart Using Inhalant Anesthesia for Maintenance

#### 6.D.5.1    Premedication
Hydromorphone: 0.1 mg/kg with acepromazine 0.05 mg/kg SQ or IM.
Meloxicam: 0.1 mg/kg SQ.

#### 6.D.5.2    Induction
Ketamine: 4–6 mg/kg with midazolam or diazepam (0.35–0.50 mg/kg) IV.

#### 6.D.5.3    Maintenance
Inhalant anesthesia as needed.

## 6.D   Sample Anesthetic Protocols (*Continued*)

| Weight (lbs) | Weight (kg) | Acepromazine (1 mg/ml) SQ or IM (ml) | Hydromorphone (2 mg/ml) SQ or IM (ml) | Ketamine (100 mg/ml) IV (ml) | Midazolam/ Diazepam (5 mg/ml) IV (ml) | Meloxicam (5 mg/ml) SQ (ml) |
|---|---|---|---|---|---|---|
| 2 | 0.9 | 0.10 | 0.10 | 0.05 | 0.05 | 0.02 |
| 3 | 1.4 | 0.10 | 0.10 | 0.08 | 0.08 | 0.03 |
| 4 | 1.8 | 0.10 | 0.10 | 0.11 | 0.11 | 0.04 |
| 5 | 2.3 | 0.10 | 0.10 | 0.14 | 0.14 | 0.05 |
| 6 | 2.7 | 0.20 | 0.20 | 0.16 | 0.16 | 0.05 |
| 7 | 3.2 | 0.20 | 0.20 | 0.19 | 0.19 | 0.06 |
| 8 | 3.6 | 0.20 | 0.20 | 0.22 | 0.22 | 0.07 |
| 9 | 4.1 | 0.20 | 0.20 | 0.24 | 0.24 | 0.08 |
| 10 | 4.5 | 0.20 | 0.20 | 0.27 | 0.27 | 0.09 |
| 11 | 5.0 | 0.50 | 0.30 | 0.30 | 0.30 | 0.10 |
| 12 | 5.4 | 0.50 | 0.30 | 0.30 | 0.30 | 0.12 |
| 15 | 6.8 | 0.50 | 0.30 | 0.40 | 0.40 | 0.14 |
| 20 | 9.1 | 0.50 | 0.40 | 0.60 | 0.60 | 0.18 |
| 25 | 11.4 | 0.70 | 0.50 | 0.70 | 0.70 | 0.20 |
| 30 | 13.6 | 0.70 | 0.65 | 0.80 | 0.80 | 0.30 |
| 35 | 15.9 | 0.10 | 0.75 | 1.00 | 1.00 | 0.30 |
| 40 | 18.2 | 0.10 | 0.85 | 1.10 | 1.20 | 0.35 |
| 45 | 20.5 | 0.10 | 1.00 | 1.10 | 1.50 | 0.40 |
| 50 | 22.7 | 0.10 | 1.10 | 1.20 | 1.80 | 0.45 |
| 55 | 25.0 | 0.10 | 1.20 | 1.30 | 2.00 | 0.50 |
| 60 | 27.3 | 0.10 | 1.30 | 1.40 | 2.40 | 0.55 |
| 65 | 29.5 | 0.10 | 1.40 | 1.50 | 2.60 | 0.60 |
| 70 | 31.8 | 0.10 | 1.50 | 1.60 | 2.90 | 0.65 |
| 75 | 34.1 | 0.10 | 1.60 | 1.70 | 3.40 | 0.70 |

Source: Data from Humane Alliance.

# References

1 Griffin, B., Bushby, P.A., McCobb, E. et al. (2016). The Association of Shelter Veterinarians' 2016 veterinary medical care guidelines for spay-neuter programs. *Journal of the American Veterinary Medical Association* **249** (2): 165–188.

2 Hart, B.L., Hart, L.A., Thigpen, A.P., and Willits, N.H. (2014). Long-term health effects of neutering dogs: comparison of Labrador retrievers with golden retrievers. *PLoS ONE* **9**: e102241.

3 American Society of Anesthesiologists (2014) ASA physical status classification system. https://www.asahq.org/resources/clinical-information/asa-physical-status-classification-system (accessed 24 January 2018).

4 Woodbridge, P.D. (1963). The components of general anesthesia. A plea for the blocking of sensory pathways. *The Journal of the American Medical Association* **186**: 641–655.

5 Chen, Y., Cai, A., Fritz, B.A. et al. (2016). Amnesia of the operating room in the B-unaware and BAG-RECALL clinical trials. *Anesthesia and Analgesia* **122** (4): 1158–1168.

6 Dutton, R.C., Maurer, A.J., Sonner, J.M. et al. (2002). Isoflurane causes anterograde but not retrograde amnesia for pavlovian fear conditioning. *Anesthesiology* **96** (5): 1223–1229.

7 Gaskell, A.L., Jephcott, C.G., Smithells, J.R., and Sleigh, J.W. (2016). Self-administered methoxyflurane for procedural analgesia: experience in a tertiary Australasian centre. *Anaesthesia* **71** (4): 417–423.

8 Purdon, P.L., Sampson, A., Pavone, K.J., and Brown, E.N. (2015). Clinical electroencephalography for anesthesiologists: Part I: background and basic signatures. *Anesthesiology* **123** (4): 937–460.

9 Wagner, B.K., O'Hara, D.A., and Hammond, J.S. (1997). Drugs for amnesia in the ICU. *American Journal of Critical Care* **6** (3): 192–201.

10 Brodbelt, D. (2009). Perioperative mortality in small animal anaesthesia. *The Veterinary Journal* **182** (2): 152–161.

11 Li, G., Warner, M., Lang, B.H. et al. (2009). Epidemiology of anesthesia-related mortality in the United States, 1999–2005. *Anesthesiology* **110** (4): 759–765.

12 Williams, L.S., Levy, J.K., Robertson, S.A., Cistola, A.M., Centonze, L.A. (2002). Use of the anesthetic combination of tiletamine, zolazepam, ketamine, and xylazine for neutering feral cats. *Journal of the American Veterinary Medical Association* **220** (10): 1491–1495. Available at https://doi.org/10.2460/javma.2002.220.1491

13 Yadav, K.K., Clark, L., Tamminen, M., et al. (2016). Comparison between two different injectable anaesthetic techniques: effects on physiological variables, including SpO$_2$. AVA Spring Meeting, Lyon, France (20–22 April 2016).

14 McMillan, M. and Darcy, H. (2016). Adverse event surveillance in small animal anaesthesia: an intervention-based, voluntary reporting audit. *Veterinary Anaesthesia and Analgesia* **43** (2): 128–135.

15 Rigotti, C.F., Jolliffe, C.T., and Leece, E.A. (2015). Effect of prewarming on the body temperature of small dogs undergoing inhalation anesthesia. *Journal of the American Veterinary Medical Association* **247** (7): 765–770.

16 Moola, S. and Lockwood, C. (2011). Effectiveness of strategies for the management and/or prevention of hypothermia within the adult perioperative environment. *International Journal of Evidence-Based Healthcare* **9** (4): 337–345.

17 Bruniges, N., Taylor, P.M., and Yates, D. (2015). Injectable anaesthesia for adult cat and kitten castration: effects of medetomidine, dexmedetomidine and atipamezole on recovery. *Journal of Feline Medicine and Surgery* **18**: 860–867.

18 Sinclair, M.D. (2003). A review of the physiological effects of alpha2-agonists related to the clinical use of medetomidine in small animal practice. *The Canadian Veterinary Journal* **44** (11): 885–897.

19 Hasiuk, M.M., Brown, D., Cooney, C. et al. (2015). Application of fast-track surgery principles to evaluate effects of atipamezole on recovery and analgesia following ovariohysterectomy in cats anesthetized with dexmedetomidine-ketamine-hydromorphone. *Journal of the American Veterinary Medical Association* **246** (6): 645–653.

20 Riviere, J. and Papich, M. (2009). Veterinary Pharmacology and Therapeutics. Ames: Wiley Blackwell.

**21** Valtolina, C., Robben, J.H., Uilenreef, J. et al. (2009). Clinical evaluation of the efficacy and safety of a constant rate infusion of dexmedetomidine for postoperative pain management in dogs. *Veterinary Anaesthesia and Analgesia* **36** (4): 369–383.

**22** Slingsby, L.S., Murrell, J.C., and Taylor, P.M. (2010). Combination of dexmedetomidine with buprenorphine enhances the antinociceptive effect to a thermal stimulus in the cat compared with either agent alone. *Veterinary Anaesthesia and Analgesia* **37** (2): 162–170.

**23** Houghton, K.J., Rech, R.H., Sawyer, D.C. et al. (1991). Dose-response of intravenous butorphanol to increase visceral nociceptive threshold in dogs. *Proceedings of the Society for Experimental Biology and Medicine* **197** (3): 290–296.

**24** Lascelles, B.D. and Robertson, S.A. (2004). Antinociceptive effects of hydromorphone, butorphanol, or the combination in cats. *Journal of Veterinary Internal Medicine* **18** (2): 190–195.

**25** Benitez, M.E., Roush, J.K., KuKanich, B., and McMurphy, R. (2015). Pharmacokinetics of hydrocodone and tramadol administered for control of postoperative pain in dogs following tibial plateau leveling osteotomy. *American Journal of Veterinary Research* **76** (9): 763–770.

**26** Cagnardi, P., Villa, R., Zonca, A. et al. (2011). Pharmacokinetics, intraoperative effect and postoperative analgesia of tramadol in cats. *Research in Veterinary Science* **90** (3): 503–509.

**27** Virk, M.S., Arttamangkul, S., Birdson, W.T., and Williams, J.T. (2009). Buprenorphine is a weak partial agonist that inhibits opioid receptor desensitization. *Journal of Neuroscience* **29** (22): 7341–7348.

**28** Lutfy, K., Eitan, S., Bryant, C.D. et al. (2003). Buprenorphine-induced antinociception is mediated by mu-opioid receptors and compromised by concomitant activation of opioid receptor-like receptors. *Journal of Neuroscience* **23** (32): 10331–10337.

**29** Shih, A.C., Robertson, S., Isaza, N. et al. (2008). Comparison between analgesic effects of buprenorphine, carprofen, and buprenorphine with carprofen for canine ovariohysterectomy. *Veterinary Anaesthesia and Analgesia* **35** (1): 69–79.

**30** Slingsby, L.S., Taylor, P.M., and Waterman-Pearson, A.E. (2006). Effects of two doses of buprenorphine four or six hours apart on nociceptive thresholds, pain and sedation in dogs after castration. *Veterinary Record* **159** (21): 705–711.

**31** Ko, J.C., Freeman, K.J., Barletta, M. et al. (2011). Efficacy of oral transmucosal and intravenous administration of buprenorphine before surgery for postoperative analgesia in dogs undergoing ovariohysterectomy. *Journal of the American Veterinary Medical Association* **238** (3): 318–328.

**32** Warne, L.N., Beths, T., Holm, M. et al. (2014). Evaluation of the perioperative analgesic efficacy of buprenorphine, compared with butorphanol, in cats. *Journal of the American Veterinary Medical Association* **245** (2): 195–202.

**33** Grubb, T.L., Greene, S.A., and Perez, T.E. (2013). Cardiovascular and respiratory effects, and quality of anesthesia produced by alfaxalone administered intramuscularly to cats sedated with dexmedetomidine and hydromorphone. *Journal of Feline Medicine and Surgery* **15** (10): 858–865.

**34** Tamura, J., Ishizuka, T., Fukui, S. et al. (2015). Sedative effects of intramuscular alfaxalone administered to cats. *Journal of Veterinary Medical Science* **77** (8): 897–904.

**35** Tamura, J., Ishizuka, T., Fukui, S. et al. (2015). The pharmacological effects of the anesthetic alfaxalone after intramuscular administration to dogs. *Journal of Veterinary Medical Science* **77** (3): 289–296.

**36** Tamura, J., Ishizuka, T., Fukui, S. et al. (2016). The pharmacological effects of intramuscular administration of alfaxalone combined with medetomidine and butorphanol in dogs. *Journal of Veterinary Medical Science* **78** (6): 929–936.

**37** Le, A. and Patel, S. (2014). Extravasation of noncytotoxic drugs: a review of the literature. *Annals of Pharmacotherapy* **48** (7): 870–886.

**38** Michou, J.N., Leece, E.A., and Brearley, J.C. (2012). Comparison of pain on injection during induction of anaesthesia with alfaxalone and two formulations of propofol in dogs. *Veterinary Anaesthesia and Analgesia* **39** (3): 275–281.

**39** Keates, H. and Whittem, T. (2012). Effect of intravenous dose escalation with alfaxalone and propofol on occurrence of apnoea in the dog. *Research in Veterinary Science* **93** (2): 904–906.

**40** Muir, W., Lerche, P., Wiese, A. et al. (2008). Cardiorespiratory and anesthetic effects of clinical and supraclinical doses of alfaxalone in dogs. *Veterinary Anaesthesia and Analgesia* **35** (6): 451–462.

**41** Muir, W., Lerche, P., Wiese, A. et al. (2009). The cardiorespiratory and anesthetic effects of clinical and supraclinical doses of alfaxalone in cats. *Veterinary Anaesthesia and Analgesia* **36** (1): 42–54.

**42** Gieseg, M., Hon, H., Bridges, J., and Walsh, V. (2014). A comparison of anaesthetic recoveries in cats following induction with either alfaxalone or ketamine and diazepam. *New Zealand Veterinary Journal* **62** (3): 103–109.

**43** Doebeli, A., Michel, E., Bettschart, R. et al. (2013). Apgar score after induction of anesthesia for canine cesarean section with alfaxalone versus propofol. *Theriogenology* **80** (8): 850–854.

**44** Ramoo, S., Bradbury, L.A., Anderson, G.A., and Abraham, L.A. (2013). Sedation of hyperthyroid cats with subcutaneous administration of a combination of alfaxalone and butorphanol. *Australian Veterinary Journal* **91** (4): 131–136.

**45** Hellebrekers, L.J., van Herpen, H., Hird, J.F. et al. (1998). Clinical efficacy and safety of propofol or ketamine anaesthesia in dogs premedicated with medetomidine. *Veterinary Record* **142** (23): 631–634.

**46** Fletcher, D.J., Boller, M., Brainard, B.M. et al. (2012). RECOVER evidence and knowledge gap analysis on veterinary CPR. Part 7: clinical guidelines. *Journal of Veterinary Emergency and Critical Care (San Antonio)* **22** (Suppl. 1): S102–S131.

**47** Mathews, K., Kronen, P.W., Lascelles, D. et al. (2014). Guidelines for recognition, assessment and treatment of pain. *Journal of Small Animal Practice* **55** (6): E10–E68.

**48** Williams, A.C. and Craig, K.D. (2016). Updating the definition of pain. *Pain* **157** (11): 2420–2423.

**49** Bourne, S., Machado, A.G., and Nagel, S.J. (2014). Basic anatomy and physiology of pain pathways. *Neurosurgery Clinics of North America* **25** (4): 629–638.

**50** Morton, C.M., Reid, J., Scott, E.M. et al. (2005). Application of a scaling model to establish and validate an interval level pain scale for assessment of acute pain in dogs. *American Journal of Veterinary Research* **66** (12): 2154–2166.

**51** Reid, J., Nolan, A.M., Hughes, J.M.L. et al. (2007). Development of the short-form Glasgow composite measure pain scale (CMPS-SF) and derivation of an analgesic intervention score. *Animal Welfare* **16** (Suppl. 1): 97–104.

**52** Brondani, J.T., Mama, K.R., Luna, S.P. et al. (2013). Validation of the English version of the UNESP-Botucatu multidimensional composite pain scale for assessing postoperative pain in cats. *BMC Veterinary Research* **9** (1): 143.

**53** de Oliveira, F.A., Luna, S.P., do Amaral, J.B. et al. (2014). Validation of the UNESP-Botucatu unidimensional composite pain scale for assessing postoperative pain in cattle. *BMC Veterinary Research* **10**: 200.

**54** Taffarel, M.O., Luna, S.P., de Oliveira, F.A. et al. (2015). Refinement and partial validation of the UNESP-Botucatu multidimensional composite pain scale for assessing postoperative pain in horses. *BMC Veterinary Research* **11**: 83.

**55** Calvo, G., Holden, E., Reid, J. et al. (2014). Development of a behaviour-based measurement tool with defined intervention level for assessing acute pain in cats. *Journal of Small Animal Practice* **55** (12): 622–629.

**56** Slingsby, L.S. and Taylor, P.M. (2008). Thermal antinociception after dexmedetomidine administration in cats: a dose-finding study. *Journal of Veterinary Pharmacology and Therapeutics* **31** (2): 135–142.

**57** Martins, T.L., Kahvegian, M.A., Noel-Morgan, J. et al. (2010). Comparison of the effects of tramadol, codeine, and ketoprofen alone or in combination on postoperative pain and on concentrations of blood glucose, serum cortisol, and serum interleukin-6 in dogs undergoing maxillectomy or mandibulectomy. *American Journal of Veterinary Research* **71** (9): 1019–1026.

**58** Benitez, M.E., Roush, J.K., McMurphy, R. et al. (2015). Clinical efficacy of hydrocodone-acetaminophen and tramadol for control of postoperative pain in dogs following tibial plateau leveling osteotomy. *American Journal of Veterinary Research* **76** (9): 755–762.

**59** Brondani, J., Loureiro Luna, S.P., Beier, S.L. et al. (2009). Analgesic efficacy of perioperative use of vedaprofen, tramadol or their combination in cats undergoing ovariohysterectomy. *Journal of Feline Medicine and Surgery* **11** (6): 420–429.

**60** Steagall, P.V., Taylor, P.M., Rodrigues, L.C. et al. (2009). Analgesia for cats after ovariohysterectomy with either buprenorphine or carprofen alone or in combination. *Veterinary Record* **164** (12): 359–363.

**61** Staffieri, F., Centonze, P., Gigante, G. et al. (2013). Comparison of the analgesic effects of robenacoxib, buprenorphine and their combination in cats after ovariohysterectomy. *Veterinary Journal* **197** (2): 363–367.

**62** Kamata, M., King, J., Seewald, W. et al. (2012). Comparison of injectable robenacoxib versus meloxicam for peri-operative use in cats: results of a randomised clinical trial. *Veterinary Journal* **193** (1): 114–118.

**63** Ko, J. and Berman, A.G. (2010). Anesthesia in shelter medicine. *Topics in Companion Animal Medicine* **25** (2): 92–97.

# 7

# Regional Anesthesia and Local Blocks

*Carolyn McKune[1] and Amanda Shelby[2]*

[1]*Affiliated Veterinary Specialists, Orange Park Specialty Center, Orange Park, FL 32073, USA*
[2]*Jurox Animal Health, Avon, IN 46123, USA*

*We shall not cease from exploration, and the end of all our exploring will be to arrive where we started and know the place for the first time.*

T.S. Eliot

## 7.1 Introduction

Veterinary medicine has a foundation in large animal medicine, where production and, therefore, profitability were improved for the working class farmer through better care of their stock. In animals so large, local anesthetics coupled with sedation were often the *only* option for an invasive intervention, owing to the high mortality of, and lack of equipment (at that time) for, large animal anesthesia. As the field changed and small animal medicine and surgery rose in popularity, veterinary anesthesia experienced a shift toward general anesthesia and local anesthesia lost favor. However, our human counterparts have revealed the stark cost of excluding a local block, with an increased dependence on pain medication resulting in a major increase in opioid abuse [1]. This, as well as ethical obligations to reduce pain, has driven the emergence of subspecialties in the human arena, such as acute pain teams, who utilize various tools (including local blocks) to reduce perioperative pain, with the intention of reducing the amount of acute pain necessitating treatment and therefore the necessity of opioid analgesia. Although this is a different foundation for local anesthetic use, the goal of reducing the necessity of opioid analgesia aligns nicely with the limited ability of opioids (and in some cases *any* injectable analgesia) in the field (see Chapter 6). Additional benefits of local analgesic techniques include reduced requirements of other anesthetic agents and a lack of controlled substance requirements. However, it is remiss not to point out some of the concerns of local anesthetics:

- Respect the toxic dosage ranges for local anesthetics.
- Accidental injection of bupivacaine in an artery or vein could be fatal. *Always* aspirate before injection of local anesthetic!
- Infection and inflammation at the site of the block may reduce the effectiveness of the block.
- Do not use a local anesthetic block in regions where malignant cells may be spread along the needle track.
- Allow sufficient time for local anesthetic to desensitize the target nerves before attempting to perform the intended procedure.

This chapter is divided into three sections: universal blocks (recommended blocks for all field settings), select blocks (recommended blocks suitable in some circumstance), and reserved blocks (extremely useful blocks but which may be technically difficult or require optimum sterility and equipment).

## 7.2 Universal Blocks

Universal blocks are blocks with all the possible advantages of local anesthetics and minimal

*Field Manual for Small Animal Medicine*, First Edition. Edited by Katherine Polak and Ann Therese Kommedal.
© 2018 John Wiley & Sons, Inc. Published 2018 by John Wiley & Sons, Inc.

consequences. They are blocks suitable to virtually every field situation. Equipment is often minimal and includes local anesthetic, syringes, and small-gauge (25 g) needles, as well as the ability to prepare the site for a local block in a cleanly manner.

### 7.2.1 Digital (Three-point) Block or Ring Block

*Uses*

Procedure requiring desensitization distal to the carpus (e.g. of distal branches of radial, ulnar, and median nerve for areas).

*Practical Points*

- A ring block is alternatively performed for this block. Infuse local anesthetic circumferentially around the distal aspect of the limb by connecting the "blebs" similar to the line block.
- Divided the calculated volume between the two paws (0.9% NaCl is added to increase volume if needed). Deposit a quarter of the volume of local anesthetic for each paw at each site.
- Avoid diluting bupivacaine below 0.25% (2.5 mg/ml), as it may result in a poor block.

---

**Textbox 7.1 Digital radial/ulnar/medial nerve block**

Technique

1) Prepare the site appropriately. (Remember to avoid alcohol for preparation if LASER declaw method is used.)

2) Insert a 25-g needle at the level of the first digit, below the carpal pad. This will allow desensitization of the median nerve (which courses down the medial, palmar aspect of the paw) and the palmar branch of the ulnar nerve.

3) The radial nerve is desensitized in a similar fashion on the dorsal medial aspect of the paw, just above the first digit.

4) To desensitize the dorsal branch of the ulnar nerve (located on the palmar side of the paw), place a 25-g needle dorsal to the carpal pad, laterally.

---

5) Finally, another quarter volume is placed on the dorsal side of the paw at the level of the fifth digit where the ulnar nerve courses over the lateral side.

6) Repeat this procedure on each limb undergoing surgery (Figure 7.1).

Radial/ulnar/median nerve block (Distal)

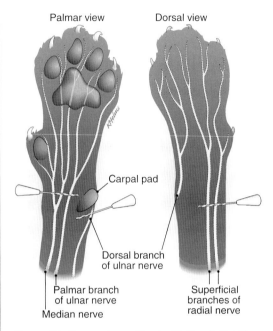

**Figure 7.1** Nerves desensitized with the digital (three point) block or ring block. Source: Courtesy of Teton New Media.

### 7.2.2 Infiltrative or Splash Blocks

*Uses*

Infiltrative blocks are performed before an incision to locally desensitize an area for minor surgical procedures. Splash blocks are performed before closure of an incisional site to provide local analgesia to the incised tissue.

*Practical Points*

- Due to its longer length (up to 3.5 in.), use of a 22-g spinal needle is preferred for infiltrative blocks, to cover a longer distance with a single insertion point.

---

**Textbox 7.2 Infiltrative or splash blocks**

Infiltrative technique

1) An infiltrative block involves the subcutaneous distribution of local anesthetic into tissue surrounding a mass or area of incision.

Splash technique

1) Splash block involves "splashing" local anesthetic on a site after closure of the muscle layer, but before closure of the skin (essentially bathing that area in local anesthetic). Maintaining sterility is important, so the solution is given sterilely to the surgeon or splashed sterilely into incision without contamination by the anesthetist.

---

**Textbox 7.3 Intratesticular block**

Technique

1) Grasp the testicle in the nondominant hand and insert a 25-g needle attached to a lidocaine syringe into the testicle with the dominant hand.

2) For this block in particular, it is critical to aspirate.

3) Inject the appropriate volume into the testicle.

4) Repeat this procedure on the other testicle.

---

### 7.2.3 Intratesticular Block

*Uses*

Lidocaine is, and has been, used for field castration for ages, but like many local blocks, it has fallen out of favor with the advent of general anesthesia. However, studies examining intratesticular block document significantly lower maximum values for both heart rate and mean arterial pressure for dogs receiving a local intratesticular block [2]. Although not statistically significant, it may be clinically significant that only 7 out of 21 dogs in the lidocaine block group required rescue analgesia and 12 out of 21 dogs in the control group required rescue analgesia.

*Practical Points*

- Lidocaine, *not bupivacaine*, is suitable for this block due to the high risk of vascular injection.
- Some surgeons note that there is a change in the appearance of the testicle and that it distorts the anticipated anatomy.
- In general, the amount of local anesthetic is not dosed by weight but by average size of the animal. After calculating the safe dosage of lidocaine for the patient, to ensure we do not exceed this, we will administer roughly 0.5 ml/testicle in cats and small dogs and 1.0 ml/testicle in medium to large dogs.

## 7.3 Select Blocks

Blocks in this section retain all the possible advantages of local anesthetics blocks, but also may have negative consequences if performed in less than ideal circumstances (lacking proper equipment, knowledge, monitoring, etc.). These blocks are often best performed with additional equipment such as a nerve stimulator or an ultrasound unit.

### 7.3.1 Femoral and Sciatic Nerve Block

*Uses*

Hind limb procedures at the level of the stifle and below. Note: for structures distal to stifle (i.e. the hock and below), only the sciatic portion of this nerve block is necessary.

*Practical Points*

- Puncture of the femoral vein or artery, when is not addressed, may result in profound hemorrhage.
- This block is best performed with a nerve stimulator and a 20- to 22-g insulated needle, described below.
- There is a case report series suggesting that this is effective when combined with sedation as a way to avoid general anesthesia for a hind limb procedure [3].
- The femoral and sciatic nerve block is comparable with an epidural for stifle procedures [4].

---

**Textbox 7.4 Femoral and sciatic nerve block**

Technique

1) *Femoral nerve block.* The author prefers the animal in lateral recumbency, with the limb for blockade up. The limb is extended slightly medial and caudally with access to the medial side of the thigh by the nondominant hand, as operator stands near the patient's dorsum. Palpate for the femoral artery in the femoral triangle with the nondominant hand. The femoral nerve courses cranial to the femoral artery, in the femoral triangle (composed of the pectineus, Sartorius, and iliopsoas muscles). The fingers of the nondominant hand gently pull the pulsing artery away from the nerve; introduce the insulated needle. Assess for the twitch of the quadriceps muscle/extension of the stifle at 1 mA. When present, decrease the mAs to 0.4 to ensure the twitch ceases, lending support to positioning the needle perineural rather than intraneural. Aspirate and then deposit local anesthetic.

2) *Sciatic nerve block.* With the patient in lateral recumbency, and the operator against the patient's dorsum, palpate the ischiatic tuberosity. Grasp the biceps femoris with the nondominant hand and elevate this muscle gently to expose the sciatic as it courses between the biceps femoris and semimembranosus/semitendinosus muscles. Insert the insulated needle just below the tuberosity, between the muscle bellies. The nerve stimulator elicits either dorsiflexion or plantar foot extension at 1.0 mAs. Again, assess for twitch at 1 mA. When present, decrease the mAs to 0.4 to ensure the twitch ceases, lending support to positioning the needle perineural rather than intraneural. Aspirate and then deposit local anesthetic.

---

### 7.3.2 Oral Nerve Blocks

*Uses*

Regional blocks of the maxilla and mandible prevent sensation to the teeth and lips (specific to which block is used).

*Practical Points*

- Infection in the oral cavity may reduce the effectiveness of local blocks.
- Due to anatomical limits, the amount of drug administered is often based on the total volume each site requires (0.5–1.0 ml) as opposed to the patient weight; however, especially for smaller patients, toxic doses based on weight are calculated and not exceeded.
- In cats, some of these foramens (such as the infraorbital foramen) are very short; place the needle at the opening of the foramen rather than in the canal to avoid complications.

#### 7.3.2.1 Infraorbital Nerve Block

*Uses*

Procedures of the maxillary dental arcade.

---

**Textbox 7.5 Infraorbital nerve block**

Technique

1) The infraorbital foramen is palpable above the second premolar, on the buccal side of the maxilla.

2) The index finger assists with guiding the needle into the opening of the foramen. Inserting the needle deeper into foramen increases chance of injecting into the nerve.

3) Inject local anesthetic solution around opening of and slightly within the foramen. When correctly placed, there should be very little resistance.

---

#### 7.3.2.2 Mandibular Nerve Block

*Uses*

Procedures of the mandibular dental arcade.

**Textbox 7.6 Mandibular nerve block**

Technique

1) The mandibular foramen is palpable along the curve of the caudal ramus, on the lingual side, roughly behind the last molar. The foramen is palpable both internally on the lingual side of the ramus and externally (see Figures 7.2 and 7.3).

2) With the nondominant hand, palpate the mandibular foramen.

3) With the dominant hand, introduce the 25-g needle either externally (by targeting the curve of the ramus and then "walking it off" the lingual edge of the ramus) or internally (by visualizing the region of the foramen). A 1-ml syringe of local anesthetic is attached, aspiration is performed, and local anesthetic is injected if no blood is present.

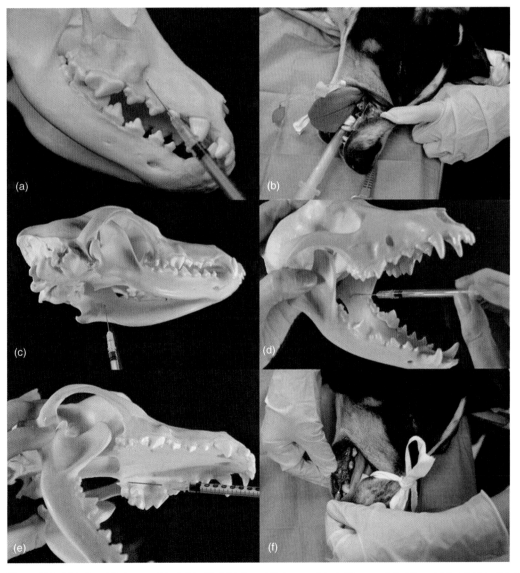

**Figure 7.2** (a) Infraorbital nerve block (skull), (b) infraorbital nerve block (live model), (c) and (d) mandibular nerve block (skull; two alternative approaches), (e) maxillary nerve block (internal approach), (f) mental nerve block (live model). Note: This is canine anatomy. Source: Courtesy of Anderson de la Cunha.

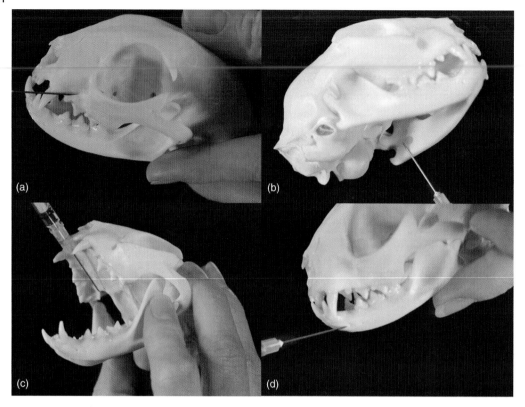

**Figure 7.3** (a) Infraorbital nerve block, (b) mandibular nerve block, (c) maxillary nerve block, (d) mental nerve block. Note: This is feline anatomy. Source: Courtesy of Anderson de la Cunha.

### 7.3.2.3 Maxillary Nerve Block

*Uses*

Procedures involving the maxilla, upper teeth, and lip.

---

**Textbox 7.7  Maxillary nerve block**

Technique (inside mouth approach)

1) Using the nondominant hand, palpate on midline of the hard palate and locate the caudal nasal spine of the palate, medial to the last molar. The pterygopalatine fossa and pterygoid process lie laterally to this caudal nasal spine, and the maxillary nerve passes through the pterygoid fossa.

2) Use the dominant hand to guide a 25-g needle into the area near this pterygoid fossa. See Figures 7.2 and 7.3.

3) Exercise caution to aspirate; apoptosis of eye can occur with laceration of the maxillary artery.

Technique (from outside mouth)

1) Use the nondominant hand to palpate the ventral border of the zygomatic process and approximately 0.5-cm caudal to lateral canthus of eye.

---

2) The dominant hand will direct a 25-g needle through the skin over this ventral border and perpendicular to the arch. The target is in close approximation to the pterygopalatine fossa but not to make direct contact.

3) Deposit 1–2 ml of local anesthetic (staying within the dosage limits for the patient; see Table 7.1).

Table 7.1 Dosage limits for use in field blocks.

| Species | Local anesthetic | Dosage (mg/kg) |
|---------|------------------|----------------|
| Feline | Bupivacaine | 2.0 |
| Canine | Bupivacaine | 3.0 |
| Feline | Lidocaine | 4.0 |
| Canine | Lidocaine | 6.0 |

#### 7.3.2.4 Mental Nerve Block

*Uses*

Procedures involving rostral lower lip of the mandible, mandibular canine and incisor teeth, and the mandibular symphysis.

---

**Textbox 7.8 Mental nerve block**

Technique

1) Use the nondominant hand to palpate the mental foramen on the buccal side of the mandible (just rostral the second premolar tooth).

2) With the dominant hand, insert a 25-g needle in front of the mental foramen; aspirate and inject.

---

### 7.3.3 Retrobulbar Blocks

*Uses*

Enucleation.

*Practical Points*

- Multiple approaches with different complications are described; this approach is one of many.
- Proptosis of the eye may result from unintentional laceration of the vessel.
- Subarachnoid injection/optic sheath injection will result in seizures and possibly death; if there is resistance to injection, DO NOT INJECT.

---

**Textbox 7.9 Retrobulbar block inferior temporal palpebral technique**

Technique

1) Some operators will curve the needle to conform to the orbit.

2) The needle is inserted at approximately the 7 o'clock position, below the eyelid, allowing the needle to traverse along the bony orbit to (which assists with avoiding puncturing the globe and/or blood vessels).

3) The position of the globe will rotate caudally until the conjunctival sac is penetrated, after which the globe will rotate back to a standard position.

4) If resistance is felt, back needle out slightly.

5) It is critical to aspirate for blood, fluid, or resistance. A test dosage (0.5 ml or less) of local anesthetic is administered if no resistance is present. If the test dose is smooth, and patient remains stable, continue with the rest of the injection (Figure 7.4).

---

### 7.3.4 Radial, Ulnar, Median, and Musculocutaneous (RUMM) Block

*Uses*

Desensitization of the elbow and below (including the paw and carpus).

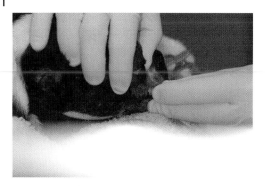

Figure 7.4 Retrobulbar block.

*Practical Points*

- Much of the complications associated with the brachial plexus block (see Reserved blocks) are avoided with the use of the RUMM block, and a majority of the same area is desensitized.

---

**Textbox 7.10 RUMM block**

Technique

1) *Radial nerve.* The author prefers the animal in lateral recumbency, with the limb for blockade up. The operator stands on the patient's ventral side. The nondominant hand will grasp the brachialis muscle and separate it from the lateral head of the triceps distally and laterally on the humerus. This will expose the radial nerve as it courses between the two muscle bellies. Using an insulated, stimulating needle, set to 1 mA current, evaluate for extension of the carpus. When present, decrease the mAs to 0.4 to ensure the twitch ceases, lending support to positioning the needle perineural rather than intraneural. Aspirate and then deposit local anesthetic.

2) *Ulnar, median, and musculocutaneous.* With the patient in lateral recumbency, and the operator on the patient's ventral side, palpate for the brachial artery distally on the humerus, on the medial side of the limb. Using the tips of the fingers of the nondominant hand, gently retract the artery away from the nerve and protect the artery from puncture. Introduce the insulated stimulating needle in close proximity to one's

---

fingertips, using caution to avoid the artery. The nerve stimulator elicits extension, flexion, and pronation of the antebrachium, at 1 mA. Once present, decrease the mAs to 0.4 to ensure the twitch ceases, lending support to positioning the needle perineural rather than intraneural. Aspirate and then deposit local anesthetic (Figure 7.5).

## 7.4 Reserved Blocks

Reserved blocks have all the possible advantages of local anesthetics but can result in harm without prior training or conditions. These blocks are often best performed with additional equipment such as a nerve stimulator or an ultrasound unit, as well as by an experienced individual.

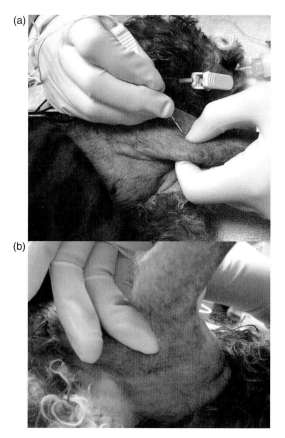

Figure 7.5 RUMM block. (a) Radial nerve puncture site, (b) brachial artery palpation.

### 7.4.1 Bier Block or Intravenous Block

*Uses*

Distal limb procedures less than 90 min in duration.

*Practical Points*
- Complications of this block may include tourniquet pain (often manifested as tourniquet-induced hypertension, secondary to tourniquet pain) and hypoperfusion of the limb distal to the tourniquet.
- Additionally, as one will note in the textbox below, once lidocaine is injected, the tourniquet has a minimum time before it may be removed. Removing the tourniquet too early results in hypotension from rapid systemic absorption of a large dose of local anesthetic.
- Tourniquet is not used for longer than 90 min.
- When the procedure is complete, the tourniquet is released slowly and the patient is monitored for hypotension and negative effects of rapid systemic absorption of lidocaine.
- Bupivacaine is *not* suitable for intravenous injection and is *never* used in this block. Lidocaine is the local anesthetic of choice.

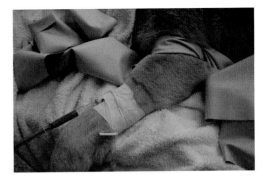

**Figure 7.6** Bier block technique.

### 7.4.2 Brachial Plexus Block

*Uses*

Forelimb procedures below mid-humerus with nerve location guidance; hence, this is how this block will be described.

*Practical Points*
- Blockade of both forelimbs is contraindicated, as patients may lose motor function and therefore ability to ambulate in the front half of the body.
- One possible complication is the puncture of the thoracic cavity, resulting in a possible pneumothorax. Aspiration for negative pressure is just as important in as aspiration for blood with this block.

---

**Textbox 7.11 Bier block technique**

Technique

1) A cephalic intravenous catheter is placed distal to (and directed towards) the proposed area for blockade.

2) After catheter placement, wrap the limb with an Esmarch bandage to exsanguinate it, beginning at the distal aspect of the digits. Once at the level of the elbow, tie off the tourniquet, or use a blood pressure cuff attached to a sphygmomanometer pressurized to 200 mmHg to prevent blood flow to and from the limb.

3) Once blood flow is occluded, begin unwrapping the tourniquet (up to the level of the elbow) to expose the catheter.

4) Administer 2–3 mg/kg lidocaine via the IV catheter.

5) Onset of analgesia is within 5–10 min. Note, *do not remove* the occlusion to blood flow before this, or serious hypotension could result.

6) The maximum duration the tourniquet is left in place is 90 min, although analgesia lasts for ~30 more min following the release of the tourniquet. Muscle and nerve damage are possible complications if the tourniquet is left in place too long (Figure 7.6).

**Textbox 7.12  Brachial plexus block**

Technique

1) Locate the scapulohumeral joint ("point of the shoulder").

2) Insert the spinal needle through the skin, just below the point of the shoulder.

3) Maintain the needle parallel to the thoracic cavity and lateral to the chest wall/medial to the scapula. The needle is also parallel to the transverses processes of the cervical vertebrae with appropriate placement. As one advances the needle, it is directed toward the scapula to avoid entering the thorax. The target location is approximately caudal to the second rib.

4) With the nerve finder and insulated locator needle technique, one lead is placed on the skin and the other on the needle. With the needle caudal to the second rib, the current begins relatively high (1.0–2.0 mA) and the needle is slowly advanced and retracted until a strong twitch is located. Reduced the current to the lowest possible setting with a detectable twitch (usually about 0.4 mA).

5) Connect syringe of drug to needle and aspirate. A small volume is injected; it is normal for twitching to disappear during injection. To ensure effectiveness, some anesthesiologists advocate depositing local anesthetic as the needle is slowly removed (Figure 7.7).

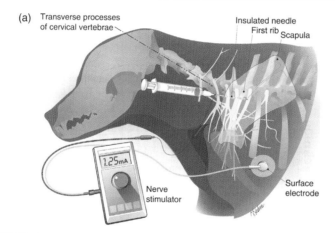

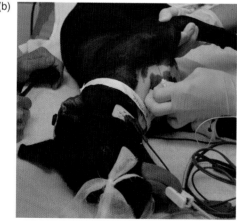
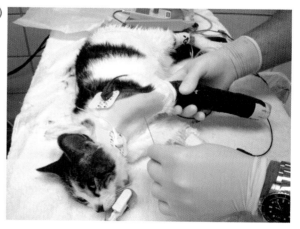

Figure 7.7 (a) Brachial plexus block, (b) brachial plexus block (canine), (c) brachial plexus block (feline). Source: Courtesy of Teton New Media & Anderson de la Cunha.

Note: With a blind technique, the needle is inserted in the same fashion until it is caudal to the second rib. Attach the drug syringe, aspirate, and if no blood or air is present, one-third of the drug volume is deposited in this region. The needle is withdrawn a short distance (1–2 cm), and this process of aspirating and injecting is repeated continues until all drug is administered. This is less reliable in terms of area covered.

### 7.4.3 Epidural

*Uses*

Procedures of the caudal abdomen, hind limb, or thorax. Epidurals containing morphine, in addition to local anesthetic, may provide a long duration (12–24 h) of analgesia. Epidurals are also used to reduce the amount of maintenance anesthetics required.

*Practical Points*

- Complications are variable. Hypotension, cardiovascular collapse, and a reduction in sympathetic tone can result from local anesthetic agents administered epidurally too rapidly. Hypoventilation and apnea may result from systemic uptake of epidural morphine. Urinary retention may result from an increase in antidiuretic hormone secondary to use of morphine epidurally (which is also possible when systemic morphine is administered); it is wise to express the bladder following a procedure in which epidural morphine is administered and monitor an animal for any urinary retention overnight.

Other complications such as delayed hair growth and pruritus are reported as well [5].

- Epidural administration is reserved for use in only in systemically healthy patients. Patients with skin infections, sepsis, hypovolemia, neurological deficits, and coagulopathies should not receive an epidural, due to the inherent risks. The author prefers not to use an epidural for patients undergoing a urinary tract surgery due to possible urinary retention if morphine is included in the epidural. Use good judgment in cases of abnormal epidural space confirmation (e.g. pelvic fracture); although a more experienced anesthetist may have success with the epidural in these cases, this is unlikely for the novice.
- For cranial abdominal or thoracic procedures, use only morphine; advancing local anesthetics past the thoracolumbar region risks the possibility of desensitizing the sympathetic trunk, which branches off in that region, and therefore obliterating sympathetic tone. Bradycardia and hypotension are evident when this occurs and may not be reversible.
- Preservative-free (PF) drugs formulations are indicated.
- It is important to respect total volume calculation for an epidural. In general, the author uses 1 ml per 10 kg for perianal procedures, 1 ml per 7 kg for hind limb procedures, and 1 ml per 5 kg for thoracic (*morphine only*) and abdominal procedures. Avoid total volumes over 6–8 ml. Sterile 0.9% NaCl is used to add volume if desired.

---

**Textbox 7.13 Epidural performed in lateral recumbency**

Technique

1) The anesthetized patient is placed in sternal or lateral recumbency and hind limbs are pulled forward (ventrally).

2) After opening gloves, the inside of the glove paper is used as sterile field to place necessary materials.

3) Palpate the wings of the ilium with the nondominant hand's thumb and middle finger; it helps the anesthetist to stand on the same side of the patient as is the anesthetist's nondominant hand, when the patient is sternal. Use the index finger of this nondominant hand to palpate the lumbosacral junction. This is typically just caudal to a line drawn between the two iliac wings.

4) Midline is located visually (note that the tail is often helpful in maintaining perspective for where midline runs). In the canine, insert the needle perpendicular to the skin, approximately half way between the spinous process of L7 and the sacrum. In the feline, the junction lies slightly more caudal. After inserting the needle below the skin, remove the stylet from hub and place enough drug to form a meniscus at the hub.

5) As one is advancing the needle, they are "feeling" for two "pops" (overcoming resistance abruptly). The first of these pops is minor, as we pass through muscle fascia. A more prominent pop signifies passing through the ligamentum flavum. A tail twitch is occasionally seen in cats.

6) Bone is often encountered while advancing the needle. Withdraw the needle to just below the surface of the skin, re-assess location, and redirect the needle if no blood is present in the needle hub. If blood is present, withdraw the needle and use an alternative analgesic technique.

7) After penetrating the ligamentum flavum, inspect the hub of the needle for cerebral spinal fluid (CSF) or blood. If CSF is present, reduce the dose of drugs by 50%; some anesthetists will withhold local anesthetics as well. Obtaining CSF is more likely in the feline patient as their spinal cord ends (L7) more caudally than in dogs.

8) Add 1 ml of air to the drug syringe to help confirm that the needle remained in the epidural space. That is, during injection of drugs, the air bubble should not collapse. Some anesthesiologists will aspirate before drug injection for blood or CSF. Inject drugs slowly over 60–90 s. This should go smoothly with no resistance.

9) The author advocates rotating the animal and placing the affected limb down, for epidurals in a sternal position, to encourage epidural spread to that region when local anesthetics are used (Figure 7.8).

(a)

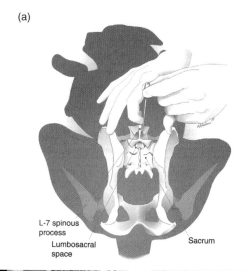

L-7 spinous process

Lumbosacral space

Sacrum

(b)

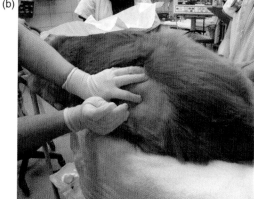

(c)

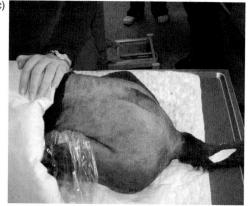

**Figure 7.8** (a) Epidural landmarks, (b) epidural in a laterally recumbent patient, (c) epidural in a sternal patient. Source: Courtesy of Teton New Media & photo courtesy of Anderson de la Cunha.

### 7.4.4 Intra-articular Block (Joint Block)

*Uses*

Patient undergoing a procedure where the joint capsule is incised.

*Practical Points*

- Typically, this block is done during surgery as the surgeon directly visualizes site for blockade.

- If this performed not in conjunction with a surgical procedure, adhere strictly to aseptic technique to prevent joint contamination.
- Differing opinions exist on what is suitable for use within a joint. Expression of μ receptors in inflamed joint cartilage makes PF morphine (0.1–0.3 mg/kg) a suitable choice [6].

---

**Textbox 7.14 Intra-articular block of the stifle before surgery**

Technique

1) Flex the joint.

2) Insert the needle lateral to the patellar ligament, on midline (imagine advancing between the femoral epicondyles).

3) Aspirate and examine for joint fluid; if present, inject drug solution.

---

## References

1 Ling, W., Mooney, L., and Hillhouse, M. (2011). Prescription opioid abuse, pain and addiction: clinical issues and implications. *Drug and Alcohol Review* **30** (3): 300–305.

2 Huuskonen, V., Hughes, J.M., Estaca Banon, E., and West, E. (2013). Intratesticular lidocaine reduces the response to surgical castration in dogs. *Veterinary Anaesthesia and Analgesia* **40** (1): 74–82.

3 Campoy, L., Martin-Flores, M., Ludders, J.W., and Gleed, R.D. (2012). Procedural sedation combined with locoregional anesthesia for orthopedic surgery of the pelvic limb in 10 dogs: case series. *Veterinary Anaesthesia and Analgesia* **39** (4): 436–440.

4 Campoy, L., Martin-Flores, M., Ludders, J.W. et al. (2012). Comparison of bupivacaine femoral and sciatic nerve block versus bupivacaine and morphine epidural for stifle surgery in dogs. *Veterinary Anaesthesia and Analgesia* **39** (1): 91–98.

5 Troncy, E., Junot, S., Keroack, S. et al. (2002). Results of preemptive epidural administration of morphine with or without bupivacaine in dogs and cats undergoing surgery: 265 cases (1997–1999). *Journal of the American Veterinary Medical Association* **221** (5): 666–672.

6 Keates, H.L., Cramond, T., and Smith, M.T. (1999). Intraarticular and periarticular opioid binding in inflamed tissue in experimental canine arthritis. *Anesthesia & Analgesia* **89** (2): 409–415.

# 8

# Nonsurgical Fertility Control

*Valerie A.W. Benka*

*Alliance for Contraception in Cats & Dogs, 11145 NW Old Cornelius Pass Rd., Portland, OR 97231, USA*

## 8.1 Introduction

The twenty-first century has witnessed the first extended-duration, and even permanent, nonsurgical fertility control for companion animals. These first products add to the toolbox of innovations to increase the capacity to spay/neuter safely, humanely, and in sufficiently high numbers to reduce numbers of homeless and unwanted cats and dogs. This is especially true when working in the field.

Research on nonsurgical fertility control for companion animal species dates back multiple decades [1,2]. However, it has proven difficult to develop technologies offering permanent or multiyear fertility suppression in a single dose, while being simultaneously safe for the animal and human providing treatment, plus affordably priced.

Efforts have persisted, and 2008 marked the launch of the Michelson Prize & Grants in Reproductive Biology program (MP&G). The program brings essential funds to advance this field for cats and dogs. As of this writing, MP&G has committed over $14 million to more than 30 projects worldwide. It has also established a $25 million prize for the first entity to develop a long-lasting (10-to-20-year), single-dose, nonsurgical treatment that meets requirements for safety, animal welfare, field application potential, cost, and capacity for U.S. Food & Drug Administration (FDA) approval, and that is effective for both male and female cats and dogs [3].

Nonsurgical fertility control offers choice to owners, caretakers, communities, and veterinarians. As more products become available, they will increasingly enhance practicing veterinary medicine in a way that is best for individual animals, people, and communities in light of surgical and economic resources, veterinary training, and owner/caretaker preferences.

This chapter discusses what nonsurgical fertility control entails, nonsurgical approaches and methods, specific options currently available commercially or in an experimental phase, and considerations for using nonsurgical fertility control.

## 8.2 What is Nonsurgical Fertility Control?

Nonsurgical fertility control prevents reproduction without surgical alteration or removal of reproductive organs. The Alliance for Contraception in Cats & Dogs (ACC&D) defines nonsurgical sterilization as permanent and nonsurgical contraception as temporary and/or reversible; these definitions are used throughout this chapter. The length of contraception varies, ranging from an oral contraceptive requiring multiple doses per week to a single vaccine with promise for multiyear contraception. Future options will ideally extend the duration of efficacy, potentially to lifetime, with a single dose.

This is where the simplicity ends. The reproductive system is wonderfully complex, and the following is a brief outline. There are three major components of the reproductive systems of dogs and cats:

1) *The brain.* Neurons in the hypothalamus secrete pulses of gonadotropin-releasing hormone

*Field Manual for Small Animal Medicine*, First Edition. Edited by Katherine Polak and Ann Therese Kommedal.
© 2018 John Wiley & Sons, Inc. Published 2018 by John Wiley & Sons, Inc.

(GnRH). GnRH controls the release of major reproductive hormones by acting directly on the second major component: the pituitary gland.

2) *The pituitary gland.* GnRH binds receptors in the pituitary gland, causing the secretion of gonadotropins luteinizing hormone (LH) and follicle-stimulating hormone (FSH) into the blood.

3) *The gonads.* LH and FSH bind to receptors in the ovaries and testes. In the female, LH and FSH are essential for the estrous cycle and production of estrogen and progesterone. In the male, LH and FSH contribute to maturation of sperm and production of testosterone.

Reproductive hormones operate through a negative feedback system. When estradiol and testosterone are secreted, they travel in the blood to the brain and suppress secretion of GnRH. A decrease in these hormone levels prompts secretion of more GnRH pulses.

## 8.3 Nonsurgical Approaches and Methods

The reproductive system offers multiple potential targets for fertility suppression. While all approaches discussed below prevent reproduction, they have various modes of action, and some but not all suppress sex hormones. The primary contraception or sterilization methods that are currently in use, or that are being explored in a research stage, are treatment with synthetic sex steroids (hormones), intratesticular injections causing permanent sterility, GnRH agonists/antagonists, and immunocontraception. These general categories are introduced in this section. Products currently available for dogs and/or cats are discussed in Section 8.4.

### 8.3.1 Intratesticular Injections

To date, approaches directly targeting the gonads are limited to intratesticular injections. In dogs, these have been found to cause fibrosis or sclerosis of the testes and render dogs sterile by interfering with sperm production and transport [4,5].

Multiple intratesticular injection formulations have been studied and, as might be expected, not all are created equal. They have demonstrated varied safety, application techniques, modes of action, effects on testosterone levels, and efficacy. Zinc-gluconate- and calcium-chloride-based formulas are presently being used to induce permanent sterility and are discussed in this chapter.

It is often assumed that an intratesticular injection is painful. Although pain can vary with the administration technique, speed, and solution, pain upon injection is not inevitable. Namely, afferent nerve endings associated with pain sensation are located on the scrotal skin and in the capsule of the testis rather than within the testicular and epididymal parenchyma [6].

### 8.3.2 GnRH Agonists/antagonists

GnRH agonists mimic the hormone GnRH, which is the main hormone controlling reproduction. These drugs have been studied in both male and female dogs and cats. When a GnRH agonist is administered as an implant, it initially binds pituitary GnRH receptors like GnRH, and thus results in secretion of LH and FSH. Prolonged continuous release of the agonist desensitizes the receptors and suppresses hormone secretion [7]. This, in turn, suppresses both fertility and testosterone and estradiol secretion, which may result in suppression of hormone-driven sexual behaviors. Due to the mechanism of action, a GnRH agonist must be continuously administered in order to have contraceptive effect; in cats and dogs, the most feasible way to do this is a long-lasting implant, or depot application.

GnRH antagonists have been developed for human therapies for endometriosis; they also prevent fertility by blocking GnRH receptors on pituitary cells. Relative to GnRH agonists, research on GnRH antagonists for companion animals is limited [8].

### 8.3.3 Immunocontraception

Immunocontraception is defined as vaccination with an antigen that stimulates the body's production of antibodies, and in some cases a cell-mediated response, to proteins involved in reproduction. Immunocontraceptive vaccines targeting GnRH and zona pellucida proteins have been approved by the U.S. Environmental Protection Agency (EPA) for female white-tailed deer, wild horses, and wild burros.

GonaCon™, a GnRH immunocontraceptive vaccine approved for these wildlife species, has also been investigated in cats. A single injection was found to cause a median contraceptive duration of at least 39.7 months in female cats in a laboratory setting [9]. ACC&D subsequently studied GonaCon in a simulated free-roaming colony to see if these promising results could be replicated in a more "real-world" setting. The pregnancy rate was higher than in the laboratory cats and exceeded the benchmark for continuing the study past 12 months. (Each cat was spayed early in her pregnancy and adopted.) Reasons for these results are inconclusive. In dogs, GonaCon formulations have caused severe injection site reactions [10,11].

Challenges of immunocontraceptive vaccines are that they may require "boosters" to sustain antibody titers needed for efficacy, and as with any vaccine, not every individual will develop an equally strong immune response, particularly in stressed, undernourished, or immunocompromised animals (L. Rhodes, personal communication).

### 8.3.4 Synthetic Sex Steroids (Hormones)

Synthetic progesterone analogues (also called progestins, progestogens, or progestagens) are believed to suppress fertility through multiple mechanisms: [12–14]

1) Negative feedback to the brain and/or pituitary gland leading to suppression of GnRH, FSH, and LH secretion and, in females, failure of folliculogenesis and/or ovulation
2) Altered motility of the female reproductive tract leading to failed gamete transport and fertilization
3) Altered receptivity of the endometrium resulting in implantation failure.

Although widely used in human contraception, progestins have significant limitations when used in cats and dogs. Shortcomings include administration route, safety profile, and treatment timing, and they arguably make progestins a nonviable alternative to surgical sterilization. Limitations are significantly amplified in the context of field use.

Androgenic drugs are an alternative form of synthetic sex steroids, which have been studied in companion animals; they are not discussed in this chapter.

## 8.4 Nonsurgical Products/compounds

The following section discusses products and formulations that are currently approved for use in dogs and/or cats in one or more countries. Information is also provided on calcium chloride, which is being promoted for use in dogs but does not have regulatory approval, and should therefore be considered experimental.

### 8.4.1 Zeuterin™/EsterilSol™/Infertile® (Zinc-gluconate-based Intratesticular Injections)

A small number of zinc-gluconate-based intratesticular injectable sterilants have regulatory approval for sterilization of male dogs. One of these is Infertile, approved, registered, and launched in Brazil in 2009, and manufactured by Rhobifarma Indústria Farmacêutica Ltda. Another product, zinc gluconate neutralized with L-arginine, was approved for sale by the U.S. FDA for male dogs under the name Neutersol™ and subsequently sold by Ark Sciences as Zeuterin. This same proprietary formula was also registered in Colombia and Mexico under the name EsterilSol. This section focuses on Zeuterin/EsterilSol due to the quantity of data on and use of this product, although as of this writing, Zeuterin/EsterilSol is off the market.

There are limited anecdotal reports of zinc gluconate neutralized with L-arginine use in cats, and it is approved for this species in Colombia. Due to the absence of published data, use in cats is not discussed.

#### 8.4.1.1 Zeuterin/EsterilSol Product Profile
The FDA restricts the use of Zeuterin "by or on the order of a licensed veterinarian" [15,16]. The product causes atrophy of the testicles, epididymides, and seminiferous tubules due to the formation of scar tissue that prevents sperm from moving from the seminiferous tubules to the epididymis [15,16]. There is also some reduction in the size of the prostate gland in treated dogs [15].

Zeuterin is presently approved in the United States for use in male dogs aged 3–10 months, with testicular widths of 10.0–27.0 mm. In Mexico, EsterilSol was approved for dogs over 3 months of age. Zeuterin is a sterile liquid that is supplied in 3.5 ml sterile vials. It can be stored at a controlled room temperature of 15–30 °C (59–86 °F) [16]. The product is supplied with a caliper to measure the width of each testicle, and dosage is calculated based on that width: between 0.4 and 1.0 ml of formula per testicle. The product is injected using a 1 ml syringe with a 28-gauge, 1/2" needle [16].

There are published data on use in dogs over 10 months of age [4, 17–19], plus anecdotal use without complications in dogs with larger testicles [4,18].

### 8.4.1.2 Efficacy

The Zeuterin label reports a 99.6% efficacy rate based on attempts to collect semen from 224 owned male dogs of various breeds and mixes 6 months after treatment [15]. Smaller clinical studies in Beagles aged 4 or 6 months at the start of the study measured efficacy over periods up to 24 months [15], although it is worth noting that these studies did not consistently use doses indicated on the product label for dogs. In the 24-month clinical study, semen analysis and progeny testing results indicated sterility (although a minority of treated males tied with females, none resulted in pregnancy), as did histology of reproductive organs [15]. The product label advises separating treated dogs from females in heat for at least 60 days following treatment because Zeuterin may not kill sperm present at the time of injection [16].

### 8.4.1.3 Administration and Safety

Use of Zeuterin carries some risk of adverse reactions requiring veterinary intervention. The following data on administration of Zeuterin and adverse reactions associated with its use are drawn from studies submitted for FDA registration, plus independent research using the product [4,15,17,20].

In a study with 270 dogs, 2.5% exhibited pain during injection, and 6.3% showed signs of scrotal pain in the days immediately following treatment; systemic reactions included neutrophilia (6.3%), vomiting (4.4%), anorexia (4.0%), and lethargy (2.2%) [15]. The most common postinjection reaction was testicular and scrotal swelling, peaking approximately 48 h following injection [15]. Monthly evaluations of body weight, body temperature, complete blood counts, and serum chemistries, performed for 1 year following treatment identified no long-term pattern of adverse effects [15].

It is important that veterinarians using Zeuterin be trained in injection techniques to minimize adverse effects. Because the liquid causes tissue necrosis, if the

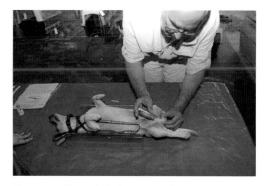

**Figure 8.1** Zeuterin being injected. Source: Courtesy of Dr. Weedon, Ark Sciences.

same needle is used to withdraw the liquid from the vial and inject the testicle, the small amount of liquid on the outside of the needle can cause severe necrosis of the scrotal tissue surrounding the injection site. Side effects are minimized by changing the needle following withdrawal from the vial and slow injection to avoid leakage from the testicle; sedation is also important to minimize movement during injection (Figure 8.1).

Necrotizing tissue reactions at the injection site have been reported [4,15,20]. In one study, 0.3% of dogs (1/270) developed a scrotal ulceration, and 0.3% (1/270) developed a scrotal infection [15]. In another, 3.9% (4/103) had necrotizing zinc gluconate injection site reactions [4]. Dogs in these studies were of varied breeds, ages, and sizes. Dogs with reactions were treated with medical therapy, orchiectomy, surgical debridement, and/or scrotal ablation; all recovered. In early studies conducted for FDA registration, scrotal ulcers or testicular necrosis were also observed and thought to be related to improper or suboptimal injection technique [15]. Veterinary training is now required by Ark Sciences prior to use.

FDA guidelines state that dogs should be prevented from biting or licking the scrotal area for at least 7 days after injection [15]. Dogs must be monitored for adverse reactions and receive prompt veterinary care if reactions develop. For this reason, ACC&D strongly recommends that dogs only be sterilized with Zeuterin if there is a person to monitor them posttreatment (the same recommendation applies to surgical sterilization) and that skilled veterinary care be available in the days following the procedure. Administration of an injectable nonsteroidal anti-inflammatory drug (NSAID) can minimize post-injection discomfort.

#### 8.4.1.4 Treatment Impact on Hormone Levels

Two studies, one a 24-month study with 40 male Beagle dogs aged 6 months when treated with Zeuterin and the other a 6-month study with 118 Chilean free-roaming dogs of varied breeds and ages, evaluated testosterone of Zeuterin-treated dogs relative to intact and/or sterilized animals. The data indicated that the treatment, on average, does not reduce testosterone to the same low level as surgical castration [15,18]. Individual variation in testosterone was also observed, with some dogs' dropping to levels comparable to surgically castrated animals, and others remaining in the same range as their intact counterparts [15,18]. Both studies took a single sample of blood for evaluation at a particular time point; given the variability of circulating testosterone, it is not surprising that large variability was seen in the results (see Section 8.5.6 for additional information on sex hormone measurement).

### 8.4.2 Calcium Chloride Dihydrate in Ethyl Alcohol

No product using calcium chloride is approved for veterinary use. Beginning in the late 1970s, studies evaluated various calcium chloride dihydrate ($CaCl_2$) concentrations, diluents, dosages, and administration techniques in dogs, cats, and other species [2,5, 21–24]. Different formulations and dosages are associated with different outcomes in terms of efficacy and safety, including the impact on blood testosterone levels, semen analyses, and adverse reactions.

Due to variations in formula, experimental design, injection technique, and characteristics of dogs treated, it is difficult to compare data from various studies. Leoci et al. [24] suggest that $CaCl_2$ at 20% concentration in 95% ethyl alcohol (ethanol), in the authors' opinion, best balances safety and efficacy. This recommendation is based on a 12-month evaluation in shelter dogs receiving $CaCl_2$ at 20% concentration in ethyl alcohol ($n = 21$) and lidocaine ($n = 21$), plus a prior dose-finding study of $CaCl_2$ at different concentrations in saline [5,24]. As of this writing, the 20% $CaCl_2$ concentration in 95% ethyl alcohol is being championed for use in male dogs and cats by U.S.-based Parsemus Foundation and U.S.-based SpayFIRST!. A Canadian-based company, CaClCa, sells sterile vials of $CaCl_2$ to veterinarians in the appropriate quantity to create the $CaCl_2$-ethanol formulation, and a limited number of veterinarians and spay/neuter programs that have incorporated this nonsurgical sterilant into their operations. These entities offer additional information on their websites:

- www.parsemusfoundation.org
- www.calciumchloridecastration.com
- www.spayfirst.org
- www.calchlorin.org

The following discussion of $CaCl_2$-based sterilization focuses on the $CaCl_2$–ethanol formulation. As there is no peer-reviewed literature on this formulation in cats, other formulations are referenced when appropriate, and formula differences are specified.

---

**Textbox 8.2 A word of caution about CaCl₂**

Unlike other nonsurgical contraceptives and sterilants discussed in this chapter, no CaCl₂-based sterilant solution has undergone regulatory review in any country. Published clinical studies provide data on different formulations, dosages, and injection techniques; although outside of one early anecdotal report [2], there is only one peer-reviewed study on the CaCl₂-ethanol formulation [24]. In 2015, Parsemus Foundation funded a prize to incentivize those treating dogs and cats with CaCl₂–ethanol to share learnings and best practices. Although these resources are valuable, they offer limited data on dogs and even fewer data on cats. Field data are anecdotal. Unlike products that have been evaluated by a regulatory agency with review of data on short- and long-term efficacy, safety, formulation consistency, manufacturing, and adverse events, CaCl₂ formulations have limited information to allow veterinarians and owners to evaluate their risk/benefit. Due to the cost of regulatory approval and low profit potential of a CaCl₂-based formula, it is unlikely that any company will pursue regulatory approval.

From a user standpoint, this means that a veterinarian cannot purchase a CaCl₂-based sterilant guaranteed to have been manufactured according to established standards for a particular country. At present, one way to acquire the CaCl₂–alcohol solution is through compounding. To be sure, many veterinarians have a trusted compounding pharmacy, but compounded drugs are not required to undergo the rigorous safety, efficacy, and manufacturing testing required for drugs with regulatory approval, or to provide information about drug stability or purity under different storage and use conditions [25]. Moreover, compounded pharmaceuticals do not require labels to guide the veterinarian on appropriate use and known side effects, nor do they have a standardized mechanism to report adverse events so the frequency of adverse events is not tracked [25]. CaClCa is, in essence, a compounding company, which provides 4 g CaCl₂ in a sterile bottle, to which the veterinarian adds 20 ml of 95% pharmaceutical grade ethanol. It is the veterinarian's responsibility to then handle the solution to maintain sterility, generally by using a syringe filter.

The absence of regulatory approval places the onus on the veterinarian to determine the legality, safety, ethics, and advisability of use in a particular country and condition.

---

### 8.4.2.1 CaCl₂-Based Sterilant Profile

Researchers believe that injection of a CaCl₂-based formula into the testicles causes edema, leading to necrosis and fibrosis of the testicular tissue, plus degeneration of seminiferous tubules and some of the interstitial (Leydig) cells [22, 23]. Some Leydig cell function is retained as Leydig cells produce testosterone, and testosterone in treated dogs does not reach levels seen in surgically castrated dogs (see Section 4.2.4).

As of this writing, information and instructions on performing the procedure, dosing, efficacy, aftercare, and management of adverse reactions were based on use of the CaCl₂–ethyl alcohol formulation and available on the aforementioned websites. SpayFIRST! [26] recommends injecting dogs with well-formed testicles and scrotums (i.e., no puppies younger than 16 weeks of age).

---

**Textbox 8.3 Why consider CaCl₂?**

One reason for interest in CaCl₂ is that it can be made from inexpensive and readily available ingredients; CaClCa reports that the cost of sterilization with the product is under $1.00 USD per animal [27].

---

### 8.4.2.2 Efficacy

Studies of efficacy using CaCl₂ have lasted a maximum of 12 months. They have not included breeding trials and instead used other fertility indicators. One study observed dogs 2–6 years of age and weighing 18–28 kg for 12 months. At 2, 6, and 12 months following treatment, the 21 dogs treated with 20% CaCl₂ in 95% ethyl alcohol were azoospermic; all dogs in this treatment group also had 0% sperm motility 1 year after treatment. Results of CaCl₂ in lidocaine were less promising [24].

Small studies in cats, each with a duration of 60 days, have used varied CaCl₂ concentrations in either saline or saline with 1% lidocaine hydrochloride. Higher concentrations of CaCl₂ were correlated with lower sperm counts compared to lower concentrations of CaCl₂ [23,28]. There are no efficacy studies using CaCl₂–ethanol in cats.

Based on research with other intratesticular injections and/or with other species, there can be a 4–6 week delay to infertility following treatment, most likely due to residual sperm in the epididymis prior to injection [29].

### 8.4.2.3 Administration and Safety

The safety profile of $CaCl_2$ and adverse reactions associated with it are based on peer-reviewed research and field use; adverse reactions have not been systematically collected outside of clinical research studies, and these studies have not been designed specifically to evaluate safety. Research that has recorded adverse reactions has used a variety of $CaCl_2$ concentrations and diluents; adverse reactions for each formulation may be different.

Limited canine and feline studies, using varied formulations that include the $CaCl_2$–ethanol formula in dogs, have reported either no or mild pain during injection [5,23,24,28]. A slight increase in firmness of testes on palpation in dogs receiving $CaCl_2$–ethanol was reported beginning 24 h after injection and continuing for 3–4 days [24]. Swelling or soreness was also noted with other formulations and in cats, although not always in this same timeframe [5,23,28]. The canine study using the $CaCl_2$–ethanol formula evaluated physiological data (e.g., respiratory rate, appetite, rectal temperature), response to palpation, posture, vocalization, and behaviors indicating pain or discomfort and reported no changes in these measures during the first 2 weeks after treatment [24].

As with zinc gluconate, it is important that veterinarians using a $CaCl_2$–ethanol solution be trained in injection techniques to minimize adverse effects. Care must be taken to prevent solution from leaking from the testicle, which can lead to abscess formulation and severe necrosis of tissue, and any solution that touches skin and/or mucosal surfaces must be removed immediately. Preventing licking of the treatment site is also important [30], and light-to-moderate sedation is recommended [26].

The most serious reported side effects in peer-reviewed literature are scrotal ulcer and testicular fistula in dogs treated with 30% or 60% $CaCl_2$ in saline; 8 of 20 (40%) dogs developed these reactions, which required anti-inflammatory drugs, antibiotics, and surgical castration or scrotal ablation [5]. No adverse effects in dogs were noted in the study using 20% $CaCl_2$ in alcohol [24].

There are no published studies of $CaCl_2$ at 20% concentration in 95% ethyl alcohol in cats, and, therefore, there is no information regarding adverse reactions to treatment with this formula.

**Textbox 8.4 Example of CaCl₂ use in the field**

Amici Cannis provides spay/neuter and veterinary care services in the small community of Cotacachi, Ecuador. The organization uses 20% $CaCl_2$ in 95% ethyl alcohol, with the $CaCl_2$ purchased in sterile vials from CaClCa, to neuter male dogs. The organization neutered 107 male dogs during one of its first campaigns; the majority (102) were brought by owners or guardians to the clinic, and volunteers brought in the other five. Dogs were released the same day of treatment. Volunteers monitored the five community dogs for up to 1 week post-treatment, and the remainder were monitored by owners/guardians. Complications were seen in 4/107 dogs (3.7%); scrotal dermatitis subsequent to licking occurred in two dogs 3–4 days postinjection, and sterile abscesses were observed in the other two dogs 5–7 days following injection. With veterinary intervention, each dog was completely normal by 12–14 days postinjection.

Amici Cannis treats dogs under light-to-moderate sedation to minimize movement, which is, in turn, believed to reduce the likelihood of formula leaking into the scrotum and consequent adverse reactions. The program also emphasizes the need to educate owners/guardians on the importance of preventing licking and to expect swelling of testicles and scrotum following treatment. To reduce the possibility of contamination, a vial is discarded at the end of the day, even if formula remains, which the organization can afford to discard because of the low cost of the sterilant (H. Steyn, personal communication).

As with zinc gluconate, given the potential for serious and potentially life-threatening (if left untreated) adverse reactions, it is recommended that only trained veterinary practitioners use this sterilant, caretakers be committed to observing animals posttreatment, and a veterinary surgeon be accessible if complications arise.

### 8.4.2.4 Treatment Impact on Hormone Levels

In dogs 1 year after treatment, mean serum testosterone of sexually mature dogs treated with 20%

CaCl$_2$ in ethyl alcohol was 63.6% lower than the mean pretreatment baseline testosterone of this cohort; testosterone levels remained at the low end of the physiological range throughout the study and decreased relative to both baseline and the intact control group. Treatment with human chorionic gonadotropin (hCG) prior to measuring plasma testosterone at each time step was designed to stimulate the animal's production of testosterone. (See Section 5.6 for discussion of hormone measurement.) Dogs that received CaCl$_2$–lidocaine had initially reduced testosterone levels that returned to baseline at the end of the study [24].

There is no published data on testosterone in cats treated with the CaCl$_2$–ethyl alcohol solution.

Different concentrations of CaCl$_2$ in saline with 1% lidocaine yielded dose-dependent reductions in serum testosterone over a 60-day study, with the largest dose yielding a 73% reduction compared to control cats [23]. It is not known whether testosterone levels would have increased had the study been longer.

### 8.4.3 Suprelorin® (Deslorelin Acetate)

Suprelorin is an implant whose active ingredient is deslorelin acetate, a peptide GnRH agonist drug. It is manufactured by Virbac and approved in New Zealand, Australia, and the European Union (EU) for the induction of temporary infertility of male dogs. The product has been studied in female dogs and cats of both sexes but has not been approved for these uses. This section focuses on use in male dogs, but also discusses research in cats and female dogs.

#### 8.4.3.1 Suprelorin Product Profile

Suprelorin is commercially produced as implants containing 4.7 or 9.4 mg of deslorelin. The 4.7 mg implant is approved for sale in Australia, the EU, and New Zealand for sexually mature male dogs. Australia and the EU have also approved sale of the 9.4 mg implant for male dogs.

Suprelorin slowly releases a continuous low dose of deslorelin. Deslorelin initially acts on the pituitary to stimulate the release of luteinizing and FSHs into the bloodstream. Prolonged stimulation of pituitary GnRH receptors by deslorelin leads to desensitization of these receptors, which, in turn, suppresses the reproductive endocrine system ("downregulation") [7]. This downregulation results in suppression of pituitary gonadotroph production and secretion of LH and FSH, which then results in suppression of testosterone production in males and decrease in estradiol in females.

In males, testosterone suppression stops sperm production and may reduce libido and testosterone-related behaviors [31, 32]. In females, Suprelorin has been found to suppress estrus and prevent pregnancy.

Suprelorin is stored refrigerated (2–8 °C) and should not be frozen; its shelf life as packaged for sale is 2 years [31].

#### 8.4.3.2 Efficacy

Suprelorin is indicated for the induction of temporary infertility in healthy, noncastrated, sexually mature male dogs, for a minimum of 6 months with the 4.7 mg implant and for a minimum of 12 months with the 9.4 mg implant. The contraceptive has been shown to have an above-99.9% rate of efficacy in contracepting adult male dogs [31]. The key variable observed is duration of fertility suppression; a single implant may suppress fertility for longer than 6 or 12 months (in studies using the 4.7 mg implant, over 80% of dogs returned to pretreatment testosterone levels within 12 months and 98% within 18 months) [31]. Although timing may vary, males will likely eventually return to fertility if not reimplanted. For continued, uninterrupted suppression of fertility, dogs should receive another implant within the 6- or 12-month period, depending on dose [31].

It is important to reiterate that Suprelorin is not approved for bitches or for cats, and research is limited in these animals. Studies that have taken place indicate a promising response to the implant and a highly variable duration of efficacy.

Female dogs have long periods of anestrus and come into estrus (heat) at variable times, making it challenging to evaluate the duration of fertility suppression after treatment. Small clinical studies evaluating deslorelin implants in bitches of varied ages indicate that Suprelorin can cause suppression of

**Textbox 8.5 Suprelorin use in the field for dog population control**

The Dogs With No Names™ (DWNN) initiative provides Suprelorin implants to female dogs to prevent unwanted litters in Canada's remote First Nations communities. Between 2009 and 2012, DWNN conducted a pilot study in two Alberta communities using 9.4 mg implants in free-roaming bitches, targeting lactating and prepubescent (4-to-6-month old) individuals. In this study, 96 dogs were implanted a first time; 44 were reimplanted at 12-to-24-month intervals. Results in monitored animals were promising: no reimplanted dog gave birth, and no animal became pregnant within the 2 months following her first implant (during the "stimulation phase" that can be seen with the initial stimulation of hormones). One female produced a litter after 9 months, indicating poor response to or failure of the implant [33]. DWNN has measured efficacy based on litters born, whereas clinical studies have monitored return to estrus (Figure 8.2).

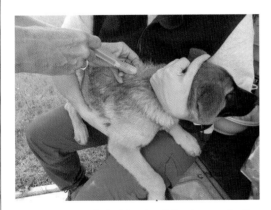

Figure 8.2 Suprelorin injection following application of Carbocaine to numb the application site. Source: Courtesy of Judith Samson-French.

estrus, but response is variable and potentially shorter than seen in male dogs. A study in 10 bitches concluded that the 4.7 mg implant may work well if administered at approximately 4.5-month intervals, and although a 9.4 mg implant lasted longer, efficacy

may still not be full 12 months [34]. In another preliminary study using one 4.7 mg implant, bitches came into heat an average of 10.2 months (range: 2.1–23.3 months) after implantation [35]. In a study of 102 bitches treated between one and five times with a 4.7 mg implant, it was observed that younger dogs had a higher treatment success of estrus suppression than older [36]. Additional, large controlled studies will be required to more fully understand efficacy and duration of fertility suppression in bitches.

Limited long-term clinical studies in cats have also shown extended, but variable, duration of efficacy. In females, queens ($N = 20$) who received a 4.7 mg implant were infertile for approximately 22 months on average (range: 16 to >37 months) [37]. Another study found that a 9.4 mg implant successfully suppressed estrus behavior and fecal estradiol secretion in 18/21 queens [38].[1] In male cats ($N = 7$), a 4.7 mg implant suppressed fertility for an average of approximately 19 months (range: 15–25 months) [39].

Deslorelin has been studied in prepubertal dogs and cats of both sexes and was shown to delay puberty [40–42].

Suprelorin treatment can result in a "stimulation phase" caused by the initial stimulation of hormones. It is recommended that male dogs be separated from females in heat for 6 weeks following their first Suprelorin treatment [31]. (This separation does not apply to retreatments within the specified period of efficacy.) In a small study in male tomcats, an increase in sexual behavior (libido, mountain, mating) was observed in 8 of 10 cats until day 16 after implantation [43].

In clinical studies of sexually mature female dogs and cats treated with Suprelorin, investigators have observed frequent induced estrus within approximately 2 weeks of treatment [34,37,38,44–46]. This induced estrus should be assumed fertile. Due to the downregulation that occurs, this estrus is followed by suppression of fertility.

Methods to reduce the likelihood of induced estrus have been explored. Some studies in bitches and queens suggest that induced estrus varies based on

1 Peptech Animal Health did not manufacture a 9.5 mg implant, but rather 9.4 mg.

the stage in the estrous cycle in which the female is treated [7,34,47]. Some research has shown that if progesterone levels are high enough at implantation, the treatment does not produce an induced estrus [34,48]. DWNN has targeted lactating and pre-pubescent dogs and has not reported problems with induced estrus, although the study was not designed to observe for or detect estrus [33].

Short-term administration of progestins to prevent induced estrus has been studied in bitches and queens on a limited basis and with varied protocols. Results in dogs have been inconsistent [7,47,49]. In one study, a protocol using the progestational drug megestrol acetate (MA) showed promise in queens [38]. Pro-gestins are also used for a short time before and after Suprelorin implantation when treating captive wild-life, with good results at avoiding an induced estrus (C. Asa, personal communication).

### 8.4.3.3 Administration and Safety

The Suprelorin label for male dogs calls for sub-cutaneous implant in the loose skin between the lower neck and lumbar area; sedation is not needed [31].

Studies submitted for regulatory approval have found Suprelorin to be safe and well tolerated in sexually mature male dogs. There are reports of moderate swelling at the implantation site within 2 weeks after treatment, and/or mild local reactions (e.g., inflammation, hardening) for up to 3 months; these resolve naturally [31]. Safety in prepubescent male dogs has not been studied.

Studies in female dogs have not been specifically designed to evaluate safety. In a study that surveyed owners and practitioners of bitches treated between one and five times with a 4.7 mg implant, researchers found metropathies (uterine disease) reported in 16/102 animals (15.7%); older bitches were significantly more likely to be affected than younger [36]. Addi-tional randomized, controlled studies are warranted to understand the safety of Suprelorin in bitches.

Studies in cats have similarly not been designed to evaluate safety. Adult tomcats and queens appear to tolerate Suprelorin well. Cats have shown little or no local reactions (e.g., swelling or scratching) at the insertion site [37,38,43]. Clinical examinations, blood counts, and serum biochemistry during treat-ment have been found to remain in the normal range [32]. Further studies are needed to better understand safety.

If Suprelorin were to be used off-label in females, it is possible (or likely) that pregnant or lactating bitches or queens would be implanted. Safety data for pregnant or lactating animals, including survival of pups or kittens born to pregnant females inadver-tently treated, are very limited. In a clinical study with dogs, bitches implanted with varying doses of deslor-elin during pregnancy produced normal litters and raised healthy pups to weaning [48]. In the DWNN studies, implanting pregnant or lactating bitches did not appear to compromise lactation or the health of puppies, and bitches were not subsequently observed in heat for at least 12 months, although the study was not designed to observe for these outcomes [33]. In a case report, a queen who was mismated 1 week before receiving a Suprelorin implant showed little interest in kittens and had inadequate lactation [50]. Similar to the queen, captive wildlife treated while pregnant have been observed to give birth to normal litters but not produce sufficient milk to support offspring (C. Asa, personal communication).

---

**Textbox 8.6 Suprelorin use in field settings**

A key challenge of Suprelorin, particularly in free-roaming animals and field settings, is a "stimulation phase," during which reproductive hormone con-centrations increase. This has been widely reported in both species and sexes, and animals should be assumed fertile during the stimulation phase. It is recommended that male dogs be separated from females in heat for 6 weeks after the first Suprelorin treatment [31]. Recommendations are not available for female dogs or cats of either sex.

---

### 8.4.3.4 Treatment Impact on Hormone Levels

Suprelorin has been shown to dramatically suppress levels of reproductive hormones after the first weeks of treatment. In male dogs, studies have shown reduced serum testosterone levels, reduced testicle size, decreased libido, and decreased spermatogenesis while the implant is effective [31]. Studies in male cats have also shown decreases in serum testosterone similar to those seen after surgical castration, with physical (e.g., disappearance of penile spines, decreased testis size) and behavioral (e.g., sexual behavior, urine marking) characteristics similar to those expected of a surgically sterilized male [32,43]. In female cats, estradiol concentrations decreased to basal levels in concert with treatment and suppression of fertility [37,38].

## 8.4.4 Synthetic Progesterone Analogues

Progesterone analogues are manufactured steroids with a structure and biological effect similar to that of progesterone. They have been studied and used for contraception of female dogs and cats for more than five decades, in several instances a by-product of contraceptive development for humans. Progesterone analogues are variously called progestins, progestogens, and progestagens.

This contraceptive category includes multiple active ingredients, which have been approved for use in animals in various countries. Those most commonly used in dogs and cats are as follows [12]:

- MA, whose brand names in various countries include Megecat®, Ovaban®, Ovarid®, Felipil®, MiniPil®, Estropill®, and others
- Medroxyprogesterone acetate (MPA), whose brand names include Depo-Promone®, Promone-E®, Perlutex®, and Depo-Provera®
- Proligestone (PR), whose brand names include Covinan® and Delvosteron®.

Due to space constraints, this section does not detail specific commercial products; rather, it provides an overview of this contraceptive category, brief summaries of MA, MPA, and PR, and factors to consider regarding use. The ranges seen in treatment timing, dosages, treatment frequencies, and treatment durations pose a challenge in describing research on progestins in dogs and cats, and those considering using one of these drugs are advised to research product-specific details.

No progestin drugs have been approved by regulatory bodies for use in male dogs or cats and are not advised for this sex [8]. Limited data in male dogs suggest that lower doses of MA and MPA do not have a significant effect on sperm quality and that the MPA dose required to have an effect on sperm production and quality was high [51,52]. Higher doses can be expected to be associated with higher rates of side effects [8]. In male cats, use of progestins is discouraged for fertility control based on lack of efficacy and risks of mammary

hypertrophy and diabetes [53] and other side effects also seen in queens [8].

### 8.4.4.1 Synthetic Progesterone Analogue Profile

There are multiple mechanisms through which progestins are believed to suppress fertility:

1) Negative feedback on the brain leading to suppression of GnRH, FSH, and LH secretion and, in females, failure of folliculogenesis and/or ovulation
2) Altered motility of the female reproductive tract leading to failed gamete transport and fertilization
3) Altered receptivity of the endometrium resulting in implantation failure [12–14].

Progestins can be given orally or via a long-acting depot injection, depending on the compound.

---

**Textbox 8.7 Disadvantages to the use of progestins**

While at first glance progestins may seem very attractive, they are not a viable option for permanent sterilization or even long-term contraceptive use, but rather a potential option for very temporary suppression or postponement of estrus. They may also have a role in combination with Suprelorin: short-term progestin treatments have been studied in dogs and cats in conjunction with Suprelorin to prevent the induced estrus [7,38,47,49].

Use in free-roaming animals carries particular limitations and risks. Although the duration of efficacy varies among progestins, maximum duration is months, not years, and the risk of adverse effects increases with repeat treatments and higher doses. Ensuring proper dosing of oral progestagen drugs is also difficult if not impossible in a field context, such as a community or feral cat colony.

Lastly, there are well-known contraindications for use; if examinations cannot be performed and medical history and estrous details are unknown, an individual animal is placed at a higher risk of adverse side effects from use.

---

### 8.4.4.2 Efficacy

Duration of efficacy varies according to the compound used, method of treatment (oral or depot injection), and when in the estrous cycle treatment is started. Progestins are used for acute suppression of an ongoing cycle, temporary postponement of an imminent cycle, and protracted or permanent postponement of cycles [12]. Treatment regimens vary not only by product but also by when in the cycle treatment is initiated [13].

MA is an oral progestagen that was first marketed in the 1970s and is the shortest acting progestin available for veterinary use. It is approved for sale for dogs and cats, with variation by country [12,53]. Studies have used varied doses, frequencies of treatment, and durations of treatment. Studies using different doses and dosing frequencies, and started at different stages of the estrous cycle have shown high rates of fertility suppression (>90%) in both dogs and cats [54,55], although in dogs the study lasted a maximum of 32 days [54]. Higher doses of MA, as defined by greater dosing at each treatment, more frequent treatment, or longer treatment, are associated with an increased risk of side effects [53].

Anecdotally, those who have used MA to control reproduction in free-roaming cat populations report few adverse events and few litters born in treated colonies; however, there have been no studies with rigorous data collection and analysis [56]. Moreover, observations of adverse events in this population are limited by the fact that sick cats will likely not be seen. It is important to emphasize that this compound suppresses or postpones estrus, but it cannot provide the long-term contraception that is needed for population control purposes, particularly in field contexts.

MPA is available in long-acting injectable or short-acting oral forms [6]. It is approved for sale for dogs and cats, with variability by country. As with other progestins, there is significant variability in recommendations regarding dosing, treatment frequency, and duration for safe use of MPA [53]. In female dogs, injectable MPA given during anestrus is estimated to be 85–90% effective at suppressing fertility if repeated every 6 months, and up to 98% effective if repeated every 5 months [12]. However, MPA use has been associated with pronounced cystic endometrial hyperplasia, with many dogs developing pyometra [8]. One early study found a daily low oral dose to be nearly 100% effective at suppressing estrus in cats over 12 months, but compromised health of the first litter of kittens born following treatment [53]. Higher

MPA doses given by injection for longer duration of efficacy have also been studied and demonstrated a high incidence of side effects, leading some researchers to advise against use of MPA in cats [6,53,57]. Other researchers emphasize the need to be attentive to dosing rather than avoid the product altogether [53], and MPA has a user base for cats in Europe [14].

Proligestone has weaker progestational activity than other progestins [6]. It is marketed as an injectable contraceptive for female dogs and cats, with variation by country. It has been reported to prevent, delay, or suppress estrus in bitches when given subcutaneously in three doses over 7 months [6] and marketed for cats in Europe with treatment every 5 months [53]. PR is reported to have less effect on the uterus and mammary glands than do other progestins; there are indications that this reduces the incidence of certain side effects [6,53].

### 8.4.4.3 Administration and Safety

Progestins have been associated with numerous side effects in both dogs and cats. They are reported to alter glucose metabolism, suppress adrenal cortical function, and promote growth of the mammary gland [13]. Serious, potentially fatal side effects include, but are not limited to, cystic endometrial hyperplasia-pyometra complex, mammary tumors and fibroadenomatosis, hypertrophies, uterine tumors, mammary cancers, and insulin resistance causing diabetes mellitus [6,12–14]. Weight gain, lethargy, and restlessness have also been reported [6]. Risk is greater in animals predisposed to certain diseases, treated for an extended period, or treated with high doses [12,14,53].

Generally speaking, it is wise to interpret reports and data on adverse effects with care, as certain complications associated with one progestin may not be generalizable to all progestins, and dosage and treatment frequency have been shown to affect side effects. Further, in many cases, well-documented safety studies have not been done. These variables make it difficult to speak to the relative benefit versus risk of a particular progestin at a specific dose.

Precautions that may limit side effects include starting treatment in anestrus/avoiding starting treatment in diestrus; not treating prepubescent, pregnant, or pseudopregnant bitches or queens; and not treating individuals with a history of reproductive pathologies, mammary tumors, or diabetes, in addition to using a minimum effective dose and duration of treatment [12,14,53,58]. These precautions to reduce the incidence of adverse effects in supervised pets cannot be taken with free-roaming animals who have unknown histories or cannot receive a complete physical exam, making the use of progestins in community/feral cat populations or free-roaming dogs much riskier than in pets. In combination, contraindications make progestins an unviable alternative to permanent sterilization and a difficult-to-manage option for field use, particularly for an extended period (versus, e.g., in combination with the Suprelorin implant or for a short time while building surgical capacity).

#### 8.4.4.4 Treatment Impact on Hormone Levels

For their duration of efficacy, progestins suppress the release of GnRH from the brain, and, therefore, inhibit FSH and LH release from the pituitary and sex steroids from the gonads [13]. Careful studies of steroid levels following treatment have not been conducted.

## 8.5 Considerations Regarding Use of Nonsurgical Fertility Control

Nonsurgical fertility control options expand the tools available to veterinarians to use in various locations and situations. As new options emerge, they will likely offer particular value in field contexts. Risk–benefit analyses will no doubt vary according to product, objectives, and circumstances. Below are broad topics that veterinarians and animal welfare professionals might find helpful to consider while evaluating the potential role of nonsurgical fertility control in their work.

### 8.5.1 Safety and Risk–Benefit Considerations in Field Settings

Every nonsurgical contraceptive/sterilant will have its own safety profile. For products that have been reviewed by regulatory agencies, extensive safety data is required for approval. Treatments that are used off-label often have minimal species- or sex-specific safety data available.

The safety profile and incidence of adverse events, available resources, and product efficacy (both

numbers of animals successfully contracepted and expected duration of fertility suppression) help develop a robust risk–benefit analysis for use of any approach.

When reviewing data on adverse reactions, it is important to keep in mind the following:

- Rates and types of adverse reactions and their welfare implications should be considered relative to both surgical and no sterilization, as well as the particulars of where one works – surgical resources, surgical training of veterinary practitioners, anesthesia used, body condition and health of animals, capacity to hold animals for recovery, and available postoperative monitoring and follow-up care.
- The numbers of treatments performed, and methods for recording adverse reactions, vary among nonsurgical products and are the results of factors such as regulatory approval, breadth of research, and frequency of use. It is generally not accurate to directly compare reported adverse reactions from one treatment to another.

It is also important to consider the following to maximize the safety of any nonsurgical option:

- Animals may need posttreatment monitoring, as with surgery; guidelines will vary by product.
- Improper use of nonsurgical options can pose adverse health and welfare consequences. It is essential that any procedure be performed by a professional who has product-specific training.
- Some nonsurgical procedures may require access to a veterinary surgeon in case of emergency. For example, some synthetic progestins have been associated with pyometra, and adverse reactions following intratesticular injection may require surgical castration or even scrotal ablation.

### 8.5.2 Logistics (Infrastructure, Resources, and Time)

Nonsurgical options available today, and those anticipated for the future, require less infrastructure than surgery: no drapes or gowns, autoclave, spay packs, suture material, or general anesthesia. Although there are currently no permanent nonsurgical sterilization options for female dogs or cats, use of Zeuterin in male dogs, for example, could allow limited surgical resources to be used for female dogs and cats of both sexes.

A vaccine, intratesticular injection, or implant requires less treatment time than surgery, in turn, allowing veterinary professions to reach more animals. The amount of time required for the logistics around treatment is also relevant; for example, in free-roaming cat colonies, it may be possible to trap and treat free-roaming cat colonies on-site, thereby eliminating the need to transport animals or hold overnight for recovery.

### 8.5.3 Cost

Careful analysis will be needed to understand if surgical or nonsurgical options are the best use of financial resources in a given context. The cost of nonsurgical options relative to surgery will vary based on the nonsurgical option being used and cost of surgery in a particular location. An accurate comparison requires accounting for the time, infrastructure, and ancillary products needed for each procedure, as well as the duration of action of a nonsurgical product.

As one reference point, the MP&G program's $25 million USD prize seeks a product price tag of less than $25 USD per dose when manufactured commercially. For products sold to veterinarians (prescription products), pricing will reflect what the market will bear and will need to return a fair profit to the companies willing to take on the research and development to achieve regulatory approval.

Compounded products such as calcium-chloride-based sterilants may cost less than nonsurgical sterilants that have regulatory approval. Without the regulatory approval process, however, there is no guarantee of robust safety and efficacy data.

### 8.5.4 Ethics of Use

Although discussion of ethics is beyond the scope of this chapter, it bears mention that any intervention used to manage populations of cats and dogs, whether surgical or nonsurgical, can prompt ethical questions.

Ethical dilemmas may be created by unknowns regarding the use of certain nonsurgical methods, including the safety profile of a treatment without regulatory approval. Decisions around where and how to field trial new technologies also have ethical

underpinnings. There are undoubtedly situations in which animals cannot be closely or reliably observed following a treatment that carries some risk of side effects (this is also true for surgery). These are but three probable situations that raise questions about how to proceed most ethically and that require weighing risks and benefits from multiple perspectives, both human and animal, and both individual and population.

Due to ease of application, including no surgical incision or general anesthesia, nonsurgical methods in particular risk being abused through treating animals covertly or without owner/caretaker consent. It is worth emphasizing that this is both unethical and unsafe and that receiving consent to treat an animal is imperative for any population control intervention.

### 8.5.5 Regulatory Approval

Commercial use of a nonsurgical product requires regulatory approval in the country of use; the approval status of individual products is discussed in the product profiles.

> **Textbox 8.8 Regulatory approval**
>
> Although requirements differ by country, in the United States, for example, the process of regulatory approval by the U.S. Food & Drug Administration (FDA) for drugs for dogs and cats can require 5–10 years of research and development and cost from approximately $8–12 million USD [25]. This approval process is essential for ensuring that the product is manufactured under standards that ensure consistency and sterility and that the product provides effective fertility control and has an acceptable safety margin for animals, humans, and the environment. It is one reason why promising new technologies may take years to become commercially available.

Compounded nonsurgical sterilants or contraceptives have not undergone regulatory approval. As discussed above in the context of $CaCl_2$-based sterilants, compounded formulations are not evaluated by a regulatory agency on measures such as efficacy, dosing, safety, formulation consistency, manufacturing, adverse events, storage conditions, or stability.

Those using the formula can only rely on peer-reviewed and/or anecdotal data regarding the compounded drug. The onus is on the veterinarian or user to determine legality of use in a given country. The onus is also on the veterinarian and/or population management program to evaluate the risk/benefit ratio for use, which will vary based on location, alternative available options with regulatory approval, program and community resources, and individual tolerance for risk, among other factors.

### 8.5.6 Sex Hormone Measurement and Hormone-correlated Behaviors

When reading the literature, it is important to account for methods of hormone measurement. It can be difficult though to compare and contrast data on circulating sex hormones following various fertility control treatments. Hormone levels can vary by individual animal, season, day, and even time of day. To help standardize measurements, animals can be treated with GnRH or hCG prior to measuring plasma hormones. This may be useful for measuring hormones such as testosterone, which is normally released in a pulsatile manner; hCG was used, for example, in measuring testosterone levels in dogs following treatment with $CaCl_2$ in ethyl alcohol [24]. This stimulation then does not measure an animal's inherent circulating levels of testosterone, but his capacity to be stimulated to release that hormone when treated with GnRH or hCG.

Much attention has been devoted to correlations between sex hormone levels and behaviors such as urine marking, sexual mounting, roaming, fear, anxiety, excitability, and various manifestations of aggression. Until recently, studies of sex-hormone-related behavior have usually compared surgically sterilized and intact animals, often using retrospective owner reports on pet behavior before and after spaying or neutering. A common hypothesis is that spaying or neutering "improves" behavior by reducing hormone production. However, research results have varied regarding the relationship between surgical sterilization (yielding a complete suppression of sex hormones) and behavior [59]. Not surprisingly, a general finding has been that surgical sterilization most commonly affects sexually dimorphic behaviors: those that vary between sexes and are likely to be at least partially mediated by sex hormones [59].

One study has compared behavior of free-roaming owned male dogs in three groups (surgically sterilized ($n = 39$), nonsurgically sterilized using EsterilSol ($n = 36$), and intact ($n = 44$)) using objective measures [19]. Following treatment, surgically castrated dogs had significantly decreased serum testosterone; dogs treated with EsterilSol had more varied testosterone levels [18]. The study found no consistent association between serum testosterone concentrations and behavior in any group [19]. The authors also noted no change in sexual activity or home range (roaming) in either surgically or chemically sterilized dogs, and no decrease in dog aggression among surgically sterilized dogs. Chemically sterilized dogs in this study exhibited an increase in dog-directed aggression for which there is no clear explanation, but it was not correlated with testosterone levels of this treatment group [19]. It can be concluded that further work is needed in other dog populations, but this research indicates that there is not a clear relationship between serum testosterone and specific behaviors, including aggression.

What to make of these behavior and hormone data? There is a lot that has not been quantitatively assessed, particularly in free-roaming populations. Findings regarding relationships between hormones and behaviors in cats are generally consistent in that sexually dimorphic behaviors are reduced with sterilization and suppression of sex hormones. Pet dogs show certain behavioral trends, but with abundant exceptions and often contradictory data. Behavior of pet dogs should not necessarily be extrapolated to free-roaming populations. Ultimately, it can be concluded that suppression of sex hormones may not improve undesirable behaviors in an individual dog, but for cats, sexual behaviors seem to be more related to sex steroid levels.

### 8.5.7 Identification of Treated Animals

It is important to be able to identify animals that are sterilized (surgically or non-surgically) or have received a contraceptive. This is particularly true for free-roaming or community populations. Identification shows that an animal is not contributing to unwanted dog or cat populations and prevents unnecessary retreatment, which wastes resources and, in the case of nonsurgical options, could increase the risk of side effects. For temporary contraception, there is additionally a need to convey retreatment timing.

Considerations for selecting a method to mark and identify dogs and cats include the amount and type of information that must be conveyed, duration required for identification, visibility required for identification, the number of animals who must be marked, degree of handling required to create and detect the mark, invasiveness and humaneness of the marking procedure, expense of the technology, and the risks or consequences associated with not having proof of spay/neuter.

There are a variety of methods used to mark animals, and many have been used to identify surgically sterilized dogs or cats in field campaigns. Visible methods intended to be permanent include ear tipping, ear notching, tattooing (ear or abdominal, using an electric tattooing needle or tattoo clamp/forceps), or ear tagging with products sold primarily for livestock and wildlife. Photographing animals and observing individual markings has also been used on small scales. Other identification methods that are not simultaneously visible *and* permanent include microchipping, collars, and nontoxic paint. Freeze branding has been studied in dogs but does not appear to be used in sterilization efforts [60,61]. These methods are summarized in Table 8.1.

Current permanent marking options can present challenges for surgical sterilization efforts, among them risk of infection or blood loss, need for skilled personnel, and legal, cultural, and social barriers to physically altering the appearance of an animal. Challenges are amplified for nonsurgical options. Permanent visible marking methods (ear tipping, ear notching, livestock or wildlife ear tags, tattooing) require anesthesia, yet field-friendly nonsurgical fertility control should require at most sedation. The need to convey a necessary retreatment timeframe if using a contraceptive adds yet further complexity (Figure 8.3).

In 2013, ACC&D launched an initiative to develop a means to visually identify free-roaming animals that have been temporarily contracepted or permanently sterilized without surgery. A novel ear marker design emerged as the top contender, and a partnership between a multidisciplinary Cornell University team and ACC&D, along with consultants in body piercing and ophthalmology, yielded a prototype ear marker that might be possible to use humanely with topical anesthesia or sedation [63,64]. The prototype includes solution-dyed acrylic fabric, selected due to its weight, breathability, color-fastness, and durability, that is affixed to the ear with a thin polypropylene nylon "fastener" like those used to attach price tags to clothing. A hypodermic-like needle is used to for application. There is precedent for this nylon fastener and its associated applicator in other species [65]. Work is ongoing, and the design and application process presently show greater potential for cats than for dogs (Figure 8.4).

## 8.6  Conclusion

The field of nonsurgical fertility control is exciting, complex, and challenging. Looking toward the future, there is potential to enhance existing technologies through, e.g., extending the duration of GnRH agonists or immunocontraceptive vaccines. It is also quite possible that novel approaches, such as gene silencing/gene therapy or targeted delivery of cytotoxins (to kill specific cells necessary for reproduction) will someday become available for widespread

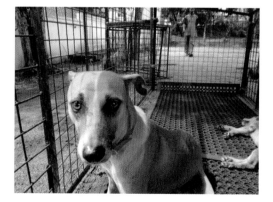

**Figure 8.3** Sterilized dog in Sri Lanka with an ear notch and collar. Source: Courtesy of Dr. Katherine Polak.

Table 8.1 Summary of methods currently used to mark and identify dogs and cats [60,61].

| | Observation of natural markings, including photography | Collars | Paint | Microchips | Freeze branding | Tattoos | Commercial ear tag (manufactured for livestock or wildlife) | Ear tip or notch |
|---|---|---|---|---|---|---|---|---|
| Species | Small-scale study in cats; more common in wildlife | Dogs and cats, many additional species | Dogs, many additional species | Dogs and cats, plus livestock species | Limited use in dogs, more common in livestock | Dogs and cats | Dogs | Dogs and cats |
| Type of information | Individual | Individual or population | Population | Individual | Individual or population | Individual or population | Individual or population | Population |
| Invasiveness | None | None (assuming correct fit) | Minor | Moderate (chip implanted under skin) | Moderate (destroys melanocytes in skin, fur must be clipped) | Moderate | High (attached to ear via hole made in ear or metal clip) | High (requires removal of ear tissue) |
| Pain | None | None (assuming correct fit) | None | Minimal | Moderate | None to high (depending on anesthesia) | High (requires anesthesia) | High (requires anesthesia) |
| Animal welfare and health concerns | None | Low (assuming correct fit, not embedded, etc., and that collar loss does not put animal at risk) | None (assuming proper application (e.g., no spray in eyes) and nontoxic) | Minimal-to-moderate brief pain | Limited data. Potential to cause pain. Time required for application could cause stress | None if tattooed under general anesthesia. Concerns if tattooed while conscious | | |
| Sedation or anesthesia required? | No sedation or anesthesia required | No sedation or anesthesia required | No sedation or anesthesia required | No sedation or anesthesia required | Study in dogs performed under sedation [62] | Sedation or general anesthesia | Commonly applied under anesthesia | General anesthesia |
| Skill required to apply | High (careful note taking, system to organize and access images) | Low (safe handling of conscious animal and proper collar application) | Low (safe handling of conscious animal) | Moderate (safe handling of conscious animal and knowledge of microchip application technique) | High (experience with branding technique; coolant materials are dangerous if handled improperly) | High (experience with application technique) | High (experience with application technique) | High (experience with application technique) |

(continued)

**Table 8.1** (Continued)

| | Observation of natural markings, including photography | Collars | Paint | Microchips | Freeze branding | Tattoos | Commercial ear tag (manufactured for livestock or wildlife) | Ear tip or notch |
|---|---|---|---|---|---|---|---|---|
| Skill and resources to detect | High (careful observation, indexed referencing system) | None | None | Moderate (proper use of reader to detect, access to registry) | None | Moderate (safe handling of conscious animal, detection of tattoo) | None | Moderate |
| Quantity of information that can be conveyed | High (requires recording or indexing system) | Varied (can convey binary info; colors, patterns, or tags can show more) | Low (binary info) | High (requires database to convey more than binary info) | Low (detailed symbols/patterns difficult to create) | Low to high (depends on type of tattoo, coding system) | Low to high (at minimum binary info; can number or color-code) | Low (binary info) |
| Duration | Lifetime | Variable (high likelihood of loss or removal) | Short (days). Mostly useful for short-term capture-mark-recapture | Lifetime | Lifetime (results not seen until hair grows back) | Lifetime | Variable (due to possible loss or removal) | Lifetime |
| Visibility | None (differentiating physical features difficult in cats and dogs) | High | High | None (requires scanner to detect) | High | Low (handling likely required) | High | Moderate |
| Expense | Variable (depends on technology used for observation) | Low/moderate | Low | High | Moderate | Low/moderate (depending on tattoo method) | Low | Low |

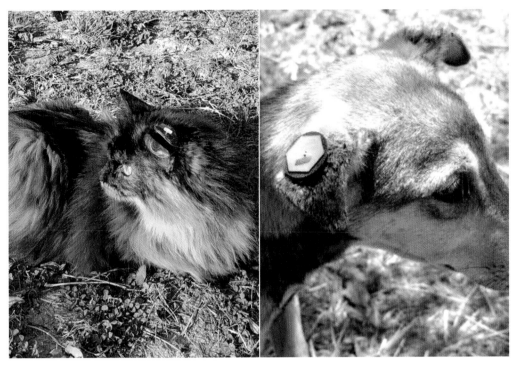

Figure 8.4 Dog and cat with prototype ear tag. Note that a future study will reduce the size of the feline ear tag from a 3 to 2 cm diameter. Source: Courtesy of Valerie Benka/ACC&D and Amy Fischer.

use. In fact, the Michelson Prize & Grants Program has committed significant funding to such research. New products will provide choice and new options to owners, caretakers, communities, and veterinarians, particularly as new, field-friendly options become available. This has the potential to create a sea of change in animal welfare, particularly in vulnerable animal populations, if used to their fullest potential.

## Acknowledgments

Many thanks go to Elaine Lissner and Stefano Romagnoli for providing feedback on sections of the manuscript and to Linda Rhodes and Joyce Briggs for reviewing and improving its quality.

## References

1 Harris, T. and Wolchuk, N. (1963). The suppression of oestrus in the dog and cat with long term administration of synthetic progestational steroids. *American Journal of Veterinary Research* **24**: 1003–1006.

2 Koger, L.M. (1978). Calcium chloride castration. *Modern Veterinary Practice* **59**: 119–121.

3 Found Animals Foundation (2016). Michelson prize criteria. http://www.michelsonprizeandgrants .org/michelson-prize/criteria (accessed 18 November 2016).

4 Levy, J.K., Crawford, P.C., Appel, L.D., and Clifford, E.L. (2008). Comparison of intratesticular injection of zinc gluconate versus surgical castration to sterilize male dogs. *American Journal of Veterinary Research* **69**: 140–143.

5 Leoci, R., Aiudi, G., Silvestre, F. et al. (2014). A dose-finding, long-term study on the use of

calcium chloride in saline solution as a method of nonsurgical sterilization in dogs: evaluation of the most effective concentration with the lowest risk. *Acta Veterinaria Scandinavica* **56**: 63.

6 Kutzler, M. and Wood, A. (2006). Non-surgical methods of contraception and sterilization. *Theriogenology* **66**: 514–525.

7 Fontaine, E. and Fontbonne, A. (2010). Clinical use of GnRH agonists in canine and feline species. *Reproduction in Domestic Animals* **46**: 344–353.

8 Alliance for Contraception in Cats & Dogs (2013). Contraception and fertility control in cats & dogs. http://www.acc-d.org/resource-library/e-book/ (accessed 18 November 2016).

9 Levy, J.K., Friary, J.A., Miller, L.A. et al. (2011). Long-term fertility control in female cats with GonaCon™, a GnRH immunocontraceptive. *Theriogenology* **76**: 1517–1525.

10 Griffin, B., Baker, H., Welles, E., et al. (2004). Response of dogs to a GnRH-KLH conjugate contraceptive vaccine adjuvanted with AdjuVac™ [abstract]. 2nd International Symposium on Nonsurgical Methods for Pet Population Control, Breckenridge, CO (24–27 June). http://www.acc-d.org/docs/default-source/2nd-symposium/2004-symposium-proceedings-final.pdf (accessed 1 October 2016).

11 Massei, G., Fagerstone, K., Dhakal, I.P., et al. (2013). Testing GonaCon for female dogs in Nepal: preliminary results [abstract]. 5th International Symposium on Non-Surgical Contraceptive Methods of Pet Population Control, Portland, OR (20–22 June). http://www.acc-d.org/docs/default-source/5th-symposium/massei_nepal_abstract.pdf (accessed 1 October 2016).

12 Romagnoli, S. and Concannon, P. (2003). Clinical use of progestins in bitches and queens: a review. In: *Recent Advances in Small Animal Reproduction* (ed. P. Concannon, G. England, J. Verstegen and C. Linde-Forsberg). Ithaca, NY: International Veterinary Information Service.

13 Munson, L. (2006). Contraception in felids. *Theriogenology* **66**: 126–134.

14 Goericke-Pesch, S., Wehrendi, A., and Georgiev, P. (2014). Suppression of fertility in adult cats. *Reproduction in Domestic Animals* **49** (Suppl. 2): 33–40.

15 U.S. Food & Drug Administration (2003). Freedom of information summary. NADA 141-217: Neutersol® Injectable Solution for Dogs. http://www.fda.gov/downloads/AnimalVeterinary/Products/ApprovedAnimalDrugProducts/FOIADrugSummaries/ucm118024.pdf (accessed 1 October 2016).

16 Ark Sciences (2015). (Zinc Gluconate Neutralized by Arginine) Manufacturer: Ark Sciences, New York (Package insert).

17 Esquivel LaCroix, C.F. (2006). Report on field use in 10,000 dogs in Mexico. Third International Symposium on Non-Surgical Contraceptive Methods Pet Population Control. Alexandria, VA: Alliance for Contraception in Cats & Dogs. http://www.acc-d.org/docs/default-source/3rd-symposium/esquivel_abstract_ppt.pdf (accessed 16 November 2016).

18 Vanderstichel, R., Forzán, M.J., Pérez, G.E. et al. (2015). Changes in blood testosterone concentrations after surgical and chemical sterilization of male free-roaming dogs in southern Chile. *Theriogenology* **83**: 1021–1027.

19 Garde, E., Pérez, G.E., Vanderstichel, R. et al. (2016). Effects of surgical and chemical sterilization on the behavior of free-roaming male dogs in Puerto Natales, Chile. *Preventive Veterinary Medicine* **123**: 106–120.

20 Forzán, M.J., Garde, E., Pérez, G.E., and Vanderstichel, R.V. (2014). Necrosuppurative orchitis and scrotal necrotizing dermatitis following intratesticular administration of zinc gluconate neutralized with arginine (Esterilsol) in 2 mixed-breed dogs. *Veterinary Pathology* **51**: 820–823.

21 Samanta, P.K. (1998). Chemosterilization of stray dogs. *Indian Journal of Animal Health* **37**: 61–62.

22 Jana, K. and Samanta, P.K. (2007). Sterilization of male stray dogs with a single intratesticular injection of calcium chloride: a dose-dependent study. *Contraception* **75**: 390–400.

23 Jana, K. and Samanta, P.K. (2011). Clinical evaluation of non-surgical sterilization of male cats with single intra-testicular injection of calcium chloride. *BMC Veterinary Research* **7**: 39.

24 Leoci, R., Aiudi, G., Silvestre, F. et al. (2014). Alcohol diluent provides the optimal formulation for calcium chloride non-surgical sterilization in dogs. *Acta Veterinaria Scandinavica* **56**: 62.

25 Rhodes, L. (2015). Put a label (claim) on it: getting non-surgical contraceptives approved for use in cats and dogs. *Journal of Feline Medicine and Surgery* **17**: 783–789.

26 SpayFIRST (2014). Calcium chloride dihydrate in alcohol for male dogs and cats. http://www.

spayfirst.org/wp-content/uploads/2014/10/CaCl-formulation-and-dosing-chart-with-photos-for-website-English.pdf (accessed 10 October 2016).

27 Calcium Chloride Castration (2016). Chemical castration of stray dogs and feral cats using calcium chloride. http://www.calciumchloridecastration .com/calcium-chloride-castration-stray-dogs-feral-cats/ (accessed 10 October 2016).

28 Baran, A., Ozdas, O.B., Gulcubuk, A., et al. (2010). Pilot study: intratesticular injection induces sterility in male cats [abstract]. 4th International Symposium on Non-Surgical Methods of Pet Population Control, Dallas, TX (8–10 April). http://www.acc-d.org/docs/default-source/4th-symosium/baran_abstract.pdf (accessed 1 October 2016).

29 Kutzler, M.A. (2015). Intratesticular and intraepididymal injections to sterilize male cats: from calcium chloride to zinc gluconate and beyond. *Journal of Feline Medicine and Surgery* **17**: 772–776.

30 SpayFIRST (2015). Complications that may occur. http://www.spayfirst.org/wp-content/uploads/2015/09/CaCl-Possible-Complications.pdf (accessed 1 October 2016).

31 European Medicines Agency (2010). Annex I: summary of product characteristics. http://www .ema.europa.eu/docs/en_GB/document_library/ EPAR_-_Product_Information/veterinary/000109/ WC500068835.pdf (accessed 1 July 2016).

32 Fontaine, C. (2015). Long-term contraception in a small implant: a review of Suprelorin (deslorelin) studies in cats. *Journal of Feline Medicine and Surgery* **17**: 766–771.

33 Samson-French, J. and Rogers, L. (2013). The use of contraceptive implants (Suprelorin) to control unwanted dog populations on First Nations reserves – a retrospective study. 5th International Symposium on Non-Surgical Contraceptive Methods of Pet Population Control, Portland, OR (20–22 June). http://www.acc-d.org/docs/default-source/5th-symposium/samson-french_deslorelin_abstract.pdf (accessed 13 April 2016).

34 Romagnoli, S., Stelletta, C., Milani, C. et al. (2009). Clinical use of deslorelin for the control of reproduction in the bitch. *Reproduction in Domestic Animals* **44** (Suppl. 2): 36–39.

35 Fontbonne, A., Fontaine, E., Mir, F., et al. (2012). GnRH agonist implants results in oestrus induction and oestrus suppression. 7th

International Symposium on Canine and Feline Reproduction, Whistler, Canada (26–29 July). http://www.ivis.org/proceedings/iscfr/2012/195. pdf (accessed 15 October 2016).

36 Palm, J. and Reichler, I. (2013). May deslorelin acetate be used safely in bitches for contraception? A retrospective clinical study. 5th International Symposium on Non-Surgical Contraceptive Methods of Pet Population Control, Portland, OR (20–22 June). http://www.acc-d.org/docs/default-source/5th-symposium/reichler_abstract.pdf (accessed 13 April 2016).

37 Goericke-Pesch, S., Georgiev, P., Atanasov, A. et al. (2013). Treatment of queens in estrus and after estrus with a GnRH-agonist implant containing 4.7 mg deslorelin; hormonal response, duration of efficacy, and reversibility. *Theriogenology* **79**: 640–646.

38 Toydemir, T.S.F., Kilicarslan, M.R., and Olgaç, V. (2012). Effects of the GnRH analogue deslorelin implants on reproduction in female domestic cats. *Theriogenology* **77**: 662–674.

39 Goericke-Pesch, S., Georgiev, P., Antonov, A. et al. (2014). Reversibility of germinative and endocrine testicular function after long-term contraception with a GnRH agonist implant in the tom – a follow-up study. *Theriogenology* **81**: 941–946.

40 Carranza, A., Faya, M., Lopez Merio, M. et al. (2014). Effect of GnRH analogs in postnatal domestic cats. *Theriogenology* **82**: 138–143.

41 Schäfer-Somi, S., Kaya, D., Gültiken, N., and Aslan, S. (2014). Suppression of fertility in pre-pubertal dogs and cats. *Reproduction in Domestic Animals* **49** (Suppl. 2): 21–27.

42 Kaya, D., Schäfer-Somi, S., Kurt, B. et al. (2015). Clinical use of deslorelin implants for the long-term contraception in prepubertal bitches: effects on epiphyseal closure, body development, and time to puberty. *Theriogenology* **83**: 1147–1153.

43 Goericke-Pesch, S., Georgiev, P., Antonov, A. et al. (2011). Clinical efficacy of GnRH-agonist implant containing 4.7-mg deslorelin, Suprelorin, regarding suppression of reproductive function in tomcats. *Theriogenology* **75**: 803–810.

44 Fontaine, E., Mir, F., Vannier, F. et al. (2011). Induction of fertile oestrus in the bitch using Deslorelin, a GnRH agonist. *Theriogenology* **76**: 1561–1566.

45 Von Heimendahl, A. and Miller, C. (2012). Clinical evaluation of deslorelin to induce oestrus,

ovulation and pregnancy in the bitch. *Reproduction in Domestic Animals* **47** (Suppl. 6): 398–399.

46 Zambelli, D., Bini, C., Küster, D.G. et al. (2015). First deliveries after estrus induction using deslorelin and endoscopic transcervical insemination in the queen. *Theriogenology* **84**: 773–778.

47 Lucas, X. (2014). Clinical use of Deslorelin (GnRH agonist) in companion animals: a review. *Reproduction in Domestic Animals* **49** (Suppl. 4): 64–71.

48 Trigg, T., Wright, P., Armour, A. et al. (2001). Use of a GnRH analogue implant to produce reversible long-term suppression of reproductive function in male and female domestic dogs. *Journal of Reproduction and Fertility* **57** (Suppl): 255–261.

49 Sung, M., Armour, A.F., and Wright, P.J. (2006). The influence of exogenous progestin on the occurrence of proestrous or estrous signs, plasma concentrations of luteinizing hormone and estradiol in deslorelin (GnRH agonist) treated anestrous bitches. *Theriogenology* **66**: 1513–1517.

50 Goericke-Pesch, S., Georgiev, P., Atanasov, A., and Wehrend, A. (2013). Treatment with Suprelorin in a pregnant cat. *Journal of Feline Medicine and Surgery* **15**: 357–360.

51 Wright, P.J., Stelmasiak, T., Black, D., and Sykes, D. (1979). Medroxyprogesterone acetate and reproductive processes in male dogs. *Australian Veterinary Journal* **55**: 437–438.

52 England, G.C. (1997). Effect of progestogens and androgens upon spermatogenesis and steroidogenesis in dogs. *Journal of Reproduction and Fertility* **51**: 123–138.

53 Romagnoli, S. (2015). Progestins to control feline reproduction: historical abuse of high doses and potentially safe use of low doses. *Journal of Feline Medicine and Surgery* **17**: 743–752.

54 Burke, T. and Reynolds, H. Jr. (1975). Megestrol acetate for estrus postponement in the bitch. *Journal of the American Veterinary Medical Association* **167**: 285–287.

55 Oen, E.O. (1977). The oral administration of megestrol acetate to postpone oestrus in cats. *Nordiskveterinaermedicin* **29**: 287–291.

56 Greenberg, M., Lawler, D., Zawistowski, S., and Jöchle, W. (2013). Low-dose megestrol acetate revisited: a viable adjunct to surgical sterilization in free roaming cats? *The Veterinary Journal* **196**: 304–308.

57 Jackson, E. (1984). Contraception in the dog and cat. *The British Veterinary Journal* **140**: 132–137.

58 Romagnoli, S. (2006). Control of reproduction in dogs and cats: use and misuse of hormones. In: 2006 World Congress WSAVA/FECAVA/CSAVA, 701–706. Ithaca, NY: International Veterinary Information Service.

59 Kustritz, M.V.R. (2012). Effects of surgical sterilization on canine and feline health and on society. *Reproduction in Domestic Animals* **47** (Suppl. 4): 2014–2222.

60 World Society for the Protection of Animals (2014). Identification methods for dogs and cats. http://www.icam-coalition.org/downloads/ Identification%20methods%20for%20dogs%20and %20cats.pdf (accessed 1 November 2016).

61 Alliance for Contraception in Cats & Dogs (2013). Methods of marking and identification for dogs and cats. http://www.acc-d.org/docs/default-source/think-tanks/markingmethodsreview.pdf (accessed 20 October 2016).

62 Leoci, R., Aiudi, G., Silvestre, F., et al. (2013). A comparison of the humaneness and large-scale application potential of two visual identification methods for stray dogs. 5th International Symposium on Non-Surgical Contraceptive Methods of Pet Population Control, Portland, OR (20–22 June). http://www.acc-d.org/docs/default-source/5th-symposium/leoci_marking_abstract.pdf (accessed 20 October 2016).

63 Benka, V. (2013). ACC&D Think Tank and Innocentive® challenge results. 5th International Symposium on Non-Surgical Contraceptive Methods of Pet Population Control, Portland, OR (20–22 June). http://www.acc-d.org/docs/default-source/5th-symposium/benka_abstract.pdf (accessed 20 October 2016).

64 Benka, V. (2015). Ear tipsto ear tags: marking and identifying cats treated with non-surgical fertility control. *Journal of Feline Medicine and Surgery* **17**: 808–815.

65 Kitagaki, M. and Shibuya, K. (2004). Nylon ear tags for individual identification of guinea pigs. *Journal of the American Association for Laboratory Animal Science* **43**: 16–20.

# 9

# Spay/Neuter Surgical Techniques

## 9.1

# Orchiectomy and Ovariohysterectomy

*Lori Bierbrier[1] and Hillary Causanschi[2]*

[1]American Society for the Prevention of Cruelty to Animals, 424 East 92nd Street, New York, NY 10128, USA
[2]Bucks County Society for the Prevention of Cruelty to Animals, 60 Reservoir Road, Quakertown, PA 18951, USA

### 9.1.1 Introduction

Sterilization, or spay/neuter, is a commonly performed elective procedure for dogs and cats. In the field, sterilization is the cornerstone of catch–vaccinate–neuter–return (CVNR) and trap–neuter–return (TNR) programs. There are many potential reasons for sterilization including the following:

- Prevention of diseases of the reproductive tract and associated hormonal related conditions
- Prevention of reproduction
- Potential reduction of undesirable behaviors
- Part of a population management program

Although neuter is a general term for sterilization, in veterinary medicine, it is customarily defined as

- Spay or ovariohysterectomy (OHE) for female animals
- Neuter or castration for male animals.

Many veterinary textbooks detail the techniques to perform spay/neuter procedures [1,2]. Although there are specific aspects to each surgery that must be performed, there is a wide variation in acceptable techniques and surgeon's preferences.

The advent of high-quality high-volume spay/neuter (HQHVSN) has further refined these techniques to streamline the surgical process so as to maximize surgical efficiency [3]. HQHVSN techniques include reducing the incision size and ligating vessels in a more efficient manner. This benefits the patient by reducing surgery and anesthesia time, and minimizes tissue handling. These techniques are particularly advantageous in the field setting where one may be working in challenging conditions and where maximizing the number of animals who can receive surgery safely in a day is paramount. In addition, HQHVSN techniques are particularly useful for free-roaming animals that will be returned to the field with limited to no postoperative monitoring after clinic discharge.

Although surgical techniques will be described in this chapter, the ideal way to learn HQHVSN techniques is to receive hands-on training or watch surgery (either in person or via video).

The ASPCA Spay/Neuter Alliance (www.aspcapro .org/about-programs-services/aspca-spayneuter-alliance), has many e-learning and in-person training opportunities. The online Yahoo group HQHVSNvets also offers additional peer support.

This chapter focuses specifically on the spay/neuter surgical procedure itself. The procedure can however only be safely and effectively performed if there is appropriate patient selection and perioperative care, well-maintained surgical instruments and supplies, and adequate site support (see Chapter 5). Surgical sterilization may not be appropriate for every situation, especially if the availability of resources cannot ensure that minimum acceptable standards of care are met. In the future, nonsurgical fertility control techniques may become available that are better suited for such situations.

### 9.1.2 Surgical Preparation

#### 9.1.2.1 Surgeon Sterilization and Preparation Techniques

Proper sterile technique involves multiple preparations: the surgical packs, patients, and surgeon. The surgeon should always be aware of his/her sterility. Regardless of clinic location and setup, the minimum level of appropriate surgical attire that the surgeon should be wearing is a cap, a mask that covers the mouth and nose, and new sterile gloves for each patient. The surgeon's surgical scrub should be performed via acceptable techniques as outlined in surgical texts and in Chapter 11 [1,2]. Hands should be dried with a sterile hand towel, and a pair of sterile gloves should be put on immediately following the surgical scrub. Each surgery warrants a new pair of sterile gloves without exception. Gowning should be based on local laws first and foremost.

Waterless antimicrobial products (e.g. Avagard™ D) are an alternative to traditional scrub brushes with antimicrobial products. When using a waterless product, it is still recommended that the surgeon thoroughly clean his or her hands and forearms prior to application. The waterless products can be especially useful in clinic settings with limited access to running water [1].

HQHVSN surgeons maintain sterility but do not generally rescrub between each surgery. Any small break in sterility (e.g. a tear in a glove) can be managed either through the use of a topical waterless disinfectant product or through rescrubbing the hands. A large break in sterility warrants complete rescrubbing.

---

**Textbox 9.1.1 Surgeon sterility tip**

Sterility is easily maintained if the surgeon keeps his/her gloves on in between surgeries (and does not remove them or touch things with his/her bare hands) and changes gloves immediately before the next surgery.

---

### 9.1.2.2 Surgical Packs for Spay/Neuter

Spay/neuter surgical packs, also known as surgical kits in many parts of the world, can be made very simply. First, one must decide upon the type of pack wrap and drape material that is best for the clinic (reusable drape or nonreusable materials). While the initial cost for reusable materials is generally higher, long-term cost may be comparable. When deciding between the two materials, consider the following: reusable materials will require that the clinic has regular access to a washing machine and that there

is a way to preclean or soak the pack wraps and drapes during the day to keep them from becoming blood stained. This can be challenging in alternative clinic models such as mobile army surgical hospital (MASH)-style or mobile clinics. Additionally, if a clinic decides to use reusable drapes and pack wraps, the clinic will need to keep double the number of pack wraps and drapes on hand so that instruments can be wrapped and packed during the clinic day, autoclaved, and ready for the next day. Reusable materials require daily laundry washing. If this is challenging given the clinic setup, the clinic may want to choose disposable materials. In both cases, be aware that the minimum thread count for pack wraps is 270 [1, 3].

When constructing a surgical pack, consider what the surgeon needs and what might work best for the support staff. Technicians and veterinary assistants (and sometimes volunteers) are generally responsible for cleaning, packing, wrapping, and autoclaving surgical packs in the clinic setting. Having many different types of packs (e.g. different packs for canine spays, feline spays, canine neuters, and feline neuters) may put additional strain on support staff and be more time consuming for them in what is already a very fast paced, busy day. Consider streamlining the clinic pack system so that one pack fits all surgeries. The author recommends one pack type that can be used for a feline spay, canine spay, and canine neuter and another pack type that can be used for feline neuters.

### 9.1.2.3 Primary Surgical Packs

As mentioned in the previous section, one pack can be constructed for both feline and canine spays and canine neuters. The instrument makeup of the pack needs to work for the surgeon and the clinic. There are certain instruments that should be standard including a spay hook, thumb forceps, a needle driver, Metzenbaum scissors, and towel clamps (Table 9.1.1). Hemostats (Kelly and mosquito) are also necessary components of the spay/neuter pack.

The decision to use curved or straight instruments is entirely surgeon dependent. If the clinic has many veterinarians or utilizes rotating volunteers, consider having one of each in the pack. Additionally, if the clinic tends to do a significant number of large breed and giant dogs, consider adding an additional Carmalt forceps to the surgical packs.

**Table 9.1.1** Suggested surgery pack for routine spay surgical procedures.

| Number | Instrument |
|---|---|
| 1 | Olsen-Hagar needle driver (or Mayo-Hagar) |
| 1 | Spay hook |
| 1 | Brown-Adson tissue forceps |
| 1 | Metzenbaum scissors |
| 2 | Kelly hemostats |
| 2 | Mosquito hemostats |
| 2 | Towel clamps (optional) |
| 1 | Carmalt forceps |
| +/− 1 | Mayo scissors (if the packs contain disposable patient drapes or Mayo-Hagar needle drivers) |

Besides instruments, a surgical pack includes the following necessary items:

- Stack of gauze of known number
- Autoclave indicator strip that is compatible with the clinic's autoclave (i.e. use a steam indicator strip for steam sterilization)
- Patient drape (with the exception of the feline neuter packs).

### 9.1.2.4 Feline Neuter Packs

Feline neuter packs can be easily assembled using hemostats and gauze. Multiple hemostats can be placed in a single feline neuter pack to facilitate minimizing the number of packs needed for feline neuters. Care must be taken by the surgeon to remove instruments and gauze from the pack for each surgery and keep the remaining instruments/gauze sterile. In the author's experience, this works well by using the surgical glove wrap as a sterile field to place items needed for the individual surgery.

Kelly hemostats (either curved or straight) or mosquito hemostats (either curved or straight) would be appropriate for the pack and instrument selection can be dependent on what the clinic has and/or what the surgeon's preference is. The number of instruments used for the neuter pack is entirely up to the surgeon and clinic needs. Within the neuter pack, aim for about a ratio of 2:1 for gauze to instruments and include an indicator strip within the pack as well (Figure 9.1.1).

It is prudent to keep spare autoclaved instruments individually packed in pouches in case they are needed. The authors recommend that the clinic have at least 2 of each type of instrument individually packaged and autoclaved (mirroring what is in the pack). It is also recommended that the clinic have individually autoclaved patient drapes, hand towels, and pouches of autoclaved gauze.

Another important factor when constructing surgical packs is to make sure that all instruments are cleaned thoroughly prior to sterilization. Refer to Chapter 11 on sanitation and surgical asepsis for further information.

### 9.1.2.5 Suture and Needle Selection

Many types of suture and surgical needles are available. A detailed description of the wide variety of products available is beyond the scope of this text, but can be found in a comprehensive veterinary surgery textbook [4]. Suture selection may be influenced by surgeon preference and local availability of products.

#### 9.1.2.5.1 Suture

The surgeon should assess several variables when selecting appropriate suture.

- *Behavior in the tissue.* Absorbable versus non-absorbable
- *Structure.* Braided versus monofilament
- *Packaging.* Individual packaged suture versus bulk cassette.

In the author's opinion, monofilament absorbable suture is preferable for spay/neuter surgery (e.g. poliglecaprone 25/Monocryl® and polydioxanone/PDS®). This type of suture works well in soft tissue and it generally causes minimal tissue reaction during absorption. Absorbable sutures also have the advantage that they can be used to place intradermal skin sutures that do not require removal. This eliminates the need for follow-up skin suture removal, which may be impractical or impossible in the field. Tables 9.1.2 and 9.1.3 describe the characteristics of both absorbable and non-absorbable sutures, when their use is appropriate, and strength retention times.

Regarding strength retention, PDS retains its strength longer than plain catgut, chromic catgut, and Monocryl [5]. The author prefers Monocryl to

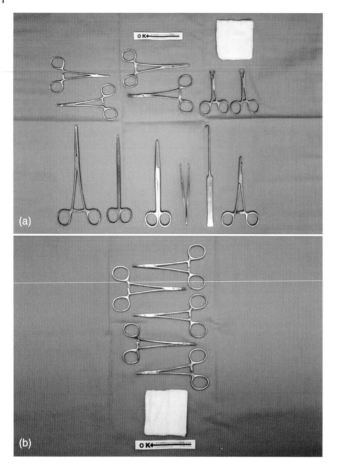

Figure 9.1.1 (a) Instruments, gauze, and sterile indicator strip for a spay/neuter surgery pack and (b) feline neuter pack. Source: Courtesy of Thomas Newberger and the ASPCA.

PDS, given that it is absorbed more rapidly in the body than the latter.

Braided suture (e.g. Polyglactin 910/Vicryl®) is not the preferred suture choice as it is more likely to cause unnecessary inflammation during reabsorption and may harbor bacteria [4]. However, Vicryl is used commonly in field situations due to its cost and wide availability.

Surgical gut suture is another absorbable suture material used for spay/neuter surgery. Although it is

Table 9.1.2 Suture characteristics: absorbable versus non-absorbable.

| Absorbable | Non-absorbable |
| --- | --- |
| More reactive in the short-term; less reactive in the long-term | Less reactive in the short-term |
| Used when the suture will be buried under the skin | Used for removable skin sutures |
| Can be used in the skin (may take up to 60 days for complete absorption) | Used when holding strength is important after typical absorption time has been exceeded |
| Ideal for catch–vaccinate–neuter–return (CVNR) and trap–neuter–return (TNR) programs when return to the clinic for suture removal is unlikely | Rarely used in field programs |

Source: Fossum 2007 [4]. Reproduced with permission of Elsevier

Table 9.1.3 Characteristics of commonly used absorbable suture.*

| Suture material | Strength retention profile | Complete absorption |
| --- | --- | --- |
| Catgut (plain) | 90% loss at 7–10 days | 70 days (Unpredictable) |
| Chromic surgical catgut | 50% loss at 7 days; 100% loss by 21 days | 80–120 days (Unpredictable) |
| Vicryl (polyglactin 910) | 35% loss at 14 days, 60–70% loss by 21 days | 70 days |
| Monocryl (poliglecaprone 25) | 50% loss at 7 days; 100% loss by 21 days | 90–120 days |
| PDS (polydioxanone) | 14% loss at 14 days; 40% loss by 30 days | 180 days |

* Note values included here are estimates as loss of tensile strength and absorption may vary depending on the suture material used and tissue.
Source: Adapted from ASPCA Spay/Neuter Alliance Veterinary Reference Guide [5].

not the author's preferred choice, it can be used for the ovarian pedicles and uterine body, as well as for the spermatic cord. Gut suture should not be used to close the body wall, subcutaneous tissue, or intradermal layers.

Stainless steel suture, a non-absorbable product, may also be used effectively although it is not the author's preference. It requires a somewhat different technique from other non-metallic sutures, which must be mastered prior to use.

Clips such as hemoclips may be used for vessel ligation [4]. They are not commonly used in high-quality, high-volume spay/neuter surgery.

If the surgeon chooses suture with swaged-on needles (individually suture packets with the needle attached), it should be of a type that is appropriate for all components of the surgery, so that one packet (ideally) can be used for the entire surgery. If the surgeon uses bulk cassette suture (larger cartridges with suture that are meant for multiuse), the surgeon can more easily and less wastefully use multiple types of suture for one patient. If cassettes are used, the clinic will also have to have sterilized needles of varying size on hand to use with the suture.

### 9.1.2.5.2  Suture Size
The choice of suture size is based on surgeon preference.

> **Textbox 9.1.2  General suture size recommendations**
>
> - Cats and small dogs. 2–0 USP or 3–0 USP
> - Small dogs > 10 lbs (22 kg) but < 30 lbs (66 kg): 2–0 USP
> - Dogs > 30 lbs (66 kg): 0 USP.

> **Textbox 9.1.3  Suture selection take-home points**
>
> - Monofilament absorbable suture is preferred for spay/neuter surgery.
> - Medical-grade, sterilized suture and needles should be used for each surgical patient.
> - Bulk cassette suture is far less expensive than swaged-on suture.
> - Cable ties should never be used as a ligature. Toxic substances are released during their degradation and their use may result in abscess or tumor formation [4].
> - Suture should not be soaked in disinfectants and reused.

### 9.1.2.5.3  Needles
Many types of surgery needles are available. The following two are main categories for HQHVSN:

- Swaged end versus eyed end
- Cutting versus taper end.

Individual suture packets with swaged-on needles are very convenient for the surgeon. These tend to be costlier than suture on a cassette but regional variation necessitates that this be evaluated on an individual basis. In addition to the convenience for the surgeon, they offer the benefit that each package is sterile until the time of opening. In a mobile or MASH setting where materials are repeatedly packed/unpacked, this benefit is important. Another benefit is that there is no need to autoclave surgical needles separately.

Although taper point needles are less traumatic to tissue, a cutting needle is required for intradermal closure. A HQHVSN surgery can typically be performed using a single packet of this suture. If individually packaged suture is being used, the needle selection should be a cutting needle to allow for effective intradermal closure. The product that the authors use has a reverse-cutting needle, which causes less tissue trauma and is stronger than a traditional cutting needle [4,6].

If using suture from a cassette, it is imperative to remove suture from the cassette in a sterile manner. If the surgeon is unsure whether the protruding end of suture on the cassette is sterile, it must be removed.

---

**Textbox 9.1.4 How to remove suture from cassette in a sterile manner**

- The assistant holds onto the unsterile suture end and pulls out a small amount of suture.
- The surgeon cuts this suture off using sterile scissors.
- The surgeon then proceeds to pull out the needed amount of suture.

---

### 9.1.2.6 HQHVSN Surgical Techniques

One of the most effective ways to improve spay/neuter speed and efficiency is to appropriately place the incision and minimize its size. Small incisions decrease surgery time and accelerate healing by reducing tissue trauma [2].

---

**Textbox 9.1.5 Techniques to improve spay/neuter efficiency**

- Adjust the number of clamps used (it is rare to utilize the "three-clamp technique").
- Reduce use of towel clamps.
- Reduce use of ties for positioning the patient – use V trays, sand bags, or similar ones to hold the animal in position.
- Use alternative ligature techniques including the ovarian pedicle tie, Miller's knot, and figure-eight knot.
- In the author's opinion, reducing the number and size of knots can reduce postsurgical suture reaction and increase surgical efficiency.

---

### 9.1.2.7 Tissue Adhesive

Surgical tissue adhesives (cyanoacrylates) such as Vetbond™ can be placed on the incision after the intradermal skin closure. When using tissue adhesives, it is extremely important to gently squeeze the skin edges together and place the tissue adhesive over top of the incision. If the tissue adhesive is placed *in* the incision (rather than *on* the incision), it can cause a foreign body reaction and potentially impede healing.

Tissue adhesives can also be placed on the skin after a tattoo is placed. The author has seen non-veterinary glue products being used in spay/neuter clinics (e.g. Krazy® glue). This is not recommended as one cannot be assured of their sterility and they are a potential irritant to the skin.

### 9.1.2.8 Antibiotics

The use of antibiotics in routine spay/neuter procedures is controversial. Antibiotics should really only be given under certain situations, such as a break in sterility or in an animal with a pre-existing infection such as a pyometra [3]. Furthermore, antibiotics are not a replacement for adherence to sterile surgical technique, use of sterile instruments, and suture and effective shaving/patient preparation [7]. Ultimately, the decision on whether to give a long-acting pre-operative, intraoperative, or postoperative is at the doctor's discretion but all efforts should be made to improve hygiene to eliminate the need for routine administration of antibiotics.

### 9.1.2.9 Local Anesthetic Blocks

Local blocks are very useful for pain management in spay/neuter surgeries and should be incorporated when available. See Chapter 7 for additional information on local blocks.

## 9.1.3 Identifying Previously Altered Animals

In addition to identifying the sex of the animal during presurgical examination, it is also imperative to determine, when possible, whether the animal has previously been sterilized.

For female dogs and cats, there is no absolute external anatomical indicator to identify an animal as sterilized. That being said, it is important to shave the animal's

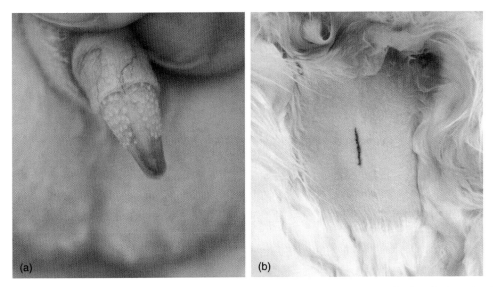

**Figure 9.1.2** (a) Spines on male cat penis (b) Abdominal skin tattoo to permanently identify the animal as sterilized. Source: Courtesy of Thomas Newberger and the ASPCA.

abdomen and look for a midline scar consistent with the location of a spay scar (caudal to the umbilicus). If a scar is found, then further discussion with the owner or caretaker is needed to determine whether this animal may have had abdominal surgery previously (e.g. caesarian section, foreign body removal). If a surgeon is working in an area in which flank spays are more common, he or she should also consider shaving the lateral abdomen to look for a scar (see the section on flank spays for anatomic location). In addition, the surgeon should also examine the vulva and mammary glands. An enlarged vulva is more likely found in an intact animal, whereas lack of mammary development in an adult animal would be consistent with previous sterilization surgery. Often an exploratory surgery is needed to confirm the presence or absence of reproductive tissue.

In male dogs, the lack of testicles in the scrotum may be consistent with previous neuter. This is not 100% confirmatory however, as it is possible that the animal is bilaterally cryptorchid. It may be beneficial to shave the prescrotal area to find a scar, although a scar may not be visible depending on the size and how long ago the animal was neutered. If there are no testicles in the scrotum nor in the inguinal area (for a bilateral inguinal cryptorchid dog), then abdominal exploratory surgery is required to confirm the presence or absence of testicles.

In male cats, there is a definitive means of identifying whether they are neutered or a bilateral cryptorchid. Unneutered male cats have small spines present on the penis. These spines are testosterone dependent and will atrophy within 6 weeks of neuter [2].

In some cases, a tattoo may have been placed on the animal to indicate that he/she was sterilized. This is an extremely valuable and highly recommended practice as for most animals it is not obvious whether they have been sterilized (Figure 9.1.2).

Blood tests are available to measure sex hormone levels as a means of assessing whether an animal is altered, but these are impractical in the field and are excluded here.

### 9.1.3.1 Tattoo

Tattooing is a valuable procedure done at the time of spay/neuter surgery to identify sterilized animals. It can prevent an animal of unknown reproductive status from unnecessary future surgery to confirm sterilization. This is especially beneficial for animals who had this procedure performed at an early age and may have a very small scar on their skin.

A common technique for tattooing is to place a thin "line" of tattoo ink near or in the incision. Several types of tattoo ink are available, both in a liquid and paste form. In the author's opinion, the paste form (e.g. Ketchum brand) is very user–friendly and cost–effective.

---

**Textbox 9.1.6 Abdominal tattoo techniques**

- *Tattoo in the incision*. Place tattoo ink in the incision after intradermal closure.
- *Tattoo lateral to incision*\*. Perform a small (half inch) partial thickness skin incision lateral to the incision; instill tattoo ink in this line.

\*This is the author's preferred method so that the tattoo ink is not incorporated into the area of full-thickness incisional healing. Should the animal need further abdominal surgery, either on the same day or in the future, the tattoo area will then not be compromised.

---

A small amount of ink can be placed either on the unused, dull end of the scalpel or on the edge of the sterile indicator strip and then carefully applied into the incision. It is important not to use the sharp end of the used scalpel blade so as not to contaminate the ink. A small amount of tissue adhesive is placed over the tattoo.

Many field programs use tattoo pliers to tattoo a combination of letters and numbers in the animal's ear, indicative of specific information related to the animal such as location and year of surgery. This is commonly performed in areas where ear notching is forbidden.

Tattoo machines are also available. These are not preferable as they require electricity, user skill to operate, and it is impossible to maintain sterility between patients.

### 9.1.3.2 Ear Tipping

Ear tipping is an effective, humane, and universally accepted method used to identify spayed/neutered free-roaming cats. This is a preferred identification method as it can be difficult to get close to free-roaming cats and identification must be visible from a distance. Free-roaming cats may interact with a variety of caretakers, veterinarians, and animal control personnel during their lives so immediate visual identification is necessary to prevent an unnecessary second trapping and surgery.

Ear tipping is performed under anesthesia by removing no more than 1 cm of the tip of an adult cat's left ear

in a straight line (and a proportionately smaller amount in a kitten) (Figure 9.1.3). There is little or no bleeding when done properly, it is relatively painless, and the ear tip does not significantly alter the cat's appearance.

---

**Textbox 9.1.7 Ear tipping technique**

1) Place a clean, straight hemostat across the tip of the cat's left ear, exposing no more than 1 cm of the ear tip for adult cats and proportionally less for kittens.
   Use new, clean hemostat for each cat.
2) Using sterile scissors or sterile blade, cut the tip off of the ear, leaving the hemostat on the ear. Use new sterile scissors or new sterile blade for each cat.
3) Apply small amount of styptic powder to the cut edge of the ear.
4) To reduce bleeding, keep the hemostat on the cat's ear until just before returning the cat to trap [8].

---

Ear tipping can be a more challenging form of identification in very cold areas where cats may already have damaged ear pinnae from frostbite. Ear notching rather than tipping is routinely done on community dogs given the lack of uniformity of ear types in dogs.

## 9.1.4 Practical Techniques for Routine Spay/Neuter Surgery

### 9.1.4.1 Canine Spay (Ovariohysterectomy)

Canine spays can be somewhat more challenging than feline spays given the anatomical differences of the uterus in each of the species (e.g. the associated fat within the broad ligament and the tension of the suspensory ligament). There are some techniques that will help make the approach easier.

#### 9.1.4.1.1 Incision Placement
Start by looking at the dog and estimating her age:

- If the patient is a pediatric (2–5 months old), place the skin incision midway between the umbilicus and pubis.
- If the patient is over 1 year old, the incision should be placed closer to the umbilicus (the incision can be placed anywhere from directly at the umbilicus

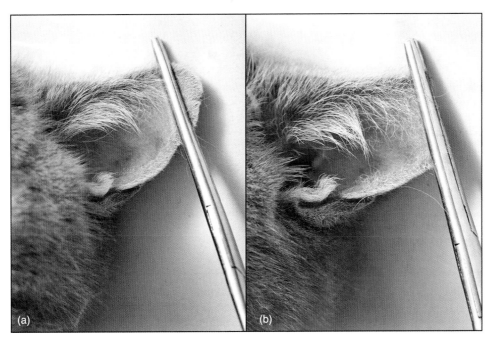

**Figure 9.1.3** Ear tipping technique for cats. (a) Placement of hemostat on the left ear (b) Remove the ear tip using sterile scissors or surgical blade. Source: Courtesy of Thomas Newberger and the ASPCA.

to two-finger widths caudal to the umbilicus, depending on surgeon preference).

Patients between 5 months and 1 year of age are slightly more challenging, and incision placement is more difficult. Placement can be variable and dependent on a number of factors: large breed versus small breed, deep chested versus barrel chested, etc.

#### 9.1.4.1.2 Canine Spay Procedure
The procedure should be performed as follows:

- Once the skin incision has been placed, take the time to clear the fat off of the linea as needed through a combination of blunt and sharp dissection, so that the linea can be confidently identified. The incision should be approximately 1 inch long, but the size will vary depending on the age and size of the dog.
- Once the linea is identified (which will appear as a white line, of variable width, and may even appear as a slight indentation in the body wall), grasp the linea with thump forceps (tent the linea) and make a stab incision with a surgical blade. For safety, face the sharp side of the blade upward away from the abdomen when making the stab incision. The author prefers a #10 surgical blade for dog spay surgeries,

but a #15 blade is also a good option. This is very important to avoid accidentally incising through abdominal organs, which may be just under the body wall such as the spleen or the urinary bladder.
- Slide the thumb forceps into the hole made by the blade. Lift the linea upward with the thumb forceps and extend the incision cranially and caudally with either a blade or scissors.
- Once the linea incision is complete, lift the body wall on the right side of the abdomen using the thumb forceps to allow the spay hook to slide into the abdomen (also on the right side) with ease.
- Advance the spay hook down along the body wall (with the hook facing laterally) until the dorsal abdomen has been reached. Placing the spay hook in this manner will avoid contact with abdominal organs. Searching for the uterus on the right side will prevent trauma to the spleen.
- Turn the hook so that it is facing medially and sweep the spay hook toward the midline, then bring the hook upward out of the abdomen. If the uterus has been grabbed in the spay hook, there will be a slight amount of tension as the spay hook is brought out of the abdomen. If there is significant amount or lack of tension, then it is unlikely that the uterus is in the spay hook and

the tissue should be released. Repeat the process until the uterus has been successfully exteriorized with the spay hook.

 – Alternatively, the surgeon may choose to advance the finger into the abdomen and use it to scoop up the uterus (as if the finger was a spay hook). The finger can scoop from the midline laterally and can start beneath the bladder, where the uterus is anatomically positioned (between the bladder and the colon), in order to more easily locate it.

---

**Textbox 9.1.8 Tips for finding the uterus**

When using the spay hook, there is a very specific feel of moderate resistance when the uterine tissue is being retracted from the abdomen.

- Too little resistance – likely mesentery
- Too much resistance – likely pancreas, colon, or other organ

---

- Once the uterus is in the spay hook (or the surgeon's finger), bring the horn out of the abdomen and trace it cranially to the ovary.
- Apply tension to the proper ligament; this will allow the surgeon to exteriorize the ovary. Then the surgeon should advance his/her fingers into the abdomen to break down the suspensory ligament. The suspensory ligament will have some tension to it and will angle craniodorsally from the ovary.
- Strum the suspensory ligament to break it down in order to get full visualization of the pedicle. Options for this process include the following steps:
 – The surgeon keeps his/her index finger on one side of the suspensory ligament and thumb on the other. The surgeon then uses the index finger against the thumb to break it down.
 – The surgeon puts gentle, even pressure on the ligament moving the thumb and fingers in the opposite direction. This does a good "controlled" break. Using this technique allows the surgeon to put pressure on the ligament going in both directions.
- Once the pedicle can be exteriorized adequately, there are a couple of approaches that can be used for ligation:
 – Ligate the pedicle before transecting: although surgery textbooks describe a three-clamp

technique, one does not necessarily have to have three clamps in place to safely ligate a pedicle. One to two clamps can be sufficient and less cumbersome to work around, using either a Kelly or Carmalt on the pedicle itself.
 – The "cut-away technique" (cut first, ligate second): Place hemostats on the ovarian pedicle (in this case three clamps may be warranted), cutting between the two closest to the ovary so that the pedicle is separated from the ovary prior to ligation. A ligature is then placed in the crush of the most proximal clamp (the deeper of the two clamps).

---

**Textbox 9.1.9 Ligature selection**

There are multiple options for the type of ligature placed on a pedicle, including an encircling ligature with surgeon's knot, a Miller's/modified Miller's knot, or a transfixation. The author prefers the Miller's knot and has found that transfixation is very rarely necessary as one Miller's knot is usually sufficient to provide complete hemostasis in most patients.
 To perform a Miller's knot [2]:

- Place the suture below the tissue, encircling the tissue and pulling it below the tissue again to form a loose loop.
- Place the needle driver through the loop and then place the first throw of a square knot. Tighten carefully to evenly incorporate the initial loop.
- Place a second throw to complete the square knot.
- Continue to place 2–3 additional square knots.

---

- Once the right pedicle has been ligated and transected, trace the right uterine horn caudally until the uterine body and left uterine horn appear. If the uterine body is not easily exteriorized in the process, one technique the author has found beneficial is to apply tension to the body wall at the caudal aspect of the incision while applying gentle tension to the uterus. If that does not work, the surgeon may need to extend the incision to safely exteriorize the uterus. Trace the left uterine horn cranially to the ovary and repeat the above process on the left ovarian pedicle.
- Once each pedicle has been sufficiently ligated, break down the broad ligament using blunt dissection. In the author's experience, it is rare for the

broad ligament to require ligation and the determination to place a ligature on the broad ligament should be based on whether or not it appears particularly vascular (for example, in a patient actively in heat, you might notice more prominent vessels within the broad ligament) or the surgeon is operating in an area endemic with diseases that make a patient more prone to bleeding intraoperatively (e.g. *Ehrlichia* spp. endemic areas).

- Once the broad ligament is broken down, proceed with ligation of the uterine body using one of the abovementioned ligatures. The author has found that in most cases (with normal, healthy tissue), the Miller's or modified Miller's knot is sufficient without the need for additional ligatures or transfixation (Figure 9.1.4). Additional ligatures may be necessary in the case of a uterus that is enlarged (such as in heat, pregnant, pyometra, or hydrometra).
- The abdominal wall may be closed with a simple interrupted, cruciate, or simple continuous pattern. The simple continuous pattern is efficient and results in minimal number of knots. It is the author's opinion that knots are a source of potential tissue reaction during reabsorption. Minimizing the number of knots and placing the appropriate number of throws (4–6) is important in preventing such postoperative complications. The choice of suture pattern for abdominal wall closure may also depend on the size of the incision. A simple continuous pattern may be selected for a larger incision, such as that of a canine spay. In the author's opinion, if the linea alba incision is relatively small, the cruciate pattern may be a more efficient means of abdominal closure; however, this ultimately depends on the size of the incision and surgeon preference.
- Following complete closure of the abdominal wall, proceed with closure of the subcutaneous and intradermal layers. In patients with minimal subcutaneous fat, closing the intradermal layer alone is

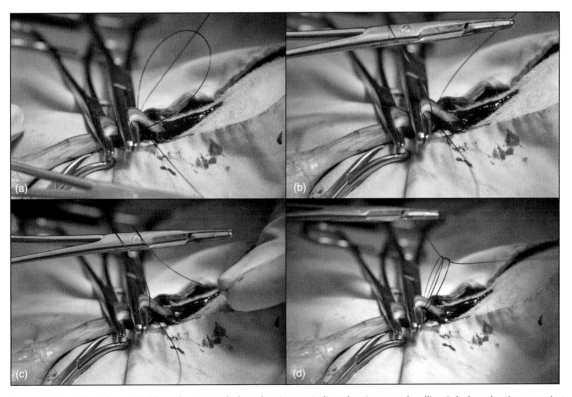

**Figure 9.1.4** Miller's knot. (a) Place the suture below the tissue, circling the tissue and pulling it below the tissue again to form a loose loop. (b) Place the needle driver through the loop. (c) Place the first throw of a square knot. (d) Tighten carefully to evenly incorporate the initial loop. Place a second throw to complete the square knot. Continue to place 2–3 additional square knots. Source: Courtesy of Thomas Newberger and the ASPCA.

likely adequate. Otherwise, the surgeon will want to proceed with closures of both subcutaneous and intradermal layers. These layers can be closed independently of each other.

- The subcutaneous tissue may also be closed in all methods noted for the abdominal wall. It is common practice to close the subcutaneous tissue with a simple continuous pattern. Surgeons vary in opinions as to whether to close the subcutaneous layer in cats. The author has seen surgeries with both subcutaneous layer closed and not closed with little variation in outcome.
- An approach that has worked for the authors is to incorporate the subcutaneous and intradermal closure together. This reduces the number of knots and creates an efficient and effective closure.

---

**Textbox 9.1.10 Steps for closing the subcutaneous and intradermal layers**

1) Begin as if burying a knot at one end of the incision (starting deep to superficial within the subcutaneous fat on one side of the incision and superficial to deep on the other) on the surgeon's left-hand side, leaving a tail of suture.
2) Commence with a simple continuous pattern within the subcutaneous fat from until the other end of the incision has been reached.
3) Without placing a knot, begin the intradermal pattern and proceed back to the other side of the incision (where the subcutaneous pattern began).
4) As the final bite, place a superficial-to-deep throw in the subcutaneous tissue and ligate it to the tail that was left initially. (Note: The first two throws of that knot should be made snug, but do not apply excess tension to those throws, otherwise the incision will cinch together. On the third throw, it should be possible to apply more tension to the knot without causing the accordion effect.)
5) If further assistance is needed in burying the knot following your final throw, prior to cutting the needle off the suture, place the needle into the incision, through the subcutaneous tissue and exiting through the skin adjacent to the incision, there should be a slight pop as the knot slides under the skin.

---

- The tattoo should then be placed adjacent to the incision as described previously.

It is recommended to minimize handling of the skin with surgical instruments such as forceps. Any tissue trauma to the skin can interfere with wound healing.

One technique favored by the author is to hold the skin tight with the opposite (non-suturing) hand by gently pulling in the opposite direction that the suture is being placed when placing intradermal sutures. This slight tension on the skin makes using skin forceps unnecessary. That being said, some surgeons prefer to use Brown-Adson tissue forceps.

Alternatively, the skin can be closed with skin sutures, simple interrupted or cruciate suture patterns, rather than intradermal closure. This is not the preferred method by the author as this requires suture removal, which may be impractical or impossible in the field. Non-absorbable skin sutures, if placed, should be removed at 10–14 days postsurgery if incisional healing appears normal.

### 9.1.4.2 Feline Spay (Ovariohysterectomy)

The feline spay (midline approach) is performed in much the same way as the canine spay.

- The skin incision is made midway between the umbilicus and pubis. Once a surgeon is proficient at spay surgeries, a small incision (approximately ½ inch long) is all that is needed. If the patient is found to have an unexpectedly large uterus (pyometra, hydrometra) or enlarged ovaries (tumor, cysts) that will not fit through this size incision, the incision can be extended as needed.
- The spay hook is an invaluable tool in HQHVSN given the small incision size. It is preferred to retrieve the right ovary first to avoid placing the spay hook on the left side of the abdomen close to the spleen. The spay hook is inserted with the curved end toward the abdominal wall. It is carefully lowered into the abdomen along the body wall, avoiding abdominal organs. It is then rotated 180° and gently retracted while also moving toward the midline. This approach will usually "catch" the uterine tissue. Never force the spay hook.
- Once the uterine horn and ovary have been exposed, either a ligature or pedicle tie can be placed.
  - The pedicle tie is an efficient method for ligating the ovarian pedicle in cats [3]. The pedicle tie is

**Figure 9.1.5** Cutting the suspensory ligament for feline ovarian pedicle tie. The ovarian pedicle and associated blood vessels/suspensory ligament are very prominent because this cat is pregnant. Source: Courtesy of Thomas Newberger and the ASPCA.

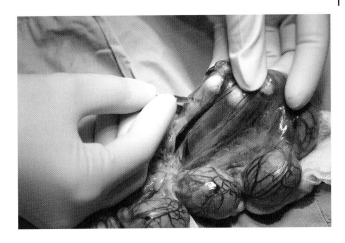

an autoligation, similar to the spermatic cord tie used in male cats, which when used can significantly reduce the time needed to perform a cat spay. This technique is not performed on dogs, as canine ovarian pedicles tend to have more fatty tissue, which does not lend itself to autoligation.

  - There are several techniques described for how to perform a pedicle tie [2]. One key point to note is that once the ovary has been located, the suspensory ligament MUST be cut in order to readily perform a pedicle tie (Figure 9.1.5).
- Once the suspensory ligament has been cut, a window is made in the broad ligament as would be done for a canine spay.
- While gently holding the ovary, the surgeon will place a curved mosquito hemostat perpendicular to the abdomen (point facing down) and rotate around the ovarian vessel in a manner similar to a half-hitch knot used for a cat neuter.
- The ovarian vessel is then clamped with this hemostat and the ovary is transected.
- The knot is gently pushed off the end of the hemostat and secured.
  - If a hemostat is placed on the ovarian pedicle, a single secure ligature may be placed. It is also recommended to minimize the use of hemostats (i.e. "three-clamp technique," as the added clamps often will get in the way or damage friable tissue). Use hemostats on an as-needed basis, rather than on every patient regardless of the size, etc. of the uterus.
- In general, the broad ligament is not ligated, unless there are prominent vessels or fat [1].

- The uterus is traced to the other horn and the left ovary is ligated in a similar manner.
- The body of the uterus is ligated below the bifurcation. A single Miller's knot is usually sufficient, although additional ligatures including ligating each uterine artery separately may be needed if the uterine body is enlarged, thickened, or edematous.
- There is no need to place excessive pressure on the uterine body in an attempt to remove "all" of the uterus. Given that we remove the uterus proximal to the cervix, there will always be some uterus remaining. Such animals are at no risk of a stump pyometra as long as both ovaries are removed. After the ligature(s) are placed, the uterine body is transected and observed for hemorrhage.
- Closure is then done in either two layers (body wall and intradermal) or three layers (body wall, subcutaneous, and intradermal). The choice is based on surgeon preference. A small feline spay incision may warrant only a single cruciate suture for closure of the body wall.

---

**Textbox 9.1.11 Tip from the field**

The ovarian pedicle tie is a time-saving technique in cats once mastered. However, when first learning this technique, it will likely slow down rather than speed up surgery time.

---

### 9.1.4.3 Canine and Feline Pediatric Spay

The surgical procedure is similar to that of the adult patient. Surgical incision placement is one of the most

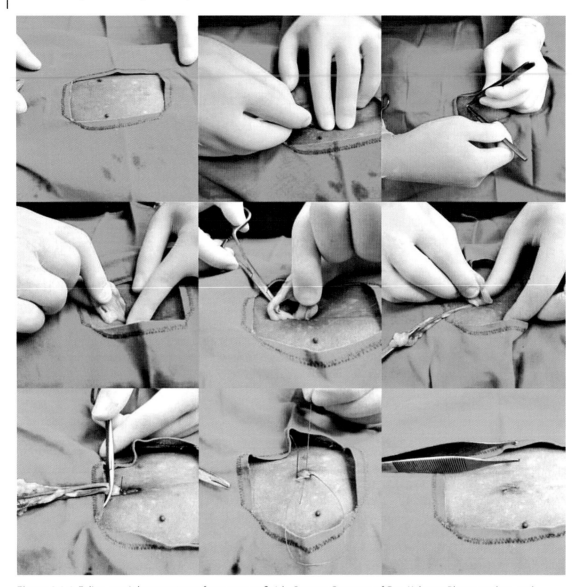

**Figure 9.1.6** Feline ovariohysterectomy from start to finish. Source: Courtesy of Drs. Kalyarat Phonnongkun and Ularn Kanyook.

important considerations when performing pediatric spay/neuter. The incision is best positioned on the midline at the midpoint between the umbilicus and pubis (as with an adult feline spay) in both puppies and kittens (Figure 9.1.6).

The uterus in both puppies and kittens should be easily identified using a spay hook in the same technique used for an adult animal, and the tissue should be able to be exteriorized with adequate visibility of all necessary structures to perform spay as with for any other patient. Care must be taken to handle pediatric tissue, as it can be more friable than the adult uterus. Gentle soft tissue handling is the key.

### 9.1.4.4 Umbilical Hernia

Occasionally an umbilical hernia may be present. This may be repaired at the time of body wall closure. Please consult other surgical texts for further descriptions on how to repair.

### 9.1.4.5 Animals in Estrus (Heat)

Animals in estrus should be spayed. They tend to have more prominent blood vessels, however, and may ooze more when the skin/subcutaneous incision is made. As well, the uterus of dogs and cats in estrus tends to be larger, thicker, and more edematous. The associated blood vessels may also be enlarged. This can present challenges with ligation, particularly, of the uterine stump. For animals with a thickened uterus, it may be necessary to place additional ligatures on each uterine artery independent of the uterine tissue. If these additional ligatures are not placed, the circumferential ligature (Miller's knot or otherwise) may loosen as the uterine tissue contracts postsurgery. In the author's experience, postoperative bleeding from in-estrus pregnant and pyometra surgeries has typically been from the uterine stump likely due to this reason.

### 9.1.4.6 Pregnant Animals

The surgical approach to the pregnant patient should be similar to that of the non-pregnant patient. Incision size will have to be large enough to safely exteriorize the gravid uterus without rupturing it. The author tends to find the procedure runs more smoothly if the entire uterus is exteriorized prior to ligating either pedicle or uterine body.

The uterus and associated vessels will appear greatly enlarged. Additional ligatures may be warranted. The spay procedure should be approached as the surgeon would approach that of the non-pregnant uterus.

When a spay surgery is performed on a pregnant dog or cat and the fetuses are aborted, it is necessary to ensure that the fetuses are handled in a manner that eliminates fetal suffering. This can best be accomplished by keeping the uterus closed and clamping off the open end. The fetuses should remain undisturbed inside the uterus. The uterus should be set aside ideally for 30 min. Some argue that the administration of euthanasia solution is unnecessary [9]. Others prefer to gently administer intraperitoneally an injection of a barbiturate or other appropriate anesthetic drug in late-term fetuses to ensure humane euthanasia.

Pregnant patients require additional supportive care, specifically fluid therapy. At a minimum, pregnant patients should receive subcutaneous fluids postoperatively. Intravenous fluids are recommended for pregnant patients; however, in the absence of intravenous fluid therapy, subcutaneous fluids are adequate in the author's opinion. Given that these procedures tend to be slightly longer than a routine spay, thermal support intraoperatively and postoperatively is particularly necessary. In the author's opinion, the use of nonsteroidal anti-inflammatory drugs (NSAID)s in third-trimester pregnant patients should be evaluated on a case-by-case basis, with special attention to the patient's hydration status.

Careful monitoring postoperatively is also a key. Pregnant animals are the patients that tend to have postoperative hemorrhage. Careful monitoring after surgery will allow the surgeon and staff to catch a complication such as a postoperative hemorrhage in a timelier fashion so that the surgeon can intervene. Patients with postoperative hemorrhage will have the following signs:

- Prolonged recovery
- Pale mucous membranes
- Hypothermia
- Tachycardia
- +/− blood on abdominal tap.

Pale mucous membranes and prolonged recovery can also be from hypothermia alone, so in the cases in which the surgeon does not have a positive abdominocentesis, the surgeon must use his/her judgment combined with the clinical picture to make a determination as to whether or not the patient requires surgical intervention. If surgical intervention is necessary, the author recommends that the surgeon set up for an autotransfusion (see Section 15.6.22.6.2) prior to surgery in addition to placing the patient on intravenous fluids.

---

**Textbox 9.1.12 Tips and tricks for pregnant spays**

- Individually ligate uterine arteries in animals with a large, thick uterus.
- Careful monitoring postoperatively will allow the surgeon to catch potentially life-threatening complication of a hemoabdomen after a pregnant spay.
- Pregnant spay procedures can be approached in the same way as non-pregnant procedures, but may require additional ligatures.
- At a minimum, pregnant patients should receive subcutaneous fluids postoperatively.

### 9.1.4.7 Pyometra

The approach to the clinically ill patient with pyometra differs from that of the clinically stable patient. A patient may present clinically symptomatic with a known pyometra or clinically asymptomatic but the surgeon uncovers that the patient has a pyometra during his/her surgical procedure. In asymptomatic patients, the surgeon should be able to proceed with the standard anesthetic approach; however, in the clinically ill patient, the surgeon should use his/her best judgment as to whether or not the anesthetic protocol can safely be used or if the protocol should be adjusted.

Clinically ill patients (and potentially those that are not clinically ill, but have diagnosed with a pyometra) should receive fluid therapy. Clinically ill patients should ideally receive injectable antibiotics prior to or at the time of surgery and a second dose can be given postoperatively before release. Some patients will require hospitalization. If the clinic is not able to provide this level of care, it might be in the patient's best interest to be spayed at another clinic that can provide postoperative care.

The surgical approach should be the same as animals with a normal, healthy uterus. Care should be taken when entering the abdomen. The surgeon should tent the linea both while making the stab incision and while extending the incision so that they do not cause an iatrogenic rupture of the uterus. The incision in the linea should be large enough to allow the surgeon to easily exteriorize the organ and the tissues should be handled with care.

Proceed with a routine spay. In cats, this means that you may still be able to do pedicle ties. The surgeon should use his/her best clinical judgment to determine if this is appropriate. If the patient is not already receiving fluids prior to surgery, subcutaneous or intravenous fluids should be administered postoperatively.

Heat support is crucial for these patients, as the surgeries can be longer than that of the healthy uterus.

### 9.1.4.8 Hydrometra

Hydrometras are typically an incidental finding at the time of surgery. The uterus itself will appear turgid and the lumen will contain a clear fluid. Uterine vessels will appear more prominent; however, these findings should not preclude the surgeon from using techniques outlined for a standard spay. In a cat, a pedicle tie is still an option for ligation of the ovarian pedicles. The surgical approach in these patients will be the same as a healthy uterus.

Postoperatively, these patients require no additional interventions or antibiotics as long as surgery proceeds without complication.

### 9.1.4.9 Postpartum

The postpartum uterus in both cats and dogs can be very friable. Extra care is required when handling the tissues. It is of particular importance to minimize the use of clamps as the uterus may tear simply from clamp placement. As well, it may be valuable to use a slightly larger suture size to avoid the guillotine-like effect of very thin suture, which could slice through the fragile tissue as the ligature is being placed.

### 9.1.4.10 Uterus Unicornis

Uterus unicornis is the congenital absence of one horn of the uterus [2]. This malformation occurs during embryologic development and the cause is unknown. It is usually an incidental finding at the time of spay and can occur in both cats and dogs. Even though the animal does not have a developed uterine horn, there is always an ovary present and this must be removed. The ovary is found at the usual location, although it may be slightly more cranial in the abdomen.

Animals with uterus unicornis may also be missing the kidney on the same side as the missing uterine horn. If possible, the presence or absence of this kidney may be assessed at the time of surgery by slightly increasing the abdominal incision and visualizing/palpating the area near the ovary.

---

**Textbox 9.1.13 Tip from the field**

Animals with uterus unicornis always have two ovaries. The ovary associated with the absent uterine horn must be removed. Animals with uterus unicornis may be missing a kidney on the side with the absent horn.

### 9.1.4.11 Uterine/Ovarian Pathology

There will be times during which an unsuspecting surgeon will stumble upon uterine or ovarian pathology. Ovarian and uterine tumors, previous uterine ruptures, and adhesions to the uterus and/or ovary can be seen in animals that appear otherwise healthy. In the cases of ovarian or uterine tumors that are incidental findings at the time of surgery, care should be taken to remove the entire area of affected tissue. When adhesions are present, care should be taken to gently break down the adhesions using blunt dissection. If omental adhesions are particularly vascular, consider placing a ligature around the omental tissue involved to prevent excessive hemorrhage after the adhesions are broken down. Offering histopathology to a client whose animal has uterine or ovarian pathology is always a good idea when it is available. The client may decline, and in such cases, document this information in the patient record. When there is not access to a laboratory to perform these tests, you must still advise the clients of the presence of a mass or abnormality so they are aware of the issue.

### 9.1.4.12 Ovarian Remnant Syndrome

When a surgeon performs spay/neuter on a regular basis, he or she is bound to come across a dog or cat who had been previously spayed and is showing signs of estrus. This phenomenon is known as ovarian remnant syndrome. This can occur when either all of the ovarian tissue was not removed at the time of spay or if there is ectopic ovarian tissue that the surgeon did not identify at the time of surgery (and thus did not remove). A 2010 article published in the Journal of the American Veterinary Medical Association (JAVMA) noted that ectopic ovarian tissue is generally found on the right side, which is the side that one might expect to have an issue given that this ovary is the more cranial ovary and can be more challenging to exteriorize [10].

Patients with this syndrome will present with signs of estrus: female dogs may have an enlarged vulva and/or bloody vulvar discharge, female cats may vocalize excessively or may be described as more needy than normal and may present their hind ends. Owners may misinterpret signs, thinking their pet has a urinary tract infection or other ailment.

---

> **Textbox 9.1.14 Confirmation of ovarian remnants**
>
> Diagnosis of ovarian remnants involves a combination of history/clinical suspicion. Tests can be performed to confirm the diagnosis:
>
> - *Vaginal cytology.* If a microscope is available, the surgeon may want to perform vaginal cytology to add weight to his/her clinical suspicion.
> - *Hormone testing.* To confirm elevated progesterone levels
> - *Surgical abdominal exploration.* In the absence of a microscope or the ability to perform laboratory tests such as the abovementioned hormone tests, the only option to confirm the presence or absence of ovarian tissue may be through surgical intervention.
>
> Always rule out exogenous estrogen exposure (i.e. through exposure to owner medications) before considering surgical exploration.

If all signs point to an ovarian remnant and surgery is the only available method for diagnosis, the author recommends performing an abdominal exploration. While it may be the easiest to find ovarian tissue while the animal is actively showing signs of heat, it may be logistically impossible to coordinate the timing of the surgery. Therefore, the surgery can be performed at any time. It is important to check the sites of both pedicles and also explore the rest of the abdomen, as if a piece of ovary inadvertently fell back into the abdomen during the spay procedure and became revascularized, it may be anywhere. If the surgeon truly suspects a patient has an ovarian remnant, it must be removed as that patient is at a risk of a stump pyometra.

### 9.1.4.13 Ovariohysterectomy (OHE) Versus Ovariectomy (OE)

Ovariohysterectomy (OHE) has been the standard of care in North America for sterilization of female dogs and cats [11]. Ovariectomy (OE) refers to the removal of both ovaries while leaving the uterus otherwise intact and is an alternative technique for sterilization. In reality, when OHE is performed there is always a small amount of the uterus remaining proximal to the cervix. As long as both ovaries are fully removed in either type of surgery, the patient is not at a risk of a stump pyometra or pregnancy. Either technique is acceptable unless there is preexisting uterine pathology.

In the author's opinion, there is not a significant advantage to OE versus OHE, except in selected situations where manipulation of the uterus and associated vessels is undesirable. An example of this could include an animal with abdominal adhesions including the uterus from a previous trauma or illness where manipulating the uterus could be difficult and prolong surgical time.

## 9.1.5 Canine Neuter

### 9.1.5.1 Adult Male

The canine neuter can be performed via a prescrotal or scrotal incision. The author prefers the prescrotal approach for adult dogs to minimize any contact and potential irritation to the scrotal tissue. Recent articles discussed a comparison of two approaches [12,13]. Although these articles show preference for the scrotal technique, it is the author's opinion that the choice of technique falls on surgeon preference rather than one technique being clearly superior to the other. A closed technique (no incision in the vaginal tunic surrounding the testicle) versus open technique is preferred regardless of the approach taken by the surgeon [8].

- Apply pressure to the skin to advance one testicle into the prescrotal area [1]. Do not make the prescrotal skin incision without moving the testicle into this area first so as to prevent injury to subcutaneous tissues or penis. Gently continue the incision through the subcutaneous tissue as needed.
- The testicle is exteriorized (to minimize the incision size, expose from pole to pole vs. side to side) by stripping away excess tissue. Once exteriorized, place a Miller's or modified Miller's knot while leaving a tissue tag to ensure no slippage of the suture. A single ligature is typically sufficient. A transfixing ligature (pass needle between the cord and vessel) can be used in place of the modified Miller's knot if preferred, but it may not be as efficient.
- This is repeated on the opposite testicle.
- Closure can be accomplished by placing a simple continuous pattern in the subcutaneous and intradermal tissues by using the method previously described in the suture pattern section of this chapter. Surgical tissue adhesive is placed on the incision.

#### 9.1.5.1.1 Prevention of Scrotal Hematomas

For adult dogs with large, pendulous scrotums, extra care should be taken during surgery to avoid a postsurgical scrotal hematoma. Should a patient develop a scrotal hematoma, these can usually be managed medically with rest, warm compresses, and anti-inflammatory medication. A scrotal hematoma that does not resolve may require scrotal ablation surgery [8].

---

**Textbox 9.1.15 Tips for preventing scrotal hematomas**

- Pay strict attention to hemostasis during the neuter, being particularly mindful of small subcutaneous vessels, which may ooze during recovery.
- Avoid excessive tissue handling during surgery in order to reduce inflammation.
- Apply a few drops of dilute phenylephrine directly into the scrotal incision prior to subcutaneous/ skin closure to aid in vasoconstriction.
- Consider placing a scrotal wrap using vet wrap-type cohesive bandage immediately after surgery to minimize the dead space within the scrotum. The scrotal wrap should remain on for 20–30 min and must be removed prior to discharging the patient (Figure 9.1.7).
- Apply a cold compress to the surgical area directly after surgery for 15–20 min.
- Modify postoperative instructions to include supplemental oral NSAIDs to reduce inflammation as needed.
- If the dog has an owner, provide him or her with clear discharge instructions stressing the importance of limiting the patient's activity during the postoperative period.

---

Application of dilute phenylephrine into the scrotal incision prior to skin closure is a simple, cost–effective way to prevent scrotal hematomas. Textbox 9.1.16 includes a recipe for dilution [8].

### 9.1.5.2 Pediatric Canine Neuter: Scrotal Approach

Pediatric canine neuters are often easier to perform via a scrotal approach given the lack of scrotal development and small size of the testicles (Figure 9.1.8). An additional benefit of this technique is that it requires a single mosquito hemostat, rather than a full surgical pack and it does not require suture. Perform the procedure as follows:

- Isolate one testicle between your fingers.
- Incise on the midline over that testicle.
- Exteriorize the testicle and autoligate the cord using either a half-hitch or figure-eight knot (as outlined in the feline neuter section).

- Isolate the second testicle in your fingers and exteriorize it through the same skin incision as the first testicle (this will require that the surgeon incise over the subcutaneous tissue ventral to the testicle) and autoligate the cord using the same technique as the previous testicle.
- Roll the skin ends together, blot any residual blood off of the incision and place a small volume of surgical glue over the incision (alternatively, the surgeon may leave the incision open).
- Tattoo the dog lateral to the prepuce (in the same area where the tattoo would be placed in an adult male dog).

### 9.1.5.3 Feline Neuter

There are several ways to neuter a cat. Approaches include open and closed castration, and the steps to perform both approaches are listed in Table 9.1.4. Both are acceptable and can be accomplished quickly. In both approaches, the surgeon makes one or two incisions through the skin of the scrotum to expose the testicle (some surgeons prefer exteriorizing the testicles through a single incision and some prefer exposing them through separate incisions). Once the

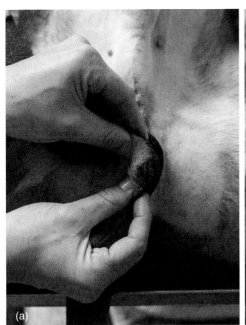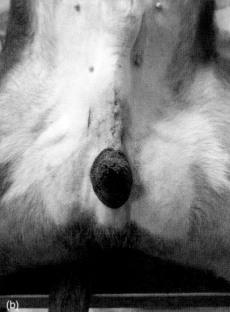

**Figure 9.1.7** Scrotal wrap. (a) Wrap a cohesive bandage (vet-wrap type) fully around scrotum immediately after surgery to minimize the dead space within the scrotum. (b) The scrotal wrap should remain on for 20–30 min and must be removed prior to discharging the patient. Source: Courtesy of Thomas Newberger and the ASPCA.

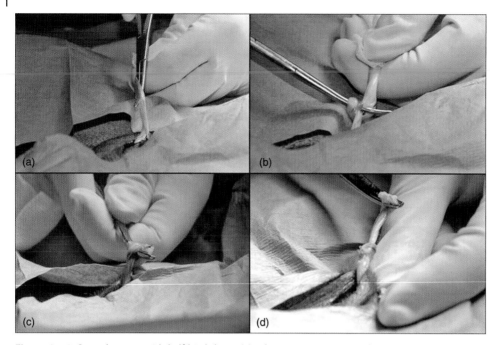

**Figure 9.1.8** Scrotal neuter with half-hitch knot. (a) A hemostat is positioned parallel to the spermatic cord with the tip of the hemostat pointing toward the scrotum. Place the tip of the hemostat under the spermatic cord. (b) The surgeon then rotates his/her wrist around so that the tip of the hemostat now points toward the surgeon's body, opens the hemostat and grabs the spermatic cord in the hemostat. Close the hemostat and clamp down on the cord. (c) Cut the cord between the hemostat and the testicle. (d) With either a piece of gauze or gloved fingers, slide the loop of the spermatic cord over the tip of the hemostat to make a knot. Tighten the knot down as far as it will go without pulling on the spermatic cord. Release the hemostat from the cord and allow the cord and surrounding tissue to go back into the scrotum. Source: Courtesy of Bucks County SPCA.

**Table 9.1.4** How to tie half-hitch and figure-eight knots.

| Half-hitch knot | Figure-eight knot |
| --- | --- |
| • The surgeon holds the testicle in his/her non-dominant hand.<br>• Take a hemostat and position it parallel to the spermatic cord with the tip of the hemostat pointing toward the scrotum.<br>• Place the tip of the hemostat under the spermatic cord.<br>• The surgeon then rotates his/her wrist around so that the tip of the hemostat now points toward the surgeon's body, opens the hemostat and grabs the spermatic cord in the hemostat.<br>• Close the hemostat and clamp down on the cord.<br>• Cut the cord between the hemostat and the testicle.<br>• With either a piece of gauze or gloved fingers, slide the loop of spermatic cord over the tip of the hemostat to make a knot.<br>• Tighten the knot down as far as it will go without pulling on the spermatic cord.<br>• Release the hemostat from the cord and allow the cord and surrounding tissue to go back into the scrotum. | • The surgeon holds the testicle in his/her non-dominant hand.<br>• Start with the hemostat perpendicular to the spermatic cord.<br>• Wrap the spermatic cord once around the hemostat.<br>• Turn the hemostat so that the tip is now pointing toward the scrotum.<br>• Place the tip of the hemostat under the spermatic cord.<br>• The surgeon then rotates his/her wrist around so that the tip of the hemostat now points toward the surgeon's body, opens the hemostat and grabs the spermatic cord in the hemostat.<br>• Close the hemostat and clamp down on the cord.<br>• Cut the cord between the hemostat and the testicle.<br>• With either a piece of gauze or gloved fingers, slide the loop of spermatic cord over the tip of the hemostat to make a knot.<br>• Tighten the knot down as far as it will go.<br>• Release the hemostat from the cord and allow the cord and surrounding tissue to go back into the scrotum. |

testicle has been exposed, commence with one of the following procedures:

### 9.1.5.3.1 Feline Neuter – Open Castration

- Incise over the testicle itself, opening the tunic.
- Exteriorize the testicle.
- Separate the tunic from the testicle gently using your fingers.
- Identify the spermatic cord and the vessels. Separate the spermatic cord from the testicle and begin tying square knots (loop and pull as if tying the initial throw in shoelaces). Tighten each knot down after each throw. Once 6–8 throws have been completed, sever the remaining length of the spermatic cord, vessel, and testicle.

### 9.1.5.3.2 Feline Neuter – Closed Castration

- Exteriorize the testicle, pull with gentle, even pressure until two clicks/pops are felt or there is an ample cord exposure to place a knot with ease.

- Using a Kelly or mosquito hemostat, tie a half-hitch knot or figure-eight knot (Figure 9.1.9).
- Transect the cord distal to the knot (between the hemostat and the testicle).
- Tighten the knot sufficiently.
- Using a blade, cut the remaining length of the spermatic cord, vessel, and testicle.

In both cases (closed and open castration), it is recommended that there is about 0.5 cm of tissue remaining as a tag distal to the knot to help ensure that the knot does not slip off. The skin incision is left open. Care must be taken to ensure that the spermatic cord and any associated fascia and/or fat are guided back into the scrotum and not left protruding from the skin incisions.

A tattoo should be placed centered on the ventral midline between the umbilicus and pubis to signify that the patient is now neutered. Placement of the tattoo in this location is helpful in case the cat is either mischaracterized as a bilateral cryptorchid or

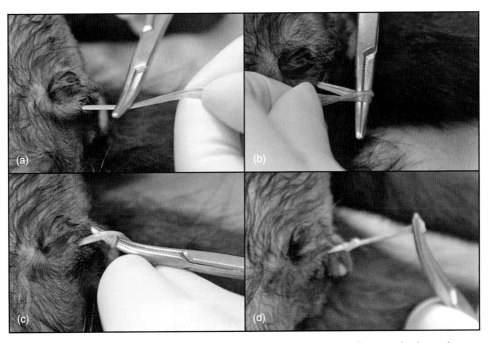

**Figure 9.1.9** Cat neuter with figure-eight knot. (a) A hemostat is positioned perpendicular to the spermatic cord. (b) Wrap the spermatic cord once around the hemostat. (c) Turn the hemostat so that the tip is now pointing toward the scrotum. Place the tip of the hemostat under the spermatic cord. The surgeon then rotates his/her wrist around so that the tip of the hemostat now points toward the surgeon's body, opens the hemostat and grabs the spermatic cord in the hemostat. Close the hemostat and clamp down on the cord. Cut the cord between the hemostat and the testicle. (d) With either a piece of gauze or gloved fingers, slide the loop of spermatic cord over the tip of the hemostat to make a knot. Tighten the knot down as far as it will go. Release the hemostat from the cord and allow the cord and surrounding tissue to go back into the scrotum. Source: Courtesy of Bucks County SPCA.

accidentally identified as female in the future and his abdomen is shaved to find a spay scar.

### 9.1.5.4 Cryptorchidism

Cryptorchidism is defined as the failure of one or both testicles to descend into the scrotum [1,2]. During the presurgical examination of male animals, the surgeon should palpate the scrotum for the presence of both testicles. If one or both testicles are absent from the scrotum, the surgeon should then palpate the adjacent area to see if the testicle is in the subcutaneous inguinal area. If the surgeon cannot palpate the testicle in the inguinal area, the surgeon should repeat palpation once the patient is anesthetized, as it is often easier to palpate the inguinal area in a relaxed, anesthetized patient. When palpating the inguinal area, it is important to differentiate between inguinal fat/lymph nodes and an apparent testicle. If the testicle cannot be located in the inguinal area or scrotum, then it is assumed to be abdominal. Cryptorchid testicles are typically smaller in size that the scrotal testicle and are at an increased risk of becoming cancerous.

It is best practice to remove the cryptorchid testicle first and then remove the scrotal testicle. In the event that the cryptorchid testicle cannot be located, the scrotal testicle should be left in place so as to not give the false impression that the dog is neutered.

Abdominal cryptorchid surgery may be very challenging. Although there is a risk of the undescended testicle developing cancer, there are also risks to the patient if a surgeon is inexperienced with this procedure. The author recommends that the cryptorchid testicle always be removed at the time of neuter surgery. But if a surgeon is unsure of his/her ability with this surgery, the author recommends the surgeon seek assistance from a surgeon who has greater expertise in this procedure.

#### 9.1.5.4.1 Inguinal Cryptorchid Neuter

An inguinal cryptorchid testicle is located in the subcutaneous tissue of the inguinal area. It may be covered with a layer of subcutaneous fat.

- Make an incision through the skin over the inguinal testicle.
- Use blunt dissection of the subcutaneous fat if warranted.
- Locate the testicle, ligate the associated vessels, and remove the testicle.
- Close the subcutaneous tissue and skin in the standard manner as described for the standard neuter technique.

#### 9.1.5.4.2 Abdominal Cryptorchid Neuter

##### 9.1.5.4.2.1 Canine

Due to the location of the prepuce in dogs, there are two approaches for retrieving an abdominal cryptorchid testicle, each with their own advantages and disadvantages (Table 9.1.5).

In either approach, a spay hook can be used to locate the spermatic cord of the abdominal testicle. This allows for a smaller abdominal incision and minimal abdominal tissue handling. Use the spay

**Table 9.1.5** Comparison of approaches to retrieve a cryptorchid testicle.

| Ventral midline incision cranial to prepuce | Incision lateral to prepuce |
| --- | --- |
| <ul><li>The approach into the abdomen is similar to that for spay.</li><li>This approach will allow easy access to both sides of the abdomen, which may be beneficial in a bilateral cryptorchid dog.</li><li>If the testicles did not descend at all from the origination point (caudal to the kidney), they will be easily accessible via this approach.</li><li>The downside of this approach is that it is difficult to access the caudal abdominal area, especially of concern if the testicles are caught in the inguinal ring.</li></ul> | <ul><li>The incision is made lateral to the prepuce on the side of the suspected abdominal cryptorchid testicle. Care must be taken to avoid the caudal superficial epigastric artery, which runs lateral to the prepuce. Once the skin incision has been made and the blunt dissection through the subcutaneous fat, an incision can be made through the ventral midline by gently pushing this tissue medially. This avoids incising through the abdominal wall musculature, which can result in bleeding.</li><li>The benefit of this approach is that there is better access to the caudal abdomen.</li><li>One challenge to this approach is that it does not give great access to both sides of the abdomen should the patient be bilateral cryptorchid.</li></ul> |

hook in a similar manner as one would in a female animal, although the surgeon may have to search more caudally or cranially depending on the location of the abdominal testicle.

If the testicle cannot be found using this method, then a large abdominal incision can be made and the testicle can be located by visualizing the testicle. It may be necessary to gently manipulate the urinary bladder to locate the spermatic cord and trace it to the testicle.

If the testicle is trapped in the inguinal ring, extend the body wall incision as needed to allow better access to this area. Blunt dissection of the inguinal ring area may free the entrapped testicle. If that is unsuccessful, a very small incision may be made in the inguinal ring using Metzenbaum scissors to free the testicle. This incision in the inguinal ring generally does not need to be closed [1].

There may be a time when the spermatic cord is located but it cannot be traced to a testicle. In that case it is likely that the testicle is actually in the inguinal area. Visualize whether the spermatic cord travels caudally toward the inguinal ring. One technique to locate the inguinal testicle is to have the surgeon gently tug on the spermatic cord while an assistant observes the inguinal area for movement. If there is movement in the inguinal area, the surgeon may have to extend the existing incision or make an additional incision in the inguinal area to locate the testicle.

Once the testicle is found (either abdominal or subcutaneous), it can be removed in the standard manner. The body wall, subcutaneous, and skin incisions can be closed routinely subsequent to the removal of the testicle.

---

**Textbox 9.1.17 Tips for canine cryptorchid testicle removal**

- Palpate the inguinal area once the patient is anesthetized to locate inguinal testicle (if not obvious during presurgical exam).
- To determine which testicle has descended, push on the testicle toward the inguinal area. It will become apparent which "side" the testicle came from.
- Remove the cryptorchid testicle before removing the scrotal testicle.
- If the cryptorchid testicle cannot be located, do not remove the scrotal testicle.

---

### 9.1.5.4.2.2 *Feline*

In cats, the approach to find the abdominal cryptorchid testicle is through an incision on the ventral midline midway between the umbilicus and the pubis. The location is similar to where one would make an incision for a cat spay, although slightly more caudal over the area of the urinary bladder. The remainder of the surgery is the same as described for the dog.

---

**Textbox 9.1.18 Tips for feline cryptorchid testicle removal**

- A spay hook is effective in locating the cryptorchid testicle. Use it as you would to find a uterine horn.
- Remove the cryptorchid testicle first. If the cryptorchid testicle cannot be located, do not remove the scrotal testicle. If the scrotal testicle was removed, it would give the false impression that the animal is neutered.

---

## 9.1.6 Special Considerations with Spay/Neuter Surgeries

As with any surgical procedure, surgeons should be familiar with special considerations that may require adjustments in surgical technique, fasting times, and anesthetic protocols. Table 9.1.6 describes surgical considerations for commonly observed conditions.

### 9.1.6.1 Pediatrics

Pediatric spay/neuter surgery should be approached similarly to all other spay/neuter surgeries. There are

---

**Textbox 9.1.19 Special considerations for recovering pediatric patients**

- *Body temperature.* Pediatric patients will get cold regardless of the duration of surgery, providing adequate heat support throughout the procedure and in recovery is very important.
- *Blood glucose level.* Pediatric patients may become hypoglycemic when food is withheld.
  - Provide a small meal in the morning on the day of surgery.
  - Apply a small amount of clear corn syrup or dextrose to the gums while patients are recovering.
  - Once the patient is fully awake, provide another small meal.

Table 9.1.6 Summary of medical conditions and surgical considerations.

| Condition | Anesthetic considerations | Surgical approach | Antibiotics? | Postoperative supportive care |
|---|---|---|---|---|
| Pregnancy | Can use normal protocol | Same as normal OHE, but larger incision; may want to individually ligate uterine vessels | Not necessary | Heat support, fluids Consider withholding NSAIDs in late-term pregnancy |
| Pyometra | May want to adjust protocol for clinically ill patient (depending on the clinic's protocol) | Same as normal OHE, but larger incision | Recommended | Heat support, fluids |
| Hydrometra | Can use normal protocol | Same as normal OHE, but may require a larger incision depending on size | Not necessary | Heat support, +/− fluids |
| Postpartum | Can use normal protocol | Same as normal OHE, use caution when handling the tissue (usually more friable) | Not necessary | Heat support, fluids if lactating |
| Heat (estrus) | Can use normal protocol | Same as normal OHE | Not necessary | Heat support |

some minor differences in how these patients should be managed prior to surgery. Food should not be withheld overnight for patients 4 months of age and younger. These patients should also receive a small meal in the morning hours prior to surgery to avoid potential hypoglycemia in these patients.

### 9.1.6.2 Hermaphrodites/Pseudohermaphrodites

Occasionally, a cat or dog may be found to have ambiguous external genitalia. These patients may be a true hermaphrodite (both ovarian and testicular tissue are present) or a pseudohermaphrodite (primary sex characteristics of one sex, but secondary sex characteristics that differ from what would be expected based on the gonadal tissue).

Regardless of the unusual presentation, the gonadal tissue should be surgically removed as it is not known

whether these animals are fertile. Surgery should proceed in the usual manner for the apparent gender.

### 9.1.6.3 Feral/Community Cats

Spay and neuter procedures for feral/community cats do not differ from handleable cats. Anesthetic protocols should allow the staff to administer all drugs without having to handle the awake patient (i.e. an intramuscular protocol should be used). This is for the safety of the staff and patients. They should receive all treatments that are otherwise given to handleable patients. A left ear tip should be performed so that the spayed or neutered community cat can be identified from a distance and a tattoo should be placed on the ventral abdomen (either lateral to the spay incision or between the umbilicus and pubis in males) for further confirmation in the event that the ear tip is either missed or difficult to recognize.

### 9.1.6.4 Previous Abdominal Illness or Trauma

Occasionally spay surgery will be performed on a patient who has a history of abdominal illness or trauma. If this illness or trauma occurred recently, the surgery should be postponed to allow time for proper healing. For animals with unknown history, previous abdominal illness or trauma may not be apparent until surgery begins.

---

**Textbox 9.1.20 Examples of pseudohermaphrodites**

- A female dog with an enlarged clitoris and an os penis-like structure
- A male cat with a large urogenital opening with testicles located on either side of this apparent vaginal cleft.

---

**Textbox 9.1.21 Common findings due to previous abdominal insult**

- Abdominal adhesions
  - This can occur subsequent to peritonitis, inflammation (e.g. pancreatitis), infection (e.g. parvovirus), or trauma.
  - In most cases, the adhesions can be manually broken down and the surgery can proceed.
  - The tissue may be more friable, and there may be some minor bleeding when the adhesions are addressed.
- Diaphragmatic hernia
  - The author has managed several patients who had no external signs of respiratory difficulty until placed under anesthesia.
  - Stabilize the patient and do not proceed with surgery.
  - Further evaluation may confirm the presence of a diaphragmatic hernia.
- Uterine rupture
  - Trauma can result in a uterine rupture that then healed.
  - If the patient is pregnant at the time of the trauma, it is possible that fetuses could travel into the abdomen from the rupture site. These will typically become mummified or be reabsorbed fully/partially.
  - If fetuses are noted in the abdomen during OHE, it is necessary to remove them.

---

## 9.1.7 Management of Complications Related to Spay/Neuter

A summary of the prevention and management of complications related to spay/neuter is summarized in Table 9.1.7 [3]. The authors strongly encourage all veterinarians new to high-quality high-volume spay/neuter work to familiarize themselves with these types of complications.

**Table 9.1.7** Management suggestions for surgical complications.

| Complication | Medical management | Surgical intervention | Additional considerations |
|---|---|---|---|
| Hemorrhage | n/a | Manage by surgical exploration to find the source of bleeding and control; autotransfuse if significant blood loss. | It is always better to prevent hemorrhage through careful surgical technique. |
| Iatrogenic organ laceration | n/a | Spleen – carefully suture capsule if large laceration<br>Urinary bladder – suture bladder wall with 3-0 absorbable suture, taper needle. | Careful surgical technique can prevent these complications:<br><br>– For the spleen, gently advancing the spay hook on the right side of the body with the hook facing laterally will help avoid this complication.<br>– For the urinary bladder, expressing the bladder prior to surgery and tenting the linea up and incising the linea with the blade facing upside down will help to avoid this complication. |
| Incisional seroma | Warm compress, +/− NSAIDs, +/− antibiotics | Not necessary, but can explore fluid pocket | n/a |
| Suture reaction | Warm compress, +/− NSAIDs | Not necessary | n/a |
| Incisional dehiscence (linea, skin, or both) | n/a | Surgical repair required | Postoperative pain management and antibiotics may be necessary; if skin incision has opened, consider flushing area with sterile saline prior to closure. |
| Scrotal hematoma | NSAIDs, warm compress | If severe or unresolving, may require scrotal ablation | Ensure patient is rested if this occurs/ is not overactive while healing. |

## 9.1.8 Conclusion

Safe and effective spay/neuter surgery can be performed in settings outside of the traditional veterinary practice. Regardless of the location, the surgeon should adhere to the strict sterile technique and careful tissue handling. HQHVSN surgical skills will make for effective and efficient surgery.

Although spay/neuter surgery may be thought of as "routine," it can be far from that as described in this chapter. The surgeon should be prepared to manage each surgery on a case-by-case basis.

## References

1 Fossum, T.W. (2012). Surgery of the reproductive and genital systems. In: Small Animal Surgery, 4e, St. Louis, Mo: Mosby Elsevier.

2 Bushby, P.A. (2013). Surgical techniques for spay/neuter. In: Shelter Medicine for Veterinarians and Staff, 2e, eds. L. Miller and S. Zawistowski), 625–645. Wiley.

3 Griffin, B., Bushby, P., McCobb, E. et al. (2016). The Association of Shelter Veterinarians' 2016 veterinary medical care guidelines for spay-neuter programs. *Journal of the American Veterinary Medical Association* **249**: 165–188.

4 Fossum, T.W. (2007). Biomaterials, suturing and hemostasis. In: Small Animal Surgery. Elsevier Mosby, Inc.

5 ASPCA Spay/Neuter Alliance (2016). Veterinary reference guide. https://www.aspcapro.org/sites/default/files/wysiwyg-uploads/asna_vet_reference_guide.pdf (accessed 16 March 2018).

6 Ethicon (2016). Selection & use of surgical needles. http://www.agnthos.se/media/pdf_technical/ETHICON_Surgical_Needles.pdf (accessed 22 August 2016).

7 International Fund for Animal Welfare. IFAW's companion animal field manual – primary veterinary health care standards. Food and Agriculture Organization. http://www.fao.org/fileadmin/user_upload/animalwelfare/asset_upload_file726_61605.pdf (accessed 2 September 2016).

8 American Society for the Prevention of Cruelty to Animals (2016). Manual of Standard Operating Procedures. New York: NYC Mobile Clinics.

9 White, S.C. (2012). Prevention of fetal suffering during ovariohysterectomy of pregnant animals. *Journal of the American Veterinary Medical Association* **240**: 1160–1163.

10 Ball, R.L., Birchard, S.J., May, L.R. et al. (2010). Ovarian remnant syndrome in dogs and cats: 21 cases (2000–2007). *Journal of the American Veterinary Medical Association* **236**: 548–553.

11 Detora, M. and McCarthy, R.J. (2011). Ovariohysterectomy versus ovariectomy for elective sterilization of female dogs and cats: is removal of the uterus necessary? *Journal of the American Veterinary Medical Association* **239**: 1409–1412.

12 DiGangi, B.A., Johnson, M., and Isaza, N. (2016). Scrotal approach to canine orchiectomy. *Clinicians Brief*, http://www.cliniciansbrief.com/article/scrotal-approach-canine-orchiectomy (accessed 9 September 2016).

13 Woodruff, K., Bushby P., Brestle, K., and Wills, R. (2015). Scrotal castration versus prescrotal castration in dogs. Is the scrotal castration technique as safe and efficient as the commonly taught prescrotal technique? The results of this study might surprise you http://veterinarymedicine.dvm360.com/scrotal-castration-versus-prescrotal-castration-dogs (accessed 22 Nov 2016).

## 9.2

# Ovariohysterectomy – Flank Approach

*J.F. Reece*

*Help in Suffering, Maharani Farm, Durgapura, Jaipur, 302018, Rajasthan, India*

### 9.2.1 Introduction

The lateral flank approach is an alternative to the standard ventral midline approach for ovariohysterectomy (OHE) in dogs and cats. In many countries, this approach is considered the conventional one, particularly in canine catch–vaccinate–neuter–return (CVNR) and feline trap–neuter–return (TNR) programs. Many believe this approach allows stray animals to be returned to their environment quicker following surgery and allows for better monitoring of the incision site. The flank approach is also useful in patients with excessive mammary gland development due to lactation or hyperplasia. The various advantages and disadvantages of this technique are summarized in Table 9.2.1.

This section provides a practical description of how to perform an OHE using a flank approach by an experienced author. Note that the procedure described here and materials listed are those used by the author in India.

### 9.2.2 Surgical Packs – What Instruments Are Needed?

The following instruments and supplies are recommended when performing canine OHEs using the flank approach (Table 9.2.2).

#### 9.2.2.1 Additional Instruments and Supplies to Include in the Surgical Pack

- One plastic sheet 37 in. × 26 in. (92 × 65 cm) with a fenestration 6.5 in. (17 cm) square. This prevents wicking of infection from the underlying skin and hair through wet patches on cloth drapes.
- One surgical drape 32 in. × 28 in. (80 × 70 cm) with an asymmetric fenestration of 2.5 in. × 4 in. (6 × 10 cm). The fenestration is placed so that its left-hand border is in the midline of the drape. This enables an adult dog's hind feet to be fully draped by a moderate-sized drape. The fenestration's long axis runs craniocaudally when placed on the positioned female dog. Initially, the author had rectangular fenestrations as described above. More recently, however, the author's organization has been using drapes with elliptical fenestrations of similar dimensions to those given above. These appear to last longer and do not fray at the corners of the fenestration as easily as rectangular ones. Drapes are of surgical green cotton and can be made locally. It is better to have extra sterile drapes available during an operation in case of accidental contamination, etc.
- One cloth trolley (instrument stand) drape of suitable dimensions to cover fully the instrument trolley. One trolley drape is used to wrap the surgical instruments; the other one is placed on the instrument trolley to receive the wrapped instruments. Trolley drapes are of surgical green cotton and are unfenestrated.
- Five to six gauze sponges per operation. These can be homemade from surgical gauze by cutting several thicknesses of gauze into rectangles of about 9 in. × 7 in.. These are then folded to produce surgical sponges of approximately 2 in. square. When folding gauze every effort is made to ensure that all outer, cut edges of gauze are folded to be within the

*Field Manual for Small Animal Medicine*, First Edition. Edited by Katherine Polak and Ann Therese Kommedal.
© 2018 John Wiley & Sons, Inc. Published 2018 by John Wiley & Sons, Inc.

Table 9.2.1 Advantages and disadvantages of the flank approach.

| Advantages | Disadvantages |
|---|---|
| 1) Able to monitor the incision from a distance.<br>2) Topical medication can be more easily applied to the incision site in fractious animals.<br>3) The incision is not under the weight of the abdominal contents. Healing time may be reduced due to less tension on the incision site and increased vascularity.<br>4) Animals may be able to be released earlier in CVNR/TNR programs.<br>5) Evisceration is less likely if the body wall incision breaks down.<br>6) Surgical time is minimized as the ipsilateral ovary and uterine horn lie immediately below the incision, minimizing time necessary to locate the ovary. | 1) Incising through three muscle layers causes bleeding, which may obscure the surgical field and lead to increased risk of post-operative infection.<br>2) Recovery of a dropped or bleeding pedicle can be difficult.<br>3) Exposing the opposite (contralateral) ovary and uterine bifurcation may prove challenging if the original incision was incorrectly placed.<br>4) For animals that are pregnant or have uterine distension, the initial incision may or may not provide sufficient exposure to manipulate the uterus. |

Table 9.2.2 Suggestions for a basic OHE flank-approach surgical pack.

| Number | Instrument |
|---|---|
| 4 | Towel clamps |
| 1 | Rat tooth forceps |
| 1 | Scalpel handle |
| 1 | Mayo scissors |
| 4 | Allis tissue clamps |
| 4 | 5-in. Kelly hemostats |
| 2 | 7-in. Kelly hemostats |
| 4 | Small mosquito hemostats |
| 1 | Spay hook |
| 1 | Needle holder |
| 1 | Mayo scissors (for cutting sutures) |
| 1 | Metzenbaum scissors |
| 1 | Tissue forceps |

sponge. Careful folding results in effective sponges that do not shed pieces of cotton fiber into the surgical field.

## 9.2.3 Suture Material

The following suture materials are commonly used in the field for performing canine OHEs using a flank approach. Catgut is used here partly due to surgeons' preference but also because the material is readily available and cheap, which are important considerations in a field setting. More modern, expensive suture materials could no doubt be used to equal effect.

- 6 metric (2 USP) chromic catgut
- 5 metric (1 USP) chromic catgut
- 3 metric (3/0 USP) chromic catgut
- 3 metric (3/0 USP) braided coated polyglycolide-co-L lactide/vicryl.

## 9.2.4 Surgical Preparation

The surgical field should be clipped craniocaudally from the 10th rib to the femur, and dorsoventrally from the transverse spinal processes to the abdominal midline.

In places where electric clippers cannot be properly maintained or sourced, the site is clipped using safety razors (from which the lateral bars had been removed) and chlorhexidine solution is often used (to wet the fur and facilitate clipping). The site is then prepared for surgery with povidine–iodine solution or similar product in a conventional manner. See Chapter 11 for additional information.

### 9.2.4.1 Patient Positioning

In a flank approach, the animal can be positioned in either right or left lateral recumbency. The author prefers the right flank approach as it allows for better exposure of the more cranial right ovary.

(a)

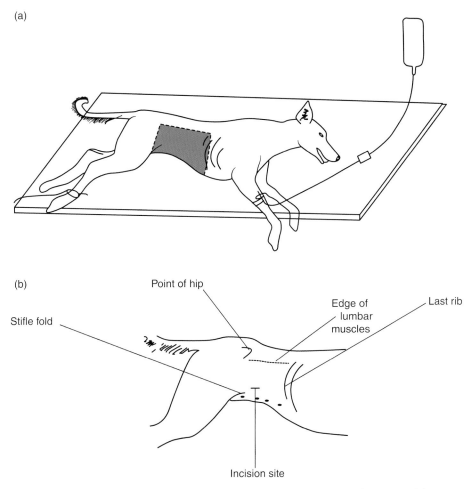

(b)

Point of hip

Edge of
lumbar
muscles

Last rib

Stifle fold

Incision site

**Figure 9.2.1** (a) Area to be prepared for a right lateral flank approach. (b) Placement of the incisional site in an adult dog for a flank approach.

Female dogs are positioned on the operating table in left lateral recumbency. The right hind limb is tied to the table and the dog stretched in a craniocaudal direction. The left stifle is extended caudally and hooked behind the right hock (Figure 9.2.1).

## 9.2.5 Surgical Technique

A craniocaudal incision is made at a position ventral to the iliac crest, and at the level of the fold of skin connecting the stifle to the abdominal wall, the stifle fold. In young dogs, the incision should be placed slightly more caudally, otherwise there is a risk that the uterine bifurcation cannot be exteriorized. In a study undertaken by the author and colleagues, the average incision length was 2.2 cm (0.86 in.), slightly less if the incisions of pregnant female dogs were excluded. The incision is made craniocaudally because this allows it to be extended easily should this be necessary, for example, in pregnant dogs or those with cystic ovaries. The incision can be made more dorsally, but this tends to mean each muscle layer is thicker and hemorrhage more likely. Exposure will then be more difficult through a deep, small hole [1].

The external oblique muscle, or its aponeurosis, is exposed by blunt dissection through the fascia. The

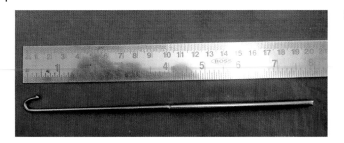

**Figure 9.2.2** Custom-made spay hook.

muscle is grasped with Allis clamps, incised using scissors, and then split along the fibers by blunt dissection. The internal oblique muscle is grasped and cut in a similar manner, and the incision edges are isolated with Allis clamps. The rectus abdominis muscle is thus revealed. This is elevated and incised in a similar manner. The elevation and incision is done very carefully and with a very small initial incision to avoid the possibility of unintentional injury to the underlying abdominal organs, which may be inadvertently grasped along with the muscle. Once incised and found to be free from the underlying structures, the incision edges of the rectus abdominis and peritoneum are enlarged through blunt dissection and isolated with Allis clamps. Failure to grasp the edges of the incisions through both the internal oblique and rectus muscles can result in considerable difficulty in relocating these tissues during wound closure. Academic surgeons have expressed dislike in using Allis clamps due to the trauma they cause. The author and his colleagues have not experienced any obvious difficulties in using them for the short duration of a standard flank spay.

With a spay hook, the right uterine body is exteriorized. The hook is run dorsally along the peritoneum of the body wall until the transverse spinal processes and at about 1 o'clock position from the incision. As it is then removed it will usually bring the uterine body or the mesometrium exterior to the incision where it may be grasped manually. By gentle manual tension on the uterus, broad and round ligament, the ovary is also exteriorized. If the initial incision is in the correct place, the uterus will often be immediately accessible. The author uses custom-made spay hooks as he has found commercially available spay hooks being too short and the hook too broad. Some are also too sharply pointed, thereby risking damage to the abdominal organs while finding the uterus. It is, in the author's opinion, the use of the spay hook that allows the incision to be small whether a midline or flank approach is used. Most surgeons use two fingers to find and extract the uterus and thus the incision needs to be at least the width of the surgeon's two fingers. The spay hook means that the incision need be only the width necessary for the removal of the ovary, its bursa and the uterus (Figure 9.2.2).

A small hole is made in the broad ligament and mesometrium. The ovary and ovarian bursa are isolated using the standard triple-clamp method across the ovarian pedicle. While many high-volume spay neuter surgeons are moving away from using the three-clamp technique, the author routinely uses it with few complications.

An encircling ligature of 6 metric (2 USP) chromic catgut or a similar suture material is placed around the ovarian pedicle. At the surgeon's discretion, a second or transfixing ligature may be placed. The ovarian pedicle is cut between the two clamps and checked for hemorrhage, and the excised structure examined to ensure complete excision of ovarian tissue. The ligated pedicle is then returned to the abdominal cavity (Figure 9.2.3).

The dependent ovary is then located by following the right uterine horn caudally to the uterine bifurcation, which is drawn into the incision site.

From the uterine bifurcation, the left uterine horn is exteriorized, and the left ovary exteriorized and removed in a similar manner to that of the right. In older dogs, or those with a lot of abdominal fat, it is sometimes easier to remove the cervical stump after the first ovary. Returning the ligated stump and associated mesometrium and fat to the abdominal cavity effectively makes the incision bigger through which to draw the remaining ovarian bursa and ovary.

Following the removal of both ovaries, the whole reproductive tract is exteriorized. A window is made

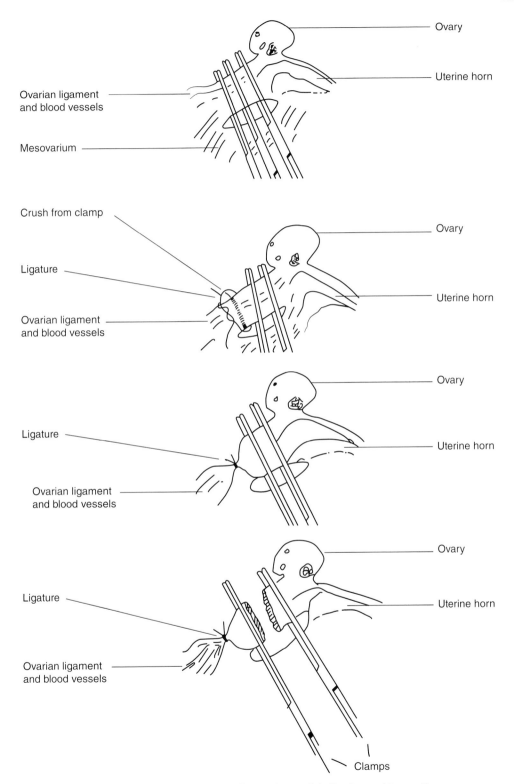

**Figure 9.2.3** Standard three-clamp technique for ovarian pedicle ligation and transection.

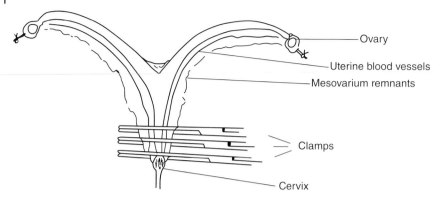

**Figure 9.2.4** Standard three-clamp technique for ligation of the uterine body.

in each mesometrium. This is extended through controlled tearing and breaking, from the free ovarian edge, caudally along the reproductive tract close to the uterine vasculature to the level of the cervix. The fatty structures are returned to the abdominal cavity. Normally, these do not need ligating; but if large vessels are present, an encircling ligature can be placed. The freed uterine body and vasculature are isolated just cranial to the cervix using the triple-clamp method (Figure 9.2.4).

The uterine body is ligated using 6 metric (2 USP) chromic catgut or a similar suture material, and the uterine body then excised. A second, or transfixing ligature, is placed at the surgeon's discretion before excision. The uterine stump is examined for hemorrhage and returned to the abdomen.

If at any point in the procedure it is felt necessary to extend the incision this is done at the surgeon's discretion in a craniocaudal direction to facilitate the safe removal of the uterus and ovaries. Experience suggests that there is little to be gained in "milking" structures through a small incision. Very rarely however is it necessary to make an incision longer than 3.0 cm (1.18 in.).

The incision is closed using 5 metric (1 USP) chromic catgut or a similar suture material. Horizontal mattress sutures are placed in each of the three muscle layers. The peritoneum is incorporated into the closure of the rectus abdominis. In puppies and young dogs, the peritoneum, rectus abdominis, and internal oblique muscles are closed together at the discretion of the surgeon. Allis clamps are left on the rectus muscle edge throughout surgery to facilitate identification of layers. Before suturing the various layers, it is good practice to identify and isolate the adjacent layer outward to that being sutured to avoid confusion and misalignment. In longer incisions, a Ford interlocking pattern can be used to close muscle layers. The subcutaneous fat and fascia are closed with 3 metric (3/0 USP) chromic catgut. The skin is closed using 3 metric (3/0 USP) "Vicryl" equivalent in a continuous intradermal pattern terminated with a buried Aberdeen knot.

Following or prior to surgery, free-roaming animals should always be permanently identified to indicate that they have been sterilized and rabies vaccinated.

## 9.2.6 Special Feline Flank Considerations

The flank approach is commonly used in cats with significant mammary development. In cats, the incision is traditionally made in a dorsoventral direction starting just caudal to the midpoint between the last rib and iliac crest. Some advocate for the incision to be located two-finger-widths behind the last rib and one finger-width below the vertebral transverse process. The length of the incision is typically about 2 cm (0.78 in.).

When closing, the body wall can generally be closed in a single layer using one or two simple interrupted or crucial sutures. Bites can be taken through all three layers of the musculature. The subcutaneous layer and skin can be closed according to surgeon preference. Intradermal suture patterns are recommended in feral or fractious cats to avoid the need for suture removal.

### 9.2.7 Surgeries with Special Considerations When Using a Flank Approach

#### 9.2.7.1 Puppies

There are a few special considerations when performing juvenile surgeries.

- Place the skin and muscle incision further caudally to allow the uterine bifurcation to be found easier.
- Reproductive structures in puppies can be very small. Therefore, consider using a suture material smaller than what would normally be used on an adult animal.
- The body wall is closed in two layers, not three.

#### 9.2.7.2 Pyometra

In a high volume street dog control program, pyometra cases may not be recognized before surgery. In adult dogs, pyometra must be considered if the uterus cannot be exteriorized in the normal easy manner. The pyometric uterus may be more friable than usual. A large incision is thus advisable.

#### 9.2.7.3 Postpartum

The postpartum uterus is often large and more friable than normal. If in doubt, make the incision larger.

#### 9.2.7.4 In Heat

Female dogs in heat pose no special risks using a flank approach. Estrogen may have effects on the clotting mechanism however. At certain stages of estrus, the uterus is turgid; clamps need to be well spaced along the structure to avoid tearing that may occur if they are placed too close together.

#### 9.2.7.5 Pregnancy

If the program objective is population control, it would seem counterproductive to not spay pregnant bitches. First trimester pregnancies pose no special problems. Late-term pregnancies require a longer body wall incision, and consideration must be given to the enlarged mammary vasculature in late pregnancy. These vessels can often be seen on their course across the flank. It is helpful if the first uterine horn can be exteriorized by localizing and pulling at the ovary using the spay hook, rather than exteriorizing from mid-uterine horn. This may be achieved by directing the spay hook rather more cranially than is normal. Ovarian pedicles will often be stretched and relaxed. Light pressure on the abdomen can help eject the dilated uterus through the incision. In late pregnancies, care must be taken to ensure a fetus is not left caudal to the cervical ligature. In very late pregnancies, the surgical team may euthanize, on humane grounds, fetuses in-utero once removed from the dog. Transfixing sutures are used more frequently in mid or late pregnancies especially at the cervical stump.

### Reference

1 Reece, J., Nimesh, M., Wyllie, R. et al. (2012). Description and evaluation of a right flank, mini-laparotomy approach to canine ovariohysterectomy. *Veterinary Record* **171**: 248–248.

# 10

# Ancillary Surgical Procedures

*Field Manual for Small Animal Medicine*, First Edition. Edited by Katherine Polak and Ann Therese Kommedal.
© 2018 John Wiley & Sons, Inc. Published 2018 by John Wiley & Sons, Inc.

## 10.1

# Forelimb, Hindlimb, and Digit Amputation

*Tatiana Motta¹ and Lawrence Hill²*

¹College of Veterinary Medicine, Clinical Sciences, The Ohio State University, 601 Vernon Tharp St., Columbus, OH 43210, USA
²College of Veterinary Medicine, Clinical Sciences, The Ohio State University, 232 Veterinary Medical Center, 601 Vernon Tharp St., Columbus, OH 43210, USA

### 10.1.1   Introduction

This chapter describes simple, practical, and efficient steps involved in the limb or digit amputations. The authors focus on definitions and clear descriptions of the procedure, as well as advise regarding perioperative patient care. Most of the procedures can be performed with a traditional surgery pack. If bone transection is involved, as described for the pelvic limb amputation section, a Gigli wire, osteotome, bone saw, or sterile hacksaw blade are needed.

### 10.1.2   Thoracic Limb Amputation

#### 10.1.2.1   Indications

Common indications for thoracic limb amputation in the field environment include fracture complications such as delayed union, nonunion, malunion, open fractures, and muscular contraction as a result of inappropriate fracture healing, degloving injury, infection, neoplasia and nerve injury, unmanageable joint disease (severe osteoarthritis, luxations), and congenital limb defects. The decision to amputate should be carefully considered based on the overall health of the animal and a consideration of the environment in which the animal will be placed following surgery. Most small animals adapt extremely well and present good functional ambulation on three legs following limb amputation[1]. However, in certain patients with additional pathologies, amputation of the thoracic limb may be contraindicated. These include multiple limb involvement, obesity, or other neurological deficits. Also, if neoplasia is the indication for amputation, the possibility of metastasis should be considered and discussed with the owner, as this may be associated with a poor prognosis.

In the authors' experience, it is also advisable to stabilize the patient for a few hours prior to the procedure. Due to the highly invasive nature of the surgery, correcting for dehydration, providing perioperative antibiotics, and pain management should be considered if at all possible.

#### 10.1.2.2   Anatomic Considerations

The following are anatomic structures that will be encountered during this surgery. It is not critical that the surgeon is able to identify each individual structure, with exception of the axillary artery and vein and the brachial plexus.

The extrinsic muscles to be transected include the brachiocephalicus, omotransversarius, trapezius, rhomboideus, serratus ventralis, and latissimus dorsi. All located in the lateral aspect of the limb. Medially, the superficial pectoral and deep pectoral are transected. The vasculatures to be located, dissected, and ligated are the axillary artery and vein. Nerves to be located and blocked before transection are all part of the brachial plexus and include suprascapular, subscapular, axillary, thoracodorsal, musculocutaneous, radial, median/ulnar, pectoral. The prescapular (superficial cervical) and axillary lymph nodes are in great proximity to the surgical site and should not be excised (Figure 10.1.1).

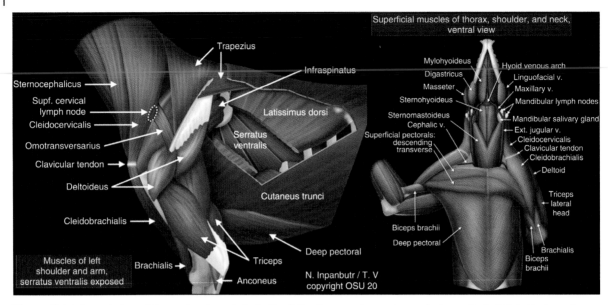

**Figure 10.1.1** Lateral view of the canine thoracic limb. The following muscles are transected near their distal attachments: brachiocephalicus, omotransversarius, trapezius, rhomboideus, serratus ventralis latissimus dorsi, superficial pectoral, and deep pectoral. For a thoracic limb amputation, it is not critical that the surgeon is able to identify each individual structure, with the exception of the axillary artery and vein and the brachial plexus. Source: Courtesy of Dr. Nong Inpanbutr and Mr. Tim Vojt, Ohio State University.

### 10.1.2.3  Patient Preparation

In the field, it is important to take a few, simple, but important steps to decrease the likelihood of complications due to infection. After the patient is stabilized and anesthetized, the limb should be clipped from just below the carpus to dorsal midline over all aspects of the limb. In the authors' experience, it is best to then suspend the limb, allowing for 360° access during prepping. An IV fluid pole or other stable structure is recommended for this purpose. The limb can be secured to the pole using medical tape, or a towel clamp can be attached to the distal limb. At this stage, any infected or compromised tissues should be covered to allow for a more sterile limb prep. A 2% chlorhexidine surgical scrub is the authors' preferred solution; however, any product labeled as surgical scrub can be used. Once the limb is aseptically prepped, the surgeon should drape the patient, and the limb should either be wrapped with sterile bandaging tape ("Vet Wrap"), or, alternatively, the limb can be grasped with a sterile surgical towel or drape and fully wrapped and secured using towel clamps (Figure 10.1.2).

### 10.1.2.4  Procedure

Based on the authors' experience, amputating the limb to include the scapula is more practical and technically less demanding. Alternatively, the scapulohumeral joint can be disarticulated if there is no scapular lesion; however, this can be more technically demanding and time-consuming and is not associated with improved outcome [2]. The authors prefer to create a crescent-shaped incision, starting just below dorsal midline over the proximal aspect of the scapula, with the incision extending medially and distally to the axillary region.

The concave aspect of the incision is on the caudal aspect, while the convex portion of the incision will be on the cranial aspect of the limb. The reason why this approach is chosen over other approaches is to minimize the need to resect redundant skin upon completion of the amputation, while respecting lines of tension. Closure of the incision parallel to the lines of tension improves healing outcome, by minimizing tension forces throughout the surgical wound. Excessive removal of skin should be avoided for similar reasons. In addition, while transecting extrinsic muscles, the surgeon should aim to stay close to the bony aspect of the scapula and humerus to provide ample muscular tissue for closure over the exposed thoracic wall and brachial plexus.

The spine of the scapula is palpated, and a towel clamp is placed on this structure to provide retraction of the scapula away from the thoracic wall. Once the scapula is retracted, the dorsal rim of the scapula is

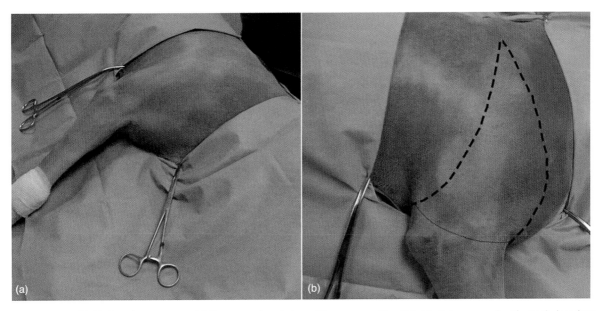

**Figure 10.1.2** (a) Limb to be amputated fully prepped and draped for surgery. The distal limb is wrapped with sterile bandage since this is a challenging area for proper aseptic preparation. (b) Skin incision for thoracic limb amputation, lateral view. The incision is crescent-shaped with the concave aspect on the caudal side, while the convex portion of the incision will on the cranial aspect of the limb. This incision is parallel to the lines of tension, improving healing outcome by minimizing tension forces during the healing phase. The thick striped lines represent the incision on the lateral aspect of the limb, while the thin dotted lines indicate the incision on the medial aspect of the limb.

easily palpated. Begin sharply incising the muscular attachments to the scapula along the contour of the bone. Dissection of the scapula away from the thoracic wall should be done in such a manner that the cranial and caudal aspects are transected alternately to ensure safe exposure of the brachial plexus. Careful, gentle blunt dissection of the brachial plexus will readily expose the vascular bundle. Once the brachial plexus is exposed, the axillary artery and vein are isolated and ligated. To minimize blood loss, first the axillary artery is visualized, dissected, clamped, and ligated.

Once the vessel is transected, two circumferential ligatures are placed proximally (patient side of the vessel), and one circumferential ligature is placed distally (amputated side of the vessel). The axillary vein is ligated next in a similar manner. The suture of choice for the authors is chromic gut due to its superior knot security; however, any absorbable suture can be used. Prior to severing the brachial plexus, identifiable nerves can be injected with 0.5% bupiva-caine or 2% lidocaine if available. A sufficient amount should be injected to create a slight enlargement in the transected nerve [3]. If the indication for amputation is neoplasia, then any visible lymph nodes encountered during dissection should also be removed. At this

point, any additional soft tissue attachments to the medial aspect of the humerus can be transected and the limb removed from the surgical field.

Muscle atrophy will occur within a few months following surgery, so it is critical to protect the site by overlapping the cranial and caudal muscle bellies over the thoracic wall and the brachial plexus. This can be done using a variety of suture patterns. Most commonly, simple interrupted or cruciate patterns are used for this purpose. Upon completion of this step, the skin is evaluated for wound tension. If excess skin is present, it can be trimmed for a more cosmetic skin closure. Be cautious to avoid excess tension on the skin closure, as this can result in necrosis and wound dehiscence. Sub-cutaneous tissues can be closed with absorbable syn-thetic or chromic gut suture by using a simple continuous suture pattern. The skin can be closed with suture or staples, depending on availability (Figure 10.1.3).

## 10.1.3 Pelvic Limb Amputation

### 10.1.3.1 Indications

Common indications for thoracic limb amputation in the field environment include fracture complications

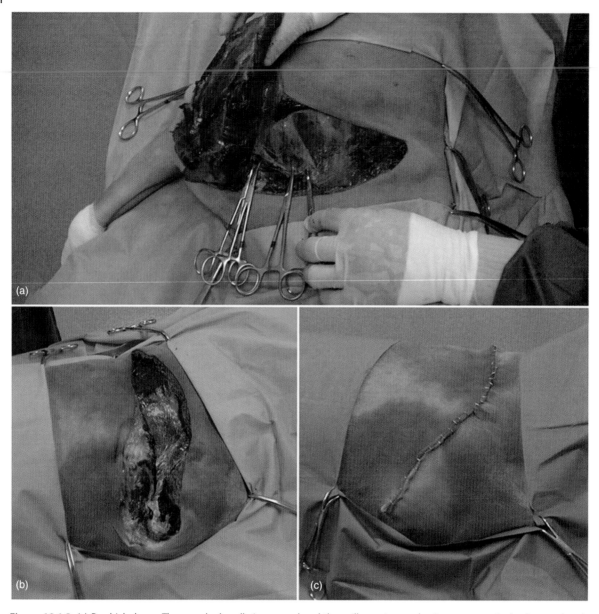

**Figure 10.1.3** (a) Brachial plexus. The vascular bundle is exposed and the axillary artery and vein are, respectively, dissected and ligated. Two circumferential ligatures are placed proximally (patient side of the vessel), and one circumferential ligature is placed distally (amputated side of the vessel). The axillary artery is ligated before the axillary vein. (b) Limb is removed from surgical field and the surgical site must be protected by overlapping the cranial and caudal muscle bellies over the thoracic wall and the brachial plexus. (c) After subcutaneous closure is performed, the skin can be closed with simple continuous suture or staples.

such as delayed union, nonunion, malunion, open fractures, muscular contraction as a result of inappropriate fracture healing, degloving injury, infection, neoplasia and nerve injury, unmanageable joint disease (severe osteoarthritis, luxations), and congenital limb defects. The decision to amputate should be carefully considered based on the overall health of the animal and a consideration of the environment in which the animal will be placed following surgery. Most small animals do extremely well following a pelvic limb amputation [1, 4]; however, in certain patients with additional pathologies amputation of the pelvic limb may be contraindicated. These include multiple limb involvement, obesity, or other neurological deficits. Also, if neoplasia is the indication for amputation, the possibility of metastasis should be considered and discussed with the owner, as this may be associated with a poor prognosis.

In the authors' experience, it is also advisable to stabilize the patient for a few hours prior to the procedure. Due to the highly invasive nature of the surgery, correcting for dehydration, providing perioperative antibiotics and pain management should be considered if at all possible.

### 10.1.3.2 Anatomic Considerations

The following are anatomic structures that will be encountered during this surgery. It is not critical that the surgeon is able to identify each individual structure, with exception of the femoral artery and vein.

The muscles to be transected include quadriceps femoris, biceps femoris, semitendinosus, semimembranosus, adductor, gracilis, and sartorius. The vasculatures to be located, dissected, and ligated are the femoral artery and the femoral vein, medially. Nerves to be located and blocked before transection are the saphenous nerve associated with the femoral vessels and the sciatic nerve on the caudolateral aspect of the femur (Figure 10.1.4).

### 10.1.3.3 Patient Preparation

In the field, it is important to take a few, simple, but important steps to decrease the likelihood of complications due to infection. After the patient is stabilized and anesthetized, the limb should be clipped from just below the tarsus to dorsal midline over all aspects of the limb. In the authors' experience, it is best to then suspend the limb, allowing for 360° access during prepping. An IV fluid pole or other stable structure is recommended for this purpose. The limb can be secured to the pole using medical tape, or a towel clamp can be attached to the distal limb. At this stage, any infected or compromised tissues should be covered to allow for a more sterile limb prep. A 2% chlorhexidine surgical scrub is the authors' preferred solution; however, any product labeled as surgical scrub can be used. Once the limb is aseptically prepped, the surgeon should now drape the patient, and the limb should either be wrapped with sterile bandaging tape ("Vet Wrap"), or, alternatively, the limb can be grasped with a sterile surgical towel or drape and fully wrapped and secured using towel clamps.

### 10.1.3.4 Procedure

Based on the authors' experience in the field, it is quicker and easier to perform an osteotomy on the

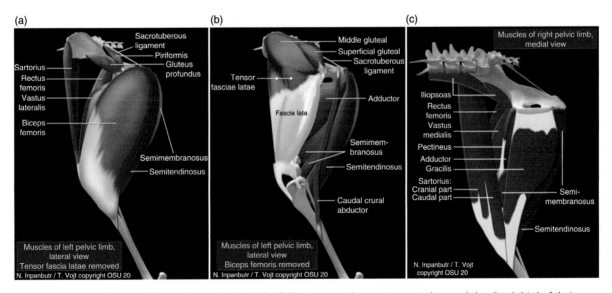

**Figure 10.1.4** Lateral view of the canine pelvic limb. The following muscles are transected around the distal third of their muscle bellies: quadriceps femoris, biceps femoris, semitendinosus, semimembranosus, adductor, gracilis, and sartorius. For a pelvic limb amputation, it is not critical that the surgeon is able to identify each individual structure, with the exception of the femoral artery and vein and the sciatic and saphenous nerve. Source: Courtesy of Dr. Nong Inpanbutr and Mr. Tim Vojt, Ohio State University.

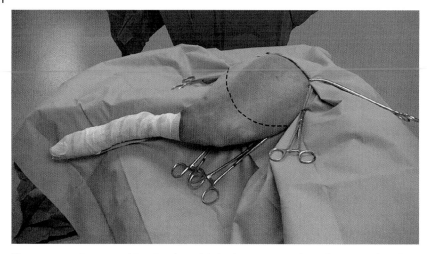

**Figure 10.1.5** Drapes and incision for pelvic limb amputation, lateral view. Limb to be amputated is fully prepped and draped for surgery. The distal limb is wrapped with sterile bandage since this is a challenging area for proper aseptic prep. This circumferential skin incision is performed just proximal to the stifle joint.

proximal third of the femur as opposed to a coxofemoral disarticulation. It is recommended to make the lateral incision fairly distal, while the medial aspect of the incision is carried more proximally. Starting laterally, a circumferential incision is performed just proximal to the stifle joint (Figure 10.1.5).

The incision is continued medially, and the skin is undermined to the level of the pectineus muscle. This muscle is readily palpated in the inguinal region as a firm triangular structure, with the femoral artery and vein located just cranial to this muscle (Figure 10.1.6).

To minimize blood loss, first the femoral artery is visualized, dissected, clamped, and ligated. Once the vessel is transected, two circumferential ligatures are placed proximally (patient side of the vessel), and one circumferential ligature is placed distally (amputated side of the vessel). The femoral vein is ligated next in a similar manner. The suture of choice for the authors is chromic gut due to its superior knot security; however, any absorbable suture can be used. The craniolateral musculature is transected around the stifle joint, while the caudomedial musculature is

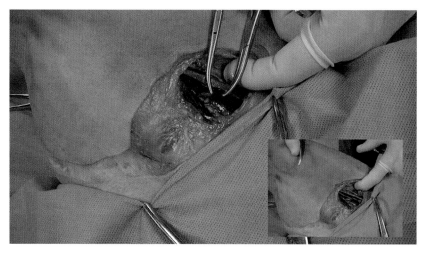

**Figure 10.1.6** Femoral artery. The femoral artery and vein are palpated cranial to the pectineus muscle. Once located, the artery and vein are, respectively, dissected and ligated. Two circumferential ligatures are placed proximally (patient side of the vessel), and one circumferential ligature is placed distally (amputated side of the vessel). The femoral artery is ligated before the femoral vein.

transected at the level of the proximal third of the femur. While transecting the lateral musculature of the thigh, the sciatic nerve will be seen.

Prior to severing the sciatic nerve, it can be injected with 0.5% bupivacaine or 2% lidocaine if available. A sufficient amount should be injected to create a slight enlargement in the transected nerve [3]. Once the musculature has been transected and the dissection continued proximally, the proximal third of the femur is exposed in preparation for the osteotomy. An osteotomy can be performed using a Gigli wire, a bone saw, or a previously sterilized hacksaw blade. In the authors' experience, the use of osteotomes often leads to additional fracturing or fissuring of the proximal end of the femur. At this point, any additional soft tissue attachments to the distal femur can be transected and the limb removed from the surgical field.

Significant muscle atrophy will occur within a few months following surgery, so it is critical to protect the osteotomy site by overlapping the craniolateral and caudomedial muscle bellies around the exposed end of the femur. This can be done using a variety of suture patterns. Most commonly, simple interrupted or cruciate patterns are used for this purpose. Upon completion of this step, the skin is evaluated for wound tension. If excess skin is present, it can be trimmed for a more cosmetic skin closure. Be cautious to avoid excess tension on the skin closure, as this can result in necrosis and wound dehiscence. Subcutaneous tissues can be closed with absorbable synthetic or chromic gut suture by using a simple continuous suture pattern. The skin can be closed with suture or staples, depending on availability (Figure 10.1.7).

## 10.1.4 Digit Amputation

### 10.1.4.1 Indications

Common indications for digit amputation in the field environment include fracture, infection, neoplasia, nerve injury (ulnar nerve injury affecting the fifth digit), and unmanageable joint disease (severe osteoarthritis, luxations of the digit). The decision to amputate should be carefully considered based on the overall health of the animal and a consideration of the environment in which the animal will be placed following surgery. Most small animals do extremely well following digit amputation [5]; however, in certain patients with additional pathologies, digit amputation may be contraindicated.

These include multiple limb involvement, obesity, or other neurological deficits. Digits III and IV are the primary weight-bearing digits; therefore, if multiple amputations of digits on the same limb are necessary, a whole limb amputation could be indicated, depending on the size of the patient and the digits involved. Also, if neoplasia is the indication for amputation, the possibility of metastasis should be considered and discussed with the owner, as this may be associated with a poor prognosis.

### 10.1.4.2 Patient Preparation

In the field, it is important to take a few, simple, but important steps to decrease the likelihood of complications due to infection. After the patient is anesthetized, the limb should be clipped from just above the carpus/tarsus distally, encompassing the entire circumference of each digit. Remove as much hair as possible with special attention to removing debris between pads, between digits, and in nail beds. In terms of prepping the distal limb, it is convenient and practical to simply hang the paw over the edge of the surgical table. Other options include having an assistant suspend the distal limb using a towel clamp through the nail of the affected digit, or using an IV fluid pole or other stable structure to suspend the limb.

Refer to Section 10.1.2 for details regarding prepping a suspended limb. A 2% chlorhexidine surgical scrub is the authors' preferred solution; however, any product labeled as surgical scrub can be used. Once the limb is aseptically prepped, the surgeon should now drape the distal limb by wrapping a sterile drape around the area just below the carpus/tarsus, and secure the drape using towel clamps. Any instruments that are used during the prepping phase should be removed as the surgeon drapes the patient. The limb can remain suspended over the edge of the table for the procedure as is demonstrated in Figure 10.1.8. Alternatively, the limb can be repositioned to be on the surgical table, in which case the prepped area should be placed on a sterile drape.

### 10.1.4.3 Procedure

Based on the authors' experience, we do not recommend amputating the last phalanx/nail only. Amputation at this level would have to be accompanied by preservation of the digital pad in order to avoid pressure

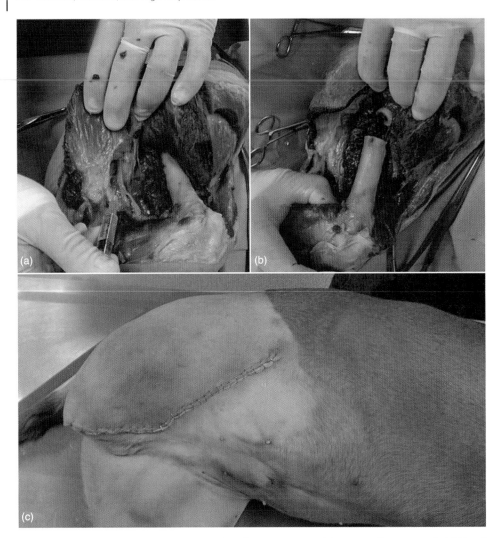

Figure 10.1.7 (a) Sciatic nerve. Prior to severing the sciatic nerve, inject a small amount of 0.5% bupivacaine or 2% lidocaine. Inject enough to create a slight enlargement in the transected nerve. (b) Femoral osteotomy. The proximal third of the femur is exposed and transected with a Gigli wire, a bone saw, or a previously sterilized hacksaw blade. An osteotome can also be used but can lead to additional fracturing or fissuring of the proximal end of the femur. (c) Closure. Protect the osteotomy site by overlapping the craniolateral and caudomedial muscle bellies around the exposed end of the femur. This can be done using a variety of suture patterns. Most commonly, simple interrupted or cruciate patterns are used for this purpose. After subcutaneous closure is performed, the skin can be closed with simple continuous suture or staples.

sores caused by the distal aspect of the middle phalanx. Although this can be accomplished, it is technically more demanding compared to amputation more proximally. To avoid this complication, the authors prefer to amputate at the level of the metacarpophalangeal/metatarsophalangeal joint space even for very distal lesions.

Before starting the skin incision, a sterile towel clamp should be placed in the nail of the affected digit. If the nail is not present, then the clamp can be placed on the most distal phalanx that is available. At this stage, the surgeon should try to minimize manipulation of the aseptically prepped nails and pads, as these structures still are a significant source of contamination.

To perform the amputation, begin by palpating the affected digit to localize the distal aspect of the metacarpus/metatarsus. Begin the skin incision dorsally and slightly distal to this landmark and carry it

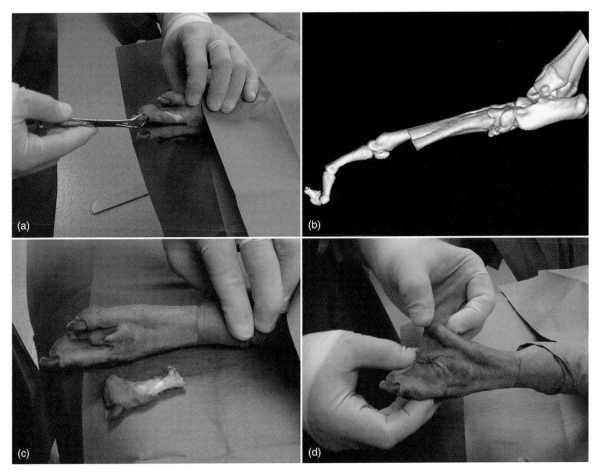

**Figure 10.1.8** (a) The limb is clipped from just above the carpus/tarsus distally, encompassing the entire circumference of each digit. Remove as much hair as possible with special attention to removing debris between pads, between digits, and in nail beds. The limb can remain suspended over the edge of the table for prepping and for the procedure. A skin incision is made dorsally and slightly distal to the metacarpo/tarsophalangeal joint and carry it distally in an elliptical fashion to the level of the proximal digital pad. (b) Bony anatomy of the metatarsophalangeal joint. This joint should be palpated and is an important landmark for the skin incision. Flexion and extension of the digit will assist the surgeon in locating the joint space. Amputations at the level of this joint are associated with lower complications rates compared to amputations performed distal to this joint. (c) Once the joint space is clearly identified, a scalpel is used to perform the disarticulation. It is technically easier to place the joint in flexion while approaching the dorsal aspect of the joint. Once the blade has entered the joint space, sharp transection of the tendons, ligaments and joint capsule is continued medially and laterally until reaching the palmar/plantar aspect of the joint. This completes the disarticulation, and the affected digit is removed from the surgical field. (d) Closure. To close the wound, simple interrupted or cruciate patterns can be used for this purpose. Generally, there is not an indication to perform a subcutaneous layer closure due to minimal presence of connective tissues in this area. If enough subcutaneous tissues are available, a two-layer closure can be performed. When performing the skin closure, it is important to achieve adequate apposition of the skin edges to ensure a good seal as the surgical wound will be immediately in contact with the ground.

distally in an elliptical fashion to the level of the proximal digital pad (Figure 10.1.8a). Continue dissection of the subcutaneous tissues to expose the ligaments and tendons associated with the metacarpophalangeal/metatarsophalangeal joint. Flexion and extension of the digit will assist the surgeon in locating the joint space. Once the joint space is clearly identified, a scalpel is used to perform the disarticulation. It is technically easier to place the joint in flexion while approaching the dorsal aspect of the

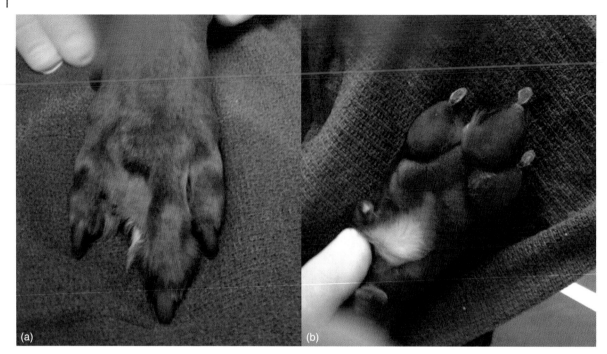

**Figure 10.1.9** Healed surgical wound.

joint. Once the blade has entered the joint space, sharp transection of the tendons, ligaments, and joint capsule is continued medially and laterally until reaching the palmar/plantar aspect of the joint. This completes the disarticulation, and the affected digit is removed from the surgical field. Hemostasis should be achieved prior to closure. In most cases, minimal hemorrhage is encountered.

To close the wound, simple interrupted or cruciate patterns can be used for this purpose. Generally, there is not an indication to perform a subcutaneous layer closure due to minimal presence of connective tissues in this area. If enough subcutaneous tissues are available, a two-layer closure can be performed. When performing the skin closure, it is important to achieve adequate apposition of the skin edges to ensure a good seal as the surgical wound will be immediately in contact with the ground Figure 10.1.8.

Once healed, the animal will have an acceptable weight distribution within the remaining digital pads (Figure 10.1.9).

## References

1 Kirpensteijn, J., van den Bos, R., and Endenburg, N. (1999). Adaptation of dogs to the amputation of a limb and their owners' satisfaction with the procedure. *Veterinary Record* **144** (5): 115–118.
2 Karen Tobias, S.J. (2012). Veterinary Surgery: Small Animal. St. Louis: W.B. Saunders Co.
3 Flor, H. (2002). Phantom-limb pain: characteristics, causes, and treatment. *The Lancet Neurology* **1** (3): 182–189.

4 Hogy, S.M., Worley, D.R., Jarvis, S.L. et al. (2013). Kinematic and kinetic analysis of dogs during trotting after amputation of a pelvic limb. *American Journal of VeterinaryResearch* **74** (9): 1164–1171.
5 Kaufman, K.L. and Mann, F.A. (2013). Short- and long-term outcomes after digit amputation in dogs: 33 cases (1999-2011) and. *Journal of the American Veterinary Medical Association* **242** (9): 1249–1254.

# 10.2

# Enucleation

*Joshua S. Eaton*

*School of Veterinary Medicine, Ocular Services on Demand (OSOD), LLC, University of California, Davis, CA 95616, USA*

## 10.2.1 Introduction

Enucleation is commonly performed in small animal practice, chiefly indicated as a palliative treatment for animals with blind and intractably painful globes. Clinical scenarios that often necessitate enucleation include the following:

- Penetrating ocular injury or globe rupture with extensive or irreparable intraocular tissue damage
- Penetrating ocular injury or globe rupture with secondary infectious endophthalmitis
- Severe traumatic proptosis with hyphema and/or loss of globe viability
- Chronic, refractory end-stage glaucoma (primary or secondary)
- Chronic refractory uveitis with retinal detachment (or other blinding complication)

Enucleation is also indicated in dogs or cats with malignant intraocular neoplasms or space-occupying intraocular tumors associated with secondary pain or loss of visual function (i.e. uveitis, secondary glaucoma).

## 10.2.2 Relevant Surgical Anatomy

Enucleation comprises surgical removal of the globe, conjunctiva, nictitating membrane (third eyelid), and eyelid margins. It is important to differentiate enucleation from *exenteration*, the latter specifying a more aggressive surgery to remove the globe and all associated orbital soft tissues. Unlike enucleation, exenteration is indicated for surgical management of refractory infectious or inflammatory orbital soft tissue disease or for resection of primary orbital neoplasms or extensive intraocular neoplasms that involve adjacent orbital tissues.

Surgical approaches to enucleation are similar in dogs and cats due to similarities in orbital anatomy between the two species. In dogs and cats, the globe and associated structures are contained within an open or "incomplete" orbit, so-named for the presence of a fibrous orbital ligament comprising the orbit's caudolateral aspect. Ventrally and laterally, the globe is supported by soft tissues including the pterygoid and masticatory muscles and zygomatic (dog) or infraorbital (cat) salivary glands. The flat bones of the skull determine the medial and dorsal limits of the orbit and, with the temporalis muscle, form the caudal limit [1].

The orbit is lined by fibrous connective tissue, continuous with fascial membranes that encase the globe, extraocular muscles, lacrimal gland, and associated blood vessels and nerves. Tenon's capsule (fascia bulbi) is the connective tissue layer immediately external to the sclera and must be surgically incised in order to access the extraocular muscles when performing an enucleation.

The eye and its associated structures are robustly vascular. The majority of the blood supply to the globe, adnexa, and orbital tissues is carried by the maxillary and external ophthalmic arteries. The internal ophthalmic artery courses along the dorsal aspect of the optic nerve and is transected with the optic nerve during enucleation surgery in both dogs and cats. It is a small artery and does not necessarily require ligation, though some surgeons will advocate

*Field Manual for Small Animal Medicine*, First Edition. Edited by Katherine Polak and Ann Therese Kommedal.
© 2018 John Wiley & Sons, Inc. Published 2018 by John Wiley & Sons, Inc.

for placement of a ligating suture or hemostatic clip following transection. The angular vein (V. angularis *oculi*) is a branch of the facial vein and is one of the major routes of venous drainage from the eye and adnexa. This vein courses superficially along the medial aspect of the dorsal orbital rim before turning to enter the orbit. Therefore, surgeons must be aware of this structure when dissecting the broad and dense medial canthal ligament and medial subcutaneous tissues. Inadvertent transection of this vessel always requires ligation to prevent untoward hemorrhage.

### 10.2.3 Pre- and Perioperative Considerations

#### 10.2.3.1 Preoperative Assessment

A complete physical examination should be performed in any animal prior to enucleation to identify abnormalities that may guide choice of anesthetic protocol or postoperative treatment plan. Furthermore, chronic uveitis or intraocular neoplasms in dogs and cats may represent clinical manifestations of a range of systemic infectious, inflammatory, and neoplastic diseases. Particularly in cases with suspected intraocular neoplasia, preoperative staging (3-view thoracic radiographs, abdominal ultrasound, and lymph node aspirations) is recommended in both species.

At the time of enucleation, complete bloodwork (complete blood count (CBC), serum biochemical profile) is generally recommended in dogs and cats older than 6–8 years. Though the risk for life-threatening hemorrhage is low during and after routine enucleation, the recommended minimum database for any patient should include measurement of packed cell volume (PCV), total solids (TS), and general assessment of renal function (i.e. Azostix™).

#### 10.2.3.2 Anesthetic and Analgesic Considerations

Enucleation in dogs and cats is a major surgical procedure and should be performed in a clean operatory or a designated surgical area with restricted foot traffic, observing all aspects of sterile surgical preparation and technique. As the primary intraoperative risk in all animals is hemorrhage, intravenous (IV) access should be obtained in all patients and crystalloid fluid therapy administered at a surgical maintenance rate.

Enucleation should be performed under general anesthesia; and once an animal has been induced, anesthesia should be maintained using endotracheal intubation and inhalant anesthetics such as isoflurane or sevoflurane. Premedication protocols in dogs and cats should include an opioid analgesic (i.e. hydromorphone, oxymorphone, buprenorphine) to enhance postoperative pain control and reduce the amount of inhalant anesthetic required during surgery. Preoperative treatment with a nonsteroidal anti-inflammatory drug (NSAID) and administration of perioperative broad-spectrum antibiotics (i.e. cefazolin at 20 mg/kg IV) are recommended in both dogs and cats.

#### 10.2.3.3 Regional Anesthesia for Enucleation

Adjunctive regional anesthesia has shown clinical efficacy in augmenting pain control after enucleation in dogs and cats. The most commonly employed anesthetics, lidocaine and bupivacaine, are amides that inhibit action potentials from nociceptive sensory nerves. Lidocaine induces anesthesia quickly (within 1–2 min), with an effect lasting 20 min to 2 h. Bupivacaine induces anesthesia within 3–6 min, with a longer effect than lidocaine, lasting 4–6 h [2]. Therefore, bupivacaine or a combination of the two agents is recommended to provide extended analgesia following enucleation.

Fortunately, toxicity associated with local anesthetics is very rare, especially since the volume required for ocular analgesia is small in dogs and cats. However, serious systemic toxicities, including cardiovascular effects (arrhythmia, hypotension, cardiac arrest) and neurological effects (seizures, obtundation, death), may occur [2, 3]. These risks are highest when the agent is administered in an excessive dose or volume, or if injected directly into a blood vessel. Intrathecal administration of an anesthetic agent (i.e. into the subarachnoid space and cerebrospinal fluid surrounding the optic nerve) is also rare, but can occur during retrobulbar injection. In dogs, local anesthetic dose should not exceed 5 mg/kg of lidocaine or 1.5 mg/kg bupivacaine [2]. In cats, use of bupivacaine is advocated, and local dose should not exceed 2 mg/kg [4].

### 10.2.3.3.1 The Inferotemporal-Palpebral Technique for Adjunctive Anesthesia in Dogs

While several techniques for periocular and orbital injections have been described in dogs, the inferotemporal-palpebral (ITP) technique is most commonly advocated by veterinary ophthalmologists. In both *in vivo* and postmortem studies in dogs, ITP injection was deemed the easiest to perform, provided the best distribution of anesthetic into the retrobulbar space immediately behind the globe, and effectively induced analgesia and anesthesia [5]. Furthermore, clinical efficacy was demonstrated in a prospective, controlled trial of dogs undergoing enucleation, reducing the need for additional postoperative analgesic medications [6].

To perform the ITP injection, a 22-gauge, 1.5″ spinal needle is used, with an approximately 20″ bend created at the needle midpoint. For an adult dog, a total volume of 2 ml of anesthetic is prepared. The procedure thereafter is as follows:

1) At a point approximately 1/3 the distance from the lateral canthus to the medial canthus, the needle is inserted through the inferior eyelid, 5–10 mm from the eyelid margin (see Figure 10.2.1).
2) The needle is gently "walked" along the underlying inferior orbital rim until it reaches the edge.
3) With the needle tip just past the edge of the orbital rim, it is slowly advanced ventral to the globe. A slight "pop" may be felt when the needle penetrates the fascial tissue of the orbital septum.

4) After penetrating the septum, the needle tip is directed slightly dorsally and nasally, aiming toward the posterior orbital apex.
5) The needle is advanced approximately 1–2 cm. After plunger withdrawal confirms that the needle tip is not intravascular, the full 2 ml volume of anesthetic is injected slowly.

### 10.2.3.3.2 Peribulbar Injection Technique for Adjunctive Anesthesia in Cats

Adjunctive regional anesthesia techniques have also been investigated for enucleation in cats. However, the relatively small feline orbit limits available routes of administration and the volume of anesthesia that can be delivered. In one *ex vivo* study, a dorsomedial peribulbar injection technique demonstrated superior distribution of an injected volume radiologically [7]. A subsequent *in vivo* study corroborated these findings and demonstrated anesthesia for 3 h following peribulbar injection [4]. It is noteworthy, however, that peribulbar injection was associated with a transient increase in intraocular pressure, so this technique should be used with caution in cats with ruptured globes [4].

For an adult cat, a total volume of 3 ml bupivacaine is used. The procedure thereafter is as follows:

1) A 5/8″, 25-gauge needle is inserted through the upper eyelid medially and advanced long the orbital wall for its entire length.

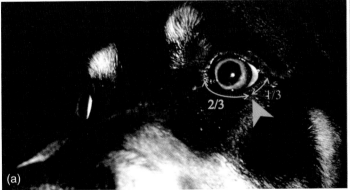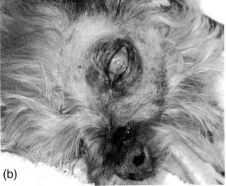

**Figure 10.2.1** (a) Approximate needle entry point (orange arrowhead) for the inferotemporal-palpebral retrobulbar injection in dogs. The needle is inserted through the inferior eyelid, at a point approximately 1/3 the distance from the lateral canthus to the medial canthus (green double-arrow), and 5–10 mm from the eyelid margin. (b) A wide clip (2–4″) of the periocular hair should be performed around the palpebral fissure. The eyelashes should also be carefully trimmed or clipped. Source: Courtesy of Ellison Bentley, DVM, DACVO, School of Veterinary Medicine, University of Wisconsin – Madison.

2) After plunger withdrawal confirms that the needle tip is not intravascular, the entire 3 ml of bupivacaine is injected slowly.

## 10.2.4 Surgical Technique

### 10.2.4.1 Aseptic Preparation of the Eye

While the eye cannot be made truly "aseptic" preoperatively, a thorough preparation of the eyelids and ocular surface should be performed prior to enucleation. For dogs and cats, a recommended aseptic preparation is as follows:

1) A wide clip (2–4 in.) of the periocular hair should be performed around the palpebral fissure. The eyelashes (cilia) should also be carefully trimmed or clipped at the eyelid margins.
2) A gross scrub of the periocular skin should be performed gently using dilute baby shampoo (i.e. 1 : 20 preparation of shampoo:distilled water) to remove any residual dirt or hair from the surgical site. If shampoo is unavailable, 0.5% iodine solution (see Step 3 below) can be used.
3) A small volume (~1 ml) of dilute (0.5%) povidone iodine aqueous *solution* (not surgical *scrub* preparation) is instilled onto the ocular surface and into the conjunctival fornices. The solution is left in place for 30 s. A sterile cotton-tipped applicator is used to gently clear the conjunctival fornices of iodine solution and residual debris, and the ocular surface is then liberally irrigated with isotonic saline or balanced salt solution (BSS). Step 3 is repeated 2–3 more times (Figure 10.2.1).

### 10.2.4.2 Positioning

Positioning of the animal for enucleation may depend on surgeon preference. Dorsal, lateral, or sternal recumbency are all acceptable positions for enucleation, regardless of species or technique used. This author's preference is dorsal recumbency for dolicho- and mesaticephalic breeds and sternal recumbency with an elevated and oblique head position in brachycephalic breeds.

### 10.2.4.3 Draping

Animals should be draped such that any unclipped periocular hair is excluded from the surgical field.

This can be done using a four-corner draping technique, a sterile fenestrated drape, or a combination of the two.

### 10.2.4.4 Surgical Instrumentation

Many of the surgical instruments included in general surgical packs can be used to perform enucleation. There are, however, several ophthalmic surgical instruments (marked with asterisks) that enhance surgical precision when manipulating gentle ocular and periocular tissues. The list of recommended instruments for enucleation in dogs and cats includes the following:

- Mayo scissors (blunt-tipped, straight or curved)
- Metzenbaum scissors (blunt-tipped, curved)
- *Stevens tenotomy scissors (blunt-tipped)
- Bard-Parker scalpel blade handle
- No. 15 blade (preferred) or No. 10 blade
- Adson tissue forceps (toothed)
- *Bishop-Harmon tissue forceps (toothed, 0.5 mm [fine])
- Backhaus towel clamp or Allis tissue forceps
- *Derf needle holders
- Hartmann mosquito hemostatic clamps (straight or curved)
- Curved hemostatic clamp (Kelly or Crile)
- 3-0 to 5-0 synthetic absorbable suture (polyglactin (Vicryl™) recommended)
- 3-0 to 5-0 synthetic non-absorbable suture (i.e. nylon, prolene)
- *Barraquer wire eyelid speculum (for subconjunctival technique)
- Small or medium hemostatic clips (i.e. HemoClip™)
- Cautery (if available) (Figure 10.2.2).

Magnification is also highly recommended for ocular or periocular surgery. Surgical magnifying loupes are often expensive, but lower-cost alternatives such as the Optivisor™ headset can provide up to 3.5X magnification.

### 10.2.4.5 Enucleation Techniques

While either of the techniques presented herein is appropriate for enucleation in dogs and cats, the *subconjunctival technique* is preferred by many surgeons as it provides better anatomical visualization

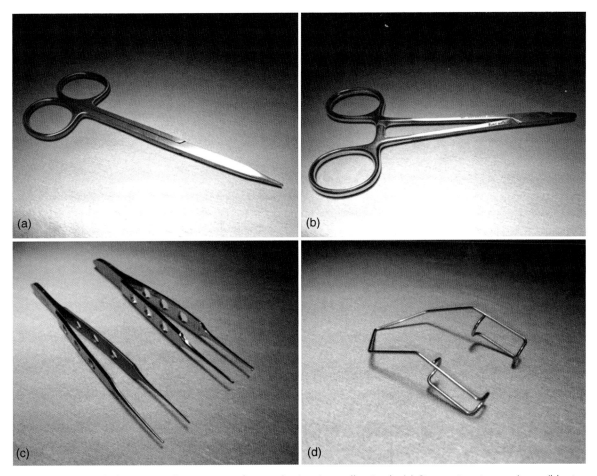

**Figure 10.2.2** Ophthalmic surgical instruments for enucleation in small animals. (a) Stevens tenotomy scissors (blunt-tipped, straight blades) are excellent for safe, precise dissection of adnexal and conjunctival tissue. (b) Derf needle holders are useful for handling smaller sutures (4-0 to 5-0) with small jaws and serrated blade surfaces. (c) Toothed Bishop-Harmon tissue forceps (delicate (0.3 mm) tip on the left, fine (0.5 mm) tip on the right) are used for handling ocular tissues. Both tip sizes are appropriate for conjunctival tissue, but only fine tip should be used for handling of eyelid tissue. (d) A Barraquer wire eyelid speculum is required to provide adequate exposure of the ocular surface when performing a subconjunctival enucleation.

intraoperatively, facilitating dissection of the extra-ocular muscles and ocular soft tissue attachments. It does, however, require surgical entry into the orbit via the ocular surface (i.e. through the conjunctiva), which carries an increased risk of microbial contamination. Therefore, it is best reserved for the removal of globes without ocular surface infections, infectious endophthalmitis, or ocular injuries from penetrating trauma.

When performing the *transpalpebral technique*, the initial dissection/surgical plane is not established at the ocular surface, but instead initiated through the eyelids. This technique is associated with more tissue dissection, limited visualization of the extraocular muscles, and potentially more hemorrhage. However, it does avoid surgical penetration through the conjunctival tissue or fornix thereby minimizing the risk of orbital contamination intraoperatively. This is preferred when active infection is present on the ocular surface or within a ruptured globe at the time of surgery. Also, *en bloc* removal of the globe with intact conjunctival tissue, third eyelid, and eyelid margins minimizes the risk of leaving secretory tissue in the orbit postoperatively.

### 10.2.4.5.1 Subconjunctival Technique

1) Ensure that the correct eye has been prepared for surgical removal.
2) A Barraquer wire eyelid speculum is placed to provide exposure of the ocular surface.
3) A 10 to 20 mm lateral canthotomy is performed using a #10 or #15 blade and/or Metzenbaum scissors to enhance exposure of the conjunctival fornix and globe.
4) The bulbar conjunctiva is grasped 1–2 mm from the limbus with Bishop-Harmon forceps. A 360° peritomy (full-thickness incision through the conjunctiva, circumferentially around the cornea/limbus) is made with tenotomy scissors. *Note: If Bishop-Harmon forceps are unavailable, toothed Adson thumb forceps are a reasonable alternative.*
5) Tenotomy scissors are used to bluntly separate the bulbar conjunctiva from Tenon's capsule. Tenon's capsule is incised and bluntly separated from the underlying extraocular muscles.
6) Each extraocular muscle is transected to mobilize the globe. To minimize hemorrhage, each muscle should be bluntly undermined and transected anteriorly at its scleral insertion.
7) The globe is gently rotated laterally or medially to expose the retractor bulbi muscle and its insertion on the posterior globe. *Note: Excessive anterior or torsional ("twisting") traction of the globe and remaining attachments should be avoided. Excessive traction risks trauma to the optic chiasm and contralateral blindness, particularly in cats whose optic nerve is comparatively shorter. Excessive traction can also risk inducing the oculocardiac reflex.*
8) *In dogs*, the retractor bulbi muscle, optic nerve, and internal ophthalmic artery are clamped with a pair of curved hemostatic forceps, and a pair of Metzenbaum scissors used to transect those structures between the clamp and the posterior aspect of the globe. Any remaining soft tissue attachments are sharply transected to deliver the globe from the orbit. *In cats*, sharp dissection of soft tissues and delivery of the globe is performed without placement of a clamp, to minimize the risk of excessive traction on the optic nerve.
9) Before releasing the clamp, a suture ligature or hemostatic clip can be placed around the transected tissues behind it. It may be unnecessary to ligate the optic nerve in dogs and cats.
10) Digital compression with surgical sponges is used to control any residual bleeding in the orbit. Handheld cautery can also be used if available.
11) The third eyelid and its gland are identified, bluntly and sharply dissected from the underlying orbital tissue using tenotomy scissors, and excised.
12) The eyelid margins are excised using a scalpel blade and Metzenbaum scissors, including 4–5 mm of perimarginal skin, to ensure complete removal of the Meibomian glands.
13) Remaining fibrous and connective tissues are apposed across the orbital surface with a simple continuous pattern using 3-0 or 4-0 absorbable suture (i.e. Vicryl).
14) The edges of the excised eyelids are apposed in two layers. Secure wound closure can be achieved using a continuous subcutaneous or subcuticular layer with 4-0 or 5-0 absorbable suture, followed by interrupted or cruciate skin sutures using non-absorbable suture (or absorbable for aggressive dogs, or those in which follow-up cannot be performed).
15) Whenever possible, the globe should be fixed in formalin and submitted for histopathology (Figure 10.2.3).

### 10.2.4.5.2 Transpalpebral (en bloc) Technique

1) Ensure that the correct eye has been prepared for surgical removal.
2) The eyelids are apposed using 3-0 to 5-0 non-absorbable suture to close the palpebral fissure and isolate the ocular surface from the rest of the surgical dissection.
3) Using a #10 or #15 scalpel blade, an elliptical skin incision is made circumferentially around the closed palpebral fissure, remaining 5–8 mm from the eyelid margins.
4) Through the incision, the subcutaneous tissues are bluntly and sharply dissected from the adjacent subcutaneous tissue using Metzenbaum or tenotomy scissors, exposing the external aspect of the conjunctival membranes (the subconjunctival submucosa). Dissection is performed toward the orbital rim until it can be easily

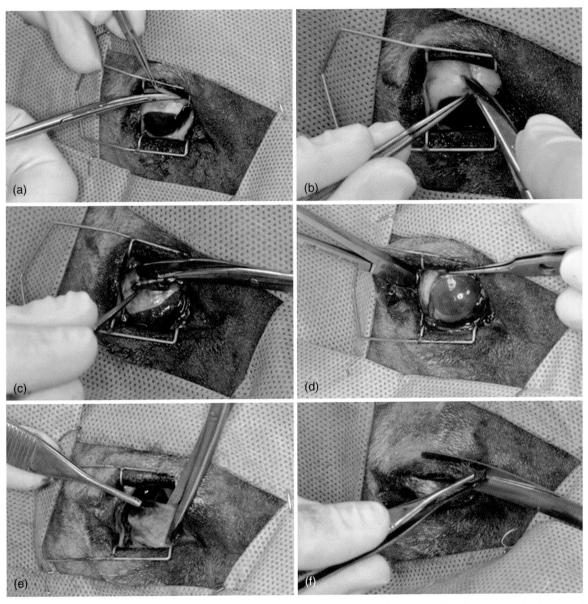

Figure 10.2.3 Subconjunctival enucleation. (a) A wire eyelid speculum is placed. The perilimbal bulbar conjunctiva is grasped with Bishop-Harmon forceps, and tenotomy scissors used to initiate a peritomy, approximately 4–5 mm from the limbus. (b) Tenotomy scissors are used to continue the peritomy circumferentially around the limbus, completely exposing Tenon's capsule. Where still intact following the peritomy, Tenon's capsule is sharply incised and bluntly dissected away from the underlying extraocular muscles. (c) The extraocular muscles identified are transected at their anterior insertions using tenotomy scissors. In this image, a muscle hook is used to elevate the dorsal rectus muscle and facilitate identification of the insertion. (d) After transection of all extraocular muscles and anterior soft tissue connections, the globe is rotated medially or laterally, and the retractor bulbi muscle, optic nerve, and internal ophthalmic artery are clamped with a pair of curved hemostatic forceps and a pair of Metzenbaum scissors used to transect those structures between the clamp and the posterior aspect of the globe. Any remaining soft tissue attachments are sharply transected to deliver the globe, eyelid margins, third eyelid, and conjunctiva from the orbit. In cats, a clamp is not placed to minimize the risk of optic nerve traction. (e) Following delivery of the globe, the nictitating membrane (third eyelid) is grasped with thumb forceps, protracted, and excised using Metzenbaum surgical scissors. Care is taken to ensure that the entire gland at the membrane's base is removed in its entirety. (f) Gauze is placed in the orbit to provide hemostasis. The eyelids and remaining conjunctiva are excised using Metzenbaum scissors, remaining at least 4–5 mm from the eyelid margins to ensure complete removal of the Meibomian glands. Gauze is removed prior to the closure of the surgical site. Source: Courtesy of Christa Corbett, DVM, MS, DACVO, Upstate Veterinary Specialties, Latham, NY.

palpated and observed in at least several locations around the circumferential dissection plane. *Note: Manipulation of the apposed eyelid margins using Allis tissue forceps or a Backhaus towel clamp can facilitate circumferential dissection around the apposed eyelids.*

5) The medial and lateral canthal ligaments (which join eyelid margins to the orbital rim or orbital ligament) are identified and transected to improve exposure and globe mobilization. The long, thin lateral canthal ligament is usually easy to identify and transect using tenotomy scissors. The medial canthal ligament is broader, thicker, and extends deeper. Though its short course makes it difficult to see intraoperatively, it can be palpated between the medial canthus and orbital rim. The medial canthal ligament can be safely transected halfway between the globe and orbital rim carefully using a scalpel blade. It is noteworthy that the medial canthal ligament is adjacent to the medial orbital rim near the course of the angular vein (branch of the facial vein). *If this vein is transected, it should be surgically ligated to minimize serious hemorrhage both intraoperatively and postoperatively.*

6) At the level of the orbital rim, remaining connective tissue overlying the sclera is sharply incised and bluntly dissected around the globe circumferentially to exposure the underlying extraocular muscles. The extraocular muscles are identified and transected. Performing all soft tissue dissection at the level of the orbital rim keeps the conjunctiva intact and the ocular surface enclosed.

7) The globe is gently rotated laterally or medially to expose the retractor bulbi muscle and its insertion on the posterior globe. *Note: Excessive anterior or torsional ("twisting") traction of the globe and remaining attachments should be avoided. Particularly in cats whose optic nerve is comparatively shorter, excessive traction risks trauma to the optic chiasm and possible contralateral blindness. Excessive traction can also risk inducing the oculocardiac reflex.*

8) *In dogs,* the retractor bulbi muscle, optic nerve, and internal ophthalmic artery are clamped with a pair of curved hemostatic forceps and a pair of Metzenbaum scissors used to transect those structures between the clamp and the posterior

aspect of the globe. Any remaining soft tissue attachments are sharply transected to deliver the globe, eyelid margins, third eyelid, and conjunctiva from the orbit. *In cats,* sharp dissection of soft tissues and delivery of the globe and these tissues is performed without placement of a clamp, to minimize the risk of excessive traction on the optic nerve.

9) Before releasing the clamp in dogs, a suture ligature or hemostatic clip can be placed around the transected tissues behind it. It may be unnecessary to ligate the optic nerve in dogs and cats.

10) Digital compression with surgical sponges can be used to control any residual bleeding in the orbit. Handheld cautery can also be used if available (Figure 10.2.4).

11) Remaining fibrous/connective tissue is apposed with a simple continuous pattern using 3-0 or 4-0 absorbable suture (i.e. Vicryl).

12) The edges of the excised eyelids are apposed in two layers. Secure wound closure can be achieved using a continuous subcutaneous or subcuticular layer with 4-0 or 5-0 absorbable suture, followed by interrupted or cruciate skin sutures using non-absorbable suture (or absorbable for aggressive dogs, or those in which follow-up cannot be performed).

13) Whenever possible, the globe should be fixed in formalin and submitted for histopathology (Figure 10.2.5).

### 10.2.4.6 The Oculocardiac Reflex

While uncommonly encountered in dogs and cats, surgeons and anesthetists should be aware of the oculocardiac reflex. Surgical manipulation of the globe, traction of the extraocular muscles, and stimulation of orbital sensory nerves can stimulate various branches of the ophthalmic division of the trigeminal nerve (V) (and in some cases CN III, IV, and VI), leading to an efferent reaction mediated by the vagus nerve (X). The effects may include respiratory depression, arrhythmias, or bradycardia. In most cases, the effect is temporary, requiring momentary cessation of surgical manipulations and an increase in anesthetic depth. If recurrent or refractory, IV atropine or glycopyrrolate can be administered to counteract bradycardia; a positive chronotropic effect, however, may be variable [8].

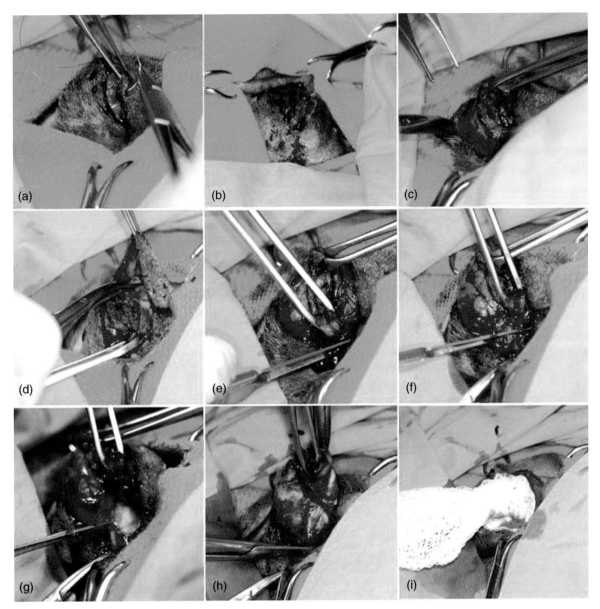

**Figure 10.2.4** Transpalpebral enucleation. (a) The eyelids are apposed using 3-0 to 5-0 non-absorbable suture to close the palpebral fissure and enclose/isolate the ocular surface from the rest of the surgical dissection. (b) An elliptical skin incision is made circumferentially around the closed palpebral fissure, 5–8 mm from the eyelid margins. (c) Allis tissue forceps (or a Backhaus towel clamp) can be used to grasp and handle the eyelid margins during surgical dissection. (d) Via the incision, the subcutaneous tissues are dissected from the adjacent subcutaneous tissues, exposing (but not penetrating through) the external aspect of the conjunctival membranes. (e, f) The medial canthal ligament is broad, thick, and extends deep to its insertion on the orbital rim. It is often difficult to view during dissection but can be palpated extending from the medial canthus. It can be transected halfway between the globe and orbital rim with a scalpel blade, taking care to avoid transecting the angular vein which courses nearby along the medial orbital rim. (g) Taking care to stay posterior to the conjunctival membranes, connective tissue is circumferentially dissected away from the globe to expose the sclera and extraocular muscles. All extraocular muscles are transected. (h) The retractor bulbi muscle, optic nerve, and internal ophthalmic artery are clamped with a pair of curved hemostatic forceps, and a pair of Metzenbaum scissors used to transect those structures between the clamp and the posterior aspect of the globe. Any remaining soft tissue attachments are sharply transected to deliver the globe, eyelid margins, third eyelid, and conjunctiva from the orbit. In cats, a clamp is not placed to minimize the risk of optic nerve traction. (i) Digital compression with surgical sponges can be used to control any residual bleeding in the orbit.

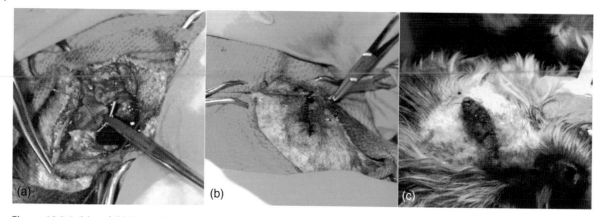

**Figure 10.2.5** (a) and (b) Remaining connective tissue is apposed with a simple continuous pattern using 3-0 or 4-0 absorbable suture, followed by a continuous subcutaneous or subcuticular layer with 4-0 or 5-0 absorbable suture. (c) Interrupted or cruciate skin sutures are placed using non-absorbable suture. Source: Courtesy of Ellison Bentley, DVM, DACVO, School of Veterinary Medicine, University of Wisconsin – Madison.

Preventive preoperative IV administration of an anticholinergic agent is controversial, but generally considered unnecessary for routine enucleations. In brachycephalic breeds or those with higher resting vagal tone, however, a prophylactic perioperative dose may be advantageous.

## 10.2.5 Postoperative Management

Immediate postoperative treatment in dogs and cats should be aimed at reducing tissue swelling and controlling pain. During postoperative recovery, cold compressing of the surgical site for 10–15 min (or as long as tolerated) is recommended in both dogs and cats to minimize swelling. Opioids can also be used as needed IV for animals exhibiting greater signs of discomfort (high heart and respiratory rate, restlessness).

As soon as it is safe for the animal, a hard Elizabethan collar should be placed to prevent self-trauma and minimize the risk for dehiscence or infection of the surgical site. Elizabethan collars should remain in place at all times for 10–14 days or until the animal is presented for recheck examination and external suture removal.

All animals should be discharged with a pain management plan, typically for 3–5 days postoperatively. NSAIDs and synthetic opioid medications (i.e. tramadol) are commonly prescribed in dogs following enucleation. However, a recent randomized, masked clinical trial suggested that an NSAID such as carprofen may provide more effective postoperative analgesia compared to tramadol [9]. In cats, NSAIDs should be used with caution postoperatively given the risks for renal or hepatic adverse effects. Alternatively, buccal (oral transmucosal) buprenorphine can be administered at 0.02 to 0.03 mg/kg q6h–q8h for 3–5 days postoperatively.

Postoperative broad-spectrum antibiotics are recommended following enucleation of eyes with documented or suspected infection. If no infectious disease process is suspected and aseptic surgical technique is observed, postoperative antibiotics are not indicated.

### 10.2.5.1 Postoperative Complications

#### 10.2.5.1.1 Swelling and Hemorrhage
Swelling and contusion are not uncommon at the surgical site postoperatively, but should resolve within 3–5 days. Owners should also be aware that hemorrhage at the nostril ipsilateral to the enucleation site may be observed in the first 3–5 days postoperatively. Patency of the nasolacrimal duct system between the orbit and nasal cavity, however, will be lost during the first week following surgery. A small amount of hemorrhage may also be observed along the suture line of the surgical site, but should also resolve within 3–7 days postoperatively.

Major hemorrhage is rare postoperatively, but owners should monitor for sudden and excessive swelling and/or bleeding at the surgical site. If bleeding persists despite compression of the site, the animal should be seen urgently, as surgical revision may be necessary.

#### 10.2.5.1.2 Infection

Infection is rare following enucleation, but may be observed following the removal of an infected globe, if surgical closure is incomplete, if a conjunctival remnant is left behind, or if intraoperative sterility was compromised. Postsurgical infections are most commonly observed within 7–10 days after surgery, and animals often present with swelling, pain, and/or warmth of the surgical site, purulent discharge at the surgical site, dehiscence of the surgical site, or systemic signs of illness (lethargy, fever, inappetence). Swabs of purulent discharge should be submitted for aerobic and anaerobic culture and sensitivity, and broad-spectrum antibiotic therapy should be instituted. If infection persists despite therapy, surgical revision will likely be necessary.

#### 10.2.5.1.3 Orbital Cysts/Mucoceles and Orbital Emphysema

Orbital cysts or mucoceles have been reported following enucleation surgery, most commonly following subconjunctival enucleation [10]. The cause is retention of secretory conjunctival or adnexal tissue (i.e. nictitating membrane) within the orbit. In most cases, the surgical site must be revised to remove the cyst and identify and excise any offending secretory tissue (Figure 10.2.6).

Emphysema of the surgical site (orbital pneumatosis) has been reported but is generally rare, most commonly observed in brachycephalic dog breeds [11–14]. The proposed mechanism is reflux of air through the nostrils and nasolacrimal ducts into the surgical site. It typically presents as nonpainful crepitus or "crackling" of the skin overlying the surgical site. In many cases, this resolves as the nasolacrimal ducts lose patency postoperatively; but in some dogs, surgical revision and ligation of the nasolacrimal duct must be pursued.

#### 10.2.5.1.4 Contralateral Blindness

Contralateral irreversible blindness is rarely encountered postoperatively, provided that excessive

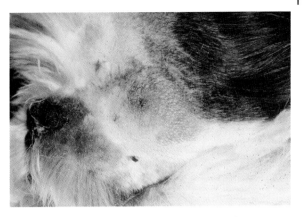

**Figure 10.2.6** A dog with a postoperative orbital cyst inferior to the healed incision line. The orbital cyst developed as a result of retained secretory conjunctival tissue following routine subconjunctival enucleation. Source: Courtesy of Paul Miller, DVM, DACVO.

traction was not placed on the globe and optic nerve intraoperatively [15, 16]. Excessive traction on the optic nerve risks physical trauma to the optic chiasm, thereby blinding the contralateral eye. This risk is particularly higher in cats where the distance between the optic nerve's entry into the globe and the chiasm is shorter.

#### 10.2.5.1.5 Wound Contracture and Skin Sinking

The most common complication of enucleation in dogs and cats is "sinkage" of the skin overlying the surgical site, occurring in weeks to months following enucleation. While not a true complication, this can be cosmetically unacceptable to some owners. A cosmetic silicone prosthesis can be placed in the orbit prior to surgical closure to minimize contracture. However, this is contraindicated following enucleation of a globe with proven or suspected infection or neoplasia, and not practical in field situations.

## 10.2.6 Special Considerations

### 10.2.6.1 Enucleation of Proptosed Globes

Traumatic proptosis of the globe is a common sequel to blunt head trauma in dogs and cats. In any animal, the prognosis for return of vision is guarded to poor following proptosis [17]. The prognosis for vision and globe viability is particularly poor in dolichocephalic dog breeds and cats due to the amount of trauma required to induce proptosis. Globe rupture, hyphema, and extensive rupture of extraocular muscles are also associated with poor prognosis for vision and viability. In globes with poor long-term prognosis for viability and vision, immediate enucleation may be indicated.

In dogs and cats with proptosis, transpalpebral enucleation is exceptionally difficult as retrobulbar soft tissue swelling and contusion complicate apposition of the eyelids and the subsequent tissue dissection required in the transpalpebral technique. Therefore, the subconjunctival technique may be easier. Swelling, hemorrhage, and distortion of ocular tissues, however, may also complicate the identification of conjunctival

tissue, increasing the risk for retained conjunctival remnants. Furthermore, the risk of contamination of the orbit using the subconjunctival technique may be higher following traumatic proptosis. Therefore, thorough irrigation of the orbit with sterile saline is recommended prior to closure, as well as postoperative antibiotics.

### 10.2.6.2 Enucleation in Kittens and Puppies

In the shelter setting, ocular disease is commonly encountered, particularly in kittens affected by herpetic keratoconjunctivitis and other concurrent or secondary ocular surface infections. In affected

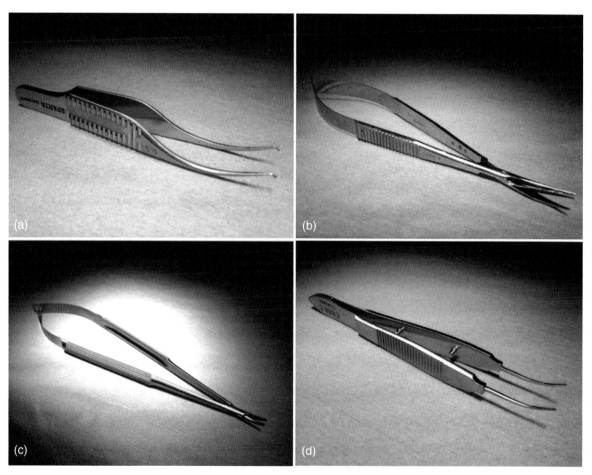

**Figure 10.2.7** Recommended ophthalmic microsurgical instruments for enucleation in puppies and kittens. (a) Colibri forceps have very fine toothed tips for handling delicate corneal and conjunctival tissues. (b) Wescott tenotomy scissors (blunt-tipped) are useful for dissection of small delicate conjunctival and orbital tissues in pediatric patients. (c) Barraquer needle holders are designed for handling of small gauge suture material (i.e. 6-0). (d) Harms tying forceps (curved blades) are essential for gentle handling and knot tying when using 6-0 suture.

kittens, severe ocular surface infections can lead to globe rupture and blinding endophthalmitis, necessitating enucleation. Tear-deficient ocular surface disease with blinding globe rupture is also commonly encountered in kittens and puppies with poor health status and particularly in brachycephalic breeds with inherently poor globe protection. Ideally, general anesthesia and enucleation will be delayed until kittens or puppies are at least 6 months of age. In cases with evidence of refractory ocular pain, however, urgent enucleation may be necessary. From a surgical standpoint, enucleation techniques in kittens and puppies are the same as those described for adults. However, precise enucleation of such small globes is best achieved using microsurgical instruments to handle and dissect delicate ocular tissues, as well as smaller suture material (5-0 to 6-0) and instruments accordingly suited to handling smaller needles (Figure 10.2.7).

### 10.2.6.3   Enucleation of Phthisical Globes

Feline post-traumatic ocular sarcoma (FPTOS) is a histologically aggressive ocular tumor, putatively originating from the lens epithelium [18]. The exact pathophysiology is unclear, but clinical scenarios that appear to precede development of this neoplasm include ocular trauma, lens surgery, and phthisis bulbi (the loss of globe volume associated with the loss of function) [19–21]. Fortunately, the average time between known ocular trauma and development of FPTOS is typically ~6 years. While phthisical globes are clinically non-painful, however, the author advocates that any feline phthisical eye should be enucleated as a preventive measure. Phthisis bulbi in dogs does not carry the same long-term risk as a canine correlate of FPTOS has not been reported.

## References

1  Murphy, C.J., Samuelson, D., and Pollock, R. (2013). The eye. In: Miller's Anatomy of the Dog, 746–785. Elsevier Saunders.

2  Giuliano, E.A. (2008). Regional anesthesia as an adjunct for eyelid surgery in dogs. *Topics in Companion Animal Medicine* 23 (1): 51–56.

3  Rubin, A. (1995). Complications of local anaesthesia for ophthalmic surgery. *British Journal of Anaesthesia* 75: 93–96.

4  Shilo-Benjamini, Y., Pascoe, P.J., Maggs, D.J. et al. (2014). Comparison of peribulbar and retrobulbar regional anesthesia with bupivacaine in cats. *American Journal of Veterinary Research* 75 (12): 1029–1039.

5  Accola, P.J., Bentley, E., Smith, L.J. et al. (2006). Development of a retrobulbar injection technique for ocular surgery and analgesia in dogs. *Journal of the American Veterinary Medical Association* 229 (2): 220–225.

6  Myrna, K.E., Bentley, E., and Smith, L.J. (2010). Effectiveness of injection of local anesthetic into the retrobulbar space for postoperative analgesia following eye enucleation in dogs. *Journal of the American Veterinary Medical Association* 237 (2): 174–177.

7  Shilo-Benjamini, Y., Pascoe, P.J., Maggs, D.J., and Kass, P.H. (2013). Retrobulbar and peribulbar regional techniques in cats: a preliminary study in cadavers. *Veterinary Anaesthesia and Analgesia* 40 (6): 623–631.

8  Gelatt, K. and Gelatt, J. (2001). Anesthesia for ophthalmic surgery. In: Small Animal Ophthalmic Surgery: Practical Techniques for the Veterinarian Oxford, 34–44. Butterworth & Heinemann.

9  Delgado, C., Bentley, E., Hetzel, S., and Smith, L. (2014). Carprofen provides better post-operative analgesia than tramadol in dogs after enucleation: a randomized, masked clinical trial. *Journal of the American Veterinary Medical Association* 245: 1375.

10  Ward, A.A. and Neaderland, M.H. (2011). Complications from residual adnexal structures following enucleation in three dogs. *Journal of the American Veterinary Medical Association* 239: 1580–1583.

11  Gornik, K.R., Pirie, C.G., and Alario, A.F. (2015). Orbital and subcutaneous emphysema following enucleation and respiratory distress in a Japanese Chin. *Journal of the American Animal Hospital Association* 51: 413–418.

12 Martin, C.L. (1971). A complication of ocular enucleation in the dog: orbital emphysema. *Veterinary Medicine, Small Animal Clinician* **66**: 986–989.

13 Bedford, P. (1979). Orbital pneumatosis as an unusual complication to enucleation. *Journal of Small Animal Practice* **20**: 551–555.

14 Barros, M., Matera, J., Alvarenga, J., and Iwasaki, M. (1984). Orbital pneumatosis in a dog. *Modern Veterinary Practice* **65** (1): 38.

15 Stiles, J., Buyukmihci, N., Hacker, D., and Canton, D. (1993). Blindness from damage to optic chiasm. *Journal of the American Veterinary Medical Association* **202** (8): 1192.

16 Cho, J. (2008). Surgery of the globe and orbit. *Topics in Companion Animal Medicine* **23** (1): 23–37.

17 Gilger, B., Hamilton, H., Wilkie, D. et al. (1995). Traumatic ocular proptoses in dogs and cats: 84 cases (1980–1993). *Journal of the American Veterinary Medical Association* **206** (8): 1186–1190.

18 Zeiss, C., Johnson, E., and Dubielzig, R. (2003). Feline intraocular tumors may arise from transformation of lens epithelium. *Veterinary Pathology Online* **40** (4): 355–362.

19 Perlmann, E., Rodarte-Almeida, A., Albuquerque, L. et al. (2011). Feline intraocular sarcoma associated with phthisis bulbi. *Arquivo Brasileiro de Medicina Veterinária e Zootecnia* **63** (3): 591–594.

20 Dubielzig, R., Everitt, J., Shadduck, J., and Albert, D. (1990). Clinical and morphologic features of post-traumatic ocular sarcomas in cats. *Veterinary Pathology* **27** (1): 62–65.

21 Naranjo, C., Southwick, J., Bentley, E. et al. (2011). Feline post-traumatic ocular sarcoma in ten cats with previous lens surgery. *Veterinary Ophthalmology* **14** (4): 279.

# 11

## Sanitation and Surgical Asepsis

*Brian A. DiGangi[1] and Ann Therese Kommedal[2]*

[1]*ASPCA, PO Box 142275, Gainesville, FL 32614, USA*
[2]*AniCura Dyresykehus Stavanger, AWAKE International Veterinary Outreach, Nedre Stokkavei 12, 4023 Stavanger, Norway*

## 11.1 Introduction

Infectious disease control is challenging in most hospital settings. Prevention of hospital-acquired disease is of major concern in human health and an area of great research focus [1]. When working in the veterinary profession hospital-acquired disease may be seen as an even greater challenge; our patients are prone to picking up pathogens from the environment as they sleep and eat on the floor, are transported in crates and carriers, are restrained by handlers and/or equipment, and groom themselves spreading whatever pathogens they are in contact with on their coat. In addition, when working in a field setting, many of the patients we serve are unvaccinated, arrive in poor health, may be malnourished, and are highly stressed. This increases the likelihood of our patients shedding harmful pathogens, with or without clinical signs of disease, and further increases the risk of hospital-acquired disease.

Given the high likelihood of pathogen shedding in this population and the multitude of opportunities for transmission during housing and handling, one might think that disease spread is inevitable in a field clinic. However, steps can be taken to ensure a comprehensive and practical sanitation plan that can reduce the overall risk. The goal of such a plan is to reduce the pathogen level to a dose that is low enough for the animal's immune system to overcome. Working in the field requires a plan to guard against infections spreading during trapping, transportation to and from the clinic, during hospitalization, and in the operating area. Aseptic technique, including the use of sterile surgical instruments and prevention of postoperative infections need to be addressed as part of this effort.

When designing a sanitation program, a few basic principles should be kept in mind. The program must:

- include sanitation methods that are appropriate for the particular setting
- include correct use and application of disinfecting agents
- consider availability of disinfection agents in different regions
- be safe for the staff and patients
- be in writing and easily accessible
- ensure adequate training for staff and volunteers

This chapter discusses commonly used disinfectants and what to consider when setting up a practical sanitation protocol for the clinic, animal handling, and surgical facility.

> It is the responsibility of all team members to provide the best possible care to every patient. An important part of that care includes providing a clean, healthy environment. Thorough cleaning limits the spread of disease and infection. There is no room for shortcuts during cleaning as this is one of the most crucial tasks to ensure the wellbeing of our patients.
>
> – HSVMA-RAVS Cleaning and Infection Control

---

**Textbox 11.1 Keeping the terms straight**

- *Sanitation*. Refers to the combination of both cleaning and disinfection.
- *Cleaning*. Includes the removal of visible contamination and dirt, including urine, fecal matter, and other organic material from the environment. Cleaning should result in visibly clean surfaces, but does not usually remove all harmful pathogens, and should be followed by disinfection.

- *Disinfection*. Results in killing of most of the contaminants in a given area.
- *Sterilization*. Refers to the destruction of all microbes, including spores, and is required for surgical instruments, surgical gloves, and other equipment necessary for sterile procedures.

---

## 11.2 Developing a Plan

Field stations and clinics are set up in various locations and facilities which can include surfaces that are more challenging to sanitize than in traditional clinic settings. Pathogens can survive for extended periods of time on different surfaces, and formation of biofilms results in adhesion and prolonged survival of pathogens on a surface. Biofilms form over time, and the longer the pathogens are allowed to remain on a surface, the more likely they are to attach. The concentration of disinfectants required to kill bacteria that adhere in biofilms may be 1000-fold higher than that required to kill freely moving bacteria of the same strain [2]. The timing of sanitation is therefore also an important consideration. Introduction of pathogens can come from a number of sources in a field setting; it is therefore imperative that the focus on sanitation protocols is not restricted to the clinic and operating areas only. The risk of a puppy contracting parvovirus is equally high in the transport crate, during handling and restraint, or in a housing unit or recovery area, as it is in an examination area or on a surgery table if adequate sanitation principles are not applied everywhere. Healthy animals should not acquire illness as a consequence of being in our care.

A practical and efficient plan is required to prevent disease and must be tailored to each particular situation. Such a plan should include all areas and equipment requiring sanitation, identification of when

sanitation protocols should be conducted, and steps for cleaning, disinfection, and drying of the items or areas of the facility. Additional considerations include the disinfectant product's spectrum of efficacy against pathogens of concern, its method of delivery, time until effect, and constraints against efficacy (e.g. many disinfectants have a reduced activity in the presence of organic matter).

## 11.3 Choosing a Disinfectant

The first step is to choose a method of disinfection. The most commonly applied methods in a clinic setting are physical and chemical disinfection.

### 11.3.1 Physical Disinfection

Physical disinfection includes the use of heat (dry or moist), drying, ultraviolet (UV) light, and other types of radiation. Heat can be applied in either dry (i.e. flame, baking) or wet form (i.e. steam). Many microbes are killed at temperatures over 158 °F (70 °C), although some of the pathogens of concern, including parvoviruses, require higher temperatures for inactivation [3]. Wet heat, most commonly used in the form of steam autoclaving, is one of the most convenient and effective means of sterilization of surgical equipment (see Section 11.5.2.2.2). A variety of environmental factors can impact the effectiveness of heat on microbial survival (Table 11.1).

Table 11.1 Impact of environmental factors on microbial heat resistance.

| Decrease microbial heat resistance | Increase microbial heat resistance |
| --- | --- |
| Increased humidity or water activity | Proteins and colloidal particles (act as protective agents) |
| pH above or below optimum growth of microbes | Large microbial populations or biofilms |

Desiccation can be an effective method of physical disinfection against some microbes, while others (e.g. feline calicivirus, parvoviruses, and dermatophytes) are able to persist for certain periods despite a dry environment. The pathogens resistant to desiccation are some of those of major concern in the veterinary field clinic; this method can therefore not be considered a reliable form of disinfection on its own.

Although UV light has several potential applications, its germicidal effectiveness and use is affected by the presence of organic matter, its wavelength, temperature, and intensity. The use of UV light as a type of physical disinfection in a clinical setting is thus limited.

### 11.3.2 Chemical Disinfection

Chemical agents are widely used for the destruction of microbes. These products have varying antimicrobial properties, and there are several factors that must be considered when choosing which one to use.

The ideal disinfectant:

- Can be used in different environmental conditions with varying surfaces, temperatures, humidity, and pH
- Maintains efficacy in the presence of organic matter
- Is compatible with other chemicals such as detergents
- Has a wide antimicrobial spectrum
- Has a high safety threshold
- Is inexpensive
- Is stable over time
- Is noncorrosive and nonstaining.

Unfortunately, the ideal disinfectant agent that fulfills all of these criteria has yet to be identified and most likely will never exist. Therefore, we are left to consider the ability of the products that are available to meet these criteria and choose those that best meet our needs (Table 11.2). The variation in the different products and clinic settings also means that no sanitation protocol will be safe if relying on a single product for all purposes.

After choosing the most appropriate disinfectant products for the intended use, it is important to ensure that they are used correctly. This includes mixing to the correct concentration for the intended spectrum of efficacy, using correct application methods, allowing sufficient contact and drying time, and rinsing when appropriate. In most field clinics, bleach is a widely available and cost–effective choice of disinfectant. See Appendix 11.A.

Tip from the Field

Some pool shock granules used for chlorinating pools have the same active ingredient, calcium hypochlorite, as commercially available disinfectants (e.g., Wysiwash®) and are often used as a more cost effective alternative:

- Before purchasing and mixing the solution, it is important to compare the active ingredients and their concentration. Not all pool shock granules are the same.
  - The product sheet for Wysiwash is available at www.wysiwash.com/pdf/wysiwash-msds.pdf
- In the following example, a product containing 78% calcium hypochlorite (i.e. POOLIFE TurboShock®) was used.
  - To make a disinfectant solution similar to commercially available products containing 60–80% calcium hypochlorite (e.g. Wysiwash), use 1/16 teaspoon powder per 1 gal (3.79 l) of water.
  - Measuring spoons for 1/16 teaspoons are readily available in most kitchen stores, but are often labeled a "pinch" rather than 1/16 teaspoon.
  - Invest in a plastic measuring spoon as the powder will likely corrode metal spoons.
- Although the contact time for calcium hypochlorite is 2 minutes at neutral pH, the use of more alkaline tap water warrants a contact time of 10 minutes.

### 11.3.3 Concentration

Many sanitation products come in concentrated form, which requires dilution at a specific concentration to ensure efficacy. Some disinfectants may even have differing spectrums of activity at different concentrations. Overdilution can result in loss of activity, while underdilution can result in harm to staff and patients. Assessing smell, color, or "eyeballing" it are not appropriate methods of preparing disinfectants. Written sanitation protocols must include clear instructions on correct product preparation. Outbreaks of infectious disease or disinfectant toxicity have been traced to something as simple as lost protocols or broken dispensers.

Table 11.2 Chemical disinfectants [3–7].

| Disinfectant product | Advantages | Disadvantages |
| --- | --- | --- |
| Accelerated hydrogen peroxide (i.e. Rescue, Accel, Oxivir) | • Good detergent activity<br>• Effective in the presence of organic material<br>• Short contact time (1–10 min depending on concentration)<br>• Efficacy against nonenveloped viruses and dermatophytes<br>• Liquid concentrate form<br>• Various application options<br>• 90-day shelf life once diluted | • Not readily available in all regions<br>• May be cost-prohibitive |
| Potassium peroxymonosulfate (i.e. Virkon®, Trifectant®) | • Completely inactivates nonenveloped viruses and dermatophytes<br>• Some detergent activity<br>• Relatively good activity in the presence of organic matter<br>• Short contact time (5–10 min depending on pathogen)<br>• Residual effect<br>• Available in tablet form convenient for travel | • Leaves visible residue on some surfaces<br>• Seven-day shelf life once diluted<br>• May be cost-prohibitive<br>• Not readily available in all regions |
| Sodium hypochlorite (Bleach) | • Completely inactivates nonenveloped viruses<br>• Effective against dermatophytes<br>• Usually inexpensive<br>• Stable for 30 days once diluted if stored correctly [4] | • Significantly inactivated by:<br>  ○ organic matter<br>  ○ exposure to light<br>  ○ extended storage<br>• *No* detergent activity<br>• Surfaces *must* be precleaned and all organic matter removed prior to disinfection<br>• Caustic at 1 : 10 dilution<br>• Respiratory irritant – animals should be removed from the environment and staff should wear PPE<br>• Corrosive to metal<br>• Stains clothing |
| Calcium hypochlorite (i.e. Wysiwash®, various pool disinfectants) | • Completely inactivates nonenveloped viruses<br>• Can be used in hose-end applicator system (specific to the different products) | • Primarily an algaecide<br>• Not reliably effective against dermatophytes<br>• Surfaces *must* be precleaned and all organic matter removed prior to disinfection<br>• Dry form is irritating to mucous membranes if inhaled |
| Sodium dichloroisocyanurate (i.e. BruClean TbC ™) | • Completely inactivates nonenveloped viruses<br>• Less corrosive to metals than bleach | • Dry form is irritating to mucous membranes if inhaled<br>• Requires multiple-step process for cleaning and disinfection via a specialized applicator |
| Quaternary ammonium compounds (i.e. Roccal®, Parvo-sol®, A33®, Maxxon®, many others) | • Some detergent activity<br>• Only moderate inactivation by organic matter (less than bleach)<br>• Low tissue toxicity when diluted correctly | • *Not* reliably effective against nonenveloped viruses or dermatophytes.<br>• Potential to be toxic causing lingual ulcers<br>• Tissue irritant at high concentration |

**Table 11.2** (*Continued*)

| Disinfectant product | Advantages | Disadvantages |
| --- | --- | --- |
| Chlorhexidine (i.e. Nolvasan®, Bactricide®) | • Very low tissue toxicity<br>• Detergent activity | • Not reliably effective against viruses or dermatophytes |
| Alcohol (i.e. ethanol, isopropyl alcohol) Most commonly used in hand sanitizers | • Less irritating to tissue than quaternary ammonium or bleach<br>• Moderately effective against calicivirus at higher concentration | • Not reliably effective against parvovirus or dermatophytes<br>• Ineffective if diluted below 50%<br>• Inactivated by organic soil<br>• Difficult to maintain sufficient contact time<br>• Hardens plastic over time |

### 11.3.4 Application

The method by which a disinfectant is applied is equally important as the product chosen. Whenever possible, use designated equipment for each area and avoid mops and buckets. When using a disinfectant that is inactivated by organic matter, the method of application is particularly crucial. For example, using a single mop in several areas and repeatedly dipping it in a bucket filled with bleach solution would set up a perfect situation for inadvertent pathogen spread. The mixture in the bucket will be increasingly contaminated by organic matter as the mop is rinsed, thus inactivating the bleach. Simultaneously, the mop will act as a vehicle to spread increasing numbers of microbes onto new surfaces. If mops and buckets are the only practical means of cleaning and disinfecting, one should choose a disinfectant with minimal inactivation by organic matter (e.g. Virkon®/Trifectant®). Contamination of the disinfectant should be minimized by rinsing the mop (or other rag) in a bucket of clean water between each application of disinfectant or, even better, use a new mop or rag for each new application of disinfectant.

The timing of application is also important as sanitation will be more effective when applied shortly after a surface has been in use. Leaving the cleaning and disinfection until just prior to the next use allows

---

**Textbox 11.2 Case study – A tale of disinfectant-induced outbreak**

A North American animal shelter was experiencing an outbreak of severe upper respiratory disease in their cats. Cats in different areas of the shelter were affected; they were of varying ages, all vaccinated, and included cats that had been in the shelter for a longer period as well as newer arrivals. Several of the cats had developed severe oral ulcerations and the ulcers were found on the planum of the nose, lips, tongues, and gums. In some of the more severely affected cats, the lesions seemed to spread into the esophagus, and a few had developed pneumonia.

Diagnostic testing did not provide a clear diagnosis. PCR testing identified a smattering of the more common upper respiratory pathogens, but there was no clear pattern in the distribution of pathogens that could help explain the outbreak and severity of the disease.

The shelter decided to call in outside help from a university shelter medicine program. A thorough examination of affected cats, necropsy of animals that succumbed to the disease, evaluation of the facility, and interviews with staff were performed.

Based on the findings, it was concluded that inappropriate cleaning practices were to blame for the suspect "outbreak." The shelter used a quaternary ammonium disinfectant, which was mixed and prepared in such a way that the concentration far exceeded the manufacturer's recommendation. As the disinfectant was used to clean cat housing areas and was left to dry on the surfaces, the cats were chronically exposed to the disinfectant, and would ingest disinfectant residues during grooming. This resulted in oral ulcerations, pain, and apparent upper respiratory disease. Affected cats were given supportive treatment, the disinfectant was replaced with a safer and more efficient product, and written protocols and training for staff were implemented. As a result, the disease outbreak quickly resolved and the surviving cats were rehomed.

any organic matter that has been transferred to the surface (through contact, sneezing, bleeding, etc.) time to dry and form biofilms.

For smaller cleaning jobs, the use of bottles with "squirt tops" rather than spray tops is ideal. These will decrease the amount of the disinfectant that is aerosolized into the environment, which can be detrimental to the respiratory health of both patients and staff. For larger areas, it is often practical to use hand-held or back-pack-style pesticide dispensers or hose-end foamers. Pesticide dispensers come in a variety of sizes and are usually convenient to transport. Some disinfectants, such as calcium hypochlorite (e.g. Wysiwash) and sodium dichloroisocyanurate (e.g. BruClean TbC), may come with specially designed dispensing equipment. These may not be as convenient for travel.

Disinfectants should be stored in the original container before dilution and as directed by the manufacturer after dilution. All disinfectants lose their efficacy over time, especially after dilution, and may also be affected by light, storage temperature, and storage method. Containers should be labeled with the name of the disinfectant, the date it was prepared, and the initials of the person preparing it; diluted disinfectant solutions should not be stored or used past their expiration date. For example, bleach that is stored in an opaque container retains its efficacy for 1 month, but will be inactivated much sooner and should be mixed freshly daily if kept in transparent containers in sunny conditions [4]. Finally, information on health, safety, and environmental hazards of any disinfectants in use should be readily available to all staff and volunteers. Material Safety Data Sheets (MSDS) for these products are easily accessible through a variety of online sources.

Having designated cleaning equipment and containers for different areas in the clinic is a simple method to reduce the risk of disease spread through sanitation. Keep designated cleaning equipment on each transport vehicle or at the drop-off point, in the receiving area, surgery area, and recovery area. This will help reduce the traffic and fomite spread of germs between the areas and facilitate early cleaning and disinfection between each animal. Squirt bottles, buckets, and other equipment should be labeled by area.

### 11.3.5 Contact Time

Contact time refers to the time a disinfectant is in contact with the application surface before it evaporates. This is generally not a problem when objects are immersed in the disinfectant, but can be more challenging when applying it to larger surfaces such as exam tables, crates, and floors as some disinfectants tend to dry quickly. If the disinfectant solution evaporates in less time than the recommended contact time, a greater volume of solution should be applied. Contact time to ensure efficacy varies by product, concentration, and desired spectrum of efficacy and may range from seconds to 10 or more minutes. Environmental temperature or level of organic contamination can increase the contact time required. Maintaining a 10-min minimum contact time is a recommended rule of thumb whenever practical [7].

### 11.3.6 Drying

Most pathogens prefer a humid environment for survival and growth, and some can persist over long periods on moist surfaces; therefore, allowing a surface to dry properly is an important and often underestimated step in the sanitation protocol. There will always be some microbes in the clinic environment that evade and survive our cleaning and chemical disinfection. These may succumb to desiccation over time helping to lower the exposure dose to a manageable level for our patients to overcome. Allowing laundry, crates, food and water bowls, litter boxes, and other equipment to dry in direct sunlight after being cleaned and disinfected, and before being used again, can be a simple and effective sanitation step in many field clinics.

## 11.4 Sanitation Consideration and Protocols

When we consider what needs to be cleaned and disinfected in a field clinic, staff tend to focus on cleaning cat cages, dog kennels, and surgical areas. While these are crucial items to include, a sanitation protocol requires close consideration of where and how pathogens are spread. Pathogens are often transported by human and animal traffic throughout facilities. They may be spread by any fomite or mechanical vector, including hands, doorknobs, clothing, exam tables, transport vehicles, bedding, litter trays, food bowls, equipment used for cleaning, and so on.

---

**Textbox 11.3 What needs to be cleaned?**

*Facilities*
- Office areas
  - Furniture
  - Computer keyboards
  - Doorknobs
- Receiving and examination area
  - Countertops/examination surfaces
  - Animal handling and restraint equipment
  - Any tools used to examine the animals
- Housing areas
  - Cages and crates
  - Bedding
  - Litter pans
  - Dishes

- Operating area
  - Operating tables
  - Surgery tools
  - Lamp handles
  - Floors
- Recovery area
- Walkways

*Transportation*
- Vehicles
- Crates and carriers
- Trapping equipment

*Staff and Volunteers*
- Clothing
- Hands
- Shoes

*Note: This is not a comprehensive list.*

---

Creating a sanitation protocol may seem like an immense task; however, some surfaces are more likely to serve as sources of pathogens compared to others. For example, a properly sanitized kennel or cage at a field clinic will only contain the pathogens belonging to the animal housed there at the time; therefore, the focus should be on sanitizing these surfaces between each animal, usually once per day. On the other hand, transport crates, staff hands and clothing, examination surfaces, or operating areas may come in contact with many animals every day and thus will require more frequent sanitation.

**Textbox 11.4 Prioritized surfaces for disinfection**

Extra care should be taken when considering cleaning and disinfection of the following areas:

- High-contact surfaces, such as hands, clothing, and countertops
- Surfaces that will be in contact with juvenile animals or those with unknown vaccination status, including trapping equipment, transport vehicles, and carriers
- Surfaces that have had contact with an ill animal, before allowing contact with a well animal, including floors, cages, countertops, and clothing and hands of those who have handled the animal.

### 11.4.1 Facilities

After removing animals from the clinic, the following sanitation steps should be applied:

1) Remove visible dirt – pick up feces, rinse off and remove urine with a squeegee, remove dry contamination (e.g. hair, grass, dirt) by sweeping, using a microfiber rag or dry mop.
2) Clean with a detergent – use a squirt bottle and rags or paper towels for smaller areas such as table surfaces, cages, and crates and a pesticide dispenser and squeegee for larger areas. The surface should appear clean before the disinfectant is applied.
3) Apply disinfectant – squirt bottles are practical for smaller areas and pesticide dispensers for larger areas. Make sure to cover all surfaces evenly and allow adequate contact time before drying.
4) Allow to dry completely before the next use – squeegee, air dry, place items in direct sunlight, use of clean rags or paper towels for smaller areas, or a combination of these as appropriate.

Receiving and examination areas have high staff and animal traffic throughout the day, making them likely areas for disease transmission. Examination surfaces should be cleaned immediately after use, between every animal, or between animals that do not cohabit together outside of the clinic. Floors should be cleaned whenever visibly soiled, when there is suspicion of contamination by an infected animal, and at the end of each shift.

---

**Textbox 11.5 Paper towels or rags**

In areas with a large tourism industry, it may be an option for shelters or animal welfare organizations to approach hotels for donations of sheets and towels that can no longer be used. These can then be cut up and used as "paper towels" to clean tables and other surfaces. Paper towels can be costly in some areas, and this can be an economical and practical option. Once used, the rags can then either be laundered or discarded.

---

#### 11.4.1.1 Operating Room

The surface of the operating table should be cleaned and disinfected between each animal, and/or clean or new table covers should be used for each animal. All surfaces that are visibly soiled with blood, feces, urine, or other contaminants need to be cleaned and disinfected as soon as possible. Floors, doorknobs, lamp handles, and other surfaces should be cleaned and disinfected at the end of every shift even if not visibly soiled. Donning of shoe covers when entering the operating area may help reduce contamination from foot traffic.

#### 11.4.1.2 Transportation Vehicles (Animal Compartments)

The animal compartments used in the transportation vehicles need to be cleaned and disinfected after each use. This should be done immediately after dropping the animal off at the clinic location and after returning patients following treatment and recovery. Sanitation equipment and products can be kept in the car (preferred) or at the drop-off point at the clinic site, to facilitate easy and efficient decontamination. Chemical containers should be clearly labeled to help separate detergents and disinfectants, and rags, paper towels or squeegees should be easily accessible. Numbering the containers so that volunteers know in

which order to use them can also be helpful. Do not reuse applicators; enough supplies should be on hand in the vehicle to ensure that fresh paper towels or clean rags are used for each housing area.

#### 11.4.1.3 Crates, Cages and Other Animal Housing Compartments

General clinic areas, including offices, break rooms and hallway floors, should be cleaned whenever visibly soiled and at the end of every day/shift. Short-term animal housing units should be cleaned immediately after use, between every animal, or between animals that do not cohabit together outside of the clinic. Smaller crates and carriers can be cleaned using the triple-basin technique. See Figure 11.1.

For long-term housing units (i.e. greater than 24 h), animals should be kept in the same enclosure throughout their stay to reduce stress and require less frequent disinfection. Daily cleaning of the enclosure is still necessary to maintain sanitary conditions. Using a "spot-cleaning method" for these cages and kennels will help reduce stress, minimize animal handling, and maintain familiar scents. During spot cleaning, animals should remain in their cage while it is being tidied and soiled materials are removed (see Appendix 11.B). The cage is thoroughly cleaned and disinfected once the animal leaves and before a new animal enters.

### 11.4.2 Staff, Tools and Equipment

All equipment coming in contact with animals should be disinfected or discarded between use with an animal or between animals that do not cohabit together outside the clinic. This includes food and water bowls, litter trays, carriers, humane traps, cleaning supplies, muzzles, gloves, bedding, medical and anesthetic equipment. Items that cannot be readily disinfected represent a risk to animals and therefore should not be used or discarded after use,

| Step 1 | Step 2 | Step 3 | Step 4 | Step 5 |
|---|---|---|---|---|
| Collect soiled items | Clean | Rinse | Disinfect | Dry |
| Remove visible dirt | Tub 1: Detergent (e.g. Dawn® dishwashing solution) | Tub 2: Warm, clean water | Tub 3: Disinfectant (e.g. 1:32 bleach solution) | Place in sunlight until items are dry |

Figure 11.1 The triple-basin technique for sanitizing.

especially if used with animals with clinical signs of infectious disease.

### 11.4.2.1 Staff and Volunteers

Untrained staff and volunteers can rapidly spread disease at a clinic or shelter. To help mitigate the risk, adequate hand sanitation should be trained and practiced. All staff and volunteers should be required to wash their hands or use a hand sanitizer before and after handling animals and fomites or use disposable gloves.

Providing hand sanitizer dispensers and disposable gloves in all areas where there are animals facilitates compliance with hand hygiene. Hand sanitizers have limited efficacy against pathogens encountered in a field setting, such as parvovirus and calicivirus, and therefore cannot be relied on as the sole means of hand sanitation. Hand washing and use of disposable gloves should be encouraged whenever there is suspicion of such pathogens. All staff and volunteers should be trained in an appropriate way to perform hand washing and use of hand sanitizers.

---

**Textbox 11.6 Proper hand hygiene techniques**

*Hand washing*
1) Wet hands with warm running water.
2) Lather with soap.
3) Scrub all surfaces for a minimum of 20 s.
4) Rinse with clean water.
5) Thoroughly dry hands. Use two single-use paper towels for 10 s each – if cloth towels are used, a fresh one must be used for each hand washing episode.

*Use of hand sanitizers*
1) Clean hands prior to use: Hand sanitizers have reduced efficacy when hands are visibly soiled or greasy.
2) Use hand sanitizers that contain 60–80% ethanol or isopropyl alcohol.
3) Apply liberally to all hand surfaces; apply enough sanitizer to ensure adequate contact time prior to drying.
4) Rub hands together for a minimum of 30 s
5) Allow to air dry.

---

Staff clothing can effectively carry pathogens even when they appear clean. Clothing should be cleaned and laundered whenever visibly soiled, at the end of every shift, and after handling an animal with a diagnosed or suspected infectious disease. Using personal protective equipment such as gowns, gloves, and shoe covers should be considered, especially when handling high-risk animals, and during cleaning, to reduce fomite spread. Using protective garments when handling especially vulnerable animals such as puppies and kittens and in the operating area is also recommended.

---

**Textbox 11.7 Key points on staff hygiene**

- Provide clearly labeled hand sanitizers in all animal areas, position them within 3 ft of animal exam stations.
- Keep in mind that there are no hand sanitizers that are effective against the most durable pathogens, such as parvoviruses or ringworm. When these pathogens are suspected, gloves and hand washing are a must.
- Consider using paper or plastic aprons that can be changed, especially when handling animals suspected to carry or exhibiting clinical signs of disease such as parvovirus or ringworm.

---

### 11.4.2.2 Foot Baths

Working in an animal clinic or kennel requires walking in and out of kennels and through areas where patients sit or lie on the floor, making feet potential vectors for pathogens. The risk of spreading disease via footwear is drastically reduced if an effective basic environmental sanitation program is in place. Additional efforts such as use of shoe covers or dedicated footwear for isolation areas will further reduce the risk.

Foot baths are commonly used as a more convenient option than using separate shoes or shoe covers. A foot bath enables all staff and volunteers to enter a given area following use of the foot bath. The major disadvantage, however, is that foot baths tend to be ineffective and may give staff a false sense of security. Foot baths are generally ineffective due to the following factors:

- All disinfectants require a minimum contact time for optimal effect that will generally not be achieved when using foot baths.

- Most foot baths are too shallow to allow for full submersion of the shoe and do not allow for the removal of organic matter, compromising the disinfectant's efficacy.
- Even when correctly used foot baths have not been shown to lead to a significant reduction in bacterial contamination of floor surfaces beyond the foot bath [8].
- Incorrectly used foot baths can increase the contamination of footwear [9].

If footbaths are to be used, it is important to ensure they are used correctly. Tips for using foot baths effectively include the following:

- Use a disinfectant that has good activity in the presence of organic matter, such as Virkon/Trifectant® or Accel®.
- Bleach is *not* an acceptable disinfectant for use in foot baths.
- Before using a foot bath, a brush should be used to remove organic matter from the bottom of the shoes.
- Make sure the foot bath is deep enough to allow complete immersion of the treads of the shoes.
- Make sure the foot bath is cleaned and changed daily and whenever it is visibly contaminated.

Following these guidelines is impractical in most field clinics, therefore, the regular use of foot baths is not recommended. Whenever infectious disease is suspected and disease transmission is a concern, the use of dedicated shoes or shoe covers is a more effective measure than foot baths. Keep shoe covers or dedicated rubber boots in a variety of sizes directly outside of the isolation rooms to facilitate ease of use.

### 11.4.2.3 Bowls and Litter Trays

Food and water bowls should be cleaned and disinfected between every animal. Commercial dishwashers are the gold standard for cleaning food and water bowls as the mechanical washing action and high temperatures destroy a majority of pathogens, although they may not destroy nonenveloped viruses such as parvoviruses. However, it is not likely that there will be access to such equipment while operating in the field, and there may not be ready access to sinks for this purpose either.

The "triple-basin technique" can be used for equipment with relatively nonporous surfaces such as food and water bowls, litter trays, carriers and crates, trapping equipment that are mobile and of size that allows immersion (Figure 11.1). With this method, large plastic tubs (basins) can be used instead of sinks, either by purchasing such tubs at the destination or utilizing transportation tubs brought to carry equipment and medication. The steps include the following:

1) Remove any visible dirt.
2) Basin 1 – Soak and clean in detergent solution.
3) Basin 2 – Rinse in clean water (preferably warm water when available).
4) Basin 3 – Soak in disinfectant solution.
5) Dry (in direct sunlight if possible).

The solutions in the basins should be changed whenever visibly soiled. Ideally, food and water receptacles should be cleaned in an area separate from litter boxes or other items contaminated by feces. When this is not feasible, the litter trays and dishes must not be cleaned at the same time in the same sink/tub. Leave the litter trays until the end and make sure to thoroughly clean and disinfect the tubs between uses.

### 11.4.2.4 Laundry

All clothing and bedding used at the clinic must be laundered and thoroughly dried between uses. Organic debris such as feces and hair should be removed from articles before laundering, and any articles that are heavily soiled should be laundered separately or discarded. Although it is not possible to sterilize clothing and bedding, in the vast majority of instances washing such articles in either a regular or commercial washing machine with hot water and bleach, and allowing them to dry, will be sufficient to prevent disease spread. Bleach (half a cup for an average household washer) or accelerated hydrogen peroxide (1 oz. per gallon of washer capacity, no additional detergent product is needed) is commonly used to launder clothes and bedding. If a dryer is not available, laundry should be hung in exposure to direct to sunlight until dry.

---

**Textbox 11.8 Laundry tips**

- Do not overload washer and dryer.
- Clothing and hands are easily contaminated when handling dirty laundry. Therefore, protective gear should be used while handling dirty laundry, or staff should change clothes and wash hands after handling dirty laundry and before handling animals or freshly laundered articles to prevent transmission of germs.

### 11.4.3 Medical and Surgical Supplies

Countless pieces of equipment and supplies come into contact with veterinary patients throughout their field clinic experience. Each of these items has the potential to harbor pathogens and transmit disease if not properly sanitized between patients. In fact, biological contamination and transmission of both bacteria and viruses have been demonstrated through needles, syringes, intravenous (IV) tubing lines, and laryngoscope blades and handles that have not been thoroughly disinfected between uses [10–15]. When contaminated items enter into the clean operating environment, they jeopardize the surgeon's ability to maintain surgical asepsis.

Recommended practices in the human health-care industry call for complete sterilization of items that come into contact with the vascular system or sterile body tissue (e.g. IV catheters, IV tubing), disinfection of items that contact mucous membranes (e.g. laryngoscope blades, masks), and thorough cleaning of items that contact intact skin (e.g. electrocardiogram leads, blood pressure cuffs) in between each use. Items such as endotracheal tubes, some breathing circuits, filters, needles, and syringes are considered single-use items to be discarded after use [16]. Many of these single-use items are commonly reused in veterinary medicine; in these cases, following the recommendations for sterilization and disinfection based on the level of patient contact described above seems prudent. Maintaining a large stock supply of these items for sanitizing once at the end of each day, utilizing disposable covers or single-use towels to protect equipment surfaces, or limiting shared use of items to groups of patients that are normally exposed to one another (e.g. animals residing in the same household or shelter housing unit) may help promote good sanitary practices without negatively impacting clinic efficiency.

## 11.5 Asepsis

### 11.5.1 Is Asepsis Really a Requirement for Field Clinic Surgery?

The goals of aseptic technique are to prevent cross contamination during surgery and to minimize the amount of microorganisms in the surgical environment, thereby preventing their entrance into the surgical wound and the associated morbidity. Maintaining asepsis is considered the standard of care for common veterinary surgical procedures and has a direct impact on patient outcome [16–18]. In most field clinic settings, there is a general lack of access to veterinary care and the logistical difficulty in providing patient follow-up (indeed these are likely the reasons the field clinic exists), making strict adherence to aseptic technique and best surgical practices even more critical.

In the human medical field, surgical site infections (SSIs) occur in 3% of all surgical procedures, make up 14–22% of all health-care-associated infections [19], and result in an estimated 9000 to 20 000 deaths each year [20, 21]. While two-thirds of human SSIs are limited to incisional infections, the majority of SSI-related deaths were attributed to infections of the internal organs or spaces [22].

Comparable data for veterinary medicine is not available; however, SSIs are the most common type of nosocomial infection reported in small animals, involving up to 24.5% of all surgical procedures [23, 24]. In one study of adult dogs undergoing elective ovariohysterectomy at a veterinary teaching hospital, SSIs made up 41.4% of all complications [25]. Other veterinary studies have indicated SSI rates of 4.5–8.5% for clean-contaminated surgical wounds in dogs and cats [24, 26–28]. One university-based spay/neuter program reported an overall complication rate of 3% [29] (Table 11.3).

### 11.5.2 Minimum Requirements for Aseptic Surgery

Broad guidelines for surgical care that are attainable in most spay/neuter programs have been established [17] and the authors have found these to be attainable in a variety of field clinic settings around the world. In most cases, these represent the minimum requirements necessary to maintain asepsis; however, veterinary surgeons should strive to practice above these requirements whenever possible to decrease the chances of wound contamination and surgical complications (Table 11.4). Programs operating below this threshold of care place their professional reputations, that of similar organizations, and most importantly, the welfare of their patients at unnecessary risk. Should these requirements be impossible to attain, reanalysis of the program mission and resource allocation is warranted.

**Table 11.3** Reported rates of surgical site infections (SSIs) in dogs and cats [24–28].

| Reference | Species | Procedure type | SSI rate (%) |
| --- | --- | --- | --- |
| Vasseur et al. [24] | Dogs and cats | Clean | 2.5 |
| | | Clean-contaminated | 4.5 |
| | | Contaminated | 5.8 |
| | | Dirty | 18.1 |
| Brown et al. [28] | Dogs and cats | Clean | 4.7 |
| | | Clean-contaminated | 5.0 |
| | | Contaminated | 12.0 |
| | | Dirty | 10.1 |
| Nicholson et al. [27] | Dogs and cats | Clean-contaminated | 5.9 |
| Eugster et al. [26] | Dogs and cats | Clean | 6.9 |
| | | Clean-contaminated | 8.0 |
| | | Contaminated | 13.7 |
| | | Dirty | 24.5 |
| Burrow et al. [25] | Dogs | Clean-contaminated | 8.5 |

#### 11.5.2.1 Operating Environment

The minimum requirements for a functional operating environment include areas designated for animal housing, anesthesia and patient preparation, a surgeon scrub sink, an operating room, and a patient recovery area. Additional areas that may enhance efficiency and promote infection control include dressing rooms, supply rooms, an instrument pack preparation room, and a designated area for donning sterile gowns and gloves. Closed doors between clean operating environments and contaminated areas of the facility will aid in infection control and the promotion of aseptic technique [30].

When designing any surgical facility, careful attention should be paid to traffic flow patterns to ensure maximum efficiency and minimize opportunities for disease transmission. One study of SSI risk in dogs and cats demonstrated a 1.3 times greater risk of SSIs for each additional person that was in the operating room [26]. To minimize this risk, only essential personnel should be allowed into the operating area and conversation kept to a minimum [31]. Overall traffic flow through the surgical clinic should be thought of as unidirectional, and, to promote compliance, the environment should be laid out such that the desired flow pattern is the most direct path for personnel and animals to follow (Figure 11.2).

Although a designated, separate working unit isolated from general facility traffic is the ideal arrangement for an operating room environment [30], many field clinics operate under conditions in which this is not possible. In such situations, priority should be given to each of the following points in order to promote asepsis and minimize the chances of cross contamination and the occurrence of SSIs [22, 30].

1) Select an area of sufficient size for necessary personnel and equipment.
2) Create physical and/or visual barriers to control and minimize traffic flow (Figure 11.3).
3) Establish a clean, uncluttered environment (e.g. remove wall posters, discard perishable items, cover ceiling fans; place a clean tarp over surfaces that cannot be removed or cleaned prior to use).
4) Select an area with constant humidity and temperature and good air flow.
5) Utilize equipment and surfaces that are amenable to cleaning and disinfection (e.g. smooth, nonporous) or cover surfaces with clean, disposable drape material.

**Table 11.4** Spectrum of aseptic practices for field clinic surgery.

| Description | Ideal | Recommended | Minimum |
|---|---|---|---|
| Operating room | Separate working unit isolated from general facility traffic | Single-purpose unit within main facility | Designated area within multipurpose room; identified with physical and visual barriers |
| *Equipment and supplies* | | | |
| Surgical instruments | Separately wrapped instrument packs for each procedure; steam, gas, or plasma sterilization utilized | Large pack of instruments for multiple surgeries; individual instruments used on a single patient; steam, gas, or plasma sterilization utilized | Liquid chemical sterilization; individual instruments used on a single patient and reprocessed |
| Suture materials | Individually packaged suture for each patient | Reeled suture, sterilely acquired for each patient | Individually packaged or reeled suture; sterile, unused portions shared between patients |
| *Surgical personnel* | | | |
| Surgical attire | Dedicated surgical attire worn by all personnel; attire not worn outside operating room; attire changed/laundered daily<br>Caps and masks worn at all times within operating room<br>Single-use, sterile, surgical gowns and gloves worn by surgeons for all operating room procedures | Surgical attire worn throughout the day; jacket/lab coat worn outside of operating room<br>Caps and masks worn while procedures are in progress<br>Single-use, sterile surgical gowns worn for all abdominal procedures; single-use, sterile gloves worn for all procedures | Surgical attire worn throughout the day<br>Caps and masks worn for all procedures except for castration of cats and pediatric puppies<br>Sterile gowns not utilized but aseptic technique is maintained; single-use sterile gloves worn for all procedures except cat castrations when single-use examination gloves are worn |
| Surgeon prep | Surgical scrub performed prior to each procedure and prior to entering operating room | Surgical scrub performed prior to a series of procedures; sterility is maintained between procedures; new single-use sterile gloves are donned prior to each procedure | Surgical scrub performed prior to individual or a series of procedures except for castration of cats and pediatric puppies |
| *Patient preparation* | | | |
| Skin scrub | Hair removal and operative site prepared after anesthetic induction and prior to entering the operating room | Hair removal and operative site prepared after anesthetic induction in designated area of operating room | Hair removal and operative site prepared within operating room |
| Draping | Complete sterile draping performed for all operating room procedures | Complete sterile draping performed for all abdominal procedures and castration of adult dogs; clean barrier draping performed for castration of cats and pediatric puppies | Complete sterile draping performed for all abdominal procedures |

### 11.5.2.2 Surgical Instruments

Aseptic surgery cannot be achieved unless each surgical instrument that contacts body tissues or blood is sterile at the time of use [17, 32]. There are three distinct components to the proper preparation of instruments for use in surgical procedures that warrant discussion: cleaning and decontamination, packaging, and sterilization.

#### 11.5.2.2.1 *Cleaning and Decontamination*

Removal of organic contamination (e.g. blood and mucous) through cleaning and decontamination of

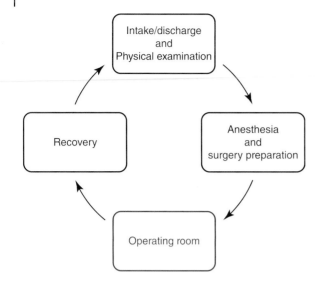

**Figure 11.2** Traffic flow through the surgical clinic should be unidirectional to minimize opportunities for contamination of the operating room. Sterile areas are indicated by red lines.

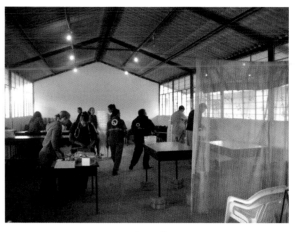

**Figure 11.3** During setup of this field clinic, a curtain has been placed as a highly visible, physical barrier separating the patient receiving area from the operating environment.

reusable surgical instruments must be undertaken prior to sterilization [16]. Organic contamination of items may inactivate or prevent penetration of chemical germicides as well as increase the bioburden of the equipment such that sterilization is not possible [33]. If allowed to dry on surgical instruments, blood, body fluids, and saline can result in corrosion, rusting, and pitting, which can also impede the sterilization process [34]. Cleaning with a detergent and water is likely the most effective as well as cost–efficient means of removing organic material [35, 36]. A pH neutral, low-foaming, free-rinsing detergent should be safe for most surgical equipment [34]. If not removed for decontamination and repackaging immediately after use, surgical instruments can be immersed in a detergent-warm water solution (80 °F–110 °F) until processing [34, 37]. Textbox11.9 describes a recommended step-by-step process for manual cleaning and decontamination of surgical instruments.

### 11.5.2.2.2 *Packaging and Sterilization*

After appropriate cleaning, decontamination and drying, surgical instruments must be packaged for processing. The choice of packaging system will depend on the type of item being sterilized and the method of sterilization being utilized [38]. For most

stainless steel surgical instruments utilized in field surgery programs, woven cotton muslin (minimum thread count 140), nonwoven SMS (spunlace–meltblown–spunbonded) materials, woven cotton/polyester-blend fabrics, or paper-plastic peel packages will be sufficient [39]. When reusable woven textiles are used, it is important they be laundered between each use, even if no visible contamination is present. In addition to its cleaning effects, laundering serves to rehydrate the material and prevent superheating during the sterilization process, which can inhibit sterilization [38]. Although probably

---

**Textbox 11.9 Manual cleaning and decontamination of surgical instruments**

- Wipe off visible organic material with a clean, moist sponge, or rag.
- Flush instrument lumens with water [34].
- Immerse in a solution of warm water (80 °F–110 °F/27 °C–43 °C) and detergent.
- Scrub instruments with purpose-designed instrument cleaning brush *(Do not use scouring pads or abrasive cleaning agents)* [37].
- Thoroughly rinse instruments with tap water to remove detergent residue and organic material.
- Rinse instruments with distilled/deionized water to prevent staining.
- Place instruments in the unlocked or open position on an absorbent, lint-free towel to dry.

unnecessary when nonwoven materials are utilized, double-wrapping surgical packs will help prevent bacterial contamination and extend shelf life of the sterilized pack [38, 39].

In the field clinic setting, sterilization of surgical instruments is most commonly accomplished through the use of liquid chemicals (i.e. "cold sterile"), dry heat, or steam. In locations or conditions where proper instrument sterilization is not feasible, consideration should be given to collaboration with human (or veterinary) hospitals and clinics that may have the necessary equipment readily available.

**Liquid Chemical Sterilization ("Cold Sterile")**  Liquid chemical sterilization is a common technique utilized in veterinary practices and field clinic settings. The active ingredients in commercially available liquid chemical sterilants include glutaraldehyde, peroxyacetic acid, hydrogen peroxide, ortho-phthalaldehyde, and phenol/phenate. It is possible to achieve sterilization with these chemicals; however, specific conditions must be met with each use [32, 33]:

1) Items to be sterilized must be clean and dry prior to immersion.
2) Complex instruments must be disassembled prior to immersion.
3) Proper immersion times must be observed; sterilization can be achieved in 6 to 12 h depending on formulation.
4) Instruments must be rinsed with sterile water and dried with sterile towels prior to use.
5) Sterilant must be changed after one "cycle" of use; reuse will result in contamination, chemical degradation, and loss of potency.

Direct immersion of surgical instruments in other solutions (e.g. alcohol, chlorhexidine, boiling water) is not an appropriate method of liquid chemical sterilization and will not result in sterilization of surgical equipment.

These requirements, along with the fact that many of the liquid chemical sterilants are known to result in significant toxicities to humans and/or animals [33, 40–43], render liquid chemical sterilization impractical in most settings and its use is generally not recommended.

**Dry Heat Sterilization**  Dry heat sterilization can be achieved through the use of dry heat sterilizers (also known as hot air ovens or hot air sterilizers). Their portability and low cost (<$100 USD depending on the model and size) may make these devices seem attractive for field clinic use. Although dry heat has good penetration and will not corrode delicate or sharp metal instruments, their use is only recommended for materials that are damaged by or impenetrable to moist heat [44]. Due to their small size, dry heat sterilizers are generally extremely limited in the number of instruments that can be sterilized in one cycle and, since they rely on the use of dry heat rather than steam, require prolonged run cycles (170 °C (340 °F) for 60 min, 160 °C (320 °F) for 120 min, and 150 °C (300 °F) for 150 min) [44]. In addition, dry heat sterilizers do not result in even distribution of heat; therefore, effective sterilization of all contents is not reliable [45].

**Steam Sterilization**  *Pressure Cookers*  Some practitioners rely on pressure cookers to sterilize surgical instruments [46] in field clinic settings. The ability of a pressure cooker to inactivate bacterial spores has been established [47], although they generally have lower pressure thresholds resulting in longer run cycles in order to achieve sterilization. In order to ensure effectiveness and operator safety, the same procedures for preparing and packaging instruments as discussed above must also be followed, instruments must not contact the water in the bottom of the cooker, and time and pressure measurements should not begin until the entire cooking chamber has filled with steam (i.e. steam rushes out of the open air vent, which is subsequently closed to start the sterilization process) [47, 48]. The number of instruments and surgical packs that can be sterilized in a pressure cooker at once may render this method impractical for some field clinics depending on the number of surgeries and available packs.

*Autoclaves*  Gravity displacement steam sterilization (e.g. use of an autoclave) is the most common method of surgical instrument preparation. In settings where there is no electricity, inexpensive ($300–600 USD) stove-top sterilizers requiring only a source of heat can be utilized; similar to pressure cookers, these generally have extremely limited load capacities. The ability of any steam sterilizer to achieve sterilization is dependent upon its ability to move air through the unit and its contents; proper packaging and loose

Table 11.5 Commonly reported minimum sterilization cycle parameters for surgical equipment in gravity displacement steam sterilizers [32, 44, 50, 51].

| Item | Temperature (°F) | Time (min) | Pressure (psi)[a] |
|---|---|---|---|
| Instruments | 250 | 15–30 | 15–17 |
| | 270 | 12–15 | 27–30 |
| | 275 | 12–25 | 27–30 |
| Textiles | 250 | 30 | 27–30 |
| | 270 | 12–25 | 27–30 |
| | 275 | 12–25 | 27–30 |
| Flash sterilization[b] | 270–275 | 3–10 | 27–29.4 |

a   For every 1000 ft of altitude, an additional 0.5 psi above 15 psi (normal atmospheric pressure at sea level) is needed.
b   Item should be unwrapped and placed in a perforated metal tray.

loading of the unit are essential to achieve this goal [32, 49]. Mechanical settings (i.e. time, temperature, and pressure) of the sterilizer must be carefully monitored to ensure sterilization is achieved. The precise settings required for sterilization will vary based on the piece of equipment to be sterilized and the sterilizer itself; however, commonly desired minimum parameters are reported in Table 11.5. After the sterilization cycle is complete, materials should be allowed to dry and cool thoroughly before removal from the sterilizer. When handled prematurely, stacked on top of one another, or placed on a cool surface, residual steam vapor can cause moisture to penetrate the packaging, resulting in loss of sterilization [32].

Additional best practices in sterilization include the use of both chemical (e.g. tape or paper sterilization indicator strips) and biological process indicators. Chemical indicators are commonly placed both inside and outside of each surgical pack and will undergo a color change in response to a threshold temperature (usually between 245 and 270 °F); however, their effectiveness is variable [32, 52]. Biological indicators are perhaps the most accurate means of assessing the sterilization process and typically consist of spore-forming bacteria contained in a glass vial that is placed within a "test pack," run through a typical sterilization cycle, and then cultured for bacterial growth.

In addition to assuring that the sterilization process itself is effective, care should be taken when storing and handling sterilized equipment to prevent contamination. Sterilized packages should be stored in closed containers, protected from moisture and aerosolized dust and debris, at a constant temperature (<75 °F/24 °C) and low humidity (<70%), and they should not be stacked on one another [39]. Handling should be limited to movement from the sterilizer to the storage container to the operating room. Excessive handling can lead to seal breakage and package damage [39]. Events and environmental changes such as these, rather than time, cause loss of sterilization. Reported recommended maximum storage times for sterilized packs range from 4 weeks (for double-wrapped woven packages) to 1 year (for plastic-peel pouches) depending on the specific packaging and storage system utilized [39].

### 11.5.2.3   Surgeon Preparation

Surgeon preparation includes donning of appropriate attire for the procedure (including caps, masks, gowns, and gloves) and the surgical hand scrub [53]. Although the use of sterile gowns is often left to surgeon discretion in veterinary practice, the use of caps, masks, and single-use sterile gloves for every procedure is an achievable best practice, a universal indication to any observer that a sterile procedure is about to be performed and a sign of respect for the client and patient.

The surgical hand scrub has three primary goals: to remove debris and transient microorganisms, to reduce the resident microbial count, and to inhibit rebound growth of microorganisms [54, 55]. These goals are typically accomplished through the use of commercially available antimicrobial soaps (i.e. an antiseptic–detergent combination) and a standardized surgical scrub procedure (e.g. anatomic timed scrub, counted brush stroke, surgical hand rub) [53].

The ideal antimicrobial soap will be rapid acting, broad spectrum, active in the presence of organic matter, nonirritating, have long-acting residual antimicrobial effects, and be economical [53, 56]. Antimicrobial soaps containing alcohol, chlorhexidine, iodine/iodophors, phenolic compounds, or some combination of these active ingredients are most common in veterinary surgical programs. The pros and cons of each antiseptic along with recommended surgical scrub contact times are presented in

**Table 11.6** Characteristics of common antiseptics found in surgical scrub solutions [55–61].

| Antiseptic | Concentration (%) | Pros | Cons | Reported effective contact times |
|---|---|---|---|---|
| Alcohol | 60–95 | Broad-spectrum bactericide Good fungicide Rapid killing activity Minimal residual activity Inexpensive | Variable efficacy against nonenveloped viruses No residual activity Loss of efficacy in the presence of organic debris | 1–5 min |
| Chlorhexidine gluconate | 0.5–4 | Broad-spectrum bactericidal Strong residual activity Maintains efficacy in the presence of organic debris | Poor efficacy against enveloped viruses Ineffective against nonenveloped viruses | 2–6 min |
| *Para*-chloro-*meta*-xylenol (PCMX) | 0.5–4 | Broad-spectrum bactericidal | Variable efficacy against nonenveloped viruses Ineffective against nonenveloped viruses Residual effects unclear | 30 s–2 min |
| Povidone iodine | 0.75–2 (free iodine) | Broad-spectrum bactericidal Moderate fungicide Sporicidal Some residual activity | Variable efficacy against nonenveloped viruses Prolonged time to effect Loss of efficacy in the presence of organic debris Staining of skin Tissue toxicity | 2–10 min |

Table 11.6. Disposable plastic brushes, soap-impregnated sponges, brushless scrub solution, and waterless scrub solutions and rubs are all acceptable and effective methods of applying antiseptic solutions to the hands [53–55, 62]. Disposable scrub brushes are not intended for repeated usage and should be discarded whenever visibly contaminated. It is important to note that not all brushless, waterless, antiseptic rubs or gels have equivalent efficacy, contact time required for surgical antisepsis is generally greater than that for purely hygienic purposes, and the technique for product application is different from that used for traditional scrub solutions [63, 64].

For a high-volume surgeon, scrubbing prior to each procedure may not be practical or possible. In these cases, it is acceptable to perform a complete surgical scrub at the beginning of the surgical period with additional scrubs occurring only after breaks in aseptic technique and after procedures lasting greater than 60 min in length. The degree of residual activity and likelihood of skin irritation of the chosen antiseptic agent should be considered when planning the frequency and duration of scrub protocols. However, in most cases, a minimum of 5 min of antiseptic contact time is recommended for the initial scrub with subsequent scrubs ensuring at least 2 min of contact time [53].

Regardless of the scrub technique utilized, it is important to ensure that the hands are fully dried prior to donning surgical gloves. Potentially pathogenic bacteria have been isolated from hospital taps and cultured from the droplets off surgeons' hands after scrubbing, setting up the potential for recontamination of properly scrubbed hands [65]. This concern may be even greater in undeveloped countries and in field clinic situations where water quality is questionable [63].

Proper hand preparation is not a substitute for the use of sterile surgical gloves. The relatively high incidence of glove perforation during surgical procedures is well established and has been directly associated with SSIs, particularly when perioperative antibiotics are not administered [66]. One multicenter veterinary study described an overall incidence of glove defects of 23% with significantly more defects found in gloves worn on the nondominant hand and those worn during procedures greater than 60 min in length. Surgeon experience was not associated with the incidence of defects [67]. Sterile surgical gloves are not intended for reuse and cannot maintain their integrity with resterilization; similarly, nonsterile examination gloves cannot be effectively sterilized for use in surgical procedures.

### 11.5.2.4 Patient Preparation

Patient preparation encompasses the removal of hair and scrubbing of the planned surgical site along with the application of appropriate barrier drapes. The goals of patient preparation are the same as those described above for the surgeon. In addition, the use of surgical drapes serves as both a physical barrier against microbes and as visual establishment of the sterile field [68], a factor of special significance in field clinic settings, when the operating area is not delineated by the walls of a sterile operating room.

Hair removal in veterinary patients can be performed through the use of electric clippers or depilatory creams. Depilatory creams (chemical hair removal agents) are less traumatic and result in a smoother skin surface than electric clippers [57, 69]; however, a mild, self-limiting inflammatory reaction has been described after using a commercial depilatory cream in rabbits [70]. Some practitioners are also adept at the use of a straight blade to prepare patients for surgery when electric clippers are not feasible.

The timing of hair removal can also contribute to the risk of SSI development. One veterinary study utilizing electric clippers for hair removal found that patients clipped 4 h or longer prior to the surgical procedure had significantly greater odds of developing an SSI than those clipped less than 4 h prior to surgery [71]; a second found that clipping of the surgical site prior to anesthetic induction resulted in a threefold increase in the likelihood of SSIs [28]. To minimize skin trauma in veterinary patients, hair clipping should be performed with an electric clipper and a sharp No. 40 clipper blade in the same direction as hair growth. In patients with dense hair coats, initially using a coarser blade (e.g. No. 10) followed by a No. 40 blade may be most effective [53]. Clipped hair should be removed from the environment with a vacuum [53]. For patients with fine hair or in locations without electricity, use of a one-sided adhesive lint roller is also effective.

Ideally, hair removal will be conducted at a location separate from the intended operating table. A general cleansing scrub prior to transporting the patient into the operating room where the sterile skin preparation takes place will help ensure that the surgical site does not become contaminated during transportation and positioning of the patient on the operating table. Alternatively, both hair removal and antiseptic preparation can be performed in one location as long as precautions are taken not to contaminate the surgical site.

Antiseptic agents useful in preparing the surgical site are similar to those described for surgeon preparation (Table 11.6). Phenolic compounds (e.g. hexachlorophene, PCMX, triclosan) and quaternary ammonium salts should not be used as they are associated with significant toxicities in animals and safe, effective alternatives are readily available [35, 53, 59, 72]. Multiple protocols for the application of antiseptics have proven effective (e.g. alternating antiseptic scrub with alcohol or saline rinse, antiseptic scrub followed by sprays or paints, antiseptic spray alone, wiping skin dry after scrubbing, leaving skin to air dry) [73–78]. Perhaps more important than the antiseptic chosen or the application protocol are the provisions that the skin surface is clean prior to beginning the surgical scrub, that the appropriate contact time for the chosen antiseptic is observed, and that application of the agent does not result in recontamination of the surgical site [78]. Figure 11.4 describes the appropriate technique for manual application of preoperative antiseptic solutions.

Once the scrub of the surgical site is complete, it should be allowed to dry thoroughly prior to draping [53]. Although wet drape material has been shown to enhance bacterial strike-through, the effectiveness of barrier drapes in protecting the patient against SSIs is the subject of debate in human surgical care [79–81]. Their role in veterinary surgery, however, seems more obvious given the relatively high risk of hair or fecal contamination of the surgical site [17] and serves as an obvious visual indication that a sterile surgical procedure is to be performed. Patient draping is generally accomplished in two layers, the true impact of the traditional two-layer draping technique in preventing SSIs is unknown [82, 83] and it is common in field clinic situations to utilize a single fenestrated drape to isolate the incision site. As long as reasonable precautions are taken to keep drape material dry and

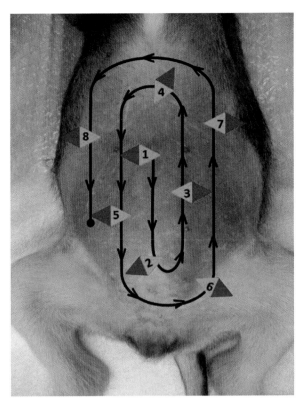

**Figure 11.4** Surgical scrubbing pattern. Once the skin surface has been cleaned, application of the antiseptic solution should proceed in gradually expanding circles from the anticipated incision site outward. Care must be taken to rotate the applicator sponge so that the contaminated "tail" end does not contact a previously scrubbed area. (GREEN = "head" of applicator sponge; RED = "tail" of applicator sponge.)

**Textbox 11.10 Patient preparation**

1) Remove hair or fur from the surgical site.
   - Use electric clippers, straight blade, or depilatory creams.
   - Patient should be anesthetized prior to hair removal to minimize trauma to the surgical site.
2) Remove clipped hair from environment.
   - Use vacuum or adhesive lint roller.
3) Apply antiseptic agent to the surgical site.
   - Antiseptic scrubs, sprays, or paints can be used with or without rinse.
   - Ensure antiseptic is applied to visibly clean surface.
   - Apply antiseptic from the intended surgical site outward.
   - Ensure adequate contact time with antiseptic.
   - If patient is to be transported to operating area after antiseptic application, protect the surgical site from contamination or repeat skin preparation in operating area.
4) Allow thorough drying of antiseptic prior to applying surgical drape.

to remain conscious of the limits of the sterile field, there is no evidence that this technique results in increased risk of SSIs. If drapes are not prefenestrated, creating a fenestration prior to applying the drape material to the patient may help prevent contamination of sterile surgical scissors by the patient's skin.

# Appendix

## 11.A    Guidelines for the Use of Bleach for Dilution and Use Instructions

### Guidelines for Using Bleach

Sodium hypochlorite is the chemical compound commonly known as bleach. Bleach is utilized as a component of the cleaning and disinfection protocol for many animal hospitals, shelters, and spay-neuter clinics. It is well-known for its ability to kill many bacteria, viruses and fungal hyphae (and at proper dilution, fungal spores). It is especially helpful for its ability to kill non-enveloped viruses, such as Canine Parvovirus, Feline Panleukopenia and Feline Calicivirus. The following guidelines should be followed when using bleach as a disinfectant to ensure its effectiveness:

1.  **Bleach must be applied to a surface that has previously been cleaned with an appropriate detergent.** Bleach is solely a disinfectant and can be inactivated by microscopic organic debris. Care must be taken to completely rinse all detergent residues and thoroughly dry the surface prior to applying bleach so as not to further dilute the bleach solution.

2.  **A 1:32 solution of regular household bleach (8.25% sodium hypochlorite) is appropriate for daily use.** Bleach solutions at concentrations less than this may not be effective. Bleach solutions at concentrations greater than this will cause facility corrosion and respiratory tract irritation in both people and animals.

    > To make a 1:32 solution, add...
    >
    > - 1/3 cup of bleach per gallon of water
    >
    > - 17 ml of bleach (1 TBSP + ½ TSP) per 32 ounce spray bottle

3.  **Bleach solutions should be stored in opaque containers and must be made fresh at a minimum of every 24 hours.** Bleach rapidly degrades in the presence of light and when mixed with water.

4.  **Bleach solutions require a full 10 minutes of contact time to ensure complete disinfection.** If bleach solution evaporates in less than 10 minutes, a greater volume of solution should be applied.

5.  **After disinfection with bleach solutions, surfaces should be rinsed and dried.** Bleach can be irritating to skin and mucous membranes, so any residue should be removed prior to returning animals to the environment.

If using bleach for periodic deep cleaning and/or for the purpose of killing fungal spores (e.g. ringworm), bleach should be diluted with water at a concentration of 1:10. *Note that studies have shown that disinfectants other than bleach may also be effective for this purpose.*

This is equivalent to:
- 1 cup of bleach per gallon of water, or
- ¼ cup of bleach per 32 ounces of water.

Animals must be removed from the area and people should wear appropriate personal protective equipment when using 1:10 bleach solutions!

Brian A. DiGangi, DVM, MS, DABVP
2015

## 11.B   Instructions for Spot Cleaning Cat Cages

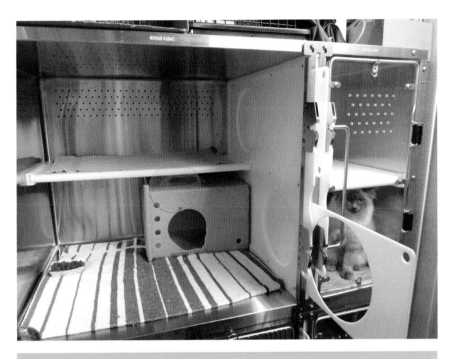

Cat Care Cleaning Tip:
Reduce cat stress by reducing noise - quietly open and close cage and room doors and make efforts to reduce the metal clang of dishes.

**Before you start**

- Look at each cat in the room for changes in health that may affect your cleaning order or who may need care
  - ○ Make sure health changes are recorded and shared with those responsible for animal health care
- Have prepared food bowls, water bowls and litter boxes as needed
  - ○ Separate cleaning supplies should be available in each cat housing room/area and not shared
  - ○ Cleaning in each room should proceed relatively uninterrupted until the room is finished.
    - This is important for reducing the risk of disease transmission into or out of a room as well as reducing stress for the cats by making cleaning time efficient
- Clean with a routine
  - ○ Changes in routine are stressful for animals - a low stress routine that is common to all staff members will help ensure a lower stress, healthier transition to the shelter environment

**Example spot cleaning protocols:**

Spot cleaning in a *double compartment cage*:

1. Put on a clean pair of gloves
2. Close the door(s) that separate the two sides of the cage
3. Quietly open the door of the compartment that the cat is NOT in
4. Examine the interior of the cage (including front bars) for organic material (feces, snot, food, etc.). Clean out the material with one time use paper towel or 'raglet' and soap and water as needed. Discard used paper towel or put 'raglet' in the laundry.
5. Depending on what is on this side remove food, water, litter box, remake bed and tidy cage. Continue to use the same bedding material unless it is wet or soiled or is dirty (some cat hair is ok). If this is the side for the food and water - replace with fresh food and water. If it is the litter box side - replace with clean litter box.
6. Close door quietly
7. Open compartment dividers that separate the two sides of the cage
8. If the cat moves to the other side on its own – great! If the cat remains on the side you need to clean try to entice it to move across or simply open the door and gently assist it through the divider door to the other side and close the divider door(s).
9. Repeat steps 4 & 5 for this compartment
10. Close cage door quietly
11. Cage has been spot cleaned!
12. Change gloves between cages if housing kittens and between banks if housing adults

Spot cleaning a *single compartment cage with friendly cat*:

1. Put on a clean pair of gloves.
2. If the cat seems friendly and unlikely to escape- open the cage door.
3. Do not handle the cat if possible or if needed gently restrain the cat with 1 gloved hand while you manage to accomplish the following:
4. Remove litter box, food and water dishes and any organic debris inside cage.
5. Examine the interior of the cage (including the front bars) for organic material (feces, snot, food) and clean with one time use paper towel or 'raglet' and soap and water as needed.
6. Tidy cage interior - make bed, etc. Continue to use the same bedding material unless it is wet or soiled or is dirty (some cat hair is ok).
7. Replace dishes with fresh food and water and place a new litter box
8. Quietly close cage door
9. Change gloves between cages if housing kittens and between banks if housing adults

Spot cleaning a *single compartment cage with unfriendly cat* (these cats should be housed in a cage with a feral box inside along with a partial to full cage cover over the cage front):

1. Put on a clean pair of gloves
2. Lift or remove cage cover
3. If cat is not already inside feral box, use safety equipment to carefully help the cat enter the feral box and close the feral box door
4. Quietly open cage door
5. Cover feral box window with towel
6. Remove litter box, food and water dishes and any organic debris inside cage
7. Examine the interior of the cage (including the front bars) for organic material (feces, snot, food) and clean with one time use paper towel or 'raglet' and soap and water as needed
8. Discard paper towel or put 'raglet' in laundry
9. Tidy cage interior- make bed, etc. Continue to use the same bedding material unless it is wet or soiled or is dirty (some cat hair is ok).
10. Replace dishes with fresh food and water and place a new litter box.
11. Remove towel covering feral box
12. Quietly close cage door
13. With safety equipment open feral box door
14. Replace cage cover
15. Change gloves between cages if housing kittens and between banks if housing adults

**Cat Care Cleaning Tip:**
Water and food dishes that spill can contribute to a messy cage for cleaning. Dishes that are 'untippable' or attach to the front of the cage can reduce spills.

Source: Used with permission from the UC Davis Koret Shelter Medicine Program

# References

1 Abreu, A.C., Tavares, R.R., Borges, A. et al. (2013). Current and emergent strategies for disinfection of hospital environments. *Journal of Antimicrobial Chemotherapy* **68** (12): 2718–2732.

2 Costerton, J.W., Stewart, P.S., and Greenberg, E.P. (1999). Bacterial biofilms: a common cause of persistent infections. *Science* **284** (5418): 1318–1322.

3 Quinn, P.J. and Markey, B.K. (2001). Disinfection and disease prevention in veterinary medicine. In: Disinfection, Sterilization and Preservation, 5ee (ed. S.S. Block), 1069–1103.

4 Rutala, W.A., Cole, E.C., Thomann, C.A., and Weber, D.J. (1998). Stability and bactericidal activity of chlorine solutions. *Infection Control and Hospital Epidemiology* **19** (5): 323–327.

5 Greene, C.E. (2011). Infectious Diseases of the Dog and Cat, 4ee. Philadelphia: Saunders Elsevier.

6 Wickstrom, M.L. Antiseptics and disinfectants. In *The Merck Veterinary Manual*. http://www. merckvetmanual.com/ (accessed 18 December 2017).

7 Hurley, K.F. (2015). Sanitation in animal shelters. https://www.sheltermedicine.com/library/ resources/?utf8=%E2%9C%93&search%5Bslug% 5D=sanitation-in-animal-shelters (accessed 18 December 2017).

8 Stockton, K.A., Morley, P.S., Hyatt, D.R., et al. (2006) Evaluation of the effects of footwear hygiene protocols on nonspecific bacterial contamination of floor surfaces in an equine hospital. *Journal of the American Veterinary Medical Association* **228**: 1068–1073.

9 Amass, S., Vyverberg, B., Beaudry, D. (2000) Evaluating the efficacy of boot baths in biosecurity protocols. *Swine Health Production* **8**: 169–173.

10 Meier, B. (2002) Reuse of needle at hospital infects 50 with hepatitis C. *The New York Times*. http:// www.nytimes.com/2002/10/10/us/reuse-of-needle-at-hospital-infects-50-with-hepatitis-c.html (accessed 22 April 2016).

11 Morell, R.C., Ririe, D., James, R.L. et al. (1994). A survey of laryngoscope contamination at a university and a community hospital. *Anesthesiology* **80** (94): 960.

12 Trepanier, C.A., Lessard, M.R., Brochu, J.G., and Denault, P.H. (1990). Risk of cross-infection related to the multiple use of disposable syringes. *Canadian Journal of Anaesthesia* **37** (2): 156–159.

13 Shulan, D.J., Weiler, J.M., Koontz, F., and Richerson, H. (1985). Contamination of intradermal skin test syringes. *The Journal of Allergy and Clinical Immunology* **76** (2): 226–227.

14 Roberts, R.B. (1973). Cleaning the laryngoscope blade. *Canadian Journal of Anaesthesia* **20** (2): 241–244.

15 Fleming, A. and Ogilvie, A.C. (1951). Syringe needles and mass inoculation technique. *British Medical Journal* **1** (4706): 543–546.

16 Association of Operating Room Nurses (2005). Recommended practices for cleaning, handling, and processing anesthesia equipment. *Association of Operating Room Nurses Journal* **81** (4): 856–870.

17 Griffin, B., Bushby, P.A., McCobb, E. et al. (2016). The Association of Shelter Veterinarians' 2016 veterinary medical care guidelines for spay-neuter programs. *Journal of the American Veterinary Medical Association* **249** (2): 165–188.

18 Hedlund, C.S. (2007) Surgery of the reproductive and genital systems. In Small Animal Surgery. (ed. T.W. Fossum), 3e pp. 702–774. Mosby Elsevier, St. Louis, MO.

19 Barie, P.S. and Eachempati, S.R. (2005). Surgical site infections. *The Surgical Clinics of North America* **85** (6): 1115–1135.

20 Klevens, R., Edwards, J., Richards, C.L. et al. (2007). Estimating health care-associated infections and deaths in U.S. hospitals, 2002. *Public Health Reports* **122** (2): 160–166.

21 Emori, T.G. and Gaynes, R.P. (1993). An overview of nosocomial infections. *Clinical Microbiology Reviews* **6** (4): 428–442.

22 Mangram, A.J., Horan, T.C., Pearson, M.L. et al. (1999). Guideline for prevention of surgical site infection, 1999. *Infection Control and Hospital Epidemiology* **20** (4): 250–280.

23 Johnson, J.A. (2002). Nosocomial infections. *The Veterinary Clinics of North America. Small Animal Practice* **32**: 1101–1126.

24 Vasseur, P.B., Levy, J.K., Dowd, E., and Eliot, J. (1988). Surgical wound infection rates in dogs and cats. Data from a teaching hospital. *Veterinary Surgery* **17** (2): 60–64.

25 Burrow, R., Batchelor, D., and Cripps, P. (2005). Complications observed during and after ovariohysterectomy of 142 bitches at a veterinary teaching hospital. *The Veterinary Record* **157**: 829–833.

26 Eugster, S., Schawalder, P., Gaschen, F., and Boerlin, P. (2004). A prospective study of postoperative surgical site infections in dogs and cats. *Veterinary Surgery* **33**: 542–550.

27 Nicholson, M., Beal, M., Shofer, F. et al. (2002). Epidemiologic evaluation of postoperative wound infection in clean-contaminated wounds: a retrospective study of 239 dogs and cats. *Veterinary Surgery* **31**: 577–581.

28 Brown, D.C., Conzemius, M.G., Shofer, F., and Swann, H. (1997). Epidemiologic evaluation of postoperative wound infections in dogs and cats. *Journal of the American Veterinary Medical Association* **210** (9): 1302–1306.

29 Isaza, N. and DiGangi, B.A. (2012). Cultivating compassion: University of Florida Merial shelter animal medicine clerkship. 2012 Maddie's Shelter Medicine Conference, Gainesville,FL: University of Florida.

30 Fossum, T.W. (2007). Surgical facilities, equipment, and personnel. In: Small Animal Surgery, 3ee (ed. T.W. Fossum), 15–18. St. Louis, MO: Mosby Elsevier.

31 Letts, R.M. and Doermer, E. (1983). Conversation in the operating theatre as a cause of airborne bacterial contamination. *The Journal of Bone and Joint Surgery* **65** (3): 357–362.

32 Fossum, T.W. (2007). Sterilization and disinfection. In: Small Animal Surgery, 3ee (ed. T.W. Fossum), 9–14. St. Louis, MO: Mosby Elsevier.

33 Favero, M.S. and Bond, W.W. (2001). Chemical disinfection of medical and surgical materials. In: Disinfection, Sterilization, and Preservation, 5ee (ed. S.S. Block), 881–917.

34 Association of Operating Room Nurses (2002). Recommended practices for cleaning and caring for surgical instruments and powered equipment. *Association of Operating Room Nurses Journal* **75** (3): 627–638.

35 Dvorak, G., Petersen, C.A., Rovid Spickler, A. et al. (2008). Disinfection 101. In: Maddie's Infection Control Manual for Animal Shelters (ed. C.A. Petersen, G. Dvorak and A. Rovid Spickler), 42–65.

36 Quinn, P.J. and Markey, B.K. (2001). Disinfection and disease prevention in veterinary medicine. In: Disinfection, Sterilization, and Preservation, 5ee (ed. S.S. Block), 1069–1103.

37 Association of Surgical Technologists (2009) Recommended standards of practice for the decontamination of surgical instruments. http://www.ast.org/uploadedFiles/Main_Site/Content/About_Us/Standard_Decontamination_%20Surgical_Instruments_.pdf (accessed 22 April 2016).

38 Association of Operating Room Nurses (2007). Recommended practices for selection and use of packaging systems for sterilization. *Association of Operating Room Nurses Journal* **85** (4): 801–812.

39 Fossum, T.W. (2007). Principles of surgical asepsis. In: Small Animal Surgery, 3ee (ed. T.W. Fossum), 1–8. St. Louis, MO: Mosby Elsevier.

40 Morinaga, T., Hasegawa, G., Koyama, S. et al. (2010). Acute inflammation and immunoresponses induced by ortho-phthalaldehyde in mice. *Archives of Toxicology* **84**: 397–404.

41 Block, S.S. (2001). Peroxygen compounds. In: Disinfection, Sterilization, and Preservation, 5ee (ed. S.S. Block), 185–204. Lippincott Williams & Wilkins.

42 Beauchamp, R.O., St. Clair, M.B., Fennell, T.R. et al. (1992). A critical review of the toxicology of glutaraldehyde. *Critical Reviews in Toxicology* **22** (3–4): 143–174.

43 Miller, J.J., Powell, G.M., Olavesen, A.H., and Curtis, C. (1973). The metabolism and toxicity of phenols in cats. 540th Meeting of the Biochemical Society University of Oxford 10 and 11, pp. 1163–1165.

44 Rutala, W.A., Weber, D.J., and Healthcare Infection Control Practices Advisory Committee (2008). Guideline for disinfection and sterilization in healthcare facilities. http://www.cdc.gov/hicpac/pdf/guidelines/disinfection_nov_2008.pdf (accessed 22 April 2016).

45 Bellissimo-Rodrigues, W.T., Bellissimo-Rodrigues, F., and Machado, A.A. (2009). Infection control practices among a cohort of Brazilian dentists. *International Dental Journal* **59**: 53–58. doi: 10.1922/IDJ_1989Rodrigues06.

46 Mulcahy, D.M. (2003). Surgical implantation of transmitters into fish. *Institute of Laboratory Animal Resources Journal* **44** (4): 295–306.

47 Expanded Program on Immunization in the Americas (1984) Using a pressure cooker as an autoclave. Expanded Program on Immunization in the Americas Newsletter, 6 (6), 5–8.

48 Frobisher, M. (1939). Disinfection in the home. *The American Journal of Nursing* **39** (1): 833–839.

49 Reuss-Lamky, H. (2012). Beating the bugs: sterilization is instrumental. AAHA Denver 2012 Yearly Conference Proceedings.

50 Sebben, J.E. (1984). Sterilization and care of surgical instruments and supplies. *Journal of the American Academy of Dermatology* **11** (3): 381–392.

51 Young, J.H. (1993). Sterilization with steam under pressure. In: Sterilization Technology (ed. R.F. Morrissey and G. Briggs Phillips), 120–151. Van Nostrand Reinhold.

52 Lee, C.H., Montville, T.J., and Sinskey, A.J. (1979). Comparison of the efficacy of steam sterilization indicators. *Applied and Environmental Microbiology* **37** (6): 1113–1137.

53 Fossum, T.W. (2007). Preparation of the surgical team. In: Small Animal Surgery, 3ee (ed. T.W. Fossum), 38–45. St. Louis, MO: Mosby Elsevier.

54 Association of Operating Room Nurses (2004). Recommended practices for surgical hand: antisepsis/hand scrubs. *Association of Operating Room Nurses Journal* **79** (2): 416–431.

55 Crabtree, T.D., Pelletier, S.J., and Pruett, T.L. (2001). Surgical antisepsis. In: Disinfection, Sterilization, and Preservation, 5ee (ed. S.S. Block), 919–934. Lippincott Williams & Wilkins.

56 Baines, S. (1996). Surgical asepsis: principles and protocols. *In Practice* **18**: 23–33.

57 Fossum, T.W. (2007). Preparation of the operative site. In: Small Animal Surgery, 3ee (ed. T.W. Fossum), 32–37. St. Louis, MO: Mosby Elsevier.

58 Hsieh, H., Chiu, H., and Lee, F. (2006). Surgical hand scrubs in relation to microbial counts: systematic literature review. *Journal of Advanced Nursing* **55** (1): 68–78.

59 Heit, M.C. and Riviere, J.E. (2001). Chemotherapy of microbial diseases. In: Veterinary Pharmacology and Therapeutics, 8ee (ed. J.E. Riviere and M.G. Papich), 783–795. Wiley Blackwell.

60 Paulson, D. (1994). Comparative evaluation of five surgical hand scrub preparations. *Association of Operating Room Nurses Journal* **60** (2): 249–256.

61 Larson, E.L., Butz, A.M., Gullette, D.L., and Laughon, B. (1990). Alcohol for surgical scrubbing? and. *Infection Control and Hospital Epidemiology* **11** (3): 139–143.

62 Parienti, J.J., Thibon, P., Heller, R. et al. (2002). Hand-rubbing with an aqueous alcoholic solution vs traditional surgical hand-scrubbing and 30-day surgical site infection rates: a randomized equivalence study. *The Journal of the American Medical Association* **288** (6): 722–727.

63 Widmer, A.F., Rotter, M., Voss, A. et al. (2010). Surgical hand preparation: state-of-the-art. *Journal of Hospital Infection* **74**: 112–122.

64 Kramer, A., Rudolph, P., Kampf, G., and Pittet, D. (2002). Limited efficacy of alcohol-based hand gels. *Lancet* **359** (9316): 1489–1490.

65 Heal, J.S., Blom, A.W., Titcomb, D. et al. (2003). Bacterial contamination of surgical gloves by water droplets spilt after scrubbing. *Journal of Hospital Infection* **53** (2): 136–139.

66 Misteli, H., Weber, W.P., Reck, S. et al. (2009). Surgical glove perforation and the risk of surgical site infection. *Archives of Surgery* **144** (6): 553–558.

67 Character, B.J., McLaughlin, R.M., Hedlund, C.S. et al. (2003). Postoperative integrity of veterinary surgical gloves. *Journal of the American Animal Hospital Association* **39** (3): 311–320.

68 Association of Operating Room Nurses (2006). Recommended practices for maintaining a sterile field. *Association of Operating Room Nurses Journal* **83** (2): 402–416.

69 Weiland, L., Croubels, S., Baert, K. et al. (2006). Pharmacokinetics of a lidocaine patch 5% in dogs. *Journal of Veterinary Medicine* **53** (1): 34–39.

70 Foley, P.L., Henderson, A.L., Bissonette, E.A. et al. (2001). Evaluation of fentanyl transdermal patches in rabbits: blood concentrations and physiologic response. *Comparative Medicine* **51** (3): 239–244.

71 Mayhew, P.D., Freeman, L., Kwan, T., and Brown, D.C. (2012). Comparison of surgical site infection rates in clean and clean-contaminated wound in dogs and cats after minimally invasive versus open surgery: 179 cases (2007–2008). *Journal of the American Veterinary Medical Association* **240** (2): 193–198.

72 Merianos, J.J. (2001). Surface-active agents. In: Disinfection, Sterilization, and Preservation, 5the

(ed. S.S. Block), 283–320. Lippincott Williams & Wilkins.

73 Moen, M.D., Noone, M.B., and Kirson, I. (2002). Povidone-iodine spray technique versus traditional scrub-paint technique for preoperative abdominal wall preparation. *American Journal of Obstetrics and Gynecology* **187** (6): 1436–1437.

74 Osuna, D.J., DeYoung, D.J., and Walker, R.L. (1990). Comparison of three skin preparation techniques. Part 2: clinical trial in 100 dogs. *Veterinary Surgery* **19** (1): 20–23.

75 Geelhoed, G.W., Sharpe, K., and Simon, G.L. (1983). A comparative study of surgical skin preparation methods. *Surgery, Gynecology & Obstetrics* **157** (3): 265–268.

76 Kutarski, P.W. and Grundy, H.C. (1993). To dry or not to dry? An assessment of the possible degradation in efficiency of preoperative skin preparation caused by wiping skin dry. *Annals of the Royal College of Surgeons of England* **75** (3): 181–185.

77 Shirahatti, R.G., Hoshi, R.M., Vishwanath, Y.K. et al. (1993). Effect of pre-operative skin preparation on post-operative wound infection. *Journal of Postgraduate Medicine* **39** (3): 134–136.

78 Association of Operating Room Nurses (2002). Recommended practices for skin preparation of patients. *Association of Operating Room Nurses Journal* **75** (1): 184–187.

79 Hadiati, D.R., Hakimi, M., and Nurdiati, D.S. (2012). Skin preparation for preventing infection following caesarean section. *Cochrane Database of Systematic Reviews* Sep 12 (9).

80 Blom, A.W., Gozzard, C., Heal, J. et al. (2002). Bacterial strike-through of re-usable surgical drapes: the effect of different wetting agents. *Journal of Hospital Infection* **52** (1): 52–55.

81 Belkin, N.L. (2002). Barrier surgical gowns and drapes: just how necessary are they? and. *Textile Rental* 66–73.

82 Owen, L.J., Gines, J.A., Knowles, T.G., and Holt, P.E. (2009). Efficacy of adhesive incise drapes in preventing bacterial contamination of clean canine surgical wounds. *Veterinary Surgery* **38** (6): 732–737.

83 Webster, J. and Alghamdi, A.A. (2015). Use of plastic adhesive drapes during surgery for preventing surgical site infection. *Cochrane Database of Systematic Reviews* Oct 17 (4).

84 DiGangi, B.A. (2015). Guidelines for Using Bleach. https://vetmed-maddie.sites.medinfo.ufl.edu/files/2011/10/Guidelines-for-Using-Bleach-updated.pdf (accessed 9 March 2018).

# 12

# Euthanasia in Veterinary Field Projects

*I. Kati Loeffler*

*Community Animals Program, International Fund for Animal Welfare, 290 Summer Street, Yarmouth Port, MA 02675, USA*

## 12.1　Introduction

Euthanasia is often one of the most difficult topics over which to come to agreement in international veterinary field projects for dogs and cats. It is wrought with religious and cultural concerns, lack of locally available and humane methods for euthanasia, social pressures regarding animal rescue, conflicted attitudes about suffering and death, and emotionally charged decision-making. This chapter describes a logical approach to the euthanasia decision that takes into account local attitudes and resource challenges. It is important that each organization – whether an animal welfare charity or veterinary clinic – develop a euthanasia policy in order to remove the need to engage in a stressful and often divisive decision-making process over every patient. The welfare of the individual patient is at the forefront of the decision and of the procedure and must be ensured regardless of cultural, religious, or resource conditions.

Appropriate and timely veterinary care is one of the fundamental welfare requirements for animals who are dependent on human guardianship. Veterinarians and nursing staff have the opportunity to represent the respect and empathy for animals that we wish to see reflected in our societies. We teach through our every action the consideration for animals that we strive to engender in communities and in the students who will rise to lead our profession. This begins with the manner in which we introduce ourselves to our patients, the skill and reassurance with which we restrain and handle them, the care that they receive in our hands, and, when necessary, the compassion with which we euthanize them.

Our demonstrated concern for the animal's emotional and physical well-being, whether in a brief encounter to vaccinate a patient, in our care for patients during hospital stays, or in the final moments of a patient's life, is paramount to professional veterinary practice and to the manner in which animals are valued in our societies.

Veterinary caregivers have the opportunity to set a strong example in communicating respect for the inherent value of individual animal lives, regardless of the commercial, aesthetic, or utilitarian worth that society may assign to an animal. We can promote veterinary professional and animal welfare standards no matter how sparse our resources may be when we work in the field, and most especially when we work in areas in which we seek to foster improved veterinary practices and attitudes of respect and compassion for animals.

In international field projects, veterinarians and veterinary nurses who have enjoyed the privilege of training to advanced standards of veterinary medicine serve as teachers in animal welfare as well as in the technical aspects of veterinary medicine and surgery. Veterinary staff who lead international field projects bear a responsibility to ensure that the subject of euthanasia is taught at all and that it is taught in a manner that will ensure both cultural sensitivity and, above all, the welfare of patients and respect for their individual lives.

Welfare standards in the slaughter of animals for food or killing animals once they have fulfilled their

*Field Manual for Small Animal Medicine*, First Edition. Edited by Katherine Polak and Ann Therese Kommedal.

role in research experiments are further very serious topics, but fall outside the scope of this chapter. In this chapter, we discuss euthanasia of companion animals in international animal welfare projects.

## 12.2 Ethical Imperatives of Euthanasia

While death permanently relieves an animal from suffering, it also eliminates the possibility of any future for positive experiences and the pleasure of existence for that individual. The question of quality of life – particularly future quality of life – is often at the center of the decision over whether or not to euthanize. We are asked to decide, on behalf of another living being who is wholly at the mercy of our decision, what constitutes a life worth living or whether sacrifice of that individual life is justifiable for a greater good.

In other instances, consideration for the quality of a patient's present and future life is rated inferior to anthropocentric positions that are based on human belief systems rather than on the inherent experience of the veterinary patient. "It is better to live a miserable life than to die a good death" is the prevalent philosophy in large regions of the world and is often combined with a fear of personal spiritual repercussion with the act of taking a life. (Passively taking lives through, for example, consuming animals that were slaughtered by someone else is usually categorized differently.) Animals are then forced to endure unacceptable degrees of terminal suffering because of human imperatives that disrespect the perspective of the patient.

Veterinarians are in the position of needing to consider the health and welfare of both animals and humans and to promote healthy and positive relationships between the two. Above all, the decision to euthanize an individual must be made on the basis of reason, with due respect for that individual life and with consideration for the ability of the people responsible for that individual life to provide adequate care.

The algorithm and accompanying discussion below guide the rational process for or against a euthanasia decision. One of the greatest challenges nonetheless may be to balance the conflicting perspectives of cultures or an animal's guardian with regard to the role or value of an animal. One may value each animal as a "subject of a life,"[1] while the animal's owner or the community may have a more utilitarian perspective. People may consider the life of a pet dog or breed dog more valuable than the life of a street dog or mongrel. Our challenge here is to determine not only the well-being of the animal in objective medical terms but also to determine the quality of life that the guardian or a community will be able to ensure for the animal. Again, our behavior toward each animal – regardless of how he or she may be valued by members of a community – and the manner in which we guide a discussion about euthanasia are critical opportunities for the change that we strive to promote in attitudes and behaviors toward animals.

The decision about euthanasia may be straightforward if the patient is suffering from illness or injury with little hope for recovery. These situations aside, many decisions about euthanasia are more about the resources with which a guardian or a community is able to care for an animal. As a welfare tool, euthanasia may be only one of a number of options to relieve an animal from the distress of a poor quality of life. Ideally, these decisions are not about whether or not to euthanize, but how to improve the animal's existence. The question then becomes one of human attitude and responsibility. A variety of human imperatives may drive the killing of animals even where termination of life is not in the best interest of the individual: convenience, disease concerns, religious or cultural beliefs, fear, and lack of resources (real or perceived). When the human element fails, where does that leave the animal who depends on humans for nutrition, health, and well-being? And is euthanasia the best option in the interest of both the

---

1 "Subject of a life" is a term popularized by the philosopher and animal rights advocate, Tom Regan, who argued that each animal has his or her personal experiences, has learned things, and has suffered and felt pleasures to develop a unique and personal life story. Similarly, Peter Singer asserted that ". . . every sentient being is capable of leading a life that is happier or less miserable than some alternative life, and hence has a claim to be taken into account." An individual's sentience necessitates that "what happens to them matters to them" (Regan), which obligates those in whose power that life lies (i.e. humans) to respect that life with the rights of a sentient individual. We ascribe value to each human being, regardless of the ability of that person to reason (e.g. infants or mentally impaired people), and argue that the same value must therefore extend to non-human lives.

animal and people? Will the termination of this animal's life improve the lives and opportunities of other animals in the community? In other words, have we learned anything from the perceived necessity to take this life?

The straightforward decision regarding a patient who is suffering without hope for relief or for animals whose welfare needs exceed available resources may not be so straightforward for people with certain cultural or religious positions against euthanasia. The ability of animals to live for long periods of time under the most abject and abusive conditions, or with chronic and painful medical problems, is sometimes used as justification to keep these individuals alive. Life in itself may be used as an argument against relieving it. In some countries, euthanasia is actually illegal, regardless of the terminal agony in which an animal may find itself.

It is our responsibility in these cases to find alternatives to relieve the prolonged suffering of the patient. Again, the issue is one of improving welfare, and where euthanasia is inappropriate for whatever reason, we must find alternatives. We can find ways to improve the living conditions of animals. We can find ways to provide relief from pain. Limited resources or availability of pain medication in some areas produce additional challenges, but even here one can be creative and figure out a way to ensure that that animal will not be left to suffer until he or she dies. Again, each opportunity is a teaching opportunity, and to do nothing at all and to leave an animal in agony is simply not an option in our collective professional effort to elevate animal welfare in veterinary medicine.

Ultimately, the question that we must be able to answer with a decision over euthanasia for each individual patient is whether our decision serves the standard to which we want our audience to be held: among our students, our colleagues, and the community in which we seek to lead by example. Would my colleagues and the public do right to disagree with my decision? Am I ashamed of my decision? Do I uphold the principle of *primum non nocere*:[2] will my decision do harm to the patient or to

other animals, or to the veterinary staff, animal guardians, and the public who are learning from me?

## 12.3 Developing a Euthanasia Policy for Your Organization

Negotiating the decision over whether or not to euthanize a patient is often an emotional experience that can disrupt an organization or psychologically exhaust the individuals who must make the decision repeatedly. In international field projects, the issue can destroy a relationship with the community if not managed with respect and consistency. It is therefore important for each organization to develop and commit to a euthanasia policy that reflects the organization's principles, communicates a consistent message of respect and rationale, and preempts the emotional anguish and inconsistency of subjective decisions.

Key stakeholders in the development of an organization's euthanasia policy include the management and trustees of the organization, the veterinarian(s), and animal care staff. Legal advice may be sought to ensure that the policy complies with local laws. Welfare advisors and other stakeholders such as government representatives and community leaders may also be asked for input. The committee meets to identify key concerns, and topics that require further research or expert input may be identified. The topic is often controversial, and discussions may benefit from an impartial facilitator to ensure that everyone is heard and to help the group come to agreement over the key points of a policy. An initial outline identifies the conditions under which euthanasia may be needed in the organization's work, and informs the first draft of an overarching policy. Definitions of certain terms that may be used in the writing of a policy (e.g. healthy, treatable) may be found in the Asilomar Accords [1]. Review by each committee member and revisions follow to ensure that everyone agrees to the principal components of the policy.

Development of a euthanasia policy provides a focused opportunity for the leaders of an organization to define the group's principles, values, and resources. These inform the position statement that heads a euthanasia policy. The position statement can come together only once the committee has been through a full and frank discussion of the perspectives and

---

2 Latin for "first, do no harm," which maxim underlies the bioethical principle of nonmaleficence in modern medicine. A version of this maxim is included in the Hippocratic Oath.

concerns of all stakeholders, and thus represents this communal agreement. Examples of position statements on euthanasia may be found in the International Companion Animal Management Coalition guidance documents [2].

Ultimately, the policy should hold up to the question of whether one would like to see it become the standard of practice. If not, then what needs to change or improve? A policy can help to identify issues in the organization's capacity or in the community that currently lead to euthanasia but that might be mitigated with a targeted effort. For example, the disproportionate occurrence of certain kinds of injuries or disease, abandonment, cruelty, or poor guardianship that often lead to euthanasia may guide an organization's strategic focus to reduce these deaths.

A policy may also identify resource needs that the group may choose to prioritize. As stated above, the most common questions in a euthanasia decision revolve around resources: most commonly space, facilities, expertise, time, money, drugs and other veterinary needs, and personnel. It may be, for example, that animals must be euthanized due to biosecurity limitations in the clinic or lack of expertise to help owners manage animal behavioral problems. Strategic priority may then be given to improving the former in the clinic and/or acquisition of the funding, training and personnel to build a dog behavior management resource for community members.

An organization's euthanasia policy is therefore a living document that provides the opportunity for regular revision that reflects advances in the organization and changes in the community.

Important considerations in developing the policy's implementation protocol include who in the organization is responsible for the final decision about whether or not to euthanize a patient and who carries out the procedure. Even with an objective decision-making guideline, and even though it is a clinical procedure that veterinarians are trained to perform, it is an emotionally costly responsibility. It may be helpful to ensure that several staff members are trained in the objective implementation of the policy so that the responsibility may be shared or rotated. Project managers should ensure that necessary support is available to help staff to cope constructively with the psychological burden of deciding and performing euthanasia.

In summary, the euthanasia policy is written to ensure the quality of life of patients, the safety of other animals, and the well-being of clinic personnel. It reflects the ethical principles of the organization and those that it seeks to exemplify in the community. It is designed to address the imperatives of animal welfare, public health, and stakeholder principles within the limits of current resources. It ensures that the procedure is carried out humanely, safely, and responsibly. As such, it is important that all of the organization's staff understand and agree to the policy and that personnel are adequately trained and supported to make euthanasia decisions and to carry out necessary procedures.

Key elements of a completed euthanasia policy may include the following:

- The organization's position statement about euthanasia.
- Who in the organization has the authority to make the decision about euthanasia for a given patient. For example: Do the staff veterinarians recommend a decision to a final decision-maker? Do two authorized staff agree on a decision, and another decision-maker is consulted only if these two cannot agree? Who is responsible if the key decision-maker is not available?
- How is the decision and procedure documented? There may be legal requirements for documentation of euthanasia. Use of certain drugs requires Schedule drug records.
- Criteria in the animal's condition or situation that may warrant euthanasia, and how these are assessed to reach a decision about whether or not euthanasia is justified. An organization may choose to list certain clinical presentations or diseases or may design a decision-making algorithm such as those presented below, but which are tailored to the resources available to the organization. It is important to be as specific as possible in defining criteria by which a decision about euthanasia may be made, but should allow some flexibility for changing resources. An example is illustrated in Textbox 12.1 (sample canine parvovirus policy).
- Method(s) for euthanasia used in the organization. This includes protocols for animal handling and restraint (e.g. ranging from obtunded to severely aggressive patients), premedication, method of euthanasia itself, and confirmation of death (method, as well as the number of witnesses and

their qualifications). Protocols may differ among species.

- Protocol for disposal of the carcass.

Committee members who develop the euthanasia policy may be tasked with responsibilities in its implementation, including communication of the policy within the organization and, as necessary, to a wider audience. Communication should ensure transparency and that public concerns are addressed effectively and in a culturally appropriate manner. The development and practice of talking points for staff members to follow when engaged by community members are often very helpful. Someone in the organization's leadership also will be responsible for the training of staff members in policy implementation and gathering feedback from staff and other stakeholders to inform regular review and revision of the policy.

---

**Textbox 12.1 Sample canine parvovirus (CPV) policy**

1) Puppies and dogs who present with a history and/or clinical signs suggestive of CPV must be tested with the SNAP-test kit.
   a) If the clinical signs suggest CPV but the SNAP test is negative, the clinical judgment of the veterinarian takes precedence.
   b) If the test is positive or the veterinarian considers the patient highly likely to have parvo, the patient may be admitted to the hospital if an isolation room is available, and if dedicated staff can be assigned to care for the patient. Staff resources may be needed for 24-h care for some patients.
      i. Those staff who are assigned to care for parvo patients will not work with other patients in the clinic.
      ii. Patient conditions that require 24-h care include dehydration, uncontrolled vomiting or diarrhea, risk of hyperthermia, high fever, pain, or hemorrhage.
   c) All conditions in 1.b. must be met; otherwise, the patient must be euthanized.
   d) The body must be removed and the examination area disinfected in a manner that ensures that other areas of the clinic are not contaminated, following procedures in the Biosecurity Protocol.

---

## 12.4 Patient Assessment Algorithms for Objective Decision-Making

Suffering may be defined as a state that compromises the animal's ability to eat, drink, or exercise normal behaviors; denies the individual positive social interactions; maintains the animal in a state of anxiety, fear, or other stress; or that maintains the animal in a state of illness and/or pain.

The reasons for which euthanasia may be considered fall into three general categories:

*Medical Issues*

- Suffering from disease, injury, or pain that is unlikely to be mitigated, given available resources.
- Infection with a pathogen that places other animals or people at significant risk that cannot be contained by available biosecurity resources and/or that results in severe suffering with nearly 100% fatality, such as rabies.
- Resources for management of medical conditions include veterinary competence or expertise, finances, biosecurity facilities and skills, drugs, equipment (diagnostic tools, surgical equipment, suitable hospital cages, etc.), and staff time.

*Behavioral Issues*

- Behavior indicating that the animal experiences a high degree of fear, distress, or anxiety, or that results in self-harm and that cannot be managed with available resources.
- Behavior that poses a risk to other animals or to people and that cannot be managed with available resources.
- Behavior that results in abuse, neglect, or abandonment of the animal and that makes it unlikely that the animal will find adequate guardianship or that the behavior can be managed successfully, given local resources. Note that this spills into the category of "failure of guardianship."
- Resources for management of behavioral issues include expertise of an animal behaviorist who can effectively and humanely relieve the animal of the problem, and space to hold the animal while waiting for behavior management.

*Failure of Guardianship*

- An animal's needs cannot be met due to lack of a guardian (or group of guardians) to provide adequate care.

**Textbox 12.2 Case study 1: Temporary euthanasia policy that was reversed once the disease outbreak was under control and resource allocation changed**

A low-cost veterinary clinic served a community in which vaccination rates for puppies were very low. Puppies frequently presented with signs of canine distemper (CDV). The small clinic had no space to dedicate an isolation ward. Distemper puppies were housed in carrier crates on the floor in the staff bathroom. The spread of pathogens could not be controlled. Staff tended to forget about the puppies during the course of their busy day, and these patients who should require the most intensive care for physiological support and pain management received the least. In addition, canine infectious tracheobronchitis (CITB) was a persistent problem in the clinic. Even routine sterilization patients who spent only a day in the clinic turned up coughing a few days later. The situation was not helping the distemper puppies and was causing harm to other patients and to the relationship of the clinic with the community. A management strategy was needed.

Among other measures, a temporary protocol was put in place for mobile clinic unit staff and the clinic intake staff to test all possible distemper patients with an antigen test before the patient was brought into the clinic. All patients who tested positive were euthanized immediately. Biosecurity efforts could thereby be focused and better managed. CITB cases in the clinic declined. Meanwhile, a Wendy house was donated and fitted as an isolation ward. A protocol was written and staff trained and assigned to work with isolation room patients. Once CDV was controlled in the clinic, the distemper euthanasia policy was lifted, and CDV patients were treated in the isolation ward with dedicated and properly trained staff.

**Textbox 12.3 Case study 2: Need for a policy to clarify an organization's objectives in saving animals**

A shelter took in street dogs, as the organization feared that the dogs would be struck by cars, poisoned, or misused by locals if they remained at large. Some of these were adult dogs who had lived their entire lives in the streets. They were not accustomed to captivity and huddled in the back of their kennels day in and day out. No one ever saw them move. They crept forth during the night to eat from the bowls that staff left for them. They lost their fur, and their skin turned black from chronic and sustained stress. The shelter staff were afraid of them, and their kennels could not be kept sanitary. The staff began to think that this behavior and appearance were normal for caged dogs, and, consequently, thought nothing of it when their own dogs at home declined in their cages. The director acknowledged that the dogs were unhappy, but felt that it was still better for them to live safely indoors than to risk the perils of street life.

This case falls into the categories of Behavior Problem and Lack of Adequate Guardianship. The shelter's treatment of the dogs also set an example of very poor animal guardianship for local people in the community. It would have been helpful for the Board of Directors to convene a committee to discuss the quality of life for the shelter's animals. A neutral facilitator would probably have been needed, as this was clearly an emotionally charged issue. A resulting position statement regarding quality of life could subsequently guide an evaluation of the organization's resources for provision of adequate care, as well as options for release of animals who could not cope in a captive environment. Discussion and agreement among stakeholders regarding the position statement would then also pave the way to a rational conversation to develop a euthanasia policy.

- Adequate care (guardianship) is defined as the provision of healthy food and water; shelter; opportunity for species-specific, natural behaviors, and social engagement; an environment in which the animal feels safe and is free from anxiety or fear; and adequate veterinary care.

Algorithms with which to navigate assessment criteria for a given patient, or for the development of a euthanasia policy are presented in Appendices 12. A–12.C. These are written with the intention that each decision is made on the basis of the unique condition and circumstances of the individual patient, with full respect for sentience and individuality. They are also written to allow flexibility in given resources and are designed to encourage constant reevaluation of the patient's condition and available resources. They provide a template from which each organization may develop its own decision tree to fit local conditions.

The guardians' concerns, input, and permission should be solicited whenever possible. Guardians may require guidance in the decision-making process, which may help them to feel more reassured that the decision was the correct one. In most regions, dogs and cats are the property of the owner, and the owner's permission to euthanize must therefore be obtained on legal grounds. This should be recorded as part of the patient's medical record. That said, there may be extreme circumstances in which the guardians cannot be reached or refuse to grant permission for a veterinary team to alleviate an animal's distress. Legal measures should be taken wherever these are supported by local legislation. It must be acknowledged that the veterinarian's professional judgment and careful documentation of rationale and procedure may take precedent in some of these situations.

The decision process begins with Question 1: Does the animal have a medical condition that is causing him or her to suffer? If the animal is suffering, then the patient's prognosis is usually the next question. The prognosis may depend, at least in part, on the resources available for treatment of the condition. These may include expertise of the veterinary staff, equipment, drugs, and personnel available to provide intensive care.

The terms "suffering" and "distress" must be defined with care and clear guidelines for the evaluation of suffering included in standard clinical protocols through pain scores, behaviors, and physiological criteria. All efforts must be made to relieve any degree of suffering as well as possible with medications, physiological stabilization, emotional support, and physical comfort. A critical question regarding resources is whether those available are sufficient to mitigate an unavoidable period of suffering to a tolerable level. Constant reevaluation of the situation is imperative in these instances.

Diseases that pose a threat to other animals or people warrant an entire arm of the decision tree

and require first of all that resources are available to protect others from exposure to pathogens. Euthanasia decisions about potentially rabid animals should follow international guidelines and local laws [3]. Again, availability of resources to provide adequate care of patients is a key question for animals that are under observation for following rabies exposure, as for patients who present with canine distemper or parvoviruses (see Textbox 12.2). Inadequate space, personnel, and ability to ensure adequate welfare of a quarantined patient are often serious restrictions.

Medical, and very often behavioral, problems may be associated with failures of guardianship. The concurrence of these factors underlines the importance of taking a careful patient history that includes information about the patient's living conditions at home and who takes responsibility for the daily care of the animal. A dog may be presented with a crushed leg, for example. Working through Question 1, one may conclude that the dog has a medical condition that is not a threat to others, and although we do not have the means to repair the bone, we can amputate the limb, control pain, and keep the dog comfortable during recovery. The period of suffering is therefore expected to be brief, but then there is the question of the dog's quality of life thereafter. What caused the leg to be crushed? Was it an accident that is unlikely to happen again? Does someone at home abuse the dog? Is the dog likely to run under the wheels of a car again? Is the dog used in dog-fighting? Alternatively, is the guardian comfortable with a three-legged dog, or will the dog be mistreated because of the abnormality? Question 3, regarding quality of guardianship, is therefore an important extension of the evaluation.

Behavioral problems must always first be evaluated for underlying medical conditions. Pain is a common cause for behaviors that are problematic for people or other animals: e.g. aggression, short temper, nipping at children, or inappropriate elimination. Pain may also cause animals to become self-destructive or depressed. If medical issues can be ruled out, the next question is whether the behavior places the animal at risk for chronic suffering or misuse at the hands of people, or if he or she is dangerous to others. Again, resources then become the critical issue: does the organization have the resources to treat the animal's problem? Resources may require the expertise and time of a skilled behaviorist, finances to support such expertise, and space in a place that ensures the welfare of the patient while under treatment. The time and willingness of the guardian to learn to work with the animal are also important, as is staff time for follow-up monitoring. If the animal is not safe at home, then resource questions arise pertaining to confiscation, sheltering, and rehoming for the patient.

---

**Textbox 12.4 Case study 3: Sometimes a clear case for euthanasia warrants a second look**

An injured dog was found in a ditch and taken to a small charity clinic. The dog was severely dehydrated, hypothermic, septic, and barely conscious. One limb had been torn off and the wound infested with maggots. The hip joint on the same side was damaged. Her jaw had been broken and many teeth knocked out. Scars and injuries identified her as having been used in the local dog-fighting rings. Clinical evaluation of her physical condition gave her a guarded prognosis, with the added complication that her medical care and surgery would be expensive. Given that she had been a fighting dog, her behavior and personality may also make it difficult to rehome her. The staff set about stabilizing her physiologically and controlling her pain while they waited for the key decision-maker to arrive at the clinic. By the time she arrived, the dog was feeling a bit stronger. She flipped her tail in a weak wag on the blanket when the director arrived, and licked her hand.

The dog's will to live and her demonstration of a favorable attitude even to strangers cast doubt on the prognosis for a poor quality of life if she could be saved. She had suffered badly, but her distress was now manageable. Her story was told as part of a campaign against dog fighting and brought a great deal of public support to the organization. She paid for her own veterinary care and beyond that with the donations that her story elicited. Here, what appeared initially to have been a clear case for euthanasia on the basis of a medical condition and potential depletion of limited resources turned out to have been reversible.

---

The objective structure of this kind of decision tree can relieve some of the emotional burden from the necessity to make a decision about euthanasia, regardless of the final choice. At the very least, it guides decision-makers through a thoughtful evaluation of the patient, as well as of the organization's facilities, staff skills, and other resources needed to care for patients effectively and responsibly. Moreover, it may help to ensure a thorough evaluation of factors that may be overlooked in a complicated case.

Nonetheless, every euthanasia decision, regardless of how objectively it may be achieved, carries its emotional toll. Support structures for those who implement the organization's euthanasia policy can make the difference between a long and productive career in animal welfare or an abbreviated and devastated one.

## 12.5 Euthanasia Methods

The performance of euthanasia requires that all efforts are made to alleviate the distress of the patient. Distress is the inability of an animal to cope with stressors and is manifested as profound physiological, emotional, and behavioral changes. By definition of the need to euthanize a patient, that patient is already suffering profound stress or even distress. The immediate conditions of handling and restraint and the method of euthanasia itself must reduce that level of distress rather than exacerbate it.

A euthanasia procedure must be properly planned and prepared to ensure that it is an experience free of distress for the patient. Euthanasia should only be attempted once the risks for potential complications are mitigated and addressed. This requires that the personnel who conduct euthanasia are well trained and thoroughly familiar with the method that will be used. It requires that all technical preparations are made before the animal is even approached. Restraint must be skilled to ensure safety and alleviation of distress. One should always ask oneself what could go wrong, and then make preparations to avoid, or effectively mitigate, those complications.

Distress of the guardian or other people participating in the euthanasia procedure must also be considered. If the patient's guardians would like to be present, they should understand what to expect at each stage of the process and be guided as to what the patient needs from them. Euthanasia should always be performed in a quiet, calm place, and if guardians are present, their privacy is imperative.

Paramount to the process of preparation for euthanasia and performance of the procedure itself are the criteria that the patient must not suffer fear, distress, pain, or discomfort from the experience. The method itself must produce rapid loss of consciousness (ideally within 7 s), followed immediately by death, and must be irreversible.

These criteria pertain to the euthanasia of single individuals, as well as to the euthanasia of groups of animals. They apply equally to an abandoned mongrel as they do to a beloved family pet. Whether a question of ethics or procedure, the immediate circumstances of the situation must never be used as a reason to relax standards or to risk suffering of an individual.

This statement may seem pedantic or even insulting to some readers. Sadly, the necessity for its expression arises from long experience by the author with international veterinary staff whose standards of practice degrade when they work in so-called developing regions. Such behavior teaches colleagues that animals do not deserve respect and that the veterinary profession operates on a sliding scale of ethics. It also trains us to lose compassion. From there, it is a rapid slide into compassion fatigue, broader unprofessional conduct, and even cruel behavior.

## 12.5.1 Preparation for Euthanasia

A quiet space that is away from other animals and unknown people is the ideal setting for euthanasia. While we do not often have the luxury of a dedicated euthanasia area, a resourceful attitude will always find or create a space that is relatively private. The patient should be protected from stressful sights, sounds, and smells. Similarly, animals must never witness the euthanasia of another animal. The process must not be a performance for people to watch unless it is organized as a structured, professional teaching experience.

Equipment that may be needed for handling and restraint should be tested to ensure that it is functional and that personnel are adept at its use (gloves, towels, leash, muzzle, cage). Further preparations will include clippers or razor, drugs, syringes, IV

catheters, needles, tape, and stethoscope. Where at all possible, drugs should be calculated on the basis of measured body weight. Necessary drugs include options for sedation or anesthesia, should these be necessary. Disposal of the remains must be planned, and arrangements prepared. If biological samples are to be collected, the sample containers, labeling supplies, and storage media must be ready. A first-aid kit must be available to deal with accidental human exposure to a euthanasia or anesthetic drug. The kit should include a card that identifies the drug(s) and its effects in the local language so that, should medical treatment of a person be necessary, local physicians can treat the exposure efficiently.

## 12.5.2 The Euthanasia Procedure

The method of euthanasia may differ among locations, species, condition of the animal, and availability of local resources. In all cases, the patient's experience must receive utmost consideration to ensure a humane death.

### 12.5.2.1 Pre-euthanasia Handling and Medication

Safe and compassionate handling of the patient is paramount. The patient should be calmed as well as possible with a quiet environment and dim lighting. Where handling alone cannot relieve a patient's fear or anxiety, sedation or an anxiolytic drug should be considered. General anesthesia may be warranted in some cases, particularly if the patient poses a significant danger to personnel, e.g. where rabies is suspected.

Standard protocols for sedation or anesthesia may be used, depending on the extent of chemical restraints necessary. The combination of an opiate (butorphanol, morphine) with a benzodiazepine (diazepam, midazolam) or an alpha-2 agonist (xylazine, medetomidine, dexmedetomidine) provides a state of sedation with analgesia (neuroleptanalgesia); the benzodiazepine combination provides a particularly good anxiolytic effect. Tranquilizers such as acepromazine must not be used with the intention of calming the patient, as it causes sedation and loss of muscle control without relieving anxiety, thereby effectively intensifying anxiety. Very fearful patients, or particularly dangerous patients (e.g. suspected of being rabid), may be fully anesthetized with an injectable anesthetic combination. Ketamine combined with a benzodiazepine and/or an alpha-2 agonist, or tiletamine–zolazepam (Zoletil, Telazol) combined with an alpha-2 agonist are commonly available for this purpose.

If the euthanasia drug(s) will be administered intravenously, an intravenous catheter (IV) should be placed as soon as the patient can be safely handled. The IV catheter ensures controlled delivery of drugs without the risk of extravascular accident. Moreover, the presence of an IV catheter allows the patient to be restrained in a more relaxed and comfortable manner than if he or she has to be held very still for insertion of a needle. While expense may be a concern, allowance for an IV catheter in the euthanasia protocol to ensure a smooth procedure is well warranted.

### 12.5.2.2 Euthanasia Methods

Table 12.1 summarizes the methods of euthanasia for dogs and cats. Intravenous injection of barbiturates (e.g. pentobarbital or products that combine

**Table 12.1** Methods of euthanasia for dogs and cats, arranged according to acceptability.

| Method | Dose and route of administration | Comment |
| --- | --- | --- |
| ***Recommended method: Best practice standard*** | | |
| Pentobarbital | 60–150 mg/kg IV | Best practice standard for euthanasia. May be used as sole agent of euthanasia, or following sedation or anesthesia. Ideally administered in a concentration of 20% solution. |
| Pentobarbital combinations (e.g. Euthasol®, Euthapent®) | Per manufacturer's instructions, IV | Products that combine pentobarbital with a local anesthetic, CNS depressant, or metabolic precursor to pentobarbital may be used as the sole agent of euthanasia, or following sedation or anesthesia. |
| ***Acceptable under certain conditions*** | | |
| Pentobarbital, IP | Double IV dose, administered IP | For very small patients, e.g. newborn kittens and puppies. Pretreatment with a neuroleptanalgesic, anesthesia, or minimally with IP lidocaine will help to relieve peritoneal discomfort. Time to loss of consciousness delayed to minutes. |
| Pentobarbital, intraorgan | Intracardiac, intrahepatic, intraosseous Double IV dose | Patients must be anesthetized to a surgical plane of anesthesia or deeper prior to administration, with the possible exception of cats (see text). Must not be performed on animals who are conscious, able to feel pain, or only sedated/tranquilized. |
| Overdose of injectable anesthetic compounds, e.g. propofol, thiopental | IV | Usually requires a large volume of drug. Perhaps suitable for patients who are already anesthetized. Risk that patient will recover. Addition of a neuromuscular blocking agent, KCl, $MgSO_4$, or pentobarbital often necessary. Great care must be taken to ensure that patient has truly deceased and will not recover. |
| Overdose of inhalant anesthetic agent, e.g. halothane, isoflurane, enflurane, sevoflurane | Inhaled | Requires high concentration to be effective and risks patient recovery. Great care must be taken to ensure that patient has truly deceased and will not recover. Perhaps suitable for patients who are already anesthetized. Addition of a neuromuscular blocking agent, KCl, $MgSO_4$, or pentobarbital is often necessary. |
| KCl, following general anesthesia | 1–2 mmol/kg (75–150 mg/kg) IV | Causes cardiac and respiratory arrest. May be used only in patients anesthetized to a surgical plane of anesthesia or deeper. May not be used in patients who are conscious, able to feel pain, or who are only sedated/tranquilized. |

**Table 12.1** *(Continued)*

| Method | Dose and route of administration | Comment |
|---|---|---|
| $MgSO_4$, following general anesthesia | 1.5–3 ml/kg of an 83% (saturated) solution = 1.25–2.5 g/kg | Causes cardiac and respiratory arrest. May be used only in patients anesthetized to a surgical plane of anesthesia or deeper. May not be used in patients who are conscious, able to feel pain, or who are only sedated/tranquilized. |
| T61, following general anesthesia | 0.3 ml/kg IV | Combination of opiate, neuromuscular blocking agent, and local anesthetic. Can cause severe pain prior to loss of consciousness, therefore may be used only in patients anesthetized to a surgical plane of anesthesia or deeper. May not be used in patients who are conscious, able to feel pain, or who are only sedated/tranquilized. |
| Exsanguination, following general anesthesia | | May be used only in patients anesthetized to a surgical plane of anesthesia or deeper. May not be used in patients who are conscious, able to feel pain, or who are only sedated/tranquilized. Considered acceptable only if there is no other humane option. Death occurs slowly. Emotionally traumatizing to personnel. |
| Bullet to the brain | | Only acceptable if performed by a trained person, with precise placement of the bullet. Considered acceptable only if there is no other humane option. Instant death if done correctly. Emotionally traumatizing and potentially dangerous to personnel. |

***Not acceptable under any conditions***

All of the following methods cause intense physical and emotional suffering and must never be used as a method of euthanasia. Some of these methods are described in the literature as acceptable under certain conditions, but in practical field application they are wrought with error and uncontrollable conditions. Therefore, these are categorized in the standards set out in this manual as unacceptable.

Burning
Carbon dioxide ($CO_2$) inhalation
Carbon monoxide (CO) inhalation
Chloral hydrate (oral or parenteral)
Crushing
Cyanide
Decompression (hypoxia)
Dismemberment
Drowning
Drugs – administration of any drugs other than those approved for euthanasia, as listed above
Electrocution
Ether (inhaled, oral, injected)
Hanging
Household chemicals
Hyperthermia

Hypothermia (freezing)
Magnesium sulfate ($MgSO_4$) without prior general anesthesia
Neuromuscular blocking agents without prior general anesthesia
Nitrogen ($N_2$), nitrogen/argon ($N_2/Ar$), or nitric oxide ($N_2O$) gas inhalation
Organophosphates and other pesticides
Potassium chloride (KCl) without prior general anesthesia
Rodenticide poison (Coumadin, warfarin, zinc phosphide)
Stabbing
Strangulation
Strychnine
Suffocation
T61 without prior general anesthesia

IV = intravenous
IP = intraperitoneal.

pentobarbital with a local anesthetic, CNS depressants, or metabolic precursors to pentobarbital) is the preferred method for dogs and cats. When administered appropriately, these products induce unconsciousness and death quickly and painlessly, without the risk of neurological excitement. Death results from cessation of breathing and cardiac arrest as a result of CNS depression, following loss of consciousness. Intravenous administration of barbiturates may therefore be used as the sole agent for euthanasia, or following sedation or general anesthesia. Pentobarbital is dosed at 60–150 mg/kg IV for euthanasia. These and other drugs sold specifically for euthanasia are usually subjected to strict licensing and accounting requirements.

If intravenous administration is not feasible due to the small size of the patient (e.g. newborns or small puppies and kittens), intraperitoneal administration of sodium pentobarbital or secobarbital is acceptable, generally dosed at twice the recommended intravenous dose. (Note: intraperitoneal administration has not been approved for pentobarbital-combination products.) Coadministration of lidocaine will help to relieve any peritoneal discomfort that has been observed in some animals with this route [4]. The disadvantage of this method is that the drug may take a few minutes rather than seconds before it is absorbed and induces unconsciousness. This effect must be weighed against the distress of handling for an alternative method (e.g. intraosseous administration or an inhaled drug).

In larger individuals for whom intravenous access is not possible, intraosseous or intraorgan administration of barbiturate products may be appropriate. With the exception of intrahepatic injection in cats, these options are appropriate only for unconscious animals, i.e. anesthetized in a deep surgical plane of anesthesia. Guidelines for the precise location of injection are illustrated in the *AVMA Guidelines for the Euthanasia of Animals* [5]. Intraosseous administration, usually accessed at the greater trochanter of the humerus, is readily achieved with a hypodermic needle in very young or very small animals. Alternatively, a Jamshidi bone marrow needle is usually suitable. An intracardiac injection is guided by the intersection of the fifth intercostal space and the point of the elbow with the animal in right lateral recumbency. Intrahepatic administration in dogs is similarly performed with the patient in right lateral recumbency, at the caudoventral point of the rib cage. If cats are comfortable being held and caressed in an upright position (spine vertical rather than horizontal), intrahepatic injection of a barbiturate product combined with lidocaine is acceptable without prior anesthesia, provided that the administrator is appropriately trained and experienced, and that the cat is calm.

Barbiturate products are not available in some regions of the world. The most reliable alternative in this case is to fully anesthetize the patient, ensuring that he or she reaches a deep surgical plane of anesthesia, with no physical or physiological response to pain (e.g. rise in heart rate or breathing in response to toe pinch), and complete loss of reflexes. Once this plane is reached, a neuromuscular blocking agent such as potassium chloride (KCl; 1–2 mmol/kg = 75–150 mg/kg IV, or 1–2 ml/kg body weight of a 10% solution) or magnesium sulfate ($MgSO_4$; 1.5–3 ml/kg of an 83% (saturated) solution) may be administered intravenously.

KCl, $MgSO_4$, and neuromuscular blocking agents such as nicotine or curariform agents cause respiratory or cardiac arrest without prior loss of consciousness. Therefore, they must never be used in conscious animals.

Overdose with other anesthetic drugs may be appropriate, provided that euthanasia can be ensured and that the process is painless and does not induce convulsions or other undesirable effects. Propofol, thiopental, or combinations of ketamine with an alpha-2 agonist are sometimes used. These options often require administration of a second drug, such as a barbiturate or a neuromuscular blocking agent, to affect death. Verification of death must be done very carefully, as an attempt at euthanasia with anesthetic overdose may result only in a very deep plane of anesthesia with a temporary cessation of respiration and heartbeat, and the animal may later wake up.

T61 is a euthanasia cocktail that is legal in some countries. It may be administered intravenously only in unconscious animals (0.3 ml/kg IV). It must not be used as the sole agent of euthanasia, as peripheral paralysis may occur prior to unconsciousness and death. For similar reasons, neuromuscular blocking agents must never be administered simultaneously with a barbiturate.

Inhaled anesthetics are not generally advised, as they often irritate the mucous membranes, and animals may struggle and panic if forced into a chamber or mask. It may be effective if administered to unconscious animals. Like overdose with injectable anesthetic drugs, overdose with inhalant anesthetics must be carefully verified to ensure that the patient is not only in a deep plane of anesthesia from which he or she may emerge.

Inhaled gases other than anesthetics are not acceptable for euthanasia. These include carbon dioxide ($CO_2$), carbon monoxide or vehicle exhaust, nitrogen-containing gases ($N_2$, nitrogen–argon combinations, nitric acid), and ether. These gases may be irritating to the mucous membranes and cause animals to express agitation and distress for a prolonged period until loss of consciousness. Death is caused ultimately by hypoxia. Sick and very young animals are often resistant to hypoxia, which prolongs time to effect even further. Administration of these gases also poses a significant hazard to personnel.

Exsanguination must be done only on fully anesthetized animals. The advantage of a physical method may be to avoid a drug residue in the carcass, but the necessity to render the animal unconscious with anesthesia prior to inducing death defeats this justification. Electrocution may, in theory, also be used for anesthetized patients, but in practice this rarely goes according to the plan, and is distressing to the administrators, and is therefore classified as unacceptable. A bullet shot to the brain may be considered an acceptable method if the administrator is properly skilled, the bullet is placed precisely, and there is no risk that the patient will move and cause the bullet to be misplaced. The risk to personnel with this method must also be considered.

It is never acceptable to kill an animal with any method that causes pain, convulsions, physiological suffering, prolonged death, injury, fear, or other forms of distress. These restrictions include drowning, suffocation, freezing, the use of household chemicals, pesticides and other poisons, drugs other than those prescribed specifically for euthanasia, strangulation, hanging, starvation, oxygen deprivation, burning, decompression, compression, or mutilation.

Unacceptable methods include neuromuscular blocking agents and other drugs that cause cardiopulmonary arrest prior to loss of consciousness or drugs such as strychnine that cause seizures and other neurologic distress. Drugs that cause an animal to die of chronic hemorrhage, such as Coumadin, must also never be used. The use of T61 without prior anesthesia is also not permissible, as it can cause severe pain and cardiopulmonary arrest prior to loss of consciousness.

### 12.5.2.3 Euthanasia of Fetuses

The question often arises as to whether fetuses that are removed in the course of an ovariohysterectomy should be left to die within the hypoxic uterus or whether they must be euthanized individually. Arguments based on estimations of when a living being achieves consciousness and sentience suggest that fetuses of altricial species such as dogs and cats do not become conscious until they first draw breath, or even later in the postnatal period, and that they do not suffer when left within the excised uterus to expire [6]. Neonates are notoriously resistant to hypoxia and may take up to an hour to die this way. More conservative perspectives suggest that responsiveness to stimuli, and therefore a certain degree of sentience, may occur already in utero and that a prolonged death by hypoxia once the uterus has been removed from the mother's circulatory system may be unacceptable if there is even a possibility that the fetuses have some level of awareness. Proponents of the latter argument suggest that fetuses older than about 4 weeks of pregnancy must be ensured humane euthanasia. The prevailing method for this is the gentle intraperitoneal injection of a barbiturate or other appropriate anesthetic drug.

### 12.5.3 Confirmation of Death

Death must be confirmed carefully for each individual patient on the basis of the loss of vital signs over a period of time that precludes survival. The loss of a single vital sign alone does not confirm death. Cessation of heartbeat by auscultation is monitored for at least a full minute, and signs of respiration for twice that long. All reflexes must cease: there must be no blink response to a tap in the medial canthus of the eye (palpebral reflex), nor a twitch in response to a firm pinch on or between the toes (pain response). Mucous membranes turn gray, and the pupil fixes in a central position. Finally, the cornea is tapped to test for a corneal reflex. (Note that the latter must never be done on an animal who is expected to live.) Ideally, two people verify each other's observations before death is declared.

---

**Textbox 12.5 Physical parameters for confirmation of death**

- No movement of the chest or other visible signs of respiration
- No heartbeat audible by auscultation for at least 60 s
- No pulse
- No palpebral reflex or toe pinch response
- Loss of mucous membrane color
- Pupil fixed centrally
- Eyes glazed
- No corneal reflex (blink)
- Rigor mortis.*

*\* If death cannot be confirmed, or if there is any doubt, wait until rigor mortis is observed before disposing of the animal's body.*

---

### 12.5.4 Disposal of Remains and Record-Keeping

Drugs that the patient may have received prior to death (e.g. antibiotics, anti-inflammatory drugs, anesthetic agents) as well the euthanasia drugs themselves can be very dangerous for scavengers who may ingest drug residues with the patient's remains. Consequent death of protected wildlife species may constitute a criminal offense by the person responsible for the drugs and the carcass. Pathogens carried by the deceased patient may spread to other animals, including wildlife and humans.

Incineration of a patient's remains is the best reassurance that scavengers and people are not at the risk of accidental exposure to drugs or pathogens. Where this is not possible, the body should be buried deeply, according to local laws or regulations. Carcasses that are picked up by other agencies for disposal must be bagged and labeled appropriately to protect personnel.

Biological samples, photographs, or other records may be needed prior to carcass disposal for testing or for forensic documentation of evidence for legal proceedings. Animals euthanized under suspicion of rabies must be submitted for testing and disposed of according to local laws. Use of any controlled drugs for euthanasia must also be recorded according to law and the organization's protocols.

## 12.6 Conclusion

Euthanasia is one of the saddest and most distressing responsibilities in our profession as we assume direct and personal responsibility for the cessation of a sentient life. Death is a devastating outcome for the patients entrusted to our care and for the animals who are loved by their people. It often feels like a failure in our competence as veterinarians and in our commitment to guardianship of life.

The option of euthanasia to relieve immutable suffering is, nonetheless, an option that is denied to human medicine and that our profession is uniquely entrusted to use with responsibility and compassion. We must, above all, do no harm, until the final moment of a patient's life.

Veterinarians and veterinary nurses personify the standard for animal welfare and attitudes toward animals in a community. When we serve among people who struggle to appreciate the sentience of animals, every interaction that we share with or about an animal can shape the manner in which a community treats its animals. In a One Welfare paradigm, our actions are thereby powerful drivers of the social and physical health of communities. The professionalism, respect, and compassion that we demonstrate for an animal in the process of ending his or her life should reflect our attitudes toward the living and for the world that we would like to see for animals and people sharing the planet.

# Appendix 12.A   Euthanasia Algorithm – Medical Conditions

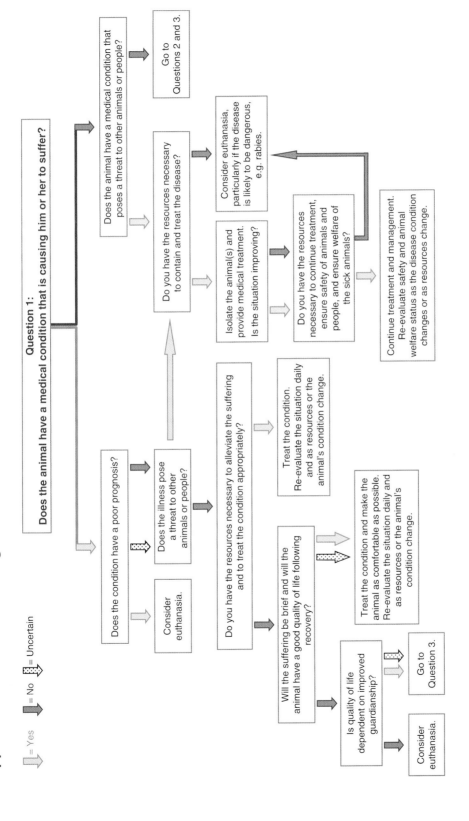

# Appendix 12.B   Euthanasia Algorithm – Behavioral Problems

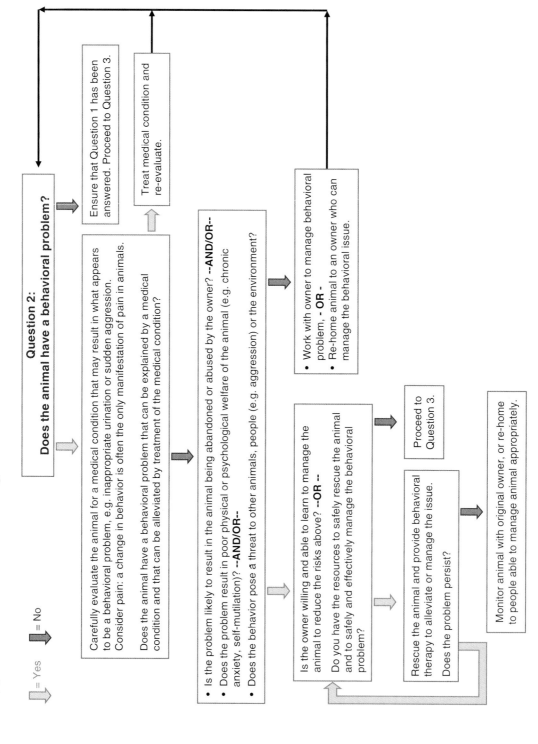

# Appendix 12.C  Euthanasia Algorithm – Inadequate Guardianship

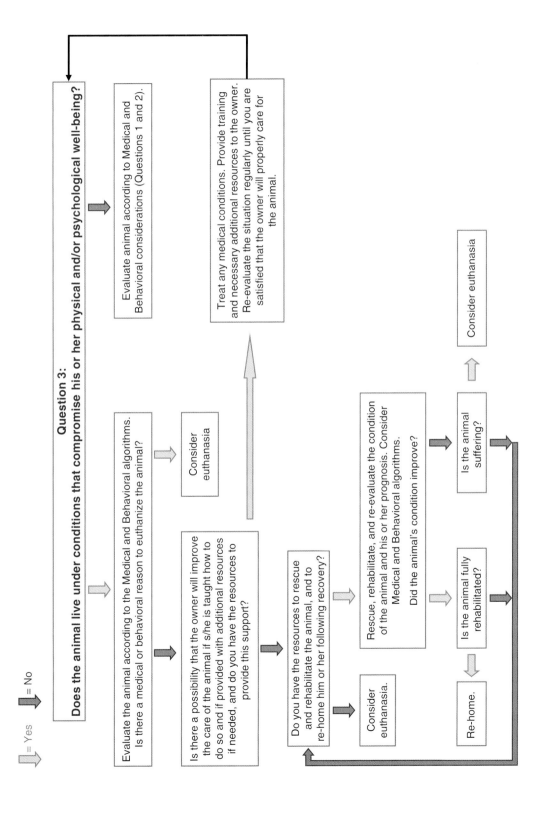

## References

1 Shelter Animals Count (2017). The Asilomar Accords. www.asilomaraccords.org (accessed 4 April 2017).

2 International Companion Animal Management Coalition (2010). The welfare basis for euthanasia of dogs and cats and policy development. http://www .icam-coalition.org/downloads/ICAM-Euthanasia% 20Guide-ebook.pdf (accessed 19 January 2017).

3 Brown, C.M., Slavinski, S., Ettestad, P. et al. (2016). Compendium of animal rabies prevention and control, 2016. *Journal of the American Veterinary Medical Association* **248** (5): 505–517.

4 National Research Council of the National Academies (2008). Recognition and Alleviation of Distress in Laboratory Animals. Washington, DC: The National Academies Press http://www.nap.edu/ catalog/11931.html (accessed 22 May 2017).

5 Leary, S., Underwood, W., Anthony, R. et al. (2013). AVMA Guidelines for the Euthanasia of Animals: 2013 Edition. Schaumburg, IL: American Veterinary Medical Association.

6 White, S.C. (2012). Prevention of fetal suffering during ovariohysterectomy of pregnant animals. *Journal of the American Veterinary Medical Association* **240** (10): 1160–1163.

# 13

## Treatment Protocols

*Katherine Polak,[1] Jennifer Landis,[2] Natasha Lee,[3] Kate Kuzminski,[4] and Ahne Simonsen[4]*

[1]Four Paws International, 11th Floor B, Gypsum Metropolitan Tower, 539/2 Sri Ayudhaya Road, Thanon Phaya Thai, Ratchathewi, Bangkok 10400 Thailand
[2]Animal Welfare Consultant, PO Box 74621, Phoenix, AZ 85087, USA
[3]Asia Animal Happiness, Jalan Kerja Ayer Lama, Ampang Jaya, Ampang, Selangor 68000, Malaysia
[4]Humane Society Veterinary Medical Association – Rural Area Veterinary Services (HSVMA-RAVS), PO Box 1589, Felton, CA 95018, USA

## 13.1 Introduction

Providing veterinary care in regions that are geographically remote or economically challenged requires a willingness to think creatively about treatment strategies. Medical conditions that are easily treatable in a traditional veterinary clinic are frequently chronic and life-threatening by the time patients present to field clinics; this is often due to a lack of routine access to veterinary care, propensity for traumatic injuries, and a lack of responsible animal guardianship in the community. Those working in limited resourced field conditions, including animal shelters, often find themselves in challenging situations attempting to manage compromised patients with a myriad of exceptionally challenging medical conditions. Clinician unfamiliarity with many of the diseases seen in field clinic settings and a need for designing treatment plans for animals unfamiliar with handling and restraint are additional complicating factors.

The treatment protocols included in this chapter are based on conditions and diseases that practitioners reported managing most frequently in the field. This is not a complete list, however. Furthermore, the authors attempted to address the lack of advanced diagnostic and treatment modalities and focus on the curative rather than preventive aspects of diseases encountered. The authors also compiled both gold standard treatment recommendations and alternative protocols, which may be more accessible, practical, economical, and welfare-conscious depending on the situation. Note that the protocols included here are derived from a variety of sources, some of which are anecdotal. The authors recognize that some treatments may be controversial, or lack clinical data to support their use. Clinicians should use their best judgment while choosing the treatment plan for their patient, given the status of the patient, available resources, owner wishes, cultural considerations, and follow-up care available.

### Abbreviations used

*Units*

| | |
|---|---|
| kg | Kilogram |
| g | Gram |
| mg | Milligram |
| µg (mcg) | Microgram |
| ng | Nanogram |
| lb | Pound |
| oz | Ounce |
| l | Liter |
| ml | Milliliter |

*Administration route*

| | |
|---|---|
| AU | Both ears |
| ID | Intradermal |
| IM | Intramuscular |
| IV | Intravenous |
| OU | Both eyes |

*Field Manual for Small Animal Medicine*, First Edition. Edited by Katherine Polak and Ann Therese Kommedal.
© 2018 John Wiley & Sons, Inc. Published 2018 by John Wiley & Sons, Inc.

| PO | Per mouth |
|----|-----------|
| SC | Subcutaneous |
| TM | Transmucosal |

*For certain drugs*

| NSAID | Nonsteroidal anti-inflammatory drug |
|-------|-------------------------------------|
| OTC | Over-the-counter |

*For certain diagnostics*

| ALP | Alkaline phosphatase |
|-----|----------------------|
| ALT | Alanine aminotransferase |
| BAL | Bronchoalveolar lavage |
| BUN | Blood urea nitrogen |
| CBC | Complete blood count |
| CSF | Cerebral spinal fluid |
| ELISA | Enzyme-linked immunosorbent assay |
| IFA | Indirect immunofluorescent assay |
| PCR | Polymerase chain reaction |
| POC | Point-of-care |
| USG | Urine specific gravity |

*For certain diseases*

| ASD | Anal sac disease |
|-----|------------------|
| CDV | Canine distemper virus |
| CIRDC | Canine infectious respiratory disease complex |
| CPV | Canine parvovirus |
| CHF | Congestive heart failure |
| FAD | Flea allergy dermatitis |
| FeLV | Feline leukemia virus |
| FIV | Feline immunodeficiency virus |
| FPV | Feline panleukopenia |
| FLUTD | Feline lower urinary tract disease |
| URI | Upper respiratory infection |

*Dosing*

| h | Hour |
|---|------|
| q8h | Every 8 hours |
| q12h | Every 12 hours |
| q24h | Every 24 hours |
| q48h | Every 48 hours |

*Physical examination*

| HR | Heart rate |
|----|------------|
| RR | Respiratory rate |
| CRT | Capillary refill time |

*Organizations and activities*

| AHS | American Heartworm Society |
|-----|----------------------------|
| NGO | Nongovernmental organization |
| TNR | Trap–neuter–return |
| USDA | United States Department of Agriculture |

## 13.2 Cardiology

### 13.2.1 Heartworm Disease

#### 13.2.1.1 General Information

Canine heartworm disease is caused by *Dirofilaria immitis*, a parasitic filarial nematode. *D. immitis* is transmitted by over 70 species of mosquitoes and has been found in more than 30 species of animals, including domestic cats, dogs, and humans [1]. Heartworm disease has been reported as an increasingly important zoonotic disease in tropical and subtropical areas [2]. The domestic dog and wild canid are the definitive host for *D. immitis*. Heartworm-infected dogs remain a significant source of infection to other susceptible hosts in the community. Disease transmission requires an appropriate mosquito vector, an infected host, and suitable climatic conditions. The disease is regionally endemic in many parts of the world including most of the United States, Central and South America, coastal Africa, southern regions of Europe, Asia, and Australia [3,4].

Mature heartworms live in the heart and pulmonary arteries and, when left untreated, can cause serious heart, lung, and systemic diseases. Clinical signs are often absent unless the worm burden becomes significant for the size of the host, the host is sensitive to the parasite, or the infected animal is very active [1]. The American Heartworm Society (AHS) classifies clinical signs into four stages [5]. The higher the class, the more severe the disease (Table 13.1).

Although migration of heartworms can cause lesions throughout the body, the primary cause of

Table 13.1 Summary of clinical signs of canine heartworm disease.

| Mild (Class 1) | Asymptomatic or occasional coughing |
|----------------|-------------------------------------|
| Moderate (Class 2) | Mild-to-moderate symptoms including occasional coughing and exercise intolerance |
| Severe (Class 3) | General loss of body condition, persistent coughing, severe exercise intolerance, syncope, and ascites |
| Caval syndrome (Class 4) | Severe lethargy, dyspnea, tachypnea, tachycardia, collapse. Anemia and hemoglobinuria often present |

Source: Adapted from American Heartworm Society 2014 [5].

disease to the host is the damage that occurs to the pulmonary arteries and lungs. The worms trigger an inflammatory response from vascular damage as well as eosinophilia, which can lead to eosinophilic pneumonitis. *Wolbachia pipientis*, an intracellular Gram-negative bacterium, has an endosymbiotic relationship with *D. immitis* and is essential for the worm's survival. *Wolbachia* likely has a critical role in the inflammatory conditions experienced in heartworm disease. Antimicrobial treatment with tetracyclines to eliminate *Wolbachia* results in sterility and eventual death of female heartworms. Doxycycline has been shown to eliminate or reduce up to 95% of *Wolbachia* organisms for 12 months [6,7].

### 13.2.1.2 Diagnostics

*Antigen testing.* The recommended screening tool is the use of antigen tests that detect a glycoprotein secreted by female heartworms. Several commercially available tests provide excellent sensitivity and specificity when at least three female heartworms are present [1,8,9]. False positives are rare.

False negatives can occur when there are:

- Low worm burdens
- Immature female heartworms
- Presence of only male heartworms or microfilariae
- Inappropriate use of test kit
- Presence of antigen–antibody complexes.

Note: Antigen tests do not detect microfilariae or male heartworms. Antigenemia may also be suppressed for up to 9 months postinfection if treated with monthly heartworm preventive. There is also no need to antigen test a dog less than 7 months of age.

*Microfilaria testing.* Another screening test involves the identification of microfilariae on blood smears by placing a drop of anticoagulated whole blood on a microscope slide and examining the sample on low power. False negatives may occur in up to 80% of heartworm-infected dogs [1]. To reduce false-negative results, use 1 ml of blood and a procedure that concentrates the blood, such as a modified Knott's test or a filtration system. This testing should be performed in tandem with antigen testing.

*Imaging.* Although likely unavailable in field situations, imaging can be a useful diagnostic. In severe disease, radiographs will show right heart enlargement and enlarged, tortuous pulmonary lobar arteries, particularly in the caudal lobes.

### 13.2.1.3 Treatment Protocols

The goal of treatment is to eliminate all life stages of the heartworm while improving the clinical status of the patient. If a patient is showing severe clinical signs of heartworm disease, it is essential to stabilize the patient before initiating heartworm treatment protocols.

Treating canine heartworm disease involves:

- Heartworm preventive
- Adulticidal therapy
- Antimicrobial therapy for *Wolbachia.*

Melarsomine, administered via deep intramuscular injection, is the only adulticidal drug approved by the Food and Drug Administration for heartworm treatment. There are two main protocols used, involving either two or three melarsomine injections. Although the AHS recommends the use of the three-dose protocol, the author recognizes that the cost and treatment timeline may be unrealistic for many agencies. These two protocols have a 90% and 98% kill rate, respectively [10, 11]. The author, therefore, recommends the following when melarsomine is available:

- Two-injection protocol for class 1 and 2 patients
- Three-injection protocol for class 3 patients.

#### 13.2.1.3.1 Gold Standard Protocols

The AHS recommends 1 month of doxycycline treatment for *Wolbachia* and 2 months of administration of a heartworm preventive before initiating adulticide therapy [5]. In field situations, this timeline may not be feasible.

1) Start treatment with monthly heartworm preventive upon diagnosis. If high microfilariae numbers, administer antihistamines or glucocorticoids before giving the first monthly preventive dose to minimize the potential for anaphylaxis from dying microfilaria. Ensure strict exercise restriction on this day.
   - Diphenhydramine (2 mg/kg IM, PO)
   - Dexamethasone (0.2 mg/kg IM, IV)
2) In highly endemic areas where animals are more likely to have significant worm burdens,

prednisone treatment should be initiated. Start treatment at 0.5 mg/kg PO q12h the first week, tapering to 0.5 mg/kg q24h the second week, and finally 0.5 mg/kg q48h for 7–14 days. Prednisone can be used in conjunction with melarsomine.

3) Administer doxycycline (10 mg/kg PO q12h) for 4 weeks for *Wolbachia* before adulticidal therapy. If doxycycline is unavailable, use minocycline at the same dose.

4) If possible, following the 4-week course of doxycycline wait 1 month before initiating melarsomine adulticide therapy. If this is not possible, begin doxycycline and prednisone at the same time the adulticide plan is initiated.

**Two-injection Protocol**  The two-injection protocol consists of two injections of melarsomine (2.5 mg/kg IM) administered 24 h apart. As described earlier, the patient should have ideally received 1 month of doxycycline and 2 months of heartworm preventive before melarsomine administration. This protocol is appropriate when there are financial constraints and mild to moderate heartworm disease.

### Day 1

**Step 1.** If the patient is not on steroid therapy, administer a nonsteroidal anti-inflammatory drug (NSAID). Options include:
- Rimadyl® (2 mg/kg SQ or PO q12h)
- Metacam® (0.1 mg/kg SQ or PO q24h).
NSAIDS should be continued for 3 days postmelarsomine injection.

**Step 2.** Prepare the patient for melarsomine injection. Sedate the patient if there is risk of movement during injection.

**Step 3.** Clip and surgically prep an area over the epaxial muscle at the level of L3–L5. Administer melarsomine 2.5 mg/kg body weight via deep IM injection into the belly of the epaxial muscle at the level of the third to fifth lumbar vertebra as shown in Figure 13.1. Change the needle between drawing up the drug and injecting it. A 22-gauge, 1.5-in. needle should be used for large dogs. Once in the muscle belly, aspirate back to ensure no blood vessel is compromised. To prevent leakage into the subcutaneous tissue, apply digital pressure over the injection site for 2 min.

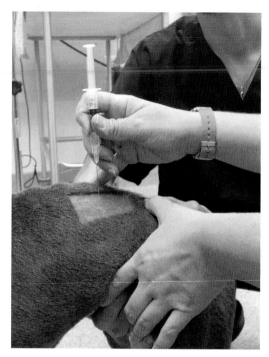

**Figure 13.1** Administration of melarsomine in the epaxial muscle at the level of L3–L5. Source: Courtesy of Dr. Brian DiGangi.

**Step 4.** Closely monitor patient for the first 24 h following adulticide treatment. Allow only short leash walks in order to urinate/defecate. Evaluate for pain, coughing/gagging, depression/lethargy, anorexia/inappetence, excessive salivation, fever, lung congestion, and vomiting.

**Day 2**  Repeat steps 2–4 using the *opposite* epaxial muscle for the melarsomine injection.

Following the second melarsomine injection, restrict patient exercise for a minimum of 1 month and repeat an antigen test in 6 months.

**Three-injection Protocol**  The three-injection protocol, also known as a split dose protocol, consists of one injection of melarsomine followed by a 30-day waiting period and then administration of two additional melarsomine injections 24 h apart. This protocol is the best approach for severe heartworm disease and should ideally occur following 1 month of doxycycline administration and 2 months of heartworm preventive.

**Day 1**  Perform steps 1–4 as described in the two-injection protocol. Restrict patient exercise until the next injection in 30 days.

**Day 30**  Repeat steps 2–4.

**Day 31**  Repeat steps 2–4 using the *opposite* epaxial muscle for the melarsomine injection.

Following the third injection, restrict patient exercise for a minimum of 30 days and repeat an antigen test in 6 months.

---

**Textbox 13.1 Recognizing signs of embolism**

Pulmonary thromboembolism (PTE) is a potential consequence of adulticide therapy. Signs of embolism include fever, cough, hemoptysis, and worsening of right heart failure. Clinical signs associated with PTE usually occur within 7–10 days of adulticide treatment but can be seen up to 4 weeks post-treatment [12]. Mild embolism may be clinically unapparent. Strict exercise restriction will reduce the risk of thromboembolic complications. If an embolic episode does occur, oxygen and steroid therapy is required.

---

#### 13.2.1.3.2 Alternative Treatment Protocols

In certain situations, especially in remote regions, adulticidal drugs (melarsomine) may be unavailable or cost prohibitive. Although not recommended by the AHS, alternative protocols have been devised to use when treatment options are limited.

**"Slow-kill" Protocol**  A "slow-kill" protocol involves the monthly administration of heartworm preventive. If used, it should be coupled with doxycycline to shorten the treatment duration. With this protocol, melarsomine is not administered and adult heartworms essentially die a natural death. This protocol is inexpensive, does not involve injections, and could result in the elimination of 95% of adult heartworms in 2–3 years [13]. However, this is not a recommended protocol in most cases as during this lengthy treatment time, infection continues and pathology may progress [14]. Exercise restriction is necessary until the heartworms have been cleared, which may be impossible given the situation.

**Step 1.**  If the patient is showing cardiac signs, stabilize before initiating heartworm treatment. If the patient is symptomatic, administer prednisone at 0.5 mg/kg PO q12h the first week and taper the dose to 0.5 mg/kg q24h the second week, followed by 0.5 mg/kg q48h for 7–14 days [5].

**Step 2.**  Administer doxycycline (10 mg/kg PO q12h) for 4 weeks. If possible, repeat every 60 days until a negative antigen test is achieved.

**Step 3.**  Start a monthly heartworm preventive such as Heartgard®. Continue for the life of the patient. Ivermectin at the heartworm preventive dose (6 μg/kg) is considered slow-kill. Slow-kill products are preferred over fast-kill products to avoid a reaction to dying microfilaria.
- Slow-kill products: Heartgard®, Revolution®, Advantage Multi®, and ProHeart 6®
- Fast-kill products: Interceptor®, Sentinel®, and Trifexis®.

An antigen test should be performed every 6 months. The patient is considered clear of disease once two negative antigen tests have been achieved 6 months apart. If the dog is still antigen positive after 1 year, repeat the doxycycline therapy. Exercise should be restricted for the duration of the treatment process.

**Ivermectin/pyrantel + Doxycycline Protocol**  Although logistically challenging in the field, a recent study found that the combination of doxycycline (10 mg/kg q24h) for 30 days and ivermectin–pyrantel (6 μg/kg of ivermectin + 5 mg/kg of pyrantel) once every 15 days for 180 days resulted in a negative microfilaria test in 90 days and antigen-negative tests in 73% of dogs [15]. This study suggests that the combination of ivermectin and doxycycline is adulticidal.

#### 13.2.1.4  Tips and Tricks from the Field

- Elective procedures including spay/neuter surgery can be safely performed on heartworm-positive dogs with absent or mild clinical signs of heartworm disease [16]. Therefore, patients should be spayed or neutered first, with administration of the first melarsomine injection immediately *after* the surgery even while the patient is still anesthetized on the surgical table. If advanced clinical signs are present, delay surgery for 6 months after the adulticide treatment.

- In absence of doxycycline or minocycline, tetracycline (10 mg/kg/day) can also be used for 30 days.
- Although not recommended by the AHS, the slow-kill protocol may be the only treatment option for many organizations. The long-term administration of a heartworm preventive, such as ivermectin, should be coupled with doxycycline whenever possible.
- Exercise restriction is mandatory following melarsomine administration to reduce the risk of PTE! This can be particularly challenging if not impossible when working with free-roaming dogs. Community caregivers or feeders can be asked to confine the patient during the post-treatment period.

---

**Textbox 13.2 Heartworm prevention**

- Start puppies on chemoprophylaxis by 8 weeks of age.
- Multiple effective heartworm preventive options exist. See Chapter 16 for cost-effective options.
- Puppies started on a heartworm preventive after 8 weeks of age should be antigen tested 6 months after the initial dose, and annually thereafter.
- Screen dogs 7 months of age and older for antigen and microfilaria before starting on a prevention program.

---

## 13.2.2 Congestive Heart Failure

### 13.2.2.1 General Information

Heart failure is a challenging condition to treat in the field as many dogs and cats lack owners to reliably provide medication, and appropriate medication and diagnostics may be unavailable. Nevertheless, congestive heart failure (CHF) is a condition that practitioners will run into from time to time and should be prepared to manage as the situation allows. Although cardiac failure is a clinically complex disease, only the basic treatment principles will be discussed here.

Heart failure by definition is a clinical syndrome in which the heart can no longer meet the circulatory demands of the body or can only meet them at high cardiac filling pressures. In dogs, mitral valve disease (MVD) and dilated cardiomyopathy (DCM) are the most common causes of heart failure [17]. Heart disease may be present without heart failure. Some cases will present with acute decompensation and others will have shown clinical signs of varying severity before presentation to the veterinarian (Table 13.2). Although CHF can be caused by many underlying disease processes, the therapeutic approach is often dictated by clinical signs and disease stage rather than by etiology.

Clinical signs of CHF will vary between cats and dogs.

#### 13.2.2.1.1 Dogs

The most common cause of heart failure in dogs is chronic degenerative MVD. Patients typically present with increased respiratory rate (RR) and effort, coughing, poor appetite, and exercise intolerance. Clinical signs are typically progressive. The respiratory signs associated with CHF must be differentiated from primary airway or respiratory disease such as

Table 13.2 Consequences of congestive heart failure.

| Low cardiac output | Left-sided congestion | Right-sided congestion |
| --- | --- | --- |
| Lethargy | Pulmonary congestion and edema (cough, tachypnea, dyspnea, orthopnea, crackles, hemoptysis, lethargy, cyanosis) | Systemic venous congestion (high central venous pressure, jugular vein distension) |
| Exercise intolerance | | |
| Weakness | | Hepatic ± splenic congestion |
| Pallor and prolonged capillary refill time | Secondary right-sided heart failure | Pleural effusion (dyspnea, orthopnea, cyanosis) |
| Syncope | Cardiac arrhythmias | Ascites |
| Prerenal azotemia | | Subcutaneous edema |
| Cardiac arrhythmias | | Cardiac arrhythmias |
| Cyanosis (poor peripheral circulation) | | Minor pericardial effusion [17] |

tracheal collapse, chronic pulmonary parenchymal disease, heartworm disease, fungal disease, and many others. Dogs with primary airway disease typically exhibit clinical signs that are intermittent or absent while resting. Dogs with CHD may have syncopal episodes and weakness. Cardiac murmurs, arrhythmias, and altered femoral pulse quality should increase the suspicion of cardiac disease.

#### 13.2.2.1.2 Cats

Primary, idiopathic hypertrophic cardiomyopathy (HCM) is the most common form of feline myocardial disease. The majority of cats with heart failure present with clinical signs relating to an impairment of left ventricular (LV) myocardial function. Physical examination of cats with CHF often reveals a systolic murmur, gallop sounds, or arrhythmias with tachypnea, dyspnea, pulmonary crackles, panting, and jugular distension [17]. In cats, other causes of pleural effusion should be ruled out including FIP (feline infectious peritonitis), trauma, heartworm disease, and lungworm infection.

#### 13.2.2.2 Diagnostics

Diagnosis is based on physical examination, auscultation, and thoracic radiographs, if available. Although ancillary diagnostics including echocardiography, electrocardiography, and blood pressure measurements are helpful, they may not be necessary to obtain a working diagnosis and design an initial treatment plan.

*Cardiovascular exam.* A thorough examination includes signalment, patient history, heart sounds (rate and rhythm), presence of murmurs, arterial pulse quality, jugular vein status (distention and pulsation), mucous membrane color, capillary refill time (CRT), and breathing pattern. In dogs with MVD or DCM, a systolic murmur can typically be heard over the left apex. Murmurs are graded from I to VI, depending on intensity.

---

**Textbox 13.3 Heart murmur grading scale [17,18]**

*Grade I*: Very soft, heard after a moment of careful listening in quiet environment
*Grade II*: Soft, easily heard
*Grade III*: Moderate intensity, easily heard
*Grade IV*: Loud, no precordial thrill
*Grade V*: Loud, palpable precordial thrill
*Grade VI*: Very loud, strong thrill, heard with stethoscope just off chest wall.

---

*Thoracic auscultation.* Careful auscultation may reveal increased bronchovesicular sounds or crackles. The point of maximal intensity (PMI) of a heart murmur may help determine the region of the defect (Table 13.3).

In dogs with MVD, the femoral pulse quality is usually normal, whereas dogs with DCM have weak or thready pulses. Jugular vein distention or pulses may be detected in cases of tricuspid valve disease, advanced MVD with pulmonary hypertension, atrial fibrillation, or DCM.

#### 13.2.2.3 Treatment Protocols

#### 13.2.2.3.1 Canine

As a general rule, all dogs with CHF due to left-sided CHF (i.e. MVD or DCM) require what is referred to as "triple therapy":

---

Table 13.3 Approximate valve locations for auscultation [17,18].

| Valve | Side | Position |
|---|---|---|
| Mitral | Left | Within the fifth intercostal space at the costochondral junction |
| Pulmonic | Left | Between the second and fourth intercostal spaces just above the sternum |
| Aortic | Left | Within the fourth intercostal space just above the costochondral junction |
| Tricuspid | Right | Between the third and fifth intercostal spaces near the costochondral junction |

Auscultation should begin at the mitral valve (M) where the PMI (point of maximal intensity) is normally located and then proceed to the aortic (A) and pulmonic valves (P).

1) Antineurohormonal drugs: ACE inhibitor (enalapril or benazepril) + spironolactone
2) Inodilator drug: pimobendan
3) Diuretic for congestion, depending on severity: furosemide.

The American College of Veterinary Internal Medicine (ACVIM) consensus statement for the treatment of heart failure in dogs with MVD offers the following general treatment guidelines [18].

Initial therapy for patients with severe disease requiring hospitalization:

- Furosemide: Initial doses of 2–4 mg/kg IV, followed by doses every 2–3 h as determined by urine output, hydration, and respiratory effort.
- Oxygen if available.
- Nitroglycerin ointment (2%) to dilate veins and lower venous pressure.
- Sedation as needed for anxious patients.
- ACE inhibitors can wait until the patient is stable and receiving oral furosemide.

Outpatient therapy[1]:

- Furosemide (1–2 mg/kg PO q12h)
- Pimobendan (0.25 mg/kg PO q12h)
- ACE inhibitor: enalapril (0.5 mg/kg PO q12h) or benazepril (0.25–0.5 mg/kg PO q24h).

### 13.2.2.3.2 Feline

Acutely decompensated cat [19]:

- Administer supplemental oxygen.
- Sedate the patient. Sedation is probably more important in cats than in dogs as they are highly prone to stress. Consider administering butorphanol (0.25 mg/kg IM).
- Furosemide IV: Initial dose no more than 2 mg/kg, every 60 min until the RRs decreases.
- Nitroglycerin ointment: One-fourth inch/cat topically applied q6–8h or 2.5 mg/24-h patch to help stabilize cats with severe pulmonary edema or effusion.
- Thoracocentesis.

Moderate congestive failure maintenance therapy:

- Furosemide (1–5 mg/kg PO q12–24h)

---

1 Note that outpatient therapy can also be used immediately for cases of mild CHF.

- Consider administering an ACE inhibitor. Benazepril (0.5 mg/kg PO q24h) should be a target dose, although dosing should be started at half this dose.
- Pimobendan (0.25–0.3 mg/kg PO q12h) appears to be helpful in the management of CHF in cats with HCM by enhancing diastolic function.

---

**Textbox 13.4 Special considerations for feline systemic thromboembolism**

Systemic thromboembolism is a common complication in cats with heart disease. A thrombus is typically formed in the left atrium and then, either in part or as a whole, dislodges and travels through the aorta distally until it reaches an artery of small enough diameter that it gets stuck. Systemic thromboembolism occurs in almost one-third of cats with heart disease. Clinical signs depend on the site of the thromboembolus. As the terminal aorta is the most common site of occlusion, most cats present for evaluation of pelvic limb paralysis or paresis. Palpation reveals that the affected limb is cool to the touch compared with the other limbs, and has firm, painful muscles. Pulses in the affected limb are typically weak or absent.

Principles of treatment include pain management, maintaining electrolyte and acid–base abnormalities, and prevention of thrombus extension. Thrombolytic therapy is controversial.

- Provide analgesia. Consider butorphanol (0.2 mg/kg SQ q8h) combined with acepromazine or epidural anesthesia
- Fluid therapy to maintain urinary output (unless pulmonary edema present)
- Antibiotic therapy with anaerobic coverage (ampicillin and amoxicillin)
- Heparin (200–300 IU/kg IV), then SQ q8h for 48–72 h

For prevention of thromboembolism, different doses of aspirin have been suggested (high dose: 40 mg/cat q72h, or low dose: 5 mg/cat q72h). More recently, clopidogrel (Plavix©) has been advocated for use over aspirin to prevent the recurrence of feline aortic thromboembolism when used at 18.75 mg PO q24h [20].

### 13.2.2.3.3 *Additional Treatment Modalities*

**Thoracocentesis** Thoracocentesis is the most effective treatment in animals with respiratory distress due to a significant volume of effusion. Perform thoracocentesis when pleural effusion is evident on radiographs, or quiet lung fields are detected on auscultation. Anxiolytic therapy should be considered for animals with severe respiratory distress secondary to CHF.

**Abdominocentesis** Ascites can lead to worsening dyspnea and discomfort. Abdominocentesis should be performed at the time of diagnosis of right heart failure if warranted. In animals with reoccurring ascites despite diuretic therapy, abdominocentesis may be performed every 1–4 weeks as needed.

**Dietary Management** Restrict salt and ensure adequate protein intake. Prescription diets for cardiac, or renal disease, and geriatric patients are best. Avoid salty table scraps and treats. A homemade diet formulated for cardiac patients may be more cost effective. See http://www.acvn.org/ for nutrition resources.

Additional considerations for any CHF patient include the following:

- Stress, excitement, and activity can be deadly in CHF patients. Consider using mild sedation or anxiolytics when indicated.
- Administer oxygen when indicated by dyspnea, mucous membrane color, and/or a low pulse oximeter reading.
- Allow the patient to assume the posture in which it is easiest to breathe.
- Maintain hydration with cautious use of IV fluids to avoid over-hydration.
- Cough suppressants should generally be avoided if coughing is due to cardiac disease.

#### 13.2.2.4 Tips and Tricks from the Field

- In general, the management is similar for non-infectious CHF regardless of the cause and in the vast majority of cases. In dogs, initiate therapy with a diuretic if indicated and begin an ACE inhibitor. Modify therapy as indicated above, which may include the addition of pimobendan.
- Many field programs are able to obtain donated cardiac medications from owners whose pets have passed away.

Table 13.4 Sedatives for CHF patients.

| | Canine dose | Feline dose |
|---|---|---|
| Butorphanol | 0.2–0.3 mg/kg SC, IM, IV | 0.2–0.25 mg/kg SC, IM, IV 0.2 mg/kg IM with acepromazine |
| Diazepam | 0.2 mg/kg IV | 0.2 mg/kg IV |
| Acepromazine (anxiolytic) | 0.025–0.03 mg/kg IV with buprenorphine | 0.05–0.1 mg/kg SC 0.1 mg/kg IM with butorphanol ≤1 mg total dose |
| Buprenorphine | 0.005–0.01 mg/kg IV with acepromazine | 0.005–0.01 mg/kg IV with acepromazine |
| Morphine | 0.1–0.5 mg/kg IM or SC | |

- Clinical signs of heart failure can be subtle. Thoracic radiography, if available, is aids in detecting left-sided heart failure.
- Allow clinical response to dictate treatment and adjustments of medication when diagnostics are unavailable.
- With very few exceptions, diseases causing CHF in dogs and cats are fatal. Patients should be assessed in the field in regard to ownership status, as well as medication availability.

Quick reference tables for CHF treatment (Tables 13.4 and 13.5).

## 13.3 Dermatology

### 13.3.1 Anal Sac Disease

#### 13.3.1.1 General Information

Anal sac disease (ASD) is the most common disease of the anal region in dogs [21]. Anal sacs are located in the subcutaneous tissues adjacent to the anus, at the 4 and 8 o'clock positions. Each sac has a corresponding duct leading to the anus and normal expression occurs during defecation. Anal sacs sometimes are erroneously referred to as anal glands [22].

Anal sac impaction is an abnormal accumulation of anal sac secretions that occurs secondary to inflammation (anal sacculitis), infection (anal sac abscess),

Table 13.5 Commonly used cardiac drugs [17–19].

| Medications by category | Canine dose | Feline dose |
| --- | --- | --- |
| *Diuretics* | | |
| Furosemide | 2–4 mg/kg IV, IM, SC q2h for acute therapy<br>2–4 mg/kg PO q8–24h | 2–4 mg/kg IV, IM, SC q2h for acute therapy<br>1–2 mg/kg PO q12–24h |
| Spironolactone | 0.5–1 mg/kg PO q12–24h | 0.5–1 mg/kg PO q12–24h |
| Chlorothiazide | 20–40 mg/kg PO q12h | 20–40 mg/kg PO q12h |
| Hydrochlorothiazide | 2–4 mg/kg PO q12h | 1–2 mg/kg PO q12h |
| *ACE inhibitors* | | |
| Enalapril | 0.25–0.5 mg/kg PO q12–24h | 0.25–0.5 mg/kg PO q12–24h |
| Benazepril | 0.25–0.5 mg/kg PO q12–24h | 0.25–0.5 mg/kg PO q12–24h |
| *Other vasodilators* | | |
| Hydralazine (for hypertension) | 0.5–3 mg/kg PO q12h | 2.5–10 mg/cat PO q12h |
| Amlodipine (alternative to hydralazine) | 0.05–0.5 mg/kg PO q12–24h | 0.3–0.6 mg/cat PO q12–24h |
| Nitroglycerin 2% ointment | ½–1½ in. (1.3–3.8 cm) cutaneously q4–6h | ¼–½ in. (0.6–1.3 cm) cutaneously q4–6h |
| Pimobendan | 0.25 mg/kg PO q12h | 1.25–1.5 mg/cat PO q12h |

or obstruction of the duct. Neoplasia is one cause of obstruction; apocrine gland adenocarcinoma is the most common type. Anal sac impaction may be bilateral, but unilateral is more common. Dogs are more commonly affected, especially small breeds. Feline anal sac impaction is rare.

The most common clinical signs include licking, biting, and chewing at anal area, sitting, scooting, and vocalizing due to pain. Hematochezia, tenesmus, and dyschezia may also be observed. In some cases, the problem becomes apparent only after the sac has ruptured.

### 13.3.1.2 Diagnostics

*Physical examination.* Impacted anal sacs are palpable externally, whereas healthy anal sacs usually are not. Rectal palpation can help confirm an impaction versus neoplasia. When sacs are ruptured, a malodorous discharge and draining track will be present in the skin of the perianal area.

An examination of anal sac material following expression can help determine the cause of ASD [23].

---

**Textbox 13.5 Gross evaluation of anal sac contents**

*Normal anal sac.* Clear or pale yellow–brown fluid
*Impacted anal sac.* Thick, brown, and pasty material
*Anal sacculitis.* Creamy, yellow–green exudate
*Anal sac abscess.* Reddish–brown, purulent exudate.

Source: Hnilica and Medleau 2011 [23]. Reproduced with permission of Elsevier.

---

*Cytology.* Infected anal sacs may have increased numbers of neutrophils, *Malassezia*, and intracellular bacteria on cytology [24]. Cytology should be used subjectively, however because there is no significant cytological difference between anal sac material in normal dogs and those with ASD [25]. A fine-needle aspirate and cytology is required to differentiate neoplasia from anal sac material.

*Culture.* A pure culture of a single bacterial species suggests anal sacculitis [26].

### 13.3.1.3 Treatment Protocols

#### 13.3.1.3.1 Gold Standard Protocols

**Manual Expression**  Whether there is a rupture or not, manual expression of both sacs is indicated. Sedation may be required as ASD is often painful, with the exception of neoplasms.

- Lifting the tail up, with a gloved, lubricated index finger, gently insert the finger into the rectum approximately 1 in. (2–3 cm) forward.
- Feel for a firm marble-sized object at the 4 and 8 o'clock positions.
- Place a towel between the dog's anus and your hand and gently milk the gland's contents outward by putting pressure on the most distant side of the gland first and continuing to squeeze towards you. Be careful to not use excessive pressure.
- Once the anal sac is emptied, flush it with an antiseptic solution such as chlorhexidine or povidone–iodine and infuse a triple antibiotic–steroid combination such as Animax® or similar product. Topical antibiotic–steroid ear medications such as Otomax® also work well. Use a curved-tip syringe, teat cannula, pipet, Tom Cat™ catheter, or similar product for flushing and infusion.
- Wipe the area clean when finished.
- In cases of ASD, apply warm compresses on the perineal area for 10 min twice daily for 2–4 days.
- Place a protective collar to prevent licking and recheck in 7 days, or sooner if not improving.
- Dispense an oral antibiotic if infection is present.

If the sac is abscessed and not yet ruptured and draining externally, it must be lanced to facilitate manual evacuation. This requires sedation or general anesthesia. If the material in the sac is hard and difficult to express, it can be softened with saline flushes and gentle massaging before expression.

**Diet**  Adding fiber to the diet increases fecal bulk which facilitates compression and emptying of the anal sacs during defecation. Fiber may come in the form of a quality commercial prescription diet such as Hill's® w/d®, pumpkin, bran, or psyllium [22].

**Anal Sacculectomy**  Surgery is typically indicated for chronic, recurring ASD, and/or neoplasia. If surgery is warranted, owners must be aware of possible complications such as fecal incontinence, fistulation, and infection [27]. Neoplasias will be readily diagnosed as such upon rectal palpation. Neoplasia should also be considered if the anal sac duct cannot be made patent for flushing, or the anal sac material cannot be expressed after multiple flushes in an attempt to loosen the material. If neoplasia is suspected, thoracic radiographs are needed to assess metastasis. Tumors are slow-growing and surgical anal sacculectomy is associated with prolonged median survival times post-surgery (>24 months) even if the local lymph nodes are affected (16 months) [28].

#### 13.3.1.3.2 Alternative Protocols

If the patient cannot be sedated to perform anal sac flushing and antibiotic infusion, start treatment with oral antibiotics (Table 13.6) and an NSAID for several days, in conjunction with warm compresses. Following several days of this protocol, flushing and infusing of the glands may be attempted in a nonsedated patient. In some cases, the author has observed resolution when only pain medication, oral antibiotics, and warm compresses were prescribed.

### 13.3.1.4 Tips and Tricks from the Field

- Diagnostically, gross examination of the anal sac material is the best guide for determining ASD and ideal course of treatment.
- Recurrent ASD is often associated with underlying food hypersensitivity or atopy.
- An otic antibiotic–corticosteroid preparation with its included applicator tip can be used as an alternative to standard antiseptic flushing supplies. The otic applicator tip is small enough to place into the anal sac duct and the medication can be used for flushing and infusing if the recommended antiseptics and saline are not available.

Table 13.6 Antibiotics used for anal sac disease.

| Antibiotic | Dosage |
| --- | --- |
| Clavamox® (amoxicillin–clavulanic acid) | 13.75 mg/kg PO q12h |
| Amoxil® (amoxicillin) | 11 mg/kg PO q12h |
| Zeniquin® (marbofloxacin) | 2.75 mg/kg PO q24h |
| Baytril® (enrofloxacin) | 5 mg/kg PO, IM q24h |

Table 13.7 Possible clinical signs associated with cuterebriasis.

| Affected organ system | Clinical signs |
| --- | --- |
| Cutaneous (the most common form) | • Excessive grooming, matted hair [32]<br>• Serosanguinous or purulent discharge may be noted at the opening, or the L2 or L3 may be visualized at the breathing pore [31,32] |
| Ophthalmic [29,31] | • Chemosis, blepharospasm, uveitis, blindness<br>• Larva may be seen in the orbit or within the globe [33] |
| Respiratory [29,31] | • Acute sneezing episodes, nasal discharge, unilateral facial swelling over the nose, swelling of the pharynx and soft palate, dyspnea |
| Neurological [30,31] | • Abnormal behavior, depression, abnormal vocalizing, head pressing, circling, vestibular signs, cranial nerve deficit, abnormal gait, unilateral or bilateral central blindness |

• Homemade warm compresses can be made from uncooked rice, oats, or beans. Place the desired volume into a tube sock, small cloth bag, or similar item and secure closed the open end. Microwave on high at 15-s intervals until desired temperature is achieved. Alternatively, fill a latex glove with warm water and tie a knot at the wrist. Warm sitz bath soaks (pet sits in a small volume of water) may be used as an alternative to warm compresses.
• In free-roaming dogs, be sure to rule out a flea allergy and other ectoparasites and endoparasites as a differential diagnosis for ASD.

### 13.3.2 Cuterebriasis

#### 13.3.2.1 General Information
Cuterebriasis is the parasitic disease that results when *Cuterebra* larva enter and migrate through a host. *Cuterebra* are a genus of Dipteran flies, otherwise known as Botflies. They are obligate parasites of lagomorphs and rodents, and there are 34 species of *Cuterebra* in North America [29]. Dogs and cats serve as accidental hosts for *Cuterebra*. It is suspected that cats may not be susceptible to the rodent infesting species of *Cuterebra* [30]. The prevalence of *Cuterebra* infection in lagomorph and rodent colonies may be as high as 30–70%, but the prevalence of infection in dogs and cats is much lower [31].

Dogs and cats often come in contact with *Cuterebra* eggs while exploring lagomorph and rodent environments and become accidental hosts while grooming. It is suspected that kittens and puppies become infected by larva stuck to the queen or bitch's fur [29]. In climates with cold winters, cases are seen mid-Summer to Fall, but in warmer climates, cases are seen year-round. Clinical signs are dependent on the location of aberrant larval migration (Table 13.7).

#### 13.3.2.2 Diagnostics
Note that there is no specific clinical or clinico-pathological test to diagnose cuterebriasis aside from visually identifying larvae. The most common presentation is a dog or cat with a subcutaneous cyst, frequently around the head or neck, which has a 2- to 4-mm opening with well-defined margins and serous discharge [29,31]. In general, larvae have the following appearance depending on their stage of development [31]:

• L1 is 1- to 1.5-mm long, skinny, and transparent.
• L2 is 5- to 15-mm long and white with black spines on the cuticle.
• L3 is 3- to 4-cm long and dark with rows of black spines on each segment.

Check each body system thoroughly for signs of cysts, swelling, and circular breathing holes.

#### 13.3.2.3 Treatment Protocols

##### 13.3.2.3.1 Gold Standard Protocols
Anesthetize the patient and surgically remove the larva (Table 13.8). Rupturing larvae may lead to a chronic foreign body reaction, secondary bacterial infection, or hypersensitivity reaction [32].

##### 13.3.2.3.2 Alternative Protocols
• Ivermectin has been shown to have efficacy against migrating larvae when used at 0.1–0.3 mg/kg. Recommended protocols include:

– 0.2–0.4 mg/kg PO, SQ q12h for two treatments [30]
– 0.4 mg/kg SQ q24h for three treatments [30]
– 0.3 mg/kg PO, SQ q48h for three treatments [30]
• Levamisole (60 mg/day) for 7 days [30]
• Complimentary treatments to medically manage the condition and prevent side effects may be required (Table 13.9).

### 13.3.2.4 Tips and Tricks from the Field

• L3 can be hard to grasp in warble and may even retreat into warble. Covering the breathing pore with petroleum jelly for 10–15 min before extraction may make removal easier [37].
• If larvae are damaged during removal or the cyst does not heal, debride the interior of the cyst, flush

**Table 13.8** Treatment options for cuterebriasis depending on organ system affected.

| Organ system | Gold standard treatment | Alternative treatment option |
| --- | --- | --- |
| Cutaneous | Carefully enlarge the breathing pore with hemostats<br>Grasp the larva with forceps and remove in one piece. Dissect carefully around early L2 larva<br>Flush the cyst with sterile saline and leave to heal by second intention | |
| Ophthalmic | Surgically remove the larva, repair ocular damage, medically manage anterior uveitis if present | If the larva is located in the anterior chamber and a skilled ophthalmic surgeon is not available, institute medical management and surgically remove the eye |
| Respiratory | Surgically remove the larva with the aid of a bronchoscope [34] | Without access to a scope, the diagnosis will be presumptive. Institute medical management or depending on severity, consider euthanasia |
| Neurological [35] | No practical treatment option exists | Without access to CT and MRI, the diagnosis will be presumptive<br>Institute medical management or depending on severity, consider euthanasia |

**Table 13.9** Complementary treatments.

| Complementary treatment | Justification |
| --- | --- |
| Diphenhydramine [30,32,35] | Premedicating with diphenhydramine (0.4 mg/kg IM) 1–2 h before ivermectin administration may prevent potential anaphylactic reactions to larval death |
| Corticosteroids [30] | The use of corticosteroids during the treatment period may prevent further inflammatory damage upon larval death.<br><br>• Prednisone (1 mg/kg PO q12h) for 3 weeks then q24h for 3 weeks<br>• Dexamethasone (0.1 mg/kg IV) at time of ivermectin administration |
| Antibiotics | Prevents secondary bacterial infections associated with larval migration. Suggested protocols include:<br><br>• Enrofloxacin (5 mg/kg PO q12h) for 14 days [35]<br>• Cephalexin (22–30 mg/kg PO q8–12h) for 21–30 days [36]<br>• Amoxicillin and clavulanate potassium (Clavamox®) (12.5–20 mg/kg PO q12h) for 21–30 days [36] |

with sterile water, and allow to heal by second intention while providing systemic antibiotics.

- Self-extraction is part of the *Cuterebra* lifecycle [29], so it is possible to find empty warbles.
- Assure owners that although humans can be accidental hosts for *Cuterebra*, they are not at risk from getting them from their dog or cat.
- Although no approved monthly preventives for *Cuterebra* exist, housing animals indoors and limiting outside access can prevent infection.

### 13.3.3 Demodicosis

#### 13.3.3.1 General Information

Demodectic mange is one of the most significant diseases of free-roaming dogs worldwide. Although most *Demodex* spp. are considered normal fauna, mite overgrowth can lead to alopecia and severe dermatitis. The most commonly identified mite in dogs is *Demodex canis*; however, *Demodex injai* can also cause disease. Demodectic mange in cats is a fairly rare condition caused by *Demodex cati* or *Demodex gatoi*. *Demodex* spp. are host-adapted mites of mammals. Mites have not been shown to cross-infest between dogs and cats, nor are they transmitted to people.

Demodicosis can result in an array of clinical signs in both dogs and cats including alopecia, erythema, scaling, comedones, seborrhea, and crusts. Pruritus is variable depending on the type of mite, extent of disease and inflammation, and presence of secondary infections.

Recent evidence indicates that treatment success is similar regardless of the mite species present [38]. The most widely accepted treatment regimen involves the administration of oral ivermectin daily, but alternative protocols can be adapted to situation.

#### 13.3.3.2 Diagnostics

*Dermatological Examination.* Determine the distribution of lesions. There are two main distribution patterns:

- *Localized.* This form usually presents as one or more small areas of alopecia seen most commonly on the head and limbs. Juvenile dogs are most commonly affected. Demodicosis should be suspected in any young dog with focal alopecia, particularly affecting the feet and face.
- *Generalized.* This form involves lesions covering either a large area of the body or disseminated areas of alopecia. Generalized demodicosis is believed to occur secondary to an underlying systemic disease or immune defect.

*Skin Scrape.* Perform a skin scrape to confirm the presence of *Demodex* mites and evaluate any secondary infection, if a microscope is available. See Chapter 14 for instructions.

#### 13.3.3.3 Treatment Protocols

##### 13.3.3.3.1 Gold Standard Protocols

Localized demodicosis – Most cases of localized demodicosis resolve spontaneously, so no treatment is warranted. Application of a rotenone-based ointment (Goodwinol) has been approved for treating localized demodicosis [39]. Local irritation may occur following application.

Generalized demodicosis – For cases of generalized demodicosis, extended and aggressive therapy is often warranted. The most widely recommended treatment course is daily administration of oral ivermectin at escalating doses using 50–100 µg/kg increments (Table 13.10). Resolution of clinical signs can be dramatic (Figure 13.2).

Some practitioners recommend remaining at the 300 µg/kg dose, whereas others recommend gradually increasing the dose to 600 µg/kg. Note that this particular treatment protocol is very time intensive and may not be practical depending on the circumstances, particularly in situations where dogs are free-roaming or fractious.

Table 13.10 Suggested ivermectin dosing.

| Day of treatment | Dose (µg/kg PO q24h) |
| --- | --- |
| 1 | 50 |
| 2–3 | 100 |
| 4–6 | 150 |
| 7–9 | 200 |
| 10–16 | 300 |
| 17+ | 400 |

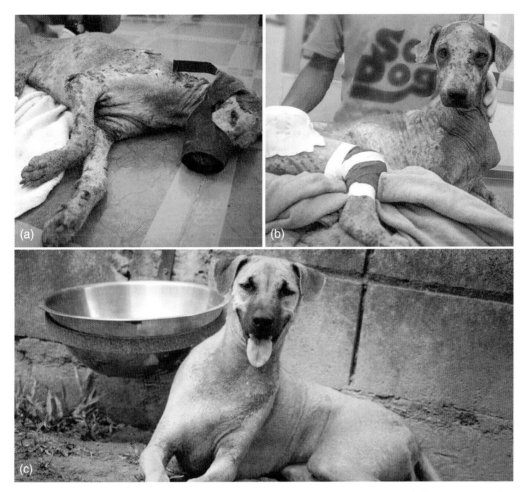

**Figure 13.2** (a) A free-roaming mixed breed dog with severe demodectic mange, pododermatitis, wounds, and pressure sores. The patient was aggressive on intake due to pain. (b) Patient at 3 weeks postintake following weekly doramectin injections and daily bandage changes. (c) Patient at 3 months postintake. Source: Courtesy of Raymond Gerritsen, Soi Dog Foundation.

Large animal ivermectin can be obtained from livestock feed stores and is used off-label to treat demodicosis, costing pennies per dose. Take care when calculating dosages as large animal formulations are much more concentrated and sold in varying concentrations.

A sample calculation using large animal ivermectin (1%) is included below.

---

**Textbox 13.6 Micrograms of ivermectin (1%) per ml**

Each ml of large animal ivermectin (1%) solution contains 10 mg/ml of ivermectin.
  Therefore, 0.1 cc = 1000 μg

---

**Textbox 13.7 Sample calculation of ivermectin dose using a 1% solution**

A 20 kg dog requires an ivermectin dose of 300 μg/kg.
  First determine the dose in micrograms,
  20 kg × 300 μg/kg = 6 000 μg ivermectin

Then determine the dose in cc's assuming a 1% solution is used.
  A 1% ivermectin solution has 10 000 μg per cc
  6 000 μg/10 000 μg = 0.6 cc ivermectin

Some dogs, particularly herding breeds, may have mutations in their *MDR1* genes making them more prone to ivermectin toxicity. There is an old veterinary saying, "White feet, don't treat", which, although somewhat outdated, still may be a good rule of thumb when practicing in the field where testing is not an option. Regardless of breed or color, all treated dogs should be monitored closely for neurological signs. If neurological signs are seen, discontinue treatment immediately.

Treatment should be administered until clinical signs resolve and no live mites can be found on skin scrape. Treatment should ideally be continued for 1–2 months after mites are no longer observed. If a microscope is available, skin scrapes should be repeated at 2- and 4-week intervals after starting treatment. Traditionally, resolution of *Demodex* infections is based on clinical improvement and two negative skin scrapes 1 month apart. Resolution of clinical signs typically precedes parasitological cure. Premature cessation of treatment is a common cause of treatment failure.

---

**Textbox 13.8 Feline demodicosis**

Demodicosis caused by *D. gatoi* is considered to be contagious to other cats. Like canine demodicosis, the feline form can result in localized or generalized disease.

*D. cati.* Clinical signs include alopecia, erythema, and crusting, with or without pruritus. Localized lesions are most commonly seen in the periocular region, head, or neck. Generalized disease is most commonly associated with an underlying systemic condition or immunosuppression. *D. cati* can also cause ceruminous otitis externa that is either localized to the ear canals or is part of generalized disease.

*D. gatoi.* Clinical signs include moderate to severe pruritus, erythema, and scaling along the dorsum, abdomen, and limbs. These clinical features are often indistinguishable from cats with allergic skin conditions or psychogenic alopecia. Miliary dermatitis or indolent lip ulcers have also been observed.

Diagnosis: See canine demodicosis.

Treatment options:

Lime sulfur: First-choice therapy for *D. gatoi* and has variable efficacy against *D. cati*.

- Apply lime sulfur solution to dry skin twice weekly and allow to dry without rinsing. Use a higher concentration (8 oz in 120 oz of water) [40]. The solution is applied to dry skin because prewetting decreases its efficacy.
- Can be applied to fractious or feral cats by restraining the cat in a wire cage and then applying the solution using a garden sprayer.
- Potential side effects: skin irritation, dry skin, and pruritus.
- Safe to use in kittens.

Ivermectin: Treatment of choice for *D. cati*. Treatment failures have been reported for *D. gatoi*.

- Anecdotal reports of efficacy using ivermectin (0.3 mg/kg SC or PO) once weekly for 4 weeks.
- For localized otic demodicosis, administer topically into the ear canal.
- Potential side effects: vomiting, diarrhea, and neurological signs.

Milbemycin oxime: Considered an effective treatment for both *D. cati* and *D. gatoi*.

- Doses range from 1 to 2 mg/kg PO q24h [40].
- For localized otic demodicosis, administer topically into the ear canal.
- Potential side effects: vomiting, diarrhea, and neurological signs.

Doramectin: Potentially an effective treatment for *D. cati*.

- Administer (600 μg/kg SQ) once weekly for no more than three injections [41].

### *13.3.3.3.2 Alternative Protocols*

- Administer doramectin (600 µg/kg SQ or PO) once weekly. Doramectin is significantly more expensive than ivermectin, but the weekly dosing schedule is far less labor intensive than daily oral ivermectin administration.
- Apply spot-on Advocate® or Advantage Multi® (imidacloprid + moxidectin) once monthly for two to four treatments per label instructions. This is one of the least time-intensive protocols but one of the most expensive. These products may also have limited availability internationally. Note that there is evidence to suggest that more frequent application (weekly to every two weeks) has a quicker time to cure [42,43]. Many free-roaming dog programs are able to procure these products through donations.
- Administer Bravecto® (fluralaner) once per label instructions. This is formulated as a chewable tablet, which has proven efficacy against generalized demodicosis, with no mites detectable in one study at 56 and 84 days following treatment [44,45].
- Administer milbemycin oxime at gradually increasing doses from 0.5 to 2 mg/kg.
- In severe, nonresponsive cases, consider using amitraz dips at 250 ppm every 2 weeks as follows:
  1) Clip the hair coat of medium- and long-haired dogs.
  2) Bathe the dog using a benzoyl peroxide shampoo and remove any crusts present.
  3) Apply protective eye ointment.
  4) Dilute one bottle (10.6 ml) of amitraz with two gallons (7.6 l) of warm water creating a 250 ppm solution. In a well-ventilated area, sponge the product thoroughly onto the dog. Allow the feet to soak if lesions on the paws are present.
  5) Allow the dog to air-dry.

  Some practitioners use amitraz dips weekly at 500 ppm to treat refractory cases but the risk of side effects increases with the concentration. If signs of toxicity occur (lethargy, hypothermia, bradycardia, and signs of hyperglycemia), administer yohimbine (0.11 mg/kg) slowly IV. Use caution if treating diabetics and asthmatics.
- *Treat secondary pyodermas.* It is necessary to treat not only the mite infection but also any secondary pyoderma that may be present.

### 13.3.3.4 Tips and Tricks from the Field

- In the author's experience, if it looks like mange it probably is mange. Treating with ivermectin is the cheapest available option.
- The standard recommendation is to wait 1 month between skin scrapes; however, in the author's experience, relapses are uncommon when two negative skin scrapes are seen 2 weeks apart.
- Do not try to perform SQ injections in fractious dogs. Injectable ivermectin can be given orally. Diluting ivermectin with fruit syrup or injecting into a meatball can mask the bitter taste.
- Spay/neuter all demodex patients to prevent reoccurrence of demodicosis during future heat cycles.
- Regardless of what treatment protocol used, remember to also treat any secondary disease processes that may be causing the demodicosis in the first place. Some underlying diseases such as endocrinopathies may or may not be treatable in a field setting.
- If a veterinarian can carry only one drug with him or her to the field, it should probably be ivermectin. A single bottle of ivermectin can cure large numbers of dogs from debilitating skin disease. If organizations can solicit donations of medications, they should ask for Bravecto due to its efficacy and single oral dosing.

## 13.3.4 Dermatophytosis

### 13.3.4.1 General Information

Dermatophytosis, also known as ringworm or fungal disease, is a highly contagious fungal infection of the skin. It is the most common infectious skin disease in cats [46]. The main species are *Microsporum canis*, *Microsporum gypseum*, and *Trichophyton mentagrophytes*, with *M. canis* being most common. Dermatophytosis is especially problematic in multi-animal environments such as catteries and animal shelters and is a significant zoonosis, especially for immunocompromised persons.

Dermatophytosis is transmitted by direct contact with infected animals, infected hair and scale in the environment, and through fomite carriage in bedding, cat trees, carriers, carpets, and furniture. Fleas from infected animals can also transmit the disease [47]. The infective portion of the dermatophyte, called arthrospores, is formed from the segmentation and fragmentation of fungal hyphae. The spores are very small and can typically survive for 3–6 months in the environment, although they can remain viable for up to 24 months. The incubation period from the time of exposure to visible lesions is 1–3 weeks [47,48].

Dermatophytes live in the superficial keratinized layer of the skin, hair, and claws where they destroy hair shafts by disrupting normal keratinization. Arthrospores cannot penetrate healthy intact skin and thus can only invade the hair shafts through compromised or traumatized skin. Self-trauma from flea infestations and clipper burn from grooming can cause the microtrauma compromising the stratum cornea. Grooming is thought to be a significant host defense mechanism [49]. Cats with reduced grooming ability such as geriatric cats or those with concurrent illness are more likely to become infected [47].

Clinical signs of dermatophytosis are varied. The classic presentation is circular, scaly lesions with hair loss. The degree of pruritus is variable. Chin acne, hyperpigmentation, erythema, and nail bed lesions are also seen. Lesions are most frequently distributed on the face, head, ears, and forelimbs and can be focal or multifocal. Excessive shedding in cats is a common owner complaint. Dermatophytosis should be a differential diagnosis for any skin reaction patterns in cats including miliary dermatitis, eosinophilic plaques, indolent ulcers, and symmetrical alopecia.

Although the infection usually is self-limiting over a 2- to 3-month period in healthy animals, immune-compromised populations such as kittens and geriatric animals are at an increased risk of overwhelming dermatophyte infections. Conditions such as diabetes, feline leukemia virus (FeLV)/Feline immunodeficiency virus (FIV), and pregnancy/lactation may also increase the risk of significant infection.

The infectious nature of the disease, cost and duration of treatment, and potential for zoonotic transmission make this disease especially noteworthy.

### 13.3.4.2 Diagnostics
Diagnosis of dermatophytosis typically requires a combination of patient signalment, history, physical examination, Wood's lamp examination, fungal culture, and/or microscopic examination of hairs (trichogram). When fungal cultures cannot be performed, treatment is often based on a Wood's lamp test, trichogram, or solely based on lesions and patient history. See Chapter 14 for more information on diagnostic techniques.

*Physical examination.* A thorough physical examination is essential for identifying potential dermatophyte lesions. The muzzle, lips, ear margins, digits, axilla, and the tail are often affected. A penlight can help identify difficult to see lesions.

*Wood's lamp.* The Wood's lamp is a useful screening tool for dermatophytosis caused by *M. canis*. Normal skin will not fluoresce while *M. canis* will often have a bright apple green fluorescence. *M. canis* will fluoresce in at least 50% of the cases under appropriate conditions, whereas *M. gypseum* and *Trichophyton* spp. do not fluoresce [48]. False negatives are possible and broken hairs can appear as fluorescent specks. False positives can occur with the presence of soaps, eye ointments, keratin scale, and oral medications such as doxycycline and pyrantel.

*Trichogram.* If a microscope is available, a trichogram is a useful tool for identifying ringworm in the field. This involves microscopically evaluating a pluck of hair from a suspicious lesion with mineral oil. Trichograms can be useful for identifying infections that do not glow on Wood's lamp testing.

*Fungal culture.* Fungal cultures are the gold standard in confirming dermatophytosis. When performed correctly, all species will grow when cultured. Although various mediums exist, dermatophyte test medium (DTM) is recommended as a red color change is often noted early, before growth becomes apparent. Consider cost, shelf life, and ease of use in the field clinic setting when selecting appropriate culture mediums.

To assess treatment efficacy, weekly fungal cultures are recommended. Colony numbers should decrease with treatment. Plate the samples at least 2 days after topical therapy. Treatment should ideally be continued until two negative culture results are obtained [50].

*Polymerase chain reaction (PCR).* Polymerase chain reaction (PCR) has been developed with excellent specificity and sensitivity for *Microsporum* spp., *M. canis*, and *Trichophyton* spp. The test is not for in-clinic use but has a turnaround time of 1–3 working days [51]. Cost and limited availability reduces its practicality in field settings.

### 13.3.4.3 Treatment Protocols

Although infection typically lasts 60–100 days, dermatophytosis is often self-limiting in healthy dogs and cats [47]. Despite the potential for self-cure, treatment is recommended to minimize disease spread to animals and humans, and to hasten the resolution of infection.

#### 13.3.4.3.1 Gold Standard Protocols

Successful ringworm treatment involves concurrent use of systemic and topical therapy, reasonable confinement to easily cleaned areas, and environmental decontamination. Treatment may take 2–3 months. Topical treatment is essential to prevent continued sporulation into the environment.

- Once dermatophytosis is suspected, bathe the patient with an antifungal shampoo that contains 0.5% climbazole, miconazole, or 1–2% ketoconazole. Leave the shampoo on for 3 min before rinsing.
- Start baths/dips with lime sulfur twice a week while awaiting disease confirmation. Mix 8 ounces of lime sulfur with 1 gallon (3.8 l) of warm water to make a 1 : 16 dilution. Place the patient on a towel and spray or wipe the animal with a sponge/towel from the neck down. For spraying, a small garden sprayer-type product with a strong mist setting is effective. Saturate the animal thoroughly and rub the lime sulfur-dip deep into the coat and onto the ears. The dip must reach the skin to be effective. Avoid the eyes and face. Physically dipping cats in the solution is not recommended, as this is stressful and can cause cross-contamination. Once complete, allow the patient to air-dry or wrap him or her in a towel. Do not rub the animal with the towel to dry. Provide supplemental heating for wet patients (e.g. heat lamp/heater and heating pads). Lime sulfur is safe for newborn puppies and kittens [47] and nursing queens. Teats should be wiped after application and before returning a queen to her kittens. Supplemental heating must be provided to wet kittens and queens.
- Once confirmed, start treatment with itraconazole (Sporanox®) (10 mg/kg PO q24h) for 21 days. After 21 days, reduce the frequency to every other week until the patient is deemed cured. It is also possible to use itraconazole on a 1-week-on, 1-week-off schedule that can reduce the drug cost by 50% [47]. Do not exceed 25 mg of itraconazole per cat per day regardless of weight. Systemic antifungal drugs should only be used when the diagnosis is confirmed, and is safe for patients as young as 3 weeks of age.
- Itraconazole and lime sulfur baths twice a week should continue until all lesions are resolved and the patient has had two negative fungal cultures.
- Clipping is not usually necessary unless the cat is long-haired and matted, and is generally not recommended as microtrauma from clippers can exacerbate lesions. If clipping is necessary, perform in a room that is easily cleaned since it causes heavy environmental contamination. Clipping should be done very gently with a #10 blade as a closer blade may cause excessive trauma. The instruments used should be carefully cleaned after use and dedicated only for that purpose!

#### 13.3.4.3.2 Alternative Protocols

- Lime sulfur continues to be the most efficacious way to remove spores on the fur. If not available, an antifungal shampoo followed by application of Pure Oxygen®, an accelerated hydrogen peroxide (AHP) leave on rinse, may be considered. Apply three times per week allowing 3-min contact time. AHP can also be applied to dry fur. A 0.5% climbazole shampoo, DOUXO® chlorhexidine/climbazole mousse, and enilconazole (Imaverol®/Clinafarm-EC®) 0.2% emulsifiable concentrate, at a dilution of 1.8 ounces (55.6 ml) in 126.2 ounces (3.73 l) of water are also possible options [47,52].
- Terbinafine is an alternative oral antifungal medication. Its efficacy is inferior to itraconazole but can be used in situations where itraconazole is unavailable. Administer terbinafine (30 mg/kg PO q24h) for 21 days in conjunction with lime sulfur dips twice a week. Dosing smaller animals may be difficult with terbinafine due to the available strengths of commercial tablets. For this reason, terbinafine is better suited to dogs and adult cats [53].
- Continue treatment until two negative culture results are obtained.

### 13.3.4.4 Environmental Decontamination

To prevent reinfection, all surfaces must be deep cleaned to remove and inactivate dermatophyte spores.

Environmental decontamination is an essential component of any treatment protocol for dermatophytosis.

1) Clean all nonporous surfaces – Ensure the mechanical removal of all hair and debris via vacuuming or sweeping and mechanical washing of surfaces with detergent and water. Swiffer®-type products are recommended over brooms.
2) Disinfect nonporous surfaces – OTC (over-the-counter) cleaners effective against *T. mentagrophytes* include:
   • Accel® (AHP 1 : 16)
   • Accel® TB (hydrogen peroxide 0.5%)
   • Enilconazole
   • Bleach diluted 1 : 32
   • Formula 409® (quaternary ammonium 0.3%)
   • Clorox Clean-Up® (sodium hypochlorite 1.84%).
   These are effective on precleaned surfaces where all organic matter has been removed. A 10-min contact time is required [54].
3) Decontaminate wood floors – Remove hair and dust daily with a vacuum cleaner, broom or Swiffer®, and then mop the floor.
4) Vacuum rugs and couches – Discard vacuum bag immediately after vacuuming. If the vacuum has a canister, dump the contents in a plastic or paper bag and discard in trash immediately. Wear gloves when handling the contents of the vacuum cleaner.
5) Decontaminate exposed bedding and toys – Wash twice in cold water for more than 14 min/wash. Discard items with hair trapped within the fibers. Bleach and hot water are not required. Do not overload the machine in order to ensure maximal agitation [55]. Wash contaminated laundry separately and transport to the laundry area in a plastic bag. Discard anything that cannot be laundered or disinfected. Decontaminate the dryer lint trap by washing in an all-purpose household detergent.
6) Clean the isolation space while the animal is under treatment.
   • The isolation room should ideally be deep-cleaned twice a week, with spot cleaning performed daily. Perform deep cleanings of cages, floors, and so on at the time of the lime-sulfur/antifungal topical application (while the animals are out of their cages).
   • Between deep cleanings, mechanically remove all hair and debris daily by wiping down surfaces

in the isolation room with a one-step cleaner such as Clorox® or Accel® wipes. A bleach solution at a 1 : 32 dilution can also be used with a rag that is immediately laundered.
• Wear clothing specific to the isolation room. Change these clothes following cleaning of the isolation area and wash with other ringworm exposed laundry.
• Once an animal has successfully been treated, perform two final rounds of cleaning and disinfection before opening the room for general access.

### 13.3.4.5 Tips and Tricks in the Field

• Gloves and gowns should be worn when handling patients with suspicious lesions. If a gown is not available, use a clean scrub shirt and change clothes after handling the patient. A large garbage bag can also be fashioned into an effective gown when needed.
• Ketoconazole has moderate efficacy against dermatophytosis in cats and dogs. Due to the potential for toxicity, use only if terbinafine or itraconazole is unavailable.
• Kittens grow rapidly. Weigh kittens weekly to ensure oral medications are being dosed accurately.
• In areas that house large numbers of cats, store bedding and supplies in closed containers or cabinets and reduce clutter.
• If infected animals are being treated in the home, limit their living space to a small area with minimal furniture and no carpeting or soft textiles. A large dog crate or bathroom works well. Keep the patient isolated until cleared of disease.
• High temperatures can destroy fungal spores. Ensure toothbrush samples are not left in hot vehicles before plating cultures.

### 13.3.5 Ear Mites

#### 13.3.5.1 General Information
Infestations of the mite, *Otodectes cynotis* can lead to highly inflammatory conditions within the ears of cats, dogs, foxes, and ferrets. Prevalence rates in the cat and dog vary, but it is estimated to be approximately 25% and 7%, respectively. Young cats are more commonly affected than older dogs [56,57]. Mixed infestations with other ectoparasites and dermatophytes are common. *O. cynotis* lives on the skin

surface of the ear as well as in the ear canal and feeds on epidermal debris. As mites feed, epithelium within the ear becomes inflamed, irritated, and prone to secondary bacterial and yeast infections. Less frequently, *O. cynotis* can also migrate to other parts of the body and be found on the neck, rump, and tail. Some animals can have a mild pruritic papular dermatitis from these mites [58]. Transmission between hosts is by direct contact.

Ear mites are more prevalent in cats than dogs and infestation is more common in juvenile than adult animals. However, recurrent issues are often seen in colonies of healthy adult cats, and adult cats can serve be asymptomatic carriers [58]. Ear mites are the leading cause of otitis externa in cats [59].

Clinical signs of ear mite infestation can include:

- Scratching the ears
- Head shaking
- Discharge and odor from the ears. Debris similar to the appearance of coffee grounds can often be seen within the ear canals. This debris contains mites, wax, inflammatory mediators, blood, and epithelial cells.
- Secondary excoriations at the base of the ear and head
- Papules on the neck, rump, or tail.

### 13.3.5.2 Diagnostics

*Physical examination.* Diagnosis is typically based on clinical signs. Infected ear canals will have significant amounts of dark, crusty debris in addition to significant pruritus.

*Pinnal-pedal reflex.* Although not pathognomonic, cats with ear mites will often have a positive pinnal-pedal reflex when infected ears are examined or swabbed.

*Cytology.* Multiple life stages of *O. cynotis* can be seen at low power when debris from an ear swab is

---

**Textbox 13.9 Diagnosing ear mites in the field**

In situations where a microscope may be unavailable for cytology, gross visual inspection of the ear canal, combined with clinical signs and lifestyle information can often be adequate to make a tenative diagnosis. If the patient is free-roaming, one must consider how appropriate follow-up care will be provided (by a caregiver or re-capture in the community).

---

suspended in a drop of mineral oil and placed on a microscope slide.

*Direct visualization O. cynotis.* Mites can be seen as moving white flecks on the hair, within the ear, and on ear swabs.

### 13.3.5.3 Treatment Protocols

The prognosis for successful treatment of *O. cynotis* infections is very good. The presence of secondary infections, excessive debris within the ear, and untreated animals in the home increases the likelihood of treatment failure. Products applied within the ear will be more successful if the ear is *gently* cleaned before starting treatment.

#### 13.3.5.3.1 Gold Standard Protocols

Use a veterinary ear cleanser to gently clean the ear canal. This will provide faster relief to the patient and remove immature mite stages present in ear exudate. Squirt a small amount of cleanser into the ear and massage at the base of the ear to soften debris and crusts. If commercial veterinary ear cleansers are not available, use warm water or saline. Allow the patient to shake his head and dry the ear with cotton balls. If using a cotton tip applicator, care must be taken to not place it too far within the canal, which can damage the tympanic membrane (TM). These should only be used to clean external debris.

Following cleaning, use *one* of the following:

- *Selamectin (Revolution®).* 6–12 mg/kg applied topically to skin at back of neck once. Repeat in 4 weeks if needed. Labeled for use in dogs and cats 8 weeks of age and older.
- *0.01% Ivermectin otic suspension (Acarexx®).* One ampule AU as per manufacturer's directions. Repeat once in 14 days if necessary. Labeled for use in cats 4 weeks of age and older.
- *Neomycin–thiabendazole–dexamethasone (Tresaderm®).* 0.125–0.25 ml AU q12h for 2–3 weeks. This is off label as the Tresaderm® label recommends using product for a maximum of 7 days.
- *0.1% milbemycin oxime solution (Milbemite® otic).* 1 ampule AU once. Labeled for cats 8 weeks of age and older.
- *Imidacloprid/moxidectin (Advantage Multi®).* 0.1 ml/kg applied topically to skin at back of the neck once. Apply a second dose in 4 weeks if needed.

#### 13.3.5.3.2 Alternative Protocols

Fipronil (0.05 ml of a 100 g/l solution) has been reported as a therapy when used directly in the ear canal as a one-time dose [60].

In the absence of veterinary products labeled for ear mites, the author recommends an efficacious and cost-effective solution using large animal ivermectin and mineral oil:

- Combine 0.1 ml of 1% ivermectin (Ivomec®) with 9.9 ml of mineral oil
- Apply one drop AU
- Repeat in 14 days.

In situations where no veterinary products are available, mineral oil is an economical and safe alternative treatment.

- Apply 1–2 drops AU once daily for 3 weeks. It is speculated that this suffocates the mites by coating the spiracles, which are the openings to the respiratory system [61].

---

**Textbox 13.10 Treating refractory cases**

If topical treatment is ineffective, consider 1% ivermectin (Ivomec®) 0.3 mg/kg PO once weekly for 4 weeks, or SQ every 10–14 days for three treatments (particularly in difficult to handle cats).

*Note: This is off-label use and should not be used in ivermectin-sensitive breeds or heartworm positive dogs.*

---

Ensure all animals in the environment are treated.

#### 13.3.5.4 Tips and Tricks from the Field

- Mites can crawl out of the ear canal and onto the fur/skin. Topical flea control that also kills mites may be necessary to prevent reinfestation. Bathing with an ascaricidal shampoo will help eliminate mites on the rest of the body. Bathing with warm water may also be helpful if it's the only option available.
- Cross-infection between cats, dogs, and people is uncommon unless the infected animal is sleeping head-to-head with another individual.
- All animals in a household must be treated at the same time to prevent reinfestation.

- Ear mites do not survive in the environment for more than 12 days. Areas where infected animals have lived should be environmentally cleaned or vacated for 12 days before introducing a new untreated cat or dog [62].

### 13.3.6 Flea Allergy Dermatitis

#### 13.3.6.1 General Information

Flea allergy dermatitis (FAD) is a pruritic condition resulting from sensitization to flea saliva. FAD is the most common allergy in dogs and cats in areas where fleas are prevalent [63]. In North America, most cases of FAD are due to the cat flea, *Ctenocephalides felis felis*. There is evidence to suggest that dogs with intermittent, rather than continuous flea exposure, appear to be at increased risk for developing FAD [64]. Both cats and dogs can develop FAD at any age.

Clinical signs typically include moderate to severe pruritus, alopecia with papules, crusts, and excoriations in both cats and dogs. Lesions are often found in the caudodorsal lumbosacral area, caudomedial thigh, abdomen, flank (dogs), and dorsal tailbase (dogs). Cats typically have lesions on the dorsal neck, dorsal lumbosacral, and ventral abdominal areas and present with miliary dermatitis.

The level of flea sensitivity is unique to each individual. While most pets are well controlled with routine use of flea prevention, some more sensitive individuals may still be hypersensitive when they come in contact with a single flea. In many parts of the world, FAD is still a problem despite very effective flea control products because:

- Owners do not believe that fleas are present as they have not observed fleas on the pet and the pet lives indoors.
- Not every pet in the household is treated with flea control products.
- The pet is exposed to wild animals and environments outside of the home area.
- There is a significant environmental flea burden.

Three categories of flea control exist: adulticides, insect growth regulators (IGR), and insect development inhibitors (IDI). Adulticides minimize exposure to flea saliva, whereas IGR and IDI disrupt egg and larval development.

### 13.3.6.2 Diagnostics

A diagnosis of FAD is typically based on clinical signs of pruritus, including characteristic lesion patterns, and the presence of fleas or flea "dirt," which is comprised of dried fecal material from the fleas. Other pruritic skin conditions such as sarcoptic mange should also be excluded.

---

**Textbox 13.11 Tip from the field**

To differentiate flea "dirt" from environmental particles, place the material on a white surface such as a paper towel or sheet and drip water onto it. Flea "dirt" will dissolve in the water and turn the paper towel red–brown in color.

---

### 13.3.6.3 Treatment Protocols

#### 13.3.6.3.1 *Gold Standard Protocols*

An integrated flea control plan is needed for treating the patient and breaking the flea life cycle. Treat all pets that come into contact with each other with a high-quality product at labeled intervals. See Chapter 16 for treatment options.

Indoor environmental control including sprays, powders, foggers, and vacuuming is recommended for heavy flea infestations. Adult fleas are not necessarily killed before they lay eggs; therefore, environmental control will be more important in FAD cases. Consider a professional exterminator if fleas persist. If a professional exterminator is not available, consider using a total release fogger (TRF), also known as bug bombs, that contains pyrethroid, pyrethrin, or both.

Anti-inflammatory doses of prednisone may be given for pruritus:

- *Dogs*. Prednisone/prednisolone (1 mg/kg PO q24h) for 1 week then taper over 2–3 weeks depending on severity.
- *Cats*. Prednisolone (1 mg/kg PO q24h) for 1 week then taper over 2–3 weeks depending on severity. Prednisolone is preferred over prednisone in cats.

Be sure to treat secondary infections.

#### 13.3.6.3.2 *Alternative Protocols*

One study determined fipronil (Frontline®) alone resulted in excellent treatment efficacy in 70% of FAD cats, and another study indicates that cats and dogs treated with selamectin (Revolution®) alone resulted in significant improvement in clinical signs of FAD [65,66]. A highly effective topical flea product may replace the traditionally recommended multi-modal treatment protocol that includes both animal treatment and environmental treatment, although treating all animals in contact with one another is still recommended to reduce the flea burden.

### 13.3.6.4 Tips and Tricks from the Field

- Flea control in free-roaming dogs and cats can be challenging, particularly if they lack an owner. In such cases, environmental control should be emphasized. Keep tall grass and bushes trimmed when practical and apply products that contain esfenvalerate, permethrin, or bifenthrin with a chemical sprayer. Be sure the product is safe for cats when indicated.
- FAD cannot be ruled out just because fleas are not seen on the patient. Cats may remove the majority of live fleas themselves when grooming.
- Consider treating animals with FAD for potential tapeworm infection. Ensure that the treatment given is effective against *Dipylidium caninum*.
- Liquid dish detergent may be used for a quick and easy method of killing fleas, especially in patients too young for other commercial products. There is no residual effect, and repeated use of this method is not recommended. Use caution in periocular areas and apply eye lubricant if available.

### 13.3.7 Myiasis (Maggots)

#### 13.3.7.1 General Information

A staggering number of free-roaming animals die every year from maggot infestations. Luckily the majority of deaths can be prevented or treated if caught at an early stage. Myiasis is the term used to describe a maggot infestation resulting from flies deliberately laying eggs in or on tissues, resulting in fly larvae growing inside the host while feeding on its tissue. Free-roaming dogs are particularly prone to myiasis as they typically live outside and their skin has a tendency to stay moist.

Commonly affected areas on the body include the ears, head, neck, and around the anus [67]. Be on the lookout for a hole in the skin of the dog or cat, and maggots crawling near the wound surface. Although the resulting lesion and smell can be quite overwhelming, treatment is quite simple and carries a high success rate.

### 13.3.7.2 Diagnostics

*Physical Examination.* Visualization of maggots on the skin or in the wound is diagnostic. Maggots may range in size but are typically slightly larger than a grain of rice. Maggot-infested wounds also have a very pungent and characteristic smell. Be sure to check for underlying wounds or skin conditions that predispose dogs to maggot infestation.

### 13.3.7.3 Treatment Protocols

There are many ways to treat maggot wounds. The mainstays of therapy consist of killing and removing the maggots and treating any secondary infections. Recommended treatment steps include the following:

1) Administer appropriate pain relief and sedation. Maggot wounds can be extremely painful and depending on the extent of the wound, maggot removal can be a lengthy procedure.
2) Shave the hair generously from the affected area. The wound size is often much larger than it appears before shaving. Prepare a set of forceps and basin for maggot removal.
3) Apply a topical product that either kills maggots or forces their migration out of tissues. Exercise caution however as many of the products commonly used in the field to kill maggots can endanger an already compromised animal's life. There are a variety of natural remedies and commercially available pharmaceutical products. Essential oils in particular are known for their ability to repel flies and maggots. Note that the majority of the products included here are used off-label for treating maggot infestations and therefore dosing instructions are based on anecdotal accounts from those working in the field. Precise dosing instructions and concentrations are unknown. These products may have limited geographic availability.
4) Manually extract all maggots once they have begun to die. Clean, sterilized blunt-ended tissue forceps and gauze work best.

---

**Textbox 13.12 Products used for extracting maggots**

- Capstar: The oral tablet can be dissolved in water and dripped in the wound.
- D-Mag spray or Topicure spray: Antimaggot sprays used extensively in India.
- Ivermectin: Some advocate using either crushed tablets dissolved in water or a dilution of the injectable product. Systemically administered ivermectin (0.2–0.4 mg/kg) may also kill maggots [36].
- Medicinal turpentine oil/Eucalyptus oil: Turpentine is an essential oil distilled from pine tree sap. Maggots will typically come out of a wound when turpentine oil-soaked gauze is used to plug the wound. This is used commonly throughout the world.
- Negasunt powder (Bayer) or Gotbac powder (Scientific Remedies Pvt. Ltd.).
- Non-alcohol-based pyrethrin or pyrethroid in dogs.
- Spot-on application of Revolution® (selamectin) or Advantage Multi®/Advocate® (imidacloprid + moxidectin) may help kill maggots. This is an off-label use [36].
- Tincture of iodine/povidone iodine (Betadine).

---

5) Copiously flush the wound. This will aid in removing any remaining maggots and fly eggs that might be present.

    Steps 3–5 may need to be repeated several times to remove all maggots.
6) Dry the wound
7) Consider applying a topical product to repel flies, promote healing, and prevent future infestation. If you are not able to dress the wound and change it at least once daily, consider applying a copious amount of antibacterial ointment.
    - Himax is an herbal veterinary skin product used widely in India, which can be applied to wounds and repels flies.
    - Scavon Vet Spray is a polyherbal formulation used commonly throughout Asia with insecticidal, antibacterial, and antimycotic properties.

8) Begin a course of systemic broad-spectrum anti-biotics if secondary infections are present. Most maggot-infested wounds should be considered infected.

- Amoxicillin and clavulanate potassium (Clav-amox®) (12.5–20 mg/kg PO q12h).

---

**Textbox 13.13 What should *not* be used to kill maggots?**

- Never apply painter's Turpentine oil, kerosene oil, alcohol, or petrol to maggot wounds.
- Never use bleach, powdered lime, boiling water, or acids. These products can be toxic and cause tissue necrosis.
- Never use a canine-specific product on a cat as many canine products have permethrin, which is toxic to cats.

---

#### 13.3.7.4 How to Prevent Maggot Infestations

- If you are lucky enough to spot a wound before a fly does, be sure to begin wound treatment immediately. Any sore or wound should be clipped, cleaned, and treated.
- Controlling flies can be difficult. Prevent flies from an area by removing all garbage and decaying material. Garbage containers should be secured. Remove standing water and wash kennel floors and walls daily to remove any waste that might attract flies.
- Botanical oils including eucalyptus, clove, peppermint, lemongrass, cinnamon, and others have been reported as fly repellents. Some working in the field report wiping down the inside of trash cans with vinegar or diluted mint oil.
- Keep dogs clean and dry and remove any fecal matter that could attract flies.

#### 13.3.7.5 Tips and Tricks from the Field

- Maggot infestations can be a cause of lameness. Be sure to check for maggots around nail beds and paw pads in limping dogs.
- The author prefers Negasunt powder for treating maggot wounds due to ease of application.
- In newborn puppies, flies are often attracted to the healing stump of the umbilical cord. Apply iodine, alcohol, or similar product to the end of the cord for antisepsis.

### 13.3.8 Notoedric Mange

#### 13.3.8.1 General Information

Feline scabies or mange is most commonly caused by the mange mite *Notoedres cati* [68]. *N. cati* is very contagious by direct contact and infested bedding. *N. cati* can also opportunistically infest dogs, rabbits, and people around the world [58]. Pruritus is severe and excoriations from scratching are commonly found on the face, periocular, and auricular areas. Crusting with alopecia can also typically be found on the neck, legs, feet, and ear margins [69]. Affected skin eventually becomes hyperpigmented and lichenified. Although the prognosis is favorable, the condition can be debilitating without treatment.

#### 13.3.8.2 Diagnostics

A diagnosis of notoedric mange is typically based on clinical signs. If a microscope is available, a skin scrape can confirm infection.

*Skin scrape.* Mites and nymphs, larvae, and eggs can be found quite easily microscopically. See Chapter 14 for additional information.

#### 13.3.8.3 Treatment Protocols

Remove crusting with gentle massaging and bathing as soon as treatment is initiated. An antiseborrheic or pyrethrin shampoo facilitates treatment.

Systemic and topical treatment options include:

- Ivermectin (0.2–0.3 mg/kg PO or SC) every 1–2 weeks for 3–4 treatments.
- Doramectin (0.2–0.3 mg/kg SC) every 1–2 weeks for 3–4 treatments.
- Use a topical scabicide on the lesions for treatment duration. Diluted lime sulfur can be used in this manner and applied weekly for 6 weeks and is safe for young animals. Other topical options include pyrethrin spray 1–2 times per week and fipronil spray every other week [70].
- As an alternative to a topical scabicide, a spot-on treatment can be used in addition to systemic treatment. Selamectin (Revolution®) and Fipronil (Frontline®) will both treat and prevent *N. cati*. Imidacloprid/moxidectin (Advantage Multi®/Advocate®) are effective as well.

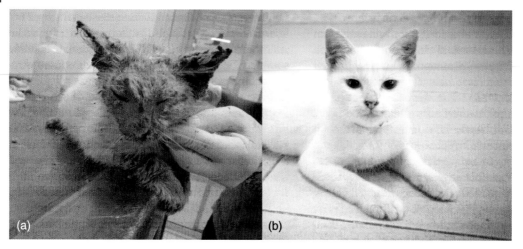

**Figure 13.3** (a) An adult domestic shorthair cat on presentation with severe notoedric mange. (b) Patient at 12 weeks post-topical and systemic therapy. Source: Courtesy of Raymond Gerritsen, Soi Dog Foundation.

Repeat skin scrapes every 1–2 weeks. The response to treatment is usually quick and cats can be considered cured following negative skin scrapings at 4–6 weeks post-treatment initiation.

Corticosteroids such as dexamethasone (0.07–0.15 mg/kg) can be used to alleviate self-mutilation and hypersensitivity reactions, but they should be given only after treatment has started [68].

Treatment can be given based on suspicion if a microscope is not available to confirm diagnosis. Use of a recommended spot-on flea/tick preventive with or without lime sulfur dips are a safe choice for treatment. Lime sulfur is a safe treatment for kittens that are too young for licensed scabicides.

#### 13.3.8.4 Tips and Tricks from the Field

- Although reported as being quite rare in the literature, in the author's experience, feline scabies can be quite common in tropical climates, particularly in Southeast Asia.
- The author has seen quick clinical resolution using the following protocol: Doramectin or ivermectin administered weekly for 3 weeks (i.e. days 1, 8, and 15) in conjunction with the application of a topical scabicide.
- All pets in a household should ideally be treated with a recommended spot-on flea/tick preventive effective against *N. cati* for the treatment duration of the infested pet. Frequent household cleaning as well as washing of bedding is important.
- *N. cati* cases make amazing before and after photos, which can be used as organizational fundraising tools! Clinical resolution is often quick and dramatic (Figure 13.3).

### 13.3.9 Sarcoptic Mange

#### 13.3.9.1 General Information

Canine sarcoptic mange, also referred to as scabies, is a highly contagious, nonseasonal zoonotic disease caused by the superficial burrowing skin mite *Sarcoptes scabiei* var. *canis*. Mites are relatively host-restricted, but humans can be affected. Disease in humans is typically self-limited. Clinical signs in dogs are usually seen anytime within 10 days to 8 weeks following infestation. The hallmark sign is intense pruritus resulting from a hypersensitivity reaction triggered by allergenic substances secreted by the mite [58]. Dogs typically become infected following direct contact with infested animals.

Early lesions typically affect thinly haired areas including the ventrum, ears, chest, and elbows. Early lesions typically include alopecia and hyperkeratosis and as the disease progresses, crusting can be seen on the elbows, ear margins, and periocular areas. In severe cases, lesions rapidly become generalized with diffuse thickening of the skin and peripheral lymphadenopathy. Intense pruritus often leads to self-mutilation and hemorrhagic lesions. Differential diagnoses include other causes of dermatological hypersensitivity (atopy, food allergy, and flea bite allergy), pyoderma, demodicosis, dermatophytosis, *Malassezia* dermatitis, and contact dermatitis [58].

Although sarcoptic mange can be difficult to diagnose, it is one of the easiest diseases to treat in free-roaming dogs.

#### 13.3.9.2 Diagnostics

Diagnosis is generally based on the patient's free-roaming status, severe pruritus, and clinical appearance.

*Pinnal-pedal reflex (ear scratch test).* A reflexive rear-leg itch induced by scratching the ear tip is present in approximately 80% of scabies cases [58].

*Skin scrape.* Mites can be difficult to find microscopically. Scrapes need to be deep and taken from several locations including the ears, elbows, and hocks.

*Response to treatment.* If no mites are observed in patients that are strong mange suspects, the patient's response to treatment can also be used as a diagnostic tool.

#### 13.3.9.3 Treatment Protocols

Treat all affected and in-contact dogs. Secondary pyodermas must be treated for as short a duration as possible to see clinical resolution. The most effective systemic treatments include:

- Selamectin (Revolution®) (6–12 mg/kg) applied every 2 weeks (a total of four applications may be most effective). Selamectin is the treatment of choice for ivermectin-sensitive breeds.
- Ivermectin (0.2–0.4 mg/kg PO or SC weekly) every 2 weeks for 4–6 weeks.
- Doramectin (0.2–0.6 mg/kg SQ) weekly for 4–6 weeks.
- Milbemycin oxime (Interceptor® and Sentinel®) (0.75 mg/kg PO q24h) for 30 days, or 2 mg/kg PO weekly for 3–5 weeks.
- Topical moxidectin/imidacloprid (Advantage Multi®) can be applied weekly every 2–4 weeks for 4–6 weeks; frequent application may lead to increased adverse effects [58]. This product can be safely used on dogs as young as 7 weeks of age.
- Fluralaner (Bravecto®) administered either orally or topically has been shown to eliminate mites and improve clinical signs.

Additional topical treatments may also be used and crusts removed using an antiseborrheic shampoo.

- Fipronil spray
  - 3 ml/kg every 2–3 weeks in puppies.
  - 6 ml/kg once weekly for at least 2 weeks in adults.
- Weekly lime sulfur dips for four to six treatments. Lime sulfur is effective and safe in puppies.
- Amitraz applied at a 0.025% solution every 1–2 weeks for 2–6 weeks [71].

Dogs that are highly pruritic may benefit from glucocorticoids such as prednisone (0.5 mg/kg PO q24h) for 5–7 days during treatment.

#### 13.3.9.4 Tips and Tricks from the Field

- Treatment may need to be based on clinical suspicion if skin scrapings are negative.
- Beware of home remedies for mange treatment. In most cases, uncomplicated mange cases can be cost effectively treated with ivermectin (0.2 mg/kg PO) every 2 weeks for two to four treatments.
- Severe clinical signs may warrant daily prednisone; however, the use of steroids may complicate empirical diagnosis.

### 13.3.10 Otitis Externa and Media

#### 13.3.10.1 General Information

Practitioners in the field are bound to see cases of otitis externa and media. Otitis externa is a common inflammatory disease of the ear, often caused by an underlying condition such as atopy, hypothyroidism, foreign body, keratinization disorders, autoimmune disease, inflammatory polyps in cats, or neoplasia [72]. Otitis in free-roaming dogs and cats is commonly caused by environmental allergies, ear mites, foreign bodies, and an overall lack of preventive care. Conformational defects can also predispose dogs to otitis due to increased moisture accumulation in the ear canal, a narrow canal, and obstruction. Certain breeds are more likely to have otitis externa such as the Cocker and Springer Spaniels, German Shepherds, Miniature Poodles, and Shar Peis [73].

Up to 50% and 89% of dogs with ear infections have concurrent otitis media [74]. This is often secondary to infection (i.e. bacterial, yeast, and fungal), neoplasia, trauma, or foreign body. Inflammatory polyps also predispose cats to otitis media. Untreated otitis media may be a perpetuating factor for chronic or recurrent otitis externa cases [75]. *Malassezia* otitis is one of the most common causes of otitis media in cats and when undiagnosed leads to chronic otitis externa.

Animals with otitis typically have a history of scratching at the ears, headshaking, or a malodorous discharge. The animal may also rub his head on various objects.

### 13.3.10.2  Diagnostics

*Physical examination.* A thorough examination of the ears should be performed to identify erythema, crusts, lichenification, or exudate. Hyperplastic tissue and stenosis of the canal are suggestive of chronic otic disease. Handheld otoscopes are extremely valuable to visualizing the TM and ear canal. Otoscopic examination may or may not be possible due to the presence of exudate, swelling, or pain.

*Microscopic examination.* Before instilling any fluid into the ear, collect a sample of exudate from the canal with a cotton-tipped applicator. After collection, roll the applicator on a glass slide and stain with a modified Wright's stain and examine under a microscope. Heat fixing the sample is unnecessary. On microscopic examination, check for keratinocytes, bacteria, yeast, and fungal hyphae, neoplastic cells, and white blood cells. On cytology, cocci are typically staphylococci or streptococci and rods are typically *Pseudomonas aeruginosa*, *Escherichia coli*, or *Proteus mirabilis* [74]. The yeast *Malassezia pachydermatis* is found in low numbers in healthy ear canals.

- *Otitis externa.* Otodectes, Malassezia, bacteria, and inflammatory cells including white blood cells may be present. The presence of neutrophils indicates a deep infection, suggestive of otitis media.
- *Otitis media.* Inflammatory cells from the middle ear and/or ruptured TM may be observed. Note that in some cases of otitis media, the TM may be intact.

*Gross examination of exudate.* Exudate should be examined for eggs, larvae, or adults of the ear mite *O. cynotis* and *Demodex* mites. Dark exudate is usually characteristic of *Malassezia* spp. overgrowth or parasitic infection.

*Diagnosing a ruptured TM.* Ruptured TMs can be difficult to diagnose if the canal is inflamed, stenotic, or if exudate is present. To help determine the integrity of the TM, one can sedate the patient and use an otoscope to place the tip of a soft rubber tube where the TM should be. If the tip cannot move farther and remains visible, then the TM is intact. If the tip can be pushed farther into the canal, moves ventrally, and is not visible, then the TM is most likely ruptured. This is also the best way to flush the middle ear, but the tube is placed ventrally into the middle ear to decrease the risk of trauma to the oval and round windows, leading to the inner ear.

Alternatively, flushing the ear canal with a non-ototoxic fluid and retrieval of all of the fluid indicate an intact TM. If the full amount of fluid is not retrieved, and drainage from the nares or swallowing occurs, a ruptured TM is likely. A bulb syringe or a soft rubber tube attached to a syringe may be used to retrieve the fluid.

### 13.3.10.3  Treatment Protocols

The ultimate key to treatment is determining the cause of the otitis and removing the underlying issue. To treat the affected ear, a multimodal approach is necessary including topical and systemic antimicrobials, glucocorticoids, and pain medications. To manage pain, tramadol can be given for 5–7 days. Glucocorticoids also help decrease swelling in the ear canal.

To increase treatment success of otitis media and for certain cases of otitis externa, the initial cleaning/flushing may need to be performed under sedation to be as thorough as possible. Subsequent cleanings for otitis externa and media are performed every 2–7 days until all debris is removed. Ears should always be cleaned before applying treatment (Table 13.11). Dry, thick exudate requires a ceruminolytic solution such as dioctyl sodium sulfosuccinate (DSS). If rods are seen on cytology, the cleaner should contain squalene.

Ceruminolytic agents contain dioctyl sodium sulfosuccinate, squalene, carbamide peroxide, or propylene glycol. Astringents are typically used after bathing and swimming. These contain isopropyl alcohol, boric acid, or salicylic acid.

Table 13.11 Otic discharge characteristics and ear cleaner recommendations.

| | Dark brown thick waxy | Pale brown moderate waxy purulent | Yellow mild waxy purulent | Green purulent hemorrhagic mucoid |
|---|---|---|---|---|
| Otitis type: | Ceruminous otits | Malassezia otitis | Staphylococcal otitis | Pseudomonal otitis |

The waxier the discharge, the more important the ceruminolytic property of the cleaner

Ceruminolytic activity ──────────────────────────────────────▶

The more purulent and mucoid the discharge, the higher the water content of the cleaner should be to flush the ear

Flushing activity ──────────────────────────────────────▶

Source: Harvey and Paterson 2014 [73]. Reproduced with permission of Taylor & Francis.

Most commercial topical otitis treatment products contain a combination of antibiotic/antifungal and steroid and require application twice daily. If the TM is ruptured, start oral antibiotics and perform ear flushing with non-ototoxic flush such as:

- Saline solution
- Vinegar/water mixture (2.5% acetic acid; mix 1 : 1 with water)
- Tris-ethylenediaminetetraacetic acid (EDTA).

Topical medications with a low probability for ototoxicity should also be chosen, including enrofloxacin and ciprofloxacin, and aqueous gentamycin [76] (Table 13.12).

Systemic therapy must be used for treating otitis media and may be used for otitis externa based on chronicity, severity, and the presence of proliferative changes of the ear canal. Systemic therapy should continue for a minimum of 4 weeks and 1–2 weeks beyond clinical resolution. Topical treatment should be continued for 7–14 days after there is no clinical or cytological evidence of active disease, which may require a minimum treatment period of 30 days. Shorter treatment times may improve but not eliminate infection. Inadequate volume of topical medication is a common reason for treatment failure [77].

Table 13.12 Topical treatment solutions when TM rupture is suspected.

| Infection | Medications | Suggested ratio |
|---|---|---|
| Bacteria | Injectable enrofloxacin (22.7 mg/ml): Synotic® otic solution | 1 : 2 |
| Yeast | Injectable enrofloxacin (22.7 mg/ml): dexamethasone sodium phosphate (4 mg/ml) | 1 : 2 |
| Mixed | Injectable enrofloxacin (22.7 mg/ml): dexamethasone sodium phosphate (4 mg/ml): 1% miconazole | 1 : 1 : 2 |

Source: Adapted from Rosychuk 2009 [76].

**Textbox 13.14 Recommended infusion volumes per ear**

Small dogs (<15 kg): 0.4–0.5 ml
Medium dogs (15–20 kg): 0.7–0.8 ml
Large dogs (>20 kg): 1.0 ml
Dogs with large, pendulous ears: 1.0 ml.

Source: Adapted from Noxon 2014 [77].

In dogs with chronic otitis, cleanings should be performed 1–2 times per week.

#### 13.3.10.4 Tips and Tricks from the Field

- Consider concurrent otitis media in cases of reoccurring otitis externa.
- Bilateral erythematous-ceruminous otitis may be the only manifestation of feline demodicosis [78]. Similarly, recurrent otitis externa has long been recognized as the only clinical sign of atopic dermatitis in dogs.
- Ideally, a commercially prepared otic medication should be used for treatment. See Chapter 20 for homemade ear cleaner recipes.
- Monitor closely for signs of irritation as substances not normally irritating to normal canals may be irritating in ears that are inflamed.
- In cases where oral antibiotics are unavailable, topical treatment alone may be sufficient for resolution of otitis externa depending on the severity and chronicity.

#### 13.3.10.5 Quick Reference Table for Otitis Treatment
See Table 13.13.

### 13.3.11 Pyoderma

#### 13.3.11.1 General Information
Canine pyoderma, a condition literally meaning pus in the skin, is common in free-roaming dogs; cats are less commonly affected. Pyodermas are typically bacterial infections that can be either simple or complex. Simple pyodermas are usually caused by a single inciting cause such as flea infestation, whereas complex infections are often caused by more complicated underlying disease processes including atopic dermatitis, metabolic diseases, or anatomic abnormalities such as excessive skin folds.

There are three classifications of canine pyoderma – surface, superficial, and deep. Surface pyodermas are very common and occur when the infection is confined to the interfollicular epidermal

Table 13.13 Medications for treating otitis [72,73,75–77].

| Drug | Canine dosage | Feline dosage |
| --- | --- | --- |
| Zeniquin® (marbofloxacin) | 5.5 mg/kg PO q24h | 5.5 mg/kg PO q24h |
| Baytril® (enrofloxacin) | 10–20 mg/kg PO, IM q24h | 5 mg/kg PO, IM q24h |
| Cipro® (ciprofloxacin) | 15 mg/kg PO q24h | 5–15 mg/kg PO q12h |
| Orbax® (orbifloxacin) | 2.5–7.5 mg/kg PO q24h | 7.5 mg/kg PO q24h |
| Keflex® (cephalexin) | 22 mg/kg PO q12h | 30 mg/kg PO q12h |
| Cefa-Drops® (cefadroxil) | 22 mg/kg PO q12h | 22 mg/kg PO q12h |
| Clavamox® (amoxicillin–clavulanic acid) | 13.75 mg/kg PO q12h | 13.75 mg/kg PO q12h |
| Antirobe® (clindamycin) | 11 mg/kg PO q12h | 11 mg/kg PO q24h |
| Ketoconazole | 5–10 mg/kg PO q12h with food | Not recommended due to toxic potential |
| Fluconazole | 5 mg/kg PO q24h with food | 10 mg/kg PO q12–24h with food; start with q24h |
| Itraconazole | 5 mg/kg PO q24h with food, or pulse 5 mg/kg PO q24h with food on 2 consecutive days each week | 5 mg/kg PO q24h with food |
| Prednisone | 0.5–1 mg/kg/day PO q24h or divided q12h for 5–10 days then taper | Use prednisolone if available |
| Prednisolone | 0.5–1 mg/kg/day PO q24h or divided q12h for 5–10 days then taper | 1–2 mg/kg/day PO for 7–14 days then taper |

layers of the skin. The most common forms of surface pyoderma are pyotraumatic dermatitis, including acute moist dermatitis (hot spots) and intertrigo (skin fold dermatitis). Superficial pyoderma is defined as a bacterial infection of the epidermis and hair follicles, resulting from infectious, allergic, inflammatory, conformational, parasitic, or neoplastic causes. Superficial pyodermas can progress to deep pyodermas, affecting the dermis.

*Staphylococcus pseudintermedius* is the primary pathogen in pyoderma cases, resulting from an overgrowth or overcolonization of normal resident or transient flora. Other bacteria can also play a role. Dogs with pyoderma frequently have papules and/or pustules, crusting, scaling, alopecia, and epidermal collarettes. Those with short hair coats often exhibit patchy alopecia with scaling. Lesions are frequently found in skin folds, axillae, ventral neck and abdomen, and interdigital areas. Pyoderma occurs commonly in dogs with atopic dermatitis, which has been shown to compromise the epidermal barrier function and increase staphylococcal colonization and adherence of lesional and nonlesional skin [79]. Furthermore, self-trauma resulting from pruritus further degrades the epidermal defenses, facilitating the inoculation of bacteria into the skin [80].

Differential diagnoses for superficial pyoderma include yeast dermatitis, demodicosis, dermatophytosis, pemphigus foliaceus, and sebaceous adenitis [81].

### 13.3.11.2 Diagnostics
Diagnosis is based primarily on clinical signs and patient history.

*Cytology.* An impression smear of exudate from the skin surface or lesions (papules, pustules, and collarettes) may reveal large numbers of cocci and degenerative neutrophils.

*Skin scraping.* Skin scrapings can be used to rule out demodicosis as an underlying cause of pyoderma.

*Bacterial culture and sensitivity.* This is typically reserved for patients that do not respond to empirical therapy or have recurring infections.

### 13.3.11.3 Treatment Protocols
The treatment of pyoderma involves the administration of topical therapy, antibiotics, and addressing underlying causes.

#### 13.3.11.3.1 *Topical Therapy*
Topical therapy alone is a desirable approach for patients with surface pyoderma, particularly when lesions are localized, and in early stages of generalized superficial pyoderma. Topical therapy two to three times a week can help most pyoderma cases initially while diagnostic procedures for primary underlying skin disease are being pursued. Topical products should contain benzoyl peroxide or chlorhexidine. If no appropriate topical products are available, or with resistant infections, sodium hypochlorite (bleach) can be carefully applied as a last resort after being diluted appropriately (see Chapter 20). Localized areas of pyoderma can be treated with antibacterial creams or ointments including mupirocin, silver sulfadiazine, and sodium fusidate.

#### 13.3.11.3.2 *Antibiotics*
Historically, canine pyoderma has been treated using empirical systemic antibiotics and minimal topical therapy. This approach is no longer reliable or recommended, especially in places where staphylococcal resistance patterns have been reported. Minimizing resistant infections in companion animals is one of the biggest challenges faced by veterinary practitioners, and conscientious use of systemic antibiotics is an important consideration in regards to both human and animal health. The empirical use of systemic antibiotic is therefore no longer recommended, particularly for surface and superficial pyodermas. Culture and sensitivity testing is recommended in patients with widespread or generalized superficial pyoderma, deep pyoderma, or recurrent pyoderma. These patients should be treated with a minimum of a 3-week course of antibiotics. All clinical lesions should be resolved for at least 7 days before discontinuing antibiotics. The criteria for antibiotic choices includes:

- Cost
- Ease of administration (oral, q24h, and q12h)
- Activity against staphylococci
- Good cutaneous penetration.

Cephalexin is among the cheapest effective antibiotics making it a routine choice for those working in the field. However, drugs given only once daily reduce necessary staff time and improve compliance

Table 13.14 Antibiotic choices for treating pyoderma [79].

| Antibiotic | Dosage |
| --- | --- |
| Keflex® (cephalexin) or Cefa Drops® (cefadroxil) | 22 mg/kg PO q12h |
| Baytril® (enrofloxacin) | 5–20 mg/kg PO, IM q24h |
| Primor® (ormetoprim/ sulfadimethoxine) (labeled for use in dogs) | 55 mg/kg PO initial dose, 27.5 mg/kg subsequent doses |
| Tribrissen® (trimethoprim/ sulfamethoxazole) | 12.5 mg/kg PO q24h |
| Zeniquin® (marbofloxacin) | 2–5 mg/kg PO q24h |
| Cipro® (ciprofloxacin) | 10–20 mg/kg PO q24h |
| Antirobe® (clindamycin) | 5.5–11 mg/kg PO q12h |
| Clavamox® (amoxicillin/ clavulanic acid) | 12.5–20 mg/kg PO q12h |

(Table 13.14). Amoxicillin, penicillin, and tetracyclines are inappropriate choices for treating pyodermas, and fluoroquinolones should ideally be reserved for more difficult to treat cases.

#### 13.3.11.4 Tips and Tricks from the Field

- Inciting causes must be identified and treated. In free-roaming dogs, be sure to perform a skin scrape to rule out the presence of mites.
- Underdosing and inappropriately short treatment courses are common reasons for treatment failure.
- Prevention of superficial pyoderma can be accomplished through regular bathing, parasite control, and management of allergic conditions that lead to self-trauma.
- An easy way to remember cephalexin dosing in dogs is to add a zero to the dog's weight in pounds. Therefore, a dog weighing 40 pounds (18.2 kg) should receive approximately 400 mg twice daily.

### 13.3.12 Wound Management

#### 13.3.12.1 General Information

Wounds are exceptionally common and challenging to manage in field settings. Severe wounds can take months to fully heal. It is therefore imperative to

consider the feasibility of any medical management plan given the logistical challenge of maintaining clean and dry bandages in field environments, as well as the challenge of arranging timely rechecks.

In order to effectively manage wounds, it is important to understand the three general phases of wound healing [32]:

- *Inflammation/debridement.* Occurs during the first 5 days post-injury and includes hemorrhage, hemostasis, vasodilation, and migration of leukocytes to the site to remove foreign debris and bacteria. This phase is associated with inflammation, edema, and pain.
- *Repair/proliferative.* Occurs from day 3 up to 4 weeks post-injury. There is a proliferation of fibroblasts, collagen synthesis, angiogenesis, formation of granulation tissue, epithelialization, and wound contraction. Healthy granulation tissue becomes obvious and exudates decrease.
- *Remodeling/maturation.* This phase is lengthy and begins around 20 days post-injury and can last for years. Wounds are healed but the underlying dermis is weak and easily damaged. Collagen continues to remodel.

At the time of presentation in the field, most wounds will be in the inflammatory or debridement phase and are often contaminated. The most critical aspects of management are:

- Stabilizing the patient and providing appropriate analgesia
- Reducing contamination/controlling infection
- Debridement
- Keeping the wound hydrated.

---

**Textbox 13.15 Common reasons for delayed/ failed wound healing**

1) Infrequent bandage changes
2) Inadequate lavage
3) Inappropriate contact layer/dressing
4) Inadequate debridement
5) Poor blood supply
6) Presence of seromas/hematomas
7) Malnutrition
8) Infection

### 13.3.12.2 Diagnostics

Clinical signs are typically diagnostic. Infected wounds may require culture and sensitivity testing, probing to assess depth and extent of wound, or radiology to detect potential foreign body.

### 13.3.12.3 Treatment Protocols

All patients should be stabilized before wound management efforts. Appropriate analgesia, fluid support, and hemostasis are priorities. Gloves should be worn when treating wounds. A routine approach to wound treatment includes the following:

**Step 1.** Assess/stabilize the patient
Evaluate the patient, considering critical parameters such as active bleeding, hypotension, hypovolemia, hypothermia, body condition, organ function, sepsis, pain, anemia, and additional injuries. Provide emergency care if required including immediate analgesia, supplemental heating, and IV fluids. If a patient is septic or infection is present, systemic antibiotics are indicated. Cover wounds with a sterile bandage or wrap while initial stabilization efforts are pursued.

**Step 2.** Evaluate the wound
- Examine the wound and surrounding area. Check for the presence of normal anatomy. A probe can be used to evaluate the depth and extent of the wound, presence of subcutaneous pockets or tracts, or foreign bodies. A sterile, blunt metal probe, cotton swab, or wound swab can be used.
- Assess tissue viability. Evaluate extent of tissue involvement, color, texture, temperature, amount of bleeding, and sensation. Hypovolemia and vasoconstriction will create pale/cold tissue and reduce blood flow to the wound. Always treat hypovolemia and hypothermia to evaluate tissue viability accurately. Use a sterile hypodermic needle to evaluate sensation.
- Develop a feasible plan for managing the wound. This should include initial lavage, antibiotics if necessary, timely debridement, analgesia, bandaging, and follow-up care. Consider the owner's ability to provide the required home care. It is not uncommon for wounds to require multiple bandage changes or surgeries.

**Step 3.** Manage the wound using the following:

*Analgesia*
Appropriate analgesia is critical when managing wounds as debridement and lavage can be painful. Nalbuphine, buprenorphine, morphine, and fentanyl are good options depending on the severity of the wound and the patient's pain.

*Lavage*
Flushing reduces bacterial counts, rehydrates tissue, and removes debris. A large volume of fluid is required at a reasonable pressure. The "dirtier" the wound, the greater the volume of flush required.

The initial lavage should remove all surface dirt. Use 500–1000 ml as a minimum volume for the lavage. In human medicine, 50–100 ml of lavage fluid per square centimeter of wound is recommended [82]. Isotonic fluids are ideal but may not be available. Lactated Ringer's, isotonic saline, ordinary drinking water, and tap water can be used. Warm the lavage fluid if possible.

Use a 35–60 ml syringe with an 18-gauge needle or a 20–30 ml syringe with a 19-gauge needle to provide enough pressure to dislodge bacteria without driving it deeper into the wound. Bulb syringes and syringes without needles do not provide adequate pressure. Direct the stream of lavage fluid at a 45° angle. A three-way stop cock and an IV fluid set attached to a bag of lavage fluids can refill syringes quickly.

Follow the initial lavage with a flush using a sterile, nontoxic solution such as saline or sterile water. Using antiseptics at low concentrations in lavage solutions can be bactericidal without being cytotoxic. They are often effective as a flush, soak, or as part of a dressing in a bandage. Most antiseptics and solutions are inactivated by the presence of organic material, so all wounds should be well lavaged before using. The addition of antibiotics to lavage solutions is *not* recommended due to lack of proven efficacy and risk of bacterial resistance.

There may be field situations where systemic antibiotics are needed but unavailable. Work in the field of human trauma has identified dilute bleach and dilute vinegar as two cost-effective solutions that have been successfully used to control infection and promote wound healing. These can be applied directly to the wound as a soak or as a dressing in a bandage. A presoaked gauze can be used as a primary layer in a wet-to-dry bandage or can simply be covered with an occlusive bandage to maintain moisture. See Chapter 20 for compounding recipes for antiseptic flushes and dressings.

*Antibiotics*

All dirty or infected wounds including punctures should be treated with broad-spectrum systemic antibiotics. Although typically not feasible in field settings, a culture of the wound is recommended to guide appropriate antibiotic therapy.

Antibiotics should provide broad coverage for both gram-positive and gram-negative bacteria, as well as aerobes and anaerobes. Bacteria commonly associated with wounds include *Streptococcus*, *Pasteurella*, *Staphylococcus*, *Actinomyces*, and *Bacteroides* species. Nonhealing wounds often contain *Pseudomonas*, *Enterobacter*, *Klebsiella*, or *E. coli* species.

Recommended broad-spectrum antibiotics for wounds include:

- Amoxicillin–clavulanic acid (Clavamox®)
- Clindamycin (Antirobe®)
- Third-generation cephalosporins such as cefpodoxime (Simplicef®) or cephalexin.

Depending on the severity of the wound and available antibiotics, additional options include:

- Cefovecin (Convenia®) + enrofloxacin (Baytril®)
- Clavulanic–amoxicillin (Clavamox®) + enrofloxacin (Baytril®)
- Enrofloxacin + metronidazole (Flagyl®).

**Step 4.** Surgical debridement

Severe wounds often require surgical management and debridement. All penetrating wounds should be surgically explored. The initial goals are to explore the wound fully, remove foreign material, control bleeding, and remove necrotic tissue. Appropriate sedation and/or general anesthesia is required during debridement and lavage.

Widely clip the area surrounding the wound (10–15 cm) to allow for thorough exploration. Place a large amount of sterile water-soluble lubricant (e.g. KY Jelly®) in the wound to prevent further contamination while clipping. Do not further traumatize the wound edges with the clipper blades. Surgically prep the area around the wound. Asepsis should be maintained during surgery. If the viability of superficial tissues is questionable, reevaluate them at a follow-up bandage change. The wound should be left as an open wound until the tissue is obviously viable, the wound is no longer contaminated, and the wound can be surgically closed without tension. Healing by second intention is appropriate in many situations.

Once the wound has been surgically explored and debrided, nonsurgical debridement is performed in open wounds using dressings and bandages. In situations where surgical debridement is not logistically possible, nonsurgical debridement through bandaging may be an option depending on the severity of the wound.

**Step 5.** Bandaging

Bandaging methods include the following:

- Modified Robert Jones bandage that uses a gauze dressing (gauze squares and lap sponges) as the primary/contact layer, cast padding for the secondary layer, and Vet Wrap®/Elastikon® for the outer tertiary layer
- Tie-over bandage for areas where traditional bandages are more difficult (e.g. inguinal region, head, flank, or chest).

---

**Textbox 13.16 Steps for placing a "tie-over" bandage**

1) Once the wound has been lavaged and debrided, place numerous "belt loop" sutures around the wound approximately 2–3 cm from the edge of the wound as depicted in Figure 13.4. Use larger monofilament nylon suture material; size 0 or 1–0 are good options depending on the size of the patient. The patient must be sedated or under general anesthesia for the sutures to be placed.
2) Place the dressing of choice on the open wound. This may be sugar, honey, or a wet-to-dry dressing.
3) Cover the dressing with a number of sterile gauze squares or lap sponges or a combination of both depending on the size of the patient and the wound. A final nonabsorbent layer (e.g. drape material) should be placed if possible.

4) Secure the entire bandage to the wound using lacing material such as umbilical tape. Thread the lacing material through the belt loop sutures in a criss-cross pattern. The laces should be pulled snug enough to hold the bandaging material in place without pulling the sutures through the skin.

Bandages should be monitored daily. Replace if wet, strike-through is present or if swelling has occurred proximally or distally to the bandage. It is critical that bandages are tight enough to provide support yet not so tight that blood flow is restricted or tissue is damaged. Bandaging strategies include the following:

1) Wet-to-dry bandaging

A wet-to-dry bandage mechanically debrides wounds. Wet a sterile gauze square with sterile saline and place on the wound bed. Provide a secondary bandage layer by placing dry gauze squares on top of the wet bandage. Wrap the

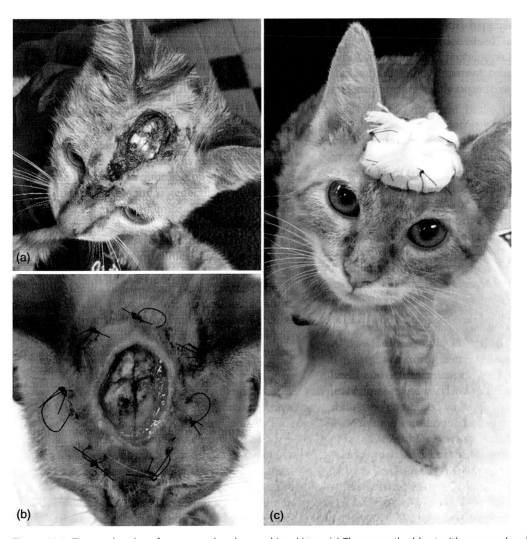

**Figure 13.4** Tie-over bandage for a severe head wound in a kitten. (a) Three-month-old cat with a severe head wound. (b) Following copious flushing of the area, belt loop sutures were placed around the periphery of the wound using 0-prolene. (c) The wound was covered with honey-soaked gauze pads (changed daily) and secured with cotton umbilical tape. Source: Courtesy of Drs. Kate Kuzminski and Jena Valdez.

secondary layer with a final layer of gauze cling followed by Vet Wrap® or Elastikon®. Change this bandage daily. A successful wet-to-dry bandage will dilute the exudate in the wound from the wet gauze and absorb it into the secondary bandage. The primary layer will dry and adhere to the wound. The wound will be mechanically debrided once the primary layer is removed at daily bandage changing. Sterile saline and solutions using chlorhexidine, povidone-iodine, acetic acid, and dilute bleach can be used to soak the primary contact layer.

2) Use of honey

Raw, unpasteurized honey has been used successfully as a dressing in severe wounds for its bactericidal effects as well as its ability to debride [83]. It is effective against *E. coli*, *Proteus*, *Pseudomonas*, *Salmonella*, *Staphylococcus*, and *Streptococcus* spp. [84]. Honey also osmotically draws fluid from tissues, which reduces edema and increases exudates. It should not be used in dry wounds.

1. Clean and dry the wound.
2. Pour unpasteurized honey onto wound or presoak sterile gauze with honey and coat the wound. Gauze strips can also be soaked in honey and wrapped around the wound.
3. Wrap/cover the honey with a secondary absorptive layer of gauze or lap sponges.
4. Change the bandage daily. The bandage should be changed before the honey is completely diluted from the exudate of the wound. Bandage changes may be possible every other day once the wound is sterile.

3) Use of sugar

The use of granulated sugar within wounds improves superficial debridement and encourages tissue growth and epithelialization [85]. It can be poured into deep wounds or made into a paste. Sugar has also been effectively used to treat *E. coli*, *Pseudomonas*, *Staphylococcus*, *Streptococcus*, and *Klebsiella* spp. [86]. Clean and dry the wound and perform the following:

1. Apply a 2–3 cm layer of sugar to coat the wound.
2. Wrap/cover the wound with a secondary absorptive layer of gauze or lap sponges.
3. Change bandages once to twice daily. Lavage the wound with body temperature tap water to remove all of the sugar. Pat dry. Replace the sugar bandage.
4. The amount of sugar present within the wound at the time of the bandage change determines the frequency of the changes. If the sugar is completely absorbed, change more frequently. If sugar is still present in the wound, lengthen the time between changes.
5. Continue using sugar bandages until all pockets are gone, a healthy bed of granulation tissue is present, and epithelialization has begun. If second intention healing is the goal, the wound can be covered at this time with an antibiotic ointment such as Furacin® or Mupirocin® using a nonadherent primary bandaging layer such as Telfa®. Bandage changes at this time can be every 2–7 days depending on the maturity of the wound [85].

#### 13.3.12.4 Tips and Tricks from the Field

- Above all do no harm. If follow-up care for a bandaged wound is not possible, do not leave the bandage on the patient without a committed plan for bandage removal.
- Elizabethan collars can be made in field clinic setting using cardboard, buckets, or towels.
- Small children's t-shirts can cover bandages and create a protective barrier from licking or chewing.
- E-collars should not be placed on animals that are free-roaming. For their safety, all patients wearing e-collars must be confined at home.
- Bandages that are placed on limbs/paws get wet quickly. Send patients home with a bag to be placed on the leg/paw when outside in damp/wet environments. Used IV fluids bags can be recycled for this purpose.

## 13.4 Gastrointestinal Parasites

### 13.4.1 Gastrointestinal Parasites Overview

Gastrointestinal (GI) parasites are frequently encountered in dogs and cats in the field, some with zoonotic potential. Although safe and effective treatments exist for the majority of internal parasites, many free-roaming animals lack access to routine preventive care. This section includes a brief overview of some of the most common parasites seen in field clinics. Although there are many commercially available deworming products on the market, it is important to keep in mind that many products may not be financially viable or available in the geographical area in which one is working (Table 13.15).

In the author's experience, most field spay/neuter clinics routinely administer either ivermectin subcutaneously or pyrantel pamoate orally in conjunction with rabies vaccination. Although ivermectin may be easier to dose particularly in fractious animals (subcutaneously versus orally), pyrantel is the safer option as there is less risk for toxicity and can be given to both pregnant and neonatal animals. Note that neither pyrantel nor ivermectin is reliably effective against whipworms.

### 13.4.2 Coccidiosis

#### 13.4.2.1 General Information

Coccidiosis in dogs and cats is commonly caused by the protozoa *Isospora*, but can also include *Cryptosporidium* and *Toxoplasma* spp. *Isospora* spp. in dogs and cats are host specific and do not infect humans. However, *Cryptosporidium* and *Toxoplasma* have zoonotic potential. Coccidia are ubiquitous parasites and asymptomatic infections are common. Younger

---

> **Textbox 13.17 Sample deworming protocol using pyrantel pamoate (50 mg/ml) for field clinics**
>
> Adult cats and dogs (>5 months old)
>
> - Administer oral dose at time of vaccination (1 ml per 10 pounds (4.5 kg) body weight).
>
> Kittens and puppies (2 weeks to 5 months old)
>
> - Administer oral dose (1 ml per 10 pounds (4.5 kg)).
> - Send one additional dose home to be administered 14 days after the initial dose.
> - If highly parasitized, a third dose can be dispensed to be given 4 weeks following the initial dose.
>
> Source: HSVMA-RAVS Vaccination Protocol [87].

---

animals are more susceptible and stress such as weaning or crowded shelter housing can trigger clinical disease.

Animals with coccidiosis have watery to mucoid diarrhea, dehydration, and weight loss.

#### 13.4.2.2 Diagnostics

Coccidiosis is diagnosed by the presence of oocysts in feces using fecal floatation and related clinical signs.

---

Table 13.15 Dewormer product summary.

| Product name | Active ingredient | Roundworms | Hookworms | Whipworms | Tapeworms |
|---|---|:---:|:---:|:---:|:---:|
| Nemex®, Strongid® | Pyrantel pamoate[a] | ✓ | ✓ | | |
| Droncit® | Praziquantel | | | | ✓ |
| Drontal® Plus | Praziquantel, pyrantel pamoate, fenbendazole | ✓ | ✓ | ✓ | ✓ |
| Panacur® | Fenbendazole | ✓ | ✓ | ✓ | ✓[b] |
| Heartgard Plus® | Ivermectin, pyrantel pamoate | ✓ | ✓ | | |
| Sentinel® | Milbemycin oxime | ✓ | ✓ | ✓ | |
| Advocate®/Advantage Multi® | Imidacloprid/moxidectin | ✓ | ✓ | ✓ | |
| Trifexis® | Milbemycin oxime/spinosad | ✓ | ✓ | ✓ | |

a) Goes by many product names.
b) Not effective against *D. caninum*.

Oocysts of nonpathogenic coccidian species found in feces are not clinically significant.

### 13.4.2.3 Treatment Protocols

Treatment options for *Isospora* infections include the following. Note that dosages for most products used for the treatment of coccidiosis in dogs and cats vary, depending on the source.

- Sulfadimethoxine (Albon®) (50 mg/kg PO) for the first day followed by 25 mg/kg q24h until the animal is asymptomatic for 2 days. Treatment may take up to 2–3 weeks.
- Sulfadimethoxine/ormetoprim (Primor®) (55 mg/kg PO) for the first day, followed by half the dose q24h until 2 days past the resolution of symptoms, or up to 21 days in dogs.
- Trimethoprim/sulfadiazine (30–60 mg/kg PO q24h) for 6 days in cats [88].
- Amprolium [89,90]
  - Dogs: (300–400 mg (total) PO q24h) for 5 days, or 110–220 mg (total) PO q24h for 7–12 days. Used in the drinking water (sole source) at 30 ml (9.6% solution)/gallon (3.8 l) for not more than 10 days
  - Cats: (60–100 mg/kg (total) PO q24h) for 7 days. Used in the drinking water (sole source) at 1.5 tbsp (23 ml) (9.6% solution)/gallon (3.8 l) for not more than 10 days
- Ponazuril (20 mg/kg PO q24h) for 1–3 days in dogs and cats.

*Cryptosporidium* are harder to treat, but these drugs have some reported success [89]:

- Paromomycin (150 mg/kg PO q24h) for 5 days in cats and dogs. Use with caution in young animals as it may cause nephropathy.
- Azithromycin (5–10 mg/kg PO q12h) for 5–7 days in dogs; 7–15 mg/kg for 5–7 days in cats.
- Tylosin (10–15 mg/kg PO q8h) for 14–21 days in cats.

### 13.4.2.4 Tips and Tricks from the Field

- Prevention is important in shelters and catteries where stressors are high. Good hygiene and prevention of food or water contamination can help prevent spread of coccidiosis as the oocysts are resistant to many disinfectants and may survive many months in the environment.

- Feces should be removed regularly as oocysts sporulate quickly.

## 13.4.3 Giardiasis

### 13.4.3.1 General Information

Giardiasis is caused by the protozoa *Giardia duodenalis* (also known as *Giardia intestinalis* or *Giardia lamblia*). It has eight "assemblages" (A–H), some of which are host specific, whereas others can infect a wide range of species including humans [91]. Dogs and cats are more commonly affected by host-specific *Giardia*, so risk of zoonotic transmission is low. Transmission of *Giardia* is via the fecal–oral route, which can be through direct contact or via contaminated water, food, or environment.

Affected animals have diarrhea or steatorrhea that can be mucoid, pale, soft and have a strong odor. Diarrhea or steatorrhea can be chronic and cause weight loss. Animals that are younger, immunosuppressed, or live in crowded environments have higher risk of being affected. However, many animals can be asymptomatically infected but still shed the protozoa.

### 13.4.3.2 Diagnostics

Giardiasis is diagnosed by identifying the trophozoites or cysts through the following:

*Direct smear.* Perform using a small sample of fresh feces mixed with saline. Lugol's iodine stain may aid identification of trophozoites.

*Fecal floatation with centrifugation.* Mix feces with floatation solution (zinc sulfate preferred) or Sheather sugar, centrifuge for 5 min at 1500–2000 rpm to detect cysts.

*Fecal ELISA.* Commercially available tests or laboratory enzyme-linked immunosorbent assay (ELISA) assays can be performed to confirm presence of *Giardia*.

### 13.4.3.3 Treatment Protocols

Treatment options include:

- Fenbendazole (50 mg/kg PO q24h) for 3–5 days in dogs and cats
- Drontal® Plus (praziquantel, pyrantel pamoate, and febantel). Given once daily for 3 days in dogs and 5 days in cats

- Metronidazole (15–25 mg/kg PO q12–24h) for 5–7 days.

#### 13.4.3.4 Tips and Tricks from the Field

- Good hygiene is essential to preventing infection. Animals should also be bathed to remove possible fecal contamination and prevent reinfection through grooming [92].

### 13.4.4 Hookworms (Ancylostomiasis)

*Ancylostoma caninum* is the primary cause of hookworm infection in dogs. Dogs are infected through ingestion of infective third-stage larvae from a contaminated environment, transmammary transmission from bitch to pups (*A. caninum*), and skin penetration.

Hookworms can cause severe disease. Immature and adult worms attach to the small intestine mucosa where they feed on blood and when the worms detach small bleeding sites occur. Clinical signs are typically related to the anemia and blood loss including pale mucous membranes and dark, tarry stools. Coughing may be observed when larvae migrate through the lungs (Table 13.16).

---

**Textbox 13.18 Hookworm infection in young puppies**

Anemia in young puppies is characteristic of hookworm infections. Hookworm infection should be taken seriously as puppies with heavy worm burdens can die from the blood loss. Clinical signs are most severe in young pups that were infected through nursing.

---

Hookworms are zoonotic and the most common cause of cutaneous larva migrans in humans.

### 13.4.5 Roundworms (Ascariasis)

Roundworms are extremely common in dogs and cats worldwide (Table 13.17). Puppies may be infected *in utero* or via nursing causing serious illness before diagnosis is even possible by fecal examination. This

**Table 13.16** Hookworm summary table.

| | |
|---|---|
| Agent | *Ancylostoma caninum, Ancylostoma braziliense, Uncinaria stenocephala* |
| Infective stages and routes of transmission | Ingestion of environmental third-stage larvae (L3), transmammary (dogs), predation of infected paratenic hosts |
| Diagnosis | Eggs by fecal flotation |
| Clinical signs | Many infected animals may be asymptomatic. Anemia, melena, and tarry feces can be observed. Coughing and nasal discharge possible during migration through the lungs |
| Treatment | • Pyrantel (5–10 mg/kg PO) is the treatment of choice<br>• Febantel (10–15 mg/kg PO q24h) for 3 days<br>• Ivermectin (0.2 mg/kg PO or SQ)<br>• Fenbendazole (50 mg/kg PO q24h) for 3 days<br>• Nitroscanate (50 mg/kg PO) given once is approved for hookworms in some countries<br>• To prevent passage of infective larvae from lactating bitches to puppies, administer fenbendazole (50 mg/kg PO q24h) from day 40 of gestation to day 14 of lactation [93] |
| Zoonotic? | Yes – Cutaneous larval migrans in humans [94] |

phenomenon is the reason puppies and kittens should be dewormed at 2 weeks of age. Prenatal infection in kittens does not occur.

Animals usually become infected from ingesting eggs from a contaminated environment, as Toxocara eggs are very hardy in the environment. Infection can also result from the consumption of larvae in the tissues of paratenic hosts (rodents). Removing eggs from a contaminated environment is extremely difficult.

Puppies infected *in utero* may fail to gain weight, appear unthrifty, and have a pot-bellied appearance. Puppies may be seen vomiting large numbers of worms and kittens appear pot-bellied and unthrifty. Death can occur in young animals as a result of hepatic and pulmonary damage by migrating larvae. Infected adult cats may have ascarids present in

**Table 13.17** Roundworm summary table.

| | |
|---|---|
| Agent | *Toxocara canis, Toxascaris leonine, Toxocara cati* |
| Infective stages and routes of transmission | Puppies are often infected with *T. canis* transplacentally before birth. Infection may result from ingesting infective eggs from the environment or paratenic hosts (rodents, rabbits, earthworms) |
| Diagnosis | Eggs by fecal flotation |
| Clinical signs | Animals with low worm burdens are typically asymptomatic, higher burden animals may display a pot-bellied appearance. Large numbers of worms can result in intestinal blockage *T. leonine* infections are usually asymptomatic |
| Treatment | • Pyrantel pamoate (5–10 mg/kg PO) is the drug of choice in young puppies<br>• Selamectin, milbemycin oxime, and moxidectin have antiascarid activity. Most deworming medications are effective against roundworms |
| Zoonotic? | Yes – visceral and ocular larval migrans in humans |

**Table 13.18** Tapeworm summary table.

| | |
|---|---|
| Agent | *Dipylidium caninum, Taenia taeniaeformis, Echinococcus multilocularis, Echinococcus granulosus* |
| Infective stages and routes of transmission | Infection occurs following ingestion of larval cysts in the tissues of intermediate hosts |
| Diagnosis | Identification of proglottids in feces or recognizing eggs on fecal flotation |
| Clinical signs | Adult tapeworms cause minimal symptoms. Cysts of *Echinococcus* spp. can cause severe disease in intermediate hosts |
| Treatment | • Praziquantel (5 mg/kg PO) is drug of choice<br>• Epsiprantel and fenbendazole are also approved for the treatment of certain tapeworm infections<br>• Only praziquantel is labeled as effective against *Echinococcus* spp. (check specific label claims to verify) |
| Zoonotic? | Yes – *D. caninum* has zoonotic potential, usually in small children. Infective *Echinococcus* and *Taenia* spp. pose a health risk to those who may inadvertently ingest the eggs |

vomitus. *Toxocara* spp. have zoonotic potential and associated syndromes include visceral larval migrans, neural larva migrans, and ocular larva migrans [95]. Puppies and kittens should be dewormed starting at 2 weeks of age, repeating every 2 weeks until 12–16 weeks of age.

### 13.4.6 Tapeworms (Cestodiasis)

Cyclophyllidean tapeworms come in two forms, each with a different intermediate host that a dog or cat must eat to become infected (Table 13.18). Infection with *D. caninum* occurs following ingestion of an infected flea, whereas infection with *Taenia* and *Echinococcus* species follows ingestion of small rodents, rabbits, or large animals such as deer or sheep [96]. Both *Dipylidium* and *Taenia* tapeworms are generally nonpathogenic in cats and dogs but may be aesthetically unpleasant to pet owners. Identifying

proglottids in the feces or eggs on a fecal float is diagnostic.

Praziquantel and epsiprantel are treatments of choice because of their efficacy against *D. caninum* and *Taenia* spp. In field clinics where animals are anesthetized, praziquantel can be administered subcutaneously as part of a comprehensive deworming protocol. Treatment of tapeworms must be combined with effective flea control and prevention of ingestion of prey species or else reinfection is likely to occur.

Echinococcosis poses a significant human health burden. Worldwide, there is an excess of one million people living with the disease. Humans are infected through ingestion of parasite eggs in contaminated food, water, soil, or through direct contact with animal hosts. Echinococcosis is a commonly cited reason for dog population management in the developing world.

**Table 13.19** Threadworm summary table.

| Agent | *Strongyloides stercoralis, Strongyloides ratti, Strongyloides felis, Strongyloides planiceps, Strongyloides tumefaciens* |
|---|---|
| Infective stages and routes of transmission | Ingestion or skin penetration of L3, transmammary, and autoinfection |
| Diagnosis | Larvae in fresh feces, Baermann technique recommended |
| Clinical signs | Mucoid and blood-tinged diarrhea, weight loss, and polyphagia. Coughing or dyspnea if larval migration |
| Treatment | • Ivermectin (0.2 mg/kg SC or PO), two doses 4 weeks apart<br>• Fenbendazole (50 mg/kg PO) for 5 days and repeated 4 weeks later. In cats, a 3-day treatment course is suggested<br>• Thiabendazole (100–150 mg/kg/day PO q24h) for 3 days, repeated weekly until resolution of infection |
| Zoonotic? | Yes – Can affect the GI, skin, and/or respiratory system |

### 13.4.7 Threadworms (Strongyloidiasis)

Threadworms or *Strongyloides* are tiny nematodes measuring about 2 mm when fully matured, making them very difficult to see on gross examination [97]. Threadworms mainly affect dogs but can occur in cats (Table 13.19).

Animals become infected through larval ingestion, skin penetration, or autoinfection. Young animals can also become infected through transmammary transmission. *Strongyloides* infections are commonly associated with warm, moist, unhygienic housing.

Clinical signs are associated with heavy worm burden. These include mucoid diarrhea with blood, weight loss, and polyphagia [98]. Coughing can be seen with visceral larval migration with patients becoming dyspneic in the advanced stages. Diagnosis is confirmed via identification of larvae on direct microscopic examination or Baermann technique using fresh feces. As with all GI parasites, fecal examinations should be performed regularly every 6 months. Prevention depends on maintaining good hygiene rather than OTC deworming products.

*Strongyloides stercoralis* is zoonotic. In immuno-compromised people, *Strongyloides* can cause a hyperinfection syndrome affecting multiple organs simultaneously.

### 13.4.8 Whipworms (Trichuriasis)

*Trichuris vulpis* is common in dogs and rare in cats. Most animals become infected after ingesting food or water contaminated with whipworm eggs. Infected animals pass eggs in their feces, which must remain in the soil for about a month before they mature and become infective. Whipworm eggs are notoriously resistant to desiccation and extremes in temperature.

Many infected animals are clinically asymptomatic and signs of infection vary with the number of worms. Some infections may result in a colitis or diarrhea containing mucous and fresh blood. Severe infections can cause anemia, weight loss, and even death (Table 13.20).

**Table 13.20** Whipworm summary table.

| Agent | *Trichuris vulpis* |
|---|---|
| Infective stages and routes of transmission | Ingesting eggs containing infective larvae (fecal–oral) |
| Diagnosis | Eggs by fecal flotation |
| Clinical signs | Infected animals are frequently asymptomatic. Weight loss, diarrhea, and poor growth is common |
| Treatment | • Drontal® Plus (febantel (25 mg/kg), pyrantel pamoate (5 mg/kg), and praziquantel (5 mg/kg)) PO single administration<br>• Panacur® (fenbendazole) (50 mg/kg PO) for 3 consecutive days |
| Control | Milbemycin, milbemycin/lufenuron, milbemycin/spinosad, milbemycin/praziquantel, and moxidectin/imidacloprid, when administered for heartworm prevention are also approved for control of *T. vulpis* infections [99] |
| Zoonotic? | Not considered zoonotic at this time |

Source: Adapted from CAPC 2016 [39] Whipworms.

When considering an anthelmintic, note that not all broad-spectrum parasiticides control adult whipworms. Drontal® Plus (febantel, pyrantel pamoate, and praziquantel) and Panacur® (fenbendazole) are effective treatments. Due to the lengthy prepatent period, some recommend that these treatments be administered at monthly intervals for 3 months [99]. Other products are also approved for treatment and the continued control of whipworms when administered for monthly heartworm prevention.

## 13.5 Infectious Disease

### 13.5.1 Babesiosis

#### 13.5.1.1 General Information

Babesiosis is a tick-transmitted disease caused by a piroplasm parasite from the genus *Babesia*. *Babesia* infects the red blood cells of various hosts including cattle, horses, sheep, goats, pigs, dogs, and cats (Table 13.21). Canine babesiosis is most commonly caused by *Babesia canis*, *B. vogeli*, or *B. rossi*. *B. gibsoni* can also affect dogs and is considered highly pathogenic. Although rare, cats can become infected with *B. felis*. Historically, *Babesia* spp. have been divided into two categories, large and small, based on the intraerythocytic form.

The incubation period varies but is usually 1–3 weeks. Dogs are infected with sporozoites via the bite of an infected tick. Sporozoites attach to erythrocytes and multiply asexually to become merozoites, which in turn rupture the red blood cells and infect other red blood cells causing a hemolytic anemia.

There have been reports of *B. gibsoni* dog-to-dog transmission through blood contamination through dog fighting, primarily in American Pit Bull Terrier-type dogs [100]. Iatrogenic infection from needles and blood transfusions is also possible.

Dogs with acute babesiosis are typically inappetant, lethargic, have pale mucus membranes, fever, splenomegaly, anemia, thrombocytopenia, and pigmenturia due to hemoglobinuria. Chronic infections can cause hyperthermia, weight loss, lethargy, and pulmonary or renal disease. More severe disease can cause progressive hemolytic anemia or hypoxic, hypotensive shock with disseminated intravascular coagulation (DIC), systemic inflammatory response syndrome, and multiple organ dysfunction syndrome. Young puppies or adults that are immunocompromised or have had a splenectomy exhibit more severe clinical signs.

In cats, babesiosis can cause inappetence, lethargy, and weakness. Clinical signs include pale mucus membranes, tachycardia and tachypnea (or dyspnea) caused by profound anemia, and sometimes icterus. Erythrocytes are typically macrocytic and hypochromic.

Many treatments do not completely eliminate the pathogen and animals that recover from clinical signs may become carriers.

#### 13.5.1.2 Diagnostics

*Complete blood count.* Thrombocytopenia is the most common finding. Macrocytic anemia and autoagglutination is variable.

*Cytology.* Acute infection can be diagnosed by microscopic identification of the organism with Giemsa

**Table 13.21** Host, vector, distribution, and severity of *Babesia* species.

| Species | Host | Vector | Distribution | Severity |
|---------|------|--------|--------------|----------|
| *B. canis* | Canine | *Dermacentor reticularis* | Europe | Mild to severe disease |
| *B. vogeli* | Canine | *Rhipicephalus sanguineus* | Southern Europe, tropical and subtropical countries worldwide | Least pathogenic. Causes mild to moderate disease, or subclinical |
| *B. rossi* | Canine | *Haemaphysalis elliptica* | South Africa, Sub-Saharan Africa | Large proportion of dogs show severe clinical disease |
| *B. gibsoni* | Canine | *Haemaphysalis longicornis, R. sanguineus* (suspected) | Africa, Asia, USA, Southern Europe, Middle East, and Australia | Most severe and highly pathogenic |
| *B. felis* | Feline | Tick-borne, exact vector unknown | Southern continent of Africa | Varying severity |

or Wright's stained blood smears. Dogs with chronic infections may have intermittent parasitemia, complicating diagnosis. Microscopic examination can differentiate between large or small *Babesia* species, but not between similar-sized species.

*PCR.* Tests can confirm disease and differentiate between the infectious species. However, low parasitemia can result in false negatives on PCR. Serological tests such as IFAT or ELISA can be used for diagnosis, although false negatives are possible if antibodies are not present.

### 13.5.1.3 Treatment Protocols

The prognosis for most *Babesia* cases is good with early diagnosis and appropriate treatment. Even with treatment however, patients may remain persistently infected yet subclinical for the remainder of their lives.

#### 13.5.1.3.1 Gold Standard Protocols

- Fluid therapy and blood transfusions should be given when necessary.
- The treatment of choice for dogs is an injection of either imidocarb dipropionate (6.6 mg/kg SC or IM) or diminazene aceturate (5 mg/kg SC or IM). Repeat treatment in 2 weeks. These drugs work best on large species of *Babesia* and are less effective on *B. gibsoni*.
- Atovaquone (13.3 mg/kg PO q8h) and azithromycin (10 mg/kg PO q24h) combination therapy for 10 days has been found useful to either eliminate or reduce parasitemia in dogs infected with *B. gibsoni* (Asian genotype) [101].
- *B. felis* in cats can be treated with primaquine phosphate (0.5 mg/kg IM or PO q24h) once [102].

#### 13.5.1.3.2 Alternative Protocols

- Pentamidine isethionate (16 mg/kg IM q24h) for two doses can be used to treat *Babesia* spp. in dogs.
- Trypan blue (10 mg/kg as a 1% solution IV) once for mild uncomplicated babesiosis.
- Drugs that reduce clinical signs (but may not eliminate the pathogen):
  – Clindamycin (25 mg/kg PO q12h) for 14 days [103]
  – Clindamycin (25 mg/kg PO q12h), metronidazole (15 mg/kg PO q12h), and doxycycline

(5 mg/kg PO q12h) combination therapy [104]. A treatment period of 10 days has been recommended.

### 13.5.1.4 Prevention

1) *Control external parasites.* Reduce the risk of infection through year-round tick control.
2) *Screen blood donors.* Prohibit dogs with a history of babesiosis from donating blood.
3) *Vaccinate.* In certain areas of the world, vaccines exist for certain species of *Babesia*, which may reduce disease severity.
4) *Eliminate dog fighting.* Prevent dog-to-dog transmission of *B. gibsoni* and promote animal welfare.

### 13.5.1.5 Public Health Considerations

*B. canis* and *B. gibsoni* are not known to infect people. *Babesia microti*, however, naturally infects rodents and can infect people through *Ixodes* ticks. Ticks are the only known vector of human infection. In humans, clinical signs are similar to those of malaria including fever, malaise, fatigue, chills, sweats, hemolytic anemia, and thrombocytopenia.

### 13.5.1.6 Tips and Tricks from the Field

- Co-infection with *E. canis* is very common in endemic areas. Simultaneous treatment for both babesiosis and ehrlichiosis should be considered.
- Babesiosis should be considered in any dog with hemolytic anemia and thrombocytopenia, living in an endemic area with a history of tick exposure.
- *Babesia* spp. can recrudesce in some dogs following stress; identification and removal of the stressor during and after treatment is important.
- Dogs living in an endemic area can develop antibodies against *Babesia* spp, conferring a degree of resistance. Dogs imported from outside the endemic area may be more susceptible to disease.

## 13.5.2 Blastomycosis

### 13.5.2.1 General Information

Blastomycosis is endemic to primarily North America but also occurs sporadically in Central America, Africa, India, Europe, and Central America [105]. North American blastomycosis is caused by the mycotic species *Blastomyces dermatitidis* and is principally located in the Mississippi, Missouri, and Ohio

River Valley areas. Dogs and humans are most commonly infected, but occasionally cats develop systemic blastomycosis. *Ajellomyces dermatitidis* is a species of pathogenic fungi that grows as mycelial (infectious) forms at room temperature and transforms into *B. dermatitidis* as a yeast (disease causing) form at body temperature. The mycelial form grows in sandy, acidic soils that contain wood debris and animal waste, and are within 400 m (1312 ft) of water [105]. Recent disruption of soil such as during housing construction and recent rainfall are important epidemiological risk factors for outbreaks in endemic regions [106].

Although focal infection is possible with direct inoculation through the skin, *Ajellomyces* is typically inhaled in the mycelial form and transforms to the yeast form once it enters the body. Pulmonary infection can lead to signs of pneumonia, or may be asymptomatic. After infecting the lungs, the organism disseminates throughout the body via the vascular and lymphatic systems and in the dog most commonly enters the skin (including toes and claws), eyes, bones, lymph nodes, subcutaneous tissues, external nares, brain, and testes. Less commonly affected sites include the mouth, nasal passages, prostate, liver, mammary gland, vulva, and heart. GI involvement is rare [105]. In cats, respiratory tract involvement is seen most frequently, followed by the central nervous system (CNS), regional lymph nodes, skin, eyes, GI, and urinary tract [107].

---

**Textbox 13.19 Clinical signs commonly associated with blastomycosis**

- Nonspecific signs: Anorexia, weight loss, and lethargy
- Fever >103 °F (39.4 °C)
- Lungs: Cough, tachypnea, cyanosis, and respiratory distress
- Lymph nodes: Enlargement of one or more peripheral lymph nodes
- Eyes: Uveitis, conjunctivitis, iridial hyperemia, aqueous flare, miosis, and corneal edema
- Skin: Granulomatous proliferative lesions and ulcerations (nasal planum, face, and nail beds)
- Bone: Solitary bone infections (particularly involving the distal limbs).

---

Clinical signs vary by organ involvement. Between 65% and 85% of dogs have pulmonary involvement, whereas others may have cutaneous and lymph node involvement, as well as pyrexia [108]. Common clinical signs include dry, harsh lung sounds, coughing, dyspnea, draining wounds, weight loss, lameness, pyrexia, lymphadenopathy, anorexia, and ocular disease. Systemic signs in cats are similar to those of dogs. Hematuria and dysuria may be seen with urinary tract involvement.

#### 13.5.2.2 Diagnosis

*Cytology or histopathology.* Identification of Blastomyces yeast remains the gold standard for diagnosis; however, other diagnostic methods are very useful in cases in which identification is unclear or sample acquisition is not feasible [109].

- Cytological identification of 5- to 20-μm-diameter broad-based budding yeast organisms on impression smears of cutaneous lesions and draining tracts, cytology of lymph node aspirates and tracheal washes (76% positivity), or bronchoalveolar lavages (BAL) [110].
- Diff-Quik® and Wright's stains turn the yeast dark blue. A productive cough will greatly increase the likelihood of collecting yeast from tracheal washes and BAL.
- Yeast may be found in the urine with prostatic involvement. The presence of pyogranulomatous inflammation is common.
- Aspirates from lymph nodes and dermal lesions are typically of higher diagnostic value than specimens obtained from other body sites; however, in cats peripheral lymph nodes are not commonly affected.

*Culture.* Not routinely performed due to the risk to laboratory personnel. Thoracic radiographs may reveal a diffuse interstitial pattern and mediastinal lymph node enlargement characteristic of mycotic pneumonitis. Bone lesions may resemble osteosarcoma [111].

*CBC/chemistry.* Chronic inflammation including leukocytosis with left shift, lymphopenia, and mild, normocytic, normochromic anemia. Blood chemistry indicates hyperglobulinemia, hypoalbuminemia, and occasionally hypercalcemia (due to granulomatous disease).

*Serology*

- Urine, serum, cerebrospinal fluid, plasma, and BAL MiraVista Diagnostics' *Blastomyces* antigen test for dogs [109]. This is not a benchside test and may be impractical for field work.
- Antigen by ELISA. Urine may be collected by mid-stream free catch, cystocentesis, or catheterization. May also use serum, plasma, cerebral spinal fluid (CSF), tracheal wash, or other body cavity effusion [112].
- Serum agar gel immunodiffusion (AGID) antibody test.[2]
- PCR may be available depending on the geographical area. The ideal sample to test depends on affected tissues. CSF, whole blood, pharyngeal/nasal swab, tracheal wash/BAL, needle aspirate/biopsy of tissue, or feces may be used [112].

### 13.5.2.3 Treatment Protocols

The prognosis for full recovery with appropriate treatment is good except in cases with severe pulmonary or CNS involvement. As 20–25% of dogs treated for blastomycosis relapse after discontinuation of treatment, confirmation of clinical, mycological, and ideally radiological cure is essential [106].

#### 13.5.2.3.1 *Gold Standard Protocols*

The aggressiveness of treatment depends on the disease severity. Hospitalization with supportive care including IV fluids, appetite and pain management, and oxygen therapy is needed for severe cases. Mildly affected patients may receive outpatient treatment. Table 13.22 describes commonly used antifungals.

Monitor closely for side effects during the first 2 weeks of therapy. Itraconazole and fluconazole have similar side effects including anorexia, vomiting, diarrhea, and hepatotoxicity. Anorexia is often the symptomatic marker for toxicity and usually occurs in the second month of treatment [114].

Treatment efficacy and relapse rates are similar for fluconazole and itraconazole. In spite of the significantly longer duration of treatment using

---

2 Antigen tests are considered superior to AGID and sensitivity increases with urine specimens [113]. Beware of cross-reactivity with *Histoplasma* organisms.

fluconazole, it is still much less expensive than itraconazole [115], and hepatotoxicity gauged by serum increases in alanine aminotransferase (ALT) is similar to itraconazole. Fluconazole is excreted in the urine, so dosage adjustments are needed in patients with renal impairment. It also crosses the blood–brain and blood–prostate barriers better than itraconazole. There is minimal data available on veterinary use of posaconazole and voriconazole.

Amphotericin B is reserved for potentially fatal disease such as severe pneumonia, severely immunocompromised patients, and CNS involvement due to its highly nephrotoxic side effects. Amphotericin B lipid complex is speculated to be 8–10 times less nephrotoxic than the deoxycholate form. As a result, higher doses may be used and the lipid complex may be more effective [116]. Antigen serology tests are ideal for monitoring remission and should be performed 4–6 weeks after stopping treatment.

#### 13.5.2.3.2 *Alternative Protocols*

- Ketoconazole is considered for dogs and cats only when the cost of preferred drugs is prohibitive. Combination with amphotericin B is recommended.
- Amphotericin B SQ might be more cost effective and easier to administer.

### 13.5.2.4 Public Health Considerations

Blastomycosis is not considered zoonotic with casual contact; however, it can be transmitted through direct inoculation from dog bite wounds and contaminated needle pricks. Dog bite avoidance, proper bite wound cleaning, and safe needle handling are very important if blastomycosis is suspected. Although undocumented, another potential concern is reversion of the yeast form to the mycelial form on bandage materials or exudates deposited in the environment. The reversion can occur within 3–4 days at room temperature, suggestive of a risk associated with contaminated surfaces or materials [114].

### 13.5.2.5 Tips and Tricks from the Field

- The combination of respiratory disease with eye, bone, or skin involvement in a young dog is suggestive of blastomycosis [108].
- A trial period of an oral azole can be started if blastomycosis is highly suspected, but will need to

Table 13.22 Blastomycosis antifungal dosing chart.

| Antifungal | Canine dosage | Feline dosage | Treatment considerations |
|---|---|---|---|
| Itraconazole | 5–10 mg/kg PO q24h, or divided q12h with food | 5–10 mg/kg PO q24h, or divided q12h with food | • Drug of choice<br>• Oral liquid formulation (10 mg/ml) available for cats<br>• Treat for at least 60 days, and for 30 days after resolution of clinical signs |
| Fluconazole | 5–10 mg/kg PO q12–24h for 4–6 months; start with lower dose q12h and adjust dose and frequency based on response | 10 mg/kg PO q24h (typically 50 mg per cat) | • Give with or without food<br>• Continue 1–3 months after clinical resolution or negative antigen test |
| Amphotericin B | 0.5 mg/kg IV every other day three times per week (diluted in D5W slow IV over 4–6 h); 9–12 mg/kg cumulative dose; keep hydrated 0.5 mg/kg SQ two to three times per week; dilute to 5 mg/ml and give dose with 350–500 ml sodium chloride 0.45%/dextrose 2.5% SQ bolus, or inject diluted dose into SQ fluid pocket; 10–15 mg/kg cumulative dose | 0.25 mg/kg every other day three times per week (diluted in D5W slow IV over 4–6 h); 6–9 mg/kg cumulative dose; keep hydrated 0.5 mg/kg SQ two to three times per week; dilute to 5 mg/ml and give dose with 350 ml of sodium chloride 0.45%/dextrose 2.5% SQ bolus, or inject diluted dose into SQ fluid pocket; 10–15 mg/kg cumulative dose | • For severe, life-threatening disease<br>• When acute clinical signs have resolved, switch to itraconazole |
| Ketoconazole | 5–10 mg/kg PO q12–24h with food | 5–10 mg/kg PO q12–24h with food | • When cost is an issue; use as a last resort treatment<br>• In dogs, continue 30 days past clinical resolution |
| Posaconazole | 5–10 mg/kg PO q12–24h after fatty meal | 5 mg/kg PO q24h or divided q12h after fatty meal | |
| Voriconazole | 5–6 mg/kg PO q12h | Not recommended | |

be given for 7–14 days, as it may take this long to see improvement.

- The bioavailability of compounded itraconazole is low and may result in treatment failure unless prepared from commercial capsules or documented bioavailability and stability data are provided [108].
- Amphotericin B may be used if oral treatment is not an option.
- To extend the shelf life of amphotericin B deoxycholate, freeze it between doses and allow it to thaw at room temperature for collection of each dose.

### 13.5.3 Brucellosis

#### 13.5.3.1 General Information

Brucellosis in dogs is most commonly caused by the bacterium *B. canis*, but dogs in contact with other animal species can be infected with other *Brucella* species including *Brucella abortus*, *Brucella suis*, or *Brucella melitensis*. The most common sign of infection is an otherwise healthy appearing female dog aborting at around 45–55 days of gestation [117]. Following abortion, prolonged vaginal discharge for up to 6 weeks may be observed. Infected male dogs may exhibit signs of orchitis, painful scrotal enlargement, scrotal dermatitis from excessive licking, testicular atrophy, and/or preputial discharge. It is important to remember that infected dogs are not necessarily clinically ill and that clinical signs can occur in both intact and neutered animals. Clinical signs, when present, can be vague and often mimic other diseases. These can include lethargy, generalized lymphadenitis, spondylitis, or uveitis. Fever is not typical of this disease.

*B. canis* infection in dogs is primarily maintained through venereal transmission. Dogs can also become infected after contact with infectious body fluids or secretions during birth or after abortion. No immunization currently exists for *Brucella* spp. in dogs or cats.

### 13.5.3.2 Diagnostics
In the field, diagnosis of *B. canis* will typically be based on clinical signs and suspicion.

*Rapid slide agglutination test (RSAT) and tube agglutination test (TAT).* These cage-side tests kits can be used to detect antibodies to *B. canis*. Two negative tests 2–3 months apart are typically needed to confirm negativity.

*Culture.* A definitive diagnosis is made most commonly through cultures of samples from the genital tract, blood, or other affected tissues.

### 13.5.3.3 Treatment Protocols
Unfortunately, no treatment protocol to date has been found to reliably eliminate *B. canis* infections. Treatment can be expensive and lengthy, typically consisting of 4 weeks depending on the drugs used and response to therapy. Treatment with antibiotics can be successful but usually requires a combination of streptomycin or gentamicin with tetracycline (Table 13.23). The combination of tetracyclines and streptomycin is thought to be the most efficacious protocol, but streptomycin can be quite limited in its availability. Before initiating therapy, one should understand that multiple treatment courses may be necessary to clear the organism. Sample treatment protocols include the following:

- Tetracycline (30 mg/kg PO q12h) or doxycycline (10 mg/kg PO q12h) for 1 month, in combination with gentamicin (5 mg/kg SQ q24h) for 7 days repeated every 3 weeks [118].
- Tetracycline (10 mg/kg PO q8h) for 30 days and streptomycin (15 mg/kg IM q24h) on days 1–7 and

**Table 13.23** Routinely used antibiotics for treating canine *Brucella* spp. infections.

| Drug[a] | Daily dose (mg/kg) | Route | Frequency of administration |
|---|---|---|---|
| Doxycycline | 10–15 | PO | q12h |
| Minocycline | 10 | PO | q12h |
| Streptomycin | 15–20 | IM | q24h |
| Dihydrostreptomycin | 10–20 | IM, SC | q12–24h |
| Gentamicin | 2.2–5 | IM, SQ | q24h |
| Enrofloxacin | 5–10 | PO | q24h |
| Trimethoprim–sulfadiazine | 30 | PO | q12h |

a) Note that combination therapy is recommended.

24–30. During one outbreak, 15 out of 20 dogs were considered cured with this protocol [119].
- Oxytetracycline (20 mg/kg IM) once weekly for 4 weeks and streptomycin (15 mg/kg IM q24h) for the first 7 days. In one study, a total of 19 out of 24 dogs had negative testing following this protocol [120].
- Minocycline (10 mg/kg PO q24h) for 14 days in conjunction with streptomycin (4.5 mg/kg IM) divided twice daily for 7 days. In one study, 83% of treated dogs were cured [121].
- Tetracycline plus streptomycin plus trimethoprim sulfadiazine – In one study, a combination of tetracycline, dihydrostreptomycin, and trimethoprim–sulfadiazine prevented abortion [122].
- Enrofloxacin (5 mg/kg PO q12h) for 4 weeks. In one study, this protected against abortions in an infected kennel [123].

Gentamicin is routinely substituted for streptomycin. Quinolone antibiotics have also been proposed as a substitute for aminoglycosides in patients with renal compromise.

### 13.5.3.4 Public Health Considerations
*B. canis* is zoonotic, but human infection is rare and disease is usually mild. It poses the highest risk to immunocompromised individuals and children.

#### 13.5.3.5 Tips and Tricks from the Field

- There are many protocols available, each varying in cost, efficacy, and duration. Choose a protocol that best fits the situation that you are working in with medications that are readily available.
- Be aware that *B. canis* infections can cause significant management dilemmas, particularly for shelters. Some may advocate for the euthanasia of infected dogs to prevent transmission.
- All infected animals should be neutered. This will minimize environmental contamination and serve as an alternative to euthanasia.

### 13.5.4 Canine Distemper

#### 13.5.4.1 General Information

Canine distemper virus (CDV) is a highly contagious, systemic, viral disease of dogs. CDV is a morbillivirus in the *Paramyxoviridae* family related to measles in humans and rinderpest in cattle. Although CDV can affect skunks, fox, raccoons, and tigers, domestic dogs are considered the reservoir species and disease is seen most frequently in areas where vaccination coverage is low [108]. There appears to be no breed or sex predilection for CDV infection, but animals <6 months of age are particularly vulnerable.

The main route of infection is contact with respiratory secretions. Fomite transmission can also occur over short distances. As an enveloped virus, CDV is relatively easy to inactivate with commonly used disinfectants. Upon infection, the virus replicates in the lymphatic tissue of the respiratory tract. A viremia then occurs, infecting the respiratory, GI, and urogenital epithelium, CNS, and optic nerves. The degree of viremia depends on the level of humeral immunity exhibited by the host.

The incubation period is usually 1–2 weeks but can be as long as 4–5 weeks. Clinical signs of canine distemper vary depending on virulence of the virus strain, environmental conditions, and host age and immune status [124]. Usually, a constellation of systemic clinical signs including vomiting, diarrhea, and/or respiratory signs is observed. These may be difficult to distinguish from other diseases such as leptospirosis and CIRDC (kennel cough).

If inadequate immunity is present at the time of infection, acute multisystemic illness typically develops 2 weeks postinfection. Initial signs include lethargy, fever, decreased appetite, mild conjunctivitis, and nasal/ocular discharge. Note that subclinical disease can occur with a strong immune response, and more than 50% of infections are probably subclinical [124]. Respiratory signs typically consist of coughing, sneezing, dyspnea, mucoid to mucopurulent nasal discharge, and tonsillitis. Ocular signs may include anterior uveitis, optic neuritis, and keratoconjunctivitis sicca (KCS) (dry eye). Later, bronchitis or bronchopneumonia may develop. GI signs typically follow, consisting of vomiting, diarrhea (often bloody), and dehydration.

In some dogs, neurological signs may develop. Clinical signs may vary depending on the affected area of the nervous system. Myoclonus (rhythmic jerking of single muscles or muscle groups), "chewing gum" fits, ataxia, cerebellar and vestibular disease, seizures, blindness, conscious proprioception deficits, tonic–clonic spasms, and paresis may be observed [108,124,125]. Neurological signs are generally not reversible and surviving dogs often have permanent CNS sequelae such as nervous "ticks," or involuntary leg movements [125]. There is no way of knowing whether or not an infected dog will develop neurological manifestations and neurological disease can be delayed for months to years. Old dog encephalitis is a slow progressive loss of neurological functions, and hard-pad disease involves hyperkeratosis of the foot pads and nose [126].

*In utero* CDV infection causes stillbirth and abortion, neurological signs at birth, and "fading puppy" syndrome during the neonatal period. Infected puppies with unerupted permanent teeth may develop enamel hypoplasia, partial eruption, oligodontia, or impaction [126].

#### 13.5.4.2 Diagnostics

Diagnosing CDV can be frustrating and difficult. In many field environments, practical diagnosis is based on clinical suspicion. CDV should be considered in any unvaccinated febrile dog with multisystemic (respiratory, GI, and neurological) disease.

*Complete blood count.* Clinicopathological findings are usually nonspecific and include lymphopenia.
*Blood smear.* Using a stained peripheral blood smear, check for characteristic inclusion bodies in lymphocytes, neutrophils, and erythrocytes.

*Immunofluorescent assay.* For viral antigen or inclusion bodies in cells from conjunctival scrapes, in urine sediment, and buffy coat. False negatives are common.

*Serology and antigen tests.* Benchside antigens are commonly used diagnostic tools internationally. See Chapter 14 for more information.

*RT PCR.* Detects virus in respiratory secretions, CSF, feces, and urine.

*Necropsy and histopathology.* Tissues from lungs, stomach, urinary bladder, lymph nodes, and brain can be submitted to a diagnostic laboratory for virus detection [108].

### 13.5.4.3 Treatment Protocols

There is no specific treatment that targets the distemper virus and the patient prognosis depends on the strain of the virus and patient immune response. CDV treatments are symptomatic and supportive, aimed at keeping the patient hydrated and limiting secondary infections. The mainstays of therapy include broad-spectrum antibiotics, fluid therapy, antipyretics, analgesics, nutrition, and anticonvulsants when needed. Sound nursing care is a must. Even with aggressive therapy, mortality rates are reported at around 50%.

#### 13.5.4.3.1 Gold Standard Protocols

General treatment principles:

- Maintain hydration with IV fluids, if possible.
- Provide adequate nutritional support. If the patient is unable to eat, consider placing an esophagostomy or gastrostomy tube.
- Avoid using steroids except as a last-ditch effort for neurological cases.

Respiratory disease:

- Consider nebulization and coupage. Some shelters will maintain a supply of nebulizers and loan them out to foster homes as needed.
- Prevent secondary infections by administering broad-spectrum antibiotics. Antibiotics with good activity against *Bordetella bronchiseptica* and mycoplasma (e.g. doxycycline) are warranted if these pathogens are suspected.
- Recommended initial antibacterial choices for bronchopneumonia include

  - Ampicillin (20 mg/kg PO, IV, SC q8h) for 7 days
  - Doxycycline (5–10 mg/kg PO q12h) for 7 days
  - Chloramphenicol (40–50 mg/kg PO, SC q8h) for 7 days
  - Florfenicol (25–50 mg/kg SC, IM q8h) for 3–5 days

Combination therapy may be indicated.

GI disease:

- Ensure the patient is dewormed.
- Provide antiemetics and gastroprotectants as needed.
- B vitamins are a nonspecific therapy to replace losses from anorexia and diuresis.
- Ascorbic acid (vitamin C) administration has anecdotally proved beneficial in CDV patients.

Neurological disease:

- Administer anticonvulsant therapy if seizures are noted. Seizures are best treated with diazepam (0.5–2 mg/kg rectally or IV). If hospitalization is not an option, consider giving the patient a loading dose of phenobarbital (10–20 mg/kg divided into smaller doses q2h) and then send home with daily oral phenobarbital (2–4 mg/kg/day q12h) for 7–14 days. Many animal shelters in the US also use Keppra (Levetiracetam), due to its noncontrolled status.
- Seizure medications should be started immediately following the observation of seizures. Such medications can prevent seizure circuits from becoming established [126].
- In dogs with neurological signs, gabapentin (10–20 mg/kg PO q8h) coupled with an NSAID is anecdotally reported to be beneficial in treating tremors.
- Ensure a well-padded environment for dogs with seizure activity.
- In some dogs, neurological signs have been variably halted following a single anti-CNS edema dose of dexamethasone (2.2 mg/kg IV). Follow-up anti-inflammatory doses may be warranted, which can be tapered over time.

KCS (dry eye):

- Patients with KCS often respond to triple antibiotic ophthalmic ointment, artificial tears, and cyclosporine ophthalmic.

### *13.5.4.3.2 Alternative Protocols*

**Newcastle Disease Vaccine** An unorthodox approach to CDV treatment was first introduced in the early 1970s and has evolved throughout the years involving the use of a live virus vaccine for Newcastle disease virus (NDV) to stimulate a dog's immune system to effectively clear CDV infection. Although this is experimental and unconventional, it has offered a glimmer of hope to a disease that typically carries a grave prognosis. Multiple protocols exist for the use of NDV vaccine, including IV injection, use of NDV-induced serum, and NDV spinal tap. This is typically used as a last-ditch treatment effort.

For more information, visit http://www.kindhearts inaction.com.

**Botulinum Toxin (Botox®)** One case report describes the safe and effective use of botulinum toxin (Botox) type A to treat debilitating myoclonus in a dog suspected of having had distemper [127]. Botox was injected into the patient's affected muscles and initial improvement of myoclonus was noted within 5 h. Repeated Botox® treatment was required 18 days later. No long-term, overt adverse side effects were reported.

**Interferon-α and Ribavirin** In laboratory tests, *in vitro* work with antiviral drugs such as interferon and ribavirin has shown promise. Such drugs are probably most effective in treating CDV during early stages of infection. Doses are largely unknown.

#### 13.5.4.4 Tips and Tricks from the Field

- Consider CDV in any young, unvaccinated dog with multifocal CNS disease with other organ involvement [108].
- Caring for distemper-infected dogs requires a serious commitment, as the general course of treatment is often months. Furthermore, infected dogs may shed virus for up to 3 months and must be kept isolated during that time.
- In a shelter environment, once distemper has been diagnosed, any dog with respiratory or GI disease must be considered a CDV-suspect.
- Dogs that appear to recover from initial respiratory illness may still develop fatal neurological disease, even months after treatment.

- Routine vaccination is a key to prevention and avoidance. Immunity following recovery from natural infection or booster vaccination typically persists for years. However, although current vaccines appear protective against most circulating strains, vaccine breaks may occur.

### 13.5.5 Canine Parvovirus

#### 13.5.5.1 General Information

Canine parvovirus (CPV) is one of the most common and deadliest diseases practitioners in the field will face. Although vaccination is highly effective, CPV is widespread in many areas due to a lack of available preventive health services. Infected dogs in the field can be particularly challenging to manage because while interventions are often effective, the cost of treatment may be financially prohibitive depending on available resources. Without treatment, parvovirus is almost always fatal due to dehydration or a severely compromised immune system.

CPV is an un-enveloped virus from the *Parvoviridae* family, making it very hardy in the environment and resistant to common disinfectants. There are two primary strains, CPV-1 and CPV-2. CPV-2 is the most common cause of the disease and is further divided into CPV-2a, CPV-2b, and CPV-2c based on genotyping. The vaccine strain CPV-2b is, however able to give cross-protection to all variants, and treatment protocols do not vary based on the strain or genotype.

CPV disease typically consists of acute GI illness in young dogs and carries a high mortality rate if left untreated. Transmission is through the fecal–oral route and incubation period ranges between 2 and 14 days, although clinical signs typically develop within 5–7 days postinfection [128]. Shedding can occur for up to 2 weeks postrecovery.

Clinical signs include profuse diarrhea, often with a characteristic smell, vomiting, lethargy, and inappetence. Other signs include pain or discomfort on abdominal palpation, dehydration, tachycardia, and hypothermia. Most patients will present between 6 weeks and 6 months of age. Differential diagnoses include foreign body obstruction, toxin ingestion, GI parasitism, *Clostridium perfringens* infection, *Campylobacter* infection, coronaviral infection, hemorrhagic gastroenteritis, and intussusception (although intussusception can occur due to severe intestinal hypermotility caused by CPV).

#### 13.5.5.2 Diagnostics

Diagnosis is typically based on clinical signs, patient age, and vaccination history.

*CBC/chemistry.* On complete blood count (CBC), a severe neutropenia and lymphopenia are often observed. On biochemistry, hypoglycemia, electrolyte imbalance (typically hypokalemia), hypoproteinemia, elevated liver enzymes, and azotemia is common.

*ELISA.* Typical confirmatory test used on diarrhetic feces. False negatives can occur both early and late in the course of disease, and voluminous feces may dilute viral particles. Recent vaccination may cause a false positive; however, anecdotally, these are typically weak in color on the test kit.

#### 13.5.5.3 Treatment Protocols

Successful treatment involves intense supportive care, sound nursing care, and prevention of secondary bacterial infections.

##### 13.5.5.3.1 Gold Standard Protocols

Although there is no one definitive treatment protocol, supportive care should attempt to the following:

- *Hydrate.* Calculate fluid loss from dehydration, ongoing losses, plus maintenance fluid needs. IV administration is normally preferred, but the SQ route can also be used.
  - Consider correcting for hypokalemia and hypoglycemia. If blood parameters cannot be measured, consider adding potassium chloride 20–40 mEq/l and dextrose 2.5–5% into the IV fluids (add 50–100 ml of 50% dextrose per liter of replacement fluids).
  - Natural (whole blood or plasma) or synthetic (i.e. hetastarch or dextran 70) colloids may be needed in severely hypoproteinemic patients.
- *Prevent sepsis due to secondary bacterial infection.* Administer broad-spectrum antibiotics to include gram-negative organisms for 3–5 days. Avoid fluoroquinolones in young puppies and use caution with aminoglycosides in dehydrated patients.
  - Combine penicillin derivatives: (ampicillin or cefazolin (22 mg/kg IV q8h)) with an aminoglycoside, enrofloxacin (5 mg/kg IM, IV q24h), or gentamicin (6 mg/kg IV q24h).
  - Other broad-spectrum antibiotics to consider: Cephalosporins (cefoxitin, ceftazidime, and cefovecin) and fluoroquinolones.

- Control vomiting with antiemetics such as maropitant (1 mg/kg IV q24h), ondansetron (0.5 mg/kg IV q8h), or metoclopramide (0.2–0.4 mg/kg SC q6–8h). Consider administering gastroprotectants cimetidine (4–10 mg/kg SC, IM, IV q6h) or ranitidine (1–2 mg/kg IV q12h).
- Provide adequate nutrition: Control food and water intake if vomiting is intense, then start with water followed by bland, easily digestible diet (e.g. Hill's® i/d, Purina® EN, or boiled chicken).
- Manage pain: For severe cases, administer buprenorphine (0.02 mg/kg SQ q6–8h). Avoid NSAIDs (renal toxicity) until dehydration is corrected.

##### 13.5.5.3.2 Alternative Protocols

**Practical Outpatient CPV Protocol** Due to the high cost of traditional CPV treatment, the following protocol has been designed to allow owners to treat animals on an outpatient basis. This protocol has shown promising results with up to 80% survival rates and, in the author's opinion, can be used as a standard treatment protocol in the field [129,130].

Before sending patients home, on presentation patients should be stabilized to return to normal cardiovascular parameters by giving an IV bolus of isotonic crystalloid over 15–20 min, correcting for severe hypoglycemia (Table 13.24).

**Table 13.24** Determination of volume of crystalloids fluids required for IV fluid resuscitation and normalization of cardiovascular parameters.

| Class | Intravascular volume loss to replace (BV = blood volume) | Clinical signs |
| --- | --- | --- |
| I | <15% BV loss (15 ml/kg IV fluid bolus) | Mild ↑ HR |
| II | 15–30% BV loss (25 ml/kg IV fluid bolus) | ↑ HR, ↑ RR |
| III | 30–40% BV loss (35 ml/kg IV fluid bolus) | ↑ HR, ↑ RR, pale mucous membranes, ↑ CRT |
| IV | >40% BV loss (45 ml/kg IV fluid bolus) | ↑ HR, ↑ RR, pale mucous membranes, ↑ CRT, cold extremities, mental dullness |

If required, 6% hetastarch (5–10 ml/kg) can also be provided as a bolus over 10–15 min. Additional isotonic crystalloid boluses can be administered as indicated by the patient's clinical status.

---

**Textbox 13.20 CPV outpatient protocol**

- Administer cefovecin (Convenia®) (8 mg/kg SC) once.
- Provide the owner with subcutaneous crystalloid fluids to be given q8h (total volume is 120 ml/kg/day plus dehydration replacement. Divide the total daily volume by 3).
- Antiemetic: Administer maropitant (Cerenia®) (1 mg/kg SC q24h) during the entire treatment period. In case of severe vomiting, administer ondansetron (0.5 mg/kg SC q8h) as needed.
- When vomiting is under control, provide a bland, easily digestible diet (e.g. Hill's® a/d) as tolerated by patient:
  - If visceral pain, administer buprenorphine (0.02 mg/kg SC q6–8h).
  - If hypoglycemic (blood glucose <80 mmol/l), provide simple syrup buccally q2–6h.
  - If hypokalemic (serum K+ <3.4 mEq/l), oral Tumil-K at 0.5–1 teaspoon per 10 lbs (4.5 kg) q4–6h.

Note that owners and caregivers must be instructed on how to administer medications appropriately before starting this protocol. If the patient worsens during outpatient treatment, consider hospitalization.

---

Patients should be bathed post-treatment to remove any infectious viral particles that might still be present on the fur. Environmental decontamination using a parvocidal disinfectant (such as bleach) is necessary as well.

### 13.5.5.4 Tips and Tricks from the Field

- Use of antidiarrheal drugs is not recommended due to the potential risk of bacterial transmigration due to retention of fecal material.
- In the field, daily SQ fluids, injectable antibiotics (i.e. cefovecin and enrofloxacin), and injectable antiemetics (i.e. maropitant) are the mainstays of therapy. IV catheters and injection ports can be difficult to maintain and are easily contaminated.
- Transfusion of hyperimmune serum from recovered or immune dogs has not shown to be beneficial [131].

- There is no evidence that oseltamivir (Tamiflu®) is effective against CPV [132].
- Use of interferon has shown some promising results to reduce mortality rates but is expensive. Interferon-ω can be used (2.5 million units/kg q24h for three consecutive days) [133].
- Isolation and biosecurity are crucial in controlling this highly contagious disease. CPV is inactivated by household bleach at 1 : 32 dilution and Virkon®/Trifectant®, with a 10-min contact time.
- Vaccination is the most effective way to prevent disease. Puppies in high-risk environments may require booster vaccinations every 2–3 weeks until they reach 18–20 weeks of age due to waning maternal antibody.

### 13.5.6 Coccidioidomycosis

#### 13.5.6.1 General Information

Coccidioidomycosis is considered one of the most severe and life-threatening systemic mycoses and is caused by *Coccidioides immitis* and *Coccidioides posadasii* [134]. The disease is also referred to as Valley Fever, San Joaquin Valley Fever, and coccidioidal granuloma. It is considered endemic in the hot, dry southwestern USA, Mexico, and Central and South America [135].

Highly infectious spores (arthroconidia) grow in soil and produce spherules in hosts. Activities that disturb the soil such as construction and postrainfall periods release the arthroconidia, which are inhaled. Once in the lung tissue, it is spread hematogenously.

Dogs are more susceptible to infection due to sniffing and digging behaviors. The incubation period is 1–3 weeks before pulmonary signs are evident. In dogs, a chronic, wet, productive, or dry, harsh cough is most common with respiratory disease, which may worsen or resolve on its own. Dyspnea, decreased appetite, weight loss, weakness, and waxing and waning pyrexia may also be present. Other commonly observed clinical signs with disseminated disease include:

- Neck or back pain
- Lameness
- Bone and soft tissue swelling – Initially only one bone may be affected, but chronic cases may involve multiple bones [135]
- Chronic wounds and draining tracts

- Ocular disease (uveitis and keratitis)
- Lymphadenopathy
- Neurological abnormalities including seizures and ataxia
- Congestive heart failure.

Infection in cats is rare. Signs are similar to those described in dogs with the exception of respiratory involvement and bone infection, which are uncommon. Skin lesions are the most common type of infection in cats, which are commonly accompanied by fever, anorexia, and weight loss [135].

#### 13.5.6.2 Diagnosis

Diagnosis is usually based on history, clinical findings, and serology.

*Cytology/histopathology.* Diagnosis can be made by microscopically identifying spherules; however, they may be difficult to find. A granulomatous inflammatory response is typically observed.

*Culture.* Due to the risk to laboratory personnel, cultures are not routinely performed if coccidioidomycosis is suspected.

*Thoracic radiographs.* Radiographs can identify a diffuse interstitial pattern with respiratory involvement, hilar lymphadenopathy, and bony lesions, which are common with disseminated disease. In the author's experience, hilar lymphadenopathy can be seen without an accompanying respiratory pattern.

*Serology*

- Serum AGID assays are the conventional screening tests that detect early IgM titers and the later IgG titers, which can be used to differentiate exposure from actual disease.
- *Coccidioides* spp. RealPCR™ test. The ideal sample for testing depends on affected tissues and may include CSF, whole blood, deep pharyngeal and/or nasal swab, tracheal wash/BAL, needle aspirate/biopsy of tissue, or feces [136].
- MiraVista Diagnostics offers a *Coccidioides* antigen test for dogs using urine, serum, cerebrospinal fluid, and plasma [109].

A positive antibody test indicates exposure or infection. Other serology considerations include the following:

- Higher titers (generally > 1:32) indicate actual infection.

- The presence of IgM antibody is an indicator of acute illness whereas IgG is more indicative of chronic illness.
- Although low positive titers to *Coccidioides* spp. have been documented in some healthy dogs that reside in endemic areas, an antibody titer ≥1 : 16 in a dog with suggestive clinical signs is suggestive of active coccidioidomycosis.
- False-negative results are rare.
- Paired titers are ideal, but may not be practical. A four-fold change in titer is considered diagnostic.

#### 13.5.6.3 Treatment Protocols

##### 13.5.6.3.1 Gold Standard Protocols

- Treatment of disseminated disease often requires at least 1 year of aggressive antifungal therapy [134]. In some cases, treatment is lifelong and is performed on an outpatient basis. Depending on the severity and specific signs, other supportive care measures may be needed including anticonvulsants, pain management, and antitussives. Consider activity restriction when there is respiratory involvement. Common antifungals include the following:
  - Ketoconazole (5–10 mg/kg PO q12–24h) – Effective and least costly, but patients must be monitored for hepatic and GI side effects.
  - Sporanox® and Itrafungol® (itraconazole) (5 mg/kg PO q12h) – May be more effective than ketoconazole with fewer side effects. Give with food.
  - Diflucan® (fluconazole) (5 mg/kg PO q12h) – Good penetration of eyes and CNS.
  - Abelcet® and Fungizone® (amphotericin B) – In dogs, 0.5 mg/kg IV every other day three times per week (diluted in D5W given slowly over 4–6 h); 9–12 mg/kg cumulative dose; keep the patient hydrated. Lipid forms are less nephrotoxic but significantly more expensive.
  - Refer to the antifungal dosing chart included in Section 13.25.3 on blastomycosis treatment for further information on antifungal drugs.
- Unless azole drugs cannot be given, amphotericin B is not generally recommended due to its nephrotoxic potential.
- Monitor titers every 3–4 months during treatment.
- Regardless of treatment, relapses are common even after many months of apparent remission [137], especially when bone is involved.

#### 13.5.6.3.2 *Alternative Protocols*

- Ketoconazole should be considered for treating infected dogs and cats only when the cost of preferred antifungal drugs is prohibitive. To increase chances of treatment success in dogs, it should be combined with amphotericin B. Amphotericin B SC is more cost effective and easier to administer. See Section 13.25.3 for dosing instructions.

#### 13.5.6.4 Public Health Considerations

Coccidioidomycosis is not considered zoonotic, but protective clothing should be worn when performing necropsies and careful bite avoidance should be practiced with suspected animals.

#### 13.5.6.5 Tips and Tricks from the Field

- Coccidioidomycosis should be considered in any dog or cat with potential exposure during the previous 3 years that presents with chronic illness, respiratory signs, lameness, lymphadenopathy, nonhealing cutaneous lesions, or neurological, ocular, or cardiac abnormalities [138].
- In the author's experience, most cases of coccidioidomycosis will improve if not completely resolve on azole antifungal treatment. Be aware that some cases will relapse and require re-treatment.
- Prednisone (0.5 mg/kg PO q12h) may improve clinical signs associated with neurological disease [139].
- To prevent infection, try to keep animals away from areas with soil disruption such as building sites.

### 13.5.7 Cryptococcosis

#### 13.5.7.1 General Information

Cryptococcus is a localized or systemic fungal disease caused by *Cryptococcus neoformans* and *Cryptococcus gattii*. Cryptococcosis occurs far more frequently in cats than in dogs and is caused by an encapsulated yeast. *Cryptococcus* spp. can be isolated from soil and bird feces, particularly pigeon droppings, and is found primarily in Australia, western Canada, and the western United States. Transmission is most commonly from inhalation of spores or wound contamination. In cats, upper respiratory disease is the most common form of cryptococcosis and younger adult cats appear at increased risk of infection.

Clinical signs in cats commonly include sneezing, nasal discharge, head shaking, flesh-colored, polyp-like masses in the nostrils, and a firm subcutaneous swelling on the bridge of the nose [140]. Cutaneous lesions consisting of papules or nodules can be found in 40% of cases. CNS disease including cranial nerve involvement and ocular disease can be observed.

Unlike cats, dogs frequently develop disseminated disease. Granulomas in multiple organs are common with the lungs, kidneys, lymph nodes, spleen, and liver being most commonly affected [141]. Clinical signs are often related to CNS and ocular involvement.

#### 13.5.7.2 Diagnostics

*Cytology.* Cytology of nasal and skin exudates or tissue aspirates is the most rapid and easiest method of diagnosis due to the characteristic appearance of the organism. Ulcerated skin lesions and nodules make excellent cytological samples for impression smears and biopsies. *C. neoformans* have a prominent capsule and narrow-necked budding on cytology.

*Necropsy.* Lesions may vary in appearance from a gelatinous mass to firm granuloma.

#### 13.5.7.3 Treatment Protocols

The disease can be self-limiting, however long-term antifungal therapy is required in cases of chronic or multisystemic disease. Antifungals are the mainstay of therapy, but depending on the protocol used, treatment can be prolonged and expensive. Most cats with nasal cryptococcosis can be cured, whereas those with ocular or CNS involvement have a guarded prognosis. Respiratory masses in particular may require surgical debulking if possible to alleviate inspiratory dyspnea.

- Fluconazole (2.5–10 mg/kg PO q24h) – Use for 6–10 months depending on response to therapy. Use fluconazole in CNS or ocular cases as it crosses the blood–brain barrier.
- Itraconazole (10 mg/kg PO q24h) – Use for 6–10 months. This is the first choice in cases without CNS or ocular involvement. Give with a high-fat diet if possible to improve absorption.
- Terbinafine (5–10 mg/kg PO q24h) for 1–3 months.
- Amphotericin B – Typically used to treat resistant and severe canine and feline cases. To reduce the

risk of toxicity, amphotericin B can be given SC 0.5–0.8 mg/kg diluted in 0.45% saline containing 2.5% dextrose. Total volume of 400 ml for cats and 500 ml for dogs <20 kg and 1000 ml for dogs >20 kg administered SC two to three times per week [142]. Amphotericin B is synergistic with flucytosine and therefore both can be used together for refractory cases.

- Flucytosine (30 mg/kg PO q8h) – Use for 6–10 months in conjunctive with itraconazole, fluconazole, or amphotericin B in refractory cases.

### 13.5.7.4 Tips and Tricks from the Field

- The anticipated duration of treatment can be anywhere from 4 months to more than 1 year. CNS disease may require lifelong treatment, whereas disseminated infections require 6–12 months of therapy.
- Animals that survive the first 2 weeks of treatment typically have a fair prognosis but relapse is possible.

## 13.5.8 Ehrlichiosis and Anaplasmosis

### 13.5.8.1 General Information

Ehrlichiosis and anaplasmosis are important tick-borne diseases in free-roaming dogs. Disease is caused by an obligate, intracellular, gram-negative bacterium that is typically transmitted through the feeding of an infected tick. Distribution and seasonality of disease depends on the tick vector associated with each *Ehrlichia* or *Anaplasma* species, but generally, the disease is found worldwide and most frequently seen during warmer seasons when ticks are abundant.

*Ehrlichia* and *Anaplasma* species infect and replicate in the host's mononuclear or granulocytic cells, with the cell type being specific to each *Ehrlichia* or *Anaplasma* species. Infected host cells circulate in the body causing vasculitis and tissue damage. Resulting clinical signs vary depending on the species of *Ehrlichia* or *Anaplasma* (Table 13.25). Co-infections with other *Ehrlichia*, *Anaplasma*, and tick-borne pathogens are common due to shared tick vectors, complicating the diagnosis.

Table 13.25 Other disease-causing *Ehrlichia* and *Anaplasma* species.

| Species | Vector | Useful facts |
| --- | --- | --- |
| *Ehrlichia chaffeensis* | *Amblyomma americanum* (the Lone Star tick) | Similar to infection with *E. canis* |
| *Ehrlichia ewingii* | *Amblyomma americanum* (the Lone Star tick) | Canine granulocytic ehrlichiosis (CGE)<br>• Infects neutrophils, basophils, and eosinophils<br>• Incubation period is 7–14 days<br>• Most common clinical signs include lethargy, fever, lameness, stiff or stilted gait, and joint effusion [143]<br>• Clinical signs tend to be acute, including vomiting, diarrhea, and vestibular signs<br>• Hemorrhage rarely seen |
| *Anaplasma phagocytophilum* (formerly classified as *Ehrlichia equi*) | *Ixodes pacificus* and *Ixodes scapularis* (the blacklegged tick) | Canine granulocytic anaplasmosis (CGA)<br>• Infects granulocytes<br>• Coinfection with *Borrelia burgdorferi* is common<br>• Incubation period for CGA is 7–21 days<br>• Clinical signs are vague and similar to CGE |
| *Anaplasma platys* (formerly classified as *Ehrlichia platys*) | *Rhipicephalus sanguineus* (the brown dog tick) | Cyclic canine thrombocytopenia (CCT)<br>• Infects platelets<br>• Co-infections common<br>• Clinical signs are vague and related to clotting deficiencies<br>• Thrombocytopenia |
| *Ehrlichia muris*-like pathogen | | First detected in 2013 in both humans and dogs [144] |

---

**Textbox 13.21 Nonspecific acute- and chronic-phase clinical signs associated with *Ehrlichia* and *Anaplasma* infection**

| **Clotting abnormalities** | **Ocular** |
|---|---|
| Weakness, pale mucous membranes, ecchymoses, bleeding, hemoptysis | Ocular discharge, corneal ulceration, KCS, uveitis, glaucoma, blindness |
| **Respiratory** | **Gastrointestinal** |
| Nasal discharge, cough, dyspnea | Vomiting, diarrhea |
| **Systemic** | **Neurological** |
| Peripheral limb edema, scrotal edema, fever, polymyositis, polyarthritis, glomerulonephritis | Muscle twitching, cranial nerve deficits, anisocoria, vestibular signs, seizures, stupor |

---

Infection with *E. canis* is termed canine monocytic ehrlichiosis (CME). Tick vectors include *R. sanguineus* (brown dog tick), which is found worldwide and *Dermacentor variabilis* (American dog tick) in the United States. *E. canis* infections have been reported in Africa, Asia, Europe, and the United States. Clinical disease presentation occurs in three phases: acute, subclinical, and chronic [145]. During the acute phase, *E. canis* replicates in the macrophages and spreads throughout the body. The incubation period is 1–3 weeks. Common acute-phase clinical signs include lethargy, anorexia, fever, dermal or mucosal petechia, epistaxis, lymphadenopathy, and splenomegaly [146]. Splenomegaly and lymphadenopathy are only seen in approximately 20% of cases, however [147]. Acute-phase clinical signs generally last 2–4 weeks and may go unnoticed.

### 13.5.8.2 Diagnostics

A definitive diagnosis is difficult to achieve regardless of available resources. Diagnosis in the field is typically based on a combination of history and clinical signs, visit to endemic location, possible tick exposure, diagnostic testing results, and response to treatment.

*Buffy coat blood smears or Giemsa-stained blood smears.* This may reveal morulae or organisms in monocytes, lymphocytes, or neutrophils. The diagnostic usefulness of evaluating a blood smear

---

**Textbox 13.22 The challenges of managing *E. canis* infections**

- Infected dogs may clear the disease without treatment, be treated successfully with antibiotics and clear the disease, or enter a chronic phase of disease with or without treatment.
- During the subclinical phase, many dogs may not exhibit overt clinical signs but will still be thrombocytopenic.
- The subclinical phase can last months to years as *E. canis* may evade the immune response by sequestration in the spleen [145–147].
- Reports exist of *E. canis* infections lasting more than 10 years, and without treatment for the lifetime of the dog [144].
- It is unknown why some dogs proceed to the chronic phase of disease and others do not.

---

depends on the pathogen species. Blood smears have much higher sensitivity for detecting *A. phagocytophilum*, whereas *E. canis* morulae are rarely seen. Chances of observing the morulae are much higher when a buffy coat smear is performed.

*CBC.* Bloodwork often demonstrates thrombocytopenia, leukopenia, pancytopenia, and/or anemia. Thrombocytopenia is the most common hematological sign, occurring in up to 90% of dogs infected with CME or canine granulocytic anaplasmosis

(CGA) [148,149]. Thrombocytopenia typically occurs 10–20 days postinfection. A blood smear can be used to detect thrombocytopenia as a screening tool for CME, CGA, or cyclic canine thrombocytopenia (CCT).

*IDEXX SNAP® 4DX.* This benchside test detects antibodies to *E. canis*, *E. ewingii*, *A. phagocytophilum*, and *A. platys.*

- A positive test does not mean active infection. Rather it means that the patient has circulating antibodies.
- A positive test result for *Ehrlichia* in a patient with either clinical signs or hematological changes is indicative of an acute or chronic infection, a persistent infection in need of longer treatment duration, or reinfection. Antibodies do not appear to be protective or play a major role in clearing the disease. Note that following treatment and resolution of clinical signs, antibodies can persist for weeks to a lifetime [150].
- False negatives can occur early in the acute phase of infection if the patient has not produced antibodies yet, is too sick to produce antibodies, or if the test is used incorrectly. Antibodies to *A. phagocytophilum* tend to be produced 8 days postinfection and antibodies to *E. canis* 12–14 days postinfection [151].

Due to the nonspecific nature and multitude of potential clinical signs, challenges of achieving definitive diagnosis, and potential for a life-threatening disease course, the author experientially recommends treating for ehrlichiosis or anaplasmosis when a patient exhibits likely clinical signs without a definitive diagnosis for another causative agent.

### 13.5.8.3 Treatment Protocols

The prognosis is generally good for acute cases, especially if treated early in the course of disease. Chronic *E. canis* cases generally carry a poorer prognosis due to pancytopenia and/or systemic involvement. However, treatment can be successful if initiated early.

#### 13.5.8.3.1 Gold Standard Protocols

- The current gold standard for treatment is doxycycline (10 mg/kg PO q24h) or (5 mg/kg PO q12h) for 28 days [145]. Doxycycline is preferred for its comparatively increased safety in growing animals, increased CNS penetration, and longer half-life than other tetracyclines. Once daily dosing is useful for ensuring client compliance; however, twice daily dosing may decrease doxycycline-related GI side effects.
- Longer treatment durations may be necessary. Use clinical and hematological signs to gauge the need for continued treatment.
- Patients not responding to treatment may have coinfections and require a change in therapy.
- Patients not responding to treatment, showing signs of immune-mediated complication, or life-threatening thrombocytopenia should be treated with prednisone (0.5–2 mg/kg/day PO) for 2–7 days, depending on response to treatment.

#### 13.5.8.3.2 Alternative Protocols

Depending on *Ehrlichia* or *Anaplasma* species, other effective antibiotics may include:

- Tetracycline (22 mg/kg PO q8h) for 28 days
- Minocycline (10 mg/kg PO q12h) for 28 days.

Severe chronic cases, especially involving pancytopenia, may take longer to show improvement, need additional treatments, or may not respond to treatment. Bone marrow regeneration may take up to 120 days postinitiation of treatment [148]. Severe chronic cases may require fluid therapy, pain management, blood transfusions, additional antibiotics such as enrofloxacin if pneumonia develops, and steroids.

Individual welfare should always be assessed during treatment. In some cases, euthanasia may be the kindest or only available option depending on the situation.

#### 13.5.8.4 Prevention

- Prevent tick attachment with appropriate tick preventive products. Transmission of *E. canis* by *R. sanguineus* occurs within 3 h of attachment [152]. The author recommends the use of Seresto® collars in endemic areas. Although a significant expense, these collars are effective for 5–8 months and tend to work when other flea/tick products fail.
- Screen blood donors and exclude dogs with a history of ehrlichiosis or anaplasmosis from being blood donors.

#### 13.5.8.5 Spay/Neuter Considerations

- In tick-borne areas, the risks and benefits of spay/neuter surgery should be considered. If delaying surgery for a day or two is a possibility, elect to do so and start the patient on doxycycline and Yunnan Baiyao. If surgery is elected that day, the author recommends collecting a presurgical PCV, administering doxycycline (10 mg/kg PO), and administering Yunnan Baiyao (one capsule for dogs <14 kg and two capsules for dogs ≥14 kg).

- Surgical techniques should include diligent hemostasis of skin and subcutaneous tissues, delicate tissue handling, and sound ligation techniques. These include:
  - double ligation of spermatic cords or ovarian pedicles
  - single ligation en bloc of the broad ligament
  - encircling ligation of the uterine body and individual ligation of uterine vessels
  - closures that decrease dead space and prevent oozing (horizontal mattress in deep subcutaneous tissue).
- Postoperatively, the author recommends belly or scrotal bandages, icing incisions, a rectal dose of Yunnan Baiyao, close monitoring of physiological trends, and potentially serial PCV collection over time in recovery. Autotransfusion should be considered in patients with significant hemorrhage intraoperatively.

### 13.5.8.6   Tips and Tricks from the Field

- Patients can present with a variety of clinical signs. The author's field team has noted elevated third eyelids and prominent mucosal vasculature in infected dogs.
- Patients with atypical signs or occult infections are frequently misdiagnosed, leading to ineffective treatments and outcomes. Common differential diagnoses include distemper, parvovirus, immune-mediated disease, and other tick-borne pathogens.
- Ehrlichiosis and anaplasmosis are not zoonotic diseases, but humans can become infected by some *Ehrlichia* and *Anaplasma* species through ticks. Animal family members can serve as sentinels to alert families of infected ticks in their area.
- Dramatic improvement in clinical signs within 24–48 h after initiating appropriate antibiotic therapy is expected. Platelet counts generally return to normal within 14 days after initiating treatment [153].

- When in doubt, administer a 28-day course of doxycycline.

### 13.5.9   Feline Immunodeficiency Virus (FIV)

#### 13.5.9.1   General Information

FIV is a contagious retrovirus found with varying prevalence rates among cats worldwide [154]. Similar to FeLV, FIV appears to be most common in cats with certain clinical conditions including oral or respiratory disease, and abscesses. Although cats of any age or gender can become infected, adult age (5–10 years), living outdoors, and intact male gender increase the likelihood for infection.

FIV is not readily spread and the main route of transmission is through bites, when saliva containing the virus is inoculated under the skin of another cat. As FIV is not durable in the environment, cats may cohabitate for years without transmitting the disease. The introduction of an FIV-positive cat with FIV-negative cats or vice versa could pose a risk due to fighting, however. There is no cure for FIV, and infected cats remain susceptible to secondary infections due to immune suppression.

Kittens born to infected mothers are at low risk for infection, but may initially test positive due to maternal antibodies. FIV-infected cats can live a good quality of life for many years before succumbing to the disease. Most cats will not typically develop signs of disease until 2–5 years after the cat was first infected. As there is no cure, infected cats should be provided good nutrition, be protected from infectious disease, and have their secondary infections managed.

FIV causes disease by infecting cells of the immune system, thereby compromising normal immune system function. Clinical signs include

- Weight loss
- Recurrent fever
- Enlarged lymph nodes
- Lethargy
- Fever
- Gingivitis and stomatitis
- Chronic or recurrent respiratory, ocular, or intestinal disease
- Neurological disease.

Clinical signs cannot be distinguished from those of FeLV infection.

At this time, routine vaccination for FIV is not recommended. See Chapter 14 for additional information.

### 13.5.9.2 Diagnostics

*Serology*. Routine tests for FIV infection are usually based on the detection of anti-FIV serum antibodies using an ELISA or rapid immunomigration (RIM). Kittens born to FIV-infected queens may test seropositive due to materially derived antibodies. As a result, kittens testing positive for FIV should be retested after 16 weeks of age. In rare cases, however, FIV antibodies could be detected for up to 6 months due to maternal antibody interference [155]. A false-negative result may be caused by acute infection when the viral load is low or is a subtype not detected by the test.

Seroconversion usually occurs 2–4 weeks postinfection, but it occasionally takes up to 16 weeks. As long as no exposure to FIV occurs after initial testing, any sick cat that tests negative should be tested a minimum of 60 days later to confirm a true negative status.

*CBC/chemistry*. A hyperproteinemia (hyperglobulinemia), lymphopenia, neutropenia, thrombocytopenia, and nonregenerative anemia may be observed.

### 13.5.9.3 Treatment Protocols

As there is no cure for FIV infection, there is really no gold standard treatment. The most important management measure is to protect FIV-infected cats from other infections. In an ideal world, infected cats should receive physical examinations every 6 months and stay indoors. Prompt supportive care and the management of secondary conditions are paramount.

- Treat stomatitis with metronidazole (10 mg/kg PO q12h) and clindamycin (12.5 mg/kg PO q12h). In some cats, stomatitis improves with prednisone (5 mg per cat PO q12h) or immunotherapy. Refractory cases may require a full mouth extraction. FIV-infected cats may benefit from preventive dental care, which may or may not be feasible in the field.

Some drugs have been reported to suppress viral activity, decrease clinical signs, or improve survival.

- Zidovudine (AZT) (5–10 mg/kg PO or SC q12h) blocks the reverse transcriptase of retroviruses. Use the higher dose with caution due to potential side effects.
- Recombinant feline IFN (Virbagen Omega®) is licensed for veterinary use in some countries. Interferons are species specific; therefore, feline interferon-ω can be used lifelong without stimulating antibody development. Feline interferon-ω is active against FIV in vitro, but there is only one study performed in field cats, which did not show significant changes in survival rate when compared with a placebo group [156].
- Erythropoietin (EPO) is a recombinant human product that has been effectively used in cats with nonregenerative anemia in chronic renal failure. In one study, when used in FIV-infected cats at 100 IU/kg SC q48h, a gradual increase in red and white blood cell counts was observed [157]. Its use in cats is strictly extra-label, and close monitoring of PCV and blood pressure is required to detect the potential development of anti-EPO antibodies.
- Lymphocyte T-cell immunomodulator (LTCI) is the first and only USDA-approved treatment aid for cats infected with FeLV and FIV and the associated symptoms of lymphopenia, opportunistic infection, anemia, granulocytopenia, and thrombocytopenia [158]. Field studies are lacking on this product.

### 13.5.9.4 Tips and Tricks from the Field

- The presence of abscesses or gingivostomatitis should trigger testing for both FeLV and FIV.
- Healthy cats should never be euthanized based on a single FIV-positive test result.
- All FIV-infected cats should be neutered to reduce the risk of fighting and transmission.
- FIV-infected cats should never be housed in a ward with cats suffering from contagious disease, such as upper respiratory infection (URI).
- In the field, retroviral prevalence can be surprisingly high. Remember, spaying and neutering is the most effective way to reduce retroviral prevalence in free-roaming populations, not selective culling of infected cats.

### 13.5.10 Feline Leukemia Virus (FeLV)

### 13.5.10.1 General Information

FeLV is a contagious retrovirus that infects domestic cats and other feline species. Similar to FIV, FeLV presents a management challenge for foster homes, shelters, and trap–neuter–return (TNR) programs due to its transmissibility and guarded prognosis. Like other viruses belonging to the family Oncovirinae, it can cause neoplasia in cats in addition to other conditions including degenerative, immunological, and proliferative disease. The most serious manifestation of FeLV infection is typically immune system impairment.

FeLV is most often transmitted via oronasal contact with infectious saliva or urine. Vertical transmission *in utero* or via nursing can also occur. FeLV is an enveloped virus, making it fragile and unlikely to survive long in the environment.

Risk factors for infection include having outdoor access, being an intact male, living in a multicat household, or having other concurrent diseases (especially respiratory or oral disease and abscesses). FeLV is an age-dependent disease where younger kittens/cats have higher risk of infection and more serious disease progression. Cats appear to develop resistance with age.

The prevalence of FeLV is low in North America and Europe ranging from 1.2% to 5.3% [159–161], whereas it is relatively high in some Asian regions such as Bangkok, Thailand (24.5%) [162], and Peninsular Malaysia (12.2%) [163].

Viremia occurs 2–4 weeks after infection. There are several possible outcomes following infection [164]:

- *Progressive.* Uninhabited viral replication causing persistent viremia and clinical signs.
- *Abortive.* Transient viremia followed by effective immune system clearance.
- *Regressive.* A good immune response is mounted and the infection is contained. The virus may still be present in some cells, but these cats rarely develop clinical disease or shed virus.
- *Focal.* Rarely, cats develop localized infections where active viral replication occurs only in specific tissues (such as bladder or mammary gland), releasing low levels of viral antigen.

Disorders caused by FeLV infection are typically due to immunosuppression and include:

- Anemia (usually nonregenerative and normochromic)
- Neoplasia (commonly lymphoma and leukemia)
- Immunosuppression (predisposing the cat to other infections)

- Immune-mediated diseases (systemic vasculitis, glomerulonephritis, or polyarthritis)
- Reproductive problems (abortion or "fading kitten syndrome")
- Chronic enteritis (feline panleukopenia (FPV) co-infection produces FPV-like syndrome)
- Peripheral neuropathies (anisocoria, mydriasis, Horner's syndrome, vocalization, and paresis).

Vaccination is generally considered noncore. However, cats with a potential risk of exposure (cats residing outdoors, living in group housing, or living with known FeLV-positive cats) should be vaccinated. Kittens should be vaccinated at 8–9 weeks of age, with a second vaccination at 12 weeks, followed by a booster 1 year later.

### 13.5.10.2 Diagnostics

FeLV is typically diagnosed using a benchside immunochromatography (ELISA) test, but immunofluorescent assay (IFA) and/or PCR testing are also used for confirmatory testing.

*ELISA.* ELISA and other point-of-care (POC) tests detect soluble FeLV p27 antigen in whole blood or serum. Such tests are typically highly sensitive and specific and do not detect previous vaccination. FeLV antigen is usually detectable in the blood within 2–3 weeks following exposure and cats can be tested at any age. See Chapter 14 for additional information on testing.

*IFA.* Tests for FeLV p27 and other structural core antigens. This test can be used on peripheral blood smear or cytological preparations of the bone marrow. IFA is typically used to confirm a positive ELISA test and is more likely to detect progressive infections. False negative with IFA can occur due to leukopenia or lack of bone marrow involvement. Discordant results between tests, such as a positive ELISA test followed by negative IFA test, can occur due to inconsistent antigen levels in the blood, technical error, or regressive infections. In such cases, the standard recommendation is to retest in 60 days using serum.

*PCR.* Testing can be performed by diagnostic laboratories using whole blood, bone marrow, or other tissues and is sensitive enough to detect regressive infections. Fine-needle aspirates of tumors, lymph nodes, body cavity fluids, or affected organs may reveal malignant lymphocytes. Cats that have cleared

FeLV from plasma will remain negative on ELISA and IFA but remain positive by PCR for DNA.

### 13.5.10.3 Treatment Protocols

There is no cure for FeLV infection and management is aimed at providing symptomatic care. Probably, the most important management measure is to protect FeLV-infected cats from secondary infections and treat them promptly should they occur. FeLV-infected cats can live several years without major disease complications with routine prophylactic care, good husbandry, minimal stress, and avoidance of secondary infections. The average survival rate is 2.4 years after diagnosis [165].

Some drugs have been reported to suppress viral activity, decrease clinical signs, or improve survival, while others are used as a last-ditch effort (Table 13.26).

### 13.5.10.4 Tips and Tricks from the Field

- In the field, a centrifuge may not be available to obtain serum. Options include using whole blood (works best on newer generation test kits), or allowing a vial of whole blood to separate on its own (~20 minutes), facilitating serum collection.
- In the field, retroviral prevalence can be surprisingly high in certain areas. Spaying and neutering is the most effective way to reduce retroviral prevalence in free-roaming animals by reducing or eliminating the primary modes of transmission including fighting and breeding. Selective culling of infected cats is not an acceptable disease management practice.

Table 13.26 FeLV therapies.

| Drug | Description | Dosage | Notes |
|---|---|---|---|
| Zidovudine/ azidothymidine (AZT) | Antiviral that blocks the reverse transcriptase of retroviruses | 5–10 mg/kg PO or SC q12h for 3 weeks | Higher doses should be used with caution due to potential side effects |
| Raltegravir | Antiviral drug used to treat HIV infections in humans | Start at 40 mg PO q12h, gradually increase to 80 mg PO q12h. Treat for 9 weeks [166] | |
| Recombinant feline interferon (Virbagen Omega®) | Displays antiviral and immunomodulatory activities | Administer $10^6$ IU/kg SC q24h for 5 consecutive days, repeated three times with several weeks between treatments | |
| Human interferon-α | Displays antiviral and immunomodulatory activities | Administer 50 IU mucosally daily for 7 days on alternating weeks for 6 months. Then break for 2 months and repeat again | |
| Propionibacterium acnes (e.g. ImmunoRegulin®) | Shown to stimulate macrophages and enhance T-cell activity. There is some evidence to suggest that it leads to clinical improvement | 0.2 mg/cat IV once or twice weekly | |
| Acemannan | Derived from the *Aloe vera* plant and has been found to improve immune function | 2 mg/kg IP once a week for at least 6 weeks [167] | Field studies are lacking |
| Lymphocyte T-cell immunomodulator (LTCI) | LTCI is the first and only USDA-approved treatment aid for cats infected with FeLV and FIV, and the associated symptoms of lymphopenia, opportunistic infection, anemia, granulocytopenia, and thrombocytopenia | 1 μg per cat SC at days 0, 7, and 14. Subsequent injections given monthly or bimonthly as needed | Field studies are lacking |

### 13.5.11 Feline Panleukopenia

#### 13.5.11.1 General Information

FPV is a highly infectious disease caused by a non-enveloped DNA parvovirus. It is exceptionally resistant to chemical and environmental degradation. Mortality rates are high, with some estimates approaching 90% in kittens [168]. FPV can be spread via fomites (stethoscopes, thermometers, shoes/clothes, etc.), bodily secretions, and feces. The virus can also be aerosolized and spread via high-pressure spray washers. Mechanical transmission is also possible via rodents or insects.

FPV has a preference for rapidly dividing cells such as those in lymphoid tissue, intestinal crypts, and bone marrow. Replication of the virus within the bone marrow results in decreased myeloid cells and causes the significant panleukopenia seen in the disease. As a result, diarrhea and immunosuppression are often present concurrently [168]. Intrauterine transmission or perinatal infection may cause disorders of the CNS, such as cerebellar hypoplasia. Clinical signs include vomiting, diarrhea, dehydration, depression, fever, and inappetence. Hemorrhagic diarrhea occurs much less frequently than it does in dogs with CPV. The disease is seen most often in under-vaccinated kittens less than 6 months of age.

There are two common forms of panleukopenia: peracute and acute.

- Peracute cases die within 12 h from septic shock, dehydration, and hypothermia. Clinical signs may not be apparent.
- The acute form is most common and often presents as a 3- to 4-day history of lethargy, pyrexia, and inappetence that can progress to vomiting and diarrhea [169].

The incubation period for FPV is 3–14 days. Most kittens display clinical signs 5–7 days following exposure. Although FPV is closely related to CPV, it does not appear to cause clinical infection in other species than cats and is not zoonotic. Although shedding of the virus from infected cats can occur 5–14 days postinfection, it usually lasts 5–7 days [169,170]. Shedding can begin as early as 3 days before the onset of clinical signs.

Large amounts of FPV can be shed in the feces during the incubation period (24–48 h postinfection). Transmission is via fecal–oral route. Once the FPV particles enter the body, the virus replicates over 24 h in the oropharyngeal lymphoid tissues. A 2- to 7-day viremia disseminates the virus throughout the body [169].

FPV is a nonenveloped virus that makes it very durable in the environment, surviving up to 1 year at room temperature [169,170].

#### 13.5.11.2 Diagnostics

The diagnosis of FPV is usually made using a combination of history/signalment, clinical signs, leukopenia on a blood smear or CBC, and a positive fecal parvovirus antigen test [168,169].

*Antigen test.* Cats showing signs of panleukopenia or with known exposure can be tested using a fecal antigen test for CPV. Although this is an off-label use, it has been shown that the SNAP® test used for detecting CPV can also detect FPV viral antigen in feline feces [170, 171]. As shedding of the disease can precede clinical signs, a negative antigen test does not rule out panleukopenia in a symptomatic patient. A patient can be infected with FPV and not shed virus particles in its feces. False negatives may occur more in cats when testing for FPV than when used for CPV. Vaccine-induced positives on the other hand are uncommon but can occur in patients that have been recently vaccinated with a modified live vaccine [170]. For additional information on testing, see Chapter 14.

*CBC/blood smear.* If a clinically ill cat has a negative antigen test, a CBC may help make a diagnosis. Microscopic evaluation of a blood smear can be used to evaluate neutrophil count in addition to or in place of a CBC. FPV causes myelosuppression and, like CPV, will result in neutropenia which can be easily identified on a stained blood smear.

*Histopathology.* Histopathology performed by a diagnostic lab is the gold standard for diagnosing FPV. In the absence of diagnostic tests, in-house necropsy may facilitate diagnosis as segmental enteritis may be evident.

#### 13.5.11.3 Treatment Protocols

Kittens with panleukopenia often die of hypovolemic shock and sepsis. Unlike CPV, treatment success rates are low. Treatment of FPV-infected animals in a field setting should only be undertaken if sufficient facilities exist to isolate patients for 14 days to minimize the risk of exposure to other cats in the population, and if there is adequate staffing and veterinary oversight to ensure humane and appropriate care. Given the high mortality rate, aggressive treatment required, highly contagious nature of the disease, and prolonged shedding period postrecovery, humane euthanasia of infected animals may be the most humane option by ultimately saving lives through minimizing disease transmission [170].

Prognostic indicators for a negative outcome include [172]

- Albumin level <30 g/l at presentation
- Potassium serum level <4 mmol/l at presentation
- Thrombocytopenia
- Severe neutropenia
- Leukocyte count <1000 $\mu l^{-1}$

### 13.5.11.3.1 Gold Standard Protocols

As no FPV-specific antiviral drug exists, supportive care is the treatment of choice. A comprehensive treatment plan effectively manages sepsis and dehydration and provides appropriate nutrition.

- IV fluid therapy:
  Hypovolemia is a significant concern in kittens with panleukopenia. Adequate fluid therapy to replace losses and maintain appropriate hydration in the face of ongoing losses is critical. Maintenance fluid rate for pediatrics is approximately 80–120 ml/kg/day.
- Four-quadrant antibiotic coverage:
  A broad-spectrum antibiotic with a proven efficacy against gram-negative and anaerobic bacteria is recommended. Suggested protocols include:
  - Ampicillin (22 mg/kg IV, SC q6–8h) **plus** Enrofloxacin (5 mg/kg IV, SC q24h)
  - Cefovecin sodium (Convenia®) (8 mg/kg SC once) **or** Cefazolin (22 mg/kg IV, IM, SC q12h) **plus** Enrofloxacin (5 mg/kg IV, SC q24h)
  - Metronidazole (30 mg/kg PO q24h) **plus** Enrofloxacin (5 mg/kg IV, SC q24h)
  - Amoxicillin/clavulanate (13.75 mg/kg PO q12h) **plus** Enrofloxacin (5 mg/kg IV, SC q24h)
- Antiemetic:
  - Maropitant (0.5–1 mg/kg SC q24h) **or**
  - Ondansetron (0.2 mg/kg slow IV, SC, IM q12–24h)

- Nutritional support:
  - Enteral feeding may be helpful but unrealistic in most field settings.
  - Consider slow syringe feeding of Hill's a/d®, RC Recovery® or another syringeable diet.
  - The stomach capacity of a kitten is approximately 4–5 ml/100 g body weight.
- Parental vitamin B complex.

### 13.5.11.3.2 Alternative Protocols

- *Subcutaneous fluids and medications.* It may not be possible to maintain a panleukopenia kitten on IV fluids in a field setting. Providing fluids and medications SC may be possible on an outpatient basis if treatments can be provided twice daily, severe dehydration is not present, the patient is stable, and can be adequately isolated.
- *Parenteral serum.* In exposed, unvaccinated kittens, 2 ml of serum from an immune cat given SC or intraperitoneal soon after exposure may provide some protection (passive immunity) [170].

---

**Textbox 13.23 Prevention of FPV**

- Subcutaneous, modified, live vaccines against panleukopenia are highly effective in preventing feline panleukopenia.
- FVRCP (feline viral rhinotracheitis, calicivirus and panleukopenia) vaccines should be administered to kittens from the age of 4–6 weeks and repeated every 2 weeks until 18–20 weeks of age in high-risk situations to ensure adequate protection.

---

### 13.5.11.4 Tips and Tricks from the Field

- Handle all kittens <6 months of age with fresh gloves.
- Vomiting often precedes diarrhea. Any vomiting kitten should be tested for FPV.
- FPV is the leading cause of sudden death in cats and kittens in shelters.
- In a field clinic setting, a medical history should include questions about other kittens in the home or in the neighborhood that have recently died or are sick.
- Treating a clinically ill, FPV-infected cat is not feasible in many field clinic situations. Humane

euthanasia should be considered in settings without appropriate isolation facilities.

- If a FPV-infected kitten has been in contact with other kittens, all exposed kittens should be quarantined for 14 days before they are introduced to any other unvaccinated cats/kittens.
- Kittens with cerebellar hypoplasia can have a very good quality of life and a normal life expectancy; these patients should be considered for rehoming rather than euthanasia if appropriate care can be provided.

### 13.5.12 Hemotropic Mycoplasmosis (Hemobartonellosis)

#### 13.5.12.1 General Information

Hemotropic mycoplasmas are parasites that attach to the outside of erythrocytes and cause a hemolytic anemia in many mammal species. They are far more clinically important in cats than dogs [173]. In cats, clinical disease is also commonly referred to as feline infectious anemia. Several hemoplasma species are of clinical significance (Table 13.27).

Hemoplasmas are most commonly transmitted by arthropod vectors such as fleas, lice, ticks, and mosquitos [174]. The transfer of infected blood (contaminated needles, surgical instruments, and blood transfusions) and vertical transmission from mother to offspring can also serve as routes of infection. Cats at highest risk for infection are those that roam outside and have flea infestations.

Hemoplasmas are capable of causing hemolytic anemia, but clinical signs can vary. In immunocompetent adult animals, infections are typically asymptomatic. The exception to this is *M. haemofelis*, which can cause illness in healthy cats. Clinical signs may include anorexia, lethargy, and pale mucous membranes.

Table 13.27 Canine and feline hemoplasma species.

| Species | Hemoplasma species |
| --- | --- |
| Canine | *Mycoplasma haemocanis*<br>*Candidatus Mycoplasma haematoparvum* |
| Feline | *Mycoplasma haemofelis*<br>*Candidatus Mycoplasma haemominutum*<br>*Candidatus Mycoplasma turicensis* |

#### 13.5.12.2 Diagnostics

*CBC.* Regenerative anemia with marked reticulocytosis due to extravascular hemolysis is typical.

*Cytology.* Traditionally, hemoplasmas are diagnosed by microscopic evaluation of blood smears. However, organisms cannot be detected in all infected animals; it is estimated that hemoplasmas are seen in less than 50% of blood smears from infected animals [175].

*PCR.* Commercially available PCR tests are available by many reference laboratories and have been shown to be a more reliable diagnostic tool than microscopic evaluation of blood smears.

#### 13.5.12.3 Treatment Protocols

Antibiotics are the mainstay of therapy, but in most cases, hemoplasmas cannot be eliminated, even with therapy. Infected animals may have recrudescence of disease during future periods of stress or illness. Treatment for asymptomatic carrier animals is not warranted.

Doxycycline or enrofloxacin are effective in reducing parasitemia and a 3-week course is typically adequate to suppress the organism. Infected animals may remain carriers for life.

Treatment considerations for acute cases include:

- Doxycycline (5–10 mg/kg PO q12h) for 14–21 days or tetracycline (20 mg/kg PO q12–24h) for 14–21 days [175]
- Enrofloxacin (5 mg/kg PO q24h) for 14–21 days
- Penicillins/amoxicillins/macrolides have not demonstrated efficacy
- Immunosuppressive doses of glucocorticoids are recommended to limit the immune destruction of red blood cells
- A blood transfusion may be warranted to resolve severe anemia.

#### 13.5.12.4 Tips and Tricks from the Field

- Neutering and effective flea control is the best way to limit potential disease transmission in cats.
- Exercise caution when evaluating blood smears as stain precipitant can mimic hemoplasmas.

### 13.5.13 Histoplasmosis

#### 13.5.13.1 General Information

Infection with the fungus *Histoplasma capsulatum* can cause a chronic, systemic, noncontagious, granulomatous disease in dogs and cats. Histoplasmosis has a worldwide distribution and is the most commonly diagnosed major systemic mycosis in dogs [176]. *H. capsulatum* thrives in warm environments and lives naturally in nitrogen-rich matter such as soil contaminated with bird or bat feces. Dogs and cats are most commonly infected after inhaling or ingesting the organism.

Clinical signs of histoplasmosis are often variable and nonspecific depending on the organ system involved [177]. Three clinical forms of histoplasmosis are recognized: pulmonary, disseminated, and GI.

In cats, disseminated disease is most common followed by the pulmonary form. Most cats present with a history of weight loss, pale mucous membranes, lethargy, lymphadenopathy, and anorexia-disseminated disease. Rarely do infected cats cough; some may present with ocular involvement.

In dogs, the disseminated form is most common, affecting the respiratory tract, liver, spleen, lymph nodes, and GI tract. In cases of canine disease, large bowel diarrhea often predominates as the main clinical sign.

#### 13.5.13.2 Diagnostics

Histoplasmosis should be suspected in any animal with weight loss, chronic diarrhea, and respiratory distress coupled with a history of travel to an endemic area.

*CBC.* Most infected animals will have a normocytic, normochromic, nonregenerative anemia.

*Cytology/histopathology.* Definitive diagnosis requires identification of the organism on cytology or histopathology. *H. capsulatum* are oval or round, 2–4 µm in diameter found within macrophages. Wright and Giemsa stains can be used. In dogs with disseminated disease, rectal scrapings, blood smears, and tissue aspirates tend to have the highest diagnostic yield. In cats, blood smears, bone marrow, and tissue aspirates tend to be most diagnostic.

#### 13.5.13.3 Treatment Protocols

Antifungal drugs are the mainstay of therapy, but depending on the protocol used, treatment can be prolonged and expensive (Table 13.28). In most cases, long-term treatment with itraconazole or ketoconazole is recommended. For severe cases, concurrent treatment with amphotericin B is recommended.

Table 13.28 Common antifungal treatments for histoplasmosis in dogs and cats.

| Drug | Formulation | Species | Dosage | Side effects |
|---|---|---|---|---|
| Itraconazole | Capsules (100 mg) and oral suspension (10 mg/ml) | Dogs<br>Cats | 10 mg/kg PO q12–24h for 4–6 months<br>5 mg/kg PO q12h for 4–6 months | • Anorexia<br>• Vomiting/diarrhea<br>• Hepatotoxicity<br>• Cutaneous vasculitis |
| Ketoconazole | Tablets (200 mg) | Dogs<br>Cats | 10–20 mg/kg PO q12h for 4–6 months<br>5–20 mg/kg PO q12h for 4–6 months | • Anorexia<br>• Lethargy<br>• Vomiting<br>• Hepatotoxicity<br>• Pancytopenia |
| Amphotericin B | Deoxycholate (50 mg/vial) | Dogs<br><br>Cats | 0.25–0.5 mg/kg IV q48h (until cumulative dose of 5–10 mg/kg is reached)<br>0.10–0.25 mg/kg IV q48h (until cumulative dose of 4–8 mg/kg is reached) | • Infusion reactions<br>• Nephrotoxicity<br>• Vomiting/diarrhea |

Source: Adapted from Guptill and Gingerich (2008) [178].

Because of the risk for disseminated infection, corticosteroids are typically contraindicated. However, airway obstruction resulting from enlarged hilar lymph nodes may be life-threatening [179]. In such cases, prednisone (2 mg/kg PO q12–24h) given for several days results in quicker resolution of clinical signs.

#### 13.5.13.4 Tips and Tricks from the Field

- In endemic areas, histoplasmosis should be considered as a differential for chronic diarrhea and unthriftiness.
- On blood smear, be sure to check the buffy coat. One study revealed that in 19.6% of cases of cats with histoplasmosis, the organism could be seen within phagocytic cells in peripheral blood smears [180].

### 13.5.14 Infectious Canine Hepatitis

#### 13.5.14.1 General Information
Infectious canine hepatitis (ICH) is a worldwide, contagious disease caused by canine adenovirus type 1 (CAV-1). Besides dogs, this virus can be found in foxes, wolves, coyotes, bears, and other carnivores. The main source of infection in dogs is the ingestion of infected urine, feces, or saliva. Transmission occurs primarily from contact with a contaminated environment rather than dog-to-dog. In recent years, the disease has become uncommon in areas where routine vaccination is performed.

Clinical signs can vary from very mild to sudden death. In young puppies, the hyperacute form may present as acute abdominal pain with death occurring shortly after. In the acute form, dogs are initially lethargic and then develop a rather unique clinical sign of tonsillitis and hyperemia of the oral mucosa. The liver is often painful and enlarged on palpation. As the liver disease progresses, coagulation abnormalities such as spontaneous hematomas or hemorrhage around deciduous teeth may be seen. A condition known as blue eye (corneal edema) often occurs due to immune complex deposition.

#### 13.5.14.2 Diagnostics
*CBC/chemistry.* Dogs will often have increased ALT, AST, bilirubin, and leukopenia. The increase in serum ALT is often disproportionately higher to the increase in serum bilirubin [181].

*Necropsy.* In acute cases of ICH, paintbrush hemorrhages can be seen on serosal surfaces. The liver may be enlarged and mottled in appearance but can also appear small and firm in chronic cases. Impression smears of the liver may reveal characteristic inclusion bodies.

*Ancillary diagnostics.* In some places, ELISA, serological, and PCR testing may be commercially available for diagnosis.

#### 13.5.14.3 Treatment Protocols
Treatment is supportive and symptomatic. The goals of therapy are to prevent secondary bacterial infections, maintain hydration, and control hemorrhage. Treatment recommendations include the following:

- Maintain fluid balance. Ringer's solution is a recommended fluid choice.
- Plasma or whole blood transfusions may be indicated to assist with the replacement of clotting factors and platelets, depending on clinical severity.
- In comatose patients, administer an IV bolus of 50% glucose (0.5 ml/kg over a 5-min period) to combat potential hypoglycemia.
- Feeding oral lactulose can help acidify colonic contents and may help reduce protein catabolism and ammonia resorption. Parental or oral potassium may also assist in correcting the metabolic alkalosis and renal absorption of ammonia [181].
- Corneal opacity (blue eye) is typically transient and will resolve without treatment. Daily atropine may assist with painful ciliary spasm.
- Systemic corticosteroids should be avoided.

#### 13.5.14.4 Tips and Tricks from the Field

- ICH is a vaccine-preventable disease. Most commercially available vaccines for puppies include a canine viral hepatitis component. Vaccines typically include the CAV-2 (infectious canine tracheobronchitis) strain rather than CAV-1 as this provides cross-protection and is less likely to induce corneal opacities.
- ICH is a nonenveloped virus, which means it is very environmentally stable. Effective disinfectants include bleach and Trifectant/Virkon.
- Exercise caution when administering injections in infected dogs as they may be prone to excessive hemorrhage due to coagulopathy.

## 13.5.15   Leishmaniasis

### 13.5.15.1   General Information

Canine leishmaniasis is a zoonotic disease typically caused by *Leishmania infantum*. Other less significant species worldwide include *Leishmania donovani*, *Leishmania mexicana*, and *Leishmania braziliensis*. Dogs are one of the main reservoirs for this zoonotic disease, however cats can occasionally be infected. Transmission of *Leishmania* spp. requires a vertebrate (dog) and insect (sand fly). Protozoa are transmitted through the bite of a female phlebotomine sand fly, although dog-to-dog transmission can occur through contaminated blood and secretions, as well as transplacentally. Leishmaniasis is endemic in much of the Mediterranean, central and southwest Asia, and South America. This disease has been reported in more than 90 countries and is found on all continents except Australia and Antarctica [182].

The incubation period can range from 1 month to several years. Many infected dogs remain asymptomatic and only about one in five dogs will develop clinical disease [183]. Skin lesions are the most common presenting sign including alopecia and exfoliative dermatitis, which can be generalized or localized around the face, ears, and limbs. Nonpruritic lesions may be ulcerative, nodular, mucocutaneous, or papular. Some dogs may also have abnormal nail growth. In the few cats that develop clinical disease, cutaneous nodules are common.

Multisystemic disease can occur, with patients presenting with exercise intolerance, emaciation, epistaxis, lymphadenopathy, splenomegaly, ocular signs, diarrhea, vomiting, melena, signs of renal failure, and lameness due to joint, bone, or muscle lesions. Differing clinical signs may be attributed to the particular immune response of the patient [183].

### 13.5.15.2   Diagnostics

In conjunction with clinical signs, leishmaniasis can be confirmed using cytology, serology, or PCR [184].

*Cytology.* Direct identification of the parasite (amastigote form) in biopsies or aspirates from the lymph nodes, spleen, liver, skin (including impression smears), bone marrow, or joint fluid can be performed. Samples can be stained using Wright-Giemsa or other quick commercial stains. Identification can be difficult however when parasite numbers are low.

*Serology.* High antibody titers with clinical signs can be diagnostic. Antibodies can be quantified using IFA, direct agglutination assay, or enzyme immunoassay (EIA). Note that false positives can be caused by vaccination or cross-reactivity with trypanosomes, particularly *T. cruzi*. The rK39 dipstick immunoassay is a rapid and simple test used to detect leishmaniasis in dogs and people [183,185].

*PCR.* PCR is the most sensitive and specific diagnostic method to detect this parasite. It can also be used to detect asymptomatic infections.

*CBC/chemistry.* Clinical laboratory abnormalities typically include anemia, thrombocytopenia, serum hyperproteinemia with hyperglobulinemia and hypoalbuminemia (decreased albumin/globulin ratio), azotemia, and proteinuria. Hyperglobulinemia without other apparent causes in dogs from endemic areas is highly suggestive of leishmaniasis.

### 13.5.15.3   Treatment Protocols

Although no treatment protocol has been shown to consistently eliminate the parasite, the treatment of choice is a combination of allopurinol with a pentavalent antimonial (meglumine antimoniate or sodium stibogluconate) or miltefosine [184,186]. Fluid and nutritional support, as well as the treatment of proteinuria or ocular lesions may also be necessary. As relapse is common and parasite eradication difficult, patients should be evaluated at 1, 3, and 6 months post-treatment and then every 6 months for life.

#### 13.5.15.3.1   Gold Standard Protocols

- Allopurinol (10 mg/kg PO q12h) for a minimum of 6 months. This drug decreases parasitemia and the likelihood of transmission. Use of this drug alone is less effective and can lead to relapses. Allopurinol should be combined with:
  - Meglumine antimoniate (Glucantime) (100 mg/kg SC q24h) for 4 weeks
  - Sodium stibogluconate (Pentostam) (30–50 mg/kg SC or IV q24h) for 4 weeks. This drug can be obtained from the CDC in the United States [187].
  - Miltefosine (2 mg/kg PO q24h) for 4 weeks.

#### 13.5.15.3.2   Alternative Protocols

Other treatment options listed below may be limited by side effects or proven efficacy. These options should be used with caution, and only when the preferred treatment is unavailable or patients are unresponsive to initial therapy:

- *Domperidone*. An inexpensive immunomodulating drug that has been used for the treatment of visceral leishmaniasis at 1 mg/kg PO q12h for 1 month [186,188]. Treatment can be repeated every 3–4 months to prevent relapse [184].
- *Aminosidine (paromomycin) combined with meglumine antimoniate.* Aminosidine (5 mg/kg SC q24h) for 3 weeks and meglumine antimoniate (60 mg/kg IM q12h) for 4 weeks. Aminosidine can cause renal and vestibular toxic effects, and should be avoided in animals with renal insufficiency [186].
- *Spiramycin and metronidazole.* Spiramycin (150,000 U/kg PO q24h) in conjunction with metronidazole (25 mg/kg PO q24h). Treat for 3 months [186].
- *Marbofloxacin.* 2 mg/kg PO q24h for 4 weeks may improve clinical signs [186].
- *Amphotericin B.* Primarily used for humans and is not recommended for canine use as it is complicated to prepare and could contribute to drug resistance [186].

### 13.5.15.4 Prevention

Prevention includes vector control through repellent insecticides. Deltamethrin-infused collars or spot-on formulations of permethrin or imidacloprid can be used to prevent the sand fly bites in dogs. Vector control is particularly important to use on ill dogs to prevent transmission. Currently, two vaccines are commercially available (Leishmune® and Can-iLeish®), which can provide modest protection against leishmaniasis [189].

### 13.5.15.5 Public Health Considerations

- In humans, leishmaniasis, also known as kala azar, is the second largest parasitic killer worldwide. Risk factors for human infection include unsanitary living conditions, malnutrition, immune compromise, and climate change, which may alter the distribution of vectors [190].
- Reservoir species are numerous and include humans, dogs, and rodents. Transmission of the disease to humans requires the sand fly as a vector. To date, there are no reported cases of direct dog-to-human transmission [183].

- In endemic areas, drugs used to treat human disease should be avoided in dogs to prevent the development of drug resistance.

### 13.5.15.6 Tips and Tricks from the Field

- To date, no drug has shown consistent efficacy for visceral leishmaniasis in dogs.
- Leishmaniasis is occasionally cited as a reason for mass dog culling as a means of disease control. However, studies show that indiscriminate culling of seropositive dogs is ineffective as a long-term disease control strategy. In fact, mass culling is counterproductive as it eliminates genetically resistant animals and replaces infected dogs with susceptible ones [191]. A more effective strategy is vector control [192].
- If previous cases of canine or human leishmaniasis were diagnosed, investigate all suspicious lesions in dogs.

## 13.5.16 Leptospirosis

### 13.5.16.1 General Information

Leptospirosis is a zoonotic bacterial disease caused by spirochetes of the genus *Leptospira*. Leptospirosis may be one of the most under-diagnosed diseases in veterinary medicine. Although found worldwide, it is most prevalent in areas with warmer climates and higher rainfall. There are over 250 serovars adapted to various domestic and wild animals including rats, pigs, cattle, skunks, and opossums. The geographic prevalence of serovars is dependent on the presence of these maintenance hosts, which serve as reservoirs for infection. Leptospires can be shed in urine for months to years and canine infection is typically the result of direct or indirect contact with urine from maintenance hosts. This can occur from urine-contaminated soil, water, food, or bedding [193]. Feline infection is rare, partially due to their natural aversion to water and apparent resistance to infection. Although the identification of infecting serovars is important from an epidemiological standpoint, treatment is the same regardless of the infecting serovar.

The incubation period of leptospirosis in dogs can be as short as a few days. Canine infection can lead to a variety of clinical signs and disease depending on the immune response, infecting strain, and geographical location [194]. Some dogs will show no signs of illness, whereas others will develop severe illness and even death. The majority of cases will present in acute renal failure (ARF), while a smaller percentage show signs of hepatic failure. Leptospirosis is the most common infectious cause of canine ARF in the world. Veterinarians should suspect leptospirosis in any dog presenting with signs of renal or hepatic failure, acute febrile illness, pulmonary hemorrhage, or uveitis.

Clinical signs can be quite varied and nonspecific [195,196]. Coagulopathies can also be seen albeit less commonly.

---

**Textbox 13.24 Clinical signs associated with leptospirosis infection**

| | |
|---|---|
| Lethargy | Fever |
| Vomiting | Vomiting |
| Diarrhea | Epistaxis |
| Anorexia | Petechiae |
| Muscle weakness | Anterior uveitis |
| Icterus | Polyuria/polydipsia or |
| Abdominal pain | oliguria/anuria |

Source: Geisen et al. 2007 [196]. Reproduced with permission of John Wiley & Sons.

---

#### 13.5.16.2 Diagnosis

Diagnosis of leptospirosis in the field can be challenging. If bloodwork and other diagnostic modalities such as serology and PCR are unavailable, therapy should be initiated based on clinical suspicion.

*CBC/chemistry.* Common laboratory findings include:
- Mild anemia
- Thrombocytopenia
- Azotemia (elevated BUN (blood urea nitrogen), creatinine)
- Leukocytosis
- Elevated alkaline phosphatase (ALP)

*Urinalysis.* Infected dogs are frequently isosthenuric or hyposthenuric.

*Serology.* Exercise caution when interpreting serology results. In acute leptospirosis cases, titers may be low initially (1 : 100–1 : 200), but a recheck test

performed 2–4 weeks later may reveal a high titer. Therefore, it is recommended that clinicians perform a follow-up test 2–4 weeks after the initial test to determine seroconversion. A four-fold change in titer supports recent infection. Use of leptospiral vaccines can also cause a low agglutinating antibody titer (1 : 100–1 : 400).

*PCR.* PCR assays are becoming more widely available through commercial laboratories. Blood is the sample of choice for PCR during the first week of illness. Organism numbers are highest in blood during the first 10 days of infection [197]. Urine may not become positive until 7–14 days postinfection.

#### 13.5.16.3 Treatment Protocols

Treatment can be divided into two major stages; the first of which is to halt the replication of leptospires and the second is to eliminate the carrier state. As many dogs initially present in renal failure, vomiting may complicate the oral administration of drugs. Therefore, IV drugs may be warranted initially. Ampicillin, amoxicillin, and penicillin are recommended choices (Table 13.29).

**Step 1.** Administer aggressive fluid therapy. Lactated ringer's solution (LRS) and 0.9% saline are appropriate choices. A fluid rate of two to three times maintenance should be used initially.

**Step 2.** Administer intravenous ampicillin (22 mg/kg IV q8h) for acute disease until oral doxycycline is tolerated. If ampicillin in unavailable, other antibiotics can be considered.

**Step 3.** If the patient will tolerate oral medications, administer doxycycline (5 mg/kg PO q12h) or amoxicillin (22 mg/kg PO q12h). To

**Table 13.29** IV drug options for the treatment of leptospirosis.

| Drug name | Dose | Frequency |
|---|---|---|
| Ampicillin | 22 mg/kg | q8h |
| Amoxicillin | 22 mg/kg | q12h |
| Penicillin G | 25 000–40 000 U/kg | q12h |

eliminate the carrier state, tetracyclines, fluoroquinolones (enrofloxacin), or newer erythromycin derivatives can also be administered. Doxycycline, when tolerated, is the treatment of choice [194].

---

**Textbox 13.25 American College of Veterinary Internal Medicine (ACVIM) consensus statement on leptospirosis**

Per the ACVIM Small Animal Consensus Statement, the recommended treatment course for dogs with leptospirosis is doxycycline (5 mg/kg PO or IV q12h) for 2 weeks. Many clinicians recommend a minimum of 3 weeks of treatment however to clear leptospires from the renal tubules.

Source: Sykes et al. 2010 [194]. Reproduced with permission of John Wiley & Sons.

---

#### 13.5.16.4 Public Health Considerations

Due to the potential for zoonotic transmission, exercise care when handling fluids from infected animals. Wear gloves when dealing with urine-soaked bedding. Rodent control, removal of standing water, and isolation of infected animals are important for controlling the spread of disease. Luckily, leptospires are very susceptible to commonly used disinfectants.

#### 13.5.16.5 Tips and Tricks from the Field

- The availability of leptospiral diagnostics are typically limited in the field. Consider treating any patient presenting with signs of acute renal or hepatic failure with doxycycline. Don't wait until a definitive diagnosis is obtained.
- Be aware of environmental contamination. Leptospires can live outside the host for several months in the right environmental conditions.
- If you have the capacity to vaccinate dogs in the field for leptospirosis, do it. Some veterinarians are reluctant to vaccinate for leptospirosis due to anecdotal reports of anaphylactic reactions, but newer vaccines pose no greater risk for adverse reaction than any other vaccine [198].
- Past recommendations for 2 weeks of daily procaine penicillin G IM injections followed by

streptomycin is not the most humane option for treatment.

### 13.5.17 Rabies

#### 13.5.17.1 General Information

Rabies is one of the most feared and deadly diseases a field worker may encounter. It is estimated that dog bites cause more than 99% of human rabies deaths worldwide [199]. Government and nongovernmental organization (NGO)-sponsored vaccination campaigns and the mandatory rabies vaccination of owned dogs have helped decrease the number of human rabies cases in many countries. However, limitations in vaccine availability, postexposure prophylaxis, and knowledge still contribute to the death of an estimated 59 000 people annually [200].

Rabies is caused by a *Lyssavirus* from the *Rhabdoviridae* family. It is a highly fatal, zoonotic disease that produces acute and progressive viral encephalomyelitis. It mainly affects dogs and to a lesser extent other carnivores and bats, although any mammal can be affected. Rabies can be divided into two epidemiological cycles, canine, and sylvatic (wildlife). Sylvatic rabies usually occurs in one major wildlife species within a geographical area. Other mammals that contract rabies within these areas are termed "spillover" cases.

The incubation period for rabies in dogs is usually 21–80 days after exposure. However, depending on the location and severity of the bite wound, it can be shorter or longer, even up to several months [199]. After rabies exposure, the virus must spread to the salivary glands for an animal to become infective. Once this happens, the virus is secreted in the saliva and is typically transmitted through bite wounds. Viral shedding occurs in the later stages of the disease; clinical signs also appear around this time, with death occurring shortly after. Dogs and cats can shed the virus in the saliva up to 6 days before the onset of clinical signs and throughout the duration of illness. Once clinical signs become apparent, death ensues within 10 days. This is the basis for mandatory 10-day quarantine periods. If a dog or cat stays healthy during the 10-day period, one can conclude that the virus could not have been in the animal's saliva at the time of the bite incident. Cats often die within 3–4 days following the appearance of clinical signs [201], whereas dogs typically succumb within 2 days [202].

Clinical signs often include acute behavior change and progressive paralysis. Rabies can clinically manifest itself in two forms:

1) *Furious form.* Infected animals show uncharacteristically pronounced aggression, although the degree of actual aggression can be variable. The animal may attack and bite other animals, people, and even objects. Other signs can include excessive salivation, pacing, twitching, disorientation, and photophobia. Young puppies may also display this form of rabies, which may be mistaken for highly playful behavior. An infected animal will eventually display ataxia, progressive paralysis, followed shortly by death.

2) *Dumb or paralytic form.* Infected animals are lethargic, ataxic, and often salivate profusely due to their inability to swallow. Some animals avoid drinking water or show a fear of water. Dogs may often drop their lower jaw, which can be mistaken for a foreign body lodged in the oral cavity. Animals exhibiting this form of rabies may also be mistaken for other diseases such as distemper. Infected animals eventually develop progressive paralysis followed by death.

Rabies is preventable with timely vaccination. The elimination of canine-mediated rabies in humans is possible via elimination of rabies in dogs. In fact, mass dog vaccination aiming for at least 70% coverage is the only humane, effective method to significantly decrease rabies incidence in dogs and humans, and ultimately eradicate the disease.

### 13.5.17.2 Diagnostics

*Fluorescent antibody testing.* Although clinical signs are highly characteristic for rabies infection, the only gold standard diagnostic test is direct fluorescent antibody testing on brain tissue. Therefore, a confirmatory diagnosis can only be performed on dead animals by an approved laboratory. Depending on the country or laboratory, the entire animal or only the head with brain stem attached should be submitted for testing. Specimens should be refrigerated rather than frozen.

*Clinical signs.* Because clinical signs are rarely definitive, animals that are strong rabies suspects should be humanely euthanized and samples sent to the laboratory for definitive diagnosis. However, if facilities are available to safely quarantine an animal, dogs that have bitten a person can be observed in strict quarantine for 10 days, rather than resorting to euthanasia. If the animal stays healthy for more than 10 days, the dog was not shedding virus at the time of the bite. A "six-step" method has been developed to help make a presumptive diagnosis of rabies in dogs [203]. Note that these clinical criteria do not constitute proper diagnostic testing and cannot diagnose rabies during the incubation period.

---

**Textbox 13.26 Suggested clinical criteria for a presumptive diagnosis of rabies [203]**

1) Age of the dog?
   a) Less than 1 month → Not rabies
   b) >1 month or not known → Go to question 2
2) Health status of the dog?
   a) Appears healthy (no clinical signs) OR sick for more than 10 days → Not rabies
   b) Sick less than 10 days or not known → Go to question 3
3) How did the illness evolve?
   a) Acute onset from normal health → Not rabies
   b) Gradual onset or not known → Go to question 4
4) How was the condition during the clinical course in last 3–5 days?
   a) Stable or improving (with no treatment) → Not rabies
   b) Symptoms and signs progressing or not known → Go to question 5
5) Does the dog show signs of "circling?"
   (He or she stumbles or walks in a circle and hits head against the wall as if blind.)
   a) Yes → Not rabies
   b) No or not known → Go to question 6
6) Does this dog show at least 2 of the 17 following signs or symptoms below during the last week of life?
   a) Yes → Rabies
   b) No or showing only one sign → Not rabies
   Clinical signs and symptoms:
   1. Drooping jaw
   2. Abnormal sound in barking
   3. Dry drooping tongue
   4. Licks its own urine
   5. Abnormal licking of water
   6. Regurgitation

7. Altered behavior
8. Bites and eats abnormal objects
9. Aggression
10. Bites with no provocation
11. Runs without apparent reason
12. Stiffness upon running or walking
13. Restlessness
14. Bites during quarantine
15. Appears sleepy
16. Imbalance of gait
17. Frequent demonstration of the "dog sitting" position.

Source: Tepsumethanon et al. 2005 [203]. Reproduced with permission of Journal of the Medical Association of Thailand.

*POC Testing.* Note that there are unlicensed POC tests available for premortem testing in the field. These are not recommended at this time due to intermittent viral shedding and questionable sensitivity and specificity.

#### 13.5.17.3 Treatment Protocols

There is no treatment for rabies in animals. If an animal is a rabies suspect, follow the recommendations outlined above. Rabies is a reportable disease in many countries. For recommendations on postexposure management of dogs and cats exposed to rabies, see Chapter 17.

*Vaccination.*

- In areas where rabies is endemic, dogs and cats should be vaccinated at 3 months of age, boostered at 1 year of age, and then revaccinated once yearly or every 3 years according to licensed vaccine manufacturer's recommendations.
- See Chapter 17 for human pre-exposure vaccination recommendations.

#### 13.5.17.4 Rabies Control Methods

Unfortunately, many countries resort to the culling of free-roaming dogs as a rabies control method. Indiscriminate culling of free-roaming dogs alone is ineffective in controlling rabies and is counterproductive to any rabies control strategy. It is estimated that lethal management strategies require the elimination of 50–80% of dogs a year, which is both expensive and unethical [204]. Vaccination is highly effective, and proper administration of postexposure prophylaxis and rabies immunoglobulin can prevent human disease.

Per the WHO and OIE's Global Framework for the Elimination of Dog-Mediated Human Rabies that aims to achieve zero human deaths by 2030, the following must be ensured [205]:

- Affordable human vaccines and antibodies
- Prompt treatment for dog bite victims
- Mass dog vaccination in at-risk areas, supported by increased communication, awareness, and education.

#### 13.5.17.5 Tips and Tricks from the Field

- WSAVA's vaccination guidelines recommend boostering dogs for rabies at 6 months of age rather than 1 year [206].
- Puppies under 3 months of age can be vaccinated successfully using high-quality inactivated rabies vaccines [207]. It is recommended that all puppies are included in a mass vaccination campaign to increase the overall vaccination coverage.
- In North America, cats are vaccinated as far distally on their right hindlimb as possible to facilitate amputation should a fibrosarcoma develop. Research into vaccination in the distal tail shows promise as tails can be easily amputated [208].
- Veterinarians and staff working with cats and dogs in endemic areas must receive pre-exposure prophylactic vaccinations and immediate postexposure treatment if exposed.
- Exercise extreme care when handling a rabid or potentially rabid animal. Use full-length gloves of a durable material that cannot be pierced by teeth or claws. Leather is a good choice. Use of eye goggles and a face shield is advised.
- Not all rabid dogs will demonstrate characteristic aggression. Anecdotally, those working in the field have reported rabies-infected dogs pawing at the face, nipping at the legs of other dogs, and attempting to eat strange objects.

## 13.6 Neurology

### 13.6.1 Tetanus

#### 13.6.1.1 General Information

Tetanus, also known as lockjaw, is the result of a specific neurotoxin produced by *Clostridium tetani*.

*C. tetani* is ubiquitous in the environment worldwide and is found with higher frequency in warmer climates.

It is typically introduced into tissues through wounds as a degree of tissue necrosis is required to provide a suitable anaerobic environment for *C. tetani* bacterial proliferation and subsequent tetanospasmin and tetanolysin exotoxin production [209]. Once released, toxins ascend peripheral nerves to the spinal cord where they block neurotransmitter release from inhibitory interneurons, resulting in tetany [210]. Tetanus is generally uncommon in dogs and cats due to their natural resistance.

Tetanus has been reported following ovariohysterectomy and parturition [209]; however, such occurrences remain poorly documented in the literature. The onset of clinical signs varies from 4–5 days to 6–8 weeks. The most common initial clinical signs in dogs include ocular and facial abnormalities [211]. Affected animals may have a 2- to 3-day history of change in behavior, relatively acute onset of generalized stiffness, lethargy, photosensitivity, and difficulty opening the mouth. Common clinical signs include:

- Stiff gait, outstretched or dorsally curved tails, extreme muscle rigidity, hypersensitivity to touch, light, and sounds
- Ears erect, lips drawn back (sardonic grin), protrusion of third eyelid, and enophthalmos
- Trismus (lockjaw), laryngeal spasm, regurgitation, megaesophagus leading to aspiration pneumonia, and seizures [212]
- Stiffness in a muscle of limb in localized tetanus.

With more severe disease, tachyarrhythmias or bradyarrhythmias along with systemic hypertension may occur. Tetanus can be easily mistaken for other diseases including CDV, toxicity (lead and strychnine), rabies, spinal trauma, and hypocalcemia.

Tetanus toxoid vaccination is routinely used in large animals due to their higher exposure and risk. A vaccine is licensed for dogs in some countries, but not in the United States. The spores of *C. tetani* are very persistent in the environment and resistant to most disinfectants with the exception of disinfectants such as 2% aqueous glutaraldehyde (Cidex), 8% formaldehyde, and 20 ppm (20 mg/l) sodium hypochlorite (household bleach) [213].

### 13.6.1.2 Diagnostics

Diagnosis is typically made based on clinical signs and history of recent trauma or surgical procedure. There is no practical confirmatory test.

*Cytology.* In cases where a wound is present, Gram-stained smears may be used to visualize the bacteria.

### 13.6.1.3 Treatment Protocols

As a general rule, the prognosis is favorable when treatment is administered early in the disease (Table 13.30). Localized tetanus carries a more favorable prognosis than generalized cases. Most patients will exhibit improvement 1 week after the initiation of treatment and a full recovery is often seen within 4 weeks, although there are reports of stiffness persisting for up to 4 months [214].

- *Minimize stimulation.* Maintain the patient in a dark, quiet area. Place cotton balls in both ear canals.
- *Wound management.* If wounds are present clean and debride early on to remove as much tetanospasmin as possible. Leave the wounds open to avoid anaerobic conditions.
- *Antitoxin.* The antitoxin for tetanus consists of equine antitetanus serum (ATS) or human tetanus immunoglobulin (TIG). ATS is given IM or IV, whereas human TIG is given IM. IV administration of antitoxin is superior to IM or SC in producing a rapid increase in circulating antitoxin. Unfortunately, IV antitoxin is associated with anaphylaxis. Therefore, before administering ATS, be sure to give an initial test dose of 0.1–0.2 ml SC or ID to monitor for anaphylaxis. If anaphylaxis is not observed, provide the therapeutic dose.
- *Sedation.* Diazepam, phenobarbital, acepromazine, and chlorpromazine are recommended sedatives.
- *Antibiotics.* Both sodium or potassium penicillin (20,000–50,000 IU/kg given slowly IV q6h) for 10 days and metronidazole (10 mg/kg PO q6–12h) for 10 days are used for antibacterial treatment of *C. tetani*. Note that this will not alleviate signs from exotoxin already bound to nerves.
- *Pain management.* Tetanus is a painful condition even without vocalization; use caution with opioids however due to respiratory depressant properties.
- *Intensive nursing care.* IV fluids, prevention of pressure sores, indwelling urinary catheter, and nasogastric tube may be required.

Table 13.30 Medications used to treat tetanus.

| Medication | Canine dosage | Feline dosage |
|---|---|---|
| *Antibiotics* | | |
| Metronidazole (first choice) | 10 mg/kg PO or IV (given over 1 h) q8h for 10 days | 10 mg/kg PO or IV (given over 1 h) q12h for 10 days |
| Penicillin G | 20,000–50,000 IU/kg slow IV q6–12h for 5 days; can give a portion of each dose IM adjacent to the wound | 20,000–50,000 IU/kg IV q6–12h for 5 days |
| *Muscle relaxation/sedation* | | |
| Acepromazine | 0.01–0.1 mg/kg titrated to desired effect; can lower dose and combine with diazepam or opioid | 0.01–0.1 mg/kg titrated to desired effect; can lower dose and combine with diazepam or opioid |
| Diazepam (anticonvulsant) | 0.1–0.5 mg/kg/h to effect (may add acepromazine) | 0.1–0.5 mg/kg/h to effect (may add acepromazine) |
| Methocarbamol | Initially, 132 mg/kg/day PO divided q8h–12h, then 61–132 mg/kg divided q8–12h. If no response in 5 days, discontinue. If unable to give oral tablets, 55–220 mg/kg IV; administer half of estimated dose rapidly until relaxation begins then continue to effect; do not exceed 330 mg/kg/day | See canine dose |
| Phenobarbital (anticonvulsant) | 2–8 mg/kg PO q12h; 10–20 mg/kg IV to effect | 2–4 mg/kg PO q12h; 10–20 mg/kg IV to effect |
| *Analgesics* | | |
| Oxymorphone | 0.1–0.2 mg/kg IV, IM, SC q1–3h | 0.05–0.1 mg/kg IV, IM, SC q1–3h; give acepromazine if dysphoria or excitement occurs |
| Hydromorphone | 0.05–0.2 mg/kg IV, IM, SC q2–4h | 0.05–0.1 mg/kg IV, IM, SC q2–4h |
| Morphine | 0.5–1 mg/kg slow IV, IM, SC q3–4h | 0.05–0.1 mg/kg IM, SC q3–4h |
| Buprenorphine | 0.005–0.02 mg/kg IV, IM, SC q6–12h | 0.01–0.03 mg/kg IV, IM, SC q6–8h 0.01–0.03 mg/kg TM q8–12h |
| Butorphanol | 0.1–0.5 mg/kg IV, IM, SC q2–4h 1–4 mg/kg q6h PO | 0.1–0.5 mg/kg IV, IM, SC q2–4h 1.5 mg/kg PO q4–8h |
| *Antacids* | | |
| Famotidine (Pepcid®) | 0.1–0.2 mg/kg PO, SC, IM, IV, PO q12h | 0.2–0.25 mg/kg PO, SC, IM, slow IV q12–24h |
| Cimetidine (Tagamet®) | 5–10 mg/kg PO, IV, IM q6h | 5–10 mg/kg PO, IV, IM q6h |
| *Antitoxins*[a] | | |
| Human tetanus immunoglobulin (TIG) | 500–2000 IU IM near wound if found [162] | 500–2000 IU IM near wound if found [162] |
| Equine antitetanus serum (ATS) | 100–1000 IU/kg[4] slow IV, monitor for signs of anaphylaxis | 100–1000 IU/kg[4] slow IV, monitor for signs of anaphylaxis |

a) Recommended procedures before administering antitoxin:

- Perform an antitoxin test injection of 0.1–2 ml SC or ID and observe for 15–30 min for anaphylaxis and/or wheal at the injection site.
- Premedicate with an antihistamine and have epinephrine on-hand just in case.

#### 13.6.1.4 Tips and Tricks from the Field

- All surgical procedures must be performed with the highest level of asepsis possible. Cold sterilization of instruments should be avoided. Following surgery, animals should be put on clean surfaces to recover.
- There is insufficient evidence to conclude that a single antibiotic injection (e.g. penicillin) at the time of surgery can prevent tetanus.
- As long as there is a prompt diagnosis, proper supportive nursing care, and clinical signs of cardiovascular disease do not develop, tetanus can be very rewarding to treat.
- Trismus is one of the most common clinical signs of tetanus, which must be distinguished from chronic masticatory myositis.
- The absence of recent surgery or wounds does not rule out tetanus.

## 13.7 Oncology

### 13.7.1 Transmissible Venereal Tumor

#### 13.7.1.1 General Information

In the field, canine transmissible venereal tumor (TVT) is one of the most commonly observed and difficult-to-treat conditions in free-roaming dogs. TVT is a contagious neoplasia transmitted through coitus or other forms of direct contact between dogs. Upon contact, tumor cells exfoliate and transplant to the abraded epithelium of a recipient. Intact epithelium can prevent the transmission of TVT cells.

TVT has a very characteristic clinical appearance. Masses are typically friable and bloody, ranging in size from small nodules of 5 mm to larger masses of over 10 cm. Due to their ulcerative nature, secondary bacterial infections are common. Tumors are most often seen on the genitalia but can also affect oral, nasal, and conjunctival mucosa. In females, tumors are most often found in the vagina, vestibule, and on vulvar lips. TVT in male dogs are most often located at the bulbus glandis, and less commonly on the shaft and at the tip of the glans penis. Up to 80% of affected dogs are 2–8 years old. Although historically it has been thought that up to two-thirds of cases were female, more recent studies do not show a gender bias [215,216].

The initial presenting sign is typically hemorrhagic preputial or vulvar discharge, or visualization of a genital mass. Affected dogs may also be seen excessively licking the tumor site. Dogs with nasal TVT may exhibit epiphora, halitosis, epistaxis, exophthalmos, lymph node enlargement, and facial deformities [217]. Metastasis is rare but when it occurs, regional lymph nodes, kidney, spleen, liver, eye, brain, pituitary, skin, maxillary bone, and peritoneum can be affected [215,218].

The typical growth cycle of TVT involves an initial development phase of 4–6 months, a stable phase, and a regression phase. In healthy, immune competent dogs, spontaneous regression may start within 3 months of implantation of TVT cells. If the tumor is over 9 months of age, self-regression is unlikely [219]. Tumors can grow rapidly in immune-compromised patients and can progress to ulceration and metastasis [220].

TVT is common in tropical and subtropical regions of the world as well as the southern United States. Free-roaming dogs are a reservoir for the disease and propagation is primarily through unrestricted breeding. Spaying and neutering reduces the prevalence of TVT [216]. Treatment typically involves an extended course of chemotherapy, an area to isolate infected dogs, and the ability to monitor dogs undergoing treatment.

#### 13.7.1.2 Diagnostics

Diagnosis in the field is based on clinical signs and microscopic examination of impression smears or fine-needle aspirates.

*Cytology.* TVT has round to oval cells, mitotic figures, chromatin clumping, one or two prominent nucleoli, and cytoplasmic vacuolation. See Chapter 14 for a detailed cytological description.

#### 13.7.1.3 Treatment Protocols

If a microscope is not available to perform cytology, a presumptive diagnosis can be made based on clinical presentation, duration of clinical signs, and patient signalment. With treatment, the prognosis for total remission is good. Metastasis to the brain or eye is a negative prognostic indicator [220].

##### 13.7.1.3.1 Gold Standard Protocols

Vincristine, a chemotherapeutic agent, is the treatment of choice. Administration of vincristine at 0.5–0.7 mg/m$^2$ IV for three to six treatments will result in complete remission in 90–95% of cases [221]. Less than 20% of dogs exhibit temporary anorexia and depression 1–2 days after vincristine administration. Chemotherapy may cause a transient leukopenia, and if the WBC drops to below 4000 mm$^3$ [217], the next vincristine dose should be delayed for 3–4 days and reduced to 25% of the initial dose.

Clinicians should utilize caution, however, as vincristine can cause tissue necrosis if extravasation occurs. Sedating the patient during catheter placement can help reduce this risk. See Chapter 20 for a table describing how to calculate body surface areas to facilitate dosing. Every patient should be evaluated for general health, hydration status, and risk of septicemia before vincristine therapy. In patients with significant ulceration and necrotic tissue, treatment with broad-spectrum systemic antibiotics is recommended.

Therapy should be continued for two treatments beyond clinical resolution of the gross tumor. A longer treatment duration may be required for older dogs, larger tumors, and situations where treatment is administered during hot and rainy months [222]. Figure 13.5 depicts the treatment progression of a large nasal tumor.

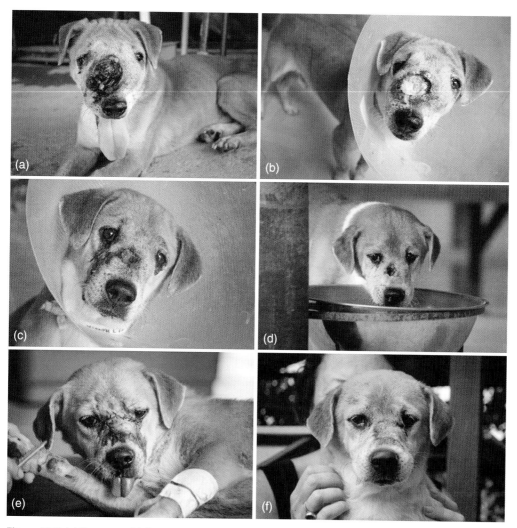

**Figure 13.5** (a) Two-year old, free-roaming, mixed breed dog presented to a shelter in Southeast Asia with a large nasal TVT. (b) Significant improvement of facial swelling following two weekly injections of vincristine. (c) Patient following four weekly injections of vincristine. (d) Patient at 6 weeks postintake. The tumor resolved and the patient is left with a defect on the dorsal muzzle. (e) A skin flap is performed to resolve the dorsal muzzle defect. (f) Patient at 3.5 months postintake. Source: Courtesy of Raymond Gerritsen, Soi Dog Foundation.

**Textbox 13.27 Sample treatment protocol for TVT patients**

1) Move the patient to a quiet area for treatment.
2) Sedate with Dexdomitor® (dexmedetomidine) (3–5 µg/kg IM) and nalbuphine (0.2 mg/kg IM). Dosing will depend on the level of arousal and clinical state of patient.
3) Place an IV catheter cleanly into the vein. This should be achieved on the first attempt and only used for the delivery of the chemotherapy. "Resticking" the vein can result in extravasation and tissue necrosis.
4) Flush the catheter with 3 ml of nonheparinized saline before administration of the vincristine. A gauze swab should be placed under the catheter hub to soak up any leaking drug.
5) Administer vincristine 0.6 mg/m$^2$ IV. Flush the catheter with 10 ml of nonheparinized saline.
6) Reverse sedation with half to full dose of Antisedan® (atipamezole) IM.
7) Remove the catheter once vincristine has been safely delivered and patient is stable/responsive. Wrap the leg after the catheter has been removed to prevent hematoma formation.
8) Note in the record which leg was used for the administration of the vincristine.

In the field, it may be prudent to administer the first vincristine injection following the spay/neuter procedure while the patient is still anesthetized.

**Textbox 13.28 Treatment precautions**

- All team members working with vincristine must wear appropriate gloves, scrub top, and eye protection.
- Hands should be washed after gloves are removed and used equipment is discarded appropriately.
- Clinicians should change into a fresh scrub top, which should be laundered once the treatment is completed.
- There should be no food or drink in areas where chemotherapy is being administered.

#### 13.7.1.3.2 Alternative Protocols

- *Doxorubicin.* If vincristine is unavailable, doxorubicin (25–30 mg/m$^2$ IV q21d) can be used for two to three cycles.
- *Surgical excision.* Surgical removal is a less desirable treatment option but may be used when vincristine is unavailable or the tumor is resistant to vincristine. Below are a few considerations:
  - High recurrence rates have been noted with surgery, largely due to tumor cell transplantation during the surgical procedure [219].
  - The use of electrocautery or cryosurgery may make the procedure safer and more effective.
  - Surgical excision is most effective on small, single, easily accessible, and noninvasive nodules [220].
  - In male dogs, damage to the penile urethra is possible.
  - If the urethral orifice is involved, an indwelling urethral catheter should be used until the site is healed.

#### 13.7.1.4 Tips and Tricks from the Field

- Dogs infected with TVT for less than 1 year are usually easily treated with vincristine. Tumors present for more than 1 year may require longer treatment periods [215].
- The probability of treatment success is reduced if the time between vincristine treatments exceeds 2 weeks [215].
- In the author's experience, nasal TVT is the most challenging to treat. Even after treatment, dogs may be left with a large defect over the dorsal muzzle or in the palate that requires grafting to close.
- Nursing dams create a special issue. To protect the puppies, the author recommends placing a diaper on the dam to protect the puppies during nursing. Because it is not known whether vincristine is excreted in milk, pups should be hand raised with mild replacer if the dam is undergoing vincristine therapy.
- The author suspects that vincristine concurs protection against reinfection during treatment. Therefore, infected dogs can be group-housed, if needed, during treatment with minimal risk of transmission.

## 13.8 Ophthalmology

### 13.8.1 Conjunctivitis

#### 13.8.1.1 General Information

The term conjunctivitis, also known as "red eye," refers to the inflammation of mucous membranes surrounding the eyelids and exposed part of the sclera. Note that conjunctivitis is a clinical description and not a diagnosis, and primary conjunctivitis should be differentiated from secondary conjunctivitis due to underlying diseases. Reaching a definitive diagnosis in the field can be challenging, but conjunctivitis must be differentiated from other causes of "red eye" such as glaucoma and uveitis.

---

**Textbox 13.29 Common causes of conjunctivitis**

Infectious (bacterial, viral, and parasitic)
Immune-mediated
Toxic or chemical
Entropion, ectropion, and distichiasis
Obstructed nasolacrimal ducts
Lymphoid follicles
Trauma/foreign body
Neoplasia
Environmental irritants
Ulcerative keratitis
KCS
Anterior uveitis
Glaucoma

---

#### 13.8.1.2 Diagnostics

A thorough ophthalmic examination is typically diagnostic. The three most common clinical signs associated with conjunctivitis include chemosis (swelling), ocular discharge, and hyperemia. Serous ocular discharge is typically associated with allergies or irritants, whereas more purulent discharge results from a bacterial infection of foreign body. Dogs typically present with blepharospasm, epiphora, and photophobia. Unilateral conjunctivitis may result from a foreign body or KCS.

#### 13.8.1.3 Treatment Protocols

Treatment should be directed at the underlying cause and may require both topical and/or systemic medications. Most cases of canine bacterial conjunctivitis should improve within 48–72 h of starting treatment, and completely resolve within a week.

---

**Textbox 13.30 Topical medications routinely used in the treatment of bacterial conjunctivitis**

Gentamicin
Tobramycin
Fusidic acid
Chloramphenicol
Oxytetracycline
Ciprofloxacin
Triple-antibiotic preparations.

---

##### 13.8.1.3.1 Feline Considerations

In cats, feline herpesvirus-1 (FHV-1) is considered the most common cause of conjunctivitis. Herpes infection is extremely common in young kittens, who often present with so much ocular discharge that their eyelids are sealed shut. It is important that kittens' eyelids are kept moistened and opened manually to both allow for drainage of secretions and administration of medication.

---

**Textbox 13.31 Treatment options for feline herpesvirus conjunctivitis**

- *Topical antibiotics for controlling secondary infections.* Given the frequency of *Chlamydophila* or *Mycoplasma* spp. involvement in the eyes of FHV-1-affected cats, systemically or topically administered tetracyclines are a good choice.
- *Topical antivirals including idoxuridine, trifluorothymidine, and vidarabine.* These medications are expensive and require administration five times daily.
- *Oral supplementation with lysine.* Lysine given at 250–500 mg daily may reduce the severity of FHV-1 conjunctivitis and keratitis [223].

---

#### 13.8.1.4 Tips and Tricks from the Field

- If the patient does not respond as expected to antibiotic therapy after several days, reconsider the diagnosis rather than the antibiotic.

- Remember to check Schirmer's tear tests (STT) for KCS as this is a common cause for secondary conjunctivitis.

## 13.8.2 Keratoconjunctivitis sicca (KCS)

### 13.8.2.1 General Information
KCS, also known as dry eye, is a commonly observed ocular disease in dogs. KCS results from a deficiency in the aqueous portion of the tear film produced by the nictitans and lacrimal glands. Causes of KCS are varied. If left untreated, KCS can result in chronic pain, globe rupture, and blindness.

Common causes of KCS include:

- Immune-mediated disease
- Drug therapy – sulphonamides, topical atropine
- Infectious – CDV
- Iatrogenic – nictitans gland removal
- Systemic – hypothyroidism, diabetes, and hyperadrenocorticism
- Neurogenic
- Trauma to the eye/orbit.

In the early stages of disease, clinical signs may include mild chemosis, conjunctival hyperemia, and intermittent ocular discharge. These patients can be easily misdiagnosed as bacterial conjunctivitis. Without appropriate treatment, the condition will progress with increasing amounts of mucopurulent discharge and discomfort observed. In cases of neurogenic KCS, a unique finding is ipsilateral nasal crusting. Other signs may include Horner's syndrome, facial paralysis, and trigeminal nerve deficits [224].

### 13.8.2.2 Diagnostics

*STT.* Obtaining a diagnosis of KCS usually only takes about a minute using a STT.
- In dogs, an STT value of >15 mm/min of wetting is considered normal.
- Eyes affected by KCS will have <10 mm/min.
- Severely affected dogs have STT results of 0 mm/min.

*Fluorescein staining.* This should also be performed to assess possible corneal ulceration. In early cases of KCS, very small areas of fluorescein uptake may be evident.

### 13.8.2.3 Treatment Protocols

#### 13.8.2.3.1 Gold Standard Protocols
Medical management is the hallmark of therapy. It typically consists of two types of long-term medications: drugs to stimulate tear production and artificial tears to wet the eye.

Tear stimulants

- Cyclosporine A (CsA) is the treatment of choice. Topical cyclosporine ophthalmic ointment should be applied every 12 h for 1 month followed by a recheck of tear production. Most patients are then maintained on once daily therapy. CsA has both anti-inflammatory and lacrimostimulant effects and an increase in tear production is usually seen within 1 month. Most canine preparations are formulated in 1% or 2% ointments. It is worth noting that Restasis®, a human preparation, has a concentration of 0.05% which is much lower than what is needed to control the disease in dogs. Cyclosporine is very expensive and in many field situations cost-prohibitive.
- Tacrolimus ointment is another topical immunomodulatory agent commonly used when compounded as a 0.02% ointment or solution. Tacrolimus is often successful in cases refractory to cyclosporine and is used twice daily [225]. Due to concerns over its potential carcinogenic risk, gloves should be worn when handling.

Tear substitutes

- Tear replacement is often needed to improve lubrication and comfort. These must be applied multiple times a day. If the frequent application of medication is not possible, petroleum-based artificial tear ointments are the best choice for coating the cornea and slowing tear evaporation. Many tear substitutes are available OTC.

#### 13.8.2.3.2 Alternative Protocols

- Broad-spectrum antibiotics should be applied four to six times daily, reducing to twice daily as conditions improve. Topical fluoroquinolones such as gatifloxacin, ofloxacin, and ciprofloxacin are good choices as they penetrate intact corneal epithelium. Avoid using antibiotic/corticosteroid drops due to the risk of corneal ulceration.

- Pilocarpine, a parasympathomimetic drug, can be given orally in cases of neurogenic KCS. It is mixed with food, one drop per 10 kg of body weight orally, twice daily. Beware of signs of toxicity including hypersalivation, vomiting, and diarrhea.

#### 13.8.2.4 Tips and Tricks from the Field

- When performing a STT, be sure to remove any mucoid discharge from the eye first, before applying the STT strip.
- Lifelong therapy is typically required, which can create an ethical dilemma for treating free-roaming dogs without a dedicated owner or caregiver.
- Use systemic sulphonamides carefully as they result in reduced tear production. Stop treatment immediately should signs of KCS be observed.
- Distemper virus is a common cause of KCS in the field. In the author's experience, these cases respond well to topical cyclosporine. If treating multiple dogs, aliquot the ointment as to not contaminate the entire tube.

### 13.8.3 Corneal Ulcer

#### 13.8.3.1 General Information

Corneal ulcers occur due to a loss of corneal epithelium and a variable amount of stroma. They are typically classified based on depth (superficial, deep, descemetocele, and perforating). The progression of the ulcer depends on the release of tissue enzymes from bacteria that digest corneal stroma. In dogs, most ulcers are superficial and are caused by physical trauma to the cornea. Ulcers can also be caused by infectious causes, eyelid or eyelash abnormalities, conjunctival foreign bodies, KCS, bullous keratopathy, and neurological dysfunction.

Clinical signs of a corneal ulcer include:

- Pain and blepharospasm
- Tearing
- Purulent ocular discharge
- Miosis
- Corneal edema/vascularization
- Stromal malacia (complicated cases).

#### 13.8.3.2 Diagnostics

A basic diagnostic approach to corneal ulcers includes an assessment of corneal and palpebral reflexes and thorough examination of the eyelids and conjunctiva.

*Ophthalmic examination.* Corneal cellular infiltrate (yellowish opacity around the ulcer) may be seen in addition to visible corneal stromal loss (defect in the cornea). Perilesional corneal edema, vascularization, and anterior uveitis (miosis, flare, and low intraocular pressure) may be observed.

*Fluorescein stain.* The uptake of fluorescein stain by exposed corneal stroma is usually diagnostic, with the exception of descemetoceles that do not stain. These will appear as a dark circle with a green boundary following staining.

*STT.* STTs help rule out KCS as a cause of the corneal ulcer.

*Cytology.* Cytology samples of the corneal epithelium can be evaluated for the presence of inflammatory cells and organisms. The presence of neutrophils may indicate infection and need for aggressive antibiotic therapy.

*Culture.* Culture can be used for unresponsive, aggressive ulcers, however it is rarely performed in the field.

#### 13.8.3.3 Treatment Protocols

##### 13.8.3.3.1 Gold Standard Protocols

The treatment of an uncomplicated corneal ulcer involves the identification and removal of the inciting cause for the ulcer, application of a topical broad-spectrum antibiotic, and prevention of self-trauma. Simple, superficial ulcers will heal in 5–7 days, provided that the underlying cause is addressed, whereas deeper ulcers involving the stroma may take 1–2 weeks to heal.

Antibiotic therapy – The frequency of instillation of antibiotic is probably more important than the specific type of medication itself. Topical triple-antibiotic ointments, chloramphenicol, oxytetracyclines, and fusidic acid are all reasonable choices.

Treatment considerations:

- Ointments should be avoided in cases where there is a risk of corneal perforation.
- In uncomplicated corneal ulcerations, topical antibiotics should be applied three to four times daily.
- Deep corneal ulcers should be medicated much more frequently (every hour for the first 1–2 days) particularly if there is uveitis or stromal loss.

- If the pupil is miotic, consider adding the topical application of atropine once daily.
- Ulcers are painful. Consider the use of tramadol or oral NSAID in addition to topical therapy.
- Never use topical steroids with ulcers.
- If an ulcer is deeper than half corneal thickness, surgery in the form of a conjunctival graft may be warranted.

Local anesthetics should never be used therapeutically for the treatment of ocular pain.

#### 13.8.3.3.2 Alternative Protocols

Other therapies include the use of cyanoacrylate adhesives (tissue glue) and autologous serum.

---

**Textbox 13.32 Use of cyanoacrylate adhesives (tissue glue) for treating corneal ulcers**

Medical grade tissue adhesive may be used in some cases as an alternative to surgery as a last-ditch effort to prevent corneal perforation [226]. It provides structural but no biological support for the ulcer. Steps for application are as follows:

1) Anesthetize the patient.
2) Gently debride the corneal wound edges.
3) Apply one very small drop of cyanoacrylate using either a 27- or 30-gauge needle. The goal is to coat the surface of the ulcer, not fill the entire defect. The glue will be naturally extruded within 2 weeks.
4) A temporary tarsorrhaphy may be performed for additional corneal protection.

---

Alternatively, autologous serum can be used to help promote ulcer healing.

---

**Textbox 13.33 Use of serum**

In patients with deep ulcers where surgery is not an option, serum can be used for its anticollagenase properties. Serum can be collected from a centrifuged venous blood sample. Samples should be stored refrigerated in a sterile vial and applied using an eyedropper as frequently as every hour. Serum should be replaced every few days.

---

#### 13.8.3.4 Tips and Tricks from the Field

- Topical antibiotics must be applied very frequently! In shelters and clinics, one must assess the staffing capacity and adjust accordingly to provide such treatment. Alternatively, consider foster homes for frequent dosing.
- If a centrifuge is available, serum is a free and effective topical treatment.
- As a general rule, when greater than two-third of the corneal thickness is affected, surgical repair in the form of a conjunctival graft is required.

## 13.9 Respiratory

### 13.9.1 Canine Infectious Respiratory Disease Complex (Kennel Cough)

#### 13.9.1.1 General Information

CIRDC, also known as kennel cough or infectious tracheobronchitis, is a contagious condition commonly affecting dogs in shelters or close confinement. Multiple pathogens can contribute, including but not limited to those listed in Table 13.31. It is important to note, however, that emerging respiratory pathogens are being routinely discovered and clinicians should stay apprised of clinical updates and discoveries [227].

The environment and host immune responses play integral roles in the disease process. Risk factors for CIRDC include overcrowding, poor ventilation, stress, lack of biosecurity, and poor cleaning practices (Table 13.32). Disease transmission is primarily

Table 13.31 Pathogens associated with CIRDC.

| Bacterial | Viral |
| --- | --- |
| *B. bronchiseptica* | Canine distemper virus (CDV) |
| *Mycoplasma* spp. | Canine parainfluenza (CPiV) |
| *Streptococcus equi* subsp. *zooepidemicus* | Canine adenovirus type 2 (CAV-2) |
| | Canine influenza virus (CIV H3N8 and H3N2) |
| | Canine respiratory coronavirus (CRCoV) |
| | Canine pneumovirus (CnPnV) |
| | Canine herpesvirus (CHV) |

**Table 13.32** Risk factors for CIRDC.

| Dog | Pathogen | Animal care |
|---|---|---|
| Age | Virulence | Crowding |
| Immune status | Incubation period | Length of stay |
| Health | Shedding period | Random comingling of dogs |
| Stress | Subclinical infection | Sanitation and environmental contamination |
| | Carrier state | |
| | Transmission routes | Ventilation |
| | Incomplete protection by vaccines | Staffing |
| | | Prompt disease recognition |
| | Vaccines lacking for new pathogens | Fomites |

Source: Adapted from Crawford 2011 [228].

through aerosolization of respiratory pathogens resulting from sneezing and coughing (>20 feet/ 6.1 m), dog-to-dog contact, or contact with contaminated fomites [228]. Similar to feline URI, CIRDC is not entirely vaccine preventable; however, routine vaccination plays a key role in mitigating disease severity and incidence.

It is important to note that preclinical shedding occurs for all CIRDC pathogens, meaning that dogs are contagious before they begin showing clinical signs. Most pathogens are shed for 7–10 days in respiratory secretions [228,229]. See Table 13.33 for additional information on incubation and shedding periods. Exceptions to this are *B. bronchiseptica* and CDV, which can be shed for weeks to months.

All of the pathogens contributing to CIRDC cause similar clinical signs early in the course of disease, resulting from inflammation of the upper airways. Coughing, sneezing, nasal/ocular discharge, and lethargy are common, but the cause of infection cannot be determined solely on clinical signs. A dry, hacking cough induced by tracheal palpation is typical. Clinical signs are usually mild and most dogs recover without complication. CDV is the major exception as many dogs die or are euthanized due to progressive disease.

### 13.9.1.2 Diagnostics

Treatment is often based on clinical signs. Bloodwork and thoracic radiographs are typically unremarkable in uncomplicated cases.

*Culture and sensitivity.* Culturing respiratory secretions is indicated during an outbreak situation or if an individual dog fails to respond to empirical therapy.

*PCR.* PCR testing has become more widely available in recent years. Nasal and/or deep pharyngeal swabs should be submitted from dogs with clinical signs for <4 days in order to detect the pathogens during their peak shedding period. Keep in mind that a positive PCR result does not necessarily

**Table 13.33** Characteristics of pathogens associated with CIRDC.

| Pathogen | Incubation period | Preclinical shedding | Duration of shedding | Subclinical infection | Persistent infection |
|---|---|---|---|---|---|
| *B. bronchiseptica* | 3–10 days | + | Weeks to months | + | Possible [230] |
| Canine parainfluenza/canine adenovirus type 2 | <1 week | + | 1 week | + | – |
| Canine distemper virus | 2 weeks | + | >1 month | + | – |
| Canine influenza virus | 2–4 days | + | 7–10 days[a] | + | – |
| Canine respiratory coronavirus | <1 week | + | 2 weeks | + | – |
| Canine herpesvirus | <1 week | + | 2 weeks | + | + |
| *Streptococcus zooepidemicus* | 1–3 weeks | + | 1–2 weeks | + | Possible |
| *Mycoplasma* spp. | 1–4 weeks | + | Several weeks | + | Possible [231] |

a) Note H3N2 strains can have prolonged shedding times of >21 days.

mean that a specific pathogen is causing disease in a particular animal. Modified live vaccines (DHPP and DH2PP) have been shown to cause false-positive PCR results as long as 3 weeks postadministration. False positives can also be seen following sample contamination and poor laboratory technique. During an outbreak in a shelter, testing a minimum of three to five dogs, or 10–30% of the affected population is recommended.

*Necropsy.* Necropsies of dogs that died or were euthanized can be a helpful diagnostic tool. Tissues for histopathology should be collected and fixed in buffered formalin (9 : 1 ratio of formalin to tissue).

#### 13.9.1.3 Treatment Protocols

##### 13.9.1.3.1 *Gold Standard Protocols*

Most cases of CIRDC are viral in origin and self-limiting with supportive care. Dogs infected with canine parainfluenza (CPiV)/CAV, canine influenza virus (CIV), and canine respiratory coronavirus (CRCoV) may appear to respond to antibiotic treatment, but in reality, these viruses have "run their course" in a time frame that coincides with duration of antibiotic therapy [228]. For dogs with evidence of bacterial disease such as fever, depression, and colored nasal/ocular discharge, antibiotic treatment is indicated. Note that antibiotics do not always reduce the severity of disease with *B. bronchiseptica* infection if clinical signs are the result of tracheal inflammation.

Antibiotic therapy – For cases requiring antibiotic therapy, administer doxycycline (5–10 mg/kg PO, IV q12–24h) for 7–10 days or until resolution of clinical signs. In severe or complicated cases, consider changing antibiotics, ideally antibiotic changes should be based on culture and sensitivity testing, see Table 13.34 for antibiotic choices for patients developing pneumonia.

Antitussive drugs – Cough suppressants are generally not indicated and can interfere with the beneficial effects of coughing. To control persistent nonproductive coughing, consider administering hydrocodone (0.25 mg/kg PO q6–12h) or butorphanol (0.05–0.1 mg/kg PO, SC q6–12h). Cough suppressants should not be used if bronchopneumonia is suspected.

Nebulization – Consider nebulization of sterile saline to improve mucociliary clearance. In severely

**Table 13.34** Antibiotic choices for canine bacterial pneumonia.

| Drug | Dosage |
|---|---|
| Amoxicillin | 22 mg/kg PO q8h |
| Ampicillin with sulbactam | 22 mg/kg IV q8h |
| Amoxicillin with clavulanate | 15–25 mg/kg PO q8h |
| Cephalexin | 20–40 mg/kg PO q12h |
| Clindamycin | 5.5–11 mg/kg PO, IV, SC q12h |
| Doxycycline | 5–10 mg/kg PO, IV q12h |
| Enrofloxacin | 5–10 mg/kg PO, IV, SC q24h |
| Marbofloxacin | 2.7–5.5 mg/kg PO q24h |
| Trimethoprim–sulfonamide | 15 mg/kg PO q12h |

affected dogs, kanamycin sulfate (250 mg) or gentamicin sulfate (50 mg) diluted in 3 ml of saline may be administered by aerosolization q12h for 3 days. For cases of bacterial pneumonia, coupage is indicated following nebulization.

Additional supportive care considerations:

- Consider elevating food and water bowls to limit sinus pressure when the dog lowers his or her head to eat.
- Offer moist food two to three times daily.
- Remove collars and use harnesses to reduce pressure on the trachea.

#### 13.9.1.4 Disease Prevention

- Reduce animal crowding and stress. Attempt to limit the amount of time a dog stays in a sheltering facility.
- Vaccinate all dogs on intake to shelters as the cornerstone for the prevention of most respiratory pathogens (*B. bronchiseptica*, CPiV, CAV-2, and CDV). All dogs should receive a modified live or recombinant subcutaneous vaccine (DHPP or DH2PP) immediately upon intake. Intranasal vaccines containing *B. bronchiseptica*, CPiV, and CAV-2 may be useful and should be used in conjunction with a subcutaneous DHPP or DH2PP vaccine. See Chapter 16 for additional vaccination recommendations.

- Reduce environmental contamination. Most pathogens associated with CIRDC are susceptible to commonly used disinfectants, with the exception of CAV-2.
- Promptly remove and isolate sick animals to reduce the infectious dose in the environment and transmission throughout a shelter.

### 13.9.1.5 Tips and Tricks from the Field

- Many facilities assume that all coughing dogs suffer from "kennel cough" due to *B. bronchiseptica* infection. Evidence suggests that most cases of CIRDC are actually viral. Be sure to rule out CDV as a cause of chronic respiratory disease.
- Once clinical signs resolve, the risk of pathogen shedding is significantly decreased. If a facility lacks isolation space, dogs whose clinical signs have resolved can usually be moved out of isolation with caution so long as all dogs have been appropriately vaccinated.

### 13.9.2 Feline Upper Respiratory Infection

#### 13.9.2.1 General Information

Feline URI, also known as cat flu, is probably the most common disease problem in cats living in shelters and overcrowded environments. In shelter cats, feline herpesvirus (FHV-1) and feline calicivirus (FCV) are the two pathogens responsible for the majority of URI cases, but disease can also be caused by *Chlamydophila felis, B. bronchiseptica*, and *Mycoplasma* spp.

Overcrowding and prolonged shelter stays are the most significant risk factors associated with URI as increased population density leads to higher contact between animals, reduced air quality, increased animal stress, and compromised animal care [232]. Clinical signs and shedding of FHV-1 have been shown to be activated by stress [233,234].

Most pathogens responsible for feline URI are shed primarily in ocular, nasal, and oral secretions and have an incubation period between 2 and 14 days. Although aerosolization and airborne transmission of pathogens can occur, fomite transmission is the most significant method of disease spread. Vaccination can reduce the severity and duration of disease; however, it does not prevent infection or development of a carrier state for URI pathogens. All shelter cats over 4–6 weeks of age should be vaccinated with a modified live FVRCP vaccine to induce immunity quickly.

Most cats with URI suffer from bouts of sneezing and ocular/nasal discharge. As a general rule, FVC-infected cats are more likely to display oral ulceration and limping, whereas FHV-1-infected cats are more likely to cause keratitis or corneal ulceration. *Chlamydophila* and *Mycoplasma* spp. are commonly associated with conjunctivitis.

Many cats enter shelters already carrying one of the viral causes of URI. In fact, these pathogens can be found in both clinical and nonclinical cats. As complete elimination of the viral causes of URI is impossible, minimization of disease impact in a facility should be the priority. Although treating the individual patient is important, consideration should be given to also developing a comprehensive sheltering plan to address overall feline well-being.

#### 13.9.2.2 Diagnostics

Diagnosis is most commonly based on clinical signs rather than the identification of a particular pathogen.

*Physical examination.* A thorough physical examination is probably the best diagnostic tool.
  - *Overall appearance.* Is the cat bright, quiet, or depressed?
  - *Hydration.* Check skin turgor between the shoulder blades.
  - *Eyes including cornea and conjunctiva.* Assess the presence of discharge, conjunctival swelling, corneal irritation or ulceration, and cloudiness in the front chamber.
  - *Nose.* Assess for discharge and degree of congestion.
  - *Mouth.* Check for oral ulcers and sores on tongue. Note that gingivitis can also be associated with FCV or FIV infection.
  - *Lungs.* Check for lower airway involvement.
  - *Temperature.* Check for fever to assess the need for fluid therapy.

Diagnostic testing is suggested when cats are displaying unusual clinical signs, during an outbreak, if there are legal implications such as the cats were confiscated from a hoarder.

*PCR.* PCR has become more widely available in recent years. Interpretation of positive results can be complicated as any of the URI-related pathogens can be isolated from clinically healthy cats.

Furthermore, PCR detects both live (field or vaccine strain) and inactivated virus.

During an outbreak situation, it is recommended that at least 10–30% of clinically affected cats be tested. The results of one PCR-positive test from an individual cat are of little significance.

*Culture and sensitivity.* These are often used for resistant infections. Samples typically consist of deep pharyngeal and/or nasal swab samples for submission to a laboratory.

*Thoracic radiographs.* Radiographs can determine lower respiratory involvement.

*Oro-nasopharyngeal examination.* When performed under anesthesia, nasopharyngeal polyps may be seen.

#### 13.9.2.3   Treatment Protocols

Stress reduction and improving feline comfort are often the most crucial elements for reducing the incidence of URI. Provide cats with adequate perching and hiding places, decrease noise exposure, and provide scratching surfaces. Consider reducing the group size of cats to two to four cats in colony rooms; large rooms can be partitioned.

In a shelter environment, the length of stay an animal spends in the facility should be minimized.

Improve air quality through increased ventilation, frequent litter box cleaning, low dust litter, and reduced population density. The presence and severity of clinical signs will dictate the treatment protocol. Tables 13.35 and 13.36 can be used to help determine when a cat needs treatment and guide treatment decisions.

#### 13.9.2.4   Tips and Tricks from the Field

- Doxycycline or minocycline tablets can cause esophagitis and subsequent esophageal strictures in cats and, if used, should be flushed with at least 6 cc of liquid. Liquid doxycycline formulations are recommended and can be compounded in-house. All compounded doxycycline should be stored in lightproof containers and used within 7 days [235].
- Most URI pathogens are inactivated by routinely used disinfectants with the exception of FCV, which can be difficult to kill. If FCV is suspected, consider using household bleach (5% sodium hypochlorite) diluted at 1 : 32 (one-half cup per gallon) or Trifectant/Virkon, and hand sanitizers containing 60–90% ethanol or propanol.

### 13.9.3   Lungworms

#### 13.9.3.1   General Information

Lungworm infection, otherwise known as verminous bronchitis, is most commonly caused by the parasite *Aelurostrongylus abstrusus* in cats. Adult worms live within the epithelium of the trachea, bronchi, and bronchioles. Adult worms produce ova that are coughed up, swallowed, and passed in the feces. Cats become infected with *Aelurostrongylus* when they eat an intermediate (snails or slugs) or paratenic host (birds, rodents, reptiles, or amphibians).

The feline immune response causes a focal interstitial pneumonia. When clinical signs are mild, the infection may be self-limiting with clinical signs spontaneously resolving within several weeks [237].

Clinical signs depend on multiple factors including the worm burden and health status of the cat. Most infected cats are clinically asymptomatic, but in heavy infections, a chronic cough, anorexia, dyspnea, and emaciation can be observed as a result of chronic bronchial disease.

#### 13.9.3.2   Diagnostics

*Baermann test.* The classic technique for identifying infection is the Baermann test. It is an inexpensive, sensitive, and noninvasive way to separate larvae from fecal material. Infection can also be confirmed by the identification of first-stage larvae using normal flotation. This is less ideal, however, as *A. abstrusus* larvae become dehydrated and damaged in hypertonic solutions, making identification more difficult. See Chapter 14 for instructions on how to perform a Baermann test.

#### 13.9.3.3   Treatment Protocols

##### 13.9.3.3.1   Gold Standard Protocols

- Fenbendazole (50 mg/kg PO q24h) for three consecutive days has an efficacy of 99% [238]. Other protocols suggest fenbendazole (20 mg/kg PO q24h) for 5 days [239].

##### 13.9.3.3.2   Alternative Protocols

- Ivermectin (400 µg/kg SC or PO), then repeated in 2 weeks.
- Other drugs including moxidectin, selamectin, and emodepside/praziquantel spot-on formulations have also shown promising efficacy against feline lungworms.

**Table 13.35** Feline URI: primary treatment in an animal shelter based on clinical signs [235].

| Category | Clinical signs | Probable interpretation | Treatment |
|---|---|---|---|
| 1a. Clear discharge | Clear discharge from eyes or nose, sneezing, squinting | Mild viral URI | Isolate. Monitor appetite and hydration status daily |
| 1b. Clear discharge | Category 1a. -AND- Fever, dehydration, anorexia, oral ulcers, congestion, depression | Moderate-to-severe viral URI | As for 1a. -AND- Administer additional treatment and supportive care as described below |
| 2a. URI with colored discharge | Category 1a. -AND- Green, brown, yellow, or bloody nasal or ocular discharge | Viral URI with secondary rhinitis and/or ocular infection | Doxycycline or minocycline (10 mg/kg PO q24h) until resolution of clinical signs. Reevaluate in 3–5 days. If no improvement, consider alternative antibiotic. If there is improvement but relapse after discontinuing antibiotic, consider testing for *Chlamydophila*. If *Chlamydophila* confirmed or suspected, treat with doxycycline for 4–6 weeks |
| 2b. URI with colored discharge fails to respond to initial therapy | Category 1b. -AND- Green, brown, yellow, or bloody nasal or ocular discharge -AND- Fails to respond to doxycycline | Viral URI with moderate-to-severe secondary bacterial infection | Enrofloxacin (5 mg/kg PO, SQ q24h) until resolution of clinical signs -OR- Other fluoroquinolone (e.g. pradofloxacin, marbofloxacin, and orbifloxacin) -OR- Azithromycin (5–10 mg/kg PO q24h) for 5 days, then q48h until resolution of clinical signs (has been shown to be ineffective in eliminating *Chlamydophila felis* in cats so do not use if this agent is suspected) |
| 3a. Ocular signs | Unilateral to bilateral ocular discharge with mild-to-moderate conjunctivitis and/or chemosis | Primary bacterial or viral ocular infection | As for 1a/b or 2a if mucopurulent discharge -AND- Erythromycin, gentamicin, or tobramycin ophthalmic OU q12h for 7 days Reevaluate after 3–5 days for response to treatment. If no improvement seen, discontinue topical treatment and provide systemic antibiotic treatment if not already done. Consider antiherpetic treatment if other causes ruled out and sufficient resources exist |
| 3b. Ocular signs, fails to respond to initial therapy | Category 3a. -AND- Persistent ocular discharge or corneal edema, corneal ulceration, blepharospasm | Severe primary viral ocular infection with or without secondary bacterial component | As for 2a. if colored ocular discharge -AND- Cidofovir 0.5% ophthalmic 1 drop OU q12h until resolution of clinical signs -OR- Idoxuridine 0.1% ophthalmic 1 drop OU q2–4h until resolution of clinical signs -OR- |

Table 13.35 (*Continued*)

| Category | Clinical signs | Probable interpretation | Treatment |
|---|---|---|---|
| | | | Idoxuridine–gentamicin–flurbiprofen (from a compounding pharmacy) 1 drop OU q8–12h until clinical signs resolve |
| 4. Systemic signs or prolonged illness | Fever >106 °F (41 °C) rapid or labored breathing, coughing, vomiting, severe diarrhea, swelling of any part of the body -OR- Failure to respond to two rounds of antibiotic therapy | Complicated URI or additional problems | Full veterinary exam Supportive care as needed for dehydration, pyrexia, pain, congestion, anorexia Perform additional diagnostic test and rule out other medical issues |

Source: Courtesy of UC Davis Koret Shelter Medicine Program.

Table 13.36 Feline URI: supportive care [235].

| Condition | Treatment |
|---|---|
| Dehydration | • <5% Subcutaneous fluids (LRS or Normosol-R) 250–500 ml q12–24h <br> • >5% Administer intravenous fluids at one to two times maintenance rate until dehydration is corrected. <br> • Vitamin B complex can be administered with fluids (1 ml/l). Cover fluid bag with a paper bag to prevent degradation of the vitamins. <br> • Add KCl to fluids for anorexic cats (20 mEq/l). |
| Congestion | • Clean nose with warm moist gauze. <br> • Nebulize for 10 min every 6 h. Use sterile saline with or without acetylcysteine and/or antibiotics (gentamicin or amikacin). <br> • As a last resort, if the cat is severely congested and not eating, try a decongestant (phenylephrine or oxymetazoline). Administer one drop q12h before feeding, in alternating nostrils. Left nostril AM and right nostril PM for no more than 3 days. The continuous use of decongestant nose drops decreases its effectiveness and may cause a rebound effect when stopped. |
| Anorexia | • Correct dehydration, treat congestion, provide analgesia, offer strong-smelling food. Consider appetite stimulants. <br> • Consider warming food slightly, offer a novel brand/flavor, encourage eating by petting. Remove food from the enclosure after 10 min. <br> • Check for oral ulcers. <br> • If above steps fail and the cat does not eat for >2 days, administer the following: <br> – Mirtazapine 15 mg tablets (1/8 tablet PO q24h)-OR- <br> – Cyproheptadine (2–4 mg per cat PO q12–24h)-OR- <br> – Midazolam (1.25 mg SC, IM) once food is present <br> • If anorexia is unresponsive to appetite stimulants and persists for >5 days, consider placing an esophageal feeding tube. Continued force-feeding may cause food aversion <br> • Monitor weight weekly. |
| Pain | • Assess pain associated with nasal, corneal, oral ulceration, or severe systemic disease. Assess renal function and hydration before administering NSAIDs. <br> • Buprenorphine SR (0.12 mg/kg SC q72h) <br> • Buprenorphine (0.01–0.02 mg/kg IM, SC, TM q4–6h or as needed) <br> • Meloxicam 0.1 mg/kg PO, SC once. For subsequent dosages, start 24 h after initial dose at 0.05 mg/kg q24h PO for 3 days [236]. <br> • Lidocaine 4% viscous. Apply directly to the affected area q6–8h as needed. |
| Fever | • If temperature > 105 °F (40.5 °C), administer crystalloid fluids (SC or IV) <br> • Rule out other systemic issues or lower respiratory tract involvement with thoracic radiographs, if possible. <br> • Antipyretic drug treatment if temperature >105 °F (40.5 °C) and fails to respond to external cooling. |

Source: Courtesy of UC Davis Koret Shelter Medicine Program.

### 13.9.3.4 Tips and Tricks from the Field

- Lungworm infection is often misdiagnosed as feline asthma. Consider lungworms in any cat with a chronic dry cough in an endemic area.

## 13.10 Theriogenology

### 13.10.1 Mastitis

#### 13.10.1.1 General Information

Canine and feline mastitis occurs frequently in postpartum bitches and less commonly in queens following estrus, or rarely during lactation with pseudopregnancy. Mastitis is associated with a bacterial infection most commonly involving *E. coli*, staphylococci, and streptococci. Sources of bacterial infection can be cutaneous (ascending), often caused by offspring, exogenous (trauma), or hematogenous (systemic infection). Infections may be acute and fulminate, or chronic and low grade, and may involve single or multiple mammary glands [240].

Early signs of disease are uncomfortable, warm, swollen mammary gland(s), galactostasis, and cutaneous inflammation. Glands become firm and purulent or hemorrhagic fluid may be expressed. Moderate cases exhibit pain, anorexia, lethargy, and reluctance to nurse. Fever can be marked and may precede other clinical signs. Severe cases can present in septic shock, with abscessed or necrotic glands [240,241].

Prevention includes environmental decontamination, keeping the mammary area clean (i.e. shaving hair from around mammary glands), minimizing the chance for trauma by trimming kitten and puppy claws, and ensuring nursing occurs from all glands [241].

#### 13.10.1.2 Diagnostics

Diagnosis can typically be made from the patient history and physical examination.

*Culture.* Milk from affected glands can be collected via fine-needle aspiration for culture/sensitivity.

*Cytology.* Cytology of the milk can be performed; however, exercise caution when interpreting as normal milk naturally contains many neutrophils, macrophages, and other mononuclear cells. In cases of septic mastitis, large numbers of free and phagocytosed bacteria and degenerative neutrophils are often present [241].

*CBC/chemistry.* One may observe neutrophilia with a degenerative left shift, or leukopenia with sepsis. Blood chemistry may reveal changes associated with sepsis (azotemia, elevated ALT and ALP, bilirubinemia, hypoglycemia, hypoalbuminemia, thrombocytopenia, and anemia) or dehydration (elevated total protein, hematocrit, blood urea, and urine-specific gravity) [242].

#### 13.10.1.3 Treatment Protocols

##### 13.10.1.3.1 Gold Standard Protocols

Administer broad-spectrum antibiotics with the understanding that there is potential passage in the milk to the offspring. Try to administer outside of normal feeding times to decrease antibiotic transfer during nursing and treat for 10–14 days past resolution of clinical signs.

Abscessed or necrotic gland(s) should be surgically debrided, flushed, and treated like an open wound. Apply warm compress to affected gland(s) three to four times daily to relieve discomfort and facilitate drainage. A 1% betadine solution can be infused into the affected gland(s) using a lacrimal cannula. While under treatment, the affected gland should be protected from trauma from nest box edges and neonatal claws [240].

Honey makes a great dressing for ruptured, infected mammary tissue. Any unpasteurized (preferably raw) honey can be used, but Manuka honey is considered superior [84].

For pain relief, narcotic analgesia in the bitch/queen is considered safer for neonates than NSAIDs. In severe cases, antiprolactin therapy may be indicated to reduce lactation; neonates will then require hand-rearing. See Table 13.37 for treatment options that are considered safe for nursing neonates.

##### 13.10.1.3.2 Alternative Protocols

- Applying cooled, raw cabbage leaves to the infected mammary gland(s) for 1–2 h twice daily will reduce swelling and pain. Monitor milk production if nursing.

#### 13.10.1.4 Tips and Tricks from the Field

- The key to treatment is to detect and diagnose mastitis early rather than having to treat a fulminant infection. Monitor mammary glands and milk throughout lactation.
- Check for mastitis if puppies or kittens are weak, crying and ill, or die.

Table 13.37 Treatment options for mastitis that are safe for nursing neonates.

| Medication | Canine dosage | Feline dosage |
| --- | --- | --- |
| *Antibiotics* | | |
| Keflex (cephalexin) | 20 mg/kg PO q8h or 30 mg/kg q12h | 20 mg/kg PO q8h or 30 mg/kg q12h |
| Amoxicillin | 10 mg/kg PO q12h | 10 mg/kg PO q12h |
| Clavamox (amoxicillin/clavulanic acid) | 14 mg/kg PO q12h | 62.5 mg/cat PO q12h |
| *For severe, systemic disease* | | |
| Ampicillin | 20 mg/kg IV q6h | 20 mg/kg IV q6h |
| Ampicillin– sulbactam | 20 mg/kg IV, IM q8h | 20 mg/kg IV, IM q8h |
| Cefazolin | 20 mg/kg IV q6h | 20 mg/kg IV q6h |
| *Analgesics* | | |
| Tramadol | 10 mg/kg/day PO, SC divided q8–12h | 2 mg/kg PO, SC q8–12h |
| Buprenorphine | 0.005–0.03 mg/kg IV, IM, SC q6–12h | 0.01–0.03 mg/kg IM, IV, TM q8h |
| Butorphanol | 0.1–0.5 mg/kg IV, IM, SC q2–4h | 0.1–0.5 mg/kg IV, IM, SC q2–4h |
| *Antiprolactin (severe cases)* | | |
| Cabergoline | 5 µg/kg PO daily | 5 µg/kg PO daily |

- Nursing should ideally be restricted from abscessed or necrotic glands. There is no evidence, however, that nursing from affected glands is problematic for neonates as they naturally tend to avoid glands that are difficult to obtain milk from anyways. Monitor nursing neonates for diarrhea due to potential bacterial enteritis.
- Nonseptic mastitis may be seen at the time of weaning. On examination, the glands are warm, swollen, and painful to the touch. Apply warm compresses four to six times daily.

## 13.11 Urinary

### 13.11.1 Feline Lower Urinary Tract Disease (FLUTD)

#### 13.11.1.1 General Information
Feline lower urinary tract disease (FLUTD) describes a collection of clinical signs that affect the bladder and urethra of cats. Affected cats typically present with a combination of the following signs:

- Straining to urinate
- Crying out while urinating
- Urinating outside the litter box
- Blood in the urine
- Frequent attempts to urinate
- Over-grooming of genital area
- Passing only small amount of urine.

A typical cat with FLUTD lives indoors, is between 1 and 10 years of age, uses a litter box, and consumes mostly dry food [243]. Environmental factors are also thought to play a role as many affected cats also have a history of negative interactions with owners or other cats in the household or have had a sudden change in their routine [244].

FLUTD can be a tricky condition to diagnose and treat. In up to 70% of FLUTD cases, a specific underlying cause cannot be identified. This is typically referred to as idiopathic FLUTD. All potential causes of lower urinary tract disease in cats must be ruled out, however, to ensure appropriate treatment.

- *Feline idiopathic cystitis (FIC).* Up to 70% of cats presenting with FLUTD clinical signs will have no specific underlying disease identified. This condition also goes by the name feline interstitial cystitis, which simply means that there is inflammation of the bladder without known cause. FIC is a diagnosis of exclusion. Cats with FIC often resolve spontaneously within a couple weeks regardless of the treatment initiated.

- *Urethral obstruction.* This is the most serious issue associated with FLUTD. Note that urethral obstruction is a medical emergency. If the bladder cannot be emptied, death will occur due to electrolyte imbalance. Time from complete obstruction to death can be as little as 24–48 h.
- *Urolithiasis.* Cats with urinary stones will present with many of the clinical signs associated with FLUTD. Radiographs or ultrasound is typically needed to make a definitive diagnosis, although an exploratory could be performed as a last resort. The two most common feline urolith types are struvite and calcium oxalate. Special stone-dissolving diets may be effective for treating cats with struvite stones. Regardless of the stone type, surgical removal is frequently warranted.
- *Urethral plugs.* Urethral plugs consist of a soft, compressible material composed of accumulated proteins, cells, and debris, which block the urethral opening.
- *Urinary tract infection (UTI).* Bacterial UTI is a relatively rare cause of FLUTD, particularly in younger cats. UTIs account for only 5–15% of all FLUTD cases. UTIs tend to be more common in older cats. Treatment with antibiotics is generally performed for 2–3 weeks, or 4–6 weeks if pyelonephritis is suspected.
- *Neoplasia.* Neoplasia is a rather uncommon cause of FLUTD, found primarily in older cats. Transitional cell carcinoma is the most frequent bladder neoplasia in cats.

### 13.11.1.2 Diagnostics

Reaching a definitive diagnosis of FLUTD can be difficult, as all possible causes must be ruled out first. Aside from a physical examination, a minimum database includes urinalysis, radiographs, and a urine culture and sensitivity.

*Urinalysis.* FLUTD cats often present with hematuria, proteinuria, crystalluria, and high specific gravity.
*Radiographs.* Radiopaque stones in the urinary bladder can be ruled out.
*Culture and sensitivity.* Urine cultures can be performed to rule out a bacterial UTI.

### 13.11.1.3 Treatment Protocols

Treatment of FLUTD depends on the underlying cause and uncomplicated cases may not require any treatment at all. Clinical signs of idiopathic cystitis usually resolve in 85% of cats within a week, with or without treatment. The mainstays of therapy include stress reduction through environmental enrichment, dietary changes, pheromone therapy, and pharmacological intervention in refractory cases. As the cause is often unknown, the goal of treatment is to reduce the severity and frequency of cystitis.

---

**Textbox 13.34 General recommendations to reduce the occurrence of FLUTD**

- *Increase water intake.* Transitioning cats to a canned diet, using water fountains, flavoring water, and adding water to a dry diet can help decrease USG and reduce the concentration of potentially noxious substances in the urine.
- *Keep a consistent diet.* Sudden changes in diet may result in recurrence of FLUTD.
- *Environmental modification.* Enrichment and frequent play can help reduce stress and FLUTD incidence. Ensure sufficient numbers of clean litter pans available in the household. The standard recommendation is $n + 1$ litter boxes; that is a household with three cats should have $3 + 1 = 4$ litter boxes.
- *Use pheromones.* Synthetic feline pheromone may help reduce anxiety-related behaviors in cats that contribute to FLUTD.
- *Eliminate conflict between cats or other animals in the household.*
- *Glucosamine.* Glucosamine has been advocated by some but has been shown to be largely ineffective in treating FIC [245].
- *Drug therapy.* May be indicated if dietary and environmental modification does not relieve clinical signs.

---

In cases of acute cystitis, pain and distress must be addressed using a combination of NSAIDs, opioids, and behavior modifying drugs.

- Acepromazine (0.05 mg/kg SC q8–12h). Acepromazine has an antispasmodic effect on the urethra.
- Buprenorphine (0.01–0.02 mg/kg PO or SC q8–12h) for 3–5 days.
- Butorphanol (0.2–0.4 mg/kg PO or SC q6h–8h).
- NSAIDs may also be beneficial for short-term pain relief.

Additional medical management options include:

- Amitriptyline (5.0–12.5 mg/cat PO q24h)
- Buspirone (0.5–1.0 mg/kg PO q12h)
- Clomipramine (0.5 mg/kg/day PO)
- Fluoxetine (1 mg/kg/day PO).

#### 13.11.1.4 Tips and Tricks from the Field

- In the vast majority of cases, cats will exhibit signs of cystitis but have no underlying cause identified. Multimodal therapy including dietary adjustment is key.
- Bacterial UTIs are rare in cats. Most FLUTD cases *do not* require antibiotics.
- Don't overlook the impact of simple environmental changes. Adding extra litterpans and changing the type of cat litter may prevent recurrence.

### 13.11.2 Urolithiasis

#### 13.11.2.1 General Information

Urolithiasis is the formation of urinary calculi in the urinary tract (kidneys, ureters, urinary bladder, and urethra). Crystalluria rarely indicates urolithiasis but plays an important role in the formation of urethral plugs and obstruction in male cats. The main factors associated with urolithiasis in dogs are UTI, diet, urine volume, frequency of urination, therapeutic agents, and genetic predisposition [246]. Clinical signs of urolithiasis may mimic those of a UTI even when one is not present and include anorexia, pollakiuria, dysuria, hematuria, inappropriate urination, and/or outflow obstruction. Note that urinary obstruction constitutes an emergency. See Table 13.38 for a quick guide to urolithiasis.

#### 13.11.2.2 Diagnostics

*Physical examination.* In many cases, examination is unremarkable although occasionally uroliths can be palpated in the urinary bladder or the animal may show signs of discomfort or pain during abdominal palpation.

*Urinalysis.* A urine specimen should be evaluated with a urine dip stick and microscopic evaluation of urine sediment. This should be done within 30 min of sampling and at room temperature. Refrigerate any samples if analysis is expected to be delayed to prevent formation of crystal or other changes.

*Microscopic evaluation of urine sediment.* This may reveal crystalluria. Although crystalluria is a risk factor for urolith formation, it can also be seen in healthy dogs and cats. Thus, urine pH and USG should be considered when interpreting crystalluria. Increased urine alkalinity and USG promotes struvite crystal formation [247].

*Urine culture and sensitivity.* Whenever possible, cultures can be used to guide UTI treatment.

*Abdominal radiographs.* If available, this should be performed in any animal with signs of urinary obstruction, and any cat with azotemia to screen for uroliths [248]. Urate and occasionally cysteine uroliths may be radiolucent.

#### 13.11.2.3 Treatment Protocols

With the exception of a few variations depending on the urolith involved, the cornerstone therapy for any treatment and management includes the following:

- *UTI treatment.* To enable successful dietary management and prevention of urolith recurrence.
- *Surgical removal.* If medical dissolution is unsuccessful or not an option. Make sure to follow up with postoperative abdominal radiographs if available to verify that all uroliths have been removed.
- *Dietary adjustments.* These can be used for both dissolution and to prevent recurrence. Different uroliths require different dietary adjustments, as described in Table 13.38.
- *Increase water intake to decrease concentration of urine.* Provide multiple sources of clean, fresh water to encourage drinking. Feeding canned food can help increase water intake.

#### 13.11.2.4 Tips and Tricks from the Field

- Antibiotic therapy for UTIs should continue for the duration of urolith dissolution due to potential liberation of bacteria from dissolving uroliths [249].
- Palpation of a urinary bladder with cystitis may be large and firm/hard; similar to a urinary bladder with a large, singular urolith.
- Oral administration of sodium chloride, historically recommended for all forms of urolithiasis,

**Table 13.38** Urolithiasis summary chart.

Canine urolithiasis overview table
Sherry Danderson, BS, DVM, PhD, Dipl AVVN Dipl ACVIM

| Parameter | Struvite | Calcium oxalate | Urate | Cysyine |
|---|---|---|---|---|
| Urine pH crystals least soluble in | Alkaline | Acidic-to-neutral | Acidic-to-neutral | Acidic |
| Typical appearance of crystals | | Dihydrate <br>Monohydrate | Ammonium urate <br>Sodium urate <br>Uric acid | |
| Commonly caused by UTI | + (majority) | − | +/− | − |
| Radiographic density<br>0 = radiolucent;<br>4+ = density of bone | + to ++++ | dihydrate ++++<br><br>monohydrate +++ | 0 to ++ | + to ++ |
| Typical radiographic appearance | Smooth, round, often very large | Dihydrate = rough (often looks like a piece of granola)<br>monohydrate = smooth, round, small | Smooth, round, small | Smooth, round, small |
| Breeds predisposed | Mn Schn, Shlh Tzu, Blchon Frise, Mn Pooles, Cocker Spanlels, Lhasa Apso | Small and miniature breeds (Mn Schn, Shih Tzu, Blchon Frise, Mn Poodles, Lhasa Apso, Yorkles) | Dalmatlans, English Bulldogs<br>also, breeds presdisposed to portosystemic shunts | English Bulldogs, French Bulldogs, Dachshunds, Newfoundlands, Corgis Mastiffs |
| Sex most commonly found in | F > M | M > F | M > F | M > F |
| Can be medically dissolved | yes | no | yes | yes |
| Recommended diet for dissolution<br>superscripts reference drugs that are needed in addition to diet to dissolve uroliths | Hill's s/d^<br>·Do not use > 6 months or when a high fat diet is contraindicated<br>Hill's c/d Multicare^<br>·Do not use when a high fat diet is contraindicated<br>Royal Canin Urinary SO^<br>·Do not use when a high fat or high sodium diet is contraindicated<br>Purina Pro Plan UR^<br>·Do not use if high fat or high sodium diet is contraindicated | None | Hill's u/d** and water added to diet<br>·do not use when a high fat diet is contraindicated | Hill's u/d ^^<br>·Some dogs with cystimuria are losing excessive amounts of carnitine in their urine and may require additional carnitine supplementation.<br>·Do not use when a high fat diet is contraindicated |
| Recommended diet for long-term management and prevention | None(unless sterile struvite stones) | • Hill's u/d*<br>• Hill's c/d Multicare*<br>• Royal Canin SO^*<br>• Purina UR^*<br>·Do not use when a high fat diet is contraindicated<br>·Do not use when a high sodium diet is contraindicated<br>Hill's w/d*<br>·Use when a high-fat diet is contraindicated (must add potassium citrate) | • Hill's u/d and water added to diet<br>·Do not use when a high fat diet is contraindicated<br><br>Royal Canin Urinary UC Low Purine | Hill's u/d<br>·Some dogs with cystimuria are losing excessive amounts of carnitine in their urine and may require additional carnitine supplementation.<br>·Do not use when a high fat diet is contraindicated<br><br>Royal Canin Urinary UC Low Purine |
| Drugs | ^Antibiotics | *Potassium citrate | **Allopurinol<br>(do not use in dogs with PSS) | ^^Thiola (2 MPG) |

Source: Courtesy of Dr. Sherry Sanderson, University of Georgia, College of Veterinary Medicine.

may promote hypercalciuria and calcium phosphate urolith formation. Therefore, oral salt therapy is not recommended to promote diuresis in dogs with uroliths containing calcium salts.

- Because soil contains high concentrations of silica, consumption of dirt and grass should be discouraged [250].

## 13.12 Renal

### 13.12.1 Renal Failure – Acute and Chronic

#### 13.12.1.1 General Information

The kidneys play numerous functions to maintain health including the excretion of toxins, maintenance of blood pressure, and production of urine. When renal health is affected, animal health can become severely compromised.

##### 13.12.1.1.1 Acute Renal Failure (ARF)

ARF is a sudden onset of kidney dysfunction and a common condition in dogs and cats. Patients often present with life-threatening renal failure with no history of urinary problems. Clinical signs of ARF and chronic kidney disease (CKD) can be variable, consisting of anorexia, lethargy, increased thirst/urination, vomiting, diarrhea, dehydration, uremic breath, and oral ulcers.

The four main causes of ARF include [251]:

1) Renal ischemia (induced by hypotension, severe dehydration, hypovolemia, hypoperfusion to kidneys, renal vessel thrombosis from DIC or other causes, avulsion of renal vessels, and hypertension)
2) Nephrotoxicity (e.g. ethylene glycol, drugs such as gentamicin, sulfonamides, and acetaminophen)
3) Primary renal diseases (pyelonephritis, leptospirosis, ICH, immune-mediated disease, and lymphoma)
4) Other systemic diseases (feline infectious peritonitis, sepsis, borreliosis, babesiosis, leishmaniasis, bacterial endocarditis, pancreatitis, DIC, heart failure, systemic lupus erythematosus, hepatorenal syndrome, hyperviscosity syndrome, hypothermia, hyperthermia, burns, and transfusion reactions).

In free-roaming animals, toxic injury and infectious disease are common causes of ARF.

##### 13.12.1.1.2 Chronic Kidney Disease (CKD)

CKD usually has gradual onset (months to years) with no clinical signs early on, making it difficult to detect until the kidney damage is advanced, with permanent loss of much of the kidney function.

Causes include hypertension, coagulopathy, hypoperfusion, glomerulonephritis, developmental defects, amyloidosis, congenital defects, pyelonephritis, neoplasia, obstructive uropathy, allergic and immune-mediated nephritis, tubular reabsorptive defects, and chronic low-grade nephrotoxicity [252].

#### 13.12.1.2 Diagnostics

Diagnosis is based on patient history, physical examination, bloodwork, urine testing, and abdominal ultrasound if available. On presentation, the clinician must establish the following:

- Is the azotemia prerenal, renal, or postrenal?
- Is the renal failure acute or chronic?

Acute and chronic cases can present in similar manner; however, both have different treatment protocols and prognoses. To answer the questions above, consider the following:

1) *History.* In ARF, patients often have a history of ingestion of toxins or nephrotoxic drugs. Cats with CRF have a history of weight loss, anorexia, and polyuria/polydipsia (PU/PD).
2) *Physical examination.* See Table 13.39 for differentiating ARF from CKD based on examination findings.
3) *Bloodwork and USG.* See Table 13.40 for how to use diagnostic testing to differentiate ARF from CKD.

Table 13.39 Physical exam findings in ARF and CKD patients.

| ARF | CKD |
| --- | --- |
| Good body condition, healthy skin and coat | Weight loss, muscle wasting, dull coat |
| Symmetrical, normal, or enlarged, often painful kidneys | Small, irregularly shaped kidneys |
| Anuria or oliguria | Polyuria/polydipsia |
| Pain on palpation of the area around the kidneys | Edema, ascites |

**Table 13.40** Diagnostic differences between ARF and CKD.

| Test | ARF | CKD |
|------|-----|-----|
| CBC | Possibly normal, elevated PCV, leukocytosis, or lymphopenia | Normocytic, normochromic, nonregenerative anemia |
| Chemistry | Moderate to severe elevation in BUN, creatinine, potassium, and phosphate<br>Variable levels of calcium and glucose<br>Elevated total protein<br>Decreased bicarbonate | Mild to moderate elevation in BUN, creatinine, potassium (or decreased), and phosphate<br>Variable levels of calcium<br>Metabolic acidosis (normal or high anion gap) |
| USG | Isosthenuria to slight hypersthenuria (1.008–1.029 in dogs, 1.008–1.034 in cats), proteinuria, casts, pyuria, WBCs, RBCs, crystals (ethylene glycol), occasionally glucosuria | Hyposthenuria to slight hypersthenuria (<1.030 in dogs and <1.035 in cats), proteinuria |

4) *Imaging.* Abdominal radiographs may demonstrate smaller (CKD) or larger (ARF) than normal kidneys.

To determine the type of azotemia present, consider the USG in light of the patient's hydration status.

- *Prerenal azotemia.* Caused by severe dehydration or other condition causing poor renal perfusion. USG is >1.035 in the cat and >1.030 in the dog. Diagnosis can be easily confirmed by a rapid response to fluid therapy.
- *Renal azotemia.* Typically the result of an insult to the kidneys. USG is between 1.007 and 1.025. The hallmark of renal azotemia is a lack of renal concentrating ability.
- *Postrenal azotemia.* Caused by an obstruction or rupture within the urinary system. This can often be diagnosed through a careful physical examination and history. USG results can be quite variable.

*Blood pressure.* Patients with CKD often have hypertension (systolic blood pressure >180 mm Hg in dogs and >200 mm Hg in cats). If hypertension is present, perform an ophthalmic exam for retinal hemorrhage and detachment, if equipment is available to do so [251].

### 13.12.1.3 Treatment Protocols

#### 13.12.1.3.1 *Acute Renal Failure*
The overall goal of treatment in AKD patients is to support the patient while the tubules repair.

- *Aggressive fluid therapy.* This is the mainstay of therapy. In addition to fluid therapy, diuretics such as furosemide and mannitol may be used to stimulate urine production.
- *Correct metabolic disturbances (acidosis).* Treat with fluid therapy and bicarbonate if needed.
- *Antiemetics and gastroprotectants.* Maropitant, sucralfate and ranitidine, or famotidine can treat nausea and vomiting in both ARF and CKD patients.
- *Antibiotic therapy.* If pyelonephritis is suspected, aggressive antibiotic therapy should be administered for 4–8 weeks. A fluoroquinolone with a β-lactam antibiotic is often effective.
- *Surgery.* If required for obstructive uropathy.

#### 13.12.1.3.2 *Chronic Renal Disease*
Nephron damage associated with CKD is usually irreversible. The goal of treatment is to reduce the kidney's workload and prevent further deterioration. Dietary modification is key. Renal-specific diets consist of reduced protein, phosphorous, sodium, and supplementation of *n*-3 fatty acids. General treatment considerations include the following:

Uremic crisis

- Antiemetics and gastroprotectants – During a uremic crisis, famotidine, maropitant, or ondansetron can help minimize vomiting and nausea.
- Potassium chloride – Administer in IV fluids or orally as needed to correct hypokalemia.

Table 13.41 Medications used for the treatment of renal failure.

| Medication | Canine dosage | Feline dosage |
|---|---|---|
| *Diuretic* | | |
| Furosemide (first choice) | 2–4 mg/kg IV, IM, SC, PO q8–12h, as needed | See canine dose. Start with lower dose |
| Mannitol | 0.25–0.5 g/kg slow IV over 5–10 min and repeat in 30–40 min to maintain diuresis; total dose ≤1.5 g/kg; discontinue if no improvement in urine flow 60 min after first dose | See canine dose |
| *Phosphate binder* | | |
| Aluminum carbonate/ hydroxide gel | 10–30 mg/kg PO q8h (with meals) | 10–30 mg/kg PO q8h (with meals) |
| Calcium citrate (Epakitin®) | 10–20 mg/kg PO per day in divided doses with meals (monitor serum calcium) | 10–20 mg/kg PO per day in divided doses with meals (monitor serum calcium) |
| *H2 antagonist* | | |
| Famotidine | 0.5 mg/kg PO q24h (CKD)<br>0.5 mg/kg PO, SC, IM, IV q12–24h | 1 mg/kg PO q24h (CKD)<br>0.5 mg/kg PO, SC, IM, IV q12–24h |
| *Antihypertensive* | | |
| Amlodipine (first choice in cats) | 0.2 mg/kg PO q24h | 0.625 mg/cat PO q24h |
| Enalapril (first choice in dogs) | 0.5 mg/kg q12h | 0.5 mg/kg PO q24h |
| *Potassium* | | |
| Potassium chloride | 1–3 mEq/kg/day PO<br>Lactated Ringer's 40 mEq KCl/l SC, or 20 mEq KCl/l IV (60 ml/kg/day fluid rate) | See canine dose |
| *Vitamin D* | | |
| Calcitriol | 2.5–3.5 ng/kg/day PO[a] (monitor serum calcium) | 0.01–0.04 µg/kg/day PO (monitor serum calcium) |
| *Alkalinizing agent* | | |
| Potassium citrate (1000 mg potassium citrate = 9.26 mEq potassium) | 0.5 mEq/kg/day PO | 0.5 mEq/kg/day PO |
| *Antiemetic* | | |
| Mirtazapine | 0.6 mg/kg PO q24h not to exceed 30 mg per day | 3–4 mg per cat PO q72h |
| Maropitant (Cerenia®) | 1 mg/kg SC q24h ≤ 5 days | 0.5–1 mg/kg SC q24h ≤ 5 days |
| Ondansetron | 0.1–0.2 mg/kg IV q6–12h, or 0.1–1 mg/kg PO q12–24h | 0.1–0.15 mg/kg slow IV q6–12h as needed<br>0.1–1 mg/kg PO |

a) ng = nanogram; 1 ng = 0.001 µg.

- Sodium bicarbonate – To correct metabolic acidosis, if needed.
- Correct clinical dehydration with isotonic, polyionic solutions such as LRS IV or SQ, as needed.

Compensated CKD

- Intestinal phosphate binders including aluminum carbonate – Aids in the correction of hyperphosphatemia.
- Antiemetics and gastroprotectants – Reduce uremic gastritis and improve appetite.
- Dietary protein reduction – Feed a strictly renal diet such as Hill's® Science Diet k/d (alkalinization, restriction of sodium, phosphorus, lipid, and calcium). If commercial diets are unavailable, homemade diets can be made. An online source for homemade recipes is www.balanceit.com.
- Oral vitamin D – May reduce uremic signs and prolong survival, particularly in dogs by preventing or correcting renal secondary hyperparathyroidism. Ideally, a baseline serum creatinine, phosphorous, calcium, BUN, and PTH level is ascertained before therapy. Serum phosphorous concentrations must be reduced to 6.0 mg/dl or lower before initiating calcitriol therapy. The product of serum calcium and phosphorous concentration should not exceed 60. The goal is to obtain a value between 42 and 50 [252].
- Erythropoietin (r-HuEPO)/iron supplementation – Therapy is indicated for non-life-threatening anemias in dogs and cats with CRF with hematocrit values below 20% and clinical signs attributable to anemia. Initial dosage of r-HuEPO is 50–100 units/kg SQ three times a week. Target hematocrit is 37–45% (dogs) and 30–40% (cats). Iron (ferrous sulfate) should be given concurrently at 100–300 mg/day (dogs) and 50–100 mg/day (cats)

orally [252]. Alternatively, iron dextran can be administered IM.
- ACE inhibitors (enalapril and benazepril) for hypertension and proteinuria. Amlodipine may be more effective in cats for lowering blood pressure.
- Ensure free-access to clean water at all times. Fluid therapy given SC should be considered for animals with intermittent signs of uremia.
- Avoid use of NSAIDs and potentially nephrotoxic drugs (aminoglycosides) (Table 13.41).

### 13.12.1.4 Tips and Tricks from the Field

- It is important to remember that degree of elevation in renal values on bloodwork does not always correlate with patient outcome. With appropriate care, patients that initially present with ARF with significant dysfunction can enjoy a favorable outcome [253].
- In the field, tick-borne disease is a common cause of ARF in free-roaming dogs, which may respond to doxycycline administration.
- Due to the contraindications of mannitol (dehydration, anuria, bleeding in the brain, certain lung diseases), risk of complications (electrolyte disturbances, fluid loss, pulmonary edema, dizziness), and requirement for close patient monitoring, furosemide may be a safer choice in field conditions [254].
- Euthanasia may be considered if therapy does not alleviate signs of uremia.
- The International Renal Interest Society is a great resource for learning more about renal disease: www.iris-kidney.com.

# References

1 Greene, C.E. (2011). Canine heartworm disease. In: *Infectious Diseases of the Dog and Cat*, 4th edn, 865–873. St. Louis, MO: Saunders Elsevier.

2 Simón, F., Siles-Lucas, M., Morchón, R. et al. (2012). Human and animal dirofilariasis: the emergence of a zoonotic mosaic. *Clinical Microbiology Reviews* **25** (3): 507–544.

3 Bowman, D.D., Little, S.E., Lorentzen, L. et al. (2009). Prevalence and geographic distribution of *Dirofilaria immitis*, *Borrelia burgdorferi*, *Ehrlichia canis*, and *Anaplasma phagocytophilum* in dogs in the United States: results of a national clinic-based serologic survey. *Veterinary Parasitology* **160**: 138–148.

4  Vezzani, D., Carbajo, A.E., Fontanarrosa, M.F. et al. (2011). Epidemiology of canine heartworm in its southern distribution limit in South America: risk factors, inter-annual trend and spatial patterns. *Veterinary Parasitology* **176**: 240–249.

5  American Heartworm Society (2014). Current canine guidelines for the prevention, diagnosis and management of heartworm infection in dogs [online]. https://www.heartwormsociety.org/veterinary-resources/american-heartworm-society-guidelines (accessed 18 December 2017).

6  Hoerauf, A., Mand, S., Fischer, K. et al. (2003). Doxycycline as a novel strategy against bancroftian filariasis-depletion of *Wolbachia* endosymbionts from *Wuchereria bancrofti* and stop of microfilaria production. *Medical Microbiology and Immunology* **192** (4): 211–216.

7  Rossi, M.I., Paiva, J., Bendas, A. et al. (2010). Effects of doxycycline on the endosymbiont *Wolbachia* in *Dirofilaria immitis* (Leidy, 1856)-naturally infected dogs. *Veterinary Parasitology* **174**: 119–123.

8  Atkins, C.E. (2003). Comparison of results of three commercial heartworm antigen test kits in dogs with low heartworm burdens. *Journal of the American Veterinary Medical Association* **222**: 1221–1223.

9  Courtney, C.H. and Zeng, Q.-Y. (2001). Comparison of heartworm antigen test kit performance in dogs having low heartworm burdens. *Veterinary Parasitology* **96**: 317–322.

10  Keister, D.M., Dzimianski, M.T., McTier, T.L. et al. (1992). Dose selection and confirmation of RM 340, a new filaricide for the treatment of dogs with immature and mature *Dirofilaria immitis*. Proceedings of the Heartworm Symposium, Austin, TX, pp. 225-229.

11  Vezzoni, A., Genchi, C., and Raynaud, J.P. (1992) Adulticide efficacy of RM 340 in dogs with mild and severe natural infections. Proceedings of the Heartworm Symposium, Austin, TX, pp. 231-240.

12  Hirano, Y., Kitagawa, H., and Sasaki, Y. (1992). Relationship between pulmonary arterial pressure and pulmonary thromboembolism associated with dead worms in canine heartworm disease. *Journal of Veterinary Medical Science* **54**: 897–904.

13  McCall, J.W., Guerrero, J., Roberts, R.E. et al. (2001) Further evidence of clinical prophylactic, retroactive (reach-back) and adulticidal activity of monthly administrations of ivermectin (Heartgard Plus®) in dogs experimentally infected with heartworms. Recent Advances in Heartworm Disease Symposium, pp. 198-200.

14  Rawlings, C.A. (1980). Acute response of pulmonary blood flow and right ventricular function to *Dirofilaria immitis* adults and microfilaria. *American Journal of Veterinary Research* **41**: 244–249.

15  Grandi, G., Quintavalla, C., Mavropoulou, A. et al. (2010). A combination of doxycycline and ivermectin is adulticidal in dogs with naturally acquired heartworm disease (*Dirofilaria immitis*). *Veterinary Parasitology* **169** (3–4): 347–351.

16  Peterson, K.M., Chappell, D.E., Lewis, B. et al. (2014). Heartworm-positive dogs recover without complications from surgical sterilization using cardiovascular sparing anesthesia protocol. *Veterinary Parasitology* **206**: 83–85.

17  Ware, W. (2011). *Cardiovascular Disease in Small Animal Medicine*, 2nd edn. London: Manson.

18  Atkins, C., Bonagura, J., Ettinger, S. et al. (2009). Guidelines for the diagnosis and treatment of canine chronic valvular heart disease. *Journal of Veterinary Internal Medicine* **23** (6): 1142–1150.

19  Fuentes, V. (2016). Management of feline heart failure [online]. http://www.ivis.org/proceedings/scivac/2007/fuentes3_en.pdf?LA=1 (accessed 20 August 2016).

20  Hogan, D. (2013). Analysis of the feline arterial thromboembolism: clopidogrel vs aspirin trial (FAT CAT). Proceedings of the American College of Veterinary Internal Medicine Forum, Seattle, WA.

21  Rubin, S. (2016). Anal sac disease: diseases of the rectum and anus. In: Merck Veterinary Manual [online]. http://www.merckvetmanual.com/mvm/digestive_system/diseases_of_the_rectum_and_anus/anal_sac_disease.html (accessed 17 March 2016).

22  Fossum, T. (2013). *Small Animal Surgery*. St. Louis, MO: Elsevier Mosby.

23  Hnilica, K. and Medleau, L. (2011). *Small Animal Dermatology*. St. Louis, MO: Elsevier Saunders.

24 Tilley, L. and Smith, F. (2011). *Blackwell's Five-Minute Veterinary Consult*. West Sussex: Wiley-Blackwell.

25 James, D., Griffin, C., Polissar, N., and Neradilek, M. (2010). Comparison of anal sac cytological findings and behaviour in clinically normal dogs and those affected with anal sac disease. *Veterinary Dermatology* **22** (1): 80–87.

26 Côté, E. (2015). *Clinical Veterinary Advisor*. St. Louis, MO: Elsevier.

27 Smeak, D. (2003). Perianal surgery in dogs. Western Veterinary Conference, Las Vegas, NV. http://www.vin.com/doc/?id=3846886 (accessed 10 December 2016).

28 Ladlow, J. (2010). Perineal masses: surgery and reconstruction. British Small Animal Veterinary Congress [online]. http://www.vin.com/members/cms/project/defaultadv1.aspx?id=4419706&pid=11304 (accessed 10 December 2016).

29 Bowman, A. (2017). Cuterebra species [online]. http://www.aavp.org/wiki/arthropods/insects/cuteribridae/cuterebra-species/ (accessed 30 April 2016).

30 James, F. and Poma, R. (2010). Neurologic manifestations of feline cuterebriasis. *The Canadian Veterinary Journal* **51**: 213–215.

31 Companion Animal Parasite Council (2012). Cuterebriasis [online] Available at. http://www.capcvet.org/capc-recommendations/cuterebriasis (accessed 2 January 2017).

32 Aiello, S. and Moses, M. (2016). *The Merck Veterinary Manual*, 11th edn. Kenilworth, NJ: Merck & Co.

33 Edelmann, M.L., Lucio-Forster, A., Kern, T.J. et al. (2014). Ophthalmomyiasis interna anterior in a dog: keratotomy and extraction of a *Cuterebra sp.* larva. *Veterinary Ophthalmology* **17** (6): 448–453.

34 Yates, J.L. and Stroup, S.T. (2011). Case report: endoscopic removal of a nasal *Cuterebra* larva from a puppy. *Compendium Continuing Education for Veterinarians* **33** (5): E1–E4.

35 Glass, E.N., Cornetta, A.M., de Lahunta, A. et al. (1998). Clinical and clinopathological features in 11 cats with *Cuterebra* larvae myiasis of the central nervous system. *Journal of Veterinary Internal Medicine* **12** (5): 365–368.

36 Côté, E. (2015). Myiasis. In: *Clinical Veterinary Advisor Dogs and Cats*. St. Louis, MO: Mosby Elsevier.

37 Moriello, K. (2013) Overview of *Cuterebra* infestation in small animals. In: Merck Veterinary Manual [online]. http://www.merckvetmanual.com/integumentary-system/cuterebra-infestation-in-small-animals/overview-of-cuterebra-infestation-in-small-animals (accessed 6 February 2017).

38 Mueller, R.S., Bensignor, E., Ferrer, L. et al. (2012). Treatment of demodicosis in dogs: 2011 clinical practice guidelines. *Veterinary Dermatology* **23**: 86–96.

39 CAPC (2016). Demodex [online] http://www.capcvet.org/capc-recommendations/demodex-mange-mite (accessed 7 March 2016).

40 Moriello, K. (2011). Treatment of demodicosis in dogs & cats. In: NAVC Clinician's Brief [online]. Available at: http://www.cliniciansbrief.com/sites/default/files/cb%20may%2011_Treatmt%20of%20Demodicosis.pdf (accessed 10 November 2016).

41 Johnstone, I.P. (2002). Doramectin as a treatment for canine and feline demodicosis. *Australian Veterinary Practitioner* **32** (3): 98–103.

42 Fourie, J., Delport, P., Fourie, L. et al. (2009). Comparative efficacy and safety of two treatment regimens with a topically applied combination of imidacloprid and moxidectin (Advocate®) against generalised demodicosis in dogs. *Parasitology Research* **105** (S1): 115–124.

43 Paterson, T., Halliwell, R., Fields, P. et al. (2014). Canine generalized demodicosis treated with varying doses of a 2.5% moxidectin 10% imidacloprid spot-on and oral ivermectin: parasiticidal effects and long-term treatment outcomes. *Veterinary Parasitology* **205** (3–4): 687–696.

44 Fourie, J., Liebebenberg, J., Horak, I. et al. (2015). Efficacy of orally administered fluralaner (Bravecto) or topically applied imidacloprid/moxidectin (Advocate®) against generalized demodicosis in dogs. *Parasite Vectors* **8** (1): 187.

45 Paterson, T., Halliwell, R., Fields, P. et al. (2009). Treatment of canine-generalized demodicosis: a

blind, randomized clinical trial comparing the efficacy of Advocate® (Bayer Animal Health) with ivermectin. *Veterinary Dermatology* **20** (5–6): 447–455.

46 Moriello, K.A. (2003). Important factors in the pathogenesis of feline dermatophytosis. *Veterinary Medicine* **98** (10): 845–855.

47 Greene, C.E. (2011). Cutaneous fungal infections. In: *Infectious Diseases of the Dog and Cat*, 4th edn, 588–602. St. Louis, MO: Elsevier.

48 Moriello, K. (2014). Feline dermatophytosis. *Journal of Feline Medicine and Surgery* **16** (5): 419–431.

49 DeBoer, D.J. and Moriello, K.A. (1994). Development of an experimental model of *M. canis* infection in cats. *Journal of Veterinary Microbiology* **42**: 289–295.

50 Frymus, T., Gruffydd-Jones, T., Pennisi, M.G. et al. (2013). Dermatophytosis in cats. ABCD guidelines on prevention and management. *Journal of Feline Medicine and Surgery* **15**: 598–604.

51 IDEXX Laboratories (2015). IDEXX Reference Laboratories introduces the Ringworm (Dermatophyte) RealPCR Panel for fast and accurate diagnosis of dermatophytosis [online]. https://www.idexx.com/files/small-animal-health/products-and-services/reference-laboratories/ringworm-pcr-panel.pdf (accessed 18 December 2017).

52 Rosenbaum, M.R. (2014). Updates in feline dermatophytosis. Atlantic Coast Veterinary Conference, Atlantic City, NJ (13–16 October 2014).

53 Moriello, K., Coyner, K., Trimmer, A. et al. (2013). Treatment of shelter cats with oral terbinafine and concurrent lime sulphur rinses. *Veterinary Dermatology* **24** (6): 618–620.

54 Moriello, K.A., Kunder, D., and Hondzo, H. (2013). Efficacy of eight commercial disinfectants against *Microsporum canis* and *Trichophyton* spp. infective spores on an experimentally contaminated textile surface. *Veterinary Dermatology* **24** (6): 621–623.

55 Moriello, K. (2016). Decontamination of laundry exposed to *M. canis* hairs and spores. *Journal of Feline Medicine and Surgery* **18**: 457–461.

56 Salib, F.A. and Baraka, T.A. (2011). Epidemiology, genetic divergence and acaricides of *Otodectes*

*cynotis* in cats and dogs. *Veterinary World* **4**: 109–112.

57 Sotiraki, S.T., Koutinas, A.F., Leontides, L.S. et al. (2001). Factors affecting the frequency of ear canal and face infestation by *Otodectes cynotis* in the cat. *Veterinary Parasitology* **96** (4): 309–135.

58 Hnilica, K. and Patterson, A. (2016). Parasitic skin disorders. In: *Small Animal Dermatology*, 4th edn. St. Louis, MO: Elsevier-Saunders.

59 Rosychuk, R. (2008). Feline otitis eternal and media. World Veterinary Congress Vancouver, BC (27–31 July 2008).

60 Coleman, G.T. and Atwell, R.B. (1999). Use of Fipronil to treat ear mites in cats. *Australian Veterinary Practitioner* **29** (4): 166–168.

61 Scherck-Nixon, M., Baker, B., Pauling, G.E., and Hare, J.E. (1997). Treatment of feline otoacariasis with 2 otic preparations not containing miticidal active ingredients. *Canadian Veterinary Journal* **38** (4): 229–230.

62 Otranto, D., Milillo, P., Mesto, P. et al. (2004). *Otodectes cynotis* (Acari: Psoroptidae): examination of survival off-the-host under natural and laboratory conditions. *Experimental and Applied Acarology* **32** (3): 171–179.

63 Thomas, R.C. (2012). Flea allergy dermatitis-why fleas are still a problem. North American Veterinary Conference, Orlando, FL (14–18 January 2012).

64 Cain, C. (2014). Flea allergy and flea control: making sense of a crowded market. North American Veterinary Conference, Orlando, FL (18–22 January 2014).

65 Medleau, L., Hnilica, K., Lower, K. et al. (2002). Effect of topical application of fipronil in cats with flea allergic dermatitis. *Journal of the American Veterinary Medical Association* **221** (2): 254–257.

66 Dickin, S., McTier, T., Murphy, M. et al. (2003). Efficacy of selamectin in the treatment and control of clinical signs of flea allergy dermatitis in dogs and cats experimentally infested with fleas. *Journal of the American Veterinary Medical Association* **223** (5): 639–644.

67 Handara, W., Karunaratne, W., Fuward, R. et al. (2016). Myiasis in dogs and cats treated in two veterinary clinics in Peradeniya, Sri Lanka. *Journal of Entomology and Zoology Studies* **4** (6): 211–215.

**68** Sivajothi, S., Sudhakara Reddy, B., Rayulu, V., and Sreedevi, C. (2013). *Notoedres cati* in cats and its management. *Journal of Parasitic Diseases* **39** (2): 303–305.

**69** Weese, J. and Fulford, M. (2011). *Companion Animal Zoonoses*. Ames, IA: Wiley-Blackwell.

**70** Moriello, K., Newbury, S., and Diesel, A. (2009). Ectoparasites. In: *Infectious Disease Management in Animal Shelters* (eds. L. Miller and K. Hurley), 275–289. Ames, IA: Wiley-Blackwell.

**71** Moriello, K., Newbury, S., and Diesel, A. (2009). *Infectious Disease Management in Animal Shelters* (eds. L. Miller and K. Hurley), 275–289. Ames, IA: Wiley-Blackwell.

**72** Hnilica, K. and Patterson, A. (2016). Diseases of the eye, ear, claws, and anal sacs. In: *Small Animal Dermatology*, 4th edn. St. Louis, MO: Elsevier-Saunders.

**73** Harvey, R. and Paterson, S. (2014). *Otitis Externa: An Essential Guide to Diagnosis and Treatment*. Boca Raton, FL: CRC Press.

**74** Fossum, T. (2013). Surgery of the ear. In: *Small Animal Surgery*, 4th edn. St. Louis, MO: Mosby-Elsevier.

**75** Griffin, C. (2010). A rational approach to otitis media. North American Veterinary Conference, Orlando, FL (16–20 January 2010).

**76** Rosychuk, R. (2009). Ten ways to maximize the benefits of ear therapy. American Animal Hospital Association Annual Meeting [proceedings], Lakewood, CO, pp. 183–187.

**77** Noxon, J. (2014). Management of chronic otitis. North American Veterinary Conference, Orlando, FL (18–22 January 2014).

**78** Moriello, K. (2004). Pruritic recurrent otitis externa in a cat. In: NAVC Clinician's Brief [online]. http://www.cliniciansbrief.com/sites/default/files/sites/cliniciansbrief.com/files/otitis%20externa_0.pdf (accessed 28 November 2016).

**79** Hnilica, K. and Patterson, A. (2016). Bacterial skin diseases. In: *Small Animal Dermatology A Color Atlas and Therapeutic Guide*, 4th edn. St. Louis, MO: Elsevier-Saunders.

**80** Mason, I.S. and Lloyd, D.H. (1989). The role of allergy in the development of canine pyoderma. *Journal of Small Animal Practice* **30** (4): 216–218.

**81** McEwan, N., Mellor, D., and Kalna, G. (2006). Adherence by *Staphylococcus intermedius* to canine corneocytes: a preliminary study comparing noninflamed and inflamed atopic canine skin. *Veterinary Dermatology* **17**: 151–154.

**82** Chisholm, C.D., Cordell, W.H., Rogers, K., and Woods, J.R. (1992). Comparison of a new pressurized saline canister versus syringe irrigation for laceration cleansing in the emergency department. *Annals of Emergency Medicine* **21** (11): 1364–1367.

**83** Mathews, K.A. and Binnington, A.G. (2002). Wound management using honey. *Compendium on Continuing Education for the Practising Veterinarian* **24** (1): 53–60.

**84** Willix, D.J., Molan, P.C., and Harfoot, C.G. (1992). A comparison of the sensitivity of wound-infecting species of bacteria to the antibacterial activity of manuka honey and other honey. *Journal of Applied Microbiology* **73** (5): 388–394.

**85** Mathews, K.A. and Binnington, A.G. (2002). Wound management using sugar. *Compendium on Continuing Education for the Practising Veterinarian* **24** (1): 41–50.

**86** Trouillet, J.L., Chastre, J., Fagon, J. et al. (1985). Use of granulated sugar in treatment of open mediastinitis after cardiac surgery. *Lancet* **2**: 180–184.

**87** HSVMA-RAVS Vaccination Protocol (2016) [online]. http://www.ruralareavet.org/PDF/Clinic_Protocols-Vaccination_Protocol.pdf (accessed 16 November 2016).

**88** Constable, P.D. (2016). Coccidiosis of cats and dogs. In: MSD Veterinary Manual [online]. http://www.msdvetmanual.com/digestive-system/coccidiosis/coccidiosis-of-cats-and-dogs (accessed 18 December 2017).

**89** CAPC. (2016) Intestinal parasites – Cryptosporidium [online]. www.capcvet.org/capc-recommendations/cryptosporidia/ (accessed 28 December 2016).

**90** Riviere, J. and Papich, M.G. (2009). Antiprotozoal drugs. In: *Veterinary Pharmacology and Therapeutics*, 9th edn, 1161–1162. Wiley-Blackwell.

**91** Heyworth, M.F. (2016). *Giardia duodenalis* genetic assemblages and hosts. *Parasite* **23**: 13.

92  Payne, P.A., Ridley, R.K., Dryden, M.W. et al. (2002). Efficacy of a combination febantel-praziquantel-pyrantel product, with or without vaccination with a commercial *Giardia* vaccine, for treatment of dogs with naturally occurring giardiasis. *Journal of the American Veterinary Medical Association* **220** (3): 330–333.

93  Côté, E. (2010). Hookworms. In: *Clinical Veterinary Advisor Dogs and Cats*. St. Louis, MO: Mosby Elsevier.

94  Bowman, D.D., Montgomery, S.P., Zajac, A.M. et al. (2010). Hookworms of dogs and cats as agents of cutaneous larva migrans. *Trends in Parasitology* **26** (4): 162–167.

95  Overgaauw, P.A. and van Knapen, F. (2013). Veterinary and public health aspects of *Toxocara* spp. *Veterinary Parasitology* **193** (4): 398–403.

96  Conboy, G. (2012). Cestodes of dogs and cats in North America. *Veterinary Clinics of North America: Small Animal Practice* **39** (6): 1075–1090.

97  Dillard, K., Saari, S., and Anttila, M. (2007). *Strongyloides stercoralis* infection in a Finnish kennel. *Acta Veterinaria Scandinavica* **49**: 37.

98  Peregrine, A. *Strongyloides* sp in small animals. In: Merck Veterinary Manual [online]. http://www.msdvetmanual.com/digestive-system/gastrointestinal-parasites-of-small-animals/strongyloides-sp-in-small-animals (accessed 18 December 2017).

99  Peregrine, A.S. Whipworms in small animals. In: Merck Veterinary Manual [online]. http://www.msdvetmanual.com/digestive-system/gastrointestinal-parasites-of-small-animals/whipworms-in-small-animals (accessed 18 December 2017).

100  Jeffries, R., Ryan, U.M., Jardine, J. et al. (2007). Blood, Bull Terriers and Babesiosis: further evidence for direct transmission of *Babesia* gibsoni in dogs. *Australian Veterinary Journal* **85** (11): 459–463.

101  Birkenheuer, M.G., Levy, M.G., and Breitschewerdt, E.B. (2004). Efficacy of combined atovaquone and azithromycin for therapy of chronic *babasia gibsoni* (Asian genotype) infections in dogs. *Journal of Veterinary Internal Medicine* **18**: 494–498.

102  Potgieter, F.T. (1981). Chemotherapy of *Babesia* felis infection: efficacy of certain drugs. *Journal of the South African Veterinary Association* **52** (4): 289–293.

103  Wulansari, R., Wijaya, A., Ano, H. et al. (2003). Clindamycin in the treatment of *Babesia* gibsoni infections in dogs. *Journal of the American Animal Hospital Association* **39** (6): 558–562.

104  Suzuki, K., Wakabayashi, H., Takahashi, M. et al. (2007). A possible treatment strategy and clinical factors to estimate the treatment response in *Babesia* gibsoni infection. *The Journal of Veterinary Medical Science* **69** (5): 563–568.

105  Greene, C. (2011). Blastomycosis. In: *Infectious Diseases of the Dog and Cat*, 4th edn. St. Louis, MO: Saunders.

106  Kristen Parker, T. (2013). Oronasal blastomycosis in a golden retriever. *The Canadian Veterinary Journal* **54**: 748.

107  Taboada, J. (2016). Blastomycosis. In: Merck Veterinary Manual [online]. http://www.merckvetmanual.com/generalized-conditions/fungal-infections/cryptococcosis (accessed 5 April 2016).

108  Tilley, L. and Smith, F. Jr. (2011). *Blackwell's Five-Minute Veterinary Consult: Canine and Feline*, 5th edn. West Sussex: John Wiley & Sons, Ltd.

109  MiraVista Diagnostics (2015). Blastomyces antigen test for dogs [online]. http://miravistalabs.com/blastomyces-antigen-test-for-dogs/ (accessed 12 April 2016).

110  Morgan, R (2016). Veterinary information network associate- blastomycosis [online] http://www.vin.com/ (accessed 10 December 2016).

111  Thrall, D. (2013). *Textbook of Veterinary Diagnostic Radiology*, 6th edn. St. Louis, MO: Elsevier-Saunders.

112  IDEXX (2016). Directory of tests and services [online]. https://www.idexx.com/smallanimal/reference-laboratories/directory-tests-services.html (accessed 12 April 2016).

113  Spector, D., Legendre, A., Wheat, J. et al. (2008). Antigen and antibody testing for the diagnosis of blastomycosis in dogs. *Journal of Veterinary Internal Medicine* **22** (4): 839–843.

114  Weese, J. (2016) Blastomycosis in a dog. NAVC Clinician's Brief. http://www.cliniciansbrief.com/article/blastomycosis-dog (accessed 9 April 2016).

115  Mazepa, A.S., Trepanier, L.A., and Foy, D.S. (2011). Retrospective comparison of the efficacy of fluconazole or itraconazole for the treatment of

systemic blastomycosis in dogs. *Journal of Veterinary Internal Medicine* **25** (3): 440–445.

116 Plumb, D. (2015). Itraconazole. In: *Plumb's Veterinary Drug Handbook*, 8th edn. Ames, IA: Wiley-Blackwell.

117 Greene, C.E. and Carmichael, L.E. (2012). Canine brucellosis. In: *Recent Advances in Canine Infectious Diseases*, 4th edn, 398–411. St. Louis, MO: Saunders Elsevier.

118 Côté, E. (2004). Brucellosis. In: *Clinical Veterinary Advisor*, 3rd edn. St. Louis, MO: Saunders.

119 Nicoletti, P. and Chase, A. (1987). The use of antibiotics to control canine brucellosis. *Compendium on Continuing Education for the Practising Veterinarian* **9**: 1063.

120 Zoha, S.J. and Walsh, R. (1982). Effect of a two-stage antibiotic treatment regimen on dogs naturally infected with *Brucella canis*. *Journal of the American Veterinary Medical Association* **180**: 1474–1475.

121 Flores-Castro, R. and Carmichael, L.E. (1981). *Brucella canis* infections in dogs: treatment trials. *Revista Latinoamericana de Microbiologia* **23**: 75–79.

122 Johnson, C.A., Bennett, M., Jensen, R.K., and Schirmer, R. (1982). Effect of combined antibiotic therapy on fertility in brood bitches infected with *Brucella canis*. *Journal of the American Veterinary Medical Association* **180** (11): 1330–1333.

123 Wanke, M.M., Delpino, M.V., and Baldi, P.C. (2006). Use of enrofloxacin in the treatment of canine brucellosis in a dog kennel (clinical trial). *Theriogenology* **66** (6–7): 1573–1578.

124 Greene, C. (2011). Canine distemper. In: *Infectious Diseases of the Dog and Cat*, 4th edn. St. Louis, MO: Saunders.

125 Thompson, M. (2014). *Small Animal Medical Differential Diagnosis*, 2nd edn. St. Louis, MO: Elsevier-Saunders.

126 Murphy, F. (1999). *Veterinary Virology*. San Diego, CA: Academic Press.

127 Schubert, T., Clemmons, R., Miles, S., and Draper, W. (2013). The use of botulinum toxin for the treatment of generalized myoclonus in a dog. *Journal of the American Animal Hospital Association* **49** (2): 122–127.

128 Mitchell, K.D. (2015) Canine parvovirus. In: The Merck Veterinary Manual [online]. http://www.msdvetmanual.com/digestive-system/diseases-of-the-stomach-and-intestines-in-small-animals/canine-parvovirus (accessed 18 December 2017).

129 Venn, E., Preisner, K., Boscan, P. et al. (2016). Evaluation of an outpatient protocol in the treatment of canine parvoviral enteritis. *Journal of Veterinary Emergency and Critical Care* **27** (1): 52–65.

130 Sullivan, L.A., Twedt, D.C., and Boscan, P.L. (2013) What is the outpatient treatment protocol utilized for the treatment of parvoviral enteritis at Colorado State University? Frequently Asked Questions Series [online]. http://csu-cvmbs.colostate.edu/documents/parvo-outpatient-protocol-faq-companion-animal-studies.pdf (accessed 1 January 2017).

131 Bragg, R.F., Duffy, A.L., Dececco, F.A. et al. (2012). Clinical evaluation of a single dose of immune plasma for treatment of canine parvovirus infection. *Journal of the American Veterinary Medical Association* **240** (6): 700–704.

132 Savigny, M.R. and Macintire, D.K. (2010). Use of oseltamivir in the treatment of canine parvoviral enteritis. *Journal of Veterinary Emergency and Critical Care* **20** (1): 132–142.

133 de Mari, K., Maynard, L., Eun, H.M., and Lebreux, B. (2003). Treatment of canine parvoviral enteritis with interferon-omega in a placebo-controlled field trial. *Veterinary Record* **152** (4): 105.

134 Tilley, L. and Smith, F. (2015). Coccidioidomycosis. In: *Blackwell's Five-Minute Veterinary Consult: Canine and Feline*, 6th edn. Ames, IA: John Wiley & Sons, Inc.

135 Greene, C. (2011). Coccidioidomycosis and paracoccidioidomycosis. In: *Infectious Diseases of the Dog and Cat*, 4th edn. St. Louis, MO: Saunders.

136 IDEXX (2016). Directory of tests and services—IDEXX reference laboratories [online]. https://www.idexx.com/smallanimal/reference-laboratories/directory-tests-services.html (accessed 20 April 2016).

137 Greene, R. and Troy, G. (1995). Coccidioidomycosis in 48 cats: a retrospective

study (1984–1993). *Journal of Veterinary Internal Medicine* **9** (2): 86–91.

138  Graupmann-Kuzma, A., Valentine, B.A., Shubitz, L.F. et al. (2008). Coccidioidomycosis in dogs and cats: a review. *Journal of the American Animal Hospital Association* **44** (5): 226–235.

139  Quigley, R., Evans, J., Plummer, S.B. et al. (2007). The neurological manifestations of coccidioidomycosis in dogs: a retrospective study of 52 cases (2000–2005). *Journal of Veterinary Internal Medicine* **21**: 591.

140  Greene, C.E. (2011). Cryptococcosis. In: *Infectious Diseases of the Dog and Cat*, 4th edn. St. Louis, MO: Saunders Elsevier.

141  O'Brien, C.R., Krockenberger, M.B., Wigney, D.I. et al. (2004). Retrospective study of feline and canine cryptococcosis in Australia from 1981 to 2001: 195 cases. *Medical Mycology* **42** (5): 449–460.

142  Taboada, J. (2016). Cryptococcosis. In: Merck Veterinary Manual [online]. http://www.merckvetmanual.com/generalized-conditions/fungal-infections/cryptococcosis (accessed 5 April 2016).

143  Cohn, L. and Breitschwerdt, E. (2012). Spotlight on Ehrlichia ewingii [online]. http://www.idexx.no/pdf/en_ie/smallanimal/snap/4dx/spotlight-on-ehrlichia.pdf (accessed 18 December 2017).

144  CAPC (2015). Ehrlichia spp. and Anaplasma spp. [online]. http://www.capcvet.org/capc-recommendations/ehrlichia-spp-and-anaplasma-spp1/ (accessed 8 May 2016).

145  Sainz, Á., Roura, X., Miró, G. et al. (2015). Guidelines for veterinary practitioners on canine ehrlichiosis and anaplasmosis in Europe. *Parasites & Vectors* **8**: 75.

146  Little, S. (2010). Ehrlichiosis and anaplasmosis in dogs and cats. *Veterinary Clinics of North America: Small Animal Practice* **40** (6): 1121–1140.

147  Alleman, A.R. (2015) More than just E. canis: the increasingly complicated story of ehrlichiosis [online]. https://michvma.org/resources/Documents/MVC/2017%20Proceedings/alleman%2002.pdf (accessed 18 December 2017).

148  Alleman, A.R. (2014) Tick-borne disease of people and pets: Anaplasma and Borrelia. Atlantic Coast Veterinary Conference, Atlantic City, NJ (16 October 2014).

149  Breitschwerdt, E.B. (2011). Treatment of canine ehrlichiosis. World Small Animal Veterinary Association World Congress, Jeju, Korea (14–17 October 2011).

150  Bartsch, R.C. and Greene, R.T. (1996). Post therapy antibody titers in dogs with ehrlichiosis: follow-up study on 68 patients treated primarily with tetracycline and/or doxycycline. *Journal of Veterinary Internal Medicine* **10** (4): 271–274.

151  Egenvall, A., Lilliehöök, I., Karlstam, E. et al. (2000). Detection of granulocytic Ehrlichia species DNA by PCR in persistently infected dogs. *Veterinary Record* **146** (7): 186–190.

152  Fourie, J.J., Stanneck, D., Luus, H.G. et al. (2013). Transmission of Ehrlichia canis by *Rhipicephalus sanguineus* ticks feeding on dogs and on artificial membranes. *Veterinary Parasitology* **197** (3–4): 595–603.

153  Neer, M.T., Breitschwerdt, E.B., Greene, R.T., and Lappin, M.R. (2002). Consensus statement on ehrlichial disease of small animals from the infectious disease study group of the ACVIM. *Journal of Veterinary Internal Medicine* **16** (3): 309–315.

154  Kornya, M., Little, S., Scherk, M. et al. (2014). Association between oral health status and retrovirus test results in cats. *Journal of the American Veterinary Medical Association* **245**: 916–922.

155  Levy, J., Richards, J., Edwards, D. et al. (2003). 2001 Report of the American Association of Feline Practitioners and Academy of Feline Medicine Advisory Panel on feline retrovirus testing and management. *Journal of Feline Medicine and Surgery* **5** (1): 3–10.

156  de Mari, K., Maynard, L., Sanquer, A. et al. (2004). Therapeutic effects of recombinant feline interferon-omega on feline leukemia virus (FeLV)-infected and feline immunodeficiency virus (FIV)-coinfected symptomatic cats. *Journal of Veterinary Internal Medicine* **18** (4): 477–482.

157  Arai, M., Darman, J., Lewis, A., and Yamamoto, J.K. (2000). The use of human hematopoietic growth factors (rhGM-CSF and rhEPO) as a supportive therapy for FIV-infected cats. *Veterinary Immunology and Immunopathology* **77** (1–2): 71–92.

158  Gingerich, D. (2008). Lymphocyte T-cell immunomodulator (LTCI): review of the

immunopharmacology of a new veterinary biologic. *Journal of Applied Research in Veterinary Medicine* **6** (2): 61–68.

159 Levy, J.K., Scott, M., Lachtara, J.P., and Crawford, P.C. (2006). Seroprevalence of feline leukemia virus and feline immunodeficiency virus infection among cats in North America and risk factors for seropositivity. *Journal of the American Veterinary Medical Association* **288**: 371–376.

160 Gleich, S.E., Krieger, S., and Hartmann, K. (2009). Prevalence of feline immunodeficiency virus and feline leukaemia virus among client-owned cats and risk factors for infection in Germany. *Journal of Feline Medicine and Surgery* **11** (12): 985–992.

161 Lee, I.T., Levy, J.K., Gorman, S.P. et al. (2002). Prevalence of feline leukemia virus infection and serum antibodies against feline immunodeficiency virus in unowned free-roaming cats. *Journal of the American Veterinary Medical Association* **220** (5): 620–622.

162 Sukhumavasi, W., Bellosa, M.L., Lucio-Forster, A. et al. (2012). Serological survey of Toxoplasma gondii, *Dirofilaria immitis*, Feline Immunodeficiency Virus (FIV) and Feline Leukemia Virus (FeLV) infections in pet cats in Bangkok and vicinities, Thailand. *Veterinary Parasitology* **188** (1–2): 25–30.

163 Bande, F., Arshad, S.S., Hassan, L. et al. (2012). Prevalence and risk factors of feline leukaemia virus and feline immunodeficiency virus in peninsular Malaysia. *BMC Veterinary Research* **8**: 33.

164 Levy, J., Crawford, C., Hartmann, K. et al. (2008). 2008 American Association of Feline Practitioners' feline retrovirus management guidelines. *Journal of Feline Medicine and Surgery* **10**: 300–316.

165 Levy, J.K., Lorentzen, L., Shields, J., and Lewis, H. (2006) Long-term outcome of cats with natural FeLV and FIV infection. 8th International Feline Retrovirus Research Symposium, Washington, DC.

166 Boesch, A., Cattori, V., Riond, B. et al. (2015). Evaluation of the effect of short-term treatment with the integrase inhibitor raltegravir (Isentress) on the course of progressive feline leukemia virus infection. *Veterinary Microbiology* **175** (2–4): 167–178.

167 Sheets, M.A., Unger, B.A., Giggleman, G.F., and Tizard, I.R. (1991). Studies of the effect of acemannan on retrovirus infections: clinical stabilization of feline leukemia virus-infected cats. *Molecular Biotherapy* **3** (1): 41–45.

168 Truyen, U., Addie, D., Belák, S. et al. (2009). Feline panleukopenia. ABCD guidelines on prevention and management. *Journal of Feline Medicine and Surgery* **11** (7): 538–546.

169 Greene, C.E. (2011). Feline parvovirus infection. In: *Infectious Diseases of the Dog and Cat*, 4th edn. St. Louis, MO: Elsevier.

170 UC Davis Koret Shelter Medicine Program (2016). Feline panleukopenia. http://www .sheltermedicine.com/library/resources/feline-panleukopenia (accessed 18 December 2017).

171 Abd-Eldaim, M., Beall, M., and Kennedy, M.A. (2009). Detection of feline panleukopenia virus using a commercial ELISA for canine parvovirus. *Journal of Veterinary Pharmacology and Therapeutics* **10** (4): E1–E6.

172 Kruse, B.D., Unterer, S., Horlacher, K. et al. (2010). Prognostic indicators in cats with feline panleukopenia. *Journal of Veterinary Internal Medicine* **24**: 1271–1276.

173 Sykes, J.E. (2003). Feline hemotropic mycoplasmosis (feline hemobartonellosis). *Veterinary Clinics of North America: Small Animal Practice* **33** (4): 773–789.

174 Greene, C.E. (2011). Hemotrophic mycoplasmosis (Haemobartonellosis). In: *Infectious Diseases of the Dog and Cat*, 4th edn, 588–602. St. Louis, MO: Elsevier.

175 Côté, E. (2014). Hemotropic mycoplasmosis, cat. In: *Clinical Veterinary Advisor*, 456. St. Louis, MO: Mosby Elsevier.

176 Greene, C.E. (2006). Histoplasmosis. In: *Infectious Diseases of the Dog and Cat*, 3rd edn, 577–584. St. Louis, MO: Saunders Elsevier.

177 Selby, L.A., Becker, S.V., and Hayes, H.W. (1981). Epidemiologic risk factors associated with canine systemic mycoses. *American Journal of Epidemiology* **113** (2): 133–139.

178 Guptill, L. and Gingerich, K. (2008) Canine and feline histoplasmosis: a review of a widespread fungus [online]. http://veterinarymedicine. dvm360.com/canine-and-feline-histoplasmosis-review-widespread-fungus (accessed 31 January 2018).

179 Schulman, R.L., McKiernan, B.C., and Schaeffer, D.J. (1999). Use of corticosteroids for treating dogs with airway obstruction secondary to hilar lymphadenopathy caused by chronic histoplasmosis: 16 cases (1979–1997). *Journal of the American Veterinary Medical Association* **214** (9): 1345–1348.

180 Davies, C. and Troy, G.C. (1996). Deep mycotic infections in cats. *Journal of the American Veterinary Medical Association* **32** (5): 380–391.

181 Greene, C. (2011). Infectious canine hepatitis, canine acidophil cell hepatitis. In: *Infectious Diseases of the Dog and Cat*, 4th edn. St. Louis, MO: Saunders.

182 CDC (2013). Parasites – Leishmaniasis. Epidemiology and risk factors [online]. www.cdc.gov/parasites/leishmaniasis/epi.htm (accessed 18 December 2017).

183 CAPC (2016). Vector-borne diseases - canine leishmaniasis [online]. www.capcvet.org/capc-recommendations/canine-leishmaniasis (accessed 18 December 2017).

184 Ferrer, L. (2016). Canine leishmaniasis. Parasitic & protozoal disease. In: Clinician's Brief.

185 Baneth, G. (2014). Overview of leishmaniasis. In: Merck Vet Manual [online]. www.merckvetmanual.com/mvm/generalized_conditions/leishmaniosis/overview_of_leishmaniosis.html (accessed 18 December 2017).

186 Oliva, G., Roura, X., Crotti, A. et al. (2010). Guidelines for the treatment of leishmaniasis in dogs. *Journal of the American Veterinary Medical Association* **236** (11): 1192–1198.

187 CDC (2016). Parasites – Leishmaniasis. Resources for health professionals [online]. www.cdc.gov/parasites/leishmaniasis/health_professionals/ (accessed 18 December 2017).

188 Gómez-Ochoa, P., Castillo, J.A., Gascón, M. et al. (2009). Use of domperidone in the treatment of canine visceral leishmaniasis: a clinical trial. *The Veterinary Journal* **179** (2): 259–263.

189 Gradoni, L. (2015). Canine Leishmania vaccines: still a long way to go. *Veterinary Parasitology* **208** (1–2): 94–100.

190 WHO (2016). Leishmaniasis fact sheet [online]. www.who.int/mediacentre/factsheets/fs375/en/. (accessed 12 January 2017).

191 Grimaldi, G., Teva, A., Santos, C.B. et al. (2012). The effect of removing potentially infectious dogs on the numbers of canine *Leishmania infantum* infections in an endemic area with high transmission rates. *The American Journal of Tropical Medicine and Hygiene* **86** (6): 966–971.

192 Vulpiani, M.P., Iannetti, L., Paganico, D. et al. (2011). Methods of control of the *Leishmania infantum* dog reservoir: state of the art. *Veterinary Medicine International* **2011**: 215964.

193 Levett, P.N. (2001). Leptospirosis. *Clinical Microbiology Reviews* **14**: 296–326.

194 Sykes, J., Hartmann, K., Lunn, K. et al. (2010). 2010 ACVIM small animal consensus statement on leptospirosis: diagnosis, epidemiology, treatment, and prevention. *Journal of Veterinary Internal Medicine* **25** (1): 1–13.

195 Harkin, K.R. (2009). Leptospirosis. In: *Kirk's Current Veterinary Therapy XIV*, 14th edn (eds. J.D. Bonagura and D.C. Twedt), 1237–1240. St. Louis, MO: Saunders.

196 Geisen, V., Stengel, C., Brem, S. et al. (2007). Canine leptospirosis infections—clinical signs and outcome with different suspected *Leptospira* serogroups (42 cases). *Journal of Small Animal Practice* **48** (6): 324–328.

197 Greenlee, J.J., Alt, D.P., Bolin, C.A. et al. (2005). Experimental canine leptospirosis caused by *Leptospira* interogans serovars pomona and bratislava. *American Journal of Veterinary Research* **66** (10): 1816–1822.

198 Moore, G.E., Guptill, L.F., Ward, M.P. et al. (2005). Adverse events diagnosed within 3 days of vaccine administration in pet dogs. *Journal of the American Veterinary Medical Association* **227** (7): 1102–1108.

199 WHO (2013). Expert Consultation on Rabies. Second Report [online]. http://apps.who.int/iris/bitstream/10665/85346/1/9789240690943_eng.pdf (accessed 18 December 2017).

200 Hampson, K., Coudeville, L., Lembo, T. et al. (2015). Estimating the global burden of endemic canine rabies. *PLoS Neglected Tropical Diseases* **9**: e0003786.

201 Rupprecht, C.E. and Childs, J.E. (1996). Feline rabies. *Feline Practice* **24**: 15–19.

202 Tepsumethanon, V., Lumlertdacha, B., Mitmoonpitak, C. et al. (2004). Survival of

naturally infected rabid dogs and cats. *Clinical Infectious Diseases* **39** (2): 278–280.

203 Tepsumethanon, V., Wilde, H., and Meslin, F.X. (2005). Six criteria for rabies diagnosis in living dogs. *Journal of the Medical Association of Thailand* **88** (3): 419–422.

204 WHO (2010). Rabies vaccines: WHO position paper–recommendations. *Vaccine* **28** (44): 7140–7142.

205 OIE (2016). Global elimination of dog-mediated human rabies. In: Report of the Rabies Global Conference [online]. http://www.oie.int/ (accessed 18 December 2017).

206 Day, M.J., Horzinek, M.C., Schultz, R.D., and Squires, R.A. (2016). WSAVA guidelines for the vaccination of dogs and cats. *Journal of Small Animal Practice* **57**: E1–E45.

207 Morters, M.K., McNabb, S., Horton, D.L. et al. (2015). Effective vaccination against rabies in puppies in rabies endemic regions. *Veterinary Record* **117**: 150.

208 Hendricks, C.G., Levy, J.K., Tucker, S.J. et al. (2014). Tail vaccination in cats: a pilot study. *Journal of Feline Medicine and Surgery* **16** (4): 275–280.

209 Mathews, K. (2006). *Veterinary Emergency and Critical Care Manual*, 2nd edn. Guelph: Lifelearn.

210 Nelson, R. and Couto, C. (2014). *Small Animal Internal Medicine*, 5th edn. St. Louis, MO: Elsevier Mosby.

211 Burkitt, J.M., Sturges, B.K., Jandrey, K.E., and Kass, P.H. (2007). Risk factors associated with outcome in dogs with tetanus: 38 cases (1987–2005). *Journal of the American Veterinary Medical Association* **230** (1): 76–83.

212 Greene, C. (2011). Tetanus. In: *Infectious Diseases of the Dog and Cat*, 4th edn. St. Louis, MO: Saunders.

213 Public Health Agency of Canada (2016). Clostridium tetani Pathogen Safety Data Sheets [online]. http://www.phac-aspc.gc.ca/lab-bio/res/psds-ftss/clostridium-tetani-eng.php (accessed 18 December 2017).

214 Sprott, K. (2008). Generalized tetanus in a Labrador retriever. *Canadian Veterinary Journal* **49** (12): 1221–1223.

215 Boscos, C.M. and Ververidis, H.N. (2004). Canine TVT – clinical findings, diagnosis and treatment. Proceedings of the 29th World Congress of the World Small Animal Veterinary Association, Rhodes (6–9 October 2004).

216 Strakova, A. and Murchison, E.P. (2014). The changing global distribution and prevalence of canine transmissible venereal tumor. *BMC Veterinary Research* **10**: 168.

217 Rogers, K.S. (1997). Transmissible venereal tumor. *Compendium on Continuing Education for the Practising Veterinarian* **19**: 1036–1045.

218 Ferreira, A.J., Jaggy, A., Varejão, A.P. et al. (2000). Brain and ocular metastases from a transmissible venereal tumour in a dog. *The Journal of Small Animal Practice* **41** (4): 165–168.

219 Das, U. and Das, A.K. (2000). Review of canine transmissible venereal sarcoma. *Veterinary Research Communications* **24** (8): 545–556.

220 Ganguly, B., Das, U., and Das, A.K. (2013). Canine transmissible venereal tumor: a review. *Veterinary Comparative Oncology* **14** (1): 1–12.

221 Withrow, S., Vail, D., and Page, R. (2012). *Withrow and MacEwen's Small Animal Clinical Oncology*, 5th edn. St. Louis, MO: Saunders.

222 Scarpelli, K.C., Valladao, M.L., and Metze, K. (2010). Predictive factors for the regression of canine transmissible venereal tumor during vincristine therapy. *Veterinary Journal* **183** (3): 362–363.

223 Stiles, J., Townsend, W.M., Rogers, Q.R., and Krohne, S.G. (2002). Effect of oral administration of L-lysine on conjunctivitis caused by feline herpesvirus in cats. *American Journal of Veterinary Research* **63** (1): 99–103.

224 Mateis, F.L., Walser-Reinhardt, L., and Spiess, B.M. (2012). Canine neurogenic keratoconjunctivitis sicca: 11 cases (2006–2010). *Veterinary Opthalmology* **15** (4): 288–290.

225 Hendrix, D.V., Adkins, E.A., Ward, D.A. et al. (2011). An investigation comparing the efficacy of topical ocular application of tacrolimus and cyclosporine in dogs. *Veterinary Medicine International* **2011**: 487592.

226 Maggs, D., Miller, P., Ofri, R., and Slatter, D. (2013). Cornea and sclera. In: *Slatter's*

*Fundamentals of Veterinary Ophthalmology*, 5th edn. Philadelphia, PA: Saunders.

227 Renshaw, R., Zylich, N., Laverack, M. et al. (2010). Pneumovirus in dogs with acute respiratory disease. *Emerging Infectious Diseases* **16** (6): 993–995.

228 Crawford, C. (2011) Canine respiratory infections in animal shelters [online]. Maddie's Shelter Medicine Program College of Veterinary Medicine, University of Florida. http://sheltermedicine.vetmed.ufl.edu/ (accessed 18 Oct 2016).

229 Gober, M. and McCloskey, R. (2013). Canine infectious respiratory disease (CIRD). Zoetis US. Management of outbreak situations [online]. https://www.zoetisus.com/ (accessed 18 October 2016).

230 Datz, C. (2003). Bordetella infections in dogs and cats: pathogenesis, clinical signs, and diagnosis. *Compendium on Continuing Education for the Practising Veterinarian* **25** (12): 896–901.

231 Chalker, V.J., Owen, W.M., Paterson, C. et al. (2004). Mycoplasmas associated with canine infectious respiratory disease. *Microbiology* **150**: 3491–3497.

232 Dinnage, J.D., Scarlett, J.M., and Richards, J.R. (2009). Descriptive epidemiology of feline upper respiratory tract disease in an animal shelter. *Journal of Feline Medicine and Surgery* **11** (10): 816–825.

233 Gaskell, R.M. and Povey, R.C. (1977). Experimental induction of feline viral rhinotracheitis virus re-excretion in FVR-recovered cats. *Veterinary Record* **100** (7): 128–133.

234 Maggs, D.J., Nasisse, M.P., and Kass, P.H. (2003). Efficacy of oral supplementation with L-lysine in cats latently infected with feline herpesvirus. *American Journal of Veterinary Research* **64** (1): 37–42.

235 UC Davis Koret Shelter Medicine Program (2015). URI sample treatment protocol [online]. http://www.sheltermedicine.com (acessed 17 January 2017).

236 Sparkes, A., Heiene, R., Lascelles, B. et al. (2010). ISFM and AAFP consensus guidelines. Long-term use of NSAIDs in cats. *Journal of Feline Medicine and Surgery* **12** (7): 521–538.

237 Traversa, D., Di Cesare, A., and Conboy, G. (2010). Canine and feline cardiopulmonary parasitic nematodes in Europe: emerging and underestimated. *Parasites and Vectors* **3**: 62.

238 Traversa, D., Milillo, P., Di Cesare, A. et al. (2009). Efficacy and safety of emodepside 2.1%/ praziquantel 8.6% spot-on formulation in the treatment of feline aelurostrongylosis. *Parasitology Research* **105**: S83–S89.

239 Hamilton, J.M., Weatherley, A., and Chapman, A.J. (1984). Treatment of lungworm disease in the cat with fenbendazol. *Veterinary Record* **114** (2): 40–41.

240 Nelson, R. and Couto, C. (2014). *Small Animal Internal Medicine*, 5th edn. St. Louis, MO: Mosby.

241 Tilley, L. and Smith, F. Jr. (2015). Mastitis. In: *Blackwell's Five-Minute Veterinary Consult: Canine and Feline*, 6th edn. Wiley-Blackwell.

242 Latimer, K., Duncan, J., and Latimer, K. (2011). *Duncan & Prasse's Veterinary Laboratory Medicine*, 1st edn. West Sussex: Wiley-Blackwell.

243 Buffington, C.A., Westropp, J.L., Chew, D.J., and Bolus, R.R. (2006). Risk factors associated with clinical signs of lower urinary tract disease in indoor-housed cats. *Journal of the American Veterinary Medical Association* **228** (5): 722–725.

244 Westropp, J.L. and Tony Buffington, C.A. (2004). Feline idiopathic cystitis: current understanding of pathophysiology and management. *Veterinary Clinics of North America: Small Animal Practice* **34** (4): 1043–1055.

245 Gunn-Moore, D.A. and Shenoy, C.M. (2004). Oral glucosamine and the management of feline idiopathic cystitis. *Journal of Feline Medicine and Surgery* **6** (4): 219–225.

246 Houston, D., Moore, A., Favrin, M., and Hoff, B. (2004). Canine urolithiasis: a look at over 16,000 urolith submissions to the Canadian Veterinary Urolith Centre from February 1998 to April 2003. *Canadian Veterinary Journal* **45** (3): 225–230.

247 Lulich, J.P. & Osborne, C.A.. (2010). Medical management of struvite disease in cats. North American Veterinary Conference, Orlando, FL (16–20 January 2010).

248 Houston, D., Moore, A., Elliott, D., and Biourge, V. (2011). Stone disease in animals. In: *Urinary Tract Stone Disease* (ed. N. Rao, G. Preminger and J. Kavanagh), 131–135. London: Springer.

249 Grauer, F. (2014). Struvite urolithiasis [online]. http://www.cliniciansbrief.com/sites/default/files/attachments/Struvite%20Urolithiasis.pdf (accessed 3 March 2017).

250 Grauer, G. (2015). Silica urolithiasis [online]. http://www.cliniciansbrief.com/article/silica-urolithiasis (accessed 3 March 2017).

251 Plunkett, S.J. (2012). *Emergency Procedures for the Small Animal Veterinarian*, 3rd edn. Saunders Ltd.

252 Sanderson, S. (2005). Use of erythropoietin and calcitriol for chronic renal failure in dogs and cats. World Small Animal Veterinary Association World Congress, Mexico City (11–14 May 2005). http://www.vin.com/apputil/content/defaultadv1.aspx?meta=Generic&pId=11196&id=3854220 (accessed 18 December 2017).

253 Brown, S. (2009). Acute renal failure: diagnosis, management, & prevention. American Animal Hospital Association Annual Meeting, Phoenix, AZ (26–29 March 2009).

254 Mathews, K. (2006). *Veterinary Emergency and Critical Care Manual*. Guelph: Lifelearn Inc.

# 14

# Diagnostic Techniques

*Field Manual for Small Animal Medicine*, First Edition. Edited by Katherine Polak and Ann Therese Kommedal.
© 2018 John Wiley & Sons, Inc. Published 2018 by John Wiley & Sons, Inc.

## 14.1

# Point-of-Care Testing

*Jennifer Bolser*

*International Veterinary Consultant, Qijiayuan Diplomatic Compound, 9 Jianwai Dajie, Chaoyang District, Beijing 100600, China*

### 14.1.1 Introduction to Point-of-Care Testing

Point-of-care (POC) testing refers to any diagnostic testing performed outside of a reference laboratory at or close to the site of patient care [1]. POC tests are often referred to as "patient-side," "in-clinic," or "bed-side" tests.

POC tests can provide rapid and valuable information for the diagnosis, treatment, and management of diseases in field settings. Globally, there are countless veterinary POC tests commercially available and in development. By far, the most common POC tests are those used to identify infectious diseases. This chapter focuses on POC tests that are the most cost–effective, practical to use, and of greatest utility in the field. These include selected infectious disease and toxicological tests, titer testing, dermatophyte detection, fecal flotation, urine test strip analysis, and the use of a portable glucometer. When choosing a POC test, one should consider test availability, handling, portability, cost, ease of use, and the medical conditions commonly found in the field area. In planning for the field work, the practitioner should consider the questions in Textbox 14.1.1.

---

**Textbox 14.1.1 Considerations when using POC tests in the field**

1) *Geographic availability.* Is the desired test available for purchase in the country/area of the field work? If not, are there potential transport restrictions for the test and/or reagents?

2) *Handling, maintenance, and disposal requirements.* What are the test storage temperature requirements? Will you need refrigeration or electricity to maintain or use the test? Will you need to bring in or buy reagents on-site? What other supplies are needed to perform the test? What is the test expiration date?

3) *Portability.* How will you travel to the field site? Is the test transportable? Are there country restrictions to outside testing agents and equipment?

4) *Cost.* What is the program budget? How do test prices compare at home versus the destination country? Do you have a local partner that can order tests? When resources are limited, will a POC test result change treatment or management decisions? Is POC testing the most effective use of resources?

5) *Ease of use.* Will there be staff with the experience and skills needed to perform and interpret the test(s)? Is there potential for testing or interpretation error? What protocols will be in place for making the decision of when and how to use the test?

6) *Conditions common in the working area.* What are the common infectious diseases, toxins, or other conditions prevalent in the working area? Will you be able to treat those conditions in the field setting?

---

*Field Manual for Small Animal Medicine*, First Edition. Edited by Katherine Polak and Ann Therese Kommedal.
© 2018 John Wiley & Sons, Inc. Published 2018 by John Wiley & Sons, Inc.

As with any diagnostic test, users should understand testing limitations when interpreting results. There is no such thing as a perfect test. Clinicians must have a basic understanding of disease pathogenesis, potential shedding times, and immunology. The overall prevalence of the disease being tested for can also affect the test's performance characteristics. Knowing a particular test's sensitivity, specificity, and what those terms mean is necessary for correct test interpretation.

*Sensitivity* (of a diagnostic test) is "the probability that a test will correctly identify patients which are infected or have a specified non-infectious condition" [2]. A test with perfect sensitivity would always detect the disease if present. The sensitivity of a test indicates how well we can trust a negative result. A test with a high sensitivity will have a low number of false negative results.

*Specificity* (of a diagnostic test) is "the probability of a test correctly identifying those patients which are not infected or which do not have the specified condition" [3]. A test with perfect specificity would *only* detect the disease being evaluated. The specificity of a test indicates how well we can trust a positive result. A test with high specificity will have a low number of false positive results.

---

**Textbox 14.1.2 Useful mnemonics for remembering the difference between sensitivity and specificity**

SNOUT: **SeN**sitive tests rule **OUT** disease
SPIN: **SP**ecific tests rule **IN** disease

---

*Prevalence* is defined as "the total number of cases of a specific disease in existence in a given population at a certain time" [4]. Ideally, practitioners would know the prevalence of specific medical conditions in their area of field work as this influences positive and negative predictive values of diagnostic tests. Given that in most field situations the prevalence of disease is unknown, further discussion is beyond the scope of this manual.

At the time of this publication, there is rapid and exciting expansion in the development of POC tests. Technological advances are allowing for a wide variety of mobile/field testing and monitoring options. Examples of new POC tests include mobile phone applications for electrocardiograph monitoring, portable ultrasound technology, and handheld biochemistry analyzers, to name a few. Practitioners will have many new POC tests to evaluate and choose from in the near future.

## 14.1.2 Selected Infectious Disease Point-of-Care Tests

There are numerous infectious disease POC tests commercially available. The most clinically relevant tests for working in the field include those for canine parvovirus (CPV), feline panleukopenia virus (FPV), canine distemper virus (CDV), feline leukemia virus (FeLV), feline immunodeficiency virus (FIV), and vector-borne diseases including ehrlichiosis, anaplasmosis, and canine heartworm. This section provides the most relevant information of each disease with regard to testing, as well as recommendations for how to best perform and interpret the various tests. A summary chart of individual test characteristics of four different manufacturers, IDEXX® SNAP®, Anigen™ Rapid (BioNote®, Inc. Korea), Zoetis® WITNESS®, and Abaxis® VetScan®, is included in Table 14.1.1. These tests were selected due to their popularity in various world markets and/or because of available clinical data.

---

**Textbox 14.1.3 Required supplies for POC testing**

- Test kits including test device, buffer/reagent solution, provided pipettes and ideally the package insert
- Refrigeration for some test kits (see details in Table 14.1.1, most tests do not require refrigeration)
- Flat and dry surface
- Disposable gloves
- Watch or timer
- Additional supplies for blood tests
  - Needles and syringes to collect blood samples
  - Ethylenediaminetetraacetic acid (EDTA) (purple top) or lithium heparin (green top) blood collection tubes.

Alternatively, syringes can be predrawn with heparin just to coat the syringe and then used to draw blood. However, a sample drop from the syringe may not be the appropriate volume as compared to the supplied pipette.

---

**Table 14.1.1** Infectious disease POC tests summary.

| Infectious disease | Test name | Storage Refrigerate approx. = 2–8°C, (35–46°F) or room temp approx. = 15–27°C, (59–80°F) | Sample type | Sample amount Drops using provided pipette | Reagent/buffer amount (Drops) | Number of times to mix or sample absorption wait time prior to adding buffer | Read time (min) | Sensitivity Reported by manufacturer (unless otherwise noted) | Specificity Reported by manufacturer (unless otherwise noted) |
|---|---|---|---|---|---|---|---|---|---|
| Canine Parvovirus Antigen Tests | SNAP Parvo [5] | Both | Feces | Swab | 5 drops of mixed sample | Mix 3 times | 8 min | 100% | 98% |
| | Anigen Rapid CPV Ag [6] | Both | Feces | Swab | 4 drops of mixed sample | Mix vigorously | 5–10 min | 100% | 100% |
| | Witness CPV [7] | Both | Feces | Swab | 3 drops of mixed sample | Mix vigorously | 10 min | Not reported | Not reported |
| | VetScan Canine Parvovirus Rapid [8] | Room | Feces | Swab | 3 drops of mixed sample | Mix 5–6 times | 10–15 min | 96.9% | 96.9% |
| Feline Parvovirus Antigen Tests | SNAP (Canine) Parvo [5, 9] | Both | Feces | Swab | 5 drops of mixed sample | Mix 3 times | 8 min | Not reported (positive predictive value 100%) | Not reported (negative predictive value 97.9%) |
| | Anigen Rapid FPV Ag [10] | Both | Feces | Swab | 4 drops of mixed sample | Mix vigorously | 10 min | 97% | 98.5% |
| | Witness CPV [7, 9] | Both | Feces | Swab | 3 drops of mixed sample | Mix vigorously | 10 min | Not reported (positive predictive value 100%) | Not reported (negative predictive value 97.4%) |
| | VetScan Canine Parvovirus Rapid [8] | Room | Feces | Swab | 3 drops of mixed sample | Mix 5–6 times | 10–15 min | Not reported | Not reported |
| Canine Distemper Virus Antigen Test | Anigen Rapid CDV Ag [11] | Both | Conjunctiva swab, urine, serum, or plasma | Conj./urine = swab Serum/plasma = 2–3 drops | 4 drops of mixed sample | Mix well | 5–10 min | 100% | 98.5% |

(continued)

**Table 14.1.1** (Continued)

| Infectious disease | Test name | Storage Refrigerate approx. = 2–8 °C, (35–46 °F) or room temp approx. = 15–27° C, (59–80 °F) | Sample type | Sample amount Drops using provided pipette | Reagent/buffer amount (Drops) | Number of times to mix or sample absorption wait time prior to adding buffer | Read time (min) | Sensitivity Reported by manufacturer (unless otherwise noted) | Specificity Reported by manufacturer (unless otherwise noted) |
|---|---|---|---|---|---|---|---|---|---|
| FeLV/FIV: Feline Retrovirus Combo Tests | SNAP Combo® ELISA kit (FeLV ag, FIV ab) [12, 13] | Refrigerate | Whole blood Serum Plasma | 3 drops | 4 drops | Mix 3–5 times | 10 min | FeLV: 96.3–98.6% FIV: 93.5% | FeLV: 98.2–100% FIV: 100% |
| FeLV – Antigen Test | Anigen Rapid FIV Ab/FeLV Ag [37] | Both | Whole blood Serum Plasma | 10 μl | 2 drops | No wait time indicated | 10 min | FeLV: 94.7% FIV: 96.8% | FeLV: 99.7% FIV: 99.6% |
| FIV – Antibody Test | WITNESS FeLV-FIV [12, 14] | Room | Whole blood Serum Plasma | 1 drop (0.05 ml) | 2 drops | Wait until sample absorbed | 10 min | FeLV: 82.9–92.9% FIV: 93.8% | FeLV: 96.5–100% FIV: 93.4% |
| | VetScan Feline FeLV/FIV Rapid [8, 12] | Room | Whole blood Serum Plasma | 1 drop | 3 drops | Wait 5–10 s for sample absorption | 10 min | FeLV: 75.6–96% FIV: 99% | FeLV: 99–100% FIV: 97% |
| *Ehrlichia* Antibody Tests | SNAP 4Dx Plus [15, 16] | Room temp for 90 days or refrigerate | Whole blood Serum Plasma | 3 drops | 4 drops | Mix 3–5 times | 8 min | 97.1% | 95.3% |
| | Anigen Rapid CaniV-4 [17, 18] | Both | Whole blood Serum Plasma | WB:20 μl S: 10 μl P: 10 μl | 3 drops | No wait time indicated | 15 min | 80% | >90% |
| | Witness Ehrlichia [19, 20] | Both | Whole blood Serum Plasma | 1 drop (0.05 ml) | 2 drops | Wait for full sample absorption | 10 min | 97% | 100% |
| | VetScan Ehrlichia Rapid [8, 21] | Both | Whole blood Serum Plasma | 1 drop | 3 drops | Wait 30–60 s for sample absorption | 8–10 min | 93.4% | 96.7% |

| | Storage | Sample | | | | Time | | |
|---|---|---|---|---|---|---|---|---|
| *Anaplasma* Antibody Tests | | | | | | | | |
| SNAP 4Dx Plus [15, 16] | Room temp for 90 days or refrigerate | Whole blood Serum Plasma | 3 drops | 4 drops | Mix 3–5 times | 8 min | 90.3% | 94.3% |
| Anigen Rapid CaniV-4 [17, 18] | Both | Whole blood Serum Plasma | WB: 20 µl S: 10 µl P: 10 µl | 3 drops | No wait time indicated | 15 min | 73.3% | >90% |
| VetScan Anaplasma Rapid [8, 22] | Both | Whole blood Serum Plasma | 1 drop | 3 drops | Wait 5–10 s for sample absorption | 8–10 min | 97.5% | 93.6% |
| Heartworm Antigen Tests | | | | | | | | |
| SNAP 4Dx Plus [15, 16] | Room temp for 90 days or refrigerate | Whole blood Serum Plasma | 3 drops | 4 drops | Mix 3–5 times | 8 min | 99% | 99.3% |
| Anigen Rapid CaniV-4 [17, 18] | Both | Whole blood Serum Plasma | WB: 20 µl S: 10 µl P: 10 µl | 3 drops | No wait time indicated | 15 min | 97.6% | >90% |
| Witness Heartworm [23] | Both | Whole blood Serum Plasma | 1 drop (0.05 ml) | 2 drops | Wait for full sample absorption | 10 min | 96.6% | 99% |
| VetScan Heartworm Rapid [8, 24] | Room only | Whole blood Serum Plasma | 1 drop | 2 drops | Wait 3–5 s for sample absorption | 8–10 min | 92% | 100% |

1) SNAP® Tests manufactured by IDEXX® Laboratories, Inc.
2) Anigen™ Rapid Tests manufactured by BioNote®, Inc.
3) Witness® Tests manufactured by Zoetis®, Inc.
4) VetScan® Rapid Tests manufactured by Abaxis®, Inc.

### 14.1.2.1 Understanding Antigen Versus Antibody Tests

Infectious disease tests detect either antigen or antibody, and it is crucial for the practitioner to know what type of test they are using in order to interpret the results appropriately. Antigen tests indicate whether or not the infectious agent is present in the patient. Note that recent vaccination (within 4–10 days) with modified live virus (MLV) vaccines may create transient false positive results in a few of the antigen tests, [25] but current opinion is that the number of such false positives is low.

Antibody tests indicate that the patient has had exposure to the infectious agent and generated antibodies. A positive antibody test is not necessarily indicative of active infection. Furthermore, most antibody tests cannot differentiate between maternally derived antibodies and those generated from natural infection. Interpret positive results with caution.

The majority of infectious disease POC tests use enzyme-linked immunosorbent assay (ELISA) technology. ELISA is a type of binding test that can measure either antigen or antibody [26]. IDEXX's SNAP technology is a commonly used example of ELISA as a POC test in veterinary medicine. For antigen tests, the patient's sample (usually blood, serum, or feces) is mixed with antibody that is conjugated to an enzyme. The mixed sample is placed into the testing well and passes over a matrix of capture antibodies specific to the antigen being tested. The "snap" technology allows bidirectional flow increasing binding, which increases sensitivity. A washing step removes unbound components, and then exposure to an enzyme substrate creates the color reaction [27].

Lateral-flow immunochromatography (also known as chromatographic immunoassay or Rapid ImmunoMigration (RIM™)) are newer technologies that developed from the foundation of ELISA [27]. Similar to ELISA, the test process relies on antigen–antibody immune complexes. The sample liquid migrates across the membrane through capillary action. For an antigen test, gold-conjugated antibodies are encountered in the sample well. The immune complexes of antigen and gold-conjugated antibodies continue migration laterally. A second antibody at the level of the test result line will bind to these complexes, immobilizing the antigen and generating a color change indicating a positive result. Excess gold-conjugated antibodies continue migration to the control line where an antibody to the gold-conjugated antibodies is waiting for binding, resulting in a color change. This technology is the basis for Anigen Rapid (BioNote), Zoetis WITNESS, and Abaxis VetScan tests.

### 14.1.2.2 Canine Parvovirus POC Tests

All CPV POC tests listed below use feces for sampling and are qualitative antigen tests. During the clinical phase of parvovirus, dogs have the highest level of virus shedding in their feces 4–7 days after infection; this often correlates with the start of clinical signs. False negative results early in the course of the disease are possible due to low antigen shedding and antigen dilution in voluminous feces; repeat testing in 1–2 days is recommended if clinical suspicion for parvovirus is high. Virus shedding in the feces starts to wane around 8 days and is often absent by 15 days postinfection [28].

Recent vaccination (within 4–10 days) with MLV vaccines may cause false positive results in some products [7]. However, in a study conducted by researchers at the University of Wisconsin evaluating 64 dogs vaccinated with six different modified live canine parvovirus-2 (CPV-2) vaccines, the SNAP Parvo Test did not detect vaccine-related canine parvovirus CPV-2 in their feces [29].

An independent study evaluating three different CPV POC tests found high specificity among all tests (>92%) but lower sensitivity (50–60%) compared with immune-electron microscopy (IEM) [30]. In general, we can consider parvovirus POC tests to be highly specific and trust a positive result. However, the potential for false negatives may be significant and should be considered when the clinical suspicion for CPV infection is high.

### 14.1.2.3 Feline Panleukopenia POC Tests

Since FPV is caused by a parvovirus, many of the CPV POC tests have been evaluated and used to test cats for this disease. Multiple studies have shown the CPV POC tests (IDEXX SNAP Canine Parvo and Witness CPV) to be useful and accurate for use in cats [9, 25, 31]. In addition, Anigen Rapid manufactured by BioNote, Inc. Korea, has developed a feline-specific parvovirus antigen test. A study evaluating postvaccination fecal parvovirus antigen testing in kittens found an overall low amount of false positive results following vaccination. However, the Symbiotics (Witness CPV) test had the highest rate of false positives [25].

### 14.1.2.4 Canine Distemper Virus POC Tests

At the time of this manual's publishing, there are no CDV POC tests available in the United States. However, there are numerous CDV POC tests available worldwide. The author has seen these tests used in many countries including China, Ecuador, Mexico, and Thailand. Considering the complex clinical course of CDV and challenge of finding independent clinical studies for CDV antigen POC tests, the reliability of these tests is questionable. Most of these tests use lateral-flow immunochromatographic technology; Anigen Rapid CDV Ag Test Kit (BioNote, Inc.) is one example. The preferred testing sample is a conjunctival swab, but urine, serum, or plasma can also be used.

#### 14.1.2.4.1 Emerging Technology

GeneReach Biotechnology Corporation has created the POCKIT™ Nucleic Acid Analyzer. This portable device uses real-time insulated isothermal polymerase chain reaction (RT-iiPCR) technology. Combined with their PETNAD™ Detection Kits for a variety of infectious diseases including CDV, this portable testing system can identify infectious agents with the accuracy of gold standard real-time PCR (RT-PCR) testing [32]. This testing system can be used patient side and the results are available in 1 h. Large-scale sheltering situations in particular may benefit from this test in the management of disease outbreaks. While this test may be out of financial reach in most field situations, it is mentioned in this chapter as an example of the exciting advancement of POC testing technology.

### 14.1.2.5 Feline Leukemia Virus and Feline Immunodeficiency POC Tests

Many of the POC tests for feline retroviruses are combination tests used for both FeLV and FIV.

#### 14.1.2.5.1 Feline Leukemia Virus

The majority of FeLV POC tests detect the presence of soluble FeLV p27 antigen. During the first 30–90 days of infection, false negative results may occur due to low amounts of detectable antigens [33]. Since this is an antigen test, there is no concern for false positive results from maternally derived antibodies. Furthermore, cats vaccinated for FeLV will not cause currently available antigen tests to be positive. Serum, plasma, and whole blood are the current preferred testing samples. Independent clinical trials for the FeLV component of all the tests listed below indicate a high level of specificity at 100%. Sensitivity was highest for the IDEXX® SNAP Feline Triple® Test (96.3%) compared to Witness FeLV-FIV Test (82.9%) and VetScan Feline FeLV/FIV Rapid Test (75.6%) [12].

#### 14.1.2.5.2 Feline Immunodeficiency Virus

The FIV component of combination FeLV/FIV tests detects the presence of antibodies against FIV proteins. Most cats will develop antibodies within 60 days of infection. Since this is an antibody test, the presence of maternal antibodies may result in a false positive result. Therefore, kittens that test positive should be retested after 6 months of age due to the possibility of maternal antibody presence [33].

Historically, it was thought that POC tests could not differentiate previously FIV-vaccinated cats from truly FIV-infected cats. However, a recent study has shown that the Witness Zoetis and Anigen Rapid BioNote immunochromatography kits accurately identify truly infected FIV cats as positive and FIV-vaccinated cats that are not infected as negative [34]. Irrespective of FIV vaccination history, the Witness Zoetis and Anigen Rapid BioNote tests can be used to determine the true FIV infection status of cats. IDEXX SNAP FIV tests cannot differentiate FIV-vaccinated cats from truly infected cats. Cats that have been FIV vaccinated will test positive on all current IDEXX SNAP FIV tests. Therefore, the lateral immunochromatography tests such as Witness Zoetis and Anigen Rapid BioNote are likely preferable to the IDEXX SNAP test for FIV testing.

### 14.1.2.6 Selected Vector-Borne POC Tests: Ehrlichiosis, Anaplasmosis, and Heartworm

There are numerous tests available for canine vector-borne infectious diseases. Some manufacturers offer combination tests that can detect up to four different agents at once. In the field, combination tests may be advantageous when working in environments where multiple diseases are a potential concern. Using one combination test decreases the number of tests required for transport to the field setting and can be more cost– and time–effective when evaluating multiple diseases. However, individual test options may be beneficial in some field environments for targeted disease surveillance, decreasing cost when evaluating for only one disease and simplifying test interpretation. In this section, the use of *Ehrlichia, Anaplasma,* and heartworm tests is discussed. Note: combination tests also include Lyme (*Borrelia burgdorferi*) antibody. Similar to the other antibody tests, this test cannot differentiate between acute/active infection and previous exposure to Lyme disease.

### 14.1.2.6.1 Tick-Borne Disease: Ehrlichiosis and Anaplasmosis

Bacterial tick-borne diseases, also known as blood parasites in many parts of the world, commonly include ehrlichiosis and anaplasmosis. The limitation of POC testing of these diseases is that commercially available tests detect antibody and a positive antibody test does not differentiate between an active infection, subclinical infection, or previous exposure. Thus, the practitioner will need to use clinical signs and other lab results (if available) to interpret these POC tests.

---

**Textbox 14.1.4 Tip from the field**

In the author's experience, a positive antibody test for *Ehrlichia* or *Anaplasma* spp. without concurrent clinical signs or classic laboratory abnormalities (thrombocytopenia and/or anemia) does not warrant treatment. If a dog tests positive on POC testing in conjunction with symptoms and/or with classic bloodwork abnormalities, treatment is warranted. A 21- or 28-day course of doxycycline is the treatment of choice.

---

Canine ehrlichiosis can be caused by multiple species of *Ehrlichia* (*E. canis, E. chaffeensis, E. ewingii*), which stimulate antibodies that cross react on POC tests. Early in the course of an acute *Ehrlichia* infection, a false negative antibody test result may occur and the practitioner may still want to initiate treatment if clinical signs are highly suggestive of ehrlichiosis. *Ehrlichia* antibodies can persist in a dog for years [33].

Canine anaplasmosis is caused by multiple species of *Anaplasma*. All of the *Anaplasma* POC tests listed in this manual detect *A. phagocytophilum* and *A. platys* (cross reacts) antibodies. A positive *Anaplasma* test does not differentiate between an active infection or previous exposure as antibodies can persist in dogs for months to years. Detection of antibodies via ELISA occurs starting 8 days after infection [35].

### 14.1.2.6.2 Canine Heartworm

POC testing for canine heartworm disease are antigen tests that detect a protein secreted by female heartworms. After a dog is exposed via the mosquito vector, a minimum of 6 months is required for an adult worm to develop from the infective larval stage. The American Heartworm Society currently recommends testing dogs starting at 7 months of age. False negative results can be observed due to a number of factors including low worm burden, male-only heartworm infection, immature female worms, and antigen–antibody complex interference [36].

### 14.1.2.7 Reading Test Results

### 14.1.2.7.1 IDEXX SNAP Tests

*Parvovirus.* Placing the sample well at the top direction, the positive control circle is at the top, negative control is on the left, and the positive parvovirus antigen result circle is on the right. If the color of the positive result circle on the right is darker than negative control circle on the left, the test is positive [5].

*FeLV/FIV.* Placing the sample well at the top direction, the positive control spot is the top circle, FIV antibody spot is on the left and FeLV antigen spot is on the right. In the FIV/FeLV Combo test, the bottom circle is the negative control spot. In the Feline Triple test, the bottom circle is for feline heartworm antigen [13].

*4Dx® Plus.* Placing the sample well at the top direction, in the result window the positive control circle is the top-left corner. Sample spots follow below clockwise with *Anaplasma* spp. at the upper middle, heartworm (*Dirofilaria immitis*) at the right middle, Lyme (*B. burgdorferi*) at the bottom and *Ehrlichia* spp. at the left-middle position (Figure 14.1.1) [15]. The clockwise pneumonic *"Ana's Heart Lies with (or to!) Ehric"* may be helpful to remember.

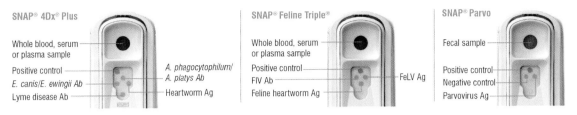

**Figure 14.1.1** IDEXX® SNAP® tests labeled. Source: Courtesy of IDEXX Laboratories, Inc.

#### 14.1.2.7.2 Anigen Rapid Tests (BioNote, Inc. Korea)

For all tests, a positive result has two color bands, one band at "T" and one band at "C," the order of appearance does not matter. A negative result has only one color band at "C." The test is invalid and should be repeated if no color band is visible or only one band is present at "T" (Figure 14.1.2) [6, 10, 11, 17, 37].

#### 14.1.2.7.3 Zoetis Witness Tests

A positive result shows a line at window "2" and window "3." A negative result shows only one line at the control window "3." Results are invalid if no lines appear or if only one line appears at window "2" [7, 14, 19, 23].

---

### Textbox 14.1.5 POC testing tips for success

#### Test Kits

- Once the test package is opened, it must be used quickly (10 min to 2 h depending on the test) [5–8, 10, 11, 13–15, 17, 19, 23, 37].
- Do not mix lot numbers of reagents and test devices.
- Sample and test should be equilibrated and run at room temperature, do not artificially heat. Allow 30 min to gently warm up if kit was refrigerated.
- Test devices need to be placed on a flat, dry surface.
- Do not touch or damage the test membranes or windows.
- Do not freeze the tests, and keep out of direct sunlight.
- Use a new swab, tube, pipette, and test for each patient.
- Hold the pipette and the solution bottles vertical for drop application into the wells.
- Mix reagent buffers gently before use.
- Discard tests that have expired.

#### Fecal Samples

- Fresh fecal samples are preferred. Refrigerated samples up to 24 h or frozen samples that have been thawed may be acceptable.
- Coat the entire swab with a thin layer of feces. Too much fecal material may cause inaccurate results.
- Avoid mucous or lubricant on the swab sample as these substances decrease the amount of potential viral antigen.

#### Blood Samples

- In the field setting the most common blood sample used will be anticoagulated whole blood (heparin-coated collection syringe, EDTA – purple top tubes, or lithium heparin – green top tubes).
- Fresh blood samples are preferred. Refrigerated samples 1–5 days old may be acceptable.
- Invert the blood sample a few times to mix prior to testing.
- Hemolytic, lipemic, and icteric samples may cause errors and/or inaccurate results with some tests.
- Use the kit's sample pipette for accurate measuring for that particular test. A drop is highly variable [23]:
  Provided pipette is typically 10–50 µl
  25 gauge needle = 8.0 µl
  22 gauge needle = 9.1 µl
  1 ml syringe hub = 31.2 µl
  3 ml syringe hub = 36.9 µl

#### Importance of Timing

- SNAP tests need to be activated at the appropriate time (when solution first enters activation circle).
- Lateral-flow immunochromatography tests and SNAP tests may develop additional colored lines/dots leading to interpretation errors if reading is delayed.

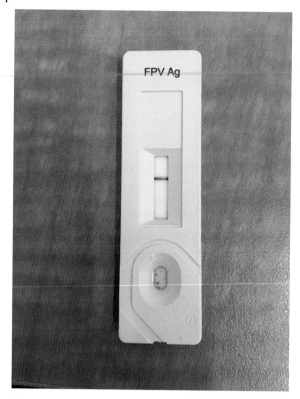

Figure 14.1.2 Anigen Rapid Feline Parvovirus Antigen negative test (BioNote, Inc.). Source: Courtesy of Dr. Jennifer Bolser.

#### 14.1.2.7.4 VetScan Rapid Tests (Abaxis)

A positive result has two colored lines, one at "C" and one at "T." The color intensity of the lines may vary, and any coloration at "T" should be considered positive. A negative result has only one line at "C." Results are invalid if no lines appear or only one line appears at "T" [8].

## 14.1.3 Toxicological POC Tests

Suspected toxicological emergencies may be encountered in field environments. Diagnosis of poisoning is often based on strong suspicion from clinical signs and exposure history. However, symptoms from poisonings can appear similar to a variety of other diseases and for many animals, medical histories are unavailable. Prompt diagnosis and initiation of treatment for these conditions is crucial for patient survival. The use of POC tests in these cases may aid the diagnosis of a suspect toxicity; however, the accuracy of many of these tests is questionable. Refer to the individual test instructions for use and chart color comparison when applicable.

### 14.1.3.1 Ethylene Glycol

Ethylene glycol (antifreeze) is one of the deadliest toxins that animals inadvertently ingest. Complete absorption occurs within 1 h of ingestion. Ethylene glycol can be detected in a patient 30 min to 12 h after exposure. However, after 6 h, the amount of ethylene glycol decreases significantly as it is converted into toxic metabolites. Thus, depending on the timing of testing postexposure and the amount ingested, test results can be affected. The serum toxic level in cats is 20 mg/dl and in dogs is 50 mg/dl [38].

There are currently two available POC tests for suspected ethylene glycol toxicity that can be used in dogs and cats, Kacey® Ethylene Glycol Diagnostic Strips and Catachem VetSpec™ Qualitative Ethylene Glycol Reagent Test Kit. The accuracy of both of these tests has been questioned with primarily a concern for false positive results. Kacey strips require plasma for testing, while the Catachem qualitative test can be performed with either serum or plasma. Animals that have received products containing propylene glycol (including activated charcoal and many injectable medications) or glycerine will have positive results for both tests [39]. Similarly, it is very important to ensure there is no alcohol contamination during blood collection.

Both tests are enzymatic based and detect ethylene glycol in the blood. Thus, these tests are most accurate in the first few hours after ingestion. Since these tests do not detect ethylene glycol metabolites, false negative results will occur if testing is done later in the disease course.

Note: Catachem has a qualitative test system (POC) and a quantitative test system that is used with automated chemistry analyzers. Data from clinical studies has suggested that accuracy of the Catachem quantitative system is relatively reliable. Even though both systems use the same enzymatic technology, there are differences between each test. The newer patient-side test (qualitative) still needs to be evaluated independently for accuracy.

There are many anecdotal reported concerns and frustrations with false positive results with the Kacey strips. Multiple clinicians have used these strips on animals with no ethylene glycol exposure and received positive results. However, one small *in vitro* study that compared the two POC systems concluded that the Kacey strips were more accurate and easier to use compared to the VetSpec Qualitative Ethylene Glycol Reagent Test Kit [40].

Use of these tests in the field is often limited due to the numerous potentials for false positives (test itself, propylene glycol exposure, alcohol contamination of the blood collection, etc.) as well as false negatives (testing too early or too late after ingestion). In addition, many field environments lack a centrifuge for plasma or serum preparation.

Additional options for field screening tests include scanning the urine, mouth, and vomitus with a Wood's lamp and/or performing a urinalysis to screen for calcium oxalate crystalluria. Sodium fluorescein dye is present in some brands of antifreeze, which may be seen with a Wood's lamp in the urine for up to 6 h postexposure. False positive and negative results can occur with Wood's lamp screening. Calcium oxalate crystalluria usually develops later, at least 6 h postexposure [38].

### 14.1.3.2 Rodenticide/Organophosphate

At the time of publication, Kacey® Diagnostics manufactures the following lateral-flow POC tests: "Rodenticide Anti-Coagulant Test Kit" and "Organo-Phosphate Diagnostic Poison Test Strips." Marketing for these tests suggest that each can detect a wide variety of toxins in their respective class. However, a study performed by Istvan et al. in 2014 showed that a lateral-flow anticoagulant test kit could only detect warfarin anticoagulant rodenticide and was unable to detect other anticoagulant rodenticides tested (pindone, chlorophacinone, brodifacoum, bromethalin, and its metabolite desmethylbromethalin) [41]. Furthermore, independent analysis of the organophosphate test strips is currently unavailable. Considering the limited available data and experience using these test strips, practitioners must evaluate the use and interpretation of test results cautiously.

### 14.1.3.3 Marijuana (THC), Opioid, Amphetamines, Barbiturates, Benzodiazepines, Cocaine

Cats and dogs are increasingly exposed either accidentally or intentionally to illicit drugs. Depending on the drug, symptoms may include unusual neurological signs (depression, stumbling, tremors, seizures), dilated or pinpoint pupils, excitability, abnormal heart rate, hyperthermia, and may lead to death. Inexpensive, rapid, easy-to-use and accessible over-the-counter human urine POC test kits can be used to help determine some of these potential drug exposures. Most of these qualitative tests are lateral-flow chromatographic immunoassays that can rapidly detect multiple drugs (or drug metabolites). These tests have been shown to be effective in identifying barbiturates, opiates, benzodiazepines, and amphetamines/methamphetamines in the urine of dogs [42]. However, false positives can occur. At this time, human urine drug screening tests are not accurate in detecting marijuana or methadone in dogs. Dogs with known marijuana exposure frequently have false negative test results. Accuracy of these screening tests in cats is currently unknown [43].

## 14.1.4 Titer Testing

### 14.1.4.1 Background

Most animals presenting to field clinics have had little to no prior veterinary care, including vaccination. In situations requiring the sheltering of large numbers of animals, this creates a high risk for an infectious disease outbreak due to an overall lack of herd immunity. New POC testing technology has made it possible to assess an individual's antibody titer for certain diseases *at a particular moment in time*. This information can be used during an outbreak to determine an individual patient's risk level for certain infectious diseases and guide decisions to manage the population while reducing the risk of further disease transmission.

During an outbreak in a shelter environment, clinically asymptomatic animals with protective antibody titers can typically be cleared for surgery and adoption, whereas those without protective antibody titers should ideally be removed, quarantined, and monitored for signs of disease. Such animals are also good candidates for foster homes. The removal of animals without protective antibodies helps protect them from disease exposure and allows them time to develop antibodies following vaccination.

In animals less than 16–18 weeks of age, titer tests can be used to assess the level of immune protection *at that moment in time.* However, these tests cannot differentiate maternal antibody from acquired immunity. Evidence of protective antibody at the time of a disease exposure, regardless if maternal or acquired, indicates the young patient likely has immune protection for that disease agent at that moment. However, if the antibody detected is maternal, the titer level will wane and the patient may eventually lose its immune protection. Appropriate vaccination protocols should be implemented to stimulate development of the young patient's own acquired immunity. Titer testing should not be used as a substitute for vaccination, in most field situations.

---

**Textbox 14.1.6 Titer testing in the field: Key points**

- Titer testing is used primarily in outbreak situations to determine which animals have the greatest risk for infection (no protective immunity) versus those that have evidence of protective immunity.
- If possible, remove animals *without* protective titers from the general population.
- Titer testing may be cost-prohibitive.
- Titer testing is for use only in clinically asymptomatic animals.
- Titers are not a substitute for vaccination.

---

### 14.1.4.2 Commercially Available Titer Test Kits

Currently two commercially available POC antibody titer test systems have been evaluated for accuracy: VacciCheck® Antibody Titer Test (Spectrum Labs) and TiterCHEK® CDV/CPV (Zoetis). VacciCheck offers a combination test system for canine adenovirus, CPV, and CDV titers. VacciCheck also offers an antibody titer test kit for FPV. TiterCHEK currently only offers testing for antibodies to canine distemper and parvovirus.

Both of these titer test systems utilize ELISA technology. Multiple studies have shown both systems to be highly specific and sensitive even in field scenarios [44–46]. These tests are portable, but require refrigeration for storage (do not freeze). Tests should be allowed to equilibrate at room temperature for 2 h prior to use. Results can be available in approximately 30 min, but

individuals unfamiliar with the test process should plan for 60 min. Each test is a series of steps and requires an individual dedicated to performing the steps with precise timing. Both kits can be used for an individual sample or batches of multiple samples at the same time. It is important for both test processes that mixing of the sample at each step is done thoroughly.

The VacciCheck system uses an ELISA spot test strip (comb tooth) for each individual sample. After the patient's sample of whole blood or serum is thoroughly mixed into the first well, the test strip is advanced through a series of preset wells with either a 5 min or 2 min incubation at each step. The test strip positive control spot, located at the top position on the strip, is assessed on the provided color chart. The color of the test spots is compared to the positive control for a semiquantitative assessment of antibody level. Any test spots that are the same color as or darker than the positive control spot are considered positive for protective antibodies. The kit can test up to 12 samples simultaneously.

The TiterCHEK process has separate antigen-coated wells for CDV and CPV. In addition to the inoculated patient sample well(s), positive and negative control wells are run at the time of testing. A maximum of 10 patient samples can be tested at the same time in one well holder. A series of four liquid reagents are added to the wells with thorough mixing, then washing and removal of liquid between each reagent step. At the end of the testing process, the positive control should change to blue color, the negative control stays clear. Any patient wells that have any blue coloration are considered positive.

The above description provides only a brief summary. Due to the detailed nature of the process for each of these tests, the author encourages practitioners to thoroughly review the test instructions provided by the manufacturer and to review YouTube videos provided by Maddie's® Institute: "Running Canine TiterCHEK CDV," "Running Canine VacciCheck Test," and "Interpreting Canine VacciCheck Test" prior to performing these tests.

Anigen Rapid (BioNote, Inc.) also manufactures CDV and CPV titer test kits. Unfortunately, at this time there is no available data on the accuracy of these tests. The author hopes that independent trials of these tests will be performed as this company's system is much simpler and easier for use in the field. The test utilizes the lateral immunochromatography system as seen in other

Anigen Rapid tests. A user-friendly color chart comparison is provided to assess titer protective level [47].

#### 14.1.4.3 Field Use Practicalities

The VacciCheck system has two main advantages over the TiterCHEK system for use in the field:

1) VacciCheck system can use whole blood or serum while TiterCHEK requires serum. In the field setting, whole blood samples may be preferred if a centrifuge to prepare serum samples is not available.
2) VacciCheck kit contains everything needed for the entire test process. TiterCHEK requires additional supplies of distilled water and plastic wash bottles to create diluted wash solution.

## 14.1.5 Fungal Culture, Trichogram, and Wood's Lamp Examination

### 14.1.5.1 General Information

Dermatophytosis (ringworm) is a fungal infection of the skin commonly encountered in field environments. Ringworm is zoonotic, highly contagious, and has the potential to cause widespread outbreaks, particularly in shelters. Early diagnosis is crucial to halt the transmission of ringworm to both people and animals. The most commonly isolated fungal organisms in dogs and cats are *Microsporum canis, Trichophyton mentagrophytes*, and *Microsporum gypseum.*

A Wood's lamp can be used for initial disease screening, but has low sensitivity (detects <50% of *M. canis* infections and does not detect *M. gypseum* nor *T. mentagrophytes)* [48]. Fungal culturing with microscopic confirmation is currently the gold standard for ringworm diagnosis. Fungal cultures are inexpensive, portable, but require 10–21 days for incubation and skill for microscopic evaluation. Dermatophyte test medium (DTM) plates are the most commonly used culture medium due to ease of inoculation and collection of colony for examination. Thus, DTM plates are generally preferred over glass jars, but either can be used. Fungal culturing can be particularly helpful when working in situations requiring the sheltering of animals such as after disasters or during hoarding responses.

---

**Textbox 14.1.7 The science of DTM plates**

DTM plates are typically a Sabouraud dextrose agar with antibacterial and antifungal compounds to inhibit contaminant overgrowth and contain phenol red as a pH indicator. Dermatophytes prefer to metabolize protein, causing them to produce alkaline metabolites. This pH change causes the color of the medium to turn from yellow to red, at the same time the dermatophyte colony starts to grow. Saprophytes (contaminants) metabolize carbohydrates during their initial growth. After the carbohydrates are depleted, saprophytes will use proteins, producing alkaline metabolites and a rapid color change later in their growth cycle (days after the original fungal growth appeared) [49]. Daily recording of the growth and color change can be helpful in assessing potential concerning colonies. Not all dermatophytes behave the same, and there are exceptions to this general rule. *Thus, microscopic evaluation for macroconidia is crucial for confirmation and identification of the fungal agent.*

---

### 14.1.5.2 Wood's Lamp Examination

A Wood's lamp emits long-wave ultraviolet light. Some *M. canis* infections (approximately 50%) will produce a tryptophan metabolite that when evaluated under this UV light fluoresces an apple green color along the hair shafts [48]. Plug-in lamps are more effective than battery-operated ones due to increased light intensity. A Wood's lamp examination can be performed in the following steps:

1) Bring the patient into a quiet room.
2) Turn on the Wood's lamp and turn off all lights. Complete darkness is needed for a Wood's lamp examination. Allow your eyes to adjust to the dark for a few minutes prior to performing the examination.
3) Hold the lamp 5–10 cm from the patient's skin and slowly move it over the entire body. Thoroughly inspect the ears, eyes, lips, chin, axilla, toes, interdigital spaces, nail beds, and the entire tail. If crusts are present, remove them to examine the hair shafts. Infected hair shafts will fluoresce apple green color. Confirm that it is the individual hair shaft that is fluorescing, not the skin.

4) Use forceps to pluck individual glowing hairs for direct microscopic examination or culture. Pluck hairs in the direction of growth and place in a folded piece of paper or red top tube for transport.

To avoid false negative Wood's lamp readings, the lamp should be turned on to warm up for at least 5 min prior to use, held over the lesion/area being inspected noting that 3–5 min of continuous light exposure to the lesion may be required for fluorescence to occur [48]. Many substances including some medications, food, dander, dermal scaling will also fluoresce under a Wood's lamp. Thus, the key is looking for individual fluorescing hair shafts. Fluorescing hair shafts are preferred for trichogram and/or fungal culturing. Note that a negative Wood's lamp screening does not necessarily mean the patient is ringworm negative.

### 14.1.5.3 Trichogram

Fluorescing hair shafts or other suspicious hairs can be plucked and examined microscopically.

1) Place a drop of mineral oil onto a microscope slide.
2) Place the plucked hair on the oil and cover with a coverslip. If a Wood's lamp was used to select the sample, use it to confirm that glowing hairs are on the slide.
3) On 10× power, move the slide on the stage until the hair is seen. If it cannot be identified, turn off the room lights and shine the Wood's lamp from beneath to help identify the fluorescence.
4) Examine the "glowing hair" under 4×, 10×, and 40×. Dermatophytosis causes the edges of hair shafts to appear swollen and "fuzzy" or frayed with an irregular outline. Hairs appear darker and wider than normal hair. The details of both the outer cortex and the inner medulla are lost. On 40×, cuffs of arthrospores/arthroconidia can be seen along the edges as tiny refractile strands or beads.

### 14.1.5.4 DTM Culture Required Supplies

- Microscope
- DTM plates
- Individually wrapped unused toothbrushes
- +/− Sterile hemostats
- Room temperature area with mild humidity (a desk drawer can suffice)
- Clear tape

- Microscope slides
- Blue dye (methylene blue, lactophenol cotton blue, or blue stain of Diff-Quick)
- Disposable gloves.

### 14.1.5.5 DTM Test Procedure

1) Wearing disposable gloves, collect hair samples for culture. There are two techniques:
   - *Hair pluck.* Use a clean hemostat to pluck hairs from around the periphery of a skin lesion. Ideally, pluck hairs that appear damaged or in areas of active crusting.
   - *Toothbrush technique.* Use a new individually wrapped toothbrush to brush over nonlesional areas first and then brush the lesions themselves. Brushing the nonlesion areas first will help avoid spreading spores to unaffected areas. If a lesion is obvious, brush it 15–20 times.
2) If refrigerated, allow the DTM plate to warm to room temperature before inoculation. Open the DTM plate upside down (to limit contamination) and gently tap the toothbrush onto the agar just hard enough to make a slight imprint but not so hard as to enter the agar. False negatives are possible if the toothbrush is pushed too hard into the medium.
3) Replace the lid and incubate the DTM plate with agar medium facing upside down (to prevent condensational damage to fungal growth). Write the animal's identification and date of the culture on the bottom of the plate.

---

**Textbox 14.1.8 How to make an incubator in the field**

Inoculated DTM plate(s) should be ideally stored in an incubator (77 to 86 °F (25 to 30 °C) with 30% humidity). An incubator can be easily made using a dark, sealed container, plastic bag, small cooler or fish tank. Place a small dish of water in the sealed container to create humidity and prevent desiccation of the gel medium. If using a small cooler, fish tank, or other covered plastic container, a light bulb or fish tank heater can be used to maintain appropriate temperature. A thermometer placed through the drain opening of a cooler or at the bottom of the container will ensure accurate temperature readings.

---

Microsporum canis

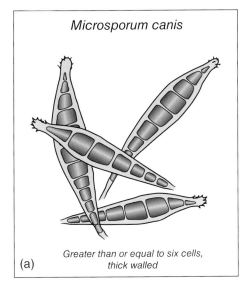

(a)  Greater than or equal to six cells, thick walled

Microsporum gypseum

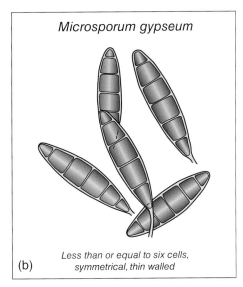

(b)  Less than or equal to six cells, symmetrical, thin walled

Trichophyton mentagrophytes

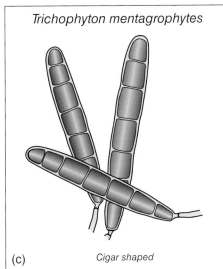

(c)  Cigar shaped

Alternaria spp

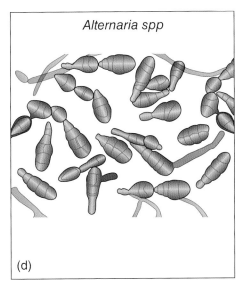

(d)

**Figure 14.1.3** Dermatophyte macroconidia.
(a) *Microsporum canis*. Macroconidia (spores) are large, thick walled, spindle shaped, with six or more internal cells. The spores typically have a terminal knob.
(b) *Microsporum gypseum*. Macroconidia are large, thin walled, spindle shaped, with six or less internal cells. The spores do not have a terminal knob.
(c) *Trichophyton mentagrophytes*. Macroconidia are long, thin walled, and cigar shaped. Microconidia (globe shaped and clustered) are often more numerous than macroconidia. Presence of spiral shaped hyphae indicates *T. mentagrophytes*.
(d) *Alternaria spp*. Alternaria is an opportunistic, saprophytic fungal infection of dogs and are not a dermatophyte. Macroconidia are irregular, often club shaped, compared to dermatophytes. Other saprophytic fungal species may not produce macroconidia but rather small spores and hyphae. These are also typically contaminant fungi and not significant ringworm species.

4) Check culture plates daily. Early subtle changes can be noted by holding the plate up to the light. If using DTM, the medium will change to red as the white, fluffy colonies begin to grow and become visible. Colony growth is typically seen in 7–10 days. *Trichophyton* sp. may need up 14–21 days to grow; therefore, it is recommended to keep all cultures for 21 days to ensure that no *Trichophyton* growth occurs. Dermatophyte colonies are typically white or pale yellow and appear fluffy. Black, gray, or green colonies can be ignored, as these are contaminant growths [48–50].

5) Evaluate any white- or pale-colored fluffy colonies microscopically using a tape-prep cytology. Place a drop of methylene/lactophenol blue on a microscope slide. Press the sticky side of a piece of clear cytology tape onto the fuzzy growth on the culture and apply the tape onto the slide, covering the drop of stain. Wipe away the excess stain. No coverslip is needed.

6) Allow the sample to absorb the stain for 5–10 min, and then scan the slide thoroughly for evidence of hyphae and macroconidia (spores). If unable to positively identify the species, return the culture plate to the incubator and retry in 2–3 days (Figure 14.1.3).

## 14.1.6 Fecal Flotation

### 14.1.6.1 General Information

Fecal flotation is an easy and inexpensive way to diagnose gastrointestinal parasites if a microscope is available. The principle behind fecal flotation is mixing feces in a solution of a higher specific gravity (density) than that of parasitic eggs, causing the eggs to float to the surface. The most common parasitic eggs have specific gravities between 1.06 and 1.20. The ideal specific gravity for a fecal flotation solution is 1.18–1.20. Solutions with too high of a density can collapse ova and float debris causing false readings [51].

Centrifugal fecal flotation with zinc sulfate solution is the most sensitive fecal examination procedure for parasitic diagnosis. In a field setting, access to a centrifuge and zinc sulfate solution will likely be limited. The simple (passive) flotation technique with a homemade solution of salt or sugar is an easier alternative procedure that may be possible in many field scenarios, but will have a higher number of false negative readings compared to centrifugal flotation. Compared to direct fecal smear examination, the simple flotation technique is superior in sensitivity.

### 14.1.6.2 Required Supplies

- Microscope
- Test tubes or 12 ml syringe cases
- Holding system to keep test tubes standing upright
- Microscope slides, +/− coverslips
- Disposable cups
- Gauze sponges or strainer
- Tongue depressors or other mixing utensils
- Gram scale and/or teaspoon, tablespoon for measuring (note: 3 teaspoons = 1 tablespoon (tbsp))
- Table salt, Epsom salt, sugar, or zinc sulfate (see recipes)
- Water
- Disposable gloves.

### 14.1.6.3 Homemade Fecal Solution Recipes

In many countries, veterinary ready-made fecal flotation solution can be purchased. In cases where such solutions cannot be easily sourced, a homemade solution can be made by mixing salt or sugar in 100 ml of hot water until dissolved (Table 14.1.2). Approximately six flotations can be performed with

Table 14.1.2 Homemade fecal solution recipes [51].

| Flotation solution | Amount to add to 100 ml water | Specific gravity |
| --- | --- | --- |
| Table salt (sodium chloride) | 40 g (approximately 2.25 tbsp) | 1.20 |
| Epsom salt (magnesium sulfate) | 50 g (approximately 5 tbsp) | 1.27 |
| Sugar (granulated) | 127 g (approximately 10 tbsp) | 1.27 |
| Sodium nitrate | 40 g (approximately 3 tbsp) | 1.18–1.20 |
| Zinc sulfate | 37 g (approximately 2 tbsp) | 1.18–1.20 |

*Note: Verifying the specific gravity of the homemade solution with a hydrometer is ideal. Hydrometers designed for car batteries are often available for purchase at auto supply stores.*

100 ml of solution. Sugar solutions should be made fresh daily.

### 14.1.6.4 Simple Flotation Test Procedure

1) Wearing gloves, place 1–3 g of feces in a clean disposable cup and add approximately 15 ml of flotation solution [51]. Mix thoroughly until solution has an even consistency. One gram of feces is approximately a cube with 1 cm (1/2 in.) sides [52].
2) Pour this mixture through straining material (gauze, tea strainer, cheesecloth) and use a tongue depressor if needed to push the liquid through into a second unused cup.
3) Pour the strained mixture into a test tube. Add additional flotation solution to the tube to create a convex meniscus.
4) Place a coverslip over the meniscus. Alternatively, if coverslips are not available, place the microscope slide directly on the meniscus.
5) Wait 15–20 min for the eggs to rise to the top of the tube and onto the coverslip/slide. Remove the coverslip and place it on a slide. Scan thoroughly under a microscope initially at 10×, followed by 40× power (Figure 14.1.4).

### 14.1.6.5 Baermann Fecal Testing

*Aelurostrongylus abstrusus* (feline lungworm), *Strongyloides stercoralis* (canine intestinal threadworm), *Angiostrongylus vasorum,* and *Crenosoma vulpis* (canine lungworms) are better identified using Baermann fecal testing because their diagnostic stage is more commonly a larva and not an egg. The L1 stage larvae are often damaged in the hypertonic fecal flotation solution. In the Baermann setup, the larvae move out of the suspended feces into the water and sink to the bottom since they cannot swim. Baermann fecal testing is most commonly used when lungworm infection is suspected. Note the capillarid lungworm species, *Eucoleus boehmi* and *Eucoleus aerophilus,* are best identified through fecal flotation testing and not Baermann testing [53].

#### 14.1.6.5.1 Required Supplies

- Fresh (not refrigerated) feces, large amount (10 g) collected immediately after defecation to avoid contamination with environmental nematodes

- Disposable gloves
- Plastic disposable wine glass with a hollow stem
- Gauze or cheesecloth to wrap and hold the fecal sample
- Material to tie the fecal package: gauze strips, rubber band, hair tie, etc.
- Stick, such as a pencil, applicator stick, tongue depressor, or chopstick
- Lukewarm water
- Syringe (1 ml) with needle or pipette
- Microscope slide and cover slip
- Lugol's iodine solution (optional)
- Microscope.

#### 14.1.6.5.2 Procedure

Note: Three-day consecutive Baermann fecal testing is recommended for optimal screening due to intermittent parasite shedding [53].

1) Fill the plastic wine glass (with hollow stem) with lukewarm tap water.
2) Wearing disposable gloves, wrap 10 g of fresh feces in gauze. Secure the pouch with a gauze loop knot or rubber band.
3) Place the stick through the gauze loop knot or rubber band. Lay the stick across the wine glass rim to suspend and immerse the fecal pouch in the water.
4) Allow the sample to sit for a minimum of 8 h, preferably overnight.
5) Remove and discard the fecal pouch. Using the needle and syringe or transfer pipette, draw a small amount of fluid from the very bottom of the hollow stem.
6) Place a few drops of the fluid on the microscope slide, apply cover slip and begin microscope examination under 40× power.
7) If larvae are highly motile, a drop or more of Lugol's iodine can be applied to the edge of the coverslip to diffuse across the sample. This will kill the larvae in a straight position, allowing easier identification.

## 14.1.7 Urine Test Strips

### 14.1.7.1 General Information

Urine test strips, also known as "dipsticks," are semi-quantitative colorimetric reagent strips used for the chemical evaluation of urine. They are inexpensive,

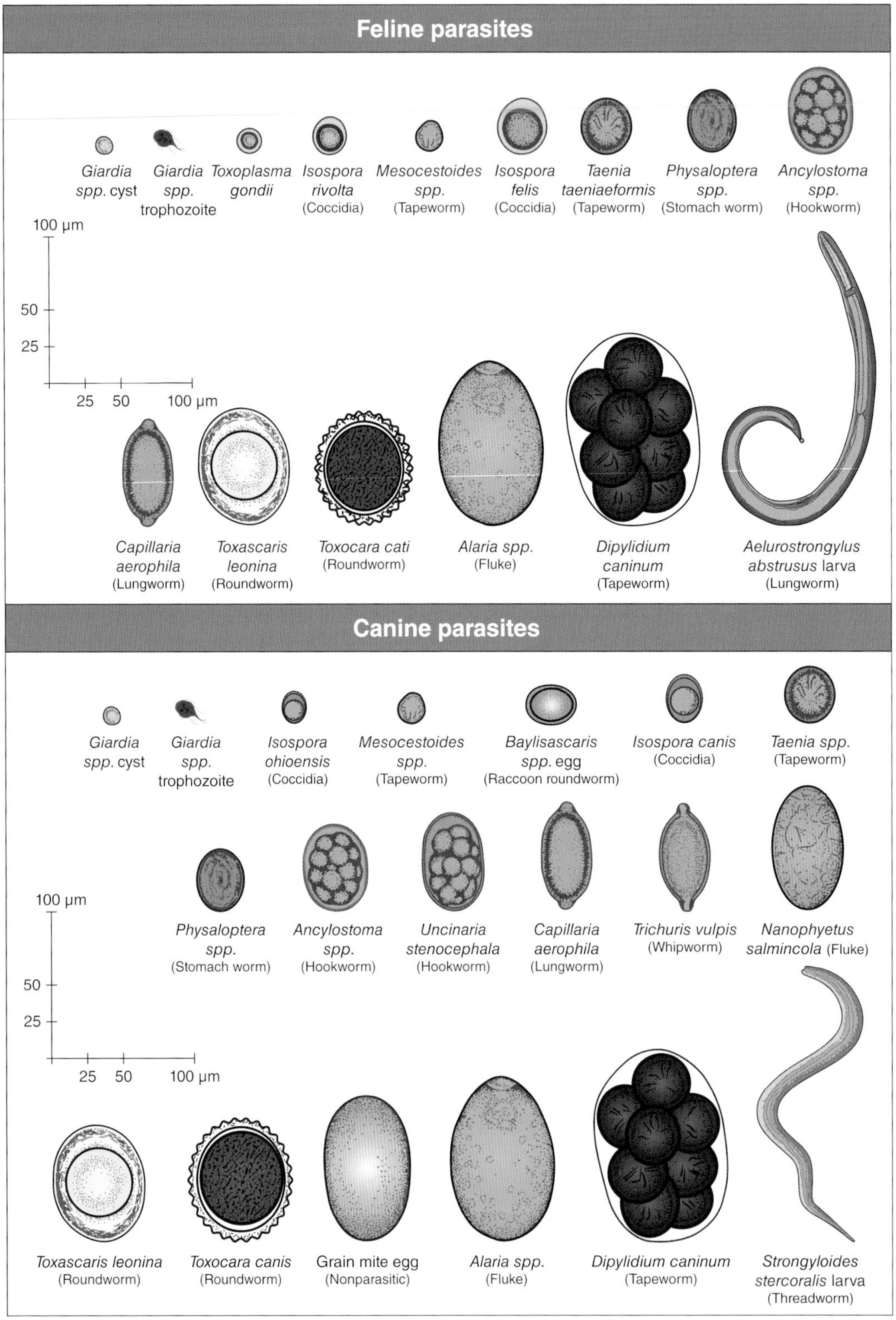

## Feline parasites

Giardia spp. cyst
Giardia spp. trophozoite
Toxoplasma gondii
Isospora rivolta (Coccidia)
Mesocestoides spp. (Tapeworm)
Isospora felis (Coccidia)
Taenia taeniaeformis (Tapeworm)
Physaloptera spp. (Stomach worm)
Ancylostoma spp. (Hookworm)

100 µm
50
25
25    50    100 µm

Capillaria aerophila (Lungworm)
Toxascaris leonina (Roundworm)
Toxocara cati (Roundworm)
Alaria spp. (Fluke)
Dipylidium caninum (Tapeworm)
Aelurostrongylus abstrusus larva (Lungworm)

## Canine parasites

Giardia spp. cyst
Giardia spp. trophozoite
Isospora ohioensis (Coccidia)
Mesocestoides spp. (Tapeworm)
Baylisascaris spp. egg (Raccoon roundworm)
Isospora canis (Coccidia)
Taenia spp. (Tapeworm)

100 µm

Physaloptera spp. (Stomach worm)
Ancylostoma spp. (Hookworm)
Uncinaria stenocephala (Hookworm)
Capillaria aerophila (Lungworm)
Trichuris vulpis (Whipworm)
Nanophyetus salmincola (Fluke)

50
25
25    50    100 µm

Toxascaris leonina (Roundworm)
Toxocara canis (Roundworm)
Grain mite egg (Nonparasitic)
Alaria spp. (Fluke)
Dipylidium caninum (Tapeworm)
Strongyloides stercoralis larva (Threadworm)

Figure 14.1.4 Fecal microscopic evaluation – Common canine and feline parasites.

portable, and easy to use. The most commonly used brand is Siemens Multistix®, which are designed for use in humans.

### 14.1.7.2 Required Supplies

- Disposable gloves.
- Test strips with storage bottle for color chart interpretation. Strips should always be stored in their container with a tight lid to keep cool and dry. Do not store in the refrigerator.
- Clean container for voided urine collection or 22 gauge needle and 3–6 ml syringe for cystocentesis.
- +/− Syringe or pipette.
- Watch or timer.

### 14.1.7.3 Test Procedure

1) Put on disposable gloves as some zoonotic diseases can be transmitted through urine.
2) Obtain a urine sample. There are two main ways to collect urine:
   - Collect a voided urine sample in a clean, dry container. Voided samples require low technical skill, are noninvasive, and have no potential for blood contamination during sampling. Disadvantages to voided samples include the potential for bacterial contamination during collection (which is mainly a concern for urine cultures, not for strip analysis).
   - Perform a cystocentesis. Cystocentesis requires moderate technical skill as complications arise from using a needle. The main advantage of this method includes the collection of a sterile sample, but there is also a risk of blood contamination.
3) Qualitatively assess the color and turbidity of the urine. A dark or highly turbid urine sample may affect certain results. Hematuria and bilirubinuria can also interfere with test results.
4) Test the urine sample within 30–60 min of collection. Refrigerated samples up to 24 h can be used, albeit less ideal, and they should be allowed to warm up to room temperature before testing. The reagent pads should not be touched, and avoid contamination with other substances or liquids. Do not use expired test strips.

   Ensure the urine sample is mixed and use a pipette or syringe to drop urine onto each reagent pad individually to avoid run-off of the reagents.

Note that the glucose reagent pad of some brands absorbs urine from the side, not the top. Alternatively, dip the strip into the urine sample, but exercise care to dab, shake, or tap off all excess urine and avoid reagent run-off into each other.

5) Align the strip in the same direction as the color comparison chart on the bottle.
6) Read the reagent pads at the time indicated by the manufacturer to avoid false results.

### 14.1.7.4 Helpful Tips Regarding Specific Urine Tests [54, 55]

- Leukocyte, nitrite, and urobilinogen reagent pads are not valid in animals and should be ignored.
- Specific gravities from urine reagent strips are often inaccurate. Specific gravity of urine should be evaluated using a refractometer.
- *pH*. The normal range is 6.0–7.0. Dogs and cats typically have slightly acidic urine. pH results on reagent strips are accurate to +/− 0.5 pH units and have minimal significance in field work.
- *Protein*. Proteinuria can be due to prerenal, renal, or postrenal causes. Increases in urine pH can cause false positive protein readings. In addition, proteinuria evaluation should be considered relative to the concentration (specific gravity) of urine. High proteinuria in a dilute urine sample is more significant than in a concentrated urine sample.
- *Glucose*. Glucosuria is an abnormal finding and can be caused by hyperglycemia (potential causes include stress, diabetes mellitus, excessive steroids, receiving glucose-(dextrose) containing intravenous fluids) or a proximal renal tubular defect. The renal threshold in dogs is 180–220 mg/dl and in cats 290 mg/dl. Stress, hyperthyroidism, some medications, acute pancreatitis, and postprandial testing can cause glucosuria from a transient hyperglycemia. Cystitis in cats and leptospirosis in dogs may also cause a false positive result.
- *Ketones*. Ketonuria is an abnormal finding and can be the result of diabetic ketoacidosis, prolonged fasting or starvation, hyperthyroidism, or eating low-carbohydrate diets (especially in cats). Ketone readings can be falsely elevated if the urine is dark-colored.
- *Bilirubin*. Low amounts of bilirubin in the urine can be normal in dogs. The presence of bilirubinuria in cats is always abnormal, suggesting a hemolytic or hepatobiliary problem.

- *Blood*. The blood reagent pad can be positive as a result of hematuria, hemoglobinuria, methemoglobinuria, or myoglobinuria. If equipment is available, centrifugation and sediment evaluation of the urine sample can differentiate hematuria if red blood cells are seen.

## 14.1.8 Portable Blood Glucose Monitor (PBGM)

### 14.1.8.1 General Information

PBGMs (glucometers) are one of the most commonly used POC tests. They are inexpensive, convenient, easy to use, and provide rapid results of blood glucose concentration. These devices work by detecting glucose via enzymatic activity through electrochemical or light detecting methods [56]. Veterinarians adopted the use of human-designed monitors for rapid blood glucose assessment in a clinic setting and for home blood glucose monitoring of diabetic patients. The application for PBGMs in the field is primarily for emergency assessment of blood glucose levels.

### 14.1.8.2 Accuracy

There are major differences among species in the distribution of glucose between red blood cells and plasma. This difference has generated concerns regarding the accuracy of using human glucometers for veterinary patients. Glucose distribution in humans is roughly equal between red blood cells (RBCs) and plasma. Dogs and cats have an uneven distribution with the majority of their glucose found in plasma (dogs 87.5%, cats 93%) [56]. However, some studies suggest that even though PBGM readings do not have exact agreement to an automated chemistry analyzer, PBGMs can be clinically acceptable for veterinary use as the differences would not alter clinical course [57]. Cohen et al. (2009) compared six PBGMs in dogs and found the lowest misclassification of results (hypoglycemic, euglycemic, or hyperglycemic) in the AlphaTrak® meter (veterinary specific) and the OneTouch meter (human) [58]. The human PBGMs consistently report blood glucose levels lower than the reference concentration, while the veterinary PBGMs may report lower or higher levels. Thus, practitioners using a human

PBGM such as OneTouch can assume that the true blood glucose concentration is higher than the reading, but this same generalization cannot be applied to the AlphaTrak system.

### 14.1.8.3 Caution Regarding Using PBGM for Diagnosis of Septic Peritonitis

A glucose concentration difference between whole blood and peritoneal fluid glucose levels greater than 20 mg/dl measured with a biochemical analyzer is often used in the diagnosis of septic peritonitis [59]. However, in a study performed by Koenig and Verlander in 2015, this concentration comparison when measured with a PBGM is not accurate in the diagnosis of septic peritonitis. Using plasma instead of whole blood with the PBGM can accurately diagnose septic peritonitis when the plasma glucose concentration to peritoneal fluid glucose concentration difference is ≥38 mg/dl [60]. Unfortunately, in the field setting, separating plasma may not be feasible, and this limits the use of a glucometer to aid in the diagnosis of septic peritonitis.

### 14.1.8.4 Required Supplies

- Glucometer kit including calibration reagent
- Test strips (unexpired) that match the glucometer
- Lancet or needle/syringe to obtain 0.3 ul to 1 ul of blood
- Note: monitors and test strips should be stored at room temperature, avoiding excessive heat and humidity.

### 14.1.8.5 Sample Test Procedure for AlphaTrak

1) Prior to use, set the date and time and calibrate according to the manufacturer's instructions. Calibration should ideally be done daily, but at a minimum whenever a new bottle of test strips is used, the battery is changed, or if the meter has been damaged [61].
2) Ensure test strips are not expired.
3) Input the appropriate code found on the bottle of strips for the species you are testing. (For OneTouch and other human devices, ensure code matches the lot number of the strips being used).
4) Insert the strip into the monitor to turn it on. The butterfly on the strip should face up and "flies into" the device.

5) Obtain a whole blood sample. For a capillary sample, use the lancet to create a small cut on the ear margin, paw pad, or inside the lip (dogs only). Alternatively, draw a venous blood sample from any accessible vein (cephalic, lateral saphenous, jugular, etc.).

6) Place only one side of the strip's collection site against the blood drop and allow the capillary action of the strip to absorb the blood. The device will "beep" and start testing once enough blood has been obtained. Only 0.3 ul of blood is needed for the AlphaTrak monitor. (In some human PBGMs the blood drop is applied to the top of the strip).

7) The results will appear within 15 s. Depending on the model, the results may be in mg/dl or mmol/l. To convert mmol/l into mg/dl multiply by 18. Values should be compared with normal reference ranges.

---

**Textbox 14.1.9  Normal blood glucose ranges**

1. Dog: 60–120 mg/dl, 3.4–6.7 mmol/l [62]
2. Cat: 75–160 mg/dl, 4.1–8.9 mmol/l

---

### 14.1.8.6  Beware of Factors Contributing to False Results

- Expired test strips should never be used.
- Input of wrong species code (veterinary models) and/or wrong lot codes (human models).
- Extreme humidity (>85%), temperature (>40 °C), and altitude.
- Extreme hypoglycemia or hyperglycemia.
- Increased packed cell volume (PCV) falsely decreases blood glucose readings.

- Decreased PCV falsely increases blood glucose readings.
- Lipemia may affect some monitors.
- Certain drugs (including tetracycline, aspirin, potassium bromide).
- Using fluoride as an anticoagulant (common in Europe, Africa, Australia) can cause lower glucose readings in some glucometers. There is no difference in results with EDTA or heparin.
- Hypertriglyceridemia (postprandial) can create a false hypoglycemia.
- Isopropyl alcohol when used on the skin should dry fully before collecting blood sample.
- Capillary blood has a 20–70 mg/dl higher glucose concentration compared to venous blood when not fasted. Fasted capillary blood sample is only 5 mg/dl higher [56].
- Whole blood and serum/plasma glucose results cannot be directly compared. Plasma sample glucose concentrations are approximately 10–15% higher than whole blood samples [56].
- The same PBGM should be used whenever making direct comparisons or monitoring trends.

### 14.1.8.7  Field-Specific Considerations

Human PBGMs and test strips are readily available through most human pharmacies. Veterinary PBGMs are only available to veterinarians through distributors. Comparing a PBGM's results with those of a chemical analyzer prior to field use can help the practitioner understand the trend and accuracy for that particular monitor. Another common use for PBGMs in the field is evaluating neonates for hypoglycemia. Note that these patients are often anemic and thus their glucose readings will be falsely elevated.

## References

1 Kost, G. (1995). Guidelines for point-of-care testing: improving patient outcomes. *American Journal of Clinical Pathology* **104**: 111–127.

2 Sensitivity Saunders Comprehensive Veterinary Dictionary, 3e. Elsevier Saunders http://medical-dictionary.thefreedictionary.com/sensitivity (accessed 1 May 2016).

3 Specificity Saunders Comprehensive Veterinary Dictionary, 3e. Elsevier Saunders http://medical-dictionary.thefreedictionary.com/specificity (accessed 1 May 2016).

4 Prevalence Saunders Comprehensive Veterinary Dictionary, 3e. Elsevier Saunders http://medical-dictionary.thefreedictionary.com/prevalence (accessed 1 May 2016).

5 SNAP® Parvo Test [package insert] (2015). IDEXX Laboratories, Inc. https://www.idexx.com/ resource-library/smallanimal/snap-parvo-pkg-insert-en.pdf (accessed 5 May 2016).

6 Anigen Rapid CPV Ag Test Kit [package insert] (2013). BioNote, Inc. Republic of Korea. http:// www.bionote.co.kr/File/Upload/2014/01/24/2014-01-24.pdf (accessed 5 May 2016).

7 Witness® CPV Test (2016). Zoetis Services LLC. https://www.zoetisus.com/products/dogs/witness-cpv-canine-parvovirus-antigen-fecal-test.aspx (accessed 5 May 2016).

8 VetScan® Rapid Tests Chart (2015). Abaxis, Inc. Union City, CA. http://www.abaxis.com/sites/ default/files/2016-02/abaxis_rapid_test_folder_kit.pdf (accessed 15 May 2016).

9 Neuerer, F., Horlacher, K., Truyen, U., and Hartmann, K. (2008). Comparison of different in-house test systems to detect parvovirus in faeces of cats. *Journal Feline Medicine and Surgery* **10** (3): 247–251.

10 Anigen Rapid FPV Ag Test Kit [package insert] (2016). BioNote, Inc. Republic of Korea. http://en.bionote.co.kr/rapid-fpv-ag-test-kit/ (accessed 19 December 2016).

11 Anigen Rapid CDV Ag Test Kit [package insert] (2013). BioNote, Inc. Republic of Korea. http:// www.bionote.co.kr/File/Upload/2014/01/24/2014-01-24(3).pdf (accessed 5 May 2016).

12 Lappin, M., Thatcher, B., Liu, J., et al. (2015). Evaluation of three in-clinic serological tests for specific detection of FeLV antigen in cats. 58th AAVLD/119th USAHA Annual Meeting. Providence.

13 SNAP® Feline Leukemia Virus Antigen-Feline Immunodeficiency Virus Antibody Test Kit [package insert] (2014). IDEXX Laboratories, Inc. https://www.idexx.com/resource-library/ smallanimal/snap-combo-package-insert-en.pdf (accessed 5 May 2016).

14 Witness® FeLV-FIV Test Kit (2016). Zoetis Services LLC. https://www.zoetisus.com/products/cats/ simplysmarterchoice.aspx (accessed 7 May 2016).

15 SNAP® 4Dx Plus [package insert] (2015). IDEXX Laboratories, Inc. https://www.idexx.com/ resource-library/smallanimal/snap-4dx-package-insert-en.pdf (accessed 7 May 2016).

16 Stillman, B., Monn, M., Liu, J. et al. (2014). Performance of a commercially available in-clinic ELISA for detection of antibodies against *Anaplasma phagocytophilum*, *Anaplasma platys*, *Borrelia burgdorferi*, *Ehrlichia canis*, and *Ehrlichia ewingii* and *Dirofilaria immitis* antigen in dogs. *Journal of the American Veterinary Medical Association* **245**: 80–86.

17 Anigen Rapid CaniV-4 Test Kit [package insert] (2015). BioNote, Inc. Republic of Korea. http:// www.bionote.co.kr/File/Upload/2015/04/17/2015-04-17(1).pdf (accessed 11 May 2016).

18 Thatcher, B., Beall, M., Liu, J., et al. (2015). Performance of the anigen rapid Caniv-4 test kit using characterized canine samples. Conference Proceedings: American College Veterinary Internal Medicine Forum.

19 Witness® Ehrlichia (2015). Zoetis Services LLC. http://diagnostics.zoetis.com/species/canine/ ehrlichia-canis/witness-ehrlichia.aspx (accessed 15 May 2016).

20 Davoust, B., Parzy, D., Demoncheaux, J.-P. et al. (2014). Usefulness of a rapid immuno-migration test for the detection of canine monocytic ehrlichiosis in Africa. *Comparative Immunology, Microbiology and Infectious Diseases* **37**: 31–37.

21 Levy, S. and Rosenfeld, A. (2015). The truth of accuracy: VetScan® Canine Ehrlichia rapid test. http://www.abaxis.com/ (accessed 10 May 2016).

22 Levy, S. and Rosenfeld, A. (2015). Performance of the Abaxis VetScan® canine anaplasma rapid test. http://www.abaxis.com/ (accessed 10 May 2016).

23 Witness® Heartworm Brochure (2013). Zoetis Services LLC. https://www.zoetisus.com (accessed 15 May 2016).

24 Aron, K., Mehra, R., Tockman, C., and Dejong, K. (2012) Canine heartworm testing – understanding low worm burden testing and a comparison of tests on the market. http://www.abaxis.com/ (accessed 11 May 2016).

25 Patterson, E., Reese, M., Tucker, S. et al. (2007). Effect of vaccination on parvovirus antigen testing in kittens. *Journal of the American Veterinary Medical Association* **230**: 359–363.

26 Kumar, S. (2015). Antigen-antibody reactions. In: Essentials of Microbiology, 112–115. London: JP Medical Ltd.

27 Day, M. and Schultz, R. (2014). Veterinary Immunology: Principles and Practice, 2e. Boca Raton, FL: CRC Press.

28 Decaro, N., Campolo, M., Desario, C. et al. (2005). Maternally-derived antibodies in pups and protection from canine parvovirus infection. *Biologicals* **33**: 261–267.

29 Schultz, R., Larson, L., and Lorentzen, L. (2008). Effects of modified live canine parvovirus vaccine on the SNAP ELISA antigen assay. In: International Veterinary Emergency Critical Symposium. Phoenix, AZ: IDEXX Laboratories http://www.idexx.no/pdf/en_ie/smallanimal/snap/parvo/parvo-abstract-vaccine-snap.pdf (accessed 1 May 2016).

30 Schmitz, S., Coene, C., König, M. et al. (2009). Comparison of three rapid commercial canine parvovirus antigen detection tests with electron microscopy and polymerase chain reaction. *Journal Veterinary Diagnostic Investigation* **21** (3): 344–345.

31 Abd-Eldaim, M., Beall, M., and Kennedy, M. (2009). Detection of feline panleukopenia virus using a commercial ELISA for canine parvovirus. *Veterinary Therapeutics* **10** (4): E1–E6.

32 Wilkes, R., Tsai, Y.-L., Lee, P.-Y. et al. (2014). Rapid and sensitive detection of canine distemper virus by one-tube reverse transcription-insulated isothermal polymerase chain reaction. *BMC Veterinary Research* **10**: 213.

33 Whitbread, T. (2015). The Merck Veterinary Manual. Kenilworth, NJ: Merck & Co., Inc. http://www.merckvetmanual.com/mvm/clinical_pathology_and_procedures/diagnostic_procedures_for_the_private_practice_laboratory/serologic_test_kits.html (accessed 5 May 2016).

34 Westman, M., Malik, R., Hall, E. et al. (2015). Determining the feline immunodeficiency virus (FIV) status of FIV-vaccinated cats using point-of-care antibody kits. *Comparative Immunology, Microbiology and Infectious Diseases* **42**: 43–52.

35 Alleman, A., Chandrashekar, R., and Beall, M. (2006). Experimental inoculation of dogs with a human isolate (Ny18) of *Anaplasma phagocytophilum* and demonstration of persistent infection following doxycycline therapy. *Journal Veterinary Internal Medicine* **20**: 763.

36 American Heartworm Society (2014). Current canine guidelines for the prevention, diagnosis, and management of heartworm (Dirofilaria immitis) infection in dogs. https:// heartwormsociety.org/images/pdf/2014-AHS-Canine-Guidelines.pdf (accessed 11 May 2016).

37 Anigen Rapid FIV Ab/FeLV Ag Test Kit [brochure] (2013). BioNote, Inc. Republic of Korea. http://www.bionote.co.kr/File/Upload/2013/03/05/2013-03-05(17).pdf (accessed 6 May 2016).

38 Richardson, J. and Gwaltney-Brant, S. (2001). Ethylene glycol toxicosis in dogs and cats. *Clinician's Brief*. http://www.cliniciansbrief.com/column/consultant-call/ethylene-glycol-toxicosis-dogs-cats (accessed 19 December 2016).

39 Little, S. (2016). August's Consultations in Feline Internal Medicine, vol. 7. St. Louis, MO: Elsevier.

40 Creighton, K., Koenigshof, A., Weder, C., and Jutkowitz, L. (2014). Evaluation of two point-of-care ethylene glycol tests for dogs. *Journal of Veterinary Emergency and Critical Care* **24** (4): 398–402.

41 Istvan, S., Marks, S., Murphy, L., and Dorman, D. (2014). Evaluation of a point-of-care anticoagulant rodenticide test for dogs. *Journal of Veterinary Emergency and Critical Care* **24** (2): 168–173.

42 Teitler, J. (2009). Evaluation of a human on-site urine multidrug test for emergency use with dogs. *Journal of American Animal Hospital Association* **45** (2): 59–66.

43 Brutlag, A (2010). Drug testing for dogs – DVM 360. http://veterinaryteam.dvm360.com/drug-testing-dogs (accessed 8 August 2016).

44 Day, M. (2013). How I treat: Serology for decision-making in core vaccination. 39th World Small Animal Veterinary Association Congress Proceedings. http://vaccicheck.com/wp-content/uploads/2012/04/WSAVA2014.pdf (accessed 9 May 2016).

45 Gray, L., Crawford, C., Levy, J., and Dubovi, E. (2012). Comparison of two assays for detection of antibodies against canine parvovirus and canine distemper virus in dogs admitted to a Florida animal shelter. *Journal of the American Veterinary Medical Association* **240** (9): 1084–1087.

46 Litster, A., Pressler, B., Volpe, A., and Dubovi, E. (2012). Accuracy of a point-of-care ELISA test kit for predicting the presence of protective canine parvovirus and canine distemper virus antibody concentrations in dogs. *Veterinary Journal* **193** (2): 363–366.

**47** Anigen Rapid CDV Ab Test Kit 2.0 [package insert] (2015). BioNote, Inc. Republic of Korea. http://www.bionote.co.kr/File/Upload/2015/04/17/2015-04-17(5).pdf (accessed 15 May 2016).

**48** Mueller, R. (2000). Dermatology for the Small Animal Practitioner. Jackson: Teton Media.

**49** Coyner, K. (2010). How to perform and interpret dermatophyte cultures. http://veterinarymedicine.dvm360.com/ (accessed 9 May 2016).

**50** Moriello, K. (2007). Fungal cultures for diagnosing dermatophytosis. *Clinician's Brief*. http://www.cliniciansbrief.com/column/procedures-pro/fungal-cultures-diagnosing-dermatophytosis (accessed 2 January 2017).

**51** Blagburn, B. (2010). Internal Parasites of Dogs and Cats Diagnostic Manual. Novartis Animal Health US, Inc.

**52** Fecal Exam Procedures (2016). CAPC Vet. http://www.capcvet.org/resource-library/fecal-exam-procedures1 (accessed 9 May 2016).

**53** Zajac, A. and Saleh, M. (2013). The Baermann test: try this parasitology test in your practice. http://veterinarymedicine.dvm360.com/ (accessed 22 August 2016).

**54** Holahan, M. (2012). The urinalysis: not just sediment and gravity. International Veterinary Emergency and Critical Care Symposium Conference Proceedings. San Antonio, TX.

**55** Alleman, R. (2014). The complete urinalysis: much more than just bladder infections. Atlantic Coast Veterinary Conference Proceedings. Atlantic City, NJ.

**56** American Society for Veterinary Clinical Pathology (2015). Quality assurance for portable blood glucose meter (glucometer) use in veterinary medicine. http://www.asvcp.org/pubs/index.cfm (accessed 10 May 2016).

**57** Johnson, B., Fry, M., Flatland, B., and Kirk, C. (2009). Comparison of a human portable blood glucose meter, veterinary portable blood glucose meter, and automated chemistry analyzer for measurement of blood glucose concentrations in dogs. *Journal of the American Veterinary Medical Association* **235** (11): 1309–1313.

**58** Cohen, T., Nelson, R., Kass, P. et al. (2009). Evaluation of six portable blood glucose meters for measuring blood glucose concentration in dogs. *Journal of the American Veterinary Medical Association* **235** (3): 276–280.

**59** Bonczynski, J., Ludwig, L., Barton, L. et al. (2003). Comparison of peritoneal fluid and peripheral blood pH, bicarbonate, glucose, and lactate concentration as a diagnostic tool for septic peritonitis in dogs and cats. *Veterinary Surgery* **32** (2): 161–166.

**60** Koenig, A. and Verlander, L. (2015). Usefulness of whole blood, plasma, peritoneal fluid, and peritoneal fluid supernatant glucose concentrations obtained by a veterinary point-of-care glucometer to identify septic peritonitis in dogs with peritoneal effusion. *Journal of the American Veterinary Medical Association* **247** (9): 1027–1032.

**61** AlphaTrak Meter Strips [package insert] (2015). Zoetis, Inc. Kalamazoo, MI. http://www.alphatrakmeter.com/PDF/Strips-2016.pdf (accessed 10 May 2016).

**62** Sodikoff, C. (2001). Laboratory Profiles of Small Animal Diseases: A Guide to Laboratory Diagnosis, 3e. St Louis, MO: Mosby.

## 14.2

# Cytology

*Laurie M. Millward*

*Department of Veterinary Clinical Sciences, College of Veterinary Medicine, 601 Vernon L. Tharp Street, Columbus, OH 43210, USA*

### 14.2.1 Introduction

This section describes the analysis of cytologic samples using minimum supplies and equipment to assist in determining accurate diagnoses and prognostic information about the patient. Techniques to maximize diagnostic yield from samples are covered. Practical interpretations of skin cytology, ear cytology, blood smears, and vaginal cytology are described to diagnose various infectious, inflammatory, neoplastic, and other pathological processes in dogs and cats. This information is presented to guide a veterinarian working in the field with limited resources to best utilize these helpful diagnostic specimens to practice high-quality medicine.

Cytology should always be interpreted in conjunction with information about the patient derived from a thorough history and physical examination. In addition, purchasing one or two cytology textbooks or picture atlases can greatly help with interpretation of cytologic specimens. The advantages of cytology are many: the necessary materials are inexpensive and readily available; you can sample a wide variety of tissues; the procedure is minimally invasive; rapid interpretation of samples can be made to establish provisional or definitive diagnoses; it can expedite decision-making with regard to triaging patients and managing infectious disease; and it helps to provide a high quality of medical care. Limitations of cytology should however be considered: it is often used as a screening tool; some neoplastic processes may require histopathology for definitive diagnosis; and diagnostic quality samples may not be easily obtained in some situations.

It is important to emphasize that your interpretation and diagnostic capabilities are only as good as your equipment. A good-quality microscope is essential. If cost is a concern, many high-performance refurbished instruments are available for sale at discounted prices. Ideally, the microscope should have 10×, 40×, and 100× objectives at a minimum. A commonly forgotten point is that a coverslip is needed for optimal viewing using the 40× objective. The microscope should be regularly cleaned and inspected to protect it from wear and tear.

In addition, purchasing appropriate stains is necessary for optimal cytology interpretation, and the stain should be maintained properly. Commonly used polychromatic aqueous Romanowsky quick stains include Diff-Quik® (Diff-Quik Differential Stain Set; Fisher Scientific, Waltham, MA, USA) and Quik-Dip™ (Mercedes Medical). These stains can be used to stain superficial skin cytology, ear cytology, vaginal cytology, blood smears, and fine needle aspirate (FNA) specimens. It is recommended that you maintain a clean stain set for blood smears, lymph node aspirates, and FNA specimens and a separate stain set for "dirty" samples that may have bacterial or fungal organisms such as dry-mount fecal cytology, ear cytology, vaginal cytology, suspected abscesses, and skin cytology. The stain should be replaced every 7 days or more frequently if it is used heavily. Diff-Quik may unreliably stain mast cell granules, basophil granules, or cytotoxic lymphocyte granules because the granule contents may be washed away by the water-diluted stain solution [1]. Interestingly, Diff-Quik is better than Wright or Giemsa stains to visualize canine distemper virus inclusion bodies in

*Field Manual for Small Animal Medicine*, First Edition. Edited by Katherine Polak and Ann Therese Kommedal.
© 2018 John Wiley & Sons, Inc. Published 2018 by John Wiley & Sons, Inc.

white and red blood cells in blood smears from infected patients [2].

The author recommends the following staining protocol for quick stains: 60 s in the fixative solution; 30 s in solution 1; 30 s in solution 2. There is no need to rinse with water between the different solutions. Water is used at the end of the staining protocol when a slow steady stream is used to gently rinse the slide for 15–20 s. The slide is then propped up vertically to allow for proper drainage, or a hair dryer can be set on low heat to dry the slide more quickly. Excess stain or smoke from the lighter can be removed from the back of the slide with alcohol-moistened gauze.

A good cytology kit to use in the field contains the items listed in Table 14.2.1. Some of the items you may already have in a field kit. Pencils are preferred

Table 14.2.1 Suggested equipment for a field cytology kit.

| Equipment | Number |
| --- | --- |
| Pencil | 2 |
| Sharpie | 1 |
| Frosted glass slides | 1 box |
| Glass coverslips | 1 box |
| #10 Scalpel blades | 10 blades |
| Skin-scraping spatula | 2 |
| Powder-free gloves | 6 pairs |
| Clear adhesive acetate tape | 1 roll |
| Lighter or matches | 1 |
| Mineral oil | 1 plastic/unbreakable vial with dropper |
| Alcohol or alcohol swabs | 1 or several packets |
| 3 ml to 6 ml syringes with 22 G needles | 12 |
| Red top tubes without serum separator | 4 |
| Purple top EDTA tubes | 4 |
| Capillary tubes | 1 box |
| Mosquito hemostats | 1 |
| Tissue forceps | 1 |
| Sterile culture swabs with test medium | 4 |
| Gauze 4 × 4 sponges | 10–20 |
| Cotton-tipped swabs | 10–20 |
| Plastic slide box (holds 3–4 slides each) | 3 |
| Syringes containing saline flush | 4 |
| Clippers with charged battery | 1 |

over Sharpies to label slides. Sharpies will often dissolve when immersed in the alcohol fixative in quick stain kits, which can cause specimens to become unlabeled. Sharpies are helpful for labeling blood tubes. Frosted glass slides are recommended over non-frosted slides so that you can quickly identify which side of the slide your sample is on for more efficient sample preparation and interpretation. Never use previously used washed glass slides. Powder-free gloves are preferred because glove powder can contaminate and produce artifacts in cytology samples. Saline flush syringes are helpful to moisten cotton-tipped swabs when obtaining certain specimens such as vaginal cytology.

## 14.2.2 Cytologic Specimens

### 14.2.2.1 Cytology of the Skin

#### 14.2.2.1.1 Sample Preparation

##### 14.2.2.1.1.1 Skin Cytology

Skin cytology is used to identify yeast, bacteria, inflammatory cells, acantholytic cells, and neoplastic cells in lesions from patients with dermatologic disease. Skin cytology specimen preparation is simple and requires a few inexpensive materials. Gloves should always be worn when sampling exudative lesions or draining tracts. Three techniques can be used to acquire skin cytology samples.

The first method is a direct impression smear of the lesion. This method is the best for moist or exudative lesions. The area of the skin that is to be sampled is gently elevated by lightly pinching the surrounding skin. A clean glass slide is gently pressed onto the skin with care being given to not break the slide by applying pressure to the center of the slide (rather than holding the slide on the edge when pressing it on the skin). The sample is gently heat fixed if it is not wet or exudative in nature and then is stained using the standard quick stain protocol. If the sample is moist in nature, allow the sample to thoroughly dry on the slide and then directly proceed with staining.

A second method involves application of clear tape or acetate tape to the lesion. This method is helpful when scaly lesions are being analyzed or when superficial mites such as *Sarcoptes scabiei* or *Cheyletiella* are a concern. If *S. scabiei* is a differential diagnosis, a superficial skin scraping is recommended as well. If you desire to stain the acetate tape sample to evaluate the cellular population, do not use the fixative step in the quick stain kit because it may ruin the tape. Proceed with the other two steps of staining as usual, and then allow the tape to dry. Place a drop of immersion oil on a clean glass slide, apply the stained acetate tape prep to the oil drop, and then view under the microscope. Alternatively, you can add one drop of the third, dark blue stain in standard quick stain kits to the glass slide and then press the tape over this drop.

The last method involves the use of a skin-scraping spatula or the dulled edge of a #10 scalpel blade. This method is useful for both moist and dry skin lesions. The skin is gently scraped in the direction of hair growth and the collected debris is gently smeared onto the center of a clean glass slide. Skin-scraping spatulas are especially helpful for areas that are tricky to sample such as nail beds, interdigital regions, and facial folds. Do not use excessive force when transferring the material to the glass slide because this may break white blood cells and make interpretation challenging. Gently heat fix skin cytology samples that are not exudative in nature and stain using the normal quick stain protocol. If samples are moist, it is best to air dry the samples prior to staining.

For all skin cytology samples, first scan the sample at low power using a 4× or 10× objective to assess where there are cellular areas of the slide and the type and behavior of cells present. Further analysis is then performed at a higher power (40× objective with coverslip or 100× objective with oil) to determine if microorganisms are present and to further analyze subtle features of the cells.

#### 14.2.2.1.1.2 Superficial Skin Scraping

Superficial skin scrapings are different from skin cytology and should be done on any pruritic patient to aid in identifying *S. scabiei* mites that live in the most superficial layer of the epithelium called the stratum corneum. Materials needed for a superficial skin scraping include a dulled #10 scalpel blade, glass slides, mineral oil, and a coverslip. Running the sharp edge of the blade over a metal surface can dull the scalpel blade prior to scraping. The skin is gently retracted and the blade is used to scrape skin and debris from areas where clinical signs are present. Usually, the ear margins, elbows, and hocks are sampled in patients with suspected *S. scabiei.*

Diagnostic yield is greatest when a large surface area of skin is sampled. The collected debris is transferred to the center of a clean glass slide. A drop of mineral oil is placed over the debris, a coverslip is placed over this material, and then the sample can be viewed using a 10× objective. The entire area under the coverslip should be examined.

#### 14.2.2.1.1.3 Deep Skin Scrape

A deep skin scrape is necessary when *Demodex* spp. infestation is a differential diagnosis. *Demodex* spp. mites live within the hair follicles, sebaceous glands, and superficial layers of the epithelium. Materials needed for a deep skin scraping include a dulled #10 scalpel blade, glass slides, mineral oil, and a coverslip. Running the sharp edge of the blade over a metal surface can dull the scalpel blade prior to scraping. The skin is scraped firmly with the dulled edge of a #10 scalpel blade until a small amount of capillary bleeding is noted. In between the scrapes, the area of skin being sampled should be firmly squeezed to move the mites out of the lumen of the hair follicles and sebaceous gland ducts. The debris is collected and then smeared onto the center of a clean glass slide. A single drop of mineral oil is then placed over the debris and a coverslip is then added. Evaluation for *Demodex* spp. mites is best performed using the 10× objective and the entire area under the coverslip should be examined.

### 14.2.2.1.2 Evaluation of Skin Cytology

#### 14.2.2.1.2.1 Normal Skin Cytology and Common Artifacts

Normal skin cytology samples contain a variable number of superficial non-nucleated squamous epithelial cells, occasional nucleated keratinocytes, keratinaceous debris, free melanin granules, and rare hair shafts. White blood cells, acantholytic cells, and parasitic organisms are not seen in health. In addition, bacteria and yeast compose normal skin flora. Bacteria or yeast can be present and are determined to be a normal finding as long as they are rare (<2 bacteria on average per oil immersion 100× objective field; <2 yeast on average per HPF (40× objective)), the patient is asymptomatic, and no white blood cells are present [3–5].

Common artifacts seen with skin cytology samples can confuse interpretation for inexperienced personnel. Scratches on the slide can occur when slides contact each other during the staining process or when the sample surface of the slide is wiped. Scratches appear as clear linear streaks in the stained background of the sample. Lubricants used for rectal examinations or ultrasound gel can create multifocal variably sized aggregates of magenta to deep purple amorphous to globular debris in the background. This material will not be seen within cells. If it is present in high enough amounts, the staining of nearby cells can be compromised since this material more readily absorbs stain. Stain precipitate is often confused for bacteria. Stain precipitate appears as a basophilic to deep purple extracellular granular material. The precipitate is of subtle variation in size and shape, whereas bacteria appear consistent in size, shape, and staining intensity. Glove powder can be confused for fungal elements or pollen. It appears as a turquoise to light blue, refractile, 30–40 µm in diameter, polyhedral to irregularly shaped structure with a distinctive cross mark in the center. Synthetic fibers can be mistaken for fungal hyphae. They appear as linear structures that vary in width and staining intensity. This is in contrast to fungal hyphae, which are of consistent width and staining intensity throughout the entire length.

#### 14.2.2.1.2.2 Noninfectious Inflammatory Processes

**Pemphigus Foliaceus**   The autoimmune skin disease Pemphigus foliaceus is characterized by the loss of intercellular adhesion of cells in the epidermis. It can occur spontaneously or secondary to chronic illness or medications. It is the most common autoimmune skin disease in dogs and cats. Patients will present with erythematous macules that turn into pustules that rupture and form crusts [6]. Lesions are usually located on the face, nose, inner pinnae, and feet, although other locations such as the neck and trunk can be involved. Patients may be febrile and lethargic, and the lesions are painful to the touch. Removing one of the crusts and making an impression smear can aid in the diagnosis of this condition. The presence of acantholytic cells is the hallmark cytologic finding. Acantholytic cells are keratinocytes that are oval in shape, stain deeply basophilic, and contain round to oval, centralized nuclei. Numerous nondegenerate neutrophils are seen. Bacteria usually are not present. Other cells such as eosinophils may be seen rarely.

**Eosinophilic Granuloma Complex**   Feline eosinophilic granuloma complex is a collection of eosinophilic cutaneous reactions that include feline eosinophilic plaque, indolent ulcers, and feline eosinophilic granulomas. These reactions are type 1 hypersensitivity reactions to allergic triggers such as insects, environmental allergens, foreign bodies, and dietary allergens. Spontaneous and idiopathic cases may also occur. Histopathology is viewed as the gold standard for a definitive diagnosis; however, skin cytology may be helpful for arriving at a working diagnosis in the field. It is important to note that these lesions can mimic other infectious and neoplastic processes such as squamous cell carcinoma or cutaneous epitheliotropic T-cell lymphoma, which are described elsewhere [6].

Feline eosinophilic plaque is an inflammatory skin disease seen in cats that has been associated with flea allergy dermatitis, cutaneous adverse food reaction, and atopic dermatitis. Clinical signs include focal or multifocal areas of hair loss that become ulcerated and erosive with exudation and crusting. The lesions are extremely pruritic and are commonly located on the head, neck, abdomen, perianal region, and medial thighs. Superficial skin cytology taken from these lesions will contain a high number of eosinophils and mast cells along with neutrophils and bacteria if secondary infection occurs. An attempt to identify and remove the allergic trigger should be made.

Indolent ulcers, also called "rodent ulcers," are focal unilateral or bilateral erosive skin lesions located on the upper lip. These lesions are associated with allergic responses to insects, foreign body reactions, or *Microsporum canis*. Indolent ulcers appear as centrally flattened to concave lesions with raised edges and are reddish-brown to yellow in color. They are usually not pruritic or painful to the patient. In the author's experience, superficial skin cytology from these lesions usually is poorly cellular and contains a low number of nondegenerate neutrophils and eosinophils. Skin cytology is also helpful in ruling out secondary yeast and bacterial infections as well as neoplastic processes.

Eosinophilic granulomas can have a variety of presentations. They may occur on the caudal thighs, chin, and footpads, as well as in the oral cavity. They too are thought to occur secondary to allergic diseases. The lesions on the caudal thighs are asymptomatic and appear yellow to rarely erythematous, linear, hard, variably alopecic, non-inflammatory swellings. Chin granulomas are firm asymptomatic swellings of the chin. Eosinophilic granulomas in the oral cavity are ulcerated and proliferative and may produce signs of dysphagia, coughing, or drooling. Superficial skin cytology of non-ulcerated eosinophilic granuloma lesions is usually nondiagnostic due to poor cellularity, and a fine needle biopsy is usually more helpful. Superficial cytology from the oral cavity eosinophilic granulomas that are ulcerated may yield sufficient cells for a working diagnosis in the field. A mixed inflammatory cell population is seen consisting of neutrophils, macrophages, lymphocytes, plasma cells, eosinophils, and mast cells. Surgical removal of focal lesions and removal of the responsible allergen are both recommended.

#### 14.2.2.1.2.3 *Infectious Inflammatory Processes*

**Bacterial Infections**  A variety of bacteria can cause bacterial skin infections or pyoderma. *Staphylococcus* spp. are the most common bacterial organisms isolated from pyoderma lesions. It is important to remember that there is likely an underlying primary cause such as allergies or endocrine disease that has allowed for the development of pyoderma. Patients with bacterial skin infections present with papules, pustules, military dermatitis, epidermal collarettes, and excessive scaling. Impression smears of exudative lesions or of a recently ruptured pustule yield the most diagnostic results. Acetate tape preparations may be more diagnostic for the cases of pyoderma that are more dry and scaly. Skin cytology cannot identify the species of bacteria that are present in lesions, but it can distinguish cocci from rod bacteria. Bacterial culture is needed to identify the bacterial species and to perform susceptibility testing. In dogs, an overgrowth of bacteria is determined when there are more than two bacteria on average per oil immersion 100× objective field [3, 5]. Exudative lesions will show a variable number of neutrophils, eosinophils, and intra- and extracellular bacteria. Deep pyodermas may have a mixed inflammatory cell population such as macrophages, lymphocytes, plasma cells, and neutrophils. Deep pyodermas frequently have a lower number of bacteria, which tend to be mostly intracellular in location on cytology. Neutrophils may exhibit degenerative changes when bacteria are present such as karyolysis, karyorrhexis, vacuolated

cytoplasm, and pyknotic nuclei. Finding intracellular bacteria within white blood cells from the lesion is strongly suggestive of a bacterial infection rather than bacterial contamination of the sample. If neutrophils or intracellular bacteria are not seen, pyoderma is less likely.

It is important to not confuse melanin granules or stain precipitate for bacteria in skin cytology samples. Melanin granules are golden brown to black in color. Stain precipitate is usually magenta to purple in color. Melanin and stain precipitate can be distinguished from bacteria because they are refractile with subtle adjustments of the fine focus. Melanin granules and stain precipitate are haphazardly arranged, whereas bacteria are arranged in clusters or chains. In addition, melanin and stain precipitate will have subtle variations in size, shape, and staining intensity, whereas bacteria will have a consistent size, shape, and color (Figure 14.2.1).

**Select Fungal Diseases**  *Malassezia* spp  As with bacterial skin infections, the majority of *Malassezia* spp. skin infections are due to an underlying primary cause such as allergies or endocrine diseases. Attempts to identify an underlying cause should be performed in addition to treating the skin infection. Patients that have *Malassezia* dermatitis are pruritic. They may present with skin that is erythematous, scaly, waxy, greasy, or crusty. A yeasty odor is often present. Patients may also present with chin acne, paronychia, and intertrigo. Chronic cases of *Malassezia* dermatitis may present with markedly lichenified and hyperpigmented skin. Many dogs with *Malassezia* dermatitis have concurrent *Staphylococcus* spp. pyoderma. *Malassezia* yeast are round to oval and may be peanut shaped if they are budding. They most often occur in clusters or are adhered to keratinocytes. In general, they measure 3–8 μm in diameter. Sources vary greatly in the definitive number of yeast organisms per high-power field to diagnose *Malassezia* dermatitis [4,7,8]. In addition, the number of yeast will vary significantly depending on the breed of dog and by location on the body [9,10]. Treatment is advised when more than two yeast on average per 40× objective field or more than one yeast per oil immersion 100× objective field are seen. Dogs with hypersensitivity reactions to *Malassezia* spp. should be treated even if rare yeast are found.

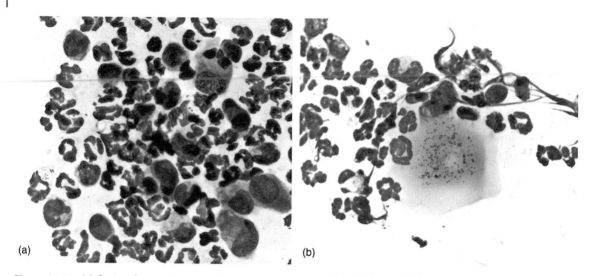

(a)

(b)

Figure 14.2.1 (a) Canine deep pyoderma – impression smear of exudate. A highly cellular sample that consists of primarily degenerative neutrophils that exhibit karyolysis and karyorrhexis. Note the intracellular cocci and rod-shaped bacteria. Rare extracellular cocci are present. There are moderate numbers of epithelioid macrophages, one of which is exhibiting leukophagia, or phagocytosis of a white blood cell. (Diff-Quik; 1000× oil). (b) Canine deep pyoderma and melanin granules – impression smear of exudate. Same case as in (a). A single non-nucleated squamous epithelial cell is in the middle. Note the abundant brownish-black melanin granules arranged haphazardly within the cell. Rare extracellular bacteria are present. Numerous degenerative neutrophils exhibiting karyolysis and karyorrhexis. Some cells are broken, which have created nuclear streaming. (Diff-Quik; 1000× oil). Source: Courtesy of Laurie. M. Millward, The Ohio State University.

***Sporothrix schenckii*** *Sporothrix schenckii* is a saprophytic fungal organism that can be associated with immunosuppression and may present in cutaneous, systemic, and cutaneolymphatic forms. It should always be a differential diagnosis for cats with non-healing fight wounds. Cats infected with *S. schenckii* may present with fight wound abscesses, draining tracts, or cellulitis. The nodular lesions usually ulcerate, rupture, drain a purulent material, and then crust over. Extensive necrosis and spread to other areas of the body are possible. It is zoonotic. Dogs usually have cutaneous nodules or ulcerated plaques with raised edges. Draining tracts may occur. The skin lesions are usually not painful or pruritic. Cytology of impression smears of the skin lesions will show marked neutrophilic, pyogranulomatous, or mixed inflammation. The yeast organisms are round, oval, or have a characteristic cigar shape and measure approximately 5–9 μm in length. They have a thin clear halo and pale blue cytoplasm. The yeast may be located intracellularly or extracellularly. They are more often seen in cases of *S. schenckii* infection in cats rather than in dogs. A working diagnosis can be made by viewing the organisms on cytology. A definitive diagnosis is made via fungal culture.

***Blastomyces Dermatitidis*** *Blastomyces dermatitidis* is a fungal infection of dogs and rarely cats that is most frequent in the Ohio and Mississippi River regions and in Canada. Clinical signs in dogs may include anorexia, weight loss, respiratory signs, lameness, skin disease/lesions, and ocular signs. Skin lesions may take the form of nodules, papules, plaques, ulcers, draining tracts, and abscesses. In cats, respiratory signs, weight loss, ocular disease (uveitis), and skin lesions are the most common clinical signs. Draining tracts, especially around the digits, are common. Cytology of impressions of the skin lesions reveals marked pyogranulomatous to granulomatous inflammation. Numerous degenerate neutrophils, macrophages, multinucleated giant cells, and lymphocytes are present. The yeast form is round to oval and measures 7–30 μm in diameter. The cell wall is thick and refractile. One can remember the description of *Blastomyces* yeast by the phrase "big, blue, broad-based budding." The yeast have broad-based budding compared to other fungal pathogens and are deeply basophilic (see Figure 14.2.2). Antigen-based urine tests, serology, tissue culture, or immunostaining of biopsy specimens can provide a definitive diagnosis.

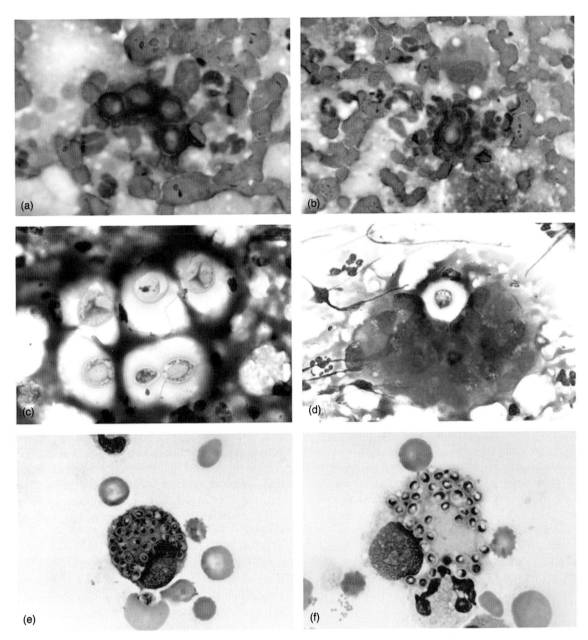

**Figure 14.2.2** (a) *Blastomyces dermatitidis* – aspirate of feline skin lesion. (a and b) Large, thickly encapsulated, deeply basophilic yeast forms of *Blastomyces dermatitidis* are demonstrating broad-based budding in a moderately hemodiluted background that contains numerous neutrophils and activated macrophages. (Wright-Giemsa; 1000× oil). (c and d) *Cryptococcus spp.* – impression smear of a feline skin lesion. (c) Multiple yeast organisms are seen taking up the majority of the field. The yeast are approximately 10–15 μm in diameter, are round to oval, and have an extremely thick nonstaining capsule surrounding them. One yeast is exhibiting the characteristic narrow-based budding that is distinctive for *Cryptococcus spp.* The background is very thick and composed primarily of red blood cells, foamy activated macrophages, and neutrophils. (Wright-Giemsa; 1000× oil). (d) Same case as in (a). One nonbudding yeast organism is seen and a multinucleated giant cell is adjacent to it and appears to be trying to engulf it. Numerous broken red blood cells and neutrophils are seen in the background. (Wright-Giemsa; 1000× oil). (e and f) *Histoplasma capsulatum* – impression smear of canine skin lesion. (e and f) Macrophages contain numerous *Histoplasma capsulatum* yeast forms that are round to oval in shape, measure 2–4 μm in diameter, and have a thin clear halo with basophilic internal contents. This patient was simultaneously infected with the extracellular red blood cell parasite, *Mycoplasma haemocanis,* which can be seen as small, 0.5–1 μm in diameter, round, basophilic structures that are free in the background. (Wright-Giemsa; 1000× oil). Source: Courtesy of Laurie. M. Millward, The Ohio State University.

*Coccidiomycosis (Valley Fever)* *Coccidioides immitis* is another saprophytic fungal organism that is endemic in the southwestern regions of the United States. Infected dogs will present with respiratory signs, fever, anorexia, weight loss, lameness, skin disease, or ocular disease. Cats may present with anorexia, fever, weight loss, respiratory signs, lameness, skin lesions, or ocular lesions. Cytology of impression smears show neutrophilic to pyogranulomatous inflammation. Thick-walled spherules may be seen on cytology. They are 20–200 µm in diameter, deeply basophilic, and contain many uninucleate round endospores. The endospores may be seen when the spherules rupture and measure 2–5 µm in diameter. The ruptured spherules may resemble *Blastomyces* and the endospores may resemble *Histoplasma*. *Coccidioides* yeast are usually much larger than *Blastomyces* yeast. Fungal culture and tissue culture are not recommended due to the risk of human infection via inhalation. Serological testing is helpful for diagnosis and for monitoring response to treatment.

*Cryptococcosis* Cryptococcosis is seen most often in tropical or subtropical regions and in locations with bird droppings. It infects both dogs and cats. Skin lesions may present as nodules, crusts, draining tracts, or erosions that commonly occur in or on the nose and face. Impression smears of the lesions reveal granulomatous inflammation that consists primarily of macrophages, lymphocytes, and multinucleated giant cells. The yeast form is approximately 4–10 µm diameter, is round to oval, and has a thick nonstaining capsule with narrow-based budding (see Figure 14.2.2). Immunostaining of biopsy specimens, latex agglutination tests, serology, or fungal culture can provide a definitive diagnosis.

*Histoplasmosis* *Histoplasma capsulatum* is another saprophytic fungal pathogen that is common in the Ohio, Missouri, and Mississippi River valleys. Clinical signs in dogs include anorexia, weight loss, fever, respiratory signs, GI signs, ocular disease, and rarely skin lesions. Skin lesions may include papules, nodules, ulcers, and draining tracts. In cats, clinical signs include anorexia, weight loss, fever, lethargy, respiratory signs, ocular signs, and skin lesions such as papules, nodules, ulcer, and draining tracts. Impression smears of skin lesions may reveal mixed inflammatory cells that consist mostly of macrophages with lesser numbers of plasma cells, lymphocytes, and multinucleated giant cells. The yeast form may be found intracellularly or extracellularly. They are round to oval in shape, measure 2–4 µm in diameter, and have a thin clear halo with basophilic internal contents and are similar in appearance to the yeast *Sporothrix*, but do not form the cigar-shape characteristic of *Sporothrix*.

**Parasitic** *Scabies* *S. scabiei* is a highly transmissible cause of nonseasonal extremely pruritic skin disease in dogs and cats. It is zoonotic. Young dogs tend to be more frequently affected. The ventral abdomen and chest, elbows, hocks, feet, face, and ear pinnae are most often affected. The lesions on the ear usually start at the tip of the pinna and then move down toward the head. Lesions begin as crusted papules and become more pruritic as they increase in number and distribution. Patients may have erythema, alopecia, thick yellow crusting, excoriations, or a diffuse papular rash. Lymphadenopathy is usually present. Asymptomatic carriers are possible. Cats may present with pruritus localized to the pinna and face, crusted papular dermatitis, pododermatitis, scale, and alopecia from overgrooming with no skin lesions.

Diagnosis is made with superficial skin scraping that involves sampling a large surface area of the affected sites on the body. Ideal locations to sample are areas that have not been excoriated. The ear margins, elbows, and hocks are most often the best areas to scrape because of the high number of mites found in these regions. A single mite, egg, or even dark brown, oval fecal pellet of *S. scabiei* is diagnostic. Eggs are oval to ellipsoid and approximately 230 µm long. Adults are approximately 300–500 µm long. The females have eight legs and the third and fourth pairs of legs have long setae. The males also have eight legs but have setae only on the third pair of legs. Both male and female adult mites have multiple large triangular spines on the dorsum. A negative cytology result does not rule out *S. scabiei* as a differential diagnosis. If *S. scabiei* mites are suspected, then a therapeutic trial of selamectin dosed at 2 week intervals for a total of three doses is recommended.

*Demodectic Mange* *Demodex* spp. mites cause dermatitis in dogs and cats when they occur in excess. These mites live in hair follicles and sebaceous gland ducts. In localized cases of canine demodicosis, the patient presents with patchy areas of partial alopecia and erythema. The lesions may or may not be pruritic. In generalized demodicosis, the patient may present with widespread numerous lesions that worsen over time. Secondary skin infections, lymphadenopathy, seborrheic changes, and follicular casts may be present. A hereditary or immune system disorder is often involved with generalized demodicosis cases. *D. gatoi*, *D. cati*, and an unnamed species, *D. sp.*, are species of *Demodex* that have been associated with skin disease and pruritus in cats. Cats may have localized or generalized lesions, and the disease can also be limited to the ears causing an extremely pruritic otitis. It is recommended that all cats with confirmed or suspected demodectic mange be tested for FeLV/FIV.

A properly performed deep skin scrape as described above is used to diagnose *Demodex* spp. infestations. Multiple sites should be examined and scraped. The absence of mites in a deep scrape sample does not rule out *Demodex* spp. as a cause for the patient's symptoms. A diagnosis of demodectic mange is made if increased numbers of immature forms of the mite such as ova, larvae, and nymphs are seen compared to adults or if large numbers of adult mites are seen. However, low numbers of mites should not be ignored because it is rare that *Demodex* spp. mites are seen when healthy skin is sampled. One must take into account history, signalment, and clinical signs in cases with low numbers of mites in order to arrive at an accurate diagnosis. The adult mites are cigar shaped and have six to eight stubby legs (see Figure 14.2.3). Canine *Demodex* species can vary in length from 180 to 210 μm for *D. canis*, 330 to 370 μm for *D. injai*, and 90 to 140 μm for *Demodex* sp. *"cornei."* Feline *Demodex* species can vary in length from 181 to 219 μm for *D. cati*, 81 to 115 μm for *D. gatoi*, and 170–174 μm for *Demodex sp.*

*Cheyletiella* *Cheyletiella* mites (otherwise known as walking dandruff) live on the surface of the skin of cats, dogs, rabbits, and humans. They cause a range of clinical signs that include an asymptomatic infestation to an intensely pruritic dermatitis. A variable amount of scaling and hair loss may also occur. Cats may have miliary dermatitis lesions and may have subtle clinical signs due to grooming and removal of mites and scale. Diagnosis can be achieved by collecting scale and debris with a scalpel or skin-scraping spatula, acetate tape, or a flea comb. The fur and scale can be evaluated in two ways to visualize Cheyletiella mites [5]. In the first method, the fur and scale are

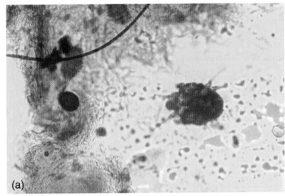

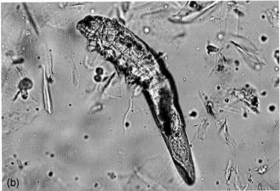

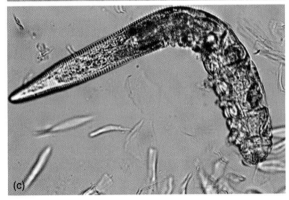

**Figure 14.2.3** *Sarcoptes* and *Demodex* mites. (a) *Sarcoptes scabiei-* superficial skin scrape of canine skin. An adult *S. Scabiei* mite is visible along with one egg (near the green arrow). The background contains keratinaceous debris and a hair. Eggs are oval to ellipsoid and approximately 230 μm long. Adults are approximately 300–500 μm long. (Mineral oil immersion; 100×). Source: Courtesy Dr. Amy Schnedeker, The Ohio State University. (b and c) *Demodex spp.* – deep skin scrape of canine skin. (b) An adult *Demodex canis* mite is present. Note the cigar-shaped body and eight stubby legs. *D. canis* ranges in length from 180 to 210 μm, and has a stubbier tail than *D. injai*. (c) An adult *D. injai* mite is present. It too has a cigar-shaped body and eight stubby legs, but it is longer in length at a range of 330–370 μm. Note the longer tail in this species of Demodex. (Mineral oil immersion; 400× for both images) Source: Courtesy of Dr. Sandra Diaz Vergara, The Ohio State University.

placed in a petri dish, immersed in mineral oil, and then visualized using a dissecting microscope. The second method involves applying 10% potassium hydroxide to the sample, immersing the solution in a warm water bath for 30 min, adding fecal flotation solution, and then centrifuging the sample at 1500-rpm for 10 min. A coverslip is placed over the solution after it is centrifuged, and then the surface solution is examined under low power for mites and eggs. In animals that ingest the mites or eggs, a fecal analysis can also be diagnostic. *Cheyletiella* eggs measure $230\,\mu m \times 100\,\mu m$, are often embryonated, and can bear a resemblance to hook worm eggs when visualized using fecal flotation [5]. Adult *Cheyletiella* mites are large, measure $500\,\mu m$ long, are visible to the unaided eye, and have large palpal claws. Lack of mites seen via a fecal analysis and microscopic examination of scale and fur do not rule out *Cheyletiella*. If the patient has clinical signs consistent with Cheyletiella infestation, then a therapeutic trial can be performed using selamectin applied at 14 day intervals for several doses.

### 14.2.2.2 Ear Cytology

Ear cytology is a valuable tool to use when patients have clinical signs of otitis externa. Clinical signs of otitis externa include scratching at the ears, shaking the head, erythema, and waxy or suppurative ear exudate. Ear mite infestations usually create a copious amount of dark brown crumbly discharge. Some cats with ear mites may have scabs in various stages of healing on the external surfaces of the base of the ear pinnae due to scratching. Bacterial infections often are associated with erythema and increased heat of the pinnae and external ear canal. Yeast otitis externa is often associated with a brown, moist, malodorous exudate. Ear cytology should always be interpreted in conjunction with the patient's clinical signs. Some otic cytology samples do not have enough material for cytologic interpretation and some do not have microscopically visible yeast or bacteria despite the patient displaying clinical signs of otitis. It is up to the discretion of the clinician whether or not to treat in such cases.

The purposes of ear cytology are to identify primary and secondary causes of otitis externa and to reduce the time to resolution of infections. Once the causes of otitis have been identified microscopically, a suitable treatment regimen can then be implemented. In addition, ear cytology is helpful in monitoring response to treatment. Recheck ear cytology samples help the clinician determine if an ear infection has resolved or if further or different treatment is warranted.

Ear cytology sample acquisition should always be performed prior to cleaning the ears. If recheck ear cytology samples are being collected, it is best to wait to collect these samples after topical ear medications have been discontinued for 2 to 3 days. It is recommended that samples are obtained from both ears, even if one ear appears normal clinically. A thorough otoscopic examination prior to sample collection is also recommended. Otoscopic examination of the ears serves to evaluate the condition of the ear; look for any masses or foreign bodies; note the presence, consistency, and color of any exudate; and evaluate the integrity and health of the tympanic membrane. Ideally, ear cytology samples should be obtained by inserting a cotton swab into an otoscope cone so that the horizontal ear canal can be visualized and sampled.

#### 14.2.2.2.1 Sample Preparation

Ear cytology sample preparation begins by obtaining a sample from the horizontal external ear canal using a cotton swab. The swabs are then gently rolled to spread the debris onto a glass slide. It is important to carefully label which sample region on the slide is from the left or right ear. There is debate over whether or not it is best to heat fix the slides prior to staining. Several publications have reported that it is not necessary to heat fix ear cytology samples in order to get a good-quality smear [11,12]. Adequate samples can also be obtained with a short period of heat fixation. The slide should be passed very quickly over the flame and not be heated excessively. Slides can then be stained with quick stains such as Diff-Quik (Diff-Quik Differential Stain Set; Fisher Scientific, Waltham, MA, USA) or Quik-Dip (Mercedes Medical) using a standard staining protocol.

It may also be useful to create a slide for Gram stain analysis to further characterize bacterial infections and a slide to see if ear mites are present. Gram staining of ear cytology samples is performed by quickly heat fixing the sample and using standard Gram stain protocol. To create a sample for ear mite detection, the otic debris is applied to a slide, a drop of mineral oil is added to the debris, and a coverslip is placed over the sample.

#### 14.2.2.2.2 Evaluation of Ear Cytology

Proper evaluation of ear cytology samples is essential for accurate diagnosis. Samples should first be examined using a low-power objective (4× or 10×) to identify the types of cells that are present and to look for parasitic organisms such as ear mites or *Demodex* spp. The samples should then be evaluated using a high-power objective (100× oil immersion objective) to assess for the presence of bacteria, intracellular bacteria in white blood cells, and yeast. Five to ten fields should be scanned, and then the average number of yeast or bacteria per high-power objective field (40× or 100× oil) should then be documented. Unfortunately, a standard number of yeast or bacteria per high-power field that constitute an infection does not exist and varies among sources [13–15]. Studies evaluating normal flora vs. the number of yeast or bacteria that are present in cases of otitis will vary in which objectives are used to quantify the organisms as well [13–15]. In addition, it is best to enumerate the average number of bacteria or yeast per HPF instead of using classification schemes such as 1+, 2+, or 3+, because no standard definition exists for how many yeast or bacteria are present in each field for 1+, 2+, or 3+ classifications. It is also important to note white blood cells and to describe what types of white blood cells are seen and how many on average are present. When inflammatory cells are present, less than one organism per high-power field is considered to be a significant finding, especially if they are found within white blood cells [5].

If the same type and number of organisms are seen with a recheck ear cytology sample, several explanations may apply. Inappropriate therapy may prevent the infection from resolving and a change in medication protocol may be needed. The clinician should also consider that an undiagnosed primary cause may exist and a thorough otic examination should be repeated or imaging studies should be performed. Poor medication techniques or lack of compliance may also be to blame.

#### 14.2.2.2.3 Pathogens

##### 14.2.2.2.3.1 *Malassezia Pachydermatis*

Yeast otitis externa in dogs and cats is most often due to the yeast *Malassezia pachydermatis*. Ear cytology can be helpful in diagnosing yeast otitis externa. The numbers of yeast per HPF that are considered to be abnormal and suggestive of infection vary among sources. Treatment is advised when ear cytology samples have an average of more than 4 yeast per 100× oil immersion objective field or an average of more than 10 yeast per 40× objective field. It is best to count the number of yeast in five randomly chosen fields and then average these numbers. The yeast organisms may vary in shape and can be round, oval, elliptical, or peanut/budding shapes. The organisms may pick up a variable amount of stain with some being dark blue to purple and some being clear with no stain uptake. Yeast are larger than bacteria and average 3–8 μm in diameter. Mixed infections that have both yeast and bacteria may occur. It is best to perform recheck ear cytology for cases of yeast otitis externa in 2–4 weeks. Severe cases of yeast otitis externa may take 3–4 weeks to resolve.

##### 14.2.2.2.3.2 *Bacterial Organisms*

Bacterial otitis externa is diagnosed when abnormal types or numbers of bacteria are seen (see Figure 14.2.4). As with yeast, the numbers of bacteria per HPF that are considered to be abnormal and suggestive of infection vary among sources. Usually, an average of more than one cocci bacteria per oil immersion 100× objective field requires treatment. Infections that have rod bacteria or inflammation present should always be treated. Cocci bacteria are usually *Staphylococcus* spp. or *Streptococcus* spp., although bacterial culture is needed for a definitive diagnosis. *Staphylococcus* spp. bacteria tend to aggregate in variably sized clusters or groupings, whereas *Streptococcus* spp. tend to form chains. Cocci bacteria are round, measure 0.5–1.5 μm in diameter, and stain dark blue to purple (with quick stains). Rod-shaped bacteria are most often *Pseudomonas aeruginosa* or *Proteus* spp. These bacteria are cylindrical and 1–3 μm in length and stain dark blue to purple (with quick stains). *Pseudomonas aeruginosa* infections can be associated with neutrophilic inflammation, the presence of rod-shaped bacteria, ulcerated ear canal epithelium, and a distinctive odor reminiscent of grapes. If rod-shaped bacteria are seen, it is advisable to submit a sample for culture and susceptibility testing if funds allow due to the high incidence of antibiotic resistance with *Pseudomonas aeruginosa*. Mixed infections that have both bacteria and yeast may occur.

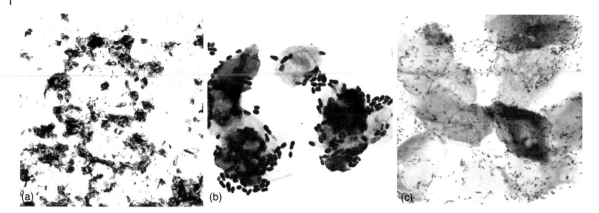

**Figure 14.2.4** Canine otitis externa. (a) Canine yeast otitis externa. Numerous angular squamous epithelial cells are present. Note the yeast organisms are visible from this magnification as deeply basophilic granular structures in the background. No white blood cells are seen. (Diff-Quik; 100×). (b) Canine yeast otitis externa. Same case as in (a). Several angular squamous epithelial cells exhibit variable staining from deeply basophilic to eosinophilic in color. There are numerous *M. pachydermatis* organisms on the surface of the epithelial cells and free in the background that are deeply basophilic and are oval to peanut (budding) shaped. (Diff-Quik; 1000× oil). (c) Canine bacterial otitis externa. Several angular squamous epithelial cells exhibit variable staining from deeply basophilic to eosinophilic in color. There are numerous mixed bacteria on the surface of the epithelial cells and free in the background. Rod-shaped bacteria are present in this sample. (Diff-Quik; 1000× oil). Source: Courtesy of Laurie. M. Millward, The Ohio State University.

Care must be taken to not confuse melanin granules for bacteria. Melanin granules are golden brown to black in color. Melanin can be distinguished from bacteria because they are refractile with subtle adjustment of the fine focus. Melanin granules are haphazardly arranged, whereas bacteria are arranged in clusters or chains.

It is best to perform recheck ear cytology for cases of bacterial otitis externa in 2–4 weeks after initiation of treatment. Oral antibiotic therapy may be needed with *Pseudomonas* spp. infections. If bacteria are persistently seen during recheck visits or if a new population of bacteria is seen, bacterial culture and susceptibility are strongly recommended.

### 14.2.2.2.3.3 Otodectes Cynotis

*Otodectes cynotis* is the most common ear mite that infests dogs and cats. It creates a brown crumbly discharge in the ear, and usually patients are extremely pruritic. Slides are best evaluated using a low-power objective field (4× or 10×), and one should scan the entire space occupied by the coverslip. Adult ear mites as well as their eggs can be seen. Adult female ear mites are about 0.4–0.5 mm and have cup-like structures at the tips of the four front legs and long setae at the tips of the four hind legs. Adult male ear mites are smaller and measure about 0.3 mm. They have cup-like structures at the tips of all eight legs. The eggs are very large, are oval in shape, contain a finely granular brownish-orange material, and measure about 0.2 mm in length.

### 14.2.2.2.3.4 Demodex spp

Rarely, *Demodex* spp. mites can be seen with otic cytology. *Demodex* spp. infestations in cats can cause extreme pruritus, head shaking, and scratching at the ears. *Demodex* spp. infestations in both dogs and cats can produce alopecia, crusting, scaling, erythema, and secondary bacterial or yeast infections. The adult mites are cigar shaped and have six to eight stubby legs. Canine *Demodex* species can vary in length from 180 to 210 μm for *D. canis*, 330 to 370 μm for *D. injai*, and 90 to 140 μm for *Demodex* sp. *"cornei."* Feline *Demodex* species can vary in length from 181 to 219 μm for *D. cati*, 81 to 115 μm for *D. gatoi*, and 170–174 μm for *Demodex sp.*

### 14.2.2.2.3.5 Ear Mass Aspirates

Fine needle aspiration of masses seen within and around the ear may produce diagnostic results. In cats, cytology of aspirates of ear masses has been shown to correlate well with histopathology results [16].

**Inflammatory Ear Polyps** Fine needle aspiration of ear polyps usually produces a highly cellular cytology sample. Mixed inflammation is present and consists of neutrophils, macrophages, lymphocytes, and a lower number of plasma cells. In addition, a variable number of multinucleated giant cells and large reactive fibroblasts due to reactive fibroplasia are seen. Squamous and secretory epithelial cells may also be present [16].

**Ceruminous Gland Adenocarcinoma**   Fine needle aspiration of ceruminous gland adenocarcinoma can produce cytology samples that contain a variable number of tightly clustered epithelial cells that have an increased nuclear-to-cytoplasmic ratio. The nuclei are round to oval, exhibit anisokaryosis, contain coarse chromatin, and have a single prominent nucleolus. Intracytoplasmic globular secretory material and melanin pigment may be present [6].

### 14.2.2.3 Vaginal Cytology

#### 14.2.2.3.1 Sample Collection

Vaginal cytology can be used to stage feline or canine patient estrous cycles and to diagnose inflammation of the vagina and neoplasia of the female reproductive tract. It is easy to perform and requires minimal materials. A saline-moistened cotton swab or a thin glass rod with a rounded end can be used to collect a cytology sample. The sampling tool is directed craniodorsally into the caudal vagina and is inserted 5–10 cm to reach the cranial portion of the vagina. The sampling tool is gently rolled several times in one direction to obtain the sample. A vaginal speculum can be helpful in directing the swab. The sample is then gently rolled onto two or three clean microscope slides, air-dried, and stained with quick stains such as Diff-Quik (Diff-Quik Differential Stain Set; Fisher Scientific, Waltham, MA, USA) or Quik-Dip (Mercedes Medical) using a standard staining protocol. Gram stain can also be utilized to further characterize bacteria. Viewing under low power using 10× magnification is suggested first to determine the types and distribution of cells. Then a closer evaluation using 40× magnification with a coverslip or 100× oil immersion can then evaluate for microorganisms and subtle cellular features. It is important to avoid the vestibule and clitoral fossa, because these areas can contaminate the sample with keratinized squamous epithelial cells, which can complicate cytologic interpretation.

#### 14.2.2.3.2 Normal Vaginal Cytology

The vagina and vestibule are not sterile structures, and it is important to remember that a variable number of mixed bacteria or normal flora can be seen in normal vaginal cytology samples. A variety of epithelial cells in different stages of maturation can be seen in a vaginal cytology sample depending on the stage of the estrus cycle the patient is in. The following epithelial cell types are in order of the most immature and deep cells to the most mature and superficial cells: basal cells, parabasal cells, intermediate cells, and superficial cells.

Basal cells are small, deeply basophilic cells with scant cytoplasm. The nuclei are round. These cells are within the deepest layer of vaginal epithelium and give rise to the more mature forms of epithelial cells. Due to their deep location, basal cells are rarely seen with vaginal cytology.

Parabasal cells are the smallest epithelial cell type. They have a high nuclear to cytoplasmic (N : C) ratio, have round nuclei that exhibit minimal to no anisokaryosis, and have scant moderately basophilic cytoplasm. These cells are seen during proestrus, diestrus, and anestrus. Vaginal cytology from sexually immature animals can have a high number of parabasal cells.

Intermediate cells are more variable in shape and size but are larger than parabasal cells. They have a lower N : C ratio and have a moderate amount of keratinized cytoplasm with round to angular cell borders. Nuclei are round and centrally located. Intermediate cells can be seen during diestrus or vaginitis and rarely are present during early proestrus.

Superficial cells are the most mature of the vaginal epithelial cell types. They have a large amount of keratinized cytoplasm, the N : C ratio is very low, and cell borders are angular or folded. The nuclei are very small and pyknotic and some superficial cells have lost their nuclei and are anucleated. These cells can be seen during early to mid-proestrus along with parabasal and intermediate cells. Superficial cells will predominate during late proestrus and estrus (Figure 14.2.5).

#### 14.2.2.3.3 Determination of Retained Ovarian Tissue

Ideally, a combination of history, physical examination findings, and hormonal testing such as anti-Müllerian hormone (AMH) testing is the most accurate way to distinguish a spayed from an intact cat or dog. AMH testing is especially helpful when there is concern for ovarian remnant syndrome after spay has been performed. It is a non-invasive test that requires a small blood sample and does not require the animal to be in heat since the ovaries are the sole source of AMH. Vaginal cytology can be helpful in identifying unspayed animals or animals with ovarian

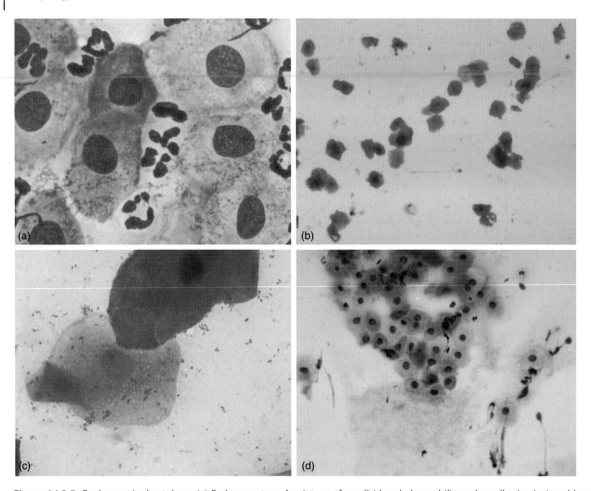

**Figure 14.2.5** Canine vaginal cytology. (a) Early proestrus: A mixture of small (deeply basophilic and smaller in size) and large (less basophilic, larger, lower N : C ratio) intermediate vaginal epithelial cells are present along with a moderate number of neutrophils. As proestrus continues, the neutrophil number will decrease. Large intermediate and superficial cells will predominate as proestrus leads to estrus. (Diff-Quick; 1000× oil) . (b) Estrus: Numerous individualized superficial vaginal epithelial cells are present. Superficial epithelial cells have a large amount of keratinized cytoplasm, the N : C ratio is very low, and cell borders are angular or folded. The nuclei are very small and pyknotic and some superficial cells have lost their nuclei and are anucleated. (Diff-Quik; 200×) . (c) Estrus – higher magnification: Superficial vaginal epithelial cells are large, with angular borders, and small, round pyknotic nuclei. There is a mixed population of bacteria adhered to the superficial epithelial cells and free in the background. (Diff-Quik; 1000× oil) . (d) Anestrus – Intermediate cells are more variable in shape and size but are larger than parabasal cells. They have a lower N : C ratio and have a moderate amount of keratinized cytoplasm with round to angular cell borders. Nuclei are round and centrally located. Intermediate cells can be seen during diestrus, anestrus, rarely during early proestrus and with cases of vaginitis. There are rare neutrophils in this image. Several cells have been broken and the nuclear contents have been smeared, which is called nuclear streaming. (Diff-Quik; 200×). Source: Courtesy of Dr. Marco Coutinho da Silva, The Ohio State University.

remnant syndrome; however, it is not completely accurate and will vary depending on the stage of the estrus cycle. It can support a diagnosis of ovarian remnant syndrome along with history, physical examination findings, and hormone testing. If an animal is presumed to be in heat and ovarian tissue is present, vaginal cytology samples will contain a high number of superficial cells. In spayed animals, noncornified epithelial cells such as parabasal cells and intermediate cells are seen.

#### 14.2.2.3.4 Transmissible Venereal Cell Tumor

Transmissible venereal tumor (TVT) is a tumor of probable histiocytic cell origin seen in both male and

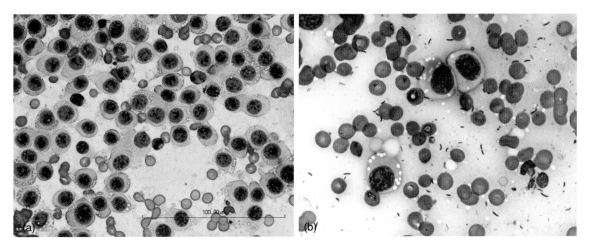

**Figure 14.2.6** Transmissible venereal tumor. (a) Impression smear of a vaginal TVT. The sample is very cellular. There are numerous large, individualized, round cells that have a low N : C ratio. The nuclei are round, eccentrically located, and contain coarse chromatin with a single prominent nucleolus. These cells have abundant lightly to moderately basophilic cytoplasm that contains a variable number of distinct punctate clear vacuoles (Diff-Quik; 60×). Source: Courtesy of Andrea Strakova, University of Cambridge. (b) Cellularity is decreased in this field, which allows for enhanced visualization of the features of the neoplastic cell population. The TVT cells are seen as round, individualized cells that have the characteristic abundant moderately basophilic cytoplasm that contains multiple punctate clear vacuoles. One prominent nucleolus is evident amidst coarse chromatin in the nucleus. Red blood cells and mixed bacteria are seen in the background. (Wright-Giemsa; 1000× oil).

female dogs in temperate regions. Affected animals are usually free roaming and sexually intact. The tumor is unique in that it is spread via the direct implantation of intact tumor cells, usually via sexual contact. These tumors have been described on the external genitalia, skin, rectum, oral mucous membranes, nasal mucous membranes, and eyes [17–21]. TVTs appear pink to red, fleshy, soft, friable, hemorrhagic, ulcerated, nodular, raised to pedunculated masses that are often necrotic and secondarily infected. An impression or fine needle aspirate of the tumor yields a highly cellular sample that consists primarily of a monomorphic population of large, individualized round cells. The nuclei are round, eccentrically located, and contain coarse chromatin with one to two prominent nucleoli. These cells have abundant lightly to moderately basophilic cytoplasm that contains a variable number of punctate vacuoles. Mitotic figures can be present. A variable number of lymphocytes, plasma cells, macrophages, and neutrophils may also be seen admixed with the tumor cells. Neutrophils will appear degenerate and contain intracellular bacteria if secondary bacterial infection is present. Metastases have

been reported but are rare [21]. Recommended treatment includes chemotherapy, surgical excision, and radiation therapy (Figure 14.2.6).

#### 14.2.2.3.5 Vaginitis

Inflammation of the vagina should be considered if abnormal vaginal discharge, dysuria, excessive vulvar licking, and dystocia are noted. Inflammation may occur with vaginal anatomic abnormalities, clitoral hypertrophy, retained fetal membranes, vaginal neoplasia, or immaturity (puppy vaginitis) [22, 23]. Samples may be obtained via swabbing the vaginal mucosa or vaginal discharge with a cotton swab and gently smearing the sample onto a glass slide. Cases of acute vaginitis will have a moderate-to-high number of neutrophils. Degenerative neutrophils along with a monomorphic population of intracellular bacteria indicate septic inflammation. The presence of a mixed population of lymphoid cells, macrophages, and neutrophils indicates chronic inflammation. Inflammation may create atypia in vaginal epithelial cells and care must be taken to not mistakenly interpret these findings as evidence of neoplasia.

## References

1  Allison, R.W. and Velguth, K.E. (2010). Appearance of granulated cells in blood films stained by automated aqueous versus methanolic Romanowsky methods. *Veterinary Clinical Pathology* **39** (1): 99–104.

2 Meyer, D.J. (2016). The acquisition and management of cytology specimens. In: Canine and Feline Cytology (eds. R. Raskin and D.J. Meyer), 1–15. St. Louis, MO: Elsevier.

3 Columbo, S. (1997). Quantitative Evaluation of Cutaneous Bacteria in Normal Dogs and Dogs with Pyoderma by Cytological Evaluation. Milan.

4 Mauldin, E.A., Scott, D.W., Miller, W.H., and Smith, C.A. (1997). *Malassezia* dermatitis in the dog: a retrospective histopathological and immunopathological study of 86 cases (1990–95). *Veterinary Dermatology* **8** (3): 191–202.

5 Miller, W.H., Griffin, C.E., and Campbell, K.L. (2013). Muller & Kirk's Small Animal Dermatology, 7e (eds. W.H. Miller, C.E. Griffin and K.L. Campbell). St. Louis, MO: Elsevier.

6 Raskin, R. (2016). Skin and subcutaneous tissue. In: Canine and Feline Cytology (eds. R.E. Raskin and D.J. Meyer), 34–90. St. Louis, MO: Elsevier.

7 Kennis, R.A., Rosser, E.J. Jr., Olivier, N.B., and Walker, R.W. (1996). Quantity and distribution of *Malassezia* organisms on the skin of clinically normal dogs. *Journal of the American Veterinary Medical Association* **208** (7): 1048–1051.

8 Plant, J.D., Rosenkrantz, W.S., and Griffin, C.E. (1992). Factors associated with and prevalence of high *Malassezia* pachydermatis numbers on dog skin. *Journal of the American Veterinary Medical Association* **201** (6): –879, 882.

9 Bond, R., Saijonmaa-Koulumies, L.E., and Lloyd, D.H. (1995). Population sizes and frequency of *Malassezia* pachydermatis at skin and mucosal sites on healthy dogs. *The Journal of Small Animal Practice* **36** (4): 147–150.

10 Bond, R. and Lloyd, D.H. (1997). Skin and mucosal populations of *Malassezia* pachydermatis in healthy and seborrhoeic basset hounds. *Veterinary Dermatology* **8** (2): 101–106.

11 Griffin, J.S., Scott, D.W., and Erb, H.N. (2007). *Malassezia* otitis externa in the dog: the effect of heat-fixing otic exudate for cytological analysis. *Journal of Veterinary Medicine Series A: Physiology Pathology Clinical Medicine* **54** (8): 424–427.

12 Toma, S., Comegliani, L., Persico, P., and Noli, C. (2006). Comparison of 4 fixation and staining methods for the cytologic evaluation of ear canals with clinical evidence of ceruminous otitis externa. *Veterinary Clinical Pathology* **35** (2): 194–198.

13 Cafarchia, C., Gallo, S., Capelli, G., and Otranto, D. (2005). Occurrence and population size of *Malassezia* spp. in the external ear canal of dogs and cats both healthy and with otitis. *Mycopathologia* **160** (2): 143–149.

14 Ginel, P.J., Lucena, R., Rodriguez, J.C., and Ortega, J. (2002). A semiquantitative cytological evaluation of normal and pathological samples from the external ear canal of dogs and cats. *Veterinary Dermatology* **13** (3): 151–156.

15 Tater, K.C., Scott, D.W., Miller, W.H. Jr., and Erb, H.N. (2003). The cytology of the external ear canal in the normal dog and cat. *Journal of Veterinary Medicine. A, Physiology, Pathology, Clinical Medicine* **50** (7): 370–374.

16 De Lorenzi, D., Bonfanti, U., Masserdotti, C., and Tranquillo, M. (2005). Fine-needle biopsy of external ear canal masses in the cat: cytologic results and histologic correlations in 27 cases. *Veterinary Clinical Pathology* **34** (2): 100–105.

17 Perez, J., Bautista, M.J., Carrasco, L. et al. (1994). Primary extragenital occurrence of transmissible venereal tumors: three case reports. *Canine Practice* **19**: 7–10.

18 Albanese, F., Salerni, F.L., Giordano, S., and Marconato, L. (2006). Extragenital transmissible venereal tumour associated with circulating neoplastic cells in an immunologically compromised dog. *Veterinary and Comparative Oncology* **4** (1): 57–62.

19 Rezaei, M., Azizi, S., Shahheidaripour, S., and Rostami, S. (2016). Primary oral and nasal transmissible venereal tumor in a mix-breed dog. *Asian Pacific Journal of Tropical Biomedicine* **6** (5): 443–445.

20 Albanese, F., Poli, A., Millanta, F., and Abramo, F. (2002). Primary cutaneous extragenital canine transmissible venereal tumour with Leishmania-laden neoplastic cells: a further suggestion of histiocytic origin? *Veterinary Dermatology* **13** (5): 243–246.

21 Park, M.S., Kim, Y., Kang, M.S. et al. (2006). Disseminated transmissible venereal tumor in a dog. *Journal of Veterinary Diagnostic Investigation: Official Publication of the American Association of Veterinary Laboratory Diagnosticians, Inc* **18** (1): 130–133.

22 Nicastro, A. and Walshaw, R. (2007). Chronic vaginitis associated with vaginal foreign bodies in a cat. *Journal of the American Animal Hospital Association* **43** (6): 352–355.

23 Snead, E.C., Pharr, J.W., Ringwood, B.P., and Beckwith, J. (2010). Long-retained vaginal foreign body causing chronic vaginitis in a bulldog. *Journal of the American Animal Hospital Association* **46**: 56–60.

# 14.3

# Blood Smear Evaluation

*Emily Walters*

*Antech Diagnostics, 17672 Cowan, Irvine, CA 92614, USA*

## 14.3.1 Blood Smear Interpretation

Interpretation of blood smears allows clinicians to quickly detect significant hematologic abnormalities including anemia, red blood cell (RBC) regenerative status, cell morphology changes indicative of disease (e.g. spherocytes with IMHA (immune mediated hemolytic anemia)), inflammation, leukopenia, thrombocytopenia, leukemia, and infectious agents. This is especially valuable in field settings as it can be accomplished with the use of a microscope in the absence of an automated hematology analyzer. Furthermore, it is also a valuable skill in a more traditional clinic setting as manual blood smear evaluation is useful for detecting errors produced by automated complete blood count (CBC) instruments, as well as certain things missed by machines (e.g. infectious organisms, low numbers of leukemic cells).

The goal of this section is to provide a step-wise approach for examining a blood smear and detecting common abnormalities. Selected infectious agents and causes of anemia seen in field work are also reviewed.

### 14.3.1.1 Sample Preparation

Blood smears should be made within a couple of hours of blood collection to prevent artifactual changes and cellular autolysis. Once blood is added to an EDTA tube, gently roll the sample to help minimize platelet clumping. Also, gently roll the sample immediately prior to use to ensure proper distribution of cells and platelets. If refrigerated, allow blood to return to room temperature before making a smear. If your slides become dusty in the field, be sure to wipe them clean before preparing the blood smear to avoid artifacts.

Steps to making a blood smear:

1) Using a microhematocrit tube, place a small drop of blood (about 4 mm diameter or the size of a peppercorn) toward one end of a glass slide on a flat surface.
2) Take a second "spreader" slide and place the short edge at about a 30–40° angle in front of the drop of blood.
3) Pull the edge of the "spreader" slide into the blood droplet and let the blood wick along the edge of the spreader slide, which occurs quickly.
4) Immediately push the "spreader" slide along the flat slide in a moderately quick, fluid motion maintaining gentle even contact.

The result should look similar to Figure 14.3.1.

The following are some common issues with obtaining a good smear:

- If the drop of blood is too large, the blood smear will extend off the end of the slide eliminating the feathered edge.
- In severely anemic samples, you may need to increase the angle of the spreader slide to create an adequate monolayer.
- In dehydrated animals with hemoconcentrated blood, you may need to decrease the angle.
- If the spreader slide is pushed too slowly, the smear may be too long and white blood cell (WBCs) may concentrate at the feathered edge.

*Field Manual for Small Animal Medicine*, First Edition. Edited by Katherine Polak and Ann Therese Kommedal.
© 2018 John Wiley & Sons, Inc. Published 2018 by John Wiley & Sons, Inc.

A properly made blood smear consists of several regions:

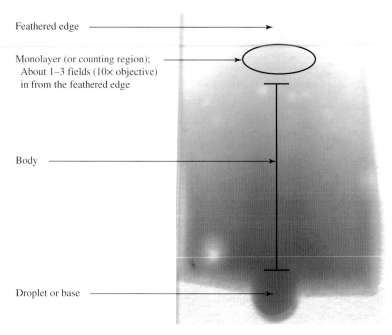

Feathered edge

Monolayer (or counting region);
About 1–3 fields (10× objective)
in from the feathered edge

Body

Droplet or base

**Figure 14.3.1** Components of a blood smear.

- If the spreader slide is pushed too rapidly, the smear may be too short.

### 14.3.1.2 How to Properly Evaluate a Blood Smear

First, examine the blood smear at low power (10× objective), then high power (50× or 100× objective). While it is important to scan all parts of the smear, the monolayer is the region where cell morphology is closely examined and cell counts are performed.

#### 14.3.1.2.1 Evaluation at 10×

Using the 10× objective, scan the feathered edge, monolayer, and several passes over the body of the smear.

*Feathered Edge.* Look for platelet clumps, abnormal cells (e.g. blasts, mast cells), and infectious agents (e.g. heartworm microfilaria, *Cytauxzoon* schizont).
*Monolayer.* Assess RBC and WBC density, look for abnormal cells and RBC agglutination.

Normal RBC density in dogs and cats is typically seen as an even distribution of RBCs in the monolayer region of the smear, where RBCs are close together but not frequently overlapping. Note, increased serum protein can result in a shorter monolayer area. Also, there may be too few RBCs for an adequate monolayer in severely anemic animals, and RBC overlap may be prominent in polycythemic animals.

With experience, WBC density can be estimated subjectively. Dogs and cats normally have approximately 15–50 WBCs/10× fields in health [1]. The following calculation can be used for a crude estimation of WBC density using the 10× objective in the *monolayer* of a well-made smear:

- WBC count $\mu L^{-1}$ = average number of WBCs in 10 fields × 300.

WBC estimates are imprecise and can be affected by uneven distribution of WBCs on the smear, but are useful in detecting marked leukocytosis and leukopenia.

*Body and Base.* Scan for abnormal cells (blasts, mast cells) and RBC agglutination. Ensure WBCs are distributed evenly and not sparse in the body but concentrated at the feathered edge, as this may occur in smears spread too slowly. Occasionally,

WBCs can aggregate together in groups (known as "leukergy") in cases of inflammation or immune stimulation.

#### 14.3.1.2.2 Evaluation at 50× or 100×

Using the 50× and/or 100× objectives, perform a WBC differential count, evaluate cell morphology, and estimate platelet numbers. It is very important to examine cells within the monolayer or "counting region" for the most accurate estimation of platelet counts and cell morphology.

*RBC Morphology.* Evaluate RBC morphology for the following changes:

- Shape (poikilocytosis):
  - *Spherocytes.* Typically seen with immune-mediated hemolysis, either primary IMHA or secondary IMHA (e.g. infection, drug, toxin, neoplasia).
  - *Acanthocytes.* May occur in patients with hemangiosarcoma, liver disease, glomerulonephritis, DIC, etc.
  - *Schistocytes.* These fragmented RBCs may occur with DIC, iron-deficiency anemia, myelofibrosis, hemangiosarcoma, glomerulonephritis, etc.
  - *Keratocytes.* Blistered or "bite" erythrocytes that can be associated with iron-deficiency anemia, liver disorder, myelodysplasia, toxins, etc.
  - *Eccentrocytes and Heinz Bodies.* Indicate oxidative damage, such as ingestion of onions or garlic, acetaminophen, prolonged propofol administration, lymphoma, etc.
  - *Echinocytes.* Commonly seen as a drying artifact (crenation). May also be present with uremia, snake bite, neoplasia, or burn victims.
  - *Target Cells.* RBCs with a central red "target" that is often seen with regenerative anemia, and less often with liver disease.
- *Size Variation.* Anisocytosis
- Color:
  - *Polychromasia.* Larger blue immature erythrocytes (increased RNA). Increased numbers of polychromatophils usually correspond with a regenerative response. A reticulocyte count is the most accurate way to characterize the regenerative status.
  - *Hypochromasia.* Pale erythrocytes due to decreased hemoglobin, typically seen with iron-deficiency anemia from chronic blood loss.
- *Inclusions.* Howell–Jolly bodies (retained nuclear fragments), basophilic stippling (RNA), siderocytes (iron).
- *Patterns.* RBC agglutination (IMHA), increased rouleaux (common in cats, horses, and animals with increased serum protein).
- *Infectious Agents.* Hemotropic *Mycoplasma*, Distemper, *Cytauxzoon*, *Babesia* spp.

*WBC Differential.* Count 100 WBCs and categorize them as segmented neutrophils, immature neutrophils (bands, metamyelocytes, or myelocytes), lymphocytes, monocytes, eosinophils, basophils, and other cells (e.g. mast cells, unclassified cells). If WBC differential counts are performed routinely, it may be worth investing in a manual cell counter (five-keys or greater). Absolute differential leukocyte counts are determined by multiplying the percentage of each cell type counted by the total WBC count (in thousands $\mu L^{-1}$).

If nucleated red blood cells (nRBCs) are present, they should be counted in a separate category and recorded as the number of nRBCs per 100 WBCs. The total WBC count should be corrected if there are significantly increased nRBCs present (>5 nRBC/100 WBCs). Corrected WBC count = (total WBC count × 100)/(100 + nRBCs per 100 WBC)[2].

*WBC Morphology.* Look for toxic changes in neutrophils, infectious agents, or abnormal cells.

- *Toxic Changes.* Develop in the bone marrow and typically indicate inflammation. Toxic changes include Döhle bodies (blue "dots" or angular inclusions within the cytoplasm consistent with retained RER), cytoplasmic basophilia, and cytoplasmic vacuolation. Toxic vacuolation is usually "wispy" and should be differentiated from prolonged storage artifact resulting in low numbers of punctate cytoplasmic vacuoles. An uncommon toxic change is toxic granulation (magenta cytoplasmic granules), which is most often seen in horses but rarely in dogs and cats. Note low numbers of Döhle bodies are normal in feline and equine neutrophils and do not indicate toxicity.

- *Reactive Lymphocytes.* Reactive lymphocytes may be intermediate to large in size (equal to or larger than a neutrophil in diameter), typically have mature clumped or sometimes stippled chromatin and often increased cytoplasmic basophilia.
- *Blast Cells.* Typically large in size with fine or stippled chromatin, often a high nuclear to cytoplasmic ratio, and visible nucleoli. Blasts may be of myeloid or lymphoid origin, or unclassified, and cannot be reliably differentiated by morphology alone. Special diagnostic tests, such as flow cytometry may be used to further classify these cells. Note that it can be difficult or impossible to differentiate reactive lymphocytes from neoplastic lymphoblasts when low numbers are present.
- *Mast Cells.* Circulating mast cells in dogs may be seen with mast cell neoplasia or non-neoplastic inflammatory/hypersensitivity conditions. However, in cats circulating mast cells are usually associated with mast cell neoplasia, and rarely other neoplasms (e.g. lymphoma) [3].
- *Infectious Agents.* Tick-borne rickettsial organisms in neutrophils, monocytes, or lymphocytes. Intracellular bacteria, yeast (e.g. *Histoplasma*), or protozoa (*Hepatozoon*).

*Platelets.* Platelet numbers should be estimated within the monolayer region of the blood smear using the 100× objective.

- *Estimated Platelet Count Per Microliter.* Count the number of platelets in 10 separate 100× fields and calculate the average number of platelets per field.

Estimated platelet count = average number of platelets per 100× fields × 15 000–20 000.

If platelet clumps are present, this may spuriously lower the platelet count and should be taken into consideration when estimating platelet mass.

Macroplatelets are large platelets, often about the size of a RBC or larger. Macroplatelets may indicate active thrombopoiesis (platelet regeneration). Macroplatelets can be considered "normal" in some breeds, such as Cavalier King Charles Spaniels (CKCS). CKCS may have a lower platelet count relative to other breeds due to inherited macrothrombocytopenia. In these dogs, the overall platelet mass remains the same as unaffected breeds, and there are

no bleeding abnormalities associated with this anomaly [4]. Some breeds have a lower reference interval for platelets, such as Greyhounds [5].

### 14.3.1.2.3 Select Infectious Organisms

Infectious organisms including bacterial, viral, protozoal, and parasitic agents may be readily identified upon blood smear evaluation, but are often missed by automated hematology analyzers. Infectious agents may be found within erythrocytes (intracellular), attached to the surface (epicellular), or free in the plasma (extracellular). A lack of identifiable organisms does not rule out these diseases as transient parasitemia or low numbers of organisms may not be visible. Additional molecular methods such as polymerase chain reaction (PCR) can be helpful to rule out infection in these cases.

#### 14.3.1.2.3.1 *Babesia*

*Babesia* spp. are intracellular erythrocyte parasites found in dogs that may be observed in two general forms, small and large. *B. gibsoni* and *B. conradae* occur as one or more small (1–3 μm) round, ring, pyriform, banded, or pleomorphic structures within RBCs. Small *Babesia* can be difficult to identify and typically require oil immersion with a high-power objective. The large (3–7 μm in length) pyriform to amoeboid shapes of *B. canis* may be found individually, in pairs, or quadruplets occupying a large portion of the RBC (Figure 14.3.2).

Multiple parasites are more likely to be detected in acute babesiosis, whereas only rare organisms may be present with chronic infection. Dogs with acute infection can present with fever, lethargy, lymphadenopathy, splenomegaly, hemolytic anemia, thrombocytopenia, neutropenia, hemoglobinuria, bilirubinemia, and bilirubinuria. Chronic infections may be subclinical or result in intermittent episodes of regenerative anemia, lymphocytosis, and other signs of chronic immune stimulation [6].

#### 14.3.1.2.3.2 *Hemotropic Mycoplasma*

Hemotropic *Mycoplasmas* are epicellular organisms found in a variety of animals, including cats and dogs. These appear as small, basophilic, coccoid, ring, or rod-shaped structures arranged individually and occasionally in chains on the surface of RBCs, and often free in the background (detached). Several species have been described, and some forms are

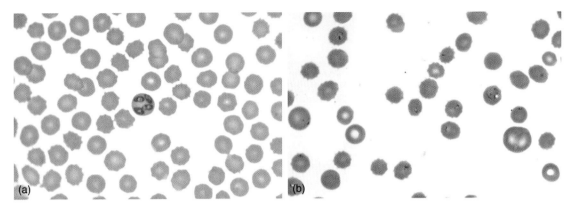

**Figure 14.3.2** (a) Four large *Babesia canis* piroplasms within a dog red blood cell. (Modified Wright stain. Original magnification 1000×.) (b) Small, more-difficult-to-visualize *Babesia gibsoni* organisms with round, banded, or amorphous shape in dog red blood cells. (Modified Wright stain. Original magnification 1000×.)

more pathogenic than others. Acute infection can result in hemolytic anemia. In cats, *Mycoplasma haemofelis* is considered the most pathologic species and is associated with feline infectious anemia (FIA), previously termed "hemobartonellosis."

Animals with immunosuppression, concurrent disease (e.g. FeLV (feline leukemia virus) infection), prior splenectomy, and concurrent infection with multiple hemoplasma species are at greater risk for developing severe acute anemia. Asymptomatic infections may occur in healthy animals [7]. PCR can be helpful to confirm the diagnosis in symptomatic animals without visible parasitemia or in instances where it is not possible to differentiate between stain precipitant and true organisms.

#### 14.3.1.2.3.3 Rickettsia

Morulae of *Ehrlichia ewingii*, *Anaplasma phagocytophilum*, and *Ehrlichia canis* are intracellular bacteria in the order Rickettsiales that may be found within canine WBCs. All three appear similar as eosinophilic to basophilic, round to oval packets of multiple small cocci. *E. ewingii* and *A. phagocytophilum* may be found within neutrophils, whereas *E. canis* morulae occur within lymphocytes and monocytes.

*E. canis* morulae are rarely detected on blood smears and usually only with acutely infected dogs. Clinicopathologic signs may include fever, thrombocytopenia, leukopenia, anemia, lymphadenopathy, splenomegaly, and/or lameness. Dogs with chronic *E. canis* infections may develop mild-to-marked lymphocytosis or eventually pancytopenia. Indirect

fluorescent antibody (IFA) and PCR tests are available for detection and speciation [8].

#### 14.3.1.2.3.4 Distemper

Canine distemper virus inclusions can occur in WBCs and/or RBCs. Inclusions are round, ovoid, or amorphous and may stain pink/red or blue depending on the stain used. Viral inclusions are variably found in infected dogs and are most prevalent during early stages of infection.

#### 14.3.1.2.3.5 Heartworm

*Dirofilaria immitis* is the causative agent for heartworm disease in dogs and cats. Microfilaria may be seen on the blood smears of infected dogs, but rarely in cats. Microfilaria can be dragged to the feathered edge of the blood smear or scattered in the body of the smear.

Although reported rarely, *Acanthocheilonema* (formerly *Dipetalonema*) *reconditum* microfilaria should be differentiated from *D. immitis* via morphology or serologic testing [9] (Figure 14.3.3).

#### 14.3.1.2.4 Select Anemias: Immune-mediated Hemolytic Anemia (IMHA) and Iron-deficiency Anemia

Anemia may occur with a wide variety of diseases. However, regenerative anemia is typically seen specifically with blood loss or hemolysis. Two specific forms of anemia are presented here because of their relative frequency (IMHA) and prevalence in patients with chronic blood loss due to intestinal parasites (iron-deficiency anemia).

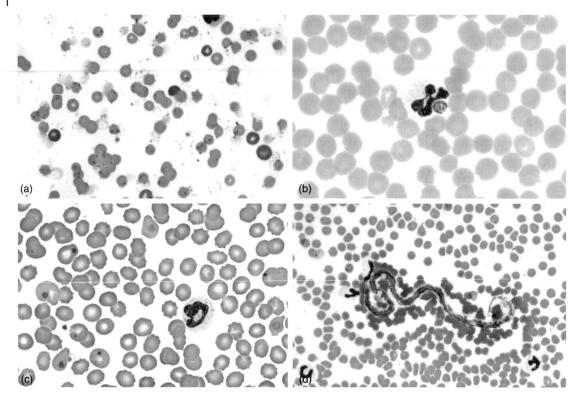

**Figure 14.3.3** (a) Cat blood smear with high numbers of small coccoid *Mycoplasma haemofelis* organisms attached to red blood cells and free in the background. Note the secondary immune-mediated hemolytic anemia (IMHA) with pale ghost erythrocytes and red blood cell agglutinates. (Modified Wright stain. Original magnification 1000×.) (b) Dog neutrophil with an intracellular morula characteristic of *Ehrlichia ewingii* or *Anaplasma phagocytophilum*. (Modified Wright stain. Original magnification 1000×.) (c) Canine distemper virus inclusions in red blood cells appear round to slightly amorphous smooth structures and may stain pale blue to pink/red. (Modified Wright stain. Original magnification 1000×.) (d) *Dirofilaria immitis* microfilaria in dog blood. (Modified Wright stain. Original magnification 500×.)

### 14.3.1.2.4.1 *Immune-mediated Hemolytic Anemia*

IMHA may be primary (autoimmune) or secondary to a variety of causes (e.g. infection, drug-related, neoplasia, bee sting, etc.). Spherocytes and/or RBC agglutinates (RBCs in grape-like bunches) are classic findings on the blood smear of affected dogs, but are not present in all cases of IMHA. Since normal feline erythrocytes do not contain significant central pallor, spherocytes are difficult to detect in cats. Other blood smear findings in patients with IMHA may include polychromasia, anisocytosis, increased Howell–Jolly bodies and nucleated RBCs, ghost erythrocytes (complement-mediated lysed RBCs), and basophilic stippling. Not all cases of IMHA are regenerative. When the immune response is targeted against RBC precursors in the bone marrow, patients may exhibit a nonregenerative anemia (precursor-directed nonregenerative IMHA). IMHA is often pro-inflammatory, and patients may exhibit neutrophilia and monocytosis, neutrophil bands, and/or neutrophil toxicity. Platelets may be increased (reactive thrombocytosis), normal, or decreased. When present, thrombocytopenia is usually due to increased consumption (DIC, vasculitis), and infrequently associated with Evan's syndrome (concurrent IMHA and IMTP).

### 14.3.1.2.4.2 *Iron-deficiency Anemia*

Iron-deficiency anemia is most commonly seen in dogs secondary to chronic blood loss. In veterinary field work, this may be observed in animals with internal and external blood-sucking parasites.

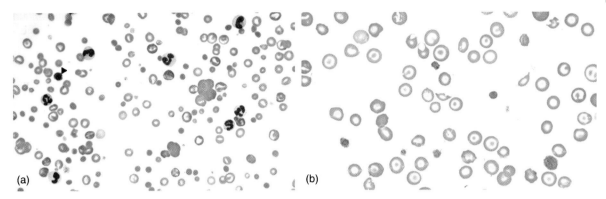

Figure 14.3.4 (a) Blood smear from a dog with immune-mediated hemolytic anemia (IMHA). There is marked polychromasia and anisocytosis. Spherocytes appear small, dense, and lack central pallor. In contrast, the immature polychromatophils appear larger with a blue hue. There are a few groups of clumped red blood cells consistent with agglutinates. A single nucleated red blood cell is present (arrowhead), attributed to the regenerative response. (Modified Wright stain. Original magnification 500×.) (b) Blood smear from a dog with iron-deficiency anemia due to chronic blood loss. Note the erythrocytes with increased central pallor and thinner outer rim of red cytoplasm (hypochromasia). There are a few keratocytes (blister cells and cells with "popped open" blisters) and schistocytes. (Modified Wright stain. Original magnification 1000×.)

However, chronic blood loss may also occur with bleeding gastrointestinal ulcers or tumors (e.g. gastrointestinal stromal tumors, leiomyosarcoma). Over time, chronic blood loss causes a microcytic (decreased mean corpuscular volume (MCV)), hypochromic (decreased mean corpuscular hemoglobin concentration (MCHC)) anemia. In the author's experience, most anemias associated with chronic blood loss are regenerative. However, nonregenerative anemia may occur in cases where iron stores are severely depleted or there is concurrent disease suppressing regeneration (e.g. anemia of inflammatory disease). Since many patients have increased numbers of larger (macrocytic) polychromatophilic RBCs associated with a regenerative response, the MCV may be within the reference interval since this is an averaged value of all RBCs analyzed. Typical findings on the blood smear include lighter staining RBCs with increased central pallor due to decreased hemoglobin content. Keratocytes and RBC fragments may be present since microcytic, hypochromic RBCs are more fragile. Many patients also have a reactive thrombocytosis with macroplatelets. Fecal evaluation for parasites, careful abdominal palpation, examination of the skin for external parasites, and abdominal ultrasound may be helpful in identifying a cause for chronic blood loss in these cases (Figure 14.3.4).

## References

1 Willard, M.D. and Tvedten, H. (2014). Small Animal Clinical Diagnosis by Laboratory Methods, 5e. St. Louis, MO: Elsevier.

2 Stockham, S.L. and Scott, M.A. (2008). Fundamentals of Veterinary Clinical Pathology, 2e. Ames: Wiley-Blackwell.

3 Piviani, M., Walton, R.M., and Patel, R.T. (2013). Significance of mastocytemia in cats. *Veterinary Clinical Pathology* **42** (1): 4–10.

4 Singh, M. and Lamb, W. (2005). Idiopathic thrombocytopenia in Cavalier King Charles Spaniels. *Australian Veterinary Journal* **83**: 700–703.

5 Zaldívar-López, S., Marín, L.M., Iazbik, M.C. et al. (2011). Clinical pathology of Greyhounds and other sighthounds. *Veterinary Clinical Pathology/ American Society for Veterinary Clinical Pathology* **40** (4): 10.

6 Birkenheuer, A.J. (2012). Babesiosis. In: Infectious Diseases of the Dog and Cat (ed. C.E. Greene), 771–784. St. Louis, MO: Saunders.

7 Messick, J.B., Tarigo, J.L., Vercruysse, J., et al. (2016). Hemotropic mycoplasmas. www .merckvetmanual.com/circulatory-system/blood-parasites/hemotropic-mycoplasmas (accessed 20 February 2017).

8 Zabolotzky, S.M. and Walker, D.B. (2014). Peripheral blood smears; White blood cell inclusions. In: Diagnostic Cytology and Hematology of the Dog and Cat (ed. A.C. Valenciano and R.L. Cowell), 482. St. Louis, MO: Elsevier.

9 American Heartworm Society (2017). Heartworm. https://www.heartwormsociety.org/ (accessed 20 February 2017).

## Additional Resources

eClinpath (2013). http://www.eclinpath.com/ hematology/hemogram-basics/blood-smear-examination/ (accessed 20 February 2017).

Harvey, J.W. (2012). Veterinary Hematology: A Diagnostic Guide and Color Atlas. St. Louis, MO: Elsevier.

Latimer, K.S. (2011). Duncan & Prasse's Veterinary Laboratory Medicine: Clinical Pathology, 5 e. Ames: Wiley-Blackwell.

## 14.4

# Neurologic Examination

*Patrick J. Kenny*

*Small Animal Specialist Hospital, Level 1, 1 Richardson Place, North Ryde, Sydney, NSW 2113, Australia*

## 14.4.1 Objectives and Neuroanatomic Correlates

The fundamental principle of clinical neurology is that it is the LOCATION of the disease within the nervous system (not the type of disease itself) that determines the clinical signs. We apply this principle when we perform and interpret our neurological examination. By determining what neurological deficits exist, we can work out *where* the problem is within the nervous system (i.e. *localizing the lesion*).

The neurological examination therefore has two aims:

1) To determine if the patient is neurologically normal or abnormal
2) To localize the lesion within the nervous system.

Certain diseases will only occur in certain parts of the nervous system, while others may occur more diffusely. Narrowing down the location of the disease shortens the list of possible causes (the differential diagnoses). This list can be further refined by interpreting the

localization alongside other clinical information such as signalment, onset, progression, symmetry of deficits, and presence or absence of pain. A concise list of differential diagnoses allows rational decision-making when formulating diagnostic and treatment plans and is particularly important if devising empirical treatment plans or attempting to prognosticate without a diagnosis due to limited resources.

*How much neuroanatomy do I need to know?* The nervous system is the most anatomically complex organ system in the body, and studying neuroanatomy can be an intimidating proposition to many students and clinicians. In the majority of clinical cases, however, the most specific neuroanatomic diagnosis will be regional, to one of the following segments:

1) Brain
   a) Forebrain
   b) Brainstem
   c) Cerebellum
2) Spinal cord
   a) C1–C5 segments
   b) C6–T2 segments
   c) T3–L3 segments
   d) L4–Cd segments
3) Neuromuscular.

The neurological examination is in essence a collection of individual tests, each assessing the functional integrity of a pathway through the nervous system. Knowledge of what structures are being tested (the neuroanatomic correlates) is required to interpret the findings of the examination and make a neuroanatomic diagnosis. A working knowledge of *regional*

---

**Textbox 14.4.1 Getting the most value out of a neurological examination**

To get the most out of our neurological exam we need two things:

1) An understanding of what each test is determining (*i.e. knowledge of the pertinent neuroanatomy*)
2) To master technique and interpretation (*i.e. practice!*).

---

Table 14.4.1 Eight main functional regions of neurolocalization.

| Region | Divisions | Functions |
|---|---|---|
| Forebrain | Cerebrum<br>Thalamus | • Cognition/behavior (cerebrum)<br>• Level of mentation<br>• Relay (thalamus) and conscious perception (cerebrum) of sensory modalities<br>• UMNs in cerebrum<br>• UMN axons projecting to the body<br>• Endocrine, thermoregulation and autonomic functions (hypothalamus) |
| Brainstem | Midbrain<br>Pons<br>Medulla<br>oblongata | • Level of mentation<br>• UMN nuclei in brainstem<br>• UMN axons projecting to the body<br>• Sensory axons (proprioception, nociception) from caudal/peripheral regions<br>• Most cranial nerve nuclei (III–XII)<br>• Autonomic functions (cardiorespiratory) |
| Cerebellum | | • Co-ordination and regulation of movement<br>• Control of Posture<br>• Vestibular projections |
| C1–C5 spinal cord | | • UMN axons projecting to all limbs and tail<br>• Sensory axons (proprioception, nociception) from caudal/peripheral regions |
| C6–T2 spinal cord | | "The cervical intumescence"<br>• LMNs innervating thoracic limbs<br>• UMN axons projecting to pelvic limbs and tail<br>• Sensory axons (proprioception, nociception) from caudal/peripheral regions |
| T3–L3 spinal cord | | • UMN axons projecting to pelvic limbs and tail<br>• Sensory axons (proprioception, nociception) from caudal/peripheral regions |
| L4–Cd spinal cord | | "The lumbar intumescence"<br>• LMNs innervating pelvic limbs and tail, urinary bladder, urethral, and anal sphincters<br>• Sensory axons (proprioception, nociception) from caudal/peripheral regions |
| Neuromuscular | Peripheral nerve<br>NMJ<br>Muscle | • LMNs in peripheral nerve: lesions of LMN, NMJ, and muscle may be hard to distinguish on examination, as together they form the final common pathway for movement – "the motor unit"<br>• Sensory axons in peripheral nerve |

UMN: Upper Motor Neuron, LMN: Lower Motor Neuron, NMJ: Neuromuscular Junction.

neuroanatomy is generally sufficient to do this (Table 14.4.1). In this chapter, neuroanatomic pathways will be referred to in broad, segmental terms, rather than to the specific tracts or nuclei contained within (though these may occasionally be mentioned). Unarguably, this is a simplification of a complex reality – but it is a useful simplification that works well in the majority of clinical cases. Acquiring a deeper understanding of functional neuroanatomy is well worthwhile – it may allow more nuanced interpretations of the examination and a more specific or narrow list of differential diagnoses to be deduced. Presenting the required detail is, however, beyond the scope of this brief chapter, and as such, the reader is referred to other excellent (and lengthier) texts [1–5].

---

**Textbox 14.4.2 Format for description of tests and regional neuroanatomic correlates in this chapter**

Technique:
Normal Response:
Pathway*: Afferent → *Central Pathway* → Efferent

*Contralateral will be explicitly stated if pathway decussates.

---

## 14.4.2 Equipment

Very little in the way of equipment is needed to perform a neurological examination. The following equipment is either useful or necessary to perform a complete neurological examination.

### A Space to Do It In

General observations are best made if the patient is free to wander around and investigate a room or area. Many cats and some dogs will seek out a hiding place; it helps to arrange the room with few places for them to take cover ahead of time. Some dogs are best examined outside – many are less stressed than when inside an examination room or hospital and will be motivated to interact with their environment (and show what they are capable of doing). Rough surfaces such as concrete or tarmac provides more traction than hospital flooring, enabling a better assessment (both seeing and hearing) of gait. Ataxic animals are often more confident on floors with some grip.

### Chair

A chair can be particularly useful when examining cats; subtle abnormalities of gait (paresis and ataxia) can be emphasized when watching a cat jump from a height and land. Placing the cat on a chair and compelling it to leap off can facilitate this.

### A Mat (e.g. A Yoga Mat or Similar)

A yoga mat is a portable surface that will provide traction for the patient when assessing postural reactions. Carpet mats may also be used, but they are more difficult to clean.

### Pleximeter/Reflex Hammer

Pleximeters (reflex hammers) are available in a range of sizes appropriate for examining small cats to large dogs. Taylor/Tomahawk reflex hammers (triangular rubber head) are most suitable for small animal patients.

### Curved Hemostats

Hemostats allow the delivery of consistent noxious stimuli.

### Q-tips/Medical Applicators

Cotton wool tipped medical applicators (Q-tips) allow the application of gentle stimuli (useful when evaluating the corneal reflex). Wooden handled medical applicators with only one end covered in cotton wool are particularly useful as the bare tip on the other end allows for a more pointed stimulus for testing sensation of other areas of the face.

### Cotton Balls

Cotton balls can be thrown and land generating little noise, hence, they can be useful in assessing vision (tracking of an object) in isolation of the other senses.

### Laser Pointer

Many cats and some dogs will follow the point of light projected from a laser pointer, and may also be used to somewhat assess vision.

### Penlight

The normal pupillary light reflex (PLR) is proportional to the intensity of the light falling on the retina. As such, a *strong* penlight is necessary to reliably assess the PLR. If the light source does not cause you to dazzle when shone into your own eye, it is not bright enough.

### Indirect Lens, or Ophthalmoscope

The penlight may also be used to perform ophthalmoscopy with an indirect viewing lens. Two advantages of this technique over direct ophthalmoscopy using an ophthalmoscope are that it is more portable and can be conducted at a safer distance in the case of fractious animals.

## 14.4.3 The Neurological Exam Itself

The neurological examination may be conceptually divided into eight parts. While much of the neurological exam can be done purely by observation, some degree of compliance is required for a complete examination. It is useful to attempt the exam in this order, as it proceeds from observation, to tests requiring some restraint and handling, to tests that may be more noxious.

### 14.4.3.1 Mentation

Assessment of mental status should include an appraisal of both the level and the quality (content) of consciousness.

> **Textbox 14.4.3 The neurological examination may be conceptually divided into eight parts:**
>
> 1) Mentation
> 2) Posture
> 3) Gait/movement
> 4) Postural reactions
> 5) Spinal reflexes
> 6) Cranial nerves
> 7) Palpation
> 8) Nociception.

**Level of Consciousness May Be Graded as Follows**

- *Alert* – Normal responsiveness to the environment and stimuli
- *Obtunded* – Decreased responsiveness to the environment and stimuli, but rousable
- *Stuporous/Semicomatose* – Responsive only to strong stimuli
- *Comatose* – Unconscious and unresponsive to all stimuli (including noxious stimuli)

Lesions of the brainstem or forebrain may affect the level of consciousness.

**Quality of Consciousness May Be Considered as Follows**

- *Normal/Appropriate*
- *Inappropriate* – Inappropriate response to the environment or to stimuli. May have abnormal or compulsive behaviors.

A change in the quality of consciousness may occur with forebrain lesions. Compulsive circling in one direction suggests a forebrain lesion on that side. The owner may be helpful in highlighting subtle changes in behavior, or abnormal behaviors not apparent at the time of examination.

### 14.4.3.2 Posture

Posture refers to the position of the limbs and carriage of the body as a whole. Abnormal head carriage may result from forebrain lesions (head pressing, or a head turn *toward* the side of the lesion) or vestibular system lesions (a head tilt *toward or away* from the side of the lesion,

depending on the location). Abnormal carriage or curvature of the spine may be due to parenchymal spinal cord disease, an abnormality of the vertebral column or pain. Certain postures indicate specific lesions' localizations, such as decerebrate rigidity (caused by an acute lesion of the rostral brainstem), decerebellate rigidity (caused by an acute cerebellar lesion), and the Schiff-Sherrington posture (caused by acute, transverse lesions of the thoracolumbar spinal cord). Animals with abnormal proprioception often have a wide-based stance. A palmigrade and/or plantigrade stance may be seen in animals with diseases of the lower motor neuron.

### 14.4.3.3 Gait/Movement

The generation of gait requires integration of many sensory and motor systems within the nervous system, acting on the musculoskeletal system to effect movement. As such, gait evaluation is one of the more complex parts of the neurological examination. Considering the movement by its constituent parts can make assessment more manageable.

- Is the gait normal or abnormal?
- What limbs are affected?
- Is there ataxia?
- Is there paresis?
- Is there lameness?
- Are there abnormal involuntary movements?

**Ataxia**
Ataxia is a lack of coordination of movement and is caused by a loss of transmission of sensory input. Ataxia may occur as one or a combination of three syndromes:

*Sensory Ataxia*

- *Sensory ataxia* (also called *proprioceptive ataxia*) is caused by loss of sense of limb and body position, often seen as wide-based stance, swaying gait, increased stride length, and dragging or scuffing of the digits. It is caused by a lesion of the afferent sensory (proprioceptive) pathways in the peripheral nerves or centrally in the spinal cord, brainstem, or forebrain.

### Cerebellar Ataxia

- *Cerebellar ataxia* is characterized by an inability to control the rate and range of movement, resulting in hypermetria/dysmetria, postural tremor, and intention tremor. Cerebellar ataxia occurs with lesions of the cerebellum or spinocerebellar tracts within the spinal cord.

### Vestibular Ataxia

- *Vestibular ataxia* caused by a unilateral lesion is seen as leaning and falling to one side. Head tilt and abnormal nystagmus are usually seen. Animals with bilateral vestibular dysfunction often adopt a crouched stance, move their head with wide side-to-side excursions, have decreased physiological nystagmus, and often no perceptible head tilt. Vestibular ataxia results from lesions of the vestibular system peripherally (receptors in the inner ear, vestibulocochlear nerve) or centrally (vestibular nuclei in the brainstem, projections to the cerebellum and thalamus).

### Paresis

Paresis is a partial loss of ability to perform voluntary movements; paralysis (plegia) refers to a total loss. It is caused by a loss of transmission of motor innervation. The syndromes of dysfunction (Upper Motor Neuron (UMN) and Lower Motor Neuron (LMN) paresis) reflect the anatomic location of the lesion in the motor pathway. Differentiation between UMN and LMN paresis cannot be made on the severity of paresis alone – muscle tone and spinal reflexes need to be assessed.

### UMN Paresis

- *UMN paresis* occurs with disease affecting the UMN in the brain or spinal cord. Quadrupedal species can have quite marked forebrain lesions and generate a normal or near-normal gait. Centers influencing extensor muscle tone and gait pattern generation are located in the brainstem and spinal cord; as such disease in the spinal cord or brainstem is likely to cause a more obvious impairment of gait than forebrain disease. Extensor muscle tone may be normal or is often increased. Chronic disease often results in spasticity. Spinal reflexes are generally normal or increased.

### LMN Paresis

- *LMN paresis* occurs with disease of the motor unit. Gait may appear stiff and short strided. May be plantigrade/palmigrade. Muscle tone is often decreased (flaccid). Spinal reflexes are generally decreased or absent.

### Lameness

Decreased weight bearing on a limb (seen as a shortened stride or limping) most commonly occurs due to pain from musculoskeletal disease, but may also be seen with acute nerve root pain ("root signature"). Painful limbs are often carried, whereas paretic limbs tend to be dragged. Animals with bilateral lameness may appear ataxic as they shift weight from side to side.

### Involuntary Movements

Involuntary movements may be associated with rest or activity and should be described in detail (type, occurrence, onset, cessation, exacerbating factors, etc.).

- *Tremors* are rhythmic, oscillatory (sinusoidal) movements.
- *Myoclonus* is characterized by sudden, brief, shock-like involuntary contractions of a muscle or group of muscles.
- *Myotonia* is the sustained contraction or delayed relaxation of muscle after the cessation of voluntary movement.
- *Myokymia* denotes rolling, rippling, and vermicular ("worm-like") contraction of muscle.
- *Tetany* is defined as sustained muscle contraction that is worsened with stimulation, but abates with relaxation.
- *Tetanus* is the sustained contraction of muscle without relaxation.

While some types of involuntary movement may have many potential causes (such as coarse, generalized tremors secondary to various toxins, or metabolic derangements), some may be pathognomonic for certain diseases (such as myoclonus associated with canine distemper encephalomyelitis, some breed-related tremor syndromes, or tetanus due to a wound infection with the tetanospasmin toxin-producing bacillus *Clostridium tetani*).

### 14.4.3.4 Postural Reactions

Postural reactions test similar pathways to gait (the proprioceptive and motor systems). As such, they are sensitive tests for nervous system dysfunction and may identify a lesion almost anywhere in the nervous system (brain, spinal cord, or neuromuscular system). Long pathways, however, mean they are nonspecific; other parts of the neurological examination (mentation, cranial nerve tests, and spinal reflexes) are needed to localize further.

The various postural reactions assess similar pathways to each other, some emphasizing the function of individual limbs (proprioceptive positioning, hopping) or groups of limbs (hemiwalking, wheelbarrowing, and extensor postural thrust).

---

**Textbox 14.4.4 Generic postural reaction pathway**[*]

(Proprioceptor[**] → Afferent Peripheral Nerve → *Spinal Cord → Brainstem → Contralateral Forebrain → Brainstem → Spinal Cord* → Efferent Peripheral Nerve (LMN) → NMJ → Muscle)

[*] Normal cerebellar function will regulate the range and rate of limb movement.
[**] Muscle Spindle and Golgi Tendon Organ.

---

Patient size and temperament may mean that performing every postural reaction test is not possible; however, completing the entire repertoire is not necessary if a confident assessment can be made using a few (usually proprioceptive positioning and hopping).

---

**Proprioceptive (Paw) Positioning**

*Technique:* Support the animal (under the thorax when testing thoracic limbs, abdomen for pelvic limbs) in a straight, standing position, then turn their paw so the dorsal surface contacts the ground ("knuckling").

*Normal Response:* The patient should immediately return the paw to the normal position.

*Pathway:* See Textbox 14.4.4.

---

**Hopping**

*Technique:* Lift the whole animal (small dogs and cats) or the contralateral limb (large dogs) and hop the animal on one limb to that side (laterally – away from their center of gravity).

*Normal Response:* Hopping on that limb in a strong and coordinated manner to keep the limb under their center of gravity.

*Pathway:* See Textbox 14.4.4.

---

**Wheelbarrowing**

*Technique:* Lift up and support the pelvic limbs off the ground and move the patient forward.

*Normal Response:* Symmetrical, strong, coordinated walking movement of the thoracic limbs.

*Pathway:* See Textbox 14.4.4.

---

**Hemiwalking**

*Technique:* Lift the thoracic and pelvic limb on one side of the animal off the ground and move the animal to the other side (away from their center of gravity).

*Normal Response:* Hopping on both limbs in a strong and coordinated manner to keep the limbs under their center of gravity.

*Pathway:* See Textbox 14.4.4.

---

**Tactile Placing**

*Technique:* Pick the patient up and either cover their eyes or extend their neck so that they cannot see the table. Move them toward the table until the dorsal surface of the paw touches the edge of the table.

*Normal Response:* The patient should place the paw onto the surface of the table.

*Pathway:* See Textbox 14.4.4.

---

**Visual Placing**

*Technique:* Similar to tactile placing, but allow the patient to see the table.

*Normal Response:* The patient should move to place the paws on the surface of the table before contact is made.

*Pathway:* See Textbox 14.4.4. This reaction also tests the visual pathways.

---

*Extensor Postural Thrust*

*Technique:* Lift the patient by the thorax, and then lower until the pelvic limbs touch the ground.
*Normal Response:* Extension of the pelvic limbs and then backward stepping movement.
*Pathway:* See Textbox 14.4.4.

---

**Textbox 14.4.5 Tip for performing postural reactions**

Though determining what is a "normal" postural reaction for different patients of various sizes and weights can take some experience, any examiner can look for asymmetrical reactions, which are often significant.

---

### 14.4.3.5 Spinal Reflexes

Spinal reflex testing allows direct assessment of the integrity of the reflex arc (Textbox 14.4.6) and indirect assessment of UMN function. The patient should ideally be placed in lateral recumbency for testing of spinal reflexes and rolled over to compare left and right limbs as they are "upside." Reflexes may be graded as absent (0), decreased (1), normal (2), increased (3), or clonic (4). Decreased reflexes may be seen with a lesion within the reflex arc but also in animals that are stressed, or have muscle fibrosis or joint contractures. A reflex should not be considered

Table 14.4.2 Reflex arcs of specific spinal reflexes.

| Reflex | Peripheral nerve | Spinal cord segments/nerve roots |
|---|---|---|
| TL Flexor | *Multiple* | C6–T2 |
| Biceps | Musculocutaneous | C6–8 |
| Triceps | Radial | C7–T2 |
| PL Flexor | Sciatic[a] | L6–S2 |
| Patellar | Femoral | L4–6 |
| Gastrocnemius | Sciatic | L6–S2 |
| Perineal | Perineal | S1–3 |

TL: Thoracic Limb, PL: Pelvic Limb.
a)  Hip flexion mediated by femoral nerve (L4–6).

decreased or absent until multiple attempts to elicit it have been made. Increased reflexes can result from a lesion of the UMN pathways cranial to the spinal segments involving the arc. The UMN normally inhibits tone in this reflex arc, so a lesion of the UMN can lead to *disinhibition*, and therefore, an increase in the reflex. Exaggerated reflexes may also be seen with excitement, or if there is a lack of antagonistic muscle tone. Reflexes should, therefore, only be interpreted in light of the rest of the patient's examination. The recumbent musculoskeletal exam may be done at the same time as spinal reflex testing for convenience Table 14.4.2.

---

**Textbox 14.4.6 Generic spinal reflex arc**

(Receptor* → Afferent Peripheral Nerve → *Spinal Cord Segment* → Efferent Peripheral Nerve (LMN) → NMJ → Muscle.)

*Stretch of the muscle spindle in the case of tendon reflexes, and stimulation of nociceptors in the case of flexor reflexes.

---

*Biceps Reflex*

*Technique:* Placing your finger around the insertion of the biceps tendon medial to the elbow, percuss finger with the pleximeter.
*Normal Response:* Contraction of the biceps muscle.
*Pathway:* See Table 14.4.2.

---

*Triceps Reflex*

*Technique:* Flex and abduct the elbow, using a pleximeter, percuss the triceps tendon just above its insertion onto the olecranon.
*Normal Response:* Contraction of the triceps muscle.
*Pathway:* See Table 14.4.2.

---

*Patellar Reflex*

*Technique:* With the pelvic limb in a partially flexed position, percuss the patellar tendon using a pleximeter.
*Normal Response:* Contraction of the quadriceps muscle and stifle extension.
*Pathway:* See Table 14.4.2.

### Gastrocnemius Reflex

*Technique:* Extend the stifle and flex the hock, using a pleximeter, percuss the common calcaneal tendon just above its insertion onto the calcaneus.
*Normal Response:* Contraction of the caudal thigh muscles.
*Pathway:* See Table 14.4.2.

### Flexor (Withdrawal) Reflex

*Technique:* Pinch the skin between the digits.
*Normal Response:* Thoracic limb – flexion of the carpus, elbow, and shoulder. Pelvic limb – flexion of the hock, stifle, and hip. Extension of the contralateral limb (*crossed-extensor reflex*) is an abnormal finding suggesting an UMN lesion.
*Pathway:* See Table 14.4.2.

### Perineal Reflex

*Technique:* Apply a stimulus to the left and right perineum (ideally with a disposable medical applicator).
*Normal Response:* Bilateral contraction of the anal sphincter.
*Pathway:* See Table 14.4.2.

### Cutaneous Trunci Reflex

*Technique:* Using hemostats to pinch the skin over the left and right flank just lateral to midline, starting at the level of the crest of the ilium and proceeding cranially. In cats, this can be done by lightly plucking guard hairs.
*Normal Response:* Bilateral contraction of the cutaneous trunci muscle.
*Pathway:* Cutaneous Nociceptors → Segmental Cutaneous Nerves → *Ipsi- and Contralateral Spinal Cord* → Ipsi- and Contralateral C8-T1 Spinal Cord and Nerve Roots → Ipsi- and Contralateral Lateral Thoracic Nerves → Ipsi- and Contralateral Cutaneous Trunci Muscle. As the pathway for this reflex runs caudally to cranially up the spinal cord, it is not necessary to continue testing cranially once the reflex is elicited – this level reflects the level of cut-off on that side.

### 14.4.3.6 Cranial Nerves

All mammals have the same 12 pairs of cranial nerves, and as such, the cranial nerve examination is comparable across species. The cranial nerve examination tests not only the afferent and efferent cranial nerves but also the areas of the brain where the central pathway of the reflex/response is located (Table 14.4.3). CN I emerges directly from the cerebrum, CN II emerges from the thalamus, CN III–XII emerge from the brainstem in increasingly caudal locations (hence the majority of the

**Table 14.4.3** Cranial nerves and their functions.

| CN | Name | Function |
| --- | --- | --- |
| I | Olfactory | Smell |
| II | Optic | Vision |
| III | Oculomotor | **Extraocular mm. (dorsal, medial and ventral rectus, ventral oblique)** *Pupillary constrictor mm.* |
| VI | Trochlear | **Extraocular mm. (dorsal oblique)** |
| V | Trigeminal | Facial sensation **Masticatory mm.** |
| VI | Abducent | **Extraocular mm. (lateral rectus, retractor bulbi)** |
| VII | Facial | Inner surface of pinna Rostral 2/3 tongue (inc. taste) **Mm. of facial expression** *Lacrimal glands* *Salivary glands (mandibular and sublingual)* |
| VIII | Vestibulocochlear | Hearing Orientation of head/balance |
| IX | Glossopharyngeal | Pharynx, caudal 1/3 of tongue (inc. taste) **Pharynx** *Salivary glands (zygomatic and parotid)* |
| X | Vagus | Sensation of caudal pharynx, larynx **Pharynx, larynx, palate** *Visceral motor and sensation (except pelvic viscera)* |
| XI | Accessory | **Trapezius, sternocephalicus and brachiocephalicus mm.** |
| XII | Hypoglossal | **Tongue mm.** |

Sensory, **Motor**, *Parasympathetic*.

cranial nerve examination tests brainstem function). Individual tests may be done in any order; however, counting through the nerves in order (as presented here) or moving through regions of the face are ways of being consistent and less likely to omit any.

## CN I – Olfactory

As there is no reliable, objective assessment of the olfactory pathways, the olfactory nerve function is not tested.

## CN II – Optic

---

### Vision

*Technique:* Observing the patient watch its environment, navigate obstacles, or track cotton balls or the point projected by a laser pointer can subjectively assess vision.

*Normal Response:* Behavioral response suggesting that the animal perceives the visual image.

*Pathway:* Retina → CN II → Optic Chiasm → *Ipsi- or Contralateral Optic Tract → Ipsi- or Contralateral Thalamus → Ipsi- or Contralateral Cerebrum.*

---

### Menace Response

*Technique:* A normal menace response involves making abrupt gestures (such as waving a hand) toward one eye or visual field, taking care not to touch the animal. Cats and stressed dogs often attenuate their menace response; performing the palpebral reflex between every few attempts at the menace response may reduce this tendency.

*Normal Response:* A blink of that (and often the contralateral) eyelid.

*Pathway:* Retina → CN II → Optic Chiasm → *Contralateral Optic Tract → Contralateral Forebrain → Cerebellum → Brainstem →* CN VII → Orbicularis oculi muscle. (This is another oversimplification, as areas of the retina project preferentially to the ipsi- and contralateral visual cortex, but the simplification appears to be clinically useful.)

---

### Pupil Size and Symmetry

Pupil size and the presence of anisocoria should be noted before performing the PLR. Subtle anisocoria is best assessed by illuminating the patient's face from a distance and looking for the tapetal reflection ("distant direct illumination"). Pupil size and symmetry should be assessed in light and dark ambient conditions, where normal response would be constricted (miotic) and dilated (mydriatic) pupils, respectively.

Pupillary construction is mediated by the parasympathetic nervous system in response to light falling on the retina (Retina → CN II → Optic Chiasm → *Ipsi- or Contralateral Optic Tract → Ipsi- or Contralateral Midbrain →* Parasympathetic CN III → Pupillary Constrictor Muscles). A lesion anywhere in this parasympathetic pathway will lead to sympathetic dominance and mydriasis.

Pupillary dilation is mediated by the sympathetic nervous system – it does not involve the visual system but is appropriate to consider here. The pathway of sympathetic innervation to the orbit is long (first-order neurons in brainstem and cervical spinal cord → second-order neurons in T1–3 spinal cord/nerve roots, thoracic sympathetic trunk and *alongside* the vagosympathetic trunk in the neck → third-order neurons in the cranial cervical ganglion adjacent to tympanic bulla and then *alongside* the ophthalmic branch of CN V → smooth muscles of orbit and pupillary dilator muscles). A lesion anywhere in this sympathetic pathway will lead to parasympathetic dominance and miosis (generally with ptosis, enophthalmus and prolapsed nictitans – **Horner's Syndrome**).

---

### Pupillary Light Reflex (PLR)

*Technique:* Shine a bright light into the eye.

*Normal Response:* Look for a reflex constriction of the stimulated (direct response) and nonstimulated (indirect/consensual response) pupil. Generally slightly greater constriction on the illuminated side (direct PLR).

*Pathway:* Retina → CN II → Optic Chiasm → *Ipsi- or Contralateral Optic Tract → Ipsi- or Contralateral Midbrain →* Parasympathetic CN III → Pupillary Constrictor Muscles. The two decussations in the pathway (optic chiasm and midbrain) generate the direct and indirect reflex.

---

---

**Dazzle Reflex**

*Technique:* Shine a bright light into the eye.
*Normal Response:* A blink or squint of both eyes, generally slightly more on the illuminated side.
*Pathway:* Retina → CN II → Optic Chiasm → *Ipsi-* or *Contralateral Optic Tract* → *Ipsi-* or *Contralateral Midbrain* → *Ipsi-* or *Contralateral Brainstem* → CN VII → Muscles of Blink.

---

**Fundic Examination**

Examination of the fundus is an important part of the neurological examination as it is the only part of the nervous system we can see directly. The optic disc is the terminus of the optic nerve, which is itself a white matter tract of the brain. Papilledema (swelling of the optic disc) may represent disease of the optic nerve specifically or increased intracranial pressure generally. Many common neurological diseases with a vascular or inflammatory etiology will also cause changes in the retina such as tortuous retinal vessels or hemorrhage or chorioretinitis, respectively.

**CN III – Oculomotor, CN IV – Trochlear, and CN VI – Abducent**

CNs III, IV, and VI are considered together as they innervate the extraocular muscles (see Table 14.4.3). Dysfunction of these nerves or nuclei will result in decreased function of these muscle groups, which may cause a **strabismus** (deviation of the eye) or ophthalmoparesis/plegia. In the early stage, hypotonus will lead to a deviation of the globe away from the direction of action of that muscle. If muscular contracture occurs over time with denervation or inflammation, deviation of the globe may be toward the direction of normal muscular action.

A positional strabismus may occur with lesions of the vestibular pathway, and will be discussed under CN VIII – Vestibulocochlear nerve.

See Pupil Size and Symmetry (CN III).
See PLR (CN III).
See Corneal Reflex (CN VI).

**CN V – Trigeminal**

The trigeminal nerve divides to three major branches: the ophthalmic branch, the maxillary branch, and the motor branch. All three branches carry sensory fibers. The autonomous zones (areas with sensory innervation by one branch and one branch only) are as follows: ophthalmic branch – cornea, maxillary branch – lip adjacent to the maxillary canine tooth; mandibular branch – lip adjacent to the mandibular canine tooth.

---

**Palpebral Reflex**

*Technique:* Touch the medial canthus.
*Normal Response:* Closure of the palpebral fissure (blink).
*Pathway:* CN V → Brainstem → CN VII.

---

**Corneal Reflex**

*Technique:* Touch the cornea using a moistened Q-tip or medical applicator.
*Normal Response:* Retraction of the globe and blink.
*Pathway:* CN V → Brainstem → CN VI (retraction of globe) + VII (blink).

---

**Nasal Stimulation**

*Technique:* Stimulation of the nasal mucosa just inside the nostril.
*Normal Response:* An aversive response (moving the head away – this is a useful test of conscious perception of noxious stimuli and therefore higher centers).
*Pathway:* CN V → Brainstem → *Contralateral Forebrain.*

---

**Jaw Function/Masticatory Muscle**

The maxillary branch supplies motor innervation to the muscles of mastication. Trigeminal lesions may result in paresis/paralysis of these muscles (a "dropped jaw" – usually requires a bilateral deficit) and/or atrophy. This atrophy is often most notable in the temporalis and masseter muscles as they are the most superficial/prominent. The pterygoid muscle is located behind the eye; atrophy of this muscle may lead to an enophthalmus.

**CN VII – Facial**

The facial nerve supplies motor innervation to the superficial muscles of the face (muscles of facial expression). Acute facial paresis/paralysis will cause a droop of that side of the face (lip, ear, and widened palpebral fissure). Chronic denervating lesions may lead to contracture and deviation toward the side of the lesion. Subtle facial asymmetries are often best appreciated at a distance. A decreased ability to blink may be detected by observing a lack of spontaneous blinking, or an inadequate menace response or palpebral reflex.

*See Menace Response.*
*See Palpebral Reflex.*

Parasympathetic fibers in CN VII supply innervation to the lacrimal glands. Dysfunction will result in decreased tear production (and potentially "dry eye"). Tear production can be quantified using Schirmer tear strips.

### CN VIII – Vestibulocochlear

The vestibulocochlear nerve has two branches: the vestibular branch and the cochlear branch.

The cochlear branch carries auditory information from the receptor (cochlea) to the brainstem. Marked, bilateral lesions of this pathway will cause apparent deafness. Subtle or unilateral lesions are difficult to detect clinically and require more objective tests of the auditory pathway (Brainstem Auditory Evoked Response – BAER).

The vestibular branch carries information regarding the position of the head in space (balance) as detected by the vestibular apparatus in the inner ear to the vestibular nuclei in the brainstem. Dysfunction of the vestibular system peripherally (vestibular receptors/apparatus and CN VIII) or centrally (vestibular nuclei, and projections to and from the cerebellum and thalamus) may cause the following.

> ### Vestibular Ataxia
> Head tilt, leaning, and falling (see description in sections on posture and gait).

> ### Positional (Abnormal) Nystagmus or Strabismus.
> Any spontaneous nystagmus should be characterized by the direction of movement and the direction of the fast phase. Positioning with neck extended in dorsal recumbency may "decompensate" an animal

coping with vestibular dysfunction and unmask a subtle nystagmus. Positional strabismus is best identified by raising the patient's head; vestibular lesions often cause a ventral positional strabismus on the side of the lesion.

> ### Decreased Physiological (Normal) Nystagmus.
> *Technique:* Rotate the patient's head (either by laterally bending the neck or picking up and rotating the whole animal (small dogs and cats)).
> *Normal Response:* Both eyes make rapid, jerking movements (conjugate saccades) toward the direction of rotation.
> *Pathway:* CN VIII → Brainstem → CNs III, IV, and VI.

### CN IX – Glossopharyngeal and
### CN X – Vagus

The glossopharyngeal and vagus nerves are sensory and motor to the pharynx.

> ### Gag Reflex
> *Technique:* Stimulation of the pharyngeal mucosa with fingers.
> *Normal Response:* The patient should gag, retch, and swallow.
> *Pathway:* CN IX and X → Brainstem → CN IX and X.

A similar response may be elicited by palpating externally dorsal to the larynx (if there is a concern, the patient may bite fingers placed in its mouth).

The vagus nerve also innervates the laryngeal musculature. Lesions may result in an ipsilateral laryngeal paresis/paralysis. The owner should be questioned carefully regarding any history of dysphagia, regurgitation, loss of bark, or stridor. The vagus also carries parasympathetic fibers that innervate the heart and gastrointestinal system.

### CN XI – Accessory

The accessory nerve supplies motor innervation to the trapezius, sternocephalicus, and brachiocephalicus muscles. As paresis or atrophy of these muscles is rarely detectable in isolation, CN XI is not assessed.

### CN XII – Hypoglossal

The hypoglossal nerve supplies motor innervation to the muscles of the tongue. The tongue should be assessed for any paresis, deviation, atrophy, or asymmetry that may suggest denervation (Figure 14.4.1).

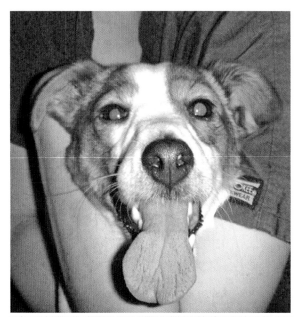

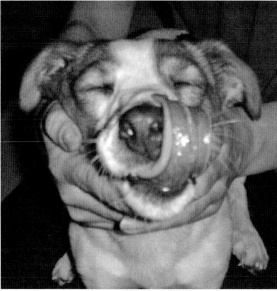

**Figure 14.4.1** Much of the cranial nerve examination can be done by observation.

### 14.4.3.7 Palpation

Palpation is potentially noxious and should be performed toward the end of the examination. Extreme care must be taken if there is history or possibility of vertebral column trauma and instability. The head should be palpated lightly for evidence of masses, swelling, muscle atrophy, or calvarial defects. This should include retropulsion of the eyes. The spine can be palpated from either end; however, if vertebral column pain is suspected from the history, it is worthwhile starting at the opposite end. Light palpation aids in detecting atrophy, swelling, masses, curvatures, or misalignments. Deep palpation segmentally to detect pain should be performed dorsally in the thoracolumbar spine and laterally in the cervical spine. The cervical spine and tail should be extended dorsally and flexed or ventrally and laterally to the limit of natural movement. Symmetry of contralateral limbs should be assessed when the patient is standing.

### 14.4.3.8 Nociception

Assessment of nociception is by definition the most noxious part of the examination and should be left until last. A hemostat should be used as it provides a consistent and reliably noxious stimulus. Pinching a fold of skin with hemostats tests "Superficial" pain perception. "Deep" pain perception is tested by compressing bone (the digits or tail). The stimulus should be initially gently applied and then gradually increased in intensity until a positive response is achieved, so as not to cause unnecessary pain. A positive response requires a behavioral response (vocalizing and turning the head). Reflex withdrawal of the limb indicates an intact reflex arc (peripheral nerves and spinal cord segments) only and is NOT a sign of conscious perception of pain (which requires transmission of the stimulus up the spinal cord to the brain). The pathways that carry this sensory modality in the spinal cord are the most resistant to damage; loss of deep pain perception indicates severe injury and has important prognostic implications. Cutaneous sensory testing of autonomous zones or dermatomes should be performed if clinically indicated. Maps of these autonomous zones are available in other texts [1–3].

---

**Textbox 14.4.7 Nociception**

Key point – Limb withdrawal (the flexor reflex) does not demonstrate an intact nociceptive pathway to the brain.

---

## 14.4.4 Putting It All Together – Clinical Problem-solving in Neurological Cases

### 14.4.4.1 Making a Neuroanatomical Diagnosis

Once the neurological examination has been completed, all deficits should be recorded and considered. If there are none, the patient may be considered neurologically normal (at least at the time of the examination). If deficits have been found, the next task is to determine where the causative lesion is within the nervous system. Deficits found on individual tests suggest a lesion within that pathway. The lesion exists on a specific part of that pathway if

1) All other parts of that pathway are deemed "normal" on the other neurological exam tests, or
2) If a deficit is found on the "intersecting pathway" of another test (i.e. the two pathways run through the same area of the nervous system).

If all deficits on the examination can be explained by a single area of localization, then a focal neuroanatomic localization is made. If a single area of localization cannot explain all the deficits, then a multifocal (multiple, noncontiguous lesions) or diffuse (extensive, contiguous lesion) neurolocalization must be made.

### 14.4.4.2 Setting Up a List of Differential Diagnoses – A Pathophysiological Approach

Diseases of the nervous system of similar pathophysiology will generally lead to similar clinical presentations, so it is often useful to consider them together as a group when initially formulating a list of differential diagnoses. Several mnemonic schemes such as DAMNITV (Table 14.4.4) and VITAMIND exist to aid in this.

### 14.4.4.3 Refining Your List of Differential Diagnoses

Of all the pieces of information we collect from the owners when we take a history, or find when we examine

**Table 14.4.4** Pathophysiological groupings of disease.

| | |
|---|---|
| **D** | Degenerative |
| **A** | Anomalous |
| **M** | Metabolic |
| **N** | Neoplastic<br>Nutritional |
| **I** | Infectious<br>Inflammatory (autoimmune)<br>"Idiopathic" conditions |
| **T** | Trauma<br>Toxic |
| **V** | Vascular |

Many diseases could be categorized in more than one group. For example, lysosomal storage diseases are congenital inborn errors of metabolism, many of which will cause neurodegeneration. Degenerative intervertebral disc disease may precipitate herniation of a disc and cause spinal cord trauma. Certain toxins (anticoagulant rodenticides) or infections (*angiostrongylus vasorum* infestation) cause a coagulopathy and spontaneous hemorrhage. The point of this exercise is not to attain the highest state of pathophysiological truth, but to have a reasonably reliable system to organize our thoughts in a consistent way when dealing with clinical cases. Knowledge of the pathophysiological and clinical characteristics of individual diseases within these groups is still necessary.

a patient, certain facts will be more pertinent to constructing and ranking our list of differential diagnoses than others (Textbox 14.4.8).

While the history and examination should obviously not be limited to these points only (the geographical location, vaccination status, diet, general health of the animal etc., must also be considered), they provide a useful prompt for remembering important details and are pertinent in almost all cases [6].

---

**Textbox 14.4.8 Six particularly useful points of clinical data**

1) Neuroanatomic localization
2) Patient signalment
3) Onset of clinical signs
4) Progression of clinical signs
5) Symmetry of clinical signs
6) Presence or absence of pain.

---

### Neuroanatomic Localization

The *key step* in clinical problem solving in neurology is making a *neurolocalization* – it is *the* piece of clinical data upon which the rest of the diagnostic plan depends. This is because specific diseases will affect only certain parts of the nervous system, and therefore certain parts of the nervous system will only be affected by specific diseases. Knowing which part of the nervous system is involved effectively rules in or out many diseases as possible causes.

Whether or not the distribution of lesions is focal, multifocal, or diffuse will also influence which differential diagnoses should be considered more or less likely. For example, infectious and inflammatory diseases often cause multifocal lesions. Degenerative and metabolic diseases generally affect the nervous system diffusely.

### Patient Signalment

Patient signalment will also determine what neurological diseases an individual has the potential to develop.

*Species* is obviously an important determinant of what diseases an animal is susceptible to.

Many neurological diseases will only affect a particular species (e.g. feline infectious peritonitis), though many important diseases can affect multiple species (e.g. rabies).

It is self-evident to any veterinary practitioner that certain diseases are over-represented within certain *breeds*. However, care must be taken in interpreting "diseases by breed" tables found in many texts: common breeds may have many diseases listed due to the size of the population of that breed, rather than a true predisposition. Many neurological diseases are also rare – single or sporadic reporting of a disease in individuals of a certain breed does not mean that breed is particularly susceptible.

Animals with congenital abnormalities, certain metabolic, or neurodegenerative conditions are more likely to present with clinical signs at a younger *age*. Intracranial or spinal neoplasms more commonly, but not exclusively, affect older animals.

With the exception of some X-linked inherited diseases, *sex* rarely increases or decreases an individual's vulnerability to neurological diseases enough to change the list of differential diagnoses.

### Onset of Clinical Signs

Ascertaining the onset of clinical signs, from first signs to maximal dysfunction (per-acute, acute, sub-acute,

chronic, and acute-on-chronic) will help determine likely causative diseases. For example, ischemic/vascular and traumatic diseases often cause a per-acute onset of signs. Neurodegenerative diseases generally lead to an insidious onset of dysfunction. Animals with intracranial or spinal neoplasia may have an acute decompensation after a period of subtle clinical signs.

### Progression of Clinical Signs

Similarly, the progression of clinical signs over time (improving, static, deteriorating, waxing and waning, episodic, or paroxysmal) will be suggestive of likely causes. For example, signs associated with many ischemic/vascular diseases may improve or resolve with time, whereas those associated with inflammatory diseases, infections, and neoplasia are likely to get worse without treatment. Neurodegenerative diseases cause unremitting deterioration over time. Metabolic disorders that affect nervous system functions often cause waxing and waning of clinical signs (Figure 14.4.2).

### Symmetry of Clinical Signs

The degree of symmetry or asymmetry of the neurological signs can be useful in determining which pathophysiological groups of diseases are more or less likely. Lateralizing forebrain signs are much more likely to reflect structural/organic brain disease than systemic diseases – metabolic derangements generally manifest themselves with symmetrical clinical signs. Strongly lateralizing spinal cord localizations are more likely to result from ischemic lesions (due to the lateralizing blood supply to the spinal cord) than compressive spinal cord lesions (where both sides of the spinal cord are likely to be functionally impaired).

### Presence or Absence of Pain*

Whether or not an animal exhibits signs of pain can also be useful in determining which pathophysiological groups of diseases are more or less likely. There are no free nerve endings within the brain or spinal cord (the CNS is "insensate"). Animals with intrinsic CNS diseases (such as neurodegenerative diseases or infarcts) will generally not present as painful. Tissues around the CNS – meninges, nerve roots, bone, ligament, intervertebral disc, articular joints, and muscle – all are innervated with free nerve endings, so any disease affecting or disrupting these tissues may result in pain. Animals with

**Figure 14.4.2** Noting the temporal nature of the disease may be useful in diagnosis as well as monitoring response to treatment.

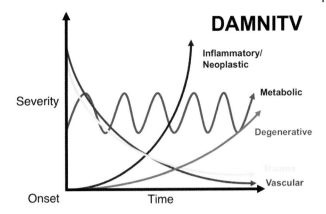

diseases that affect the surrounding tissues (e.g. meningitis, intervertebral disc herniation, bony neoplasia, polyarthritis, and abscessation) often will show signs of pain.

(*Note – here we are talking about whether an animal acts as if it is in pain. We are not talking about whether an animal has the ability to perceive painful stimuli via intact nociceptive pathways, i.e. testing nociception.*)

#### 14.4.4.4 Putting It All Together

A reasonably focused list of differential diagnoses can be constructed based on the neurolocalization, and other pertinent clinical data (as outlined above). In most cases, further diagnostic tests will be required to make a definitive diagnosis. Constructing an accurate as possible list of possible causes, ranked in order of probability, will assist in choosing the most appropriate and cost–effective diagnostic tests, or if further investigation is not possible, the most reasonable empiric treatments.

## References

1 Dewey, C.W. and da Costa, R.C. (2016). A Practical Guide to Canine and Feline Neurology, 3e. Wiley Blackwell.

2 de Lahunta, A., Glass, E., and Kent, M. (2015). Veterinary Neuroanatomy and Clinical Neurology, 4e. WB Saunders.

3 Lorenz, M.D., Coates, J.R., and Kent, M. (2010). Handbook of Veterinary Neurology, 5e. Elsevier Saunders.

4 King, A.S. (2002). Physiological and clinical anatomy of the domestic mammals. In: Central Nervous System, vol. 1. Blackwell Science.

5 Jenkins, T.W. (1972). Functional Mammalian Neuroanatomy. Lea & Febiger.

6 Cardy, T.J.A., De Decker, S., Kenny, P.J., and Volk, H.A. (2015). Clinical reasoning in canine spinal disease: what combination of clinical information is useful? *Veterinary Record* **177**: 171.

# 15

# Emergency Medicine and Procedures

*Cynthia Delany[1,2]*

[1]*Koret Shelter Medicine Program, University of California Davis, 1 Shields Avenue, CCAH, Davis, CA 95616, USA*
[2]*California Animal Shelter Friends, 34511 State Highway 16, Woodland, CA 95695, USA*

## 15.1 Introduction to Field Emergency Medicine

Veterinary professionals working in the field will often be presented with animals in critical condition, or who develop a serious medical issue while in their care. Despite the fact that the field environment can present many limitations as to the types of diagnostics and treatments that can be pursued, being prepared for emergencies can drastically improve patient outcomes.

### 15.1.1 Principles of Field Emergency Care Versus a Traditional Clinic Setting

Emergency medicine in the field is focused on diagnosing an animal's medical condition as accurately as possible and stabilizing the patient. In some cases, this will be a temporary solution until the animal can be transported to a facility with additional capabilities. In other cases, the care provided in the field will need to be as comprehensive as possible as it may be the only care that patient receives. Field emergency work may vary significantly from what would be seen in a fully equipped general or specialty practice but should still strive to address the animal's major concerns and acheive the best possible outcome for the animal.

### 15.1.2 Triage

In any setting, emergency medicine begins with triage (French meaning "to sort"). This is the process by which a quick assessment of the presenting animal is performed in an attempt to determine if the animal is in stable condition or requires immediate care. This includes gathering any available information or history on the animal – such as medical history, age, any known or suspected exposure or incidents, as well as information on the animal's living situation and husbandry.

### 15.1.3 Field Treatment Limitations

#### 15.1.3.1 Equipment – Diagnostic and Treatment

In the typical field setting, there are significant limitations in diagnostic and treatment capabilities. However, even with very little in the way of sophisticated equipment, there is a great deal of information that can be gathered and care that can be provided. In many cases, a thorough physical examination and history may be the only diagnostic tool available. Whenever possible, professionals should attempt to maximize their capacity to provide care by preparing for the most common emergencies they expect to see. Even with only basic diagnostic equipment, there is a significant amount of information that can be ascertained and used to devise treatment strategies.

#### 15.1.3.2 Expertise and Time

In addition to limited equipment, many field practitioners may find themselves limited in time and expertise, depending on the caseload, type, and severity of emergencies that present. Staffing is often limited and emergencies may exceed the typical treatment capacity of a field clinic.

*Field Manual for Small Animal Medicine*, First Edition. Edited by Katherine Polak and Ann Therese Kommedal.
© 2018 John Wiley & Sons, Inc. Published 2018 by John Wiley & Sons, Inc.

### 15.1.3.3 Ongoing and Follow-up Care

Another common limitation in the field is the ability to provide ongoing care for animals following initial stabilizing care. Veterinary care may be limited in a particular area and when visiting practitioners leave, such as during a mobile clinic, there may be few options for follow-up care. Such situations may require a degree of creativity and training of animal caretakers to ensure that animals receive continued care if needed.

## 15.2 Physical Examination

A vital component of emergency medicine is a comprehensive physical examination. Performing an examination using a body systems approach can help reduce the chances of inadvertently missing any critical information in a setting where exam findings may be the only diagnostic tool available. Developing your own systematic approach and following it consistently

---

**Textbox 15.1 Key components of a comprehensive physical examination by body system**

*General assessment.* Overall demeanor, activity/alertness level and behavior, and body temperature.

*Eyes, Ears, Nose, and Throat*

*Eyes.* Pupil size and symmetry, vision, or indications of being nonvisual, scleral color (including assess for icterus), scleral injection, hemorrhage, and globe abnormalities, including exophthalmos, buphthalmos, ectropion, entropion, foreign bodies, nictitating membrane appearance, chemosis, blepharospasm, photophobia, and nystagmus – normal/physiological vs pathology (and characterization of any seen), obvious trauma to the globe or eyelids.

*Ears.* Pinnal skin color, smell, exudate, trauma, and petechiations.

*Nose.* Airflow from each nare, any audible congestion, any discharge (and if so, characterization as serous, purulent, mucopurulent, hemorrhagic, etc.), signs of trauma, deviation, space-occupying mass effect on palpation, and sneezing.

*Oral cavity.* Mucous membrane color and capillary refill time (CRT), dental disease presence and type, foreign bodies, abnormal smell, appearance of tonsils, masses, and trauma.

*Throat.* Abnormal upper airway noise such as stertor or stridor, reverse sneezing, tracheal sensitivity on palpation, mass effect on palpation, abnormal swallowing motions, thyroid slip, and soft tissue swelling around throat.

*Lymph nodes.* Size, symmetry of palpable superficial lymph nodes, and density/firmness of each node.

*Hair coat.* Ectoparasites and missing hair (and pattern).

*Integument.* Appearance of skin, assess for petechia, color (including icterus), masses, and wounds.

*Musculoskeletal.* Gait, body condition score, musculature (including looking for symmetry), assess for lameness, full check of paws, legs, and joints, including assessing for any pain, swelling, crepitus, abnormalities of range of motion, mass effects, trauma, palpable fractures, and abnormal angulation.

*Neurological.* Assess for any deficits – cranial nerve dysfunction, gait deficits, balance deficits, abnormalities of mentation, seizures/tremors, head trauma, abnormal responses to testing reflexes, and responses.

*Cardiovascular.* Heart rate, rhythm, murmurs, pulse presence and quality, mucous membrane color and CRT, any decrease in heart sounds, and any abnormalities of distribution/shifting of heart sounds to one side of the thorax or the other.

*Respiratory.* Respiratory rate, effort, lung sounds – including increased, decreased, or absent, upper airway sounds, and evidence of chest trauma.

*Gastrointestinal.* Obvious signs of nausea, diarrhea (including type and presence of absence of blood), abdominal distension, rectal masses, abnormalities on rectal exam, abnormal palpation of intestines, obvious foreign body/mass effect, and abdominal fluid wave.

*Genital.* Appearance of external genitalia, being intact or altered, vaginal or penile discharge (and characterization of discharge), mammary gland appearance, and palpation, especially assessing for masses related to the genital system.

*Urinary.* Palpation of bladder and kidneys, appearance of urine, and ability to produce and pass urine.

with each patient will be vital to your success in the field.

## 15.3 Initial Stabilization

In the field, emphasis should be placed on treating potentially life threatening conditions. In situations where there is the possibility of the animal requiring additional care once stabilized, efforts should be focused on efficiently and effectively stabilizing the animal and transporting it to a better equipped facility. If there is no possibility for additional care, the initial focus will still be on stabilization but the practitioner will also need to develop a longer term plan for the animal to receive any additional care in the field setting.

## 15.4 Field Supplies, Equipment, and Setup

Sound preparation and planning for routine emergencies in the field is crucial for success. Compiling appropriate supplies, equipment, and a formulary of basic medications ahead of time will improve your ability to effectively deal with common emergency situations. The following tables include lists of recommended diagnostic equipment (Table 15.1), equipment and supplies for medical treatments (Table 15.2), and emergency drugs and equipment (Table 15.3).

### 15.4.1 Field Treatment Area Setup

Field treatment capabilities can be greatly impacted by the organization and setup of the treatment area.

Table 15.1 Recommended diagnostic equipment organized from basic to advanced.

| Basic | Intermediate | Advanced |
| --- | --- | --- |
| Thermometer | Microscope (and immersion oil) | Lactate machine |
| Stethoscope | Refractometer | Electrocardiograph |
| Pleximeter (for testing reflexes) | Microcentrifuge (and microhematocrit tubs, clay, packed cell volume (PCV) reading card) | Electrolyte machine |
| | | Blood chemistry machine |
| Penlight | Glucometer (and test strips) | Plain film radiographs |
| Otoscope and ear cones | Urinalysis test strips | Ultrasound |
| | Regular centrifuge | Digital radiographs |
| Ophthalmoscope | Pulse oximeter | Coagulation times machine (PT/PTT) |
| | Fluorescein strips (for corneal staining) | STAT mini blood analysis machine |
| | Schirmer tear test strips (to test tear production) | CBC machine |
| | Blood collection tubes (nonadditive, EDTA added, etc.) | Blood pressure monitor |
| | Slides (and slide stains – gram, diff-quick) | Endoscope |
| | BUN test strips | Blood gas analyzer |
| | Manual clotting time test tubes (no additive tubes with diatomaceous earth added) | Osmometer |
| | Culture swabs | Colloid oncotic pressure analyzer |
| | Formalin-containing sample collection jars | Lactate machine |
| | Esophageal stethoscope | Defibrillator (treatment/not diagnostic) |

Table 15.2 Recommended field medical equipment and supplies.

| Oxygen therapy | Fluid therapy | Nursing care | Surgical care |
| --- | --- | --- | --- |
| Oxygen flow regulator | IV catheters – various sizes – diameters and lengths | Drug formulary reference book | Surgery reference book |
| Oxygen tanks | Extension sets | Electric heating pads (or other items such as rice socks, heating discs, and access to microwave to heat up) | Surgery packs (including needle drives, hemostats, thumb forceps, surgery scissors, etc.) |
| Ambu – positive pressure ventilation bag | Male adapters and T ports to cap catheters | Oral syringes | Scalpel blades |
| Tubes for nasal insufflation | Primary fluid infusion sets | Bedding – clean towels and blankets | Suture (various types and sizes) |
| Extension sets | Syringes – various sizes include small – 1 ml, 3 ml, medium 6 ml, 12 ml and large 35 ml and 60 ml (with large syringes in both catheter tip and luer lock tip) | Cleaning and disinfecting solutions | Surgical staplers |
| Laryngoscope with blades | Three-way stopcocks | Cleaning supplies – surfaces and floors | Clippers (with additional blades, lubricant, and cleaning wash) |
| Endotracheal tubes (various sizes) | Butterfly catheters | Red rubber catheters | Laparotomy sponges |
| Tracheostomy tubes | Tape and self-adhesive wrap to secure catheters | Various width tape (½ inch (1.2 cm), 1 in. (2.5 cm)) | Sterile gauze |
| Nasal catheters | Crystalloid fluids (such as 0.9% NaCl, lactated ringers, Plasma-Lyte, and similar) | Self-adherent bandaging material | Surgical scrub |
| Bubble humidifier | Fluid additives – potassium chloride, potassium phosphate, sodium bicarbonate, dextrose | Stretch gauze rolls | Surgical solution |
| Stylet | Needles (for syringes and larger for intraosseous catheters) | Cast padding | Sterile surgery gloves |
| | Colloid fluids | Cast material | Surgery caps, masks, gowns |
| | Fluid pump | Preformed splints | Alligator forceps |
| | Syringe pump | Elastic tape (wide cotton elastic tape) | Abdominal retractors |
| | PPN (partial parenteral nutrition) solutions | Tongue depressors | Smaller bone/muscle retractors |
| | Blood products (fresh whole blood, stored whole blood, fresh frozen plasma) | | Speculum (vaginal and oral) |

- Blood collection bags (or empty IV fluid bags)
- Citrated phosphate dextrose (anticoagulant for blood transfusions)
- Hemo-Nate-type blood filters
- In-line blood filter primary set
- Pressure bag for fluids
- Fluid warmer

- Cotton-tipped applicators
- Elizabethan collars
- Cages/crates/exercise pens for patient housing
- Painting drop cloth or large durable trash bags (to create cleanable surfaces)
- Duct tape
- Bandage scissors
- Wound dressings (granulated sugar, medicinal honey, calcium alginate, nonstick wound dressings, etc.)
- Nebulizer
- Species appropriate food – dry and canned
- Liquid nutrition products (at least milk replacer–type)
- Gauze squares
- Alcohol (spray bottle or squeeze bottle)
- Hydrogen peroxide (spray bottle or squeeze bottle)
- Lubricating jelly

- Suction machine (including sterile tubes and tips)
- Cautery machine (or disposable cautery units)
- Urinary, oral and body cavity – use catheters (such as red rubber tubes, semi-rigid polypropylene "tomcat catheters," and flexible catheters – silicone or similar material – of various diameters and lengths)
- Anesthesia machine (including anesthetic agent and gas-scavenging unit)
- Vacuum for hair removal
- Waste containers
- Stomach tubes and stomach pump
- Circulating warm water blanket and/or forced air warming blankets
- Surgical lights
- Surgical table and instrument tray
- Surgical glue

Table 15.3 Emergency drug and supply recommendations.

| | | |
|---|---|---|
| Acepromazine | Epinephrine | Pentobarbital |
| Acetylcysteine | Eye lubricant | Phenobarbital |
| Activated charcoal (with and without sorbitol) | Eye medications (triple antibiotic type, with and without steroids), ocular topical atropine, etc. | Phenylephrine |
| | | Potassium chloride |
| Albuterol | Fentanyl | Potassium phosphates |
| Aminophylline | Flumazenil | Pralidoxime |
| Amiodarone | Furosemide | Prednisone |
| Antibiotics (oral and injectable) | H$_2$ antagonists (oral and injectable) | Procainamide |
| Antidiarrheal | Heparin | Proparacaine |
| Antiemetics (metoclopramide, ondansetron, etc.) | Hydrogen peroxide | Propofol |
| | Insulin | Sodium bicarbonate |
| Apomorphine (for emesis) | Ipecac (for emesis) | Terbutaline |
| Atipamezole | Ketamine (or other dissociative such as Telazol®/Zoletil®) | Theophylline |
| Atropine | Lactulose | Toxin antidotes as appropriate for region |
| B-Complex vitamins | Lidocaine | |
| Calcium gluconate | Lidocaine gel | Tropicamide |
| Citrate phosphate dextrose | Mannitol | Valium |
| Dexamethasone sodium phosphate | Methocarbamol | Vasopressin |
| Dexmedetomidine | Metoclopramide | Vitamin K |
| Dextrose M | Naloxone | Xylazine |
| Diphenhydramine | NSAIDs (nonsteroidal anti-inflammatory) – both oral and injectable | Yohimbine |
| Dobutamine | | |
| Docusate | Ondansetron (or similar antiemetic) | |
| Dopamine | Opioids (morphine, oxymorphone, buprenorphine hydromorphone, butorphanol, etc.) | |

In an ideal situation, the field hospital will resemble a traditional veterinary clinic with examination space, cages to hospitalize patients, a nonsterile care/procedure area, and separate surgery suite(s). In more austere settings, it may be necessary to create more rudimentary treatment and patient housing areas. Basic principles of sanitation, infectious disease control, and sterility for sterile procedures should still apply, regardless of the setting.

Animal transportation crates, folding panel exercise pens, collapsible playpens, and even feral cat traps can be used as housing for patients in the absence of traditional hospital cages. Any table surface covered with clean towels, housetraining pads, clean garbage bags, drop cloth, or newspaper can be used for treatment and even surgical procedures if a traditional surgical table is unavailable. A bright, focused light source can be used in lieu of traditional procedural or surgical lights, supplemented by a light source mounted on glasses or forehead of the surgeon. A portable flashlight can also provide additional light when held by an assistant during emergency procedures.

*In the field setting, creativity with a strong focus on basic principles will help provide patients with the best care possible, even in a resource-challenged setting.*

## 15.5 Supportive Care and Monitoring

In addition to providing sound medical treatment, the primary goal of supportive care in any setting is to ensure comfortable housing with minimal stress, temperature control (including appropriate heat support if indicated), and appropriate hydration and nutritional support. Other considerations to address in any medical settings include appropriate light/dark cycles and noise-control to allow animals the opportunity to sleep and rest comfortably.

Appropriate monitoring will depend on the animal's condition, how stable they are, and resources available. One of the most valuable monitoring tools is careful observations of the animal's status including eating, drinking, activity and comfort level, as well as any obvious clinical symptoms such as vomiting, diarrhea, inappetence, pain, or lethargy. Specific monitoring of basic vitals – temperature, heart rate, respiration rate, and serial physical exams to monitor all body systems is invaluable and do not require sophisticated facilities or equipment. Additional monitoring feasible in many field settings include basic blood values such as packed cell volume (PCV), total protein (TP), blood glucose, blood urea nitrogen (BUN) and urine-specific gravity and appearance. Appropriately documenting the overall patient status, vital signs, exam results, treatment plans, and diagnostic values is necessary to appropriately track patient progress or decline, and allows the clinician and support team to respond effectively.

## 15.6 Emergency Procedures

### 15.6.1 Abdominal Lavage

#### 15.6.1.1 Indications
Abdominal lavage is indicated in patients with septic abdomen or contamination of the abdominal cavity due to an externally penetrating abdominal injury or rupture/loss of integrity of some portion of the gastrointestinal (GI) tract.

#### 15.6.1.2 Setting
Abdominal lavage is performed under anesthesia whenever possible as it is considered a surgical procedure and should be done with as little additional contamination as possible. There may be instances in which a modified abdominal lavage is performed on a sedated animal if general anesthesia is not possible, or if the animal is not stable enough for general anesthesia.

#### 15.6.1.3 Equipment

1) Surgery/procedure table
2) General anesthesia, or sedation for modified lavage
3) Abdominal preparation supplies – clippers, gauze, scrub, and solution
4) Surgical equipment – basic surgery pack, scalpel blade, and suture
5) Lavage equipment – 0.9% saline or similar isotonic crystalloid fluid, warming method for bags of fluid may be microwave, warm water bath, heating pad
6) Suction or other equipment for removing fluid – suction machine, sterile suction tubes and sterile suction tips – if a suction machine not available, a good number of sterile laparotomy sponges can be used for manual removal of lavage fluid
7) Tubes without any additives – for collection of fluid samples.

#### 15.6.1.4 Procedure

1) Anesthetize and monitor the patient. If general anesthesia is not available or appropriate, sedate and monitor the patient.
2) Clip the hair coat around any penetrating injury. Do not remove any objects that may be penetrating the abdomen until you have entered the abdomen and can control hemorrhage.
3) Perform an exploratory laparotomy with appropriate hemostasis, identifying and controlling any hemorrhage.
4) Identify and debride or remove (if appropriate) any contaminated or severely damaged tissues considered nonviable.
5) Collect a sample of any abdominal fluid for further analysis and/or culture and sensitivity if possible.
6) Use copious amounts of normal saline, 0.9% NaCl, or similar isotonic crystalloid solution, warmed to just under normal body temperature to lavage the abdominal cavity.
7) If available, use a suction machine with sterile tubing and tip to remove lavage fluid from the abdominal cavity.

8) If suction machine/equipment is unavailable, sterile laparotomy sponges can be used to absorb the lavage fluid. Dispose of the saturated sponges as they are used. Continue the lavage and absorbing fluid with new sterile sponges until the fluid no longer appears contaminated.

9) Once lavage is complete, change gloves and use a new sterile surgery pack to continue the procedure.

10) In cases of severe abdominal contamination, the abdominal incision may be left partially open with a loose primary surgical closure (such as loose simple continuous body wall closure) to provide ongoing drainage and access for additional lavage. Cover the loosely closed incision with sterile laparotomy sponges, followed by cast padding and self-adhesive bandage gently wrapped around the entire abdomen.

11) If used, this abdominal wrap will need to be changed under general anesthesia or appropriate sedation every 12–24 h using aseptic technique.

12) Collect fluid from the abdomen to examine for bacterial presence. Repeat lavages until the fluid samples no longer appear contaminated at which time the incision can be fully closed under general anesthesia.

### 15.6.1.5 Possible Complications

1) General complications related to anesthesia and sedation.
2) Complications related to hemorrhage or internal damage from the primary injury.
3) Development of sepsis or severe peritonitis.
4) Development of hypoproteinemia.
5) Coexisting conditions such as poor hydration, electrolyte imbalance, poor nutritional status, surgical dehiscence, or other issues need to be taken into consideration and treated appropriately.

### 15.6.1.6 Other Considerations

1) Medical management with antibiotics and appropriate pain control is imperative.
2) Appropriate nursing care and sanitation for an animal with this type of injury, particularly if the abdominal incision is left partially open.
3) Appropriate intravenous (IV) fluid therapy, electrolyte therapy, and feeding (consider a feeding tube if prolonged inappetence/anorexia is likely).

## 15.6.2 Abdominocentesis and Diagnostic Peritoneal Lavage

### 15.6.2.1 Indications

This procedure is most commonly indicated to evaluate for free fluid within the abdomen and characterize the type of fluid. In some cases, it may have a therapeutic effect (such as in cases of severe ascites or other effusion negatively impacting respiration and comfort).

Common situations requiring this procedure include the following:

- Trauma with the suspicion of internal hemorrhage – such as blunt force trauma to the abdomen, especially in the face of findings such as a low PCV or low or decreasing TP levels not attributable to fluid support.
- Poor serosal detail on abdominal radiographs of an adult animal especially following trauma, or if free fluid is seen in the abdomen on ultrasound examination.
- Suspicion of peritonitis, or presence of abdominal fluid wave on physical examination.

### 15.6.2.2 Setting

In most cases, abdominocentesis is performed on the nonsedated/nonanesthetized patient, however where appropriate, light sedation can be utilized. When available, abdominocentesis may be performed with ultrasound guidance to locate the most appropriate sites for sampling.

### 15.6.2.3 Equipment

1) Surgery/procedure table
2) Sample site preparation supplies – clippers, gauze, scrub, and solution
3) Sampling needle/catheter (based on animal size) – typically 18- to 20-gauge needle or intravenous catheter (IVC)
4) Syringe to aspirate fluid – for diagnostic procedure a 3 ml syringe, for therapeutic a 35 ml syringe with a luer lock tip
5) For therapeutic procedures, an extension set, three-way stopcock and fluid collection bowl
6) Tubes for collecting fluid sample – with calcium ethylenediaminetetraacetic acid (EDTA)
7) In cases of suspected hemorrhage – microhematocrit tube, microcentrifuge, and PCV reading card

8) Refractometer
9) Sterile swabs or a red top/nonadditive sterile tube – for submitting bacterial cultures
10) Slides +/− stain – for microscopic evaluation
11) Sterile 0.9% saline – in case peritoneal lavage is required to obtain a sample
12) If suspicion of peritonitis – supplies to evaluate lactate and glucose content, such as a hand-held glucometer with test strips.
13) If suspicion of bladder rupture or pancreatitis – laboratory equipment to evaluate chemical properties of fluids would be ideal, but is in many cases not immediately available in a field setting.

#### 15.6.2.4 Procedure

1) Position the patient in lateral recumbency.
2) Sample sites should be clipped and aseptically prepared.
3) Sample sites include the umbilical area and the four quadrants of abdomen as needed to obtain a diagnostic sample, and as indicated based on history and clinical signs (or as guided by ultrasound visualization). In patients with a suspected or palpable splenic enlargement, the left cranial side of the abdomen should be avoided.
4) Wearing sterile gloves and following aseptic technique, gently insert a needle or catheter into the peritoneal cavity.
5) Allow fluid to drip from the inserted needle and collect sample in the collection tube (and on culture swab if indicated).
6) If no fluid is obtained passively, attach a 3-ml syringe and apply gentle suction.
7) If no fluid is obtained passively or with gentle pressure, a diagnostic peritoneal lavage may be indicated.
8) For a diagnostic peritoneal lavage the periumbilical area is prepared and infused with a local anesthetic (i.e. lidocaine). An 18- or 20-gauge, over-the-needle catheter, with additional side holes created within 1 cm of the catheter tip (using a scalpel blade), or a peritoneal lavage catheter could be used. Insert the catheter just caudal to the umbilicus in a caudodorsal direction. If no fluid is obtained passively or with light suction, infuse 10–20 ml/kg of warmed sterile saline, gently massage the abdomen or rock the patient, and collect a sample of the resulting fluid

via the catheter. In patients with respiratory distress or possible diaphragmatic hernia, exercise caution, use smaller infused volumes, or do not perform at all as the additional fluid in the abdomen can worsen breathing. When using this sampling technique the PCV and TP of the sample will be diluted.
9) Note that free blood typically will not clot. If the sample obtained clots, it may indicate entry into an organ or blood vessel during the procedure.
10) Peritoneal fluid from patients with peritonitis will typically have a higher lactate and lower glucose than serum.
11) Presence of bacteria (especially toxic or degenerate neutrophils with intracellular bacteria) indicates septic peritonitis, which is a surgical emergency.
12) Uroabdomen following injury to the urinary tract will usually result in the peritoneal fluid having a higher creatinine and potassium level than the serum.

#### 15.6.2.5 Possible Complications

1) Abdominocentesis may be contraindicated in the face of coagulopathy. It may also be contraindicated without ultrasound guidance in cases of known abdominal adhesions due to previous surgery, suspicion of pyometra or other internal abdominal abscessation, or in cases of known organomegaly.
2) False negatives may occur in patients with only small volumes of abdominal fluid, especially if negative pressure is needed to assess for fluid as viscera or omentum may occlude the needle.
3) Abdominocentesis may introduce some air into the peritoneal cavity. This should be taken into consideration if any free air is seen in the abdomen on radiographs or during ultrasonography post-abdominocentesis.
4) Complications related to anesthesia and/or sedation, can occur.
5) Complications related to hemorrhage or injury to abdominal organs can occur.
6) Contamination or infection is possible, especially if any break in aseptic technique occurs.
7) In cases of therapeutic abdominocentesis – hypovolemia, hypoproteinemia, or electrolyte imbalance can result.

#### 15.6.2.6 Other Considerations

1) When performing therapeutic abdominocentesis, appropriate IV fluid therapy, electrolyte therapy, and monitoring of blood protein levels is indicated.
2) In some cases of mild abdominal hemorrhage, if surgery is not feasible or does not yet seem indicated, placing a light compression wrap around the abdomen may aid hemostasis. Patient comfort must be monitored and any respiratory difficulties should serve as an indication to remove the wrap.
3) When removing an abdominal wrap placed to treat mild abdominal hemorrhage, the wrap should be removed slowly in stages, so as to prevent recurrence of hemorrhage with sudden decrease of pressure on the abdominal cavity.

### 15.6.3 Bandaging

#### 15.6.3.1 Indications

Bandaging is commonly used to provide appropriate treatment and protection for wounds or support for soft tissue or orthopedic injury.

#### 15.6.3.2 Setting

Bandaging can be performed in a treatment room setting, and is not typically a sterile procedure.

#### 15.6.3.3 Equipment

1) One-inch (2.5 cm)-wide tape and/or ½-inch (1.2 cm)-wide tape
2) Cast padding material
3) Stretch wrap/gauze wrap
4) Self-adherent bandage material on a roll
5) Elastic tape
6) If indicated to stabilize a known or suspect fracture – splint or equivalent (such as tongue depressors for very small/light animals) or cast material that can be used to form any splint shape and size that might be needed
7) Bandage scissors
8) Appropriate wound treatment materials and dressings – see wound care section
9) Wound cleaning supplies – including clippers, metal bowls, antiseptic scrub, antiseptic solution, and gauze pads.

#### 15.6.3.4 Procedure

1) The patient should be gently restrained standing or in recumbency, some patients require sedation to be able to appropriately treat any wounds present (see wound care).
2) In case of wounds – the fur around it should be clipped, and the area cleaned and dried before applying appropriate wound dressing (see wound care).
3) Place 1-in. (2.5 cm) tape stirrups (or ½-in. (1.2 cm) on very small animals) on either side of the appendage to be bandaged with at least ½ of the length of the tape on the appendage, the other ½ extending beyond the appendage. Use a tongue depressor to keep the loose ends from becoming stuck to other surfaces during bandaging (Figure 15.1).
4) Use cast padding to wrap circumferentially around the limb/area, always overlapping ½ of the bandage width as you proceed. Apply gentle pressure on the cast padding as you go and avoid creating folds or creases.
5) If appropriate, place a splint or tongue depressors (for very small animals) for stability (see splinting).
6) Use brown or white stretch gauze to compress the cast padding and provide additional stability to the appendage or area. As with cast padding, overlap ½ of width of material with each pass.
7) Use self-adhesive bandage to provide additional stability and durability to the bandage.
8) Use 1-in. (2.5 cm) tape or elastic tape to secure the bandage to the animal proximally and at the distal aspect of the bandage to provide additional durability to the bandage ends.
9) In some cases, your bandage will need to travel around the chest or abdomen, particularly for wounds or fractures on the proximal aspect of an appendage or on the chest/abdomen itself. In those cases, it is imperative to ensure that no significant compression occurs on any portion of the body that could cause patient discomfort, wounds, or impair breathing.
10) Whenever bandaging is considered it is important to ensure that appropriate follow-up care can be provided.
11) Animals with a bandage must be checked frequently for any complications such as bandage slipping, moisture, loosening, and tissue swelling. These issues must be addressed immediately if seen (Figure 15.1).

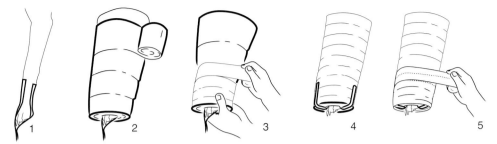

Figure 15.1 Bandaging technique: (1) Use white tape to make stirrups attached to the distal one-third of the limb and extending the same distance distal to the leg. (2) Use cotton roll to lightly wrap the leg starting distally and moving proximally, make sure the cotton overlaps itself 50% as you move up the leg. It is recommended to wrap the leg with two layers of cotton. (3) Starting at the toes tightly wrap the leg using a conforming bandage to provide compression. The bandage should appear less bulky when finishing this step. (4) Separate the tape of the stirrup, twist them so that they can be secured to the compression bandage. This prevents the bandage from slipping down. (5) The final layer is an elastic wrap such as vet wrap. Start at the toes and move proximally, making sure you get 50% coverage on itself as you move up. Source: Figure courtesy of Bernt Henrik Kommedal.

#### 15.6.3.5 Possible Complications

1) Bandages left in place for extended periods of time without removal and frequent checking can lead to complications such as pressure sores, soft tissue swelling, loss of blood supply, bandage slipping, bandage-associated wounds, which can become infected and lead to other complications.
2) In worst case situations, complications can be severe enough that the affected limb loses enough blood supply that it causes tissue death. This can result in the limb requiring amputation.

#### 15.6.3.6 Other Considerations

In situations where follow-up care is unavailable or cannot be ensured, bandaging is not advisable and the treatment plan should be modified accordingly.

### 15.6.4 Cardiopulmonary Resuscitation (CPR)

#### 15.6.4.1 Indications

Cardiopulmonary resuscitation (CPR) is indicated in patients with respiratory and/or cardiac arrest either secondary to disease process, trauma, or related to anesthesia.

#### 15.6.4.2 Setting

CPR is typically performed in a general treatment room setting. A treatment table, appropriate supplies, and ideally at least two individuals improve CPR efficiency and success. When staffing is limited, it is possible for a single individual to perform basic CPR unassisted.

#### 15.6.4.3 Equipment

In any clinic setting, a crash cart is vital to enable an effective and timely emergency response. Crash carts can be fashioned using any set of drawers or shelves on wheels, or using a small case with separate compartments to organize and label supplies.

#### 15.6.4.4 Procedure

1) If cardiac or respiratory arrest is anesthesia related, discontinue administration of anesthetic agent if possible. If gas anesthesia is used, briefly remove circuit from ET-tube, flush gas from the system, and start oxygen treatment.
2) Assess for heartbeat and pulses – if absent begin chest compressions providing 100–120 compressions/min with pressure directly over the heart with the animal in lateral recumbency.
3) Traditional CPR was based on the "ABC's" (Airway, Breathing, Circulation) of CPR – this includes first assessing for any airway obstruction and addressing these to ensure patent airways, before considering the patients circulatory system.

---

**Textbox 15.2 Sample emergency crash cart supply list**

*Documents*

CPR instructions (laminated chart)
CPR drug dosages (laminated chart)
Drug formulary

*Oxygen delivery supplies*

Oxygen tank
Pressure regulator
Oxygen delivery tubing
Ambu® bag

*IV fluid supplies*

Clippers, gauze, surgical scrub, and solution
IV catheters (range of sizes recommended including 18, 20, 22, and 25 gauge
Male adapters and/or T-ports for catheters
Tape to secure catheter
Extension sets
Crystalloid fluids (such as 0.9% NaCl or similar)
Colloids (if available)
Scalpel blades and small sterile pack (in the event venous cut down is needed to gain access)

*Thoracotomy supplies (for open chest CPR)*

Sterile surgical pack
Scalpel blades
Suture
Suction unit with sterile tubing and tips
Red rubber or other appropriate chest tube

*Intubation supplies*

Endotracheal tubes (need range of sizes – ex. sizes 2.5 mm up to 14 mm)
Stylet
Laryngoscope
Lidocaine
Syringes
Gauze or other ET tube tie-ins
Tracheostomy tubes if available

*Monitoring supplies*

Pulse oximeter
Portable electrocardiogram (EKG)
Blood pressure monitor

*Emergency drugs and supplies*

Syringes (1, 3, 6 ml)
Heparinized saline preloaded 3-ml syringes
Red rubber tubes (to deliver CPR drugs intratracheally if needed) (ex. 5 Fr, 8 Fr)
Epinephrine
Atropine
Naloxone
Atipamezole
Flumazenil
Vasopressin
Amiodarone
Lidocaine

---

4) Recent human and veterinary studies recommend that chest compressions be started immediately (the modified "CAB" sequence of circulation, airway, breathing), without delay, even if that means beginning chest compressions before securing the animal's airway.

5) Under current recommendations, once circulation has been assessed and compressions have been started, the airway should be fully evaluated and cleared if needed. The patient should then be assessed for spontaneous respiration/breathing.

6) If there are no signs of spontaneous breathing and the patient is not intubated, an endotracheal tube should be placed.

7) Begin positive pressure ventilation (PPV) with 100% oxygen (or room air via Ambu bag if oxygen is unavailable). Provide 10 breaths per minute.

8) If performing CPR without an assistant, alternate compressions and ventilation with 30 compressions followed by two breaths per cycle.

9) If possible, place monitoring equipment such as a pulse oximeter, EKG, or $CO_2$ monitor.

10) If the patient does not have an IV catheter, one should be placed while CPR is performed.

11) Based on the patients condition IV crystalloid fluid treatment should be provided.

12) Use reversal agents whenever available for the anesthetic medications used (see CPR-dosing chart for more drug doses calculated by body weight).
   a) Opioids: administer naloxone at 0.04 mg/kg.
   b) Alpha 2 agonists such as medetomidine: administer atipamezole at 100 µg/kg.
   c) Benzodiazepines such as diazepam: administer flumazenil at 0.01 mg/kg.

13) Evaluate patient for breathing, pulse, heart rate, and rhythm once every minute while performing CPR.

14) If no pulse, continue CPR, consider epinephrine (adrenaline) (at 0.01–0.1 mg/kg) and atropine (at 0.04 mg/kg). Use every other 2-min cycle of resuscitation attempts (see CPR-dosing chart below for more drug doses calculated by body weight).

15) Treat for any known or suspected complicating factors (such as hypoglycemia, acidosis, and hypocalcemia).

16) If CPR is not successful, consider open-chest CPR but be aware that the prognosis worsens if this is required. Consider thoracotomy and internal heart compressions only if reasonable given the setting, if after 5 min of CPR there is no evidence of effective CPR-associated circulation and tissue perfusion, or if after 10 min there is no spontaneous heartbeat.

### 15.6.4.5  Possible Complications

1) CPR efforts may be ineffective.

2) CPR efforts may be effective in restoring spontaneous heart rate and respiration, but anoxia or hypoxemia during the event may lead to long-term tissue damage, which could subsequently result in death.

3) Post-CPR care may be required, including oxygen supplementation, treatment and prevention of hypothermia, neurological stabilization including mannitol treatment or seizure prevention.

### 15.6.4.6  Other Considerations

1) It is important to keep in mind that CPR is ineffective in a significant number of veterinary patients.

2) The probability of success is greater in an otherwise healthy patient that arrests due to an anesthetic related event/complication.

3) CPR can lead to patient injury itself, including rib fractures, trauma to the lungs (puncture from fractured ribs, atelectasis due to recumbent compressions, alevolar ruptures from PPV), tracheal injury, and other mechanical damage.

4) An excellent resource for CPR flow charts and emergency drug-dosing charts is the Veterinary Emergency and Critical Care Society (VECCS) website. A VECCS flow chart is included in Chapter 6. It is strongly recommended that anyone practicing veterinary medicine in the field print out these resources and have them available (including the most recent CPR drug dosage charts). See Chapter 20 for a sample CPR dosing chart.

## 15.6.5  Cystocentesis

### 15.6.5.1  Indications

Cystocentesis is typically performed to obtain a urine sample for analysis or to decompress a distended bladder in the case of urethral obstruction.

### 15.6.5.2  Setting

In most cases, cystocentesis is performed on the nonsedated/nonanesthetized patient; however, where appropriate, light sedation can be used. The procedure can be performed with or without ultrasound guidance.

### 15.6.5.3  Equipment

1) Clippers, gauze, scrub, solution, alcohol spray, or squeeze bottle

2) 22-gauge needle (1–1.5 in. long)

3) For diagnostic sample – a 3 to 6 ml syringe.
4) For decompression – a 12- to 20-ml syringe, extension set, three-way stopcock and urine collection bowl.
5) Diagnostic equipment as indicated – ideally this would include a red top/nonadditive tube for bacterial cultures, a centrifuge to spin the sample and a microscope, slides and stains to evaluate urine sediments, urine test strips and a refractometer.

#### 15.6.5.4 Procedure

1) Keep the patient in dorsal recumbency or standing.
2) Generally requires two people: one to position and restrain the patient and the other to perform the sampling.
3) The sample site should be clipped and aseptically prepared for the procedure.
4) Ultrasound guided cystocentesis – visualize the bladder, insert needle into bladder and obtain sample or decompress it as indicated.
5) "Blind" cystocentesis – palpate the abdomen until you can locate the bladder. Immobilize the bladder against the ventral abdominal wall and insert the needle into the bladder. Obtain sample or decompress it as indicated.
6) The needle should be positioned to enter the bladder at an oblique angle.
7) A sample is gently aspirated, pressure on the syringe is discontinued, and the needle is removed from the abdomen.
8) For decompression, pressure is applied until the syringe is filled, the stopcock is turned, and the syringe emptied into a collection bowl. This is repeated until the bladder is soft and no longer distended (do not remove the needle during the procedure).

#### 15.6.5.5 Possible Complications

1) Bladder rupture, especially in cases of bladder distention or weakening, or other pathology compromising the integrity of the urinary bladder.
2) Hemorrhage, especially in cases of coagulopathy. Hemorrhage may enter the abdomen or collect in the bladder, resulting in free blood or clots within the abdominal cavity or bladder.
3) Other abdominal structures could be penetrated if bladder localization and needle entry are inaccurate.

4) Neoplastic cells or bacterial-contaminated material could enter the abdomen if a neoplastic mass, an abscess, or portion of the GI tract is entered.

#### 15.6.5.6 Other Considerations
Cystocentesis should only be performed by appropriately trained and experienced veterinary staff.

### 15.6.6 Cystotomy/Ruptured Bladder Repair

#### 15.6.6.1 Indications
Emergency cystotomy surgery is indicated in patients with bladder stones (cystoliths), especially if urethral stones have been retropulsed back into the bladder and need to be removed to prevent recurrence of obstruction. With similar surgical considerations, emergency bladder repair is most often indicated after traumatic or iatrogenic bladder rupture (e.g. when attempting to express the bladder preoperatively or when treating cats with urethral obstruction).

#### 15.6.6.2 Setting
These procedures require a clean surgical setting and aseptic technique.

#### 15.6.6.3 Equipment

1) Standard anesthetic induction, maintenance and monitoring, as well as a standard surgical pack (including scalpel blade and suture).
2) Sterile laparotomy sponges or carefully counted sterile gauze squares (to ensure that none are left in the abdomen).
3) Postoperative abdominal lavage may be indicated in patients with uroabdomen present initially or occurring during the procedure (see abdominal lavage).

#### 15.6.6.4 Procedure

1) Surgeons not familiar with the procedure should consult a more detailed surgical text for a full description.
2) A standard caudal ventral abdomen preparation and caudal ventral midline surgical approach is used.
3) Gently exteriorize and isolate the urinary bladder using sterile saline-soaked laparotomy sponges. Stay-sutures can be placed in the bladder wall to help stabilize and handle it.

4) Enter the lumen of the bladder with a stab incision on its ventral surface and any stones present are removed.
5) In cases of traumatic rupture, the injured area of the bladder is identified and tissue edges conservatively debrided if devitalized.
6) A single- or double-layer closure is recommended using a taper needle.
7) If uroabdomen is present, the abdomen should be lavaged with sterile crystalloid solution and suctioned (see abdominal lavage).
8) Close the abdomen using a standard ventral abdominal closure.

#### 15.6.6.5 Possible Complications

1) As with any surgical procedure hemorrhage, infection, incisional dehiscence and delayed wound healing are possible complications.
2) Uroabdomen secondary to failure of the bladder closure.
3) Hematuria may be seen postoperatively but is generally mild and resolve within days. If excessive, an additional examination and diagnostic tests should be pursued.

#### 15.6.6.6 Other Considerations

1) A sterile spoon can be used to aid in atraumatic removal of uroliths from the urinary bladder. It is imperative to ensure that all the uroliths have been removed before closing the bladder wall.
2) Placing a urinary catheter prior to opening the bladder will help flush out any uroliths located in the bladder neck or urethra. It is recommended to lavage the opened bladder copiously before closing the incision.

### 15.6.7 Endotracheal (ET) Intubation

#### 15.6.7.1 Indications

In an emergency setting, endotracheal intubation is indicated to secure the animal's airway and ensure airflow, oxygen supplementation, and possibly inhalant anesthetic administration. This procedure is also indicated to allow for PPV in the case of respiratory arrest, loss of thoracic negative pressure, or other pathology preventing effective ventilation.

#### 15.6.7.2 Setting

Intubation is typically performed in a treatment room/surgery preparation setting but can be done anywhere if a patient requires CPR.

#### 15.6.7.3 Equipment

1) Appropriately sized ET tube (typically cats will need a 2.5- to 4.5-mm tube and dogs will need a 5- to 14-mm tube based on the animal's overall body size and tracheal diameter)
2) ET tube tie-in (formed from extension set tubing, gauze, or other suitable material)
3) Laryngoscope
4) Lubricating jelly
5) Lidocain – pull up a small amount in a syringe, can be used as local anesthetic in cats with laryngospasm
6) Stylet – especially for cats and kittens. This is also helpful in animals with an oral or laryngeal mass or swelling in the oropharynx.

#### 15.6.7.4 Procedure

1) Always have a range of tube sizes available.
2) Check the air bladder of cuffed tubes ahead of time – inflate, check for leaks and deflate each bladder prior to use. Premeasure the tubes against the animal from tip of the nose to mid-cervical trachea so that they can be placed to the appropriate depth.
3) With the animal heavily sedated, anesthetized, or otherwise rendered unconscious, have an assistant support the animal in sternal recumbency with the head/neck gently outstretched.
4) Lubricate the tip of the tube with a small amount of sterile lubricant.
5) The assistant should stabilize the head by grasping the maxilla and upper lips. This will help open the mouth and enable visualization of the epiglottis.
6) Gently pull the patients tongue out, using a gauze pad will ensure a better grasp on the tongue. Apply gentle ventral force on the tongue to help further visualization of the epiglottis and airway opening.
7) If laryngospasm occurs in the cat, several drops of lidocaine can be applied to each side of the larynx, wait 1–2 min before intubation is reattempted.
8) The lubricated end of the ET tube should be directed just dorsal to the epiglottis and through the vocal folds into the trachea (Figure 15.2).

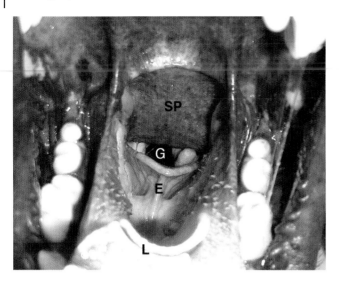

**Figure 15.2 Canine intubation.** The patient is placed in sternal recumbency and the mouth is held open by an assistant or a mouth gag. The tongue is gently pulled out and a laryngoscope (L) is used to depress the base of the tongue and epiglottis (E) if needed. The opening of the glottis (G) is clearly visible between the epiglottis and the soft palate (SP). An endotracheal tube can be passed through the glottis and into the trachea until the tip of tube is midway between the larynx and thoracic inlet. Source: Photo courtesy of Dr. Sheilah Robertson.

9) Gently follow the curve of the neck to insert the tube to an appropriate depth as determined by premeasuring. Tubes should end midway between the larynx and thoracic inlet.

10) Check for correct tube placement by palpating the neck to ensure that the tube is not palpable in the esophagus and by checking the anesthesia reservoir bag for inflation once attached to the anesthetic circuit.

11) Tie the tube in place with a tie around the distal end, being careful not to incorporate the small tube that leads to the inflatable cuff of the ET tube. Secure the ends of the tie behind the animal's ears or around the muzzle as indicated by the procedure being performed.

12) Inflate the cuff of the ET tube with sufficient air to create a good seal but not so much air as to create unnecessary pressure on the tracheal mucosa.

13) Once the tube is in place, secured with a tie and the cuff has been inflated, anesthetic gas can be administered.

14) Check for appropriate fogging of tube, movement of reservoir air bag, and lack of any noxious anesthetic gas odors.

### 15.6.7.5   Complications

1) Endotracheal intubation can result in oral, oropharyngeal, laryngeal, tracheal, and esophageal trauma.

2) Over-inflation of the lungs of an intubated patient can result in pulmonary rupture.

3) If improperly placed into the esophagus, the patient will not maintain an appropriate anesthetic depth or receive oxygen supplementation during the procedure.

### 15.6.7.6   Other Considerations

1) If inserted too deeply and thereby entering a bronchus, ventilation can be compromised in an animal that otherwise appears appropriately intubated.

2) Choosing the correct diameter ET tube is critical to avoid esophageal damage from a tube that is too large and to prevent lack of secure airway circulation from a tube that is too small.

3) While the patient is intubated, take care to always disconnect the anesthesia circuit during patient repositioning to avoid the inflated ET tube from turning in the trachea as this can cause injury or even rupture of the trachea.

4) Ensure that the ET tube cuff has been deflated before the tube is removed at the end of the procedure.

## 15.6.8   Decontamination Following Toxin Exposure (Topical and/or Oral)

### 15.6.8.1   Indications

Decontamination is typically indicated in cases of recent known or suspected toxin exposure. For topical toxins, it is important to not only remove any toxin that may be remaining on the animal but also to consider whether the topical toxin could have been accidently ingested from grooming or other incidental oral contact with the body.

Whenever possible, a toxin treatment reference or poison control hotline (phone or Internet based) should be consulted for specific information about the specific toxin the animal has been exposed to. Due to the large number and type of toxins dogs and cats can be exposed to, this reference is meant only to explain the actual decontamination procedure and not whether each is applicable to a specific toxin.

### 15.6.8.2 Setting
This procedure is performed in a treatment or exam room setting. This is not a sterile procedure.

### 15.6.8.3 Equipment

1) Examination gloves.
2) Topical toxin – Bathing equipment and gentle shampoo (or gentle liquid soap), clippers.
3) Orally ingested toxin – Agent to induce emesis (such as apomorphine, syrup of ipecac, or hydrogen peroxide).

See section on gastric lavage if indicated based on type of toxin exposure and when exposure occurred. Activated charcoal may be indicated.

### 15.6.8.4 Procedure

1) For topical toxins, make sure to wear gloves and if the toxin can be removed with water and shampoo or soap, give the animal a gentle bath. If the toxin cannot be removed with bathing, the hair coat can be clipped where the toxin is present (This is often required when cats have been treated with flea prevention products intended for dogs.).
2) For recently ingested toxins – depending on the substance, this might be within the previous 1–4 h – and if emesis is not contraindicated emesis should be induced. Inducing emesis is contraindicated in case of ingestion of caustic substances or if the animal is experiencing decreased gag reflex, respiratory distress, or severe neurological impairment.
3) Emesis can be induced with: Apomorphine (0.03 mg/kg IV, 0.04 mg/kg IM, 0.08 mg/kg SC, or 0.3 mg/kg topically into the conjunctival sac). Syrup of ipecac (1.0–2.5 ml/kg PO in dogs or 3.3 ml/kg PO in cats). Hydrogen peroxide (using 3% hydrogen peroxide dose at 1.0–2.0 ml/kg PO). Xylazine (0.4 mg/kg IM) can be used as an emetic in cats. Table salt has been used as an emetic, but this is not recommended due to an increased risk of complications.

### 15.6.8.5 Possible Complications

1) Bathing an animal following toxin exposure could result in lowering of body temperature. The patient's temperature should be carefully monitored and precautions taken to avoid this.
2) Inducing emesis can result in aspiration of vomitus, resulting in respiratory complications.
3) Some emetics can cause specific complications including GI upset, weakness, and sedation.

### 15.6.8.6 Other Considerations

1) Emesis can take 5–20 min after administration of the emetic depending on which emetic agent is used.
2) Once emesis has been successfully induced, consider giving an antiemetic before administering any oral medications or treatments.
3) If indicated, activated charcoal can be administered after emesis is complete and an antiemetic has been given. Activated charcoal is typically dosed at 1–4 g/kg. Premixed liquid formulas should be dosed as labeled depending on concentration to achieve this dose of the active ingredient.
4) Supportive care of fluid therapy, nursing care, and specific treatments based on the toxin ingested should be provided in most cases of toxin ingestion.

### 15.6.9 Enema

#### 15.6.9.1 Indications
Enema administration is indicated to address moderate-to-severe constipation or obstipation (to remove feces or other material from the colon). An enema may also be indicated as treatment in some toxicities or indicated before performing a GI contrast study or colonoscopy.

#### 15.6.9.2 Setting
Enemas are not a sterile procedure and can be performed in a treatment or exam room. Preferably they

should be done in an area that is easily sanitized, and never in the surgical area.

### 15.6.9.3 Equipment

1) Examination gloves
2) Lubricating jelly
3) Appropriately sized tubing and 20- to 60-ml syringe – typically red rubber or similar tubing
4) Enema solution – typically warm water only, warm water with lubricating jelly, warm water with lactulose, or warm water with DSS (docusate)
5) Activated charcoal – if treating for toxicity and instilling activated charcoal solution per rectum.

### 15.6.9.4 Procedure

1) Gently restrain the animal in standing position or lateral recumbency. Lubricate the enema tube and insert slowly into the rectum. Infuse the enema solution as the tube is gently advanced further into the colon. Repeated retraction and advancement of the tube, while infusing the enema solution, will help distribute the fluid evenly in the descending +/− the transverse colon.
2) Typical volumes of enema solution range from 10 to 20 ml for a small kitten to 100–200 ml for an adult cat, up to 500–1000 ml for a dog (depending on size).
3) For mild cases of constipation, the animal can then be taken to an area suitable for defecation.
4) In more severe constipation or obstipation, lubricated gloved fingers may need to be gently introduced into the rectum to help remove impacted feces. For very small animals, gentle palpation and pressure on the colon with the hand outside the rectum with the handle placed on the ventral abdomen can help to "milk" feces from the colon.
5) In very severe cases of obstipation, additional sedation, or even full anesthesia and additional gentle manual evacuation of the colon may be necessary.

### 15.6.9.5 Possible Complications

1) Injury or perforation of the colon, especially if force is used to advance tube.
2) Hemorrhage can be caused or exacerbated by this procedure.
3) If there is any injury to the lower GI tract fecal material and enema solution may enter the abdominal cavity and result in septic peritonitis.

### 15.6.9.6 Other Considerations

1) Some patients may require repeated enemas to evacuate the bowels.
2) Avoid using commercial enema products, such as products containing phosphorus in cats due to risk of hyperphosphatemia.

## 15.6.10 Feeding Tubes

A feeding tube can be used to provide enteral nutrition in patients when inappetence or inability to eat food is anticipated. In cases of mild inappetence, appropriate medical management should be attempted prior to feeding tube placement where appropriate. This could include appropriate pain medication if inappetence is related to discomfort, use of antianxiety medication if related to anxiety, or medications such as antiemetics, H2 blockers, and appetite stimulants.

Providing enteral nutrition via a feeding tube in cases where the GI tract is functional is often preferred to attempting to force-feed the animal due to the level of stress this creates as well as the risk of aspiration. A feeding tube is generally preferable in the field as opposed to providing nutrition intravenously through partial parenteral nutrition (PPN) or total parenteral nutrition (TPN) solutions. Enteral nutrition has the benefit of helping to maintain the integrity of the GI epithelium and flora and has fewer risks associated with maintaining sterility at the supplement port for PPN and TPN.

---

**Textbox 15.3 Types of feeding tubes**

1) Orogastric tube
2) Nasogastric or nasoesophageal tube
3) Esophagostomy tube
4) Percutaneous endoscopic gastrostomy (PEG) tube
5) Jejunostomy tube.

---

This section will focus on the use of orogastric, nasogastric/nasoesophageal, and esophagostomy tubes. Peg tubes, jejunostomy tubes, and other surgically implanted feeding tubes are less practical for use in the field. They require additional equipment and are higher risk surgical procedures. In general, animals requiring a longer term feeding tube should be treated at a full service veterinary clinic, rather than in a field setting.

### 15.6.10.1 Orogastric Tube

#### 15.6.10.1.1 Indications

An orogastric tube is most appropriate for a single use or intermittent feeding. This procedure can be used to instill an oral medication that requires a larger volume in patients who will not voluntarily eat the substance.

An orogastric tube is most commonly used for administration of barium for a contrast study or activated charcoal in cases of toxicity. This method may also be used for intermittent feeding of neonates. Orogastric tubes can also be used to empty stomach contents and as part of gastric lavage (see gastric lavage procedure).

#### 15.6.10.1.2 Setting

This is a nonsterile procedure. Orogastric tubing is typically performed in the nonsedated or very lightly sedated patient and is not typically considered a surgical procedure.

#### 15.6.10.1.3 Equipment

1) Feeding tube – depending on the size of animal, one may use a red rubber catheter of an appropriate diameter or an actual feeding tube. (Ex. 8 Fr may be appropriate for a small puppy or kitten up to 18 Fr for a larger adult dog.)
2) Appropriate mouth gag to prevent the animal from biting down on the feeding tube – commonly a roll of tape is used in larger animals. A syringe case can be used in smaller animals or a syringe with the plunger removed and the smaller tip cut off.
3) Liquefied, well-blended species/age/medical condition appropriate diet.
4) Appropriate infusion syringe (5–60 ml) with tip that fits on feeding tube. Alternatively the end of the feeding tube can be cut to accept syringe snuggly.
5) Bowl of room temperature water.
6) Small syringe – to test tube placement.
7) Larger syringe – to flush tube at the end of feeding/medication administration.
8) Marker or tape – to mark tube for appropriate placement.
9) Lubricating jelly.

#### 15.6.10.1.4 Procedure

1) With the animal appropriately and gently restrained in a sitting, standing or sternally recumbent position with the head elevated, measure the feeding tube from the tip of the animal's nose to the last rib. Mark the feeding tube at that level.
2) Insert the mouth gag (roll of tape, syringe casing or syringe body as above) and hold securely to prevent the animal from chewing on or trying to swallow it.
3) Lubricate the end of the feeding tube.
4) Slowly and gently insert the feeding tube – you may notice swallowing motions by the patient.
5) Insert until the mark on the tube is at the nose.
6) Check the tube for correct placement – palpate the neck to see if the tube is palpable in the esophagus, smell the open end of the tube for gastric odors, gently blow into the tube while an assistant listens for gastric bubbling, and then gently infuse a small amount of sterile saline into the tube watching for any coughing/gagging or signs of discomfort.
7) Once tube placement has been confirmed, slowly infuse the food slurry or liquid medication, continuously monitoring for any signs of breathing difficulty or distress.
8) Once the orogastric infusion is complete, use the larger syringe filled with water to gently flush the remaining food or water out of the syringe into the stomach before removing the tube.
9) Fold the end of the feeding tube over (to prevent any liquid still in the tube from entering the airway when the tube is removed) and slowly and gently remove the feeding tube.

#### 15.6.10.1.5 Possible Complications

1) Aspiration can occur if the tube is not appropriately placed into the esophagus.
2) Overfeeding or feeding too quickly can result in aspiration of food as well or cause discomfort due to excessive gastric distention.
3) If a mouth gag is not used or used incorrectly, the animal could chew through the tube, damaging the tube and allowing food/medication to leak out of the tube higher than the tube's end (increasing risk of aspiration). If the tube is fully chewed through, it will act as a foreign body in the mouth, upper airway, esophagus, or stomach.
4) Esophageal, oropharyngeal, and gastric irritation, trauma, or perforation may occur.

#### 15.6.10.1.6 Other Considerations

1) For some animals, this procedure can be stressful, and if repeated medication administrations or tube feedings are anticipated, an alternate feeding tube type should be considered.
2) This technique is generally well tolerated in underage neonates and in many cases is preferable for kittens and puppies that are not latching onto a bottle to enable accurate and efficient feeding.

### 15.6.10.2 Nasogastric or Nasoesophageal Tube

#### 15.6.10.2.1 Indications

Most commonly used for animals that are expected to be inappetent, or unable to ingest food orally for at least 12–24 h. These tubes are appropriate for patients with a functional esophagus and gastrointestinal tract including physiological motility, digestion and absorption.

The benefit of a nasogastric tube, which enters the stomach, is the ability to aspirate prior to feeding to check for evidence of gastric stasis or significant residual liquid in the stomach. However, there is some risk of gastric acid reflux/regurgitation into the esophagus as the tube placement prevents the gastroesophageal sphincter from fully closing. Nasoesophageal tubes have the benefit of decreased risk of gastric acid reflex but do not allow for checking for residual material in the stomach.

A nasogastric or nasoesophageal tube may be placed under anesthesia following procedures that are expected to reduce appetite to ensure enteral feeding (e.g. after a gastric dilatation volvulus (GDV) surgery and after gastrotomy, enterotomy, and resection/anastomosis). These types of feeding tubes should be considered in the parvovirus or panleukopenia patient to ensure enteral nutrition as this can facilitate enteral healing and speed up recovery.

#### 15.6.10.2.2 Setting

This is a nonsterile procedure that is typically performed in the unsedated or very lightly sedated animal. It is not a surgical procedure but may be performed in conjunction with surgeries with high risk of postoperative inappetence where enteral feeding would be beneficial.

#### 15.6.10.2.3 Equipment

*Tube Placement*

1) Feeding tube – depending on size of animal, one may use a red rubber catheter of an appropriate diameter or an actual feeding tube (typically 8 Fr for most dogs and 5 Fr for most cats). Tube must be small enough to enter and travel through the nasal cavity into the esophagus
2) Local anesthetic solution
3) 1-in. (2.5 cm) waterproof tape
4) Surgical stapler
5) Small syringe with water to test tube placement

*Feedings*

1) Liquefied, well-blended, species/age/medical condition appropriate diet
2) Appropriate infusion syringe (5–60 ml) with tip that fits on feeding tube, or cut end of feeding tube to accept syringe snuggly.
3) Bowl of room temperature water
4) Small syringe – to test tube placement
5) Larger syringe – to flush tube at the end of feeding/medication administration

#### 15.6.10.2.4 Procedure

*Placing the Nasogastric or Nasoesophageal Tube*

1) With the animal appropriately and gently restrained in a sitting, standing, or sternally recumbent position with the head elevated, measure the feeding tube from the tip of the animal's nose to the mid-cervical esophagus for a nasoesophageal tube and to the last rib for a nasogastric tube placement. Mark the feeding tube at the appropriate level for your chosen placement.
2) Infuse a few drops of local anesthetic into the nostril you will use for insertion with the animal's head elevated, and wait 2–3 min.
3) Lubricate the feeding tube with lidocaine gel (or regular lubricant) and gently introduce it by guiding it along the nasal cavity, along the ventromedial aspect of the nostril. The animal's head should be gently elevated in a neutral position, not held in flexion or extreme extension.
4) The person placing the tube should brace their hand against the animal's muzzle and move with the animal if they sneeze or move.
5) The tube is fed through the nasal cavity and into the esophagus to the mark on the tube.
6) Check the tube for correct placement. Palpate the neck to feel if the tube is palpable in the esophagus, smell the open end of the tube for gastric odors, gently blow into the tube while an assistant listens

for gastric bubbling, and then gently infuse a small amount of sterile saline into the tube watching for any coughing/gagging or signs of discomfort.

7) The end of the tube is then positioned at the alar notch of the nostril and the tube is run along the side of the animal's nose, onto the dorsal aspect of the nose, and onto the top of the head.

8) Using several pieces of waterproof tape each folded into a butterfly configuration (a piece of tape is folded in half with the sticky side in, the first one-third of the tape is adhered to itself, the second one-third is secured around the tube and adhered to itself, and the last one-third is adhered to itself on the other side of the tube, sandwiching the tube), tape is placed around the tube and each wing of the tape is stapled. These pieces of tape should be placed where the tube exits the nostril, on top of the nose, and on the dorsum of the head to secure the tube appropriately.

9) The tube should be capped with an appropriate male adapter port or blood sample collection tube top, to prevent air from entering the tube when it is not in use for feeding.

10) A radiograph (if available) can be used to verify appropriate tube positioning in the desired location and ensure the tube is not wrapped back on itself.

*During Feeding*

1) Gently infuse a small amount of water into the tube, watch for coughing/gagging or signs of discomfort.

2) Slowly infuse the food slurry or liquid medication, monitoring for any signs of respiratory difficulty or distress.

3) Use the larger syringe filled with water to gently flush the remaining food or water out of the tube.

*Feeding Tube Removal*

1) When the tube is no longer needed and is to be removed, remove staples holding the butterfly tape segments in place.

2) Flush the tube gently with water.

3) Fold the end of the feeding tube (to prevent any liquid still in the tube from entering the airway when the tube is removed) and slowly and gently remove the feeding tube.

### 15.6.10.2.5  Possible Complications

1) Aspiration can occur if the tube is not appropriately placed into the esophagus or stomach.

2) Overfeeding or feeding too quickly can result in aspiration of food particularly with a nasoesophageal tube, or can lead to patient discomfort from gastric distention.

3) If incorrectly measured, the tube may enter the stomach, wrap around, and exit into the esophagus, increasing the risk of aspiration pneumonia.

### 15.6.10.2.6  Other Considerations

1) Placement of the tube may be stressful for some animals and require light sedation.

2) Some animals do not tolerate nasal tubes and may repeatedly paw at their nose, develop sneezing or epistaxis.

3) Feeding tubes can become clogged. If this occurs, infuse 10–20 ml of clear carbonated beverage, wait 10–15 min, and infuse warm water to clear the clog.

4) Feeding a well-blended/liquefied diet with an appropriate liquid component can help reduce the risk of clogging.

### 15.6.10.3  Esophagostomy Tube

#### 15.6.10.3.1  Indications

Esophagostomy tube is indicated for animals that are expected to be inappetent, or unable to ingest food orally for more than 24 h. They are often used in cases where an animal will be sent home with the feeding tube in place so that an owner can continue the feedings. They are most appropriate for patients with a functioning gastrointestinal tract with appropriate motility, digestion, and absorption from the esophagus/stomach. As with the nasogastric and nasoesophageal tubes, the tube may terminate in either the stomach or the esophagus with the same risks and benefits of each placement.

#### 15.6.10.3.2  Setting

An esophagostomy tube is typically placed under general anesthesia, with a patient intubated to maintain open airways and allow easy access to the mouth, oropharynx, and esophagus without inadvertently being bitten.

#### 15.6.10.3.3  Equipment

*Tube Placement*

1) Surgery/procedure table
2) Intubated patient under general anesthesia

3) Surgical site preparation supplies – clippers, gauze, scrub, and solution

4) Surgical equipment – basic surgery pack (at least large Carmalts, thumb forceps, needle drivers, scalpel blade, and suture)

5) Feeding tube – depending on size of animal, one may use a red rubber catheter of an appropriate diameter or an actual feeding tube (typically up to 22 Fr for large dogs and 10–12 Fr for most cats and small dogs)

6) Cast padding

7) Self-adhesive bandage

8) 1-in. (2.5 cm) waterproof tape

*During Feedings*

1) Liquefied, well-blended species/age/medical condition appropriate diet

2) Appropriate infusion syringe (5–60 ml) with tip that fits on feeding tube, or cut end of feeding tube to accept the syringe snuggly

3) Bowl of room temperature water

4) Small syringe – to test tube placement

5) Larger syringe – to flush tube at the end of feeding/medication administration (Figure 15.3).

### 15.6.10.3.4 Procedure

*Placing the Esophagostomy Tube*

1) Anesthetize and intubate the patient with appropriate monitoring.

2) Clip hair coat and prepare the surgical site on the left side of the neck. Begin just caudal to the ramus of the mandible and ventral to the ear, prepare an approximately 4–6 in. (10–15 cm) square to overlay the proximal one-third of the esophagus.

3) Align the end of the tube with the mid-cervical esophagus and, extending the animal's head and neck, extend the tube so that the tip of the tube is at the level of the last rib. Make a mark on the tube where the open end of the tube hits the mid-cervical esophagus (this will be how far you want to insert the tube for gastric placement).

4) Use large curved Carmalt forceps placed into the mouth and positioned in the esophagus on the left side of the neck, aim the tip of the forceps laterally until the skin tents over the instrument's tip several inches caudal to the ramus of the mandible to the level of the mid-cervical esophagus to ensure appropriate placement.

5) Incise the skin just over the tip of the Carmalts with a scalpel blade and then extend the incision through the subcutaneous and connective tissues using blunt dissection. When only the esophageal tissue remains covering the tips of the Carmalts, make a small incision over their tip to allow entry into the esophagus until just the tip of the Carmalts can exit your incision.

6) Open the Carmalts and grasp the tip of the feeding tube with the Carmalts.

7) Pull the Carmalts (grasping the tip of the feeding tube so that it follows) out of the esophagus and out of the mouth.

8) Release the tip of the feeding tube and use your fingers to redirect it down into the mouth, through the oropharynx and down into the esophagus. At the level of your skin incision, feed the tube into the esophagus until the mark on the tube is at the level of your skin incision.

9) Check the tube for correct placement – palpate the neck to see if the tube is palpable in the esophagus, smell the open end of the tube for gastric odors, gently blow into the tube while an assistant listens for gastric bubbling, and then gently infuse a small amount of sterile saline into the tube watching for any coughing/gagging or signs of discomfort.

10) Use an overlapping interlocking suture pattern and/or waterproof tape folded into a butterfly pattern and sutured to stay sutures on the skin to secure the tube at the skin exit site.

11) Gently and loosely wrap the neck with cast padding and gently curl (without kinking) the tube before covering with a light and loose self-adhesive bandage. Tape the end of the tube to the wrap.

12) The tip of the feeding tube should be kept closed when not in use with a male adapter port, blood sample collection tube rubber tip, or other appropriate diameter implement.

13) An e-collar can be placed on the animal below the feeding tube and secured caudally to a harness to prevent the animal from using their back paws to scratch at and possibly remove or damage the feeding tube (with attachment to the harness used to prevent the e-collar from riding up and rubbing on the tube insertion site).

*During Feeding*

1) First check to make sure the tube has not obviously moved from its initial insertion depth.

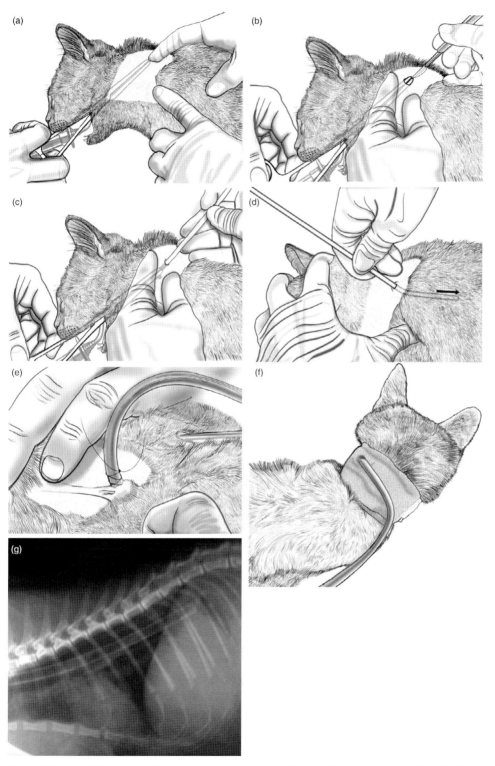

**Figure 15.3** (a–g) Placement of an esophagostomy tube (a) A pair of forceps is passed through the patient's mouth and into the cervical esophagus. (b) A small skin incision is made over the forceps jaws. (c) The esophagostomy tube is grabbed with the forceps. (d) The tube is directed aborally down the esophagus. (e) The tube is sutured in place using a finger trap suture pattern. (f) A bandage is placed around the patient's neck to cover the tube's entry point. (g) A radiograph can confirm the proper positioning of the caudal end of the tube. Source: Crow, 2009. Reproduced with permission of John Wiley & Sons.

2) Gently infuse a small amount of water into the tube, watch for coughing/gagging or signs of discomfort.
3) Slowly infuse the food slurry or liquid medication, monitoring for any signs of respiratory difficulty or distress.
4) Use the larger syringe filled with water to gently flush the remaining food or water out of the tube.

*Feeding Tube Removal*

1) Gently clean the tube entry site.
2) Remove any sutures present.
3) Flush the tube gently with water, fold the end of the feeding tube (to prevent any liquid still in the tube from entering the airway when the tube is removed), and slowly and gently remove the feeding tube.
4) Clean the tube entry site again and place one to two surgical skin staples over the insertion site.

### 15.6.10.3.5 Possible Complications

1) Complications related to anesthesia and sedation.
2) Complications related to the primary disease process necessitating placement of the feeding tube.
3) Aspiration can occur if the tube is not appropriately placed into the esophagus or stomach.

4) Overfeeding or feeding too quickly has the possibility of resulting in aspiration of food or causing patient discomfort from gastric distention.
5) If incorrectly measured, the tube may enter the stomach, wrap around, and exit into the esophagus, increasing the risk of aspiration and aspiration pneumonia.

### 15.6.10.3.6 Other Considerations

1) Most animals tolerate esophagostomy tubes fairly well and they can be maintained for extended periods of time if needed.
2) Feeding tubes can become clogged. If this occurs, infuse 10–20 ml of clear carbonated beverage, wait 10–15 min, and infuse warm water to clear the clog.
3) Feeding a well-blended, liquefied diet with an appropriate liquid component can help reduce the risk of clogging.

## 15.6.11 Fluid Therapy

This section provides an overview of emergency fluid therapy. Additional information on fluid administration is included in Chapter 20.

### 15.6.11.1 Fluid Types and Routes of Administration

Routes of administration for supplemental fluids include IV, including central or peripheral vein, intraosseous, and subcutaneous.

---

**Textbox 15.4 Fluid replacement tips for correcting dehydration**

In general, the following formula can be used to calculate the volume of fluids to administer to treat a patient for deydration:

$$\% \text{ Dehydration} \times \text{body weight(kg)} = \text{replacement volume(L)}$$

This replacement volume should be given over 12–24 h depending on the animal's condition.

In addition, patients will need to receive their normal maintenance requirement during that period and this should be continued once dehydration deficits have been replaced. See below for general calculations for daily maintenance fluids.

Note that an accurate volume is dependent on an accurate dehydration estimate. Dehydration estimates are traditionally based on physical exam findings (decreased skin turgor, tacky mucous membranes, etc.) or bloodwork findings such as hemoconcentration (elevated Hct or PCV), hyperproteinemia, and azotemia.

*Estimating dehydration with skin turgor testing:*

If return to original position is slightly delayed – dehydration is estimated at 2–5% in most cases.
If skin tenting persists and does not return to original position – dehydration is estimated at 12–15% (or higher).

*Types of Fluids*

1) *Crystalloids.* Crystalloid fluids are appropriate in most cases requiring fluid support to replace volume and electrolytes.
2) *Colloids.* In cases where hypoproteinemia is a concern, a colloid (such as hetastarch or dextran) can be used in addition to the crystalloid to help maintain colloid oncotic pressure. Colloids should be used at a maximum of 1–2 ml/kg/h to a maximum of 20–40 ml/kg/day and generally should not be administered more rapidly than 5 ml/kg IV over 10–15 min even in an emergency situation.
3) *Blood products.* Fresh whole blood (FWB), fresh frozen blood, fresh frozen plasma, and platelet-rich plasma may be indicated in special circumstances but are typically not readily available in a field setting. In most cases, the only available blood product will be FWB from an on-site donor animal (see transfusions procedure).

---

**Textbox 15.5 Shock volumes of crystalloid fluids**

For patients presenting with clinical signs of hypovolemic shock requiring rapid blood volume restoration, such as in cases of known blood, protein, or crystalloid loss, and/or when the patient presents with clinical signs of hypovolemia including poor pulse quality, low blood pressure, pale mucous membrane color, prolonged capillary refill time, shock volumes of fluid therapy may be beneficial.

Dogs: 80–90 ml/kg
Cats: 50–55 ml/kg

A helpful shortcut to estimate shock doses of fluids:

Cats – for a quarter shock dose, just add a zero to the body weight in kilograms.
Dogs – for a quarter shock dose, just add a zero to the body weight in pounds.

---

#### 15.6.11.2 Fluid Volumes

---

**Textbox 15.6 Calculating daily maintenance fluids**

For the quiet/inactive patient:

$$(97 \times \text{wt in kg}^{0.655})/24 = \text{hourly maintenance fluid rate in milliliters (this is approximately } 1 - 2\,\text{ml/kg/h})$$

For the active patient:

$$(140 \times \text{wt in kg}^{0.73})/24 = \text{hourly maintenance fluid rate in milliliters (this is approximately } 2 - 3\,\text{ml/kg/h})$$

A very general estimate of daily maintenance fluid requirements for the dog or cat:

60–75 ml/kg/day for cats/small dogs (2.5–3.1 ml/kg/h)
40–50 ml/kg/day for larger dogs (1.7–2.1 ml/kg/h)

Daily fluid requirement delivery methods:

Daily fluid requirements in animals not drinking and eating sufficiently to delivery this amount enterally can be delivered IV at a constant rate infusion by dividing by 24 to calculate an hourly rate. This can also be given via IV aliquots over the course of the day by dividing by the number of aliquots to administer, delivered as SQ fluid boluses divided into a q12h dose, or can be given partially IV with the remainder given SQ if 24 h a day fluid therapy is not an option.

---

#### 15.6.11.3 Fluid Administration

*Fluid Pumps Versus Manual Rate and Volume Monitoring*

1) Fluid pumps are the easiest method of ensuring accurate volume administration over time.

2) If a fluid pump is unavailable, counting drops per minute is needed.

3) To calculate the required drops per minute, one needs to be familiar with the drops per ml of the primary drip set being used.

4) To calculate the required drops per minute: Divide the desired fluid rate (ml/h) by 60 to get ml/min. Multiply this number (ml/min) by the number of drops per ml for the drip set in use. This will give you the number of drops per minute to be observed.

5) It is necessary to finely adjust settings on the extension set with this method and regularly recheck not only the observed drops per minute but also use tape to label your IV fluid bag with the expected rate of bag emptying.

6) To monitor fluid administration and ensure that it meets the intended rate, place tape lengthwise down the IV fluid bag and mark the current time at the current fluid level and then mark times down the tape as to where to expect the fluid level to reach based on the goal fluid administration rate. If the rate drops more quickly or slowly than planned, the infusion set settings should be re-calibrated.

#### 15.6.11.4 Fluid Supplementation

1) In situations where deficits of electrolytes such as potassium can be measured or estimated, appropriate supplementation should be added to IV fluid bags.

2) Carefully label the bags with the date and amount of any additive. Ensure even distribution by gently inverting the bag after adding supplement and prior to administering to the patient.

3) Dextrose is another supplement that can be added to the IV fluids if indicated. Ensure clearly labeling of fluid bag as described above.

4) Some patients may require medications to be added to the IV fluids, including antiemetics, pain medications, or antibiotics. Always ensure careful calculation of concentration and fluid rate, and appropriate labeling of bags and medical records.

5) If fluid rates need to be changed after adding supplements to the fluid bag, a new bag may need to be mixed or additional supplement added as needed, as changing the fluid administration rate will alter the dosing of the fluid additive.

### 15.6.12 Catheter Placement Techniques

IV catheters, central or peripheral, should be placed using aseptic technique. In addition, special techniques such as venous cutdown or intraosseous placement may be necessary in some circumstances.

#### 15.6.12.1 Cutdown Catheter Placement

##### *15.6.12.1.1 Indications*

A venous cutdown is indicated in cases where venous access is crucial but not easily obtained (often due to hypotension or attempting to catheterize a small vessel in a small animal). In these cases, a "cutdown," or incision in the skin, may be needed to successfully place an IV catheter.

##### *15.6.12.1.2 Setting*

This procedure is typically performed in a treatment or exam room setting; since a skin incision is made aseptic technique is required.

##### *15.6.12.1.3 Equipment*

1) Small sterile drape
2) Sterile scrub supplies – scrub, solution, and gauze
3) IV catheter (appropriate to size of animal) and placement supplies – sterile scalpel blade, hemostat
4) Suture and needle drivers
5) Syringe with 2% lidocaine and small amount of sodium bicarbonate (optional).

##### *15.6.12.1.4 Procedure*

1) The catheter site is clipped and prepared as for a sterile procedure.
2) The sterile drape is placed over the area.
3) The target vessel is isolated and held off proximally to increase visibility.
4) Using a sterile blade, a small longitudinal incision is made gently through the skin to avoid incising the vessel. Note that infusing the site with a small amount of 2% lidocaine and waiting 60s prior to incising the skin can improve patient comfort for the actual cutdown. Be aware however, that the infusion itself may cause some discomfort, this can be decreased by adding a small amount of sodium bicarbonate to the syringe.
5) The IV catheter is then inserted into the vessel using standard placement technique for the catheter type in use.

6) If further vessel isolation is needed prior to placement (i.e. for a jugular placement), blunt dissection with hemostats can facilitate isolation of the vessel and sutures may be placed proximal and distal to the planned insertion site to elevate the vessel during IV catheter placement.

7) The skin incision is loosely closed with suture before securing the catheter in place using standard technique.

### 15.6.12.1.5  Possible Complications

1) Care must be taken not to cut too deep when incising the skin to avoid incising the vessel itself.

2) Adherence to aseptic technique is important to minimize infection risk.

### 15.6.12.1.6  Other Considerations

1) Proper vessel and IV catheter size selection reduce the need to perform a cutdown in most patients.

2) Warming the patient and the limb to be catheterized can prevent the need to perform a cutdown by encouraging vessel dilation.

3) Whenever IV access cannot be readily obtained other fluid administration techniques should be considered as long as the patient is not in critical condition and the situation allows it.

### 15.6.12.2  Intraosseous Catheter Placement

#### 15.6.12.2.1  Indications

Intraosseous catheter placement can be used for animals where peripheral vessels are inaccessible. Most often, this procedure is used for neonatal animals or smaller animals that are severely hypovolemic or hypotensive.

#### 15.6.12.2.2  Setting

This procedure is typically performed in a treatment or exam room using aseptic technique.

#### 15.6.12.2.3  Equipment

1) Sterile preparation supplies – clippers, gauze, surgical scrub and solution

2) Appropriate size needle – typically 18- or 20-gauge

3) Tape and bandaging material – to secure in place

4) Suture and needle drivers

5) Syringe with 2% lidocaine and sodium bicarbonate

6) Scalpel blade.

#### 15.6.12.2.4  Procedure

1) The procedure must be performed with aseptic technique to avoid infection/sepsis.

2) The catheter placement site (typically the trochanteric fossa of the proximal femur, the iliac crest, or the medial side of the proximal tibia – distal to the tibial tuberosity) is clipped and prepared with aseptic technique.

3) Local anesthetic (such as 2% lidocaine, possibly mixed with a small amount of sodium bicarbonate to reduce discomfort on administration) is infused into the superficial subcutaneous tissues, then deeper into the subcutaneous and down to the periosteum of the insertion site.

4) After the site is stabilized, a small stab incision is made in the skin, and the needle is gently advanced into the medullary cavity of the bone.

5) The needle is flushed with heparinized saline and secured in place with butterfly tape and suture.

6) A light bandage should be placed to protect the site.

## 15.6.13  Foreign Body Removal

If a patient presents with a history or clinical signs suggesting a foreign body, diagnostic exploration and removal is typically indicated. The type of procedure to be performed depends on the location of the foreign body. Clinical signs can vary from scratching at the ears in case of an aural foreign body, an object protruding from under the eyelid for an ocular foreign body, draining tracts from subcutaneous and deeper foreign bodies, to gastrointestinal symptoms. A thorough history and physical exam resulting in a foreign body being included in the differential diagnoses list warrants further diagnostic exploration.

Many foreign bodies are found in orifices or superficial tissues. For orifice-associated or superficial objects, an exam room or treatment room setting is appropriate as the procedure does not require aseptic technique. For removal of internal (i.e. gastrointestinal, abdominal or intrathoracic) foreign bodies, an aseptic surgical setting is required.

Necessary equipment will depend on the type of foreign body. For many objects associated with an orifice, a good light source (direct illumination) or appropriate instrument for the specific orifice, such as an otoscope for an aural foreign body, is appropriate for visualization. Alligator forceps or curved tip hemostats are helpful when removing foreign bodies in orifices and superficial soft tissue.

Possible complications include:

1) Remnants of the foreign body left behind resulting in ongoing clinical symptoms, abscess, additional pathology due to foreign body migration
2) Iatrogenic trauma (i.e. nasal turbinate injury, ruptured tympanic membrane, corneal ulcer, hemorrhage)

In patients with a clinical suspicion of a foreign body that cannot be located, other differential diagnoses should be considered and explored. Patients may exhibit clinical symptoms persistent with a foreign body even after it has been removed or has migrated to other tissues. Ancillary medical management including antibiotic therapy and pain medication should be used as indicated.

### 15.6.13.1  Ocular Foreign Body

1) Apply proparacaine topical anesthetic to the affected eye and wait 1–2 min.
2) Gently clean any debris from around the eye and eyelids.
3) Use an eye lubricant-saturated cotton-tipped applicator to gently manipulate eyelids and/or nictitating membrane to improve access to the object.
4) Use curved tip hemostats or thumb forceps to gently remove the foreign object without making contact with the cornea.
5) Gently flush the eye with saline solution.
6) Use fluorescein stain and a black light to assess the cornea for any corneal injury from the foreign body.
7) Prescribe appropriate medications for any injury found. Ocular-associated foreign bodies often result in secondary corneal ulcers requiring treatment with antibiotic ophthalmic preparation. In cases of severe corneal ulceration, or deeper injury such as descemetocele, additional treatment, such as topical treatment with autologous serum, or surgical treatment creating a conjunctival or nictitans flap to protect the wound.

### 15.6.13.2  Aural Foreign Body

1) Sedation or general anesthesia may be necessary to fully visualize and remove a foreign body from the ear.

2) In most cases when an aural foreign body is suspected or visualized, it is beneficial to not clean the ear before removing it, as any liquids infused into the ear can make visualization and removal of the object more difficult.
3) An otoscope with ear cones appropriate for the animal's size, and that allow passage of alligator forceps, is used to examine the ear canal and visualize any foreign body.
4) Use alligator forceps to gently grasp and remove the object.
5) Following removal, additional inspection of both ears should be performed to ensure that no additional foreign bodies remain.
6) Inspect the tympanic membrane for any rupture or tears to help guide appropriate topical therapy.
7) Once the tympanic membrane is confirmed intact, the ear should be gently cleaned and appropriate medication (such as a steroid/anti-fungal/antibacterial combination) started.
8) In cases where the tympanic membrane is ruptured (or cannot be confirmed to be intact), topical medications should be used with care. In these cases, the safest approach is to avoid topical steroids and antibiotics unless labeled as safe to use in situations of known or suspected tympanic membrane rupture. The ear can be gently cleaned with saline and oral medications should be considered if indicated instead of topical medications infused into the ear.
9) If indicated, a culture could be submitted first to ensure appropriate antibiotic selection (although with most acute foreign bodies this is unnecessary).
10) Appropriate systemic therapy should be instituted – this may include pain medication such as an NSAID or an opioid, and oral antibiotics if indicated.

### 15.6.13.3  Nasal Foreign Body

1) In general, unless the object is clearly protruding from a nostril, sedation or general anesthesia is required to fully examine the nasal cavity and remove any foreign bodies.
2) Using an otoscope with an appropriately sized cone that allows alligator forceps to be used to remove the object, examine each nare for the object.

3) Due to the nasal turbinates, a thorough inspection must be performed to confirm or rule out a foreign object.
4) Once identified, the object should be gently grasped and removed at the same time the otoscope cone itself is removed from the nose to prevent the object being dislodged by trying to fit through the cone.
5) A nasopharyngeal foreign body may be visualized via the mouth – use a spay hook to gently pull the distal soft palate ventrorostrally while using a dental mirror to visualize the nasopharynx.
6) In cases where a nasal foreign body is suspected but not visualized, a nasal flush may be indicated.
7) To perform a nasal flush in an intubated animal, pack the back of the animal's mouth with gauze and gently flush warm saline into the nostril. This can help dislodge small objects/particles from deep within the nose. Keep the patients head in a lower position so that the water flows out of the oral cavity.
8) At the end of the nasal flush, ensure removal of the gauze used to pack the oral cavity, before attempting to extubate the animal.

### 15.6.13.4 Oral (Including Sublingual, Tonsillar Crypts and Oropharyngeal) Foreign Body

1) As with nasal foreign bodies, unless the object is clearly protruding from the mouth and able to be safely removed in the fully awake animal, sedation or general anesthesia with intubation is required. This allows a thorough examination of the oral cavity and removal of any foreign body.
2) Sedate or anesthetize the patient as indicated and place it in sternal recumbency.
3) The most common locations for oral foreign bodies are across the top of the mouth against the hard palate, associated with the oral labia, lodged between, lateral or medial to the teeth, under the tongue, within the tonsillar crypts, in the oral fauces, or associated with the oropharynx.
4) Most larger objects can be atraumatically removed with Carmalts and smaller objects can typically be removed with curved tip hemostats.
5) It is important to examine the entire oral cavity even once an initial foreign body is found to ensure that there are not additional objects or injuries contributing to the animal's clinical symptoms.

### 15.6.13.5 Genital (Including Vaginal and Penile Sheath) Foreign Body

1) Most genital related foreign objects can be removed with mild-to-moderate sedation for patient comfort and to aid with positioning and gentle restraint.
2) With the animal in dorsal or lateral recumbency, clip and clean around the penile sheath or vaginal labia.
3) For penile sheath-associated objects, while wearing sterile gloves gently examine the sheath and if needed extrude the penis to better visualize any foreign objects.
4) Objects protruding from the penile urethra itself should be removed while wearing sterile gloves. Also use sterile jelly with lidocaine to decrease trauma and pain from the removal.
5) Vaginal foreign bodies can be removed with the animal in sternal or lateral recumbency, using a speculum and light source, or an otoscope and appropriately sized cone. In most cases, hemostats or alligator forceps will allow you to atraumatically remove the object.

### 15.6.13.6 Rectal Foreign Body

1) With the patient standing, use a gloved hand to examine and palpate the rectum for any foreign objects.
2) The veterinarian's gloved and lubricated fingers, hemostats, or alligator forceps can be used to remove most rectal associated foreign bodies.
3) For larger objects, lubricating jelly or enema solution can be used to gently remove the object without causing trauma.

### 15.6.13.7 Subcutaneous (Including Interdigital) Foreign Body

1) Most subcutaneous foreign bodies are removed under sedation or general anesthesia.
2) The area of the known or suspected object should be clipped and surgically prepared.
3) Using sterile instruments (typically curved tip hemostats or alligator forceps) and surgical gloves, any draining tracts should be probed.
4) A curved tip syringe can be used to gently flush dilute chlorhexidine or sterile saline into the draining tract to dislodge any objects. The object

may be extruded by the flow of liquid, or as a result of the flushing, be more easily removed with an instrument.

5) In some cases, an incision may be necessary to widen a draining tract or incise any protrusion the suspect foreign body creates. Remember to use aseptic technique.

6) After removal of the foreign body, a curved tip syringe should be used to flush the area and any draining tracts.

7) If an incision has been made requiring closure, a simple interrupted suture pattern should be used to partially close it. In general, it is best to leave small draining tracts open, and leave large incisions used to remove foreign bodies partially open or place a surgical drain if sufficient dead space remains, otherwise the animal is at risk of significant abscess or seroma formation.

#### 15.6.13.8 Gastrointestinal Foreign Body

Known or suspected GI foreign bodies that require surgery will require appropriate aseptic surgical technique to perform an exploratory laparotomy, please consult appropriate surgical text books for instructions.

### 15.6.14 Luxation Reduction

Joint luxations occur most frequently secondary to trauma, and the most common luxation that responds to closed (nonsurgical) reduction includes elbow and hip/coxofemoral luxation. If at all possible, radiographs should be taken to confirm that a luxation has occurred and that it is not complicated by associated fractures to the joint. Luxations found in association with a fracture are generally not amenable to closed reduction.

Nonsurgical reduction of joint luxations usually require general anesthesia to prevent patient discomfort and ensure the muscle relaxation required to manipulate the joint.

In some smaller patients it may be possible to do a closed reduction under light sedation, while most larger patients require general anesthesia and monitoring. Larger patients may also require additional assistance from personnel and equipment (such as towels) to facilitate reduction. In many cases, the limb will need to be bandaged following reduction.

#### 15.6.14.1 Coxofemoral Luxation Reduction

1) Coxofemoral luxation usually results in a craniodorsal displacement of the femoral head (with the femoral head palpable above and in front of the normal location in the acetabulum). Ideally, radiographs are used to confirm the luxation and identify related fractures. If radiographs are not possible, careful palpation can help to confirm the location of the displaced head of the femur.

2) Place the anesthetized patient in lateral recumbency, with the unaffected limb down towards the table and affected limb off the table. Start by moving the hip through its normal range of motion to free any adhesions.

3) Have an assistant place a towel around the animal's abdomen and apply gentle and steady pressure away from the person performing the reduction.

4) To reduce the most common craniodorsal displacement – hold the leg from the mid to lower femur with one hand and with the other hand hold onto the head of the femur and greater trochanter. Gently abduct the leg (pulling away from the body) while rotating the leg cranially and medially to free the head of the femur. Apply steady and firm pressure ventrally on the head of the femur, helping it to move up and over the edge of the ilium and into the acetabulum.

5) For the less common cranioventral displacement, the femur should be rotated more caudally and medially and the pressure on the greater trochanter and head of the femur should be more lateral and dorsal.

6) If the reduction is unsuccessful on the first attempt, you can help release some tension by placing gentle traction on the limb away from the animal's body for 2–5 min and/or place a light bandage around the lower leg and suspend it from above for 2–5 min before reattempting the procedure.

7) Once reduced, move the coxofemoral joint through its range of motion keeping gentle pressure on the head of the femur in the acetabulum for 2–5 min.

8) An Ehmer sling may be placed at this point to prevent the animal from bearing weight on the leg. Ensure that the sling is placed correctly and check it frequently to make sure it is not slipping or causing any tissue swelling. It can be left in place for 10–12 days if no complications are encountered (Figure 15.4).

(a)

(b)

(c)

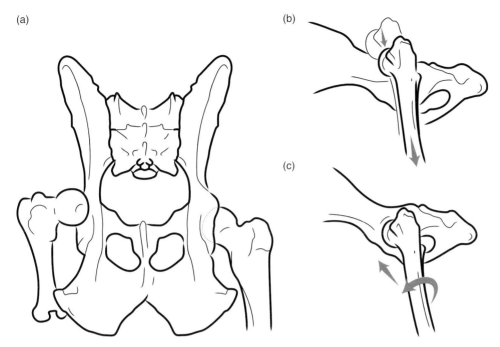

**Figure 15.4** Craniodorsal coxofemoral luxation. Reduction includes abducting the leg, applying steady and firm pressure on the head of the femur while rotating the leg cranially and medially. Source: Courtesy of Bernt Henrik Kommedal.

### 15.6.14.2 Elbow Dislocation Reduction

1) Elbow dislocation/luxation is often complicated by fracture(s). If at all possible, a dislocated elbow should be confirmed to be uncomplicated through radiographs. If radiographs are not available, careful palpation and assessment for unusual laxity or crepitus beyond what is expected with an uncomplicated dislocation should be assessed.
2) Most commonly, the radius and ulna luxate laterally.
3) Place the anesthetized patient in lateral recumbency with the unaffected limb down towards the table, and the affected limb off the table.
4) Keep the elbow flexed to 90° or slightly greater, place one hand on the mid-humerus and the other hand placed on the proximal radius/ulna.
5) Rotate the proximal radius/ulna inward/toward the animal, while applying pressure to the head of the radius until it is reduced into normal anatomical alignment.
6) Once the anconeal process is reduced, the limb is fully extended to help secure the position.

7) A support bandage, such as a modified Robert Jones, is then placed for 10–14 days.

### 15.6.14.3 Possible Complications

1) Unidentified fractures can prevent successful reduction of luxated limbs.
2) It may be impossible to reduce a chronically luxated joint.
3) Chronic changes (i.e. flattening of the acetabulum secondary to hip dysplasia, or severe soft tissue injury) may lead to reluxation within a short period.
4) Improper placement of the Ehmer sling, or unnoticed slipping of the sling, can result in reluxation of the coxofemoral joint, soft tissue swelling, and in severe cases can result in a devitalized appendage. Therefore the Ehmer sling should only be used for patients that will be appropriately monitored.

### 15.6.14.4 Other Considerations

If closed reduction is unsuccessful, surgical reduction and stabilization may be necessary, or a salvage procedure such as a FHO or amputation.

### 15.6.15 Neonatal Supportive Care

#### 15.6.15.1 Indications
In the field, neonatal patients are often in need of emergency care due to poor nutritional status, absent heat support, and/or lack of basic husbandry.

#### 15.6.15.2 Setting
Neonatal supportive care can take place in an exam room or treatment room setting as most types of basic supportive care for neonates do not require sterility.

#### 15.6.15.3 Equipment

1) Heating source – this can be heating pad, heated warming disc, or heated rice-filled socks
2) Fluid support supplies – fluid bag, large luer lock syringe needles, extension sets, +/− IV or intra-osseous catheter supplies
3) Dextrose, corn syrup, or equivalent sources of oral and injectable sugar supplementation
4) Antiparasitic treatment compounded for neonatal use
5) Bottles, formula, feeding tubes, and syringes for enteral nutrition support
6) Transfusion supplies if needed – 6-, 12-, and 20-ml syringes, Hemo-Nate® filter, and needles.

#### 15.6.15.4 Procedure

1) *Heat support.* Warming disc, rice sock, electric heating pad, see Table 15.4 for recommended environmental temperatures and Table 15.5 for physiologic rectal temperatures
2) *Fluid support.* Subcutaneous fluids, intraosseous fluids, or IV fluids.
3) *Glucose.* Can be applied to gums, given orally if swallowing, by feeding tube or intravenously.

Table 15.4 Required environmental temperature for neonatal puppies and kittens.

| Age | Temperature |
| --- | --- |
| Week 1 | 84–89 °F (28.9–31.7 °C) |
| Weeks 2–3 | 80 °F (26.7 °C) |
| Week 4 | 69–75 °F (20.6–23.9 °C) |
| Week 5 | 69 °F (20.6 °C) |

Table 15.5 Normal neonatal rectal temperatures.

| Age | Rectal body temperature |
| --- | --- |
| Week 1 | 95–99 °F (35–37.2 °C) |
| Week 2–3 | 97–100 °F (36.1–37.8 °C) |
| At weaning | 99–101 °F (37.2–38.3 °C) |

4) *Nutritional support.* Normal feeding if able to eat, syringe/trickle-feeding if able to swallow but not eating on own, tube-feeding if needed. As a general rule, a kitten should eat about 8 ml of formula per ounce of body weight per day. For example, a kitten who weighs 4 oz should eat about 32 ml of formula per day. Remember to never feed a kitten or puppy on his or her back (due to increased risks of aspiration in this position).
5) *Transfusions.* In some cases of severe anemia, basic supportive care may be inadequate and a blood transfusion is needed. See Section 15.6.22. The typical transfusion volume of fresh whole blood for a neonate is 5–30 ml.
6) *Parasite treatment.* Immediate parasite control such as nitenpyram (for immediate kill of fleas) in addition to longer acting flea control, flea removal by hand, gentle bath (unlikely most commercial flea shampoos are safe but a gentle bath with gentle soap or just warm water).

An additional recipe is included in Chapter 20.

---

**Textbox 15.7 Homemade formula for orphaned kittens**

90-ml condensed milk (or goat's milk)
90-ml water
120-ml plain yogurt (not low-fat)
Three egg yolks
The formula will be good for about 48 h if refrigerated. If the formula has been left outside the refrigerator for more than 2 h, it must be discarded.

NOTE: If using commercial milk replacer products, carefully follow package label for reconstituting (if powder form) and storage before and after reconstitution.

#### 15.6.15.5 Possible Complications

1) Not all fading neonates respond to treatment.
2) Attempting basic supportive care gives the compromised neonate the best chance of survival.

#### 15.6.15.6 Other Considerations

1) In very young neonates, appropriate diagnostics must be performed when safe for the patient.
2) Parvo/panleukopenia testing is appropriate if there is any clinical suspicion of these conditions.
3) Minimal bloodwork may be indicated and possible – PCV/TP using microhematocrit tube and blood glucose using a glucometer.
4) In general, with very young/small fading neonates, extensive bloodwork is not possible due to the small blood volume of these patients. Typical sample sizes for most full blood panels exceed what is safe to remove from most small neonatal animals and can worsen the prognosis due to exsanguination. Therefore, even when available, bloodwork diagnostics should be carefully considered and tailored to produce maximum benefit with the smallest possible sample size.

### 15.6.16 Orogastric Lavage

#### 15.6.16.1 Indications

Most commonly, orogastric lavage is indicated in cases of toxin ingestion. It may also be used in the case of gastric dilatation.

#### 15.6.16.2 Setting

Orogastric lavage is generally performed under general anesthesia in order to provide airway protection and appropriately perform the procedure. In some cases, it may be performed with only moderate sedation, but airway protection becomes more difficult.

#### 15.6.16.3 Equipment

1) General anesthesia and monitoring equipment.
2) One or two appropriately sized lavage tubes.
3) One empty bucket – to collect lavage fluid.
4) One bucket of water – to infuse into the GI tract.
5) Large infusing syringe with catheter tip to fit on lavage tube.
6) Large syringe with catheter tip to fit on lavage tube to remove fluid/contents from the stomach, or a stomach pump/large animal pump, or a vacuum/suction system as needed.
7) Activated charcoal may be infused and left in the stomach following the lavage, for additional toxin absorption.
8) Laparotomy sponge and clamp (hemostat or similar).

#### 15.6.16.4 Procedure

1) Place the anesthetized patient in sternal recumbency. Ideally the patient should be intubated and the oropharynx packed with a laparotomy sponge. The sponge should be fixed externally to prevent it from being pushed into the esophagus during the procedure.
2) Elevate the animal's head using folded towels.
3) Measure the stomach tube(s) to be used from the tip of the animal's nose to the last rib to ensure gastric placement. Mark the tube at this location to ensure appropriate placement.
4) Lubricate the end of the tube and gently pass into the oral cavity over the top of the lap sponge protecting the animal's oropharynx.
5) Confirm placement of the tube in the stomach by palpating externally, smelling for gastric contents, and listening for gastric noises.
6) Evacuate stomach contents using a syringe applied to the tube or using suction to create a siphon effect. You can begin the siphon effect by placing the end of the tube below the animal's body level and applying suction with a suction pump, bulb, syringe, or your mouth (but be careful not to apply for too long and risk-ingesting stomach contents) and then allow the stomach contents to flow out of the tube by gravity (by keeping the tip of the tube lower than the animal's body).
7) A second tube can be introduced to begin gently infusing water once the stomach has been emptied, using the first tube to continue emptying the water that has been infused. Alternatively the initial tube can be used to infuse and then suction water out of the stomach sequentially.
8) Gently repositioning the animal by rocking gently side to side can help increase the effectiveness of the lavage.
9) After thoroughly lavaging, suction, siphon, or allow passive drainage of any remaining lavage fluid.

10) If indicated, infuse activated charcoal or another appropriate treatment into the stomach.
11) Flush the tube with water before removing it from the stomach.
12) Bend the end of the tube and gently remove it from the oropharynx (this prevents contents from spilling into the airway when the tube is removed).
13) Gently clean the oropharynx and mouth after the tube has been removed.
14) Remove the lap sponge used to protect the oropharynx and ensure that the mouth/oropharynx is clean of any material/ingesta.
15) With the animal in sternal recumbency and the head elevated, allow the animal to recover from anesthesia slowly and only remove the ET tube once the swallow reflex is strongly present.
16) If not contraindicated, consider administering an antiemetic (potentially one with gastroesophageal sphincter-enhancing effects such as metoclopramide) at the end of the procedure to reduce the risk of esophageal reflux and aspiration periprocedurally (especially if activated charcoal is being administered as part of the procedure).

### 15.6.16.5 Possible Complications

1) Trauma to the oral cavity, esophagus, or stomach.
2) There is a risk of aspiration of gastric contents if the airway is not fully protected, especially in an awake or only moderately sedated animal. This can also occur during recovery or after the procedure.

### 15.6.16.6 Other Considerations

To reduce the risk of complications, use gentle technique when placing orogastric tubes and take care to not to infuse too great a volume of liquid too quickly.

## 15.6.17 Oxygen Supplementation

### 15.6.17.1 Indications

Oxygen supplementation is indicated if an animal is suffering from, or at risk of, hypoxia or poor oxygen saturation. This may be secondary to trauma or other pathology compromising the respiratory system, including patients with cardiac or pulmonary disease, or in some cases anemia.

### 15.6.17.2 Setting

Oxygen supplementation is typically provided in a basic treatment setting and is generally not considered an aseptic procedure.

### 15.6.17.3 Equipment

1) An oxygen cage is unlikely to be available in most field situations, but if available, this is often the most practical method to provide supplemental oxygen.
2) If an oxygen cage is unavailable, an oxygen tank and pressure regulator can be used as a source of supplemental oxygen.
3) Nasal insufflation – A small-diameter feeding tube, red rubber, or similar tube can be used to deliver oxygen into the proximal aspect of the nasal cavity.
4) Oxygen via mask – For unconscious, otherwise laterally recumbent, or minimally mobile animals, oxygen can be delivered by anesthesia mask held in place with a regular dog muzzle or gauze tie-in.
5) Elizabethan collar (e-collar) hood – For more active animals, an e-collar can be fitted and partially enclosed with cling wrap or other clear plastic wrap, leaving ventilation areas for expired gases. Supplemental oxygen can then be piped into the e-collar hood (Figure 15.5).
6) Fashioning an oxygen cage using a crate/transport carrier – A crate can be partially enclosed in cling/plastic wrap, leaving appropriate ventilation for expired gases. Supplemental oxygen can then be piped into the enclosure.

### 15.6.17.4 Procedure for Nasal Insufflation

1) Instill proparacaine drops into the side of the nose the tube is to be inserted into.
2) Measure from the distal tip of the nose to the medial canthus and mark this distance on the tube.
3) Gently insert the tube, aiming it ventromedially to the marked line.
4) Secure at the ventrolateral aspect of the nare with surgical staples, direct the tubing along the animal's nose, and further secure using butterfly tape and staples. Then direct it between the animal's ears and secure similarly in this location.

**Figure 15.5** Oxygen hood. A dog receiving supplemental oxygen via a homemade oxygen hood. Approximately three-fourth of the front of an Elizabethan collar is covered with clear wrap. It is essential to leave a large window to allow heat and carbon dioxide to escape. An oxygen line (black hose in photo) is taped into the back of the collar and oxygen flow rates of 100–200 ml/kg min are used. Source: Courtesy of Dr. Kate Hopper, University of California, Davis.

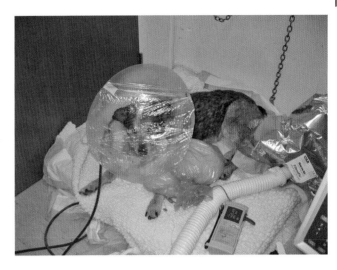

#### 15.6.17.5   Possible Complications

Animals receiving oxygen via a mask, hood, or cage must be monitored to ensure that expiratory gases can escape and that the temperature within the mask/hood/cage is appropriate (heat from expired gases and lack of fresh air circulation into the enclosure/apparatus can result in elevated temperatures and hyperthermia).

#### 15.6.17.6   Other Considerations

Appropriate oxygen flow should be maintained for the size of the animal and delivery system used. Typically, this is lower than rates required for anesthesia and appropriate supplementation can be achieved at rates approximately 50% of those that would be used for anesthesia.

### 15.6.18   Splints and Casts

#### 15.6.18.1   Indications

Splints and casts are used in the field setting as temporary, or in some cases the only treatment to stabilize fractures and dislocations. In some cases splints and casts may be used to provide support or protection to soft tissue injuries.

#### 15.6.18.2   Setting

Typically, most splints and casts are placed in a nonsterile treatment or exam room setting. In cases of open fractures or severe wounds, splinting/casting will need to be performed using aspetic technique.

#### 15.6.18.3   Equipment

1) See section on wound care if wounds are present.
2) See Section 15.6.3 for basic bandaging supplies.
3) Splints – although preformed splints are available, it is likely more economical and practical to use rolls of casting material to form custom splints as needed in the field. The benefit of using rolls of casting material is that splints (and casts) of any size and dimension that might be needed can be created as the need arises, rather than keeping a stock of various preformed splints.
4) If using casting material – prepare a stainless steel bowl, gloves, and warm water.
5) If placing a full cast – ensure that a cast saw and cast splitters are available for aftercare or at time of placement so that cast can be bivalved. Bivalving entails cutting down the full length of each side of the placed and dried cast on opposite sides after initial placement and then securely bandaging the bisected cast to the leg. Bi-valving ensures that the cast can be removed even in the absence of a cast saw.

#### 15.6.18.4   Procedure

1) If wounds are present, refer to sections on wound care and bandaging.
2) To splint or cast a fracture or other injury, first address any wounds and then begin placing the initial bandage layers including stirrup tape strips, cast padding, and stretch gauze, followed

by applying an appropriate splint. The splint should immobilize one joint below and one joint above any fractures that have been identified. (Note: if you do not immobilize the joint immediately proximal and distal to the fracture site, motion will transmit to the fracture and impair healing).

3) A customized splint can be formed from casting material cut to the appropriate length. Casting material needs to be placed in warm water, and formed into the correct length and appropriate thickness (two to three layers for light animals and five to six layers for heavier animals). This can be done by laying the material out to the appropriate length, and then doubling back to the appropriate number of layers.

4) Where appropriate, two separate lengths can be formed that overlap to create an angle.

5) Once formed, and before the cast begins to harden, place it over the cast padding covered with stretch gauze layer on the animal, hold the leg in extension or flexion as appropriate, and use stretch gauze over the splint to form it to the leg and secure it in place.

6) If placing a full cast, place the cast over the cast-padding layers and initial stretch gauze layers and then use stretch gauze to hold the cast in place and conform it to the leg.

7) If placing a full cast, it is imperative to ensure the cast can be removed when appropriate. Not all facilities will have appropriate cast removal equipment.

8) If no cast removal equipment will be available in the future, but is available at the time of placement, the cast can be placed and bivalved so that it can be removed in the future without any specialized equipment.

9) If in doubt, use a single splint, or two splints placed on opposite sides of the leg, instead of a cast.

10) Cover the stretch gauze layer with a self-adhesive bandage for durability and apply elastic tape distally and proximally to help secure the apparatus and further improve durability.

#### 15.6.18.5   Possible Complications

1) Similar to bandages, complications include slipping, moisture, and tissue swelling.

2) In some cases, a splint or a cast will fail to resolve a fracture, particularly if placed too tightly or too loosely.

3) It is imperative that patients with splints/casts are closely monitored and receive appropriate aftercare.

4) Ideally, patients with a splint/cast should be checked daily by an educated caregiver and assessed every 1–2 weeks by a veterinarian or other veterinary professional, or more frequently/sooner if any concerns are noted by the caregiver.

---

**Textbox 15.8  Word of warning**

Do not place a bandage/splint if there is no aftercare available!

---

#### 15.6.18.6   Other Considerations

1) Some areas of the body such as the elbows are prone to pressure sores when casted or splinted due to very minimal soft tissue coverage. A cutout of the cast padding, donut padding, or additional padding over these sites can reduce the risk of pressure sores.

2) Please refer to a textbook such as "Small Animal Bandaging, Casting and Splinting Techniques" (see references) for full explanations and illustrations of common techniques. This book is small, lightweight, and well worth the value of carrying in the field.

### 15.6.19   Thoracocentesis (Chest Tap)

#### 15.6.19.1   Indications

Thoracocentesis is indicated whenever there is suspicion of free fluid (pleural effusion) or air (pneumothorax) within the thorax and to drain the thorax when appropriate. For many patients, thoracocentesis has both a diagnostic and therapeutic effect. Pneumothorax or pleural effusion may cause abnormal respiratory pattern. Blunt force trauma is a common cause, but other pathologies may also lead to hemorrhage, fluid accumulation or pneumothorax, necessitating thoracocentesis.

Traumatic injury is considered the most common cause of pneumothorax in dogs and cats. Radiographic signs of pleural effusion include rounding or blunting of the lung lobe edges, border effacement with the cardiac silhouette and diaphragm, dorsal elevation of the trachea. Pneumothorax may result in elevation of the cardiac silhouette from the sternum, atelectatic lung lobes are radiopaque in contrast to the radiolucent, air-filled pleural space. Differential diagnoses for pleural effusion include pyothorax, chylothorax, and hemothorax.

In the absence of radiographs, thoracocentesis is indicated when there is a high index of suspicion of free air or fluid in the thorax based on history and physical exam findings.

---

**Textbox 15.9 Diagnostic tip**

In the dyspneic patient, one must distinguish between air and fluid in the chest; this can be accomplished through auscultation. In cases of fluid in the thorax, lung, and heart, sounds will be muffled ventrally. Patients with air in the thorax (pneumothorax) tend to have dull lung sounds dorsally.

---

#### 15.6.19.2 Setting

In most cases, thoracocentesis is performed on a lightly sedated/nonanesthetized patient. This procedure can be performed on an unsedated animal but requires a quiet setting and compliant animal to avoid complications. Ideally, thoracocentesis is performed with ultrasound guidance to help locate appropriate sites for sampling. However, this procedure is often performed without that guidance when ultrasonography is unavailable.

#### 15.6.19.3 Equipment

1) Clippers, gauze, scrub, and solution
2) 18- to 20-gauge needle or IV catheter
3) For diagnostic sampling – a 3ml syringe and a purple top tube (containing EDTA)
4) For therapeutic thoracocentesis – a 35ml luer-lock tip syringe, extension set, three-way stopcock and a bowl for collecting the fluid
5) Microhematocrit tube
6) Microcentrifuge
7) PCV reading card
8) Refractometer
9) Culture swabs or a red top/nonadditive tube (if submitting for culture)
10) Slides +/− stain and a microscope

#### 15.6.19.4 Procedure

1) Ideally performed on a treatment table with the animal in sternal recumbency if fluid is present in the thorax or in lateral recumbency in case of pneumothorax.
2) The sample sites should be clipped and aseptically prepared for the procedure. Typically, the appropriate sampling area will be between the sixth and eighth intercostal spaces on each side of the chest.
3) With the animal in sternal recumbency, a ventral needle insertion site, approximately at the costochondral junction, is used to aspirate fluid.
4) Wearing sterile gloves and following aseptic technique, insert the needle just off the cranial edge of the rib to avoid intercostal vessels. Gently insert the needle at a 30° agree to avoid pulmonary trauma.
5) Aspirate fluid from the inserted needle and collect sample in collection tube (and on culture swab if indicated).
6) Note that free blood typically will not clot. If the sample obtained clots, it may indicate entry into an organ or blood vessel during the procedure.
7) If a pneumothorax is present, clip and prepare the sampling sites as above, and with the animal in lateral recumbency, perform thoracocentesis just dorsal to the costochondral junction using the technique described above (Figure 15.6).

#### 15.6.19.5 Possible Complications

1) If the patient requires sedation or anesthesia it is important to supply oxygen to prevent hypoxemia.
2) Hemorrhage can be caused by injury of the pulmonary parenchyma or blood vessels.
3) Contamination and secondary infection, especially if there are any breaks in aseptic technique during the procedure.

#### 15.6.19.6 Other Considerations

1) Depending on pathology present, sedation and/or restraint for this procedure could worsen dyspnea.
2) The patient needs to be carefully monitored. If there are any concerns, the procedure should be stopped, the patient repositioned and monitored for improvement, and further supportive care instituted.

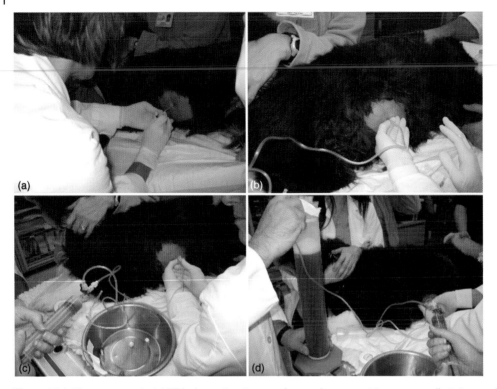

**Figure 15.6** Thoracocentesis. (a) With the patient in sternal recumbency, an 18-gauge needle is inserted into the skin over the seventh intercostal space at the level of the costochondral junction. The hub is filled with saline and the needle is slowly advanced. As the pleural space is entered, the bleb of fluid in the hub moves in or out. (b) An extension set, three-way stopcock, and syringe are attached to the needle. (c) An assistant begins to apply gentle negative pressure to the syringe plunger. (d) Aspiration continues until the syringe is full; once full, the stopcock is turned to the off position, and the contents are emptied into a large graduated cylinder. Source: Courtesy of Dr. Kate Hopper, University of California, Davis.

### 15.6.20 Thoracostomy and Chest Tube Placement

#### 15.6.20.1 Indications

Thoracostomy and placement of a chest tube is typically indicated in cases of pleural space disease involving free air or fluid within the thorax. Thoracocentesis (see above) is generally attempted before placement of an indwelling tube is considered. Most practitioners will attempt intermittent thoracocentesis up to three times and proceed to chest tube placement if there is inadequate resolution of free air/fluid in the thorax. Chest tubes can also be used to infuse medication directly into the chest and for thoracic lavage (such as in pyothorax).

#### 15.6.20.2 Setting

Chest tubes are typically placed in a treatment room or surgical setting using aseptic technique.

#### 15.6.20.3 Equipment

1) Sterile chest tube – the appropriate size depends on the patient's size and the reason for tube placement (i.e. air evacuation vs drainage of thick fluid from the chest)
2) Surgical site preparation supplies – clippers, gauze, scrub and solution
3) Appropriate sedation for the procedure – moderate sedation or general anesthesia combined with a local lidocaine block is effective
4) Sterile gloves, cap, and mask
5) Sterile surgery pack – sterile surgery drape, towel clamps, needle drivers, hemostats, Metzenbaum scissors, scalpel blade, and suture
6) Three-way stopcock and adapter
7) Large syringe – to aspirate air or fluid
8) Sample collection supplies if indicated

9) Bandaging material – sterile sponges, antimicrobial ointment, cast padding, self-adhesive bandage, and elastic tape.

### 15.6.20.4  Procedure

1) Place the sedated or anesthetized patient in lateral recumbency, aseptically prepare the lateral thorax at the level of the fifth to ninth intercostal space.

2) Perform a local block with lidocaine (infusing up to 2–3 ml of lidocaine around the site of proposed tube placement in the interdermal, subcutaneous, and muscle layers – the amount infused will be less for smaller animals).

3) Using aseptic technique (including a surgeon's cap, mask, and sterile gloves), place sterile drapes around the insertion site.

4) Make a skin incision at the level of the eighth or ninth intercostal space and use curved tip hemostats to create a tunnel under the skin from the skin incision cranially to the sixth or seventh intercostal space.

5) Place the tips of the hemostat over the caudal aspect of the intercostal space along the cranial edge of the more caudal rib (to avoid nerves and vessels that run along the caudal aspect of each rib).

6) Securing your instrument hand against the chest, rotate the hemostats until the tip is facing down toward the chest cavity. Apply gentle and steady pressure until the tip of the hemostats "pop" into the chest cavity, taking care to control your pressure so that the tips just enter the cavity without pushing deep into the thorax.

7) Without removing the first hemostat entering the thorax, use a second hemostat with the tip of your chest tube gently clamped between its jaws to insert the tube.

8) Following the tunnel created by the first hemostat, open the jaws of the first hemostat and gently insert the tip of the chest tube into the thorax by entering between the open jaws of said hemostat.

9) Open the jaws of the second hemostat and gently advance the chest tube cranially into the thoracic cavity.

10) Keep the tube in place while carefully removing both the hemostats.

11) Hold a gauze square over the exit point of the chest tube while a syringe is attached to collect a fluid sample or start therapeutic draining of gas or fluid from the thorax.

12) Place a closed three-way stopcock or other device (such as the rubber stopper of a red top tube) onto the end of the chest tube to prevent air from entering the chest. Additionally, place a tube clamp or a hemostat on the tube to prevent air or fluid leakage. The hemostats can be secured to the animal during bandaging.

13) Secure the chest tube in place using a finger trap suture pattern or by using a butterfly tape configuration secured to the chest at the tube's exit point.

14) Apply antimicrobial ointment to a gauze square and place over the drain's exit point.

15) Ensure that the drain is exiting the thorax caudally with no significant bend or kink in it, secure the tube using a light layer of cast padding and self-adhesive bandage, making sure not to apply extra tension. Apply elastic tape, (without causing significant pressure on the chest) at the cranial and caudal aspects of the bandage to prevent slippage.

16) Make sure that the distal end of the tube is left exposed through the chest wrap and then taped to the chest wrap.

17) The chest tube should be aspirated as indicated based on the animal's medical condition.

18) Local anesthetic can be infused via the chest tube periodically to increase the animal's comfort (and decrease local tissue irritation at the site where the tube lies against soft tissues within the thorax).

19) When appropriate, the chest tube should be removed using sterile technique (first cleaning the drain exit site with surgical solution), the skin incision can be stapled with surgical staples after the tube is removed and a light chest wrap placed for the first 12–24 h after tube removal to prevent subcutaneous emphysema and/or pneumothorax.

### 15.6.20.5  Possible Complications

1) Damage of the pulmonary parenchyma or blood vessels can occur during placement or maintenance of the tube.

2) Leakage of air into the chest can cause pneumothorax and/or leakage of air into the subcutaneous tissues can cause subcutaneous emphysema.

### 15.6.20.6 Other Considerations

1) Animals with a chest tube must be carefully monitored to make sure the tube is appropriately secured and closed.
2) Pain control (both systemic and local) is important to keep animals with an indwelling chest tube comfortable and calm.

## 15.6.21 Tracheostomy

### 15.6.21.1 Indications

Tracheostomy is indicated in cases of upper airway obstruction. Typically, upper airway obstruction is secondary to a foreign object, mass, soft tissue swelling, or other pathology.

### 15.6.21.2 Setting

Tracheostomy should be performed in a sterile surgical setting. In some emergencies, tracheostomies may need to be performed in a treatment, exam, or even outdoor/field setting. In all cases, employing aseptic techniques should be the goal.

### 15.6.21.3 Equipment

1) Surgical preparation supplies – clippers, gauze, scrub and solution.
2) Tracheotomy tube or modified ET tube. In an emergency setting, other equipment such as an appropriate diameter orogastric or other tube sanitized as much as possible may be employed
3) Surgical gloves, cap, and mask
4) Gauze or other material to tie the tube in place once inserted
5) Suction – electronic or manual (using a red rubber tube and large gauge syringe)
6) Small surgery pack – surgical drape, Metzenbaum scissors, hemostats, thumb forceps, towel clamps, scalpel blade, and suture material
7) Bandaging material – sterile gauze sponge, cast padding, self-adhesive bandage, and tape

### 15.6.21.4 Procedure

1) Place the lightly sedated patient in dorsal recumbency. In an emergency setting the patient may be unconscious or require anesthesia. Clip and prepare the skin of the ventral cervical area just aboral to the larynx (where aboral means away from the mouth/toward the thorax) or sufficiently aboral to whatever object, mass, or swelling that is obstructing airflow.
2) If the animal is awake or if dyspnea worsens when the animal is positioned in dorsal recumbency, the initial clipping and preparation can be done with the animal sitting up or in sternal recumbency.
3) Drape the insertion site, and using aseptic technique, make a longitudinal skin incision from the caudal aspect of the larynx to the sixth tracheal ring.
4) Use forceps to elevate the skin edges and hemostats to bluntly dissect between the muscle bellies overlying the trachea until the tracheal rings can be visualized.
5) Place a stay suture (using strong suture such as 0 or larger diameter) around the more proximal and distal tracheal rings to the proposed insertion site to elevate and stabilize the trachea. Place these as loops of suture long enough to reach externally.
6) Make a stab incision into the trachea between the third and fourth tracheal rings (or the appropriate location based on the pathology being addressed) and extend the incision horizontally just wide enough to allow tube placement.
7) If the animal is currently intubated, remove the ET tube as the tracheotomy tube is inserted with the distal end of the tube directed aborally (toward the thorax).
8) Inflate the cuff of the tracheotomy tube and begin oxygen administration via the new tube if PPV is required. If not, the cuff can be left uninflated.
9) Use simple interrupted sutures to close the majority of the skin incision around the tube to produce a loose closure.
10) Allow the stay sutures around the tracheal rings to exit the skin incision along the tube's exit point.
11) If using a tracheostomy tube designed to be sutured to the skin, apply the sutures at this point.
12) Cover the closed skin incision with sterile gauze cut to fit around the tracheotomy tube, allowing access to the stay sutures around the tracheal rings.
13) Secure the tube circumferentially around the neck using stretch gauze or extension set tubing gently tied in place without compressing the neck.
14) Place a light bandage around the neck leaving the tube's exit unobstructed.

#### 15.6.21.5 Possible Complications

1) Potential inflammation or necrosis of the tracheal tissues.
2) Infection at the insertion site or development of pneumonia due to reduced ability to cough and impairment of mucociliary elevator is possible.
3) Obstruction of the tracheostomy tube with secretions. This can be avoided with appropriate nursing care.
4) General iatrogenic tracheal trauma which can lead to secondary subcutaneous emphysema, is also possible.

#### 15.6.21.6 Other Considerations

1) The tube will need to be checked frequently and the lumen cleaned to prevent buildup of secretions/mucous that could obstruct airflow.
2) Note that specialized tracheostomy tubes can be purchased or a regular endotracheal tube can be modified with the cuffed end left intact, the anesthetic machine connection removed, the distal end of the tube cut off, and the anesthetic machine connection reattached creating a shorter tube.

### 15.6.22 Transfusions

#### 15.6.22.1 Indications

Transfusions of blood products are typically indicated as treatment for anemia due to blood loss, decreased production, or increased destruction (such as an immune-mediated hemolytic anemia/ IMHA).

#### 15.6.22.2 Setting

Transfusions generally do not require aseptic technique (other than autotransfusion), and can be performed in a treatment or exam room.

#### 15.6.22.3 Equipment

1) Blood collection equipment – large syringe or collection bag.
2) Anticoagulant – in premade collection bags or added separately to a syringe or empty bag that is used to collect the blood.
3) Hemo-Nate filter for small-volume transfusions.
4) Primary set with built-in blood filter for large-volume transfusions.
5) Ideally blood-typing cards (especially for cats).

6) If available, equipment to perform major and minor crossmatch. If unable to perform crossmatching, there is a higher risk of a potentially life-threatening reaction – especially in cats or in dogs that have previously had a transfusion.

#### 15.6.22.4 Procedure

1) Identify the blood donor – ideally a healthy animal in good condition that has been prescreened for any blood-borne diseases (appropriate screening will depend on the species and local blood-borne disease risks).
2) Confirm that the donor has a healthy PCV/TP.
3) Some donors require mild sedation. Donation is done via jugular venipuncture using a needle (needle size will depend on the animal's size but should be the largest size that can be safely used, such as 22 gauge for a kitten, 20 or 18 for a cat or small dog, and 18 or larger for a large dog) and extension set connected to a large syringe or blood collection bag with an appropriate volume of anticoagulant added.
4) Typically, the anticoagulant used is CPD (citrate phosphate dextrose) 1 ml per 9 ml of blood collected or heparin 5 units of heparin per milliliter of blood collected (it is imperative that the concentration of heparin is carefully checked prior to converting units of heparin into milliliters of heparin used for the amount of blood collected). For collecting smaller volumes of blood, you can add 2–3 ml of heparin to precoat the large syringe and then expel the excess heparin from the syringe before blood collection.
5) While collecting the blood, the bag or needle should be gently tilted back and forth to encourage distribution of the anticoagulant.
6) The donation should be given to the recipient at a slow rate initially while monitoring closely for transfusion reaction (such as facial swelling, sudden increase in temperature, and vomiting). Transfusions are often started at a rate of 0.5 ml/kg/h over the first 20–30 min, then increasing the rate if no reaction is seen so that the full transfusion is given over no more than 2–3 h. The maximum rate of infusion should be 4–5 ml/kg/h. A guideline of maximum transfusion volume is 22 ml/kg/day with the transfusion ideally completed within a 3-h period.

7) Recheck the recipient's PCV/TP 3–4 h post-transfusion to verify that you have accomplished your goals.

#### 15.6.22.5 Possible Complications

1) Transfusion reactions occur most frequently in cats with preformed antibodies against other blood types than their own. This is less likely in a dog, especially during the first transfusion as they do not have preformed antibodies.
2) Infections can be transferred from donor to recipient if the donor is not fully prescreened for blood-borne diseases.
3) Sepsis/infection is a possible concern if aseptic technique is not used during blood collection and administration.

#### 15.6.22.6 Other Considerations

In cases of IMHA, keep in mind that hemolysis of the donation may occur due to the primary disease process.

##### 15.6.22.6.1 Crossmatching

1) There are two types of crossmatching: major and minor.
2) A major crossmatch is done with donor red blood cells and patient serum, whereas a minor crossmatch is performed with donor serum and patient red blood cells.
3) In this procedure, agglutination indicates that the blood product is incompatible with the patient.
4) For full instructions on performing this procedure, consult an emergency textbook or blood banking manual.

##### 15.6.22.6.2 Autotransfusion

1) Autotransfusion refers to the process of transfusing a patient's own blood back into his or her circulation. This is particularly useful in case of significant internal hemorrhage during surgery.
2) Blood (which must not be contaminated with GI contents or other contaminants) is collected aseptically using a large bore needle and large volume syringe (such as 16 or 18 gauge).
3) The blood is administered back to the animal intravenously using a blood filter (such as a

Hemo-Nate filter – each of which can filter approximately 50 ml of blood).

4) For large blood volumes, the filter must be changed periodically or the blood should be administered through an empty IV fluid bag with an in-line blood filter.
5) Although blood in contact with abdominal serosa for greater than 1 h is considered to be defibrinated, potentially not requiring an anticoagulant, it is recommended that CPD at a volume of 1 ml per 9 ml of blood, or heparin at a volume of 5 units per milliliter of blood, is added to the blood collection syringe.
6) Coat the walls of the syringe with the anticoagulant agent before blood collection.
7) As with a donor transfusion, the syringe should be gently tilted during collection to distribute the anticoagulant appropriately.

##### 15.6.22.6.3 Sterile Collection

1) During sterile surgery, the surgeon is handed a sterile extension set, which is placed into any pooled blood in the abdomen and an assistant aspirates the free blood.
2) Blood collection should not be performed in lieu of finding and stopping the source of hemorrhage but should be performed once the hemorrhage has been addressed.

##### 15.6.22.6.4 Administration

1) With a blood filter such as a Hemo-Nate filter in place, the blood is administered to the patient through the largest gauge IV catheter that can be placed into the patient.
2) Unlike a transfusion from a donor, there is no risk of a transfusion reaction. Fresh whole blood should generally be administered no faster than 4–5 ml/kg/h; however, in an emergency setting using autotransfusion, higher rates of administration may be necessary with a maximum rate of 22 ml/kg/h or 45 ml/kg in 3 h.

---

**Textbox 15.10 How much blood to administer?**

In general, administering 2 ml/kg of FWB will increase the patient's PCV by 1%.

### 15.6.23    Urinary Catheter Placement

#### 15.6.23.1    Indications
Urinary catheters are indicated as treatment of

1) Urethral obstruction due to mucosal plugs, hematomas, crystal accumulation, or uroliths
2) Soft tissue swelling, mass effects or damage to the urethra
3) Neurological lesions preventing effective bladder emptying
4) Uroliths, mass effects or other pathology preventing emptying of the bladder
5) Nonambulatory patients, or other patients at risk of urinary retention or scalding
6) They can also be used for diagnostic purposes to obtain a urine sample or to assess for mechanical obstruction of the urethra.

#### 15.6.23.2    Setting
This procedure is usually performed in a treatment or exam setting using semi-sterile technique.

#### 15.6.23.3    Equipment

1) Sterile preparation supplies – clippers, gauze, surgical scrub, and solution.
2) Sterile gloves.
3) Appropriate urinary catheter – For a male cat, this may be a semi-rigid polypropylene "tomcat" catheter with an open end to relieve the obstruction initially, followed by placement of an indwelling flexible/less tissue-irritating catheter such as a polytetrafluroethylene or silicone "slippery sam" type or small diameter (typically 3 or 3.5 French) red rubber tube. For dogs, the appropriate diameter of Foley catheter or red rubber tube may vary from 3.5-12 French depending on the size of the dog (Textbox15.11).
4) One-inch (2.5 cm) tape, suture, and needle drivers if securing to the prepuce.
5) For emptying the bladder – extension set tubing and appropriately sized empty IV fluid bag to collect urine.

---

**Textbox 15.11  Suggested urinary catheter sizes**

Cat – 3 or 3.5 French (1 or 1.2 mm)
Small dog – 3½ or 5 French (1.2 or 1.7 mm)
Medium dog – 5 or 8 French (1.7 or 2.7 mm)
Large dog – 8, 10, or 12 French (2.7, 3.3, or 4 mm).

---

6) For collecting a sample – a 3–6 ml syringe and a red rubber tube for sample storage.
7) Sterile lubricating jelly, ideally with lidocaine.

#### 15.6.23.4    Procedure
In most male dogs, and some female dogs, sedation is not required. For cats (especially an obstructed male cat), light sedation to general anesthesia (if appropriate) may be indicated to facilitate urinary catheter placement.

##### 15.6.23.4.1    Male Dogs

1) With the dog gently restrained in lateral recumbency, clip and clean the area around the prepuce using chlorhexidine scrub.
2) Flush the prepuce with dilute chlorhexidine solution or sterile saline. Rinse the area thoroughly and gently dry.
3) Estimate how much of catheter will need to be inserted to reach the bladder by measuring from the tip of the prepuce down the length of the penis to the pelvic flexure and around to the location of the bladder. Using a marker, mark on the catheter at the likely point to which you will need to insert the catheter.
4) Have an assistant extrude the penis from the sheath.
5) Wearing sterile gloves lubricate the catheter tip and distal aspect of the catheter with sterile lubricant jelly (ideally with lidocaine).
6) Gently insert the catheter tip into the opening of the urethra and advance it slowly into the bladder.
7) If no urine is present once the catheter has been advanced to your estimated depth, use a catheter tip syringe to see if urine can be aspirated. Continue to gently advance or withdraw the catheter slightly urine can be aspirated.
8) Collect a urine sample at this point if indicated.
9) If leaving an indwelling catheter in place, connect the catheter to the extension set and a collection bag (either a special purpose urine collection bag or an empty IV fluid bag). Special catheter adapters "Christmas tree adapters" can be used to attach the system to the catheter or a 1-ml syringe can be used.
10) Use 1-in. (2.5 cm) tape in a butterfly fold around the catheter at the point where it exits the penis.

Place stay sutures in the skin of the distal prepuce to secure the catheter in place.

11) If using a Foley catheter, inflate the catheter's bladder.

12) Secure the extension set to the dog's leg or tail loosely enough that the tubing is not bent/preventing urine flow but tightly enough that the dog cannot step through the loose tubing. 1-in. (2.5 cm) tape and a self-adhesive bandage can be used.

13) Gently clean the catheter exit site every 24 h while the urinary catheter is in place.

14) Monitor (and measure if appropriate) the animal's urine output while the catheter is in place, ensuring that urine is flowing without obstruction and that the collection bag is being emptied regularly. The urine bag must be kept positioned below the animal at all times to prevent backflow of urine.

### 15.6.23.4.2 Female Dogs

1) With the dog gently restrained in sternal recumbency or standing, clip and clean around the vulva.

2) Estimate how much of the catheter will need to be inserted to reach the bladder and mark the catheter with a marker at this point.

3) Wearing sterile gloves, infuse topical anesthetic (ophthalmic or lidocaine) 3–5 cm into the vagina using a lubricated sterile tuberculin syringe without the needle.

4) Using a lubricated vaginal speculum and light source to visualize the vaginal vault, insert the speculum angling it first dorsally and then cranially, to avoid the clitoral fossa that sits on the ventral distal aspect of the vaginal vault.

5) Use the speculum and light source to visualize the urethral opening and direct the urinary catheter into the vaginal vault and the urethral opening, gently advance it into the urinary bladder.

6) Follow steps 7–14 under the male dog procedure above attaching your stay sutures to the skin of the labia.

7) Note that you can also use a nonvisual technique for catheter placement if needed – use a lubricated sterile gloved finger to palpate the urethral papilla and then pass the catheter ventral to your finger to enter the urethra.

8) Both techniques are meant to ensure that you have entered the bladder, which lies ventral to the uterus. If you deviated dorsally and entered the uterus, no urine will be observed.

### 15.6.23.4.3 Male Cats

1) With the cat appropriately secured in dorsal or lateral recumbency, clip and clean around the prepuce.

2) Wearing sterile gloves, extrude the penis with one hand and use the other sterile gloved hand to advance the lubricated catheter into the opening of the penis.

3) Note that keeping the penis parallel to the spine, rather than allowing it to deviate ventrally or dorsally will assist with inserting and advancing the catheter.

4) In some cases, especially with obese cats and those with urethral obstruction, you may need to secure your hold of the extruded penis using a curved tip hemostats over a moistened gauze square secured to the most proximal portion of the penis that can be accessed. The hemostats will be less traumatic with the gauze and should only grasp the most superficial portion of the penile tissue to prevent compression of the urethra or tissue injury.

5) In cases of urethral obstruction, the penis should be gently massaged to help extrude any distal plugs before attempting to insert or advance the catheter.

6) Using an open-end semi-rigid polypropylene "tomcat" catheter or an appropriately sized IV catheter (without the stylet), slowly infusing lukewarm water as you very gently attempt to advance the catheter can help to breakdown any obstructive plugs.

7) After collecting a urine sample, either place a closed collection system (if leaving an indwelling catheter in place following steps 9–14 in the male dog procedure) or proceed with gently flushing the bladder before placement of the closed collection system in the case of urethral obstruction.

8) To gently flush the bladder and urethra in the case of obstruction, first empty the bladder via passive flow. Do not put significant external pressure on the bladder to assist with emptying in these cases as the bladder may be injured and at risk of rupture.

9) Gently palpate the bladder to confirm that it is sufficiently empty. Slowly infuse a small amount

of lukewarm sterile saline into the bladder and allow passive emptying. Do not overfill the damaged bladder during this process. Smaller aliquots of 20–30 ml are generally recommended. The cat can be gently rotated side to side during this process to aid in bladder flushing.

10) Over the course of repeated urinary bladder lavage the returning fluid should decrease in discoloration and turbidity.

11) Gently flush the urethra itself by withdrawing the catheter slightly, gently infusing lukewarm sterile saline, and repeating this process until the catheter tip is at the end of the penis and you are flushing the length of the penile urethra with no significant obstruction or "gritty" feel. This process can be repeated several times, gently, by advancing and then withdrawing the catheter slowly as you flush.

12) Ideally, once the urethra and bladder have been appropriately flushed, an indwelling catheter, such as a silicone or other flexible material (a "slippery Sam" or other special purpose cat urinary catheter or red rubber catheter if no other option), is lightly lubricated, gently inserted, and connected to a closed collection system.

13) It is highly preferable NOT to leave a tomcat or other rigid or semi-rigid catheter in the urethra for any significant period of time and to NOT leave any catheter in place that is not connected to a closed collection system. Not doing so increases the risk of bacterial migration into the bladder.

#### 15.6.23.4.4 *Female Cats*

1) With the cat gently restrained in lateral recumbency, clip and clean around the vulva.

2) Estimate how much of the catheter will need to be inserted to reach the bladder and mark the catheter with a marker at this point.

3) Wearing sterile gloves, infuse topical anesthetic (ophthalmic anesthetic or lidocaine) 1–3 cm into the vagina using a lubricated sterile tuberculin syringe with the needle removed.

4) Lubricate the end of the catheter with sterile lubricating jelly – ideally with lidocaine-containing lubricant if available.

5) With gentle caudal and lateral traction on the vulvar lips, slide the lubricated catheter along the ventral wall of the vagina until it enters the urethra.

6) Ensure that you have entered the bladder, which lies ventral to the uterus, and that you have not deviated dorsally and entered the uterus; if in the uterus, no urine will be observed.

7) Follow steps 7–14 under the male dog procedure above attaching the stay sutures to the skin of the vulva.

#### 15.6.23.5 Possible Complications

1) Patients with indwelling catheters should wear an e-collar to prevent removal or chewing through the catheter. If the animal chews through the catheter as it exits the body, the distal part of the catheter may enter the bladder and require surgical removal.

2) Catheters may be inserted too far, resulting in looping within the urinary bladder and even exiting the bladder.

3) If not inserted far enough, the catheter may not reach the urinary bladder.

4) Ideally, a radiograph is used to confirm appropriate catheter placement.

5) Catheters can become clogged with mucous, crystals, blood, or other debris, requiring gentle flushing or even removal.

6) In patients with an obstruction or other urinary pathology, there is some risk of tissue tearing. Gentle technique, patient flushing, and slow advancement of the catheter, only when obstruction is relieved, are essential to reduce this risk.

### 15.6.24 Wound Care

#### 15.6.24.1 Indications
Appropriate wound care is indicated in all cases of injury to skin, subcutaneous tissue and mucus membranes.

#### 15.6.24.2 Setting
Wound care is typically performed in a treatment or exam room setting as a clean/contaminated surgical procedure, or in a sterile surgical setting once the basic wound preparation and cleaning has been performed in a surgical preparation area.

#### 15.6.24.3 Equipment

1) Clippers and a 40 or 50 blade
2) Antiseptic scrub and solution

3) Stainless steel bowls to prepare and hold scrub and solution
4) Gauze squares
5) Cast padding
6) Stretch gauze
7) Self-adhesive bandage
8) Elastic tape
9) One inch (2.5 cm) white tape
10) +/− surgical stapler
11) Wound dressings such as white granulated sugar, regular or medicinal grade honey, calcium alginate rope or sheets, gel foam, and nonadherent dressing (such as oil emulsion impregnated)
12) Bandage scissors.

#### 15.6.24.4 Procedure

1) Immediately on arrival, apply a sterile dressing to wounds to prevent further contamination.
2) If time permits on arrival, remove any gross debris (plant material, sand, mud, etc.) from around the wound site using copious amounts of physiological saline or tap water before placing a temporary wrap.
3) Provide light sedation, or general anesthesia depending on the type of wound and type of care being provided.
4) Pack the wound with sterile lubricant to minimize contamination.
5) Clip the hair from around the wound edges, extend this clipping to provide an appropriate sterile field and space for wound exploration and drain placement, if needed.
6) Wipe off excess hair and vacuum smaller hair clippings from the site.
7) Use wet gauze, or gauze with scrub, to remove any dried exudate or other material from the area.
8) Alternate scrub and solution to thoroughly clean the skin around the wound.
9) Gently wipe any exudate from the open wound itself.
10) Use sterile saline in a 30–35 ml syringe with an 18- to 19-gauge needle to further lavage the wound.
11) For larger wounds, consider using a three-way stopcock attached to this syringe and attached directly to a hanging bag of IV fluids to facilitate copious lavage.

12) Once the wound is thoroughly clipped, cleaned, lavaged, and prepped for surgical care, the surgeon can proceed.
13) The wound should be appropriately debrided to remove any contaminated or obviously devitalized tissues.
14) Small puncture wounds can often be left open to drain and heal.
15) Larger wounds that have been debrided to the extent that no devitalized or originally exposed tissue is present may be closed without a drain if there is no significant dead space present. Typically, a two-layer closure is performed, with simple continuous closure of the subcutaneous tissues and either a deep dermal/subcuticular closure (if the goal is to not leave any skin sutures) or surgical stapling in the most external layer.
16) Wounds with possible contamination or with significant dead space should be closed with a surgical drain in place. The more dorsal aspect of the drain should be tacked in place under the skin with a single suture (and should not exit the body). The more ventral aspect of the drain, the aspect by which you expect fluid to drain from the wound following gravity when the animal is in typical standing, sitting, or sternal position should be left exposed and tacked in place onto the surface of the skin.
17) Wounds that cannot be closed or where tissue vitality and extent of contamination is unknown may need to be managed as open wounds by placing an appropriate wound dressing, covering the wound, and checking, cleaning, and rebandaging every 12–24 h during initial wound healing.
18) White granulated sugar or raw honey are excellent wound dressings to use for the first 24–72 h for heavily contaminated wounds and can help to remove contamination, encourage autolytic debridement, prevent bacterial growth, and maintain a healthy moist environment for early wound healing.
19) Once contamination and infection of the wound is controlled, an alternate wound dressing such as calcium alginate, gel foam, or other specialty products can be used to help manage heavily exudative wounds.
20) Once a healthy granulation bed of tissue is formed and the amount of exudate begins to

reduce, a nonadherent wound dressing such as an oil-impregnated wound dressing may be used.

21) All wound dressings should be held in place with a light wrap of cast padding covered by self-adhesive bandage secured with tape.

22) When managing open wounds, it is important to ensure that the wound dressing is appropriately secured and that the wrap is not too tight, which can cause tissue swelling and devitalization.

23) As open wounds heal, the frequency of wound care/bandage changes can be decreased from every 12–24 h to every 24 h and in some cases (once a healthy bed of granulation tissue is in place) to every 48–72 h if there are no signs or significant risk of infection.

24) Bandages need to be checked frequently for strikethrough (moisture coming through the bandage that increase the risk of infection), slippage, and tissue swelling proximal or distal to the bandage.

#### 15.6.24.5 Possible Complications

1) Major complications of wound care are typically related to infection of the wound, tissue devitalization, loss of lymphatic supply/drainage, deeper tissue injury, or infection.

2) Areas with poor healing may require additional surgical and/or medical care.

#### 15.6.24.6 Other Considerations

1) In general, appropriate wound care, including exploration of puncture wounds to check for deeper tissue injury at the time of the injury will reduce the risk of complications.

2) Large wounds requiring surgical intervention and dressing must be followed up closely to ensure appropriate healing.

3) All bandaged wounds need to be monitoring closely for strikethrough, slippage, soft tissue swelling, or other complications. If ongoing care is not possible, it may be better not to bandage the wound.

### Suggested Reading

#### Textbooks

Tear, M. (2017). Small Animal Surgical Nursing, 3e. St. Louis: Elsevier.

Crow, S. (2009). Manual of Clinical Procedures in Dogs, Cats, Rabbits and Rodents, 3e. Ames: Wiley-Blackwell.

Ford, R. and Mazzaferro, E. (2012). Kirk and Bistern's Handbook of Veterinary Procedures and Emergency Treatment, 9e. St. Louis, MO: Saunders Elsevier.

Hosgood, G. and Hoskins, J. (1998). Small Animal Pediatric Medicine and Surgery. Oxford: Butterworth Heinmann.

Macintire, D., Drobatz, K., Haskins, S., and Saxon, W. (2012). Manual of Small Animal Emergency and Critical Care Medicine, 2e. Ames: Wiley-Blackwell.

Mazzaferro, E. (2010). Blackwell's Five-Minute Veterinary Consult Clinical Companion: Small Animal Emergency and Critical Care. Ames: Wiley-Blackwell.

McMichael, M. (2014). Handbook of Canine and Feline Emergency Protocols, 2e. Ames: Wiley-Blackwell.

Plunkett, S. (2012). Emergency Procedures for the Small Animal Veterinarian, 3e. London: Saunders Ltd.

Swaim, S., Renberg, W., and Shike, K. (2011). Small Animal Bandaging, Casting and Splinting Techniques. Ames: Wiley-Blackwell.

#### Online Resources

Veterinary Emergency and Critical Care Society (2012). Recover CPR initiative. http://veccs.org/recover-cpr/ (accessed 21 December 2017)

Davidson, A. (2016). Overview of management of the neonate in small animals. In: The Merck Veterinary Manual. http://www.merckvetmanual.com/management-and-nutrition/management-of-the-neonate/overview-of-management-of-the-neonate-in-small-animals (accessed 27 Dec 2016).

# 16

# Wellness and Preventive Care
*Brian A. DiGangi*

*ASPCA, PO Box 142275, Gainesville, FL 32614, USA*

## 16.1 Introduction

There has been increasing emphasis on wellness and preventive care in veterinary medicine over the past decade, and significant resources have been devoted to delivering that message to the pet owner in the developed world [1]. Prevention of physical and emotional disease is increasingly being recognized as a more efficient, cost–effective, and humane approach to animal care. The benefits of this approach may be even greater in the typical field clinic setting where geographical, cultural, and economic factors impede access to veterinary care. With this in mind, the core goal of any wellness and preventive medicine care program is to protect animal welfare and ensure a high quality of life through the prevention and mitigation of disease.

The concepts of quality of life and animal welfare and the various mechanisms by which they may be assessed are widely studied and debated [2–4]. One component of this concept that is of particular importance to the field clinic practitioner is the need to assess and define good welfare and quality of life within both a geographical and cultural context. That which is considered acceptable for animals in one culture may exceed acceptable standards for human beings in another. Similarly, environmental conditions ideal for a particular species in one physical location in the world may not be physically possible in another. It is the practitioners' role to identify such constraints and work within them to create the best possible outcome for the patient and his or her caretakers. The Farm Animal Welfare Council's five freedoms are a useful set of parameters that are widely used and applicable to assessing quality of life of animals in a variety of settings [5]. These call for the following:

1) Freedom from hunger and thirst by ready access to fresh water and a diet to maintain full health and vigor
2) Freedom from discomfort by providing an appropriate environment, including shelter and a comfortable resting area
3) Freedom from pain, injury, or disease by prevention or rapid diagnosis and treatment
4) Freedom to express normal behavior by providing sufficient space, proper facilities, and company of the animal's own kind
5) Freedom from fear and distress by ensuring conditions and treatment that avoid mental suffering.

As the five freedoms suggest, total wellness and quality of life incorporate both physical and mental health [6]. Although steps to ensure mental and emotional well-being while in the field clinic will be discussed, this chapter will focus primarily on the physical health component of total wellness and preventive care.

## 16.2 Operational Considerations

Ensuring organized and efficient clinic operations will allow for the care of more animals per unit of time at a reduced cost. Additionally, an organized clinic is perhaps the best way to demonstrate to the clients and community that their animals are valued and respected. Standard operating procedures (SOPs)

*Field Manual for Small Animal Medicine*, First Edition. Edited by Katherine Polak and Ann Therese Kommedal.

should be established, they should be written and accessible to all staff members, and staff members should be trained in their execution. Related to the provision of wellness and preventive care in the field clinic setting, SOPs should discuss the following:

- Creation and maintenance of medical records
- Mechanisms for animal identification (ID)
- Humane animal handling
- Physical examination including assessment of sterilization status
- Provision of universal preventive treatments, such as vaccination and parasite control
- Mechanisms by which to assess, teach, and encourage proper animal husbandry.

### 16.2.1 Medical Records

Accurate and timely recording of medical findings are critical for any medical operation [6]. Not only are they a source of pertinent information for the clinician that often has a direct impact on the care provided, they are a useful means of tracking organizational needs (e.g. commonly prescribed medications) and demonstrating organizational impact for fundraising, grant-writing, and otherwise developing community support. Collaborating community organizations may request or even require that particular items of information be documented; clinicians should work with local contacts to determine what requirements, restrictions, and expectations may be held for a particular clinic.

In most cases, individual animal medical records should be maintained and may be legally required. If allowed by law, group or "herd" records may be acceptable when a large number of animals are being treated at one site (e.g. a temporary animal shelter) or when services are severely limited (e.g. a single vaccination clinic operated during a specified period of time in which no services other than specific vaccinations are provided to each animal). Even in such cases, some information about the individual animals must always be recorded and any procedures or treatments outside of the scope of the clinic plan must be detailed on an individual animal medical record. At a minimum, individual animal medical records should contain one or more client identifiers, an animal identifier, animal description, and an actual or estimated age, age range, or age group (Textbox 16.1).

---

**Textbox 16.1 Minimum medical record requirements**

*Identification*

- Client identification
  - Name, physical address, phone number, community of residence
- Animal identification
  - Name, clinic-assigned identification number
- Animal description
  - Color, sex, sterilization status, species, predominant breed, and unique physical characteristics
- Age determination
  - Actual age, estimated range (e.g. 1–2 years, 3–4 years), age group (e.g. neonate, pediatric, juvenile, young adult, and geriatric)

*Background*

- Reason for presentation
- Housing and husbandry
  - Length of ownership, dietary history, lifestyle (e.g. indoor and outdoor), exposure to other animals
- Medical history
  - Existing or historical medical conditions
  - Known administration of any treatments or medications
- Existing clinical signs of illness
  - Description of signs, duration, severity, and response to any treatments provided

*Procedure Record*

- Physical examination findings
- Procedures performed
  - Description of anesthetic and surgical procedures including drug dosages, routes, suture materials and patterns
- Diagnostic test results
- Treatments administered
- Medications prescribed

*Communication*

- Caretaker instructions and recommendations
- Acknowledgment of procedural risks in native language
- Emergency and postoperative care instructions

The medical record should allow for the collection of pertinent historical information, which will vary based on the clinic. The reason for presentation, length of ownership, dietary history, lifestyle, exposure to other animals, and existing or historical medical conditions may all be useful information to record. At a minimum, known administration of any treatments or medications and existing clinical signs of illness should be documented for each patient.

Finally, medical records should contain a complete, accurate, and legible account of all procedures, diagnostic test results, treatments, prescriptions dispensed, and any instructions and recommendations provided to the caretaker. In the case of anesthetic and/or surgical procedures, medical records should also include the caretaker's acknowledgment of procedural risks in their native language along with all the details of the anesthetic and surgical procedure. Particularly for temporary field clinics, the caretaker should be provided a copy of the medical record along with information about how to handle questions or complications after the clinic's closure. Carefully designed procedure records can encourage the collection of all of this information in a concise format (see Appendix 16.A).

### 16.2.2 Animal Identification

A method of individual animal ID ensures that patients move through the clinic efficiently and minimizes the chance of errors in treatment administration. The system used should assign each animal a unique alphanumeric identifier that will be recorded on the individual animal themselves, all patient records, treatments administered, and treatments dispensed. Animals can be numbered sequentially or assigned a sequential number–letter combination to identify those from a particular location, treated on a particular date, or requiring a certain type of care (e.g. surgical vs. medical patient).

When identifying the animals themselves, a variety of methods may be considered including the use of temporary collars and tags, disposable ID bands, masking tape on the forehead of the animal, and ID microchips. Perhaps the simplest and least expensive technique is to simply write the ID number directly on the animal in semipermanent marker (Figure 16.1). If microchip identification is performed, ISO-compliant microchips should be utilized, and they should be implanted in the subcutaneous tissue of either the interscapular region or the left neck in accordance with international guidelines [7].

Whatever the identification system selected, it must be simple to use and staff members must be trained accordingly. Best practices include training staff to instinctively match an animal's ID number with that on its medical record and that recorded on any medications intended for administration prior to beginning a procedure or dispensing a medication.

### 16.2.3 Physical Examination

The physical examination is the foundation of both preventive and diagnostic medicine. In the field, practitioners must often rely on the physical examination as the primary, if not the only, source of

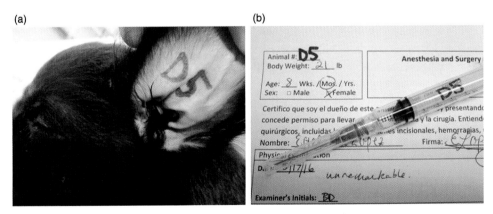

**Figure 16.1** (a) An alphanumeric code recorded on the surface of the pinna with a semipermanent marker can ensure individual animal identification throughout the field clinic. (b) The ID number can be matched to that on the medical record and on any medications prior to administration.

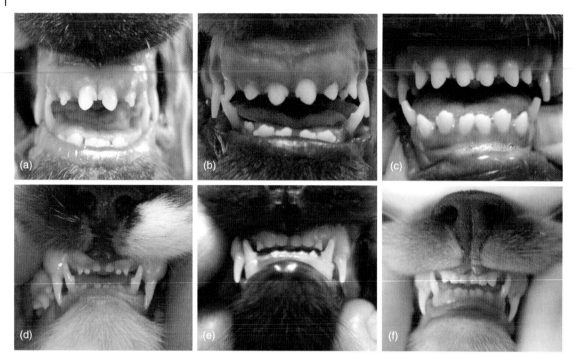

**Figure 16.2** Although dependent on overall health and nutrition status, a puppy or kitten's permanent incisors erupt at a predictable rate and can be used to estimate age. (a) Twelve-week-old puppy, (b) 14-week-old puppy, (c) 16-week-old puppy, (d) 12-week-old kitten, (e) 14-week-old kitten, (f) 16-week-old kitten.

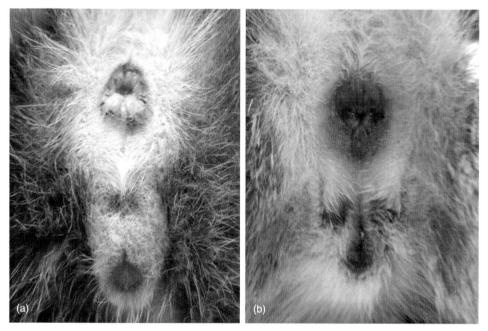

**Figure 16.3** Assessment of the shape and location of the genital opening can assist in sex determination of kittens. (a) In male kittens, the anogenital distance is longer than it is in females and the genital opening is circular in shape. (b) In female kittens, the anogenital distance is shorter than it is in males and the genital opening is long and narrow. When combined, the anal and genital openings in a male resemble a colon, while those in the female resemble a semicolon.

diagnostic information. While examination by a veterinarian is ideal, in most settings basic physical examination procedures can be performed by trained laypersons.

Complete discussion of the veterinary diagnostic physical examination is beyond the scope of this chapter, but a minimum preventive health assessment should include the following: animal description (see above); actual or estimated age (Textbox 16.2, Figure 16.2); sex and sterilization status (Figures 16.3 and 16.4); species and predominant breed or breed type; resting heart rate, respiratory rate and body temperature; general attitude and mental state; hydration status (Table 16.1); body weight and/or body condition assessment (Appendix 16.B); pain assessment; and evaluation for common signs of infectious (e.g. discharge from mucous membranes, coughing, sneezing, vomiting, and diarrhea) and noninfectious (e.g. hair loss, wounds, and abnormal growths) disease.

Additional assessment of animals presenting for anesthetic and/or surgical procedures is warranted. These should include auscultation for severe abnormalities of the heart and lungs, assessment of hemodynamic status (e.g. mucous membrane color, capillary refill time, and pulse quality), and evaluation

**Table 16.1** Estimating hydration status.

| % Dehydration | Physical examination findings |
| --- | --- |
| <5 | History/evidence of vomiting or diarrhea |
| 6–8 | Dry/tacky mucous membranes |
| 8–10 | As above plus decreased skin turgor |
| 10–12 | As above plus mental depression, sunken eyes, weak and/or rapid pulse, slow capillary refill time |

Source: Plunkett 2013 [34]. Reproduced with permission of Elsevier.

of the intended surgical site for abnormalities that may alter the procedure or impede healing (e.g. lactation and severe pyoderma). Special consideration should be given to the assessment of animals for zoonotic diseases in areas or populations known to be at particular risk (e.g. rabies, brucellosis, dermatophytosis, and infectious gastroenteritis).

### 16.2.4 Animal Handling

Due to the nature of field clinics, it is not unusual that animals presenting for care are unaccustomed to

---

**Textbox 16.2 Age estimation**

*Dentition*

- A puppy or kitten's permanent teeth erupt at a predictable rate. The incisors are the easiest to visualize and, on average, they erupt in pairs from medial to lateral at 12, 14, and 16 weeks. See Figure 16.2.
- Permanent canine teeth in both dogs and cats begin to erupt, on average, at 5 months of age. A puppy or kitten with completely erupted canine teeth is usually at least 6 months of age.

*Ophthalmologic Findings*

- Nuclear sclerosis is a common finding in aging dogs, and when seen, indicates the dog is at least 7 years of age.
- Iris atrophy and, occasionally nuclear sclerosis, can be seen in aging cats; these suggest the cat is at least 10 years of age.

*Physical Characteristics*

- Healthy kittens gain weight at a rate of approximately 1 lb per month. Therefore, a 3-pound kitten is approximately 3 months of age.
- Sexually mature cats will develop physical features such as large jowls and a thick neck at 1½–2 years of age.
- Aging dogs will often experience graying of the fur around the muzzle and around the eyes. This generally indicates a dog of at least 5 years of age.
- Aging cats will often develop an angular appearance to the head as they lose lean muscle mass and periorbital fat. A cat with this feature is usually at least 10 years of age.

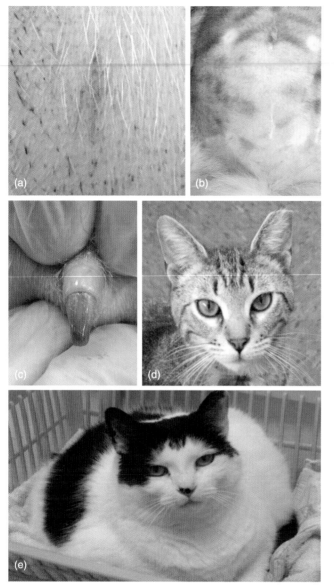

**Figure 16.4** Although not definitive, many clinical findings can indicate that a dog or cat has previously been sterilized. (a) A permanent tattoo on the ventral midline indicating surgical sterilization. (b) A ventral midline surgical scar on a female dog or cat suggests a previous surgical procedure. (c) The absence of penile spines in an adult cat indicates the absence of testosterone. *Note that the presence of penile spines in an adult cat without descended testicles suggests cryptorchidism.* (d) A cropped ear suggests progression through a trap–neuter–vaccination–return program. (e) Elevated body condition suggests the absence of reproductive hormones.

handling and restraint. For this reason, clinic staff and practitioners should be highly skilled in low stress and defensive handling techniques as well as the interpretation of canine and feline body language. In addition to protecting staff, ensuring a positive clinic experience for the patient, and enhancing clinic efficiency, respectful and appropriate animal handling is a clear demonstration of the level of care expected of the community.

Animal aggression toward humans is most commonly a consequence of fear or pain [8], therefore, clinic staff training should emphasize recognition of these states (Table 16.2). A variety of staff training resources are readily available for further discussion and self-study of this topic (Textbox 16.3).

Although it is important for staff to recognize signs of fear and pain to protect themselves and their patients from injury, steps to reduce animal stress and practice defensive handling should be a universal precaution. The handler should be cognizant of their own body language and the way in which they maintain contact with the animal. Animals should be as

---

**Textbox 16.3 Canine and feline body language training resources**

*Online*

*Canine Body Language in the Shelter*
Webinar by Dr. Sara Bennett
http://www.maddiesfund.org/canine-body-language-in-the-shelter.htm

*Canine Communications: Canine Body Language, Human Body Language and Dog Behavior, Defensive Dog Handling, Canine Communications: Dog Introductions*
Webinar Series by the American Society for the Prevention of Cruelty to Animals
http://www.aspcapro.org/webinar/canine-communications-series

*Dog Communication and Body Language*
Article by the Center for Shelter Dogs
http://centerforshelterdogs.tufts.edu/dog-behavior/dog-communication-and-body-language/

*Feline Communication*
Webinar by the American Society for the Prevention of Cruelty to Animals
http://www.aspcapro.org/webinar/2013-04-02-190000/feline-communication

Short Course by Dr. Susan Krebsbach and Dr. Laurie Peek
http://www.maddiesfund.org/feline-communication-how-to-speak-cat.htm

*Body Language Posters*

*Boogie: Doggie Language*
Illustrations by Lili Chin
http://www.doggiedrawings.net/#!freeposters/ckm8

*Cat Body Postures*
American Society for the Prevention of Cruelty to Animals
http://www.aspcapro.org/sites/pro/files/aspca_felineality_cat_body_postures_0_0.pdf

*Cat Language*
Illustrations by Lili Chin
http://www.doggiedrawings.net/#!freeposters/ckm8

*Kitty "Mood-o-meter!"*
By CATNIP
https://s-media-cache-ak0.pinimg.com/originals/af/ee/b5/afeeb587ae43af1cb83dcaf0d6217a93.gif

*Understanding Cat Behaviour*
Royal Society for the Prevention of Cruelty to Animals
http://www.rspca.org.uk/adviceandwelfare/pets/cats/behaviour/understanding

---

Table 16.2 Common signs of fear and pain in dogs and cats in the clinic.

| Dogs | | Cats | |
| --- | --- | --- | --- |
| Fear | Pain | Fear | Pain |
| Cowering | Abnormal or changing body posture | Crouched posture | Furrowed brow |
| Lip licking | Sudden change in demeanor | Dilated pupils | Squinting |
| Panting | Vocalization | Furrowed brow | Aggression |
| Furrowed brow | Extreme reaction to gentle touch | Hiding | Abnormal gait |
| Yawning | Lameness | Feigning sleep | Shifting weight |
| Hypervigilance | Reluctance to move | Tail flicking | Reduced activity |
| Salivation | Lack of appetite | Raised hackles | Lack of appetite |
| Urination or defecation | | Sudden grooming | Quiet/depressed |
| Not eating | | Hypervigilance | Hiding |
| Looking/acting sleepy | | | Vocalization |
| Sweating | | | Excessive licking |
| Displacement behaviors (e.g. scratching and sniffing) | | | Tail flicking |

Source: Mathews et al. 2014 [9]. Reproduced with permission of John Wiley & Sons.

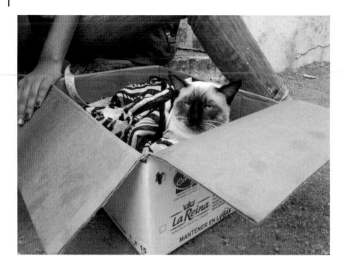

**Figure 16.5** This cat presented to a field clinic in a cardboard box which was used for confinement and gentle restraint throughout the clinic.

relaxed as possible (but controlled) prior to attempting any procedures. Restraint should be as minimal as is necessary for each individual patient and distractions and rewards (e.g. treats and toys) should be used whenever possible [10].

The equipment needed for safe and humane animal handling will depend on the socialization status of the particular patient, but in general, only a few items that are readily available in most locations should be required. Most dogs can be handled with the use of a slip leash, which can be manipulated into a harness or head halter if needed (the author prefers the use of a 6′ leather leash for its enhanced durability and maneuverability over fabric or nylon leashes) [11]. Basket or fabric muzzles should be available for use when necessary; basket muzzles are preferred in warm environments or when working with extremely stressed dogs to allow for panting and access to water. Finally, many medium and small dogs can be restrained through the use of an appropriately sized towel or blanket that is wrapped around the neck or trunk so as to prevent the dog from being able to turn its head and bite the handler.

For cats, a small box or breathable bag can be useful for both stress relief and restraint. Injectable medications can often be administered directly through such a container (Figure 16.5). A variety of methods of using towels to comfortably restrain cats along with the use of a slip leash transitioned into a harness have also been described [12]. Finally, a small capture net may be desirable in the event that a cat gets loose or hides under objects in the clinic. Once the cat is contained within the net, it can also be used for safe restraint.

When available, hinged doors can be used as a makeshift "squeeze box" for leashed dogs. The dog can be led head first up to the hinges of a closed door and the leash passed through the door itself or between the door hinges and frame. The door is then gently opened so as to restrain the dog's body in between the open door and the wall while the handler remains safely on the side of the door opposite the dog. A limited physical examination and injectable medications can be administered by approaching the restrained dog from behind (Figure 16.6).

The use of control poles, aggressive manual restraint with protective gloves, graspers, and other such devices are not recommended for use in the provision of wellness care. Animals that cannot be handled for preventive care needs with the equipment described above are candidates for chemical restraint. Chemical restraint is best utilized prior to repeated unsuccessful attempts at restraint [13]. Where chemical restraint is not available, clinic staff must decide if the risk of handling to both the patient and clinic staff is worth the intended benefits. (Note that equipment for the humane capture of wild, feral, or animals otherwise unsocialized to human interaction can be much more complicated and generally requires equipment-specific training, skill, and experience.)

### 16.2.5 Protecting Physical Health

#### 16.2.5.1 Vaccination

Vaccination is the cornerstone of protecting physical health and preventing disease. An understanding of

**Figure 16.6** Gentle compression behind a hinged door keeps this dog calm, protects the handler, and allows for the administration of injectable medications.

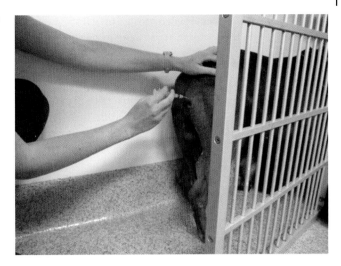

vaccine products, their pros and cons, and their administration, storage, and handling is critical to ensuring that *vaccination* actually leads to *immunization*. The many benefits of vaccination to individuals are generally well known, but in the field clinic setting, it may be their role in establishing herd immunity that is of even greater importance [14].

#### 16.2.5.1.1 Vaccine Products

Vaccine products are generally categorized as either "infectious" or "noninfectious" in nature [12]. Infectious vaccine products may be further categorized as attenuated, avirulent, modified live, or recombinant viral-vectored [15]. Table 16.3 includes the benefits and drawbacks of the different vaccine types.

---

**Textbox 16.4 Tip from the field**

Whenever possible, use modified-live vaccines in the field. Depending on the product or manufacturer, you may need to check package inserts or even call the manufacturer to determine the vaccine type.

---

A wide variety of vaccines are available around the world; product quality may vary widely. Many products contain some infectious vaccine components and some noninfectious vaccine components. Additionally, the availability of a vaccine product does not indicate its efficacy or utility in a

**Table 16.3** Benefits and drawbacks of infectious and noninfectious vaccine products.

| Infectious | | Noninfectious | |
|---|---|---|---|
| **Benefits** | **Drawbacks** | **Benefits** | **Drawbacks** |
| Rapid onset of immunity | Potential for reversion to virulence | No risk of reversion to virulence | Less able to overcome maternal antibody |
| Better able to overcome maternal antibody interference | Potential to induce clinical signs of disease | Unable to induce clinical signs of disease | Require adjuvant, may increase adverse reactions |
| Induction of immunity common after single administration | Immunity is short-lived for some pathogens | Immunity is generally long-lived | Induction of immunity generally requires multiple administrations |
| | Less stable in storage | Stable in storage | |
| May passively immunize others in population | May be contraindicated during pregnancy | Safe in immunocompromised and pregnant animals | Generally reduced degree of protection |

Source: Sykes 2013 [16]. Reproduced with permission of Elsevier.

Table 16.4 Worldwide vaccination guidelines for dogs and cats [14, 15, 17].

| Dogs | | | Cats | | |
|---|---|---|---|---|---|
| Recommended | Optional | Not recommended | Recommended | Optional | Not recommended |
| Canine distemper virus<br><br>Canine parvovirus-2<br><br>Canine adenovirus-2<br><br>Rabies | Parainfluenza virus[a]<br>*Bordetella bronchiseptica*[a]<br>*Borrelia burgdorferi*<br>*Leptospira interrogans*<br>Canine influenza virus<br>Measles | Canine coronavirus | Feline parvovirus<br>Feline herpesvirus-1<br>Feline calicivirus<br>Rabies | Feline leukemia virus[b]<br>Feline immunodeficiency virus<br>*Chlamydophila felis*<br>*Bordetella bronchiseptica* | Feline infectious peritonitis |

Note that when available, infectious vaccine products are always recommended over noninfectious products in the field clinic setting.
a) Optional for individual animals, but universally recommended in shelter-like environments.
b) Optional for individual cats and individually housed cats in shelter environments, but universally recommended for group-housed cats in shelter environments and all kittens, regardless of housing environment, up to 1 year of age.

given scenario. Practitioners should always research and identify the specific product most appropriate for their intended use. The Center for Veterinary Biologics of the Animal and Plant Health Inspection Service of the US Department of Agriculture and the Canadian Food Inspection Agency each maintain an updated list of licensed veterinary biologics, including vaccine products, on their websites.[1,2]

When choosing vaccine products for a field clinic, consider the following: product efficacy, product formulation, ease of handling and administration, target population, vaccination program design, and immunization goals (Textbox 16.5).

---

---

**Textbox 16.5 Considerations for vaccine product selection in the field clinic**

*Product Efficacy*

- Has the product demonstrated strong clinical effectiveness against the desired pathogen?
- Is the product likely to be effective in the scenario for which use is intended?

*Product Formulation*

- Is a monovalent or multivalent/combination product desired?
- Is it more cost-effective to use a combination product?

*Handling and Administration*

- Does the product require special handling accommodations (e.g. refrigeration)?
- Does the product require special administration techniques or equipment (e.g. a transdermal application system)?

*Target Population*

- Are animals at risk for the particular pathogens in the vaccine product?
- Are animals being vaccinated in order to prevent human disease (e.g. rabies)?

*Program Design*

- Can animals be safely restrained to administer injectable vaccine products?
- Will animals be handled once, or is repeat vaccination an option?

*Immunization Goals*

- Is the goal of immunization to prevent disease or reduce the duration and severity of disease?
- Is the primary purpose of the program to enhance individual animal health or to induce herd immunity?

### 16.2.5.1.2 Standard Protocols

The World Small Animal Veterinary Association along with the American Animal Hospital Association and the American Association of Feline Practitioners have published guidelines for standard vaccination practices [14, 15, 17]. Based on factors including the animal's lifestyle, likelihood of pathogen exposure, and disease severity, particular vaccinations are recommended for either all dogs and cats (i.e. "core") or are optional based on individual risk assessment (i.e. "noncore") (Table 16.4).

It is important to note that most guidelines recommend different protocols for individually owned animals versus those in shelter environments. The field clinic setting may encompass either of these scenarios. An additional consideration in many field clinics is whether or not it will be possible to obtain animals for booster vaccination; therefore, practitioners should decide the most appropriate vaccination protocol depending on the circumstances. In temporary shelters or similar scenarios where groups or large numbers of animals are to be housed, the shelter-based protocols should be followed. In general, such protocols call for initial vaccination to begin at an earlier age (e.g. 4–6 weeks) and be given immediately upon entry into the sheltering facility [14, 15, 17] In addition, secondary vaccination (i.e. "boosters") should be provided with increased frequency (e.g. every 2 weeks) until maternal antibody interference is unlikely. This vaccination protocol should also be considered outside of the shelter in the face of an infectious disease outbreak (Tables 16.5 and 16.6).

### 16.2.5.1.3 Vaccine Storage and Handling

Vaccines are sensitive to both extreme temperatures and fluctuations in temperature. When a vaccine shipment arrives at the clinic, it should be unloaded as soon as possible (i.e. within 1 h) and inspected to be sure the shipping container is intact, the product packaging is sealed, and the ice packs are cold. If any of these things are not in place, the vaccines may be compromised and should not be used.

Once unloaded, vaccines should be stored in a refrigerator maintained at 35–45 °F (2–7 °C) [16]. Temperatures higher or lower than this range can result in the death of the living vaccine organisms, leaving the vaccine ineffective [16].

---

**Textbox 16.6 Vaccination tip from the field**

Consider placing a refrigerator thermometer in each location where vaccines are stored to assure that temperatures are being maintained. Such thermometers can typically be bought at most home goods stores.

---

Temperature monitoring is especially critical in warm environments and busy clinics when the refrigerator is constantly opened and closed. A system for recording the temperature of the refrigerator at different time points throughout the day will help keep track of fluctuations and allow refrigerator settings to be adjusted to maintain a temperature within the desired range.

In many field clinics and in mobile field programs where services are provided door-to-door, refrigeration may not be possible. Such programs typically transport vaccines in coolers with ice packs. In these cases, vaccines should be administered or the ice packs replaced on a regular basis to ensure the product remains viable [15]. Whenever extended time periods away from refrigeration are anticipated, it is recommended to carry only a small supply of vaccines in the event that they are rendered nonviable.

In preparation for the day, many clinics and spay/ neuter programs will prepare vaccines in the morning and set them aside for later use, carry them in vehicles, or store them on countertops in convenient locations. All of these practices jeopardize the vaccine product's effectiveness. Although challenging, efforts should be made to ensure that vaccine products remain viable. Otherwise, resources will be wasted and even worse, use of nonviable vaccinations sets up a community for disease outbreaks and undermines program credibility.

### 16.2.5.1.4 Vaccine Administration

Vaccine products are available in two basic forms: ready-to-use, multidose vials (also known as "tanks") and single-dose vials. The only products available in multidose vials are noninfectious (or "killed") vaccines, such as those for rabies virus and the injectable canine *Bordetella bronchiseptica* vaccine. Although these products may be convenient, multidose vials carry a greater risk of contamination since the stopper is repeatedly penetrated with needles to draw out the

**Table 16.5** Sample vaccination protocol for shelter-housed dogs and cats [14, 15, 17].

| Vaccine | Initial vaccination | | Revaccination interval |
|---|---|---|---|
| **Vaccination protocol for shelter-housed dogs** | | | |
| Modified live virus | | | |
| Canine distemper virus + | Puppies | 4 weeks of age | Repeat every 2 weeks until 20 weeks of age |
| Canine adenovirus-2 + | | | |
| Canine parvovirus +/− | Adults | On admission | Repeat in 1 year |
| Canine parainfluenza virus | | | |
| Modified live virus | | | |
| Intranasal *Bordetella bronchiseptica* + | Puppies | 3 weeks of age | Repeat in 1 year |
| Canine parainfluenza virus | Adults | On admission | Repeat in 6 months |
| Inactivated | | | |
| Rabies virus | Puppies | 12 weeks of age[a] | Repeat in 1 year |
| | Adults | On admission or prior to release | Repeat in 1 year |
| **Vaccination protocol for shelter-housed cats** | | | |
| Modified live virus | | | |
| Feline viral rhinotracheitis + | Kittens | 4 weeks of age | Repeat every 2 weeks until 20 weeks of age |
| Feline calicivirus + | | | |
| Feline panleukopenia virus | Adults | On admission | Repeat in 2 weeks if possible |
| Inactivated or recombinant | | | |
| Feline leukemia virus | Kittens | 8 weeks of age | Repeat in 2 weeks |
| | Adults | On admission if group-housed | Repeat in 1 year if group-housed |
| Inactivated | | | |
| Rabies virus | Kittens | 12 weeks of age[a] | Repeat in 1 year |
| | Adults | On admission or prior to release | Repeat in 1 year |

Note: "Puppies" and "kittens" are considered to be <16 weeks of age; adults are considered to be >16 weeks of age.

a) If animals are only available for vaccination on occasions of at less than 12 weeks of age (e.g. trap–neuter–return programs), vaccination as early as 8 weeks is recommended. Such vaccination may not be legally recognized in some localities, though it is likely to provide some level of protection against disease.

product. If used, they should be gently shaken before drawing up the vaccine to ensure even distribution within the vial and they should be discarded if the rubber stopper becomes compromised [15].

Infectious vaccine products undergo a freeze-drying process known as lyophilization, and must be mixed with a sterile diluent prior to use. Using sterile technique, the sterile diluent is injected into the lyophilized vaccine product and allowed to thoroughly dissolve before drawing the product up into the syringe for administration. This process of rehydrating the vaccine is known as "reconstitution." Many types of sterile diluents are product-specific and should not be interchanged or substituted with another product or solution [16]. Once a vaccine has been reconstituted, it should be administered within 30 min and protected from temperature extremes as discussed earlier [18]. Multiple vaccine products should never be mixed with one another, and doses of vaccine should never be split between animals – kittens, puppies, and full-grown adults require the same volume of product in order to develop the expected immune response [15]. When available, empty vaccine vials should be discarded

**Table 16.6** Sample vaccination protocol for privately owned dogs and cats [14, 15, 17].

| Vaccine | Initial vaccination | | Revaccination interval |
|---|---|---|---|
| **Vaccination protocol for privately owned dogs** | | | |
| Modified live virus | | | |
|    Canine distemper virus + | Puppies | 6 weeks of age | Repeat every 4 weeks until 16 weeks of age, in 1 year, and every 3 years thereafter |
|    Canine adenovirus-2 + | | | |
|    Canine parvovirus +/− | | | |
|    Canine parainfluenza virus | Adults | On initial presentation | Repeat in 1 year, then every 3 years thereafter |
| Modified live virus | | | |
|    Intranasal *Bordetella bronchiseptica* + | Puppies | 3 weeks of age | Repeat annually |
|    Canine parainfluenza virus | Adults | On initial presentation | Repeat annually |
| Inactivated | | | |
|    Rabies virus | Puppies | 12 weeks of age | Repeat in 1 year |
| | Adults | On initial presentation | Repeat in 1 year, then every 1 or 3 years depending on product used |
| **Vaccination protocol for privately owned cats** | | | |
| Modified live virus | | | |
|    Feline viral rhinotracheitis + | Kittens | 6 weeks of age | Repeat every 4 weeks until 16 weeks of age, in 1 year, then every 3 years |
|    Feline calicivirus + | | | |
|    Feline panleukopenia virus | Adults | On initial presentation | Repeat in 4 weeks, then in 1 year, then every 3 years thereafter |
| Inactivated or recombinant | | | |
|    Feline leukemia virus | Kittens | 8 weeks of age | Repeat in 4 weeks, then annually when at risk of exposure |
| | Adults | On initial presentation | Repeat in 4 weeks, then annually when at risk of exposure |
| Inactivated | | | |
|    Rabies virus | Kittens | 12 weeks of age | Repeat in 1 year |
| | Adults | On admission or prior to release | Repeat in 1 year, then every 1 or 3 years depending on product used |

Note: "Puppies" and "kittens" are considered to be <16 weeks of age; adults are considered to be >16 weeks of age.

into a regulated medical waste container (e.g. "sharps" box) for proper disposal.

Prior to administration of any medical product, the route of administration as indicated by the manufacturer should be confirmed. Using an incorrect route can result in inactivation of the vaccine, clinical disease in the animal or at worst, severe organ damage, and death. For example, accidental injection of the intranasal *B. bronchiseptica* vaccine can cause acute, severe liver failure in dogs [19]. As a general rule, noninfectious vaccines must be administered either subcutaneously or intramuscularly, whereas infectious vaccines may be labeled for intranasal, intraoral, subcutaneous, transdermal, or intramuscular administration. Given the option, subcutaneous injection is often quicker and easier for the administrator and less painful for the animal than intramuscular injection. In addition, subcutaneous injection technique can easily be taught to individuals with minimal animal handling experience (Textbox 16.7). Cleaning the skin with an alcohol swab prior to injection is neither recommended nor necessary. Alcohol is not an effective disinfectant when used in this manner and could inactivate the vaccine if it makes contact with the infectious organisms in the product [14].

---

**Textbox 16.7 Subcutaneous injection technique**

1) Tent the skin over the desired injection site.
2) Push the needle through the skin, burying approximately $\frac{3}{4}$ the length of the needle.
3) Draw back on the plunger, if negative pressure is felt, proceed to step 4. If blood or air bubbles enter the syringe, reposition the needle under the skin prior to step 4.
4) Push the plunger to dispense the product into the subcutaneous tissue.
5) Withdraw the needle in one swift motion; gently rub the injection site to relieve discomfort.

---

In regards to choosing an injection location, using a standard site for administration of vaccinations is the best practice and, in the event of an adverse reaction, will provide a clue as to which product may have caused the reaction so future precautions can be taken. The location chosen is not as important as using a consistent location within your organization and documenting the type of vaccine and its location in the animal's medical record. Most commonly, the following sites are used:

- *Right fore leg.* Canine distemper-parvovirus and feline upper respiratory-panleukopenia
- *Right hind leg.* Rabies or combination products containing rabies
- *Left hind leg.* Feline leukemia virus or combination products containing feline leukemia.

Ideally, all products should be given as far down the leg (below the elbow or stifle) as is feasible [18]. When dealing with a fractious or fearful animal, which is often the case in the field, this may not be possible, and the interscapular region is usually the safest and easiest choice.

#### 16.2.5.2 Parasite Control

##### 16.2.5.2.1 Individual Animals

Parasiticide administration is another essential tenet of preventive care in the field. In addition to causing disease in animals, many parasites and parasite-vectored pathogens can also affect humans. Although some such parasites are isolated to distinct geographic regions, many are found worldwide. For these reasons, provisions for control of common parasites and their associated diseases should be a component of every field clinic's preventive medicine program.

The chosen parasite treatment protocol should prioritize the treatment of infestations that are common in the particular geographic region of operation as well as those that represent significant risk of zoonosis (Tables 16.7–16.9). Fecal examination (e.g. fecal flotation and direct fecal smears) is recommended when the distribution of parasites at a given clinic site is unknown, when animals present with clinical signs consistent with gastrointestinal parasite infestation (e.g. vomiting and diarrhea), or when there is lack of response to previous anthelmintic administration [22]. In the absence of a microscope, a broad-spectrum anthelmintic with efficacy against the most common and most pathogenic parasites should be administered empirically.

---

**Textbox 16.8 Deworming tip from the field**

The author generally recommends the empirical administration of pyrantel pamoate (10 mg/kg), fenbendazole (50 mg/kg), or ivermectin (0.2 mg/kg) in both dogs and cats.

---

It may be useful to explore off-label uses of products formulated for large animals (e.g. ivermectin) in order to realize significant cost savings, limit the amount of supplies that must be maintained, and ensure access to common medications in remote locations. Caution must be taken when dosing such formulations for small animals and preestablished dosage charts are recommended to minimize calculation errors. Also, note that the 0.2 mg/kg dose of ivermectin should not be used in dog breeds at risk for ivermectin sensitivity (see Appendix 16.C).

Ideally, an ectoparasiticide effective against both fleas and ticks should also be administered [23]. Infestations can diminish an individual animal's quality of life and lead to severe tick-transmitted illness. A wide variety of commercially available topical combination products are available for this purpose, some of which are effective against

Table 16.7 Common gastrointestinal parasites of cats and dogs [20, 21].

| Parasite | Distribution | Species | Zoonotic potential | Treatment options |
|---|---|---|---|---|
| Cestodes | | | | |
| *Diphyllobothrium latum* | Northern Hemisphere South America | Cats, Dogs | Yes | Praziquantel |
| *Dipylidium caninum* | Worldwide | Cats, Dogs | Yes | Praziquantel |
| *Echinococcus* spp. | Worldwide | Cats, Dogs | Yes | Praziquantel |
| *Mesocestoides* spp. | Worldwide | Cats, Dogs | No | Praziquantel Nitazoxanide |
| *Spirometra* spp. | North America South America Europe Asia | Cats, Dogs | No | Praziquantel |
| *Taenia* spp. | Worldwide | Cats, Dogs | Yes | Praziquantel Fenbendazole |
| Nematodes | | | | |
| *Aelurostrongylus abstrusus* | Worldwide | Cats, Dogs | No | Ivermectin Fenbendazole Moxidectin Emodepside |
| *Ancylostoma* spp. | Worldwide | Cats, Dogs | Yes | Fenbendazole Milbemycin Moxidectin Pyrantel |
| *Angiostrongylus vasorum* | North America Europe South America Africa | Dogs | No | Fenbendazole Levamisole Milbemycin oxime Moxidectin |
| *Aonchotheca putorii* | North America Europe New Zealand | Cats | No | Ivermectin Levamisole |
| *Baylisascaris procyonis* | North America Europe | Dogs | Yes | Fenbendazole Milbemycin Moxidectin Pyrantel |
| *Crenosoma vulpis* | North America Europe | Dogs | No | Fenbendazole Ivermectin Febantel |
| *Eucoleus* spp. | Worldwide | Cats, Dogs | Yes | Ivermectin Fenbendazole |
| *Ollulanus tricuspis* | North America Europe South America Africa Australia | Cats | No | Tetramisole |
| *Oslerus osleri* | Worldwide | Dogs | No | Doramectin |
| *Physaloptera* spp. | Worldwide | Cats, Dogs | No | Pyrantel pamoate |
| *Spirocerca lupi* | Worldwide | Dogs | Yes | Ivermectin Moxidectin Doramectin |

(*continued*)

**Table 16.7** (*Continued*)

| Parasite | Distribution | Species | Zoonotic potential | Treatment options |
|---|---|---|---|---|
| *Strongyloides* spp. | Worldwide | Cats, Dogs | Yes | Ivermectin |
| *Toxocara* spp. | Worldwide | Cats, Dogs | Yes | Fenbendazole<br>Milbemycin<br>Moxidectin<br>Pyrantel |
| *Toxascaris leonina* | Worldwide | Cats, Dogs | Yes | Fenbendazole<br>Milbemycin<br>Moxidectin<br>Pyrantel |
| *Trichuris vulpis* | Worldwide<br>Latin America<br>South America | Dogs<br>Cats | Yes | Praziquantel<br>Fenbendazole |
| *Uncinaria* spp. | North America<br>Europe | Cats, Dogs | Yes | Fenbendazole<br>Milbemycin<br>Moxidectin<br>Pyrantel |
| Protozoa | | | | |
| *Cryptosporidium* spp. | Worldwide | Cats, Dogs | Yes | Paromomycin<br>Tylosin<br>Azithromycin |
| *Giardia* spp. | Worldwide | Cats, Dogs | Yes | Fenbendazole + Metronidazole |
| *Isospora* spp. | Worldwide | Cats, Dogs | No | Sulfadimethoxine<br>Ponazuril |
| *Neospora caninum* | Worldwide | Dogs | No | Clindamycin<br>Pyrimethamine + sulfonamide |
| *Sarcocystis* spp. | Worldwide | Cats, Dogs | Yes | Pyrimethamine + sulfonamide<br>Ponazuril |
| *Toxoplasma gondii* | Worldwide | Cats | Yes | Clindamycin<br>Pyrimethamine + sulfonamide<br>Trimethoprim + sulfonamide |
| *Tritrichomonas fetus* | Worldwide | Cats, Dogs | Yes | Ronidazole<br>Metronidazole |
| Trematodes | | | | |
| *Alaria* spp. | Worldwide | Cats, Dogs | Yes | Praziquantel |
| *Cryptocotyle lingua* | Worldwide | Cats, Dogs | Yes | Praziquantel |
| *Heterobilharzia americana* | North America | Dogs | Yes | Praziquantel |
| *Nanophyetus salmincola* | North America | Cats, Dogs | Yes | Praziquantel |
| *Paragonimus kellicotti* | North America<br>South America<br>Central America<br>Africa<br>Asia | Cats, Dogs | Yes | Praziquantel |
| *Platynosomum concinnum* | North America<br>South America<br>Africa | Cats | No | Praziquantel |

**Table 16.8** Common vector-borne pathogens of cats and dogs.

| Pathogen | Distribution | Parasite vector |
|---|---|---|
| *Anaplasma* spp. | Worldwide | Ticks |
| *Babesia* spp. | Worldwide | Ticks |
| *Bartonella* spp. | Worldwide | Fleas |
| *Borrelia* spp. | Worldwide | Ticks |
| *Coxiella burnetii* | Worldwide | Ticks |
| *Dirofilaria* spp. | Worldwide | Mosquitoes |
| *Ehrlichia* spp. | Worldwide | Ticks |
| *Francisella tularensis* | Northern Hemisphere | Ticks Mosquitoes Biting flies |
| *Hepatozoon* spp. | Worldwide | Ticks |
| *Leishmania* spp. | Worldwide | Sand flies |
| *Rickettsia* spp. | Worldwide | Ticks |
| *Trypanosoma* spp. | North America South America Africa | Triatomids |
| *Yersinia pestis* | Worldwide | Fleas |

**Table 16.9** Common external parasites of cats and dogs.

| Parasite | Distribution | Species | Zoonotic potential |
|---|---|---|---|
| Fleas | | | |
| *Ctenocephalides felis* | Worldwide | Cats, dogs | No |
| *Echidnophaga gallinacea* | Worldwide | Cats, dogs | No |
| *Pulex irritans* | Worldwide | Cats, dogs | Yes |
| Flies | | | |
| *Chrysomya bezziana* | Africa India Asia | Cats, dogs | Yes |
| *Cochliomyia hominivorax* | South America | Cats, dogs | Yes |
| *Cuterebra* spp. | Western hemisphere | Cats, dogs | Yes |
| *Dermatobia hominis* | Central America South America | Dogs | Yes |

*(continued)*

**Table 16.9** *(Continued)*

| Parasite | Distribution | Species | Zoonotic potential |
|---|---|---|---|
| Lice | | | |
| *Felicola subrostratus* | Worldwide | Cats | No |
| *Trichodectes canis* | Worldwide | Dogs | No |
| Mites | | | |
| *Cheyletiella* spp. | Worldwide | Cats, dogs | Yes |
| *Demodex* spp. | Worldwide | Cats, dogs | No |
| *Lynxacarus radovskyi* | North America Caribbean Hawaii Australia | Cats | No |
| *Notoedres cati* | Worldwide | Cats | No |
| *Otodectes cynotis* | Worldwide | Cats, dogs | No |
| *Pneumonyssoides caninum* | Worldwide | Dogs | No |
| *Sarcoptes scabiei* | Worldwide | Dogs | Yes |
| *Trombiculid mites* | North America Europe | Cats, dogs | Yes |
| Ticks | | | |
| *Amblyomma* spp. | North America Latin America Africa | Cats, dogs | Yes |
| *Dermacentor* spp. | North America Europe Asia Caribbean Latin America | Cats, dogs | Yes |
| *Haemaphysalis* spp. | Worldwide | Cats, dogs | Yes |
| *Hyalomma* spp. | Europe Asia Africa | Cats, dogs | Yes |
| *Ixodes* spp. | North America Europe Africa Australia | Cats, dogs | Yes |
| *Otobius megnini* | North America South America Africa India | Cats, dogs | Yes |
| *Rhipicephalus* spp. | Worldwide | Cats, dogs | Yes |

Source: Greiner 2012 [21]. Reproduced with permission of John Wiley & Sons.

both internal and external parasites. These may seem cost-prohibitive for many field clinics; however, their broad spectrum of activity and, in many cases, the ability to purchase in bulk and distribute individual doses off-label may translate into overall cost savings (e.g. one 2 ml dose of the extra-large dog Revolution (Zoetis, Inc.) can be split to administer 0.25 ml to each of eight small cats). Their use is particularly desirable and effective in field clinics where the opportunity for repeat dosing, exact weight determination, and administration of oral medications may not be possible. Formulations, spectrum of activity, duration, and cost-effectiveness vary widely, so the practitioner is encouraged to research the products available and develop SOPs for clinic staff (Table 16.10).

Table 16.10 Topical antiparasitic products.

| Trade name | Species | Active ingredients | Indications | Dose | Supplied |
|---|---|---|---|---|---|
| Activyl® Spot-on (Merck Animal Health) | Cats Dogs | Indoxacarb (19.5%) | Fleas | 25 mg/kg 15 mg/kg | 0.51 ml/100 mg/2–9 lbs 1.03 ml/200 mg/>9 lbs 0.51 ml/100 mg/4–14 lbs 0.77 ml/150 mg/14–22 lbs 1.54 ml/300 mg/22–44 lbs 3.08 ml/600 mg/44–88 lbs 4.62 ml/900 mg/88–132 lbs |
| Activyl Tick Plus (Merck Animal Health) | Dogs | Indoxacarb (13%) + permethrin (42.5%) | Fleas Ticks | 15 mg/kg + 48 mg/kg | 0.51 ml/75 mg + 240 mg/4–11 lbs 1 ml/150 mg + 480 mg/11–22 lbs 2 ml/300 mg + 960 mg/22–44 lbs 4 ml/600 mg + 1920 mg/44–88 lbs 6 ml/900 mg + 2880 mg/88–132 lbs |
| Advantage® (Bayer Animal Health) | Cats Dogs | Imidacloprid (10%) | Fleas | Volume[a] | 0.4 ml/1–10 lbs 0.8 ml/>10 lbs 0.4 ml/1–10 lbs 1 ml/11–20 lbs 2.5 ml/21–55 lbs 4 ml/>55 lbs |
| Advantage II (Bayer Animal Health) | Cats Dogs | Imidacloprid (9.1%) + pyriproxyfen (0.46%) | Fleas Lice | Volume[a] | 0.23 ml 0.4 ml/ 0.8 ml/>9 lbs 0.4 ml/3–10 lbs 1 ml/11–20 lbs 2.5 ml/21–55 lbs 4 ml/>55 lbs |
| Advantage Multi®/Advocate (Bayer Animal Health) | Cats Dogs | Imidacloprid (10%) + moxidectin (1%) Imidacloprid (10%) + moxidectin (2.5%) | Ear mites Fleas Heartworms Hookworms Roundworms Fleas Heartworms Hookworms Mites Roundworms Whipworms | 10 mg/kg + 1 mg/kg 10 mg/kg + 2.5 mg/kg | 0.23 ml/23 mg + 2.3 mg/2–5 lbs 0.4 ml/40 mg + 4 mg/5.1–9 lbs 0.8 ml/80 mg + 8 mg/9.1–18 lbs 0.4/40 mg + 10 mg/3–9 lbs 1 ml/100 mg + 25 mg/9.1–20 lbs 2.5 ml/250 mg + 62.5 mg/20.1–55 lbs 4 ml/400 mg + 100 mg/55.1–88 lbs 5 ml/500 mg + 125 mg/88.1–125 lbs |
| Bio Spot Active Care™ (Farnam Companies, Inc.) | Cats Dogs | Etofenprox (40%) + (s)-methoprene (3.6%) Etofenprox (50%) + piperonyl butoxide | Fleas Flea eggs Mosquitoes Ticks | Volume | 1 ml/2.5–5 lbs 1.8 ml/≥5 lbs 1 ml/5–14 lbs 2.2 ml/15–30 lbs 4.4 ml/31–60 lbs |

**Table 16.10** (*Continued*)

| Trade name | Species | Active ingredients | Indications | Dose | Supplied |
|---|---|---|---|---|---|
| | | (9.1%) + *N*-octyl bicycloheptene dicarboximide) (0.91%) + pyriproxyfen (0.45%) + (*s*)-methoprene (0.23%) | | | 7.3 ml/61–150 lbs |
| Bravecto® (Merck Animal Health) | Cats / Dogs | Fluralaner | Fleas Ticks Fleas Ticks Mites | 40–93 mg/kg[a] 25–56 mg/kg[a] | 0.4 ml/112.5 mg/2.6–6.2 lbs 0.89 ml/250 mg/6.3–13.8 lbs 1.79 ml/500 mg/13.9–27.5 lbs 0.4 ml/112.5 mg/4.4–9.9 lbs 0.89 ml/250 mg/10.0–22.0 lbs 1.79 ml/500 mg/22.1–44.0 lbs 3.57 ml/1000 mg/44.1–88.0 lbs 5.0 ml/1400 mg/88.1–123.0 lbs |
| Cheristin™ (Elanco Animal Health) | Cats | Spinetoram (11.2%) | Fleas | n/a | 0.7 ml/1.8–20 lbs |
| EasySpot™ (Novartis Animal Health) | Cats | Fipronil (9.7%) | Fleas Lice Ticks | n/a | 0.5 ml/>1.5 lbs |
| EctoAdvance Plus (Virbac) | Cats Dogs | Fipronil (9.8%) + (*s*)-methoprene (11.8%) Fipronil (9.8%) + (*s*)-methoprene (8.8%) | Fleas Ticks Fleas Lice *Sarcoptes* Ticks | Volume | 0.5 ml/>1.5 lbs 0.67 ml/4–22 lbs 1.34 ml/23–44 lbs 2.68/45–88 lbs 4.02 ml/89–132 lbs |
| Effipro (Virbac) | Cats | Fipronil (9.6%) | Fleas Lice Mosquitoes Ticks | n/a | 0.5 ml |
| Effitix (Virbac) | Dogs | Fipronil (6.01%) + permethrin (44.88%) | Biting flies Fleas Lice *Sarcoptes* Mosquitoes Ticks | Volume | 0.5 ml/5–10.9 lbs 1 ml/11–22.9 lbs 2 ml/23–44.9 lbs 4 ml/45–88.9 lbs 6 ml/89–132 lbs |
| Frontline® Plus (Merial) | Cats Dogs | Fipronil (9.8%) + (*s*)-methoprene (11.8%) Fipronil (9.8%) + (*s*)-methoprene (8.8%) | Fleas Flea eggs Lice Ticks Fleas Flea eggs Lice *Sarcoptes* Ticks | Volume | 0.5 ml/>8 weeks 0.67 ml/11–22 lbs 1.34 ml/23–44 lbs 2.68 ml/45–88 lbs 4.02 ml/89–132 lbs |

(*continued*)

Table 16.10 (*Continued*)

| Trade name | Species | Active ingredients | Indications | Dose | Supplied |
|---|---|---|---|---|---|
| Frontline Spray (Merial) | Cats Dogs | Fipronil (0.29%) | Fleas Lice *Sarcoptes* Ticks | 1–2 pumps per pound[a] | 250 ml 500 ml |
| Frontline Top Spot® (Merial) | Cats Dogs | Fipronil (9.7%) | Fleas Lice *Sarcoptes* Ticks | Volume[a] | 0.5 ml 0.67 ml/<23 lb 1.3 ml/23–44 lbs 2.68 ml/45–88 lbs 4.02 ml/89–132 lbs |
| Frontline Tritak® (Merial) | Cats Dogs | Fipronil (9.8%) + etofenprox (15%) + (*s*)-methoprene (11.8%) Fipronil (9.8%) + cyphenothrin (5.2%) + (*s*)-methoprene (8.8%) | Fleas Flea eggs Lice Ticks Fleas Flea eggs Lice *Sarcoptes* Ticks | Volume | 0.5 ml/>12 weeks 0.67 ml/11–22 lbs 1.34 ml/23–44 lbs 2.68 ml/45–88 lbs 4.02 ml/89–132 lbs |
| K9 Advantix® II (Bayer Animal Health) | Dogs | Imidacloprid (8.8%) + permethrin (44%) + pyriproxyfen (0.44%) | Biting flies Fleas Lice Mosquitoes Ticks | Volume | 0.4 ml/4–10 lbs 1 ml/11–20 lbs 2.5 ml/21–55 lbs 4 ml/>55 lbs |
| Parastar™ (Elanco Animal Health) | Dogs | Fipronil (9.7%) | Fleas Lice *Sarcoptes* Ticks | Volume | 0.67 ml/4–22 lbs 1.34 ml/23–44 lbs 2.68 ml/45–88 lbs 4.02 ml/89–132 lbs |
| Parastar Plus (Elanco Animal Health) | Dogs | Fipronil (9.8%) + cyphenothrin (5.2%) | Fleas Lice *Sarcoptes* Ticks | | 0.67 ml/4–22 lbs 1.34 ml/23–44 lbs 2.68 ml/45–88 lbs 4.02 ml/89–132 lbs |
| PetArmor® (Fidopharm, Inc.) | Cats Dogs | Fipronil (9.7%) | Fleas Lice Ticks | Volume[a] | 0.5 ml/>1.5 lbs 0.67 ml/4–22 lbs 1.34 ml/23–44 lbs 2.68 ml/45–88 lbs 4.02 ml/89–132 lbs |
| PetArmor Plus (Fidopharm, Inc.) | Cats Dogs | Fipronil (9.8%) + (*s*)-methoprene (11.8%) Fipronil (9.8%) + (*s*)-methoprene (8.8%) | Fleas Flea eggs Lice Ticks | Volume | 0.5 ml/>1.5 lbs 0.67 ml/4–22 lbs 1.34 ml/23–44 lbs 2.68 ml/45–88 lbs 4.02 ml/89–132 lbs |

**Table 16.10** (*Continued*)

| Trade name | Species | Active ingredients | Indications | Dose | Supplied |
|---|---|---|---|---|---|
| Profender® (Bayer Animal Health) | Cats | Emodepside (1.98%) + praziquantel (7.94%) | Hookworms Roundworms Tapeworms | 3 mg/kg + 12 mg/kg | 0.35 ml/7.5 mg + 30 mg/2.2–5.5 lbs 0.7 ml/15 mg + 60.1 mg/5.6–11 lbs 1.12 ml/24 mg + 96.1 mg/11.1–17.6 lbs |
| Revolution (Zoetis, Inc.) | Cats Dogs | Selamectin | Ear mites Fleas Flea eggs Heartworms Hookworms Roundworms Ear mites Fleas Flea eggs Heartworms *Sarcoptes* Ticks | 6 mg/kg[b] | 0.25 ml/15 mg/<6 lbs 0.75 ml/45 mg/5.1–15 lbs 0.25 ml/15 mg/<6 lbs 0.25 ml/30 mg/5.1–10 lbs 0.5 ml/60 mg/10.1–20 lbs 1 ml/120 mg/20.1–40 lbs 2 ml/240 mg/40.1–85 lbs |
| Sentry® Fiproguard® (Sergeant's Pet Care Products, Inc.) | Cats Dogs | Fipronil (9.7%) | Fleas Ticks Lice | Volume | 0.5 ml (>8 weeks) 0.67 ml/4–22 lbs 1.34 ml/23–44 lbs 2.68 ml/45–88 lbs 4.02 ml/89–132 lbs |
| Sentry Fiproguard Max (Sergeant's Pet Care Products, Inc.) | Cats Dogs | Fipronil (9.8%) + etofenprox (15%) Fipronil (9.8%) + cyphenothrin (5.2%) | Fleas Ticks Lice | Volume | 0.5 ml (>12 weeks) 0.67 ml/4–22 lbs 1.34 ml/23–44 lbs 2.68 ml/45–88 lbs 4.02 ml/89–132 lbs |
| Sentry Fiproguard Plus (Sergeant's Pet Care Products, Inc.) | Cats Dogs | Fipronil (9.8%) + (s)-methoprene (11.8%) Fipronil (9.8%) + (s)-methoprene (8.8%) | Fleas Flea eggs Lice Ticks | Volume | 0.5 ml/>1.5 lbs 0.67 ml/4–22 lbs 1.34 ml/23–44 lbs 2.68 ml/45–88 lbs 4.02 ml/89–132 lbs |
| Vectra® (Ceva Animal Health, LLC) | Cats Dogs | Dinotefuran (22%) + pyriproxyfen (3%) | Fleas Flea eggs | Volume[a] | 0.8 ml/<9 lbs/8 weeks 1.2 ml/≥9 lbs 1.3 ml/2.5–10 lbs 2 ml/11–20 lbs 4 ml/21–55 lbs 6 ml/56–100 lbs |
| Vectra 3D® (Ceva Animal Health, LLC) | Dogs | Dinotefuran (4.95%) + permethrin (36.08%) + pyriproxyfen (0.44%) | Biting flies Fleas Flea eggs Lice Mosquitoes Ticks | Volume | 0.8 ml/5–10 lbs 1.6 ml/11–20 lbs 3.6 ml/21–55 lbs 4.7 ml/56–95 lbs 8 ml/>95 lbs |

a) Percentage of active ingredient(s) consistent across species formulations; products can be dosed by volume.
b) Dosage consistent across species; products can be dosed by concentration.

#### 16.2.5.2.2 Environmental Parasite Control

Successful ectoparasite control involves treatment of both individual animals and the environment; therefore, field clinics or other facilities that may be housing animals long-term should have a plan for environmental control of fleas and ticks. Areas surrounding the housing facility should be kept free from yard waste, grass, weeds, brush, and any points of access for wildlife to enter animal housing areas should be secured. Such measures will help discourage the presence of wildlife and/or stray domestic animals that serve as parasite hosts. Environmental acaricides (most commonly synthetic pyrethroids) can be applied around housing structures and within cracks and crevices in floors, walls, and ceilings [24]. At least two treatments per year (in spring and fall) are required to eliminate all life stages; heavy infestations may require more frequent application [25]. Care should be taken to avoid direct animal contact with such products to avoid toxicities.

### 16.2.6 Diagnostic Screening Tests

Routine diagnostic screening for common infectious diseases is an expected component of preventive veterinary care in most of the developed world. Indeed, when working with privately owned pets or animals maintained in intensive housing operations (e.g. shelters, breeding facilities, and research laboratories), this would be considered a best practice [26]. In the field clinic, however, the utility of diagnostic testing must be considered in light of the population of animals and caretakers being served, resource availability, and the program's overall mission. Some of the questions to be answered include the following:

- Does the program have enough resources (financial, staffing, equipment, and time) to conduct diagnostic screening tests?
- Does the prevalence of the disease in question in the region where the field clinic is located justify diagnostic screening?
- What screening tests are available, will they be feasible to conduct, and will they produce accurate results in the field clinic setting?
- Will the results of the screening test alter the therapeutic plan for the individual patient?

- Will the results of the screening test impact human health?
- Will the results of the screening test alter the operation of current or future clinics?
- Does the cost of conducting the screening test impact other clinic services or the clinic's effectiveness as a whole in pursuing their primary mission?
- Does conducting diagnostic testing fall within the clinic's operational mission?

If the answer to the majority of these questions is "yes," and both the risks of testing and those of not testing have been evaluated, then routine diagnostic screening may be considered. In most cases, testing for diseases that are common, highly infectious, potentially fatal, or zoonotic should be prioritized [27]. Common infectious diseases for which routine diagnostic screening testing is considered include canine heartworm disease, feline leukemia virus, feline immunodeficiency virus, and dermatophytosis.

## 16.3 Spay/Neuter

The goal of most surgical field clinics around the world is to increase the availability of elective sterilization services. In much of North America, sterilization of companion animals is a culturally expected behavior of a responsible pet owner and deemed to be an essential component of preventive care [26]. However, in many parts of Europe, the opposite is true [28]. In some cultures, sterilization is even identified as cruel, immoral, illegal, or contrary to religious belief systems [29, 30]. Given these considerations, it is important for clinic managers and practitioners to carefully consider whether or not it is appropriate to include elective sterilization as part of a given field clinic's preventive care program.

Initial evaluation for surgical sterilization can be conducted by those teams interfacing directly with animal caretakers. As with any medical procedure, there are both risks and benefits to the individual animal undergoing elective sterilization that should be discussed (Table 16.11).

In the field clinic setting, other considerations include whether or not surgical services can be provided with adequate anesthesia and analgesia, maintenance of aseptic technique, and with provisions for

Table 16.11 Benefits and risks of surgical sterilization for dogs and cats.

| Benefits | | Risks | |
|---|---|---|---|
| Dogs | Cats | Dogs | Cats |
| Increased life span | Increased life span | Increased risk of<br>  Obesity | Obesity |
| Eliminated risk of<br>  Testicular, uterine, or<br>    ovarian<br>    neoplasia<br>  Pyometra | Testicular, uterine, or ovarian<br>  neoplasia<br>Pyometra | Selected rare neoplasias<br>  Anterior cruciate ligament<br>    rupture<br>  Urinary incontinence | |
| Decreased risk of<br>  Intermale aggression<br>  Mounting<br>  Roaming<br>  Benign prostatic hyperplasia<br>  Perianal tumors<br>  Perineal hernias<br>  Mammary neoplasia | Intermale aggression<br>Roaming<br>Urine spraying<br>Mammary neoplasia | | |

Source: Root Kustritz 2012 [31]. Reproduced with permission of John Wiley & Sons.

any postprocedural care that may be required. Care must be taken not to impose one's own cultural or personal beliefs in recommending elective sterilization for a caretaker's pet or a community's animal population for which it may not be indicated to fulfill the program's mission.

## 16.4 Husbandry

A comprehensive wellness and preventive care assessment should also include evaluation of the animal husbandry provided on a regular basis. It is not uncommon for field clinic practitioners to encounter disease processes due solely to inadequate nutrition, unsanitary or otherwise inadequate living environments, and lack of appropriate grooming, breed, or age-specific care. The primary role of the practitioner is to educate animal caretakers about such needs for their particular animals. However, in underdeveloped areas, an additional role and challenge may be helping the caretaker identify the means of meeting those needs within their physical, financial, geographical, and cultural context.

A basic dietary history should be obtained to identify opportunities for caretaker education and assess the potential for nutritional deficiencies in the patient. Type and formulation of food offered, frequency and amount of administration, animal acceptance of diet, and alternate sources of caloric intake should all be assessed. Access to and availability of clean drinking water should be ensured. Animals and populations that are fed imbalanced homemade diets, diets formulated for different species, or are primarily sustained via scavenging should be assessed with particular attention to common forms of malnutrition (Table 16.12).

Finally, the preventive care clinic should be prepared to provide for and educate caretakers on the common grooming, breed-specific, and age-specific needs of their animals. Claw trimming and coat maintenance to prevent matting, urine and fecal scalding, secondary infection, and parasitic infestation should be performed and demonstrated to caretakers when necessary. When neglected, these factors can result in severe threats to physical health in addition to their negative effects on mobility, comfort, and overall quality of life [33]. Breed-specific care may include discussion of concepts such as environmental thermoregulation for brachycephalic animals, establishing an ear cleaning regimen for flop-eared breeds, and skin care for breeds with redundant skin or those prone to sunburn. Specific needs for neonatal or pediatric animals (e.g. nutritional requirements and preventive care recommendations) as well as geriatric animals (e.g. ensuring mobility and comfort) may also be discussed.

Table 16.12 Nutritional problems with imbalanced diets.

| Dietary characteristics | Species | Nutritional problem | Clinical signs |
|---|---|---|---|
| High liver content | Cats, dogs | Vitamin A toxicity | Cervical spondylosis<br>Vertebral ankylosis |
| Absence of liver, fish liver oils, or synthetic Vitamin A | Cats | Vitamin A deficiency | Conjunctivitis<br>Keratitis<br>Retinal degeneration<br>Stillbirths<br>Congenital abnormalities<br>Fetal resorption |
| High in poly-unsaturated fatty acids (e.g. marine fish oils) | Cats | Vitamin E deficiency | Steatitis<br>Anorexia<br>Muscular degeneration |
| Uncooked freshwater fish | Cats | Thiamine deficiency | Anorexia<br>Unkempt coat<br>Ventroflexion of head<br>Convulsions<br>Loss of righting reflex<br>Ataxia |
| Meat-exclusive diet (including red meat, liver, fish, poultry) | Cats, dogs | Hypocalcemia<br>Nutritional secondary hyperparathyroidism | Hyperesthesia<br>Loss of muscle tone<br>Paralysis<br>Pathologic fractures |
| High meat content<br>Saltwater fish diet | Cats, dogs | Iodine deficiency | Initial hyperthyroidism followed by hypothyroidism<br>Alopecia<br>Fetal resorption |
| Milk and/or vegetable exclusive diet | Cats, dogs | Iron deficiency<br>Copper deficiency | Anemia<br>Reddish tinge to hair coat |
| No protein diet<br>Diets formulated for dogs | Cats | Taurine deficiency | Retinal degeneration<br>Dilated cardiomyopathy |
| Low protein diet | Cats, dogs | Protein deficiency | Reduced growth rates<br>Anemia<br>Weight loss<br>Skeletal muscle atrophy<br>Dull, unkempt hair coat<br>Anorexia |
| Lack of essential fatty acids | Cats, dogs | EFA deficiency | Dry, scaly coat<br>Inactivity<br>Anestrus<br>Testicular underdevelopment<br>Lack of libido |
| High phytate content (e.g. whole grains, legumes, nuts, potatoes, and seeds) | Cats, dogs | Zinc deficiency | Emesis<br>Keratitis<br>Loss of coat color<br>Reduced growth rates<br>Emaciation |

Source: Adapted from Sanderson 2010 [32].

## 16.5   Conclusion

Providing high-quality veterinary care in a field clinic environment is not without its challenges. Facing severe infectious disease threats, treatment of diseases that have progressed due to lack of care, and the simple logistics of creating a clinic environment in an inhospitable environment, it is easy to place wellness and preventive care low on the list of priorities. However, by ensuring that things such as vaccination, parasite prevention, elective sterilization, and basic husbandry are always prioritized, the veterinary profession can lead by example. Prevention truly is the best medicine and will ensure the highest quality of life – in both the short and long term – for both the people and animals we serve.

# Appendix

## 16.A

A carefully designed medical record can capture all information pertinent to patient care in a concise, one-page format. This record is designed for use in Spanish-speaking locations.

| Animal #:_____ <br> Body Weight: _____ lb <br><br> Age: ____ Wks. / Mos. / Yrs. <br> Sex:   ☐ Male      ☐ Female | **Anesthesia and Surgery Record** | Name: _____ <br> Species: ☐ Canine    ☐ Feline <br> Breed: _____ <br> Color: _____ <br> _____ |

Certifico que soy el dueño de este animal y que lo estoy presentando en buena salud para esterilización rutina. Se concede permiso para llevar a cabo la anestesia y la cirugía. Entiendo los peligros asociados a estos procedimientos quirúrgicos, incluidas las complicaciones incisionales, hemorragias, reacciones anestésicas, y la muerte.

Nombre: _____     Firma: _____     Fecha: _____

| Physical Examination | |
|---|---|
| Date: _____ <br><br><br><br> Examiner's Initials: _____ | Microchip:  #_____ / None found <br> HR:_____   RR:_____   Temp:_____   BCS: ___/9 <br> **Males:** 2 testicles descended? **Yes / No** <br> **Females:** Spay scar or tattoo? **Yes / No** |

| Medication: | Drug(s) | Route | Amount (ml) | Time | Initials |
|---|---|---|---|---|---|
| Sedation | ☐ Acepromazine (10 mg/ml) <br> ☐ Buprenorphine  (0.3 mg/ml) <br> ☐ Dexmedetomidine (0.5 mg/ml) | IM / SC / IV | | | |
| Induction & Maintenance | ☐ Dexmedetomidine/Ketamine/Buprenorphine <br> ☐ Propofol | IM <br> IV | | | |
| Reversal | ☐ Antisedan | SC | | | |
| Analgesia | ☐ Previcox or  ☐ Rimadyl | PO / SC | ☐ Rx provided _____mg | | |
| | ☐ Lidocaine  or  ☐ Bupivacaine | Sp / Line / IT | | | |

☐ Rabies – Initials: ____; Serial #:_____; Exp: _____ ☐ FVRCP ☐ DA$_2$PP ☐ Flea/HW Preventive: _____
☐ Tattoo ☐ Antibiotics_____ ☐ Other:_____

**Anesthetic Record:**

| | Time | SpO$_2$ (%) | Heart Rate | Respiratory Rate | Depth |
|---|---|---|---|---|---|
| | | | | | |
| | | | | | |
| Pre-op temp.: _____ °F | | | | | |
| Post-op temp.: _____ °F | | | | | |

| | | Start Time | |
|---|---|---|---|
| **Surgeon** | Name: | **End Time** | |
| **Spay approach** | Midline     Left flank     Other: | | |
| • Ovarian ligatures | 0   2-0   3-0   4-0     Suture type: | Autoligation | |
| • Uterine body ligatures | 0   2-0   3-0   4-0     Suture type: | | |
| • Linea closure | 0   2-0   3-0   4-0     Suture type: | Continuous     Interrupted | |
| • Subcutaneous closure | 0   2-0   3-0   4-0     Suture type: | Continuous     Interrupted | |
| • Skin closure | 0   2-0   3-0   4-0     Suture type: | Intradermal     Adhesive | |
| • Condition | Routine     Pregnant #_____ fetuses     In heat     Lactating | | |
| **Neuter approach** | Prescrotal     Scrotal     Inguinal     Midline (Abdominal) | | |
| • Technique | Open     Closed     Modified Open | | |
| • Spermatic cord ligatures | 0   2-0   3-0     Suture type: | Autoligation | |
| • Linea closure | 0   2-0   3-0   4-0     Suture type: | Continuous     Interrupted     N/A | |
| • Subcutaneous closure | 0   2-0   3-0   4-0     Suture type: | Continuous     Interrupted     N/A | |
| • Skin closure | 0   2-0   3-0     Suture type: | Intradermal     Adhesive     None | |
| • Condition | Routine     Cryptorchid: L-Inguinal   R-Inguinal   L-Abdominal   R-Abdominal | | |
| **Notes** | | | |
| | | | |

## 16.B

The Purina nine-point body condition scoring system is a simple, widely recognized, and validated body condition assessment scale. Body condition assessment can serve as a crude indicator of welfare.

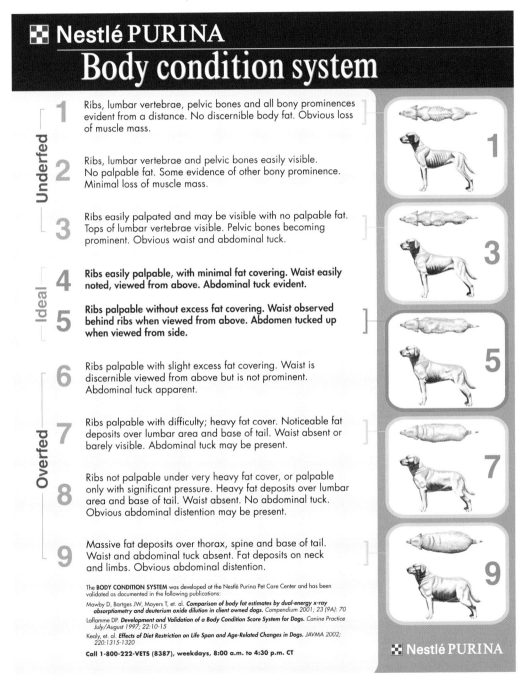

### Nestlé PURINA
# Body condition system

**Underfed**

**1** Ribs, lumbar vertebrae, pelvic bones and all bony prominences evident from a distance. No discernible body fat. Obvious loss of muscle mass.

**2** Ribs, lumbar vertebrae and pelvic bones easily visible. No palpable fat. Some evidence of other bony prominence. Minimal loss of muscle mass.

**3** Ribs easily palpated and may be visible with no palpable fat. Tops of lumbar vertebrae visible. Pelvic bones becoming prominent. Obvious waist and abdominal tuck.

**Ideal**

**4** Ribs easily palpable, with minimal fat covering. Waist easily noted, viewed from above. Abdominal tuck evident.

**5** Ribs palpable without excess fat covering. Waist observed behind ribs when viewed from above. Abdomen tucked up when viewed from side.

**Overfed**

**6** Ribs palpable with slight excess fat covering. Waist is discernible viewed from above but is not prominent. Abdominal tuck apparent.

**7** Ribs palpable with difficulty; heavy fat cover. Noticeable fat deposits over lumbar area and base of tail. Waist absent or barely visible. Abdominal tuck may be present.

**8** Ribs not palpable under very heavy fat cover, or palpable only with significant pressure. Heavy fat deposits over lumbar area and base of tail. Waist absent. No abdominal tuck. Obvious abdominal distention may be present.

**9** Massive fat deposits over thorax, spine and base of tail. Waist and abdominal tuck absent. Fat deposits on neck and limbs. Obvious abdominal distention.

The **BODY CONDITION SYSTEM** was developed at the Nestlé Purina Pet Care Center and has been validated as documented in the following publications:

Mawby D, Bartges JW, Moyers T, et. al. *Comparison of body fat estimates by dual-energy x-ray absorptiometry and deuterium oxide dilution in client owned dogs.* Compendium 2001; 23 (9A): 70

Laflamme DP. *Development and Validation of a Body Condition Score System for Dogs.* Canine Practice July/August 1997; 22:10-15

Kealy, et. al. *Effects of Diet Restriction on Life Span and Age-Related Changes in Dogs.* JAVMA 2002; 220:1315-1320

**Call 1-800-222-VETS (8387), weekdays, 8:00 a.m. to 4:30 p.m. CT**

### Nestlé PURINA

## 16.C

Off-label use of large animal formulations of common medications such as ivermectin may be cost–effective and enhance efficiency. However, preestablished dosing charts are recommended to minimize errors. *Note that food-grade propylene glycol or glycerol should be used for dilution of oral ivermectin; these can be sourced online and from most commercial food stores. Alternative diluents are not recommended.*

### Off-label use of ivermectin

**Ivermectin is available in a 1% injectable solution for use in cattle and swine (Ivomec®).** This solution can be used off-label to treat both internal and external parasites in dogs and cats.

#### Gastrointestinal parasite treatment

To treat hookworms *(0.05 mg/kg)*, roundworms *(0.2 mg/kg)*, and whipworms *(0.1 mg/kg)*, give 1% ivermectin orally or subcutaneously at a dose of **0.1 ml per 10 pounds** of body weight:

| Body weight in pounds | Volume (ml) |
|---|---|
| 10 | 0.1 |
| 15 | 0.15 |
| 20 | 0.2 |
| 25 | 0.25 |
| 30 | 0.3 |
| 35 | 0.35 |
| 40 | 0.4 |
| 45 | 0.45 |
| 50 | 0.5 |

#### External parasite treatment

To treat *Sarcoptes* mites and ear mites in dogs and cats *(0.3 mg/kg)*, give 1% ivermectin orally or subcutaneously (or topically for ear mites) at a dose of **0.15 ml per 10 pounds** of body weight:

To treat *Demodex* mites in dogs *(0.6 mg/kg)*, start at 0.1 ml per 10 pounds and gradually increase to a once daily dose of **0.3 ml per 10 pounds** of body weight:

| Body weight in pounds | Volume (ml) (0.3 mg/kg) | Volume (ml) (0.6 mg/kg) |
|---|---|---|
| 10 | 0.15 | 0.30 |
| 20 | 0.30 | 0.60 |
| 30 | 0.45 | 0.90 |
| 40 | 0.60 | 1.2 |
| 50 | 0.75 | 1.5 |

#### Heartworm prevention

To use 1% ivermectin solution as a heartworm preventive for dogs *(0.006–0.024 mg/kg)*:

**1. Dilute 1 part of 1% ivermectin solution in 9 parts of propylene glycol.**
*This will create a 1 mg/ml or 0.1% solution.*

**2. Administer 0.1 ml per 10 pounds of body weight by mouth once per month.**
*E.g., A 15 pound dog would receive 0.15 ml of diluted solution.*

| Body weight in pounds | Volume of diluted solution (mL) |
|---|---|
| <5 | 0.01 |
| 5–20 | 0.05 |
| 21–38 | 0.1 |
| 39–55 | 0.15 |
| 56–75 | 0.2 |
| 76–93 | 0.25 |

*Note: This dose is safe for all breeds of dogs, including those that are sensitive to ivermectin-related compounds (such as Collies, Australian Shepherds, Shetland Sheepdogs, and Longhaired Whippets). Dosages of ivermectin for prevention and treatment of other parasites may not be safe for ivermectin-sensitive breeds.*

*Common signs of ivermectin toxicity include dilated pupils and weakness in the hind limbs. Blindness, tremors, seizures, vomiting, and salivation can also be seen. Discontinue use and consult with your veterinarian if any of these signs are seen or suspected.*

# References

1 American Veterinary Medical Foundation. (2016) Partners for healthy pets [online]. Available at: http://www.partnersforhealthypets.org/ (accessed 15 May 2016).

2 Butterworth, A., Mench, J.A., and Wielebnowski, N. (2011). Practical Strategies to Assess (and Improve) Welfare. In: Animal Welfare, 2e (ed. M.C. Appleby, J.A. Mench, I.A.S. Olsson, et al.), 200–214. Oxfordshire: CAB International.

3 McMillan, F.C. (2013). Quality of Life, Stress, and Emotional Pain in Shelter Animals. In: Shelter Medicine for Veterinarians and Staff, 2e (ed. L. Miller and S. Zawistowski), 83–92. Ames: Wiley-Blackwell.

4 Yeates, J. (2013). Clinical Choices. In: Animal Welfare in Veterinary Practice (ed. J. Yeates), 89–112. Oxford: Wiley-Blackwell.

5 Farm Animal Welfare Council. (2009) Farm animal welfare in Great Britain: past, present, and future [online]. Available at: https://www.gov.uk/government/uploads/system/uploads/attachment_data/file/319292/Farm_Animal_Welfare_in_Great_Britain_-_Past__Present_and_Future.pdf (accessed 15 May 2016).

6 Griffin, B. (2009). Wellness. In: Shelter Medicine for Veterinarians and Staff, 2e (ed. L. Miller and S. Zawistowski), 17–38. Ames: Wiley-Blackwell.

7 World Small Animal Veterinary Association. Microchip identification guidelines [online]. Available at: http://www.wsava.org/guidelines/microchip-identification-guidelines (accessed 15 May 2016).

8 Resiner, I.R. (2016) Preventing dog bites in children. Part 1: Motivation & Myths. Today's Veterinary Practice **May/June**, 34–36. Saunders Elsevier, St. Louis.

9 Mathews, K., Kronen, P.W., Lascelles, D. et al. (2014). Guidelines for recognition, assessment, and treatment of pain. *Journal of Small Animal Practice* 55: E10–E68.

10 Yin, S. (2009a). General Handling Principles. In: Low Stress Handling, Restraint, and Behavior Modification of Dogs and Cats (ed. S. Yin), 191–230. Davis: Cattle Dog Publishing.

11 Santos, O., Polo, G., Garcia, R. et al. (2013). Grouping protocol in shelters. *Journal of Veterinary Behavior* 8: 3–8.

12 Yin, S. (2009b). Restraint for standard positions in cats. In: Low Stress Handling, Restraint, and Behavior Modification of Dogs and Cats (ed. S. Yin), 341–367. Davis: Cattle Dog Publishing.

13 Yin, S. (2009c). Handling difficult cats. In: Low Stress Handling, Restraint, and Behavior Modification of Dogs and Cats (ed. S. Yin), 387–403. Davis: Cattle Dog Publishing.

14 Day, M.J., Horzinek, M.C., Schultz, R.D. et al. (2016). Guidelines for the vaccination of dogs and cats. *Journal of Small Animal Practice* **57**: E1–E45.

15 Ford, R.B., Larson, L.J., McClure, K.D. et al. (2017). AAHA Canine Vaccination Guidelines [online]. Available at: https://www.aaha.org/guidelines/canine_vaccination_guidelines.aspx (accessed 9 March 2018).

16 Sykes, J.E. (2013). Immunization. In: Canine and Feline Infectious Diseases (ed. J.E. Sykes), 119–130. St. Louis: Saunders.

17 Scherk, M.A., Ford, R.B., Gaskell, R.M. et al. (2013). 2013 AAFP Feline Vaccination Advisory Panel report. *Journal of Feline Medicine and Surgery* **15**: 785–808.

18 Richards, J.R., Elston, T.H., Ford, R.B. et al. (2006). The 2006 American Association of Feline Practitioners Feline Vaccine Advisory Panel report. *Journal of Feline Medicine and Surgery* **299**: 1405–1441.

19 Toshach, K., Jackson, M.W., and Dubielzig, R.R. Hepatocellular necrosis associated with the subcutaneous injection of an intranasal *Bordetella bronchiseptica*-canine parainfluenza vaccine. *Journal of the American Animal Hospital Association* **33**: 126–128.

20 Zajac, A.M. and Conboy, G.A. (2012b). Detection of parasites in the blood. In: Veterinary Clinical Parasitology, 8e (ed. A.M. Zajac and G.A. Conboy), 185–211. Ames: Wiley-Blackwell.

21 Greiner, E. (2012). Diagnosis of arthropod parasites. In: Veterinary Clinical Parasitology, 8e (ed. A.M. Zajac and G.A. Conboy), 217–303. Ames: Wiley-Blackwell.

22 Zajac, A.M. and Conboy, G.A. (2012a). Fecal examination for the diagnosis of parasitism. In: Veterinary Clinical Parasitology, 8e (ed. A.M. Zajac and G.A. Conboy), 3–170. Ames: Wiley-Blackwell.

23 American Association of Veterinary Parasitologists. (2014), [online], available: www.aavp.org (accessed 15 May 2001).

24 Blagburn, B.L. and Dryden, M.W. (2009). Biology, treatment, and control of flea and tick infestations. *Veterinary Clinics of North America: Small Animal Practice* **39**: 1173–1200.

25 National Park Service. (2010) Integrated Pest Management Manual [online]. Available at: http://www.nature.nps.gov/biology/ipm/manual/ticks.cfm (27 September 2016).

26 American Animal Hospital Association-American Veterinary Medical Association Preventive Healthcare Guidelines Task Force (2011). Development of new canine and feline preventive healthcare guidelines designed to improve pet health. *Journal of the American Animal Hospital Association* **46**: 306–311.

27 Hurley, K. and Pesavento, P. Disease recognition and diagnostic testing. In: Shelter Medicine for Veterinarians and Staff, 2e (ed. L. Miller and S. Zawistowski), 329–341. Ames: Wiley-Blackwell.

28 Nolen, R.S. (2013). Study shines spotlight on neutering. *Journal of the American Veterinary Medical Association* **243**: 1218–1237.

29 Norwegian Animal Welfare Act. (2009) [online]. Available at: https://www.regjeringen.no/en/dokumenter/animal-welfare-act/id571188/ (accessed 23 May 2016).

30 Wikipedia. (2016) Religious views on neutering [online]. Available at: https://en.wikipedia.org/wiki/Neutering#Religious_views_on_neutering (accessed 23 May 2016).

31 Root Kustritz, M.V. (2012). Effects of surgical sterilization on canine and feline health and on society. *Reproduction in Domestic Animals* **47**: 214–222.

32 Sanderson, S.L. (2010) Nutritional requirements and related diseases of small animals. In: *The Merck Veterinary Manual*. (eds C.M. Kahn & S. Line), 10e, Merck.

33 Miller, L. & Janeczko, S. Canine care in the animal shelter. In: *Shelter Medicine for Veterinarians and Staff*. (eds L. Miller & S. Zawistowski), 2e, pp. 115–144. Wiley-Blackwell, Ames.

34 Plunkett, S.J. (2013). Estimating the degree of dehydration. In: Emergency Procedures for the Small Animal Veterinarian, 2e (ed. S.J. Plunkett), 475. St. Louis: Saunders Elsevier.

# 17

# Prevention Considerations for Common Zoonotic Diseases
*Amie Burling*

*University of Missouri, College of Veterinary Medicine, 900 E. Campus Dr., Columbia, MO 65211, USA*

## 17.1 Introduction

Veterinary medical personnel interface with dogs and cats in numerous scenarios that increase the risk of zoonotic disease transmission. From examining ill animals and handling diagnostic samples containing potentially infectious material to performing necropsies, the potential for animal-to-human infection exceeds most routine interactions between people and household pets. Field conditions involving a less controlled environment, limited access to equipment and supplies, and the presence of unfamiliar diseases can increase zoonotic risks considerably.

Compliance of veterinarians with recommendations to utilize personal protective equipment and adopt workplace behaviors that minimize zoonotic disease risk may have significant latitude for improvement in traditional practice [1]. Barriers to implementing these measures in field conditions could make compliance even more challenging. Demanding conditions necessitate increased attention to personal health and safety.

The goal of this chapter is to provide veterinary personnel working with dogs and cats in remote settings with two sets of information:

1) A summary of practical self-protective measures for anyone working with sick dogs and cats under varying field conditions.
2) A basic reference guide for the most common zoonotic diseases encountered in dogs and cats around the world.

Please use this chapter to make your work on behalf of animals more effective and rewarding by protecting yourself from zoonotic pathogens. For more detailed information Table 17.1 provides additional resources.

---

**Textbox 17.1  Useful compendia**

- **Compendium of veterinary standard precautions for zoonotic disease prevention in veterinary personnel: national association of state public health veterinarians: veterinary infection control committee.** (2015) Williams C.J., Scheftel J. M., Elchos B.L., et al. Journal of the American Veterinary Medical Association, **247**, 1252–1277.
- **Compendium of animal rabies prevention and control.** (2016) Brown C.M., Slavinski S., Ettestad P., et al. Journal of the American Veterinary Medical Association, **248**, 505–517.
- **Compendium of measures to prevent disease associated with animals in public settings.** (2013) National Association of State Public Health Veterinarians. Journal of the American Veterinary Medical Association, **243**, 1270–1288.

---

## 17.2 Safe Practices to Avoid Zoonotic Diseases [2]

Before you begin working with sick or high-risk dogs and cats, ask yourself:[1]

---

1 Materials adapted from Dr. Danielle Buttke, Public Health Veterinarian and One Health Coordinator, Wildlife Health Branch of the United States National Park Service.

**Table 17.1** Key sources of information on zoonotic disease prevention and management.

| | |
|---|---|
| World Organisation for Animal Health (OIE) | Provides:<br>• Transparency in global animal disease<br>• Veterinary scientific information<br>• Solidarity in the control of animal diseases<br>• Resources for national veterinary services<br>• http://www.oie.int/ |
| World Health Organization (WHO) | Directs and coordinates international health within the United Nations' system in the areas of<br>• Health systems<br>• Noncommunicable diseases<br>• Communicable diseases<br>• Preparedness, surveillance, and response<br>• http://www.who.int |
| Center for Food Safety and Public Health (CFSPH) | Provides:<br>• Information on transboundary animal diseases and zoonotic diseases<br>• Online education for veterinary students and animal health professionals<br>• Tools for infection control<br>• Resources for local, state, and federal agencies to prepare for animal emergencies<br>• http://www.cfsph.iastate.edu |
| Centers for Disease Control and Prevention (CDC) | Role:<br>• Responding to emerging health threats<br>• Using science and technology to prevent disease<br>• Promoting health and safe behaviors<br>• Training public health workforce<br>• http://www.cdc.gov |

- What are the potential disease risks or hazards in this area and/or with this species?
- What are the symptoms of these diseases in dogs, cats, and humans?
- What personal protective equipment (PPE) will I need before beginning to work?
- Do I have the necessary skills and resources?
- Do specific health concerns exist, such as pregnancy or compromised immune system?
- Is there a need for pre-exposure vaccination?
- Discuss specific health concerns with your physician.

- Do any red flags exist? Red flags include the following:
  - Multiple dead animals of unknown cause
  - Blood coming from orifices (nose, mouth rectum, etc.) without obvious signs of trauma
  - An animal exhibiting neurologic signs
- How do I properly handle, store, and ship specimens?
- Do I have contact information for everyone who may have had contact with the animal so that they can be contacted should a zoonotic disease be identified in the animal?

---

**Textbox 17.2 Tips for preventing exposure to zoonotic disease**

*Prepare.* Use available resources to identify potential zoonotic pathogens.

*Plan.* Determine potential routes of transmission.

*Execute.* Select and implement appropriate safe work practices and PPE.

---

### 17.2.1 Standard Precautions

When working with animals or potentially infectious materials, it is important to take minimum standard precautions. Always use protective barriers such as gloves and avoid bites, scratches, and physical injury. After removing gloves, wash hands thoroughly with soap and water and disinfect soiled equipment and contaminated environmental surfaces or items. Eating, drinking, or smoking is not allowed while handling animals, and it is recommended to work in well-ventilated areas when indoors and upwind of specimen when working outdoors. Make sure that samples are transported and stored properly, and avoid needle-sticks or cuts. Anyone developing clinical signs of disease must seek medical attention and inform provider of potential disease exposures.

## 17.3 Hand Hygiene [2]

Hand hygiene is an essential part of preventing disease spread [3]. All staff and volunteers should be trained to use gloves whenever indicated, as well as proper handwashing routines. Hands should be washed after touching animals or their supplies, equipment, or environment, as well as after leaving animal care areas. Whenever taking off clothing or shoes that have been in contact with animals, hand-washing is indicated. As in any setting, hands should be washed after going to the bathroom and before handling food, eating, or drinking.

## 17.4 Exposure Routes [2]

### 17.4.1 Selecting Personal Protective Equipment (PPE) Based on Routes of Exposure

Pathogens from animals are transmitted by three major routes of exposure:

I)  *Contact.* The single most common source of transmission is through contact, particularly touching eyes, nose, or mouth with contaminated hands. The most effective tool for protection is good hand hygiene:
    – Wear gloves when making contact with an animal, their fluids, or a contaminated environment.
    – Always wash hands with soap and water after removing gloves, touching potentially contaminated surfaces or tools, and before eating, drinking, smoking, or using a cell phone.
    – Hand sanitizer, while not a substitute for soap and water, can be useful in the field when you are unable to wash hands immediately.
    Contact precautions should be considered for situations where clothing or materials may be contaminated. If handling a larger animal, conducting a messy procedure, or working in a particularly contaminated environment, wear dedicated coveralls that can be laundered separately or disposable coveralls and boot covers.
    Evaluate if the activity could generate splashes or droplets. If the answer is "yes" or "I don't know," wear protective goggles or a splash guard to prevent droplets from contacting your eyes, nose, or mouth.

II) *Aerosol.* While you should always work in a well-ventilated area and work upwind of a potentially contaminated area or carcass, extra precautions against aerosol transmission are needed in a few situations. Understand the species that you are working with, the geographic range of the high-risk pathogens, and environments and activities that are likely to aerosolize these pathogens.
    – Wearing any respirator requires prior medical clearance, and half-face or face-fitting respirators require annual fit testing to ensure a proper seal is formed between the respirator and the face. Otherwise, the respirator may not be protective. Ensure filter is appropriate to the potential agent of concern and is replaced as needed.
    – Dust masks and face-fitting respirators look very similar but differ greatly in their ability to protect you against infectious agents. A respirator will typically have a "NIOSH" label on the front and two elastic straps while a dust mask only has one strap and no label (Figure 17.1).

III) *Vector.* Be especially vigilant about fleas, ticks, and vector-borne diseases when working with sick dogs or cats in outdoor settings, as these diseases may be the reason for the illness of the animal, placing you at higher risk. Remember that ticks can be active at temperatures as low as 6 °C (42.8 °F).

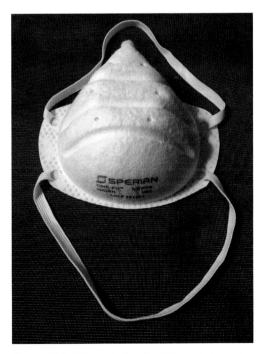

**Figure 17.1** N95 respirator. An N95 respirator is designed to block 95% of very small (0.3 micron) particles. If properly fitted, the filtration capabilities of N95 respirators exceed those of face masks.

> **Textbox 17.3 Strategies to help protect you from vector-borne disease**
>
> - Wear an insect repellent containing DEET and/or wear permethrin-treated clothing.
> - Wear long pants and sleeves and tuck pants into socks or wear dedicated or disposable coveralls with elastic wrist and ankle closures.
> - Conduct tick checks immediately following fieldwork.
> - Shower within 2 h of returning from the field.

### 17.4.2 Human Use of Mosquito and Tick Repellents

Different repellents work against different arthropods, so it is important that you select the appropriate repellent for your task. The following guidelines can help you select the right repellent (Table 17.2). All repellents should be washed from skin before sleeping for the night. Investigate repellent safety information for dogs and cats separately.

## 17.5 Personal Protective Equipment (PPE) [2]

### 17.5.1 Safe Donning of Personal Protective Equipment (PPE)

Before you begin an activity, it is recommended to define the areas you are working in according to risk:

dirty area (high risk) → Clean area (lowest risk) → Decontaminated area.

Make sure you have assembled all necessary disinfection and disposal materials, and inspect all personal protective equipment to be sure it is in working order. Then proceed to put on, or don PPE.

*Steps*

1) Put on eye protection and respirator if using these items, and ensure that a proper seal between respirator and face has formed.
2) Pull on coveralls and inspect for any holes. If coveralls have a hood, pull hood over the straps of the respirator and eye protection.
3) Pull on boot covers or boots, pulling the coverall cuffs OVER the boots or boot covers. Tape the coverall cuff/boot cover junction if there is concern about biting fleas/ticks.
4) Pull on gloves and pull coverall cuffs OVER the cuffs of the gloves. If using a second layer of gloves, the cuffs of the second layer of gloves can be pulled over the coveralls. Tape the coverall/glove juncture if there is concern about fleas/ticks.

### 17.5.2 Safe Doffing of PPE

After completing the activity, move to the decontamination area and remove (doff) PPE.

Table 17.2 Insect repellent guide.

| Repellent | Activity against ticks | Activity against mosquitos | Concentration | Contradictions |
|---|---|---|---|---|
| DEET (*N,N*-diethyl-m-toluamide)[a] | X | X | 30% | Do not use in infants under 2 months of age. Do not use concentrations over 30% on children. |
| IR3535 (3-[*N*-butyl- *N*-acetyl]-aminopropionic acid) | X | X | 20% | |
| Picaridin (KBR 3023) | | X | 5–10% for ≤2 hours; 20% for longer | |
| Oil of lemon Eucalyptus [*p*-menthane 3, 8-diol (PMD)] | X | X | 10% for ≤2 hours; 30–40 for longer | Do not use on children under 3 years old. |
| Permethrin | X | X | 0.5% | Do not apply to skin; only intended for use on clothing, shoes, bed, nets, etc. |

*a* Most products containing IR3535 and oil of lemon eucalyptus are US Environmental Protection Agency (US EPA) registered for use against ticks; however, the CDC currently recommends DEET and permethrin for protection against ticks. Be sure and read the label of any product you select for guidance on its usage. DEET concentrations above 30% do not significantly increase the level of protection, but do last longer.

*Steps for Doffing*

1) Unzip the front of the coveralls. Pull from shoulders and roll coveralls off of torso and downward toward ankles. Roll coveralls down over outside of boot covers. Remove second layer of gloves with coveralls, leaving the first layer of gloves on.

2) Step out of the boot covers into a clean zone. If you are wearing reusable boots without covers, roll the coveralls off of the boots, disinfect the boots, then step into the clean zone. Place coveralls and boot covers in disposal bag.

3) Remove the first soiled glove by gripping the palm of one gloved hand with the fingers of the other gloved hand and pulling the glove off. DO NOT slide a gloved thumb under the cuff of a glove to be removed.

4) Once the first glove has been removed, keep the removed glove in the remaining gloved hand. Slide ungloved thumb under the cuff of the gloved hand and pull down, pulling the glove inside out over the first glove. The first glove should end up in the inverted second glove. Dispose in a bag.

*Safety Tips*

- After removing PPE, wash hands thoroughly with soap and water or hand sanitizer before removing eye protection and respirator.
- Remove eye protection and respirator, taking care to use the straps to remove and not touch the exposed front areas of the eye protection and respirator.

## 17.6 Needle-Stick Injuries

Needle-stick injuries can cause physical injury resulting in loss of function, direct inoculation with infectious biologics and pharmaceuticals, or route of entry for zoonotic pathogens. It is therefore imperative to prevent these kinds of injuries [4]. This can be done by the following:

- Avoid recapping needles. If the needle must be recapped:
  - Place the cap on a horizontal surface.
  - Hold the syringe and needle.
  - Scoop up the cap without touching it.
  - Push the cap against a hard surface to secure.
- Place needles in a sturdy container that can withstand punctures and leaks.
- Avoid
  - Bending needles
  - Passing uncapped needle between people
  - Walking with an uncapped needle
  - Placing needle caps in mouth.

## 17.7 Management of Dog and Cat Bite Wounds in Humans

Whenever there is a bite incident, it is important to follow standard procedures [5]. These procedures should be familiar to all participants, whether staff or volunteers, and should be written down and easily accessible to everyone [6, 7].

When a person has been bitten, it is important to irrigate and clean the wound immediately. Flushing the wound as soon as possible can help reduce the risk of infection and can also help remove easily dislodged dirt, foreign objects, and tissue. Minor wounds can be washed thoroughly with soap and potable water. Large or contaminated wounds should be irrigated using normal saline or Lactated Ringer's Solution (LRS) copiously at a volume of 100–200 ml/in. (500 ml minimum, at least a liter on large or dirty wounds). A 16–19 gauge needle or catheter on a 35 ml or larger syringe can help to create irrigation pressure, but avoid injecting the tissue directly. Wear eye protection or a face shield to avoid contamination from the wound. Potable water can be used in the absence of sterile fluids. Appropriately immobilize and elevate the affected area and seek professional medical help for further management of the wound.

In the event of heavy bleeding, apply pressure, elevate the area if possible, and seek immediate medical treatment.

---

**Textbox 17.4 Reasons for seeking professional medical care as soon as possible following a bite**

- Minimize infection risk
- Control bleeding
- Expedite healing
- Decrease risk of requiring evacuation for advanced care
- Reduce risk of long-term loss of function
- Assess the need for rabies postexposure treatment and tetanus vaccination.

---

To aid medical personnel in ensuring appropriate care, the following information should be provided:

- Circumstances of the bite – time, location, environmental conditions, provoked, or unprovoked
- Details of the dog or cat that bit – species, breed, health status, behavior, known vaccination history, and current location
- Any wound treatment already performed including irrigation

- Bite victim's medical history – preexisting disease, allergies, immune compromise, current medications, and vaccination history including tetanus and rabies
- Preexisting medical conditions that increase the risk of infection following an animal bite in humans (i.e. diabetes mellitus, liver disease, mastectomy, prosthetic implants, splenectomy, systemic lupus erythematosus, and immune-compromise or chronic disease).

### 17.7.1 Prophylaxis

All staff and volunteers should be informed regarding the risks involved in bite incidents and potential for zoonotic disease as a consequence. It is important that you know which team members have previously received tetanus and rabies vaccines, and it may even be a consideration whether a current tetanus and rabies vaccine be required for staff and volunteers, depending on the level of risk in the region you are operating.

#### 17.7.1.1 Administration of Tetanus Prophylaxis

The Advisory Council on Immunization Practices (ACIP) issues recommendations for when tetanus prophylaxis is indicated in wound management, and this should be considered together with medical personnel whenever a bite incident has occurred.

Factors when considering tetanus prophylaxis:

- Wound contamination and severity
- Number of doses of adsorbed tetanus toxoid vaccine received previously and time since last dose.

#### 17.7.1.2 Administration of Rabies Prophylaxis

- Vaccines are used prior to exposure for those at risk and as a part of postexposure prophylaxis after a bite [8].
- Rabies immunoglobulin is used as part of postexposure prophylaxis.
- Specific recommendations are issued by the WHO and ACIP.

## 17.8 Rabies Prevention and Control

### 17.8.1 Key Points About the Rabies Virus

- Transmitted in saliva through animal bites [9].
- Incubation in domestic animals can range from a few days to 6 months but is typically 3–12 weeks.

- Virus is shed in saliva, and therefore transmittable in a bite, for only days before clinical illness develops.
- Clinical signs include dysphagia, ataxia, paralysis, altered behavior, nerve deficits, vocalization, seizures, and rapid death.
- Antiviral drugs are not effective.

---

**Textbox 17.5 Pre-exposure prophylaxis guidelines for humans**

Human pre-exposure prophylaxis is advised for those whose risk of rabies exposure is frequent, ongoing, or heightened due to occupation or location. Examples include laboratory workers handling high-risk tissues, veterinarians, other animal handlers, and travelers based on a risk assessment for exposure. Children in rabies-endemic areas are at particular risk.

The schedule for the human pre-exposure prophylaxis vaccination series listed below should be completed in the stipulated time; however, there is no need to restart the series if the doses are not given exactly on schedule.

*Intramuscular administration.* One intramuscular dose is given on each of days 0, 7, and 21 or 28. Day 0 is the date of administration of the first dose of vaccine.

*Intradermal administration.* One intradermal injection is given on each of days 0, 7, and 21 or 28. To maximize savings, sessions of intradermal pre-exposure prophylaxis should involve enough individuals to use all opened vials within 6 h.

Source: Adapted from WHO Expert Consultation on Rabies 2013 [10]

---

### 17.8.2 Diagnosis in Animals

The gold standard is the direct fluorescent antibody test. This test requires the entire intact brain to be submitted to a laboratory. Refrigeration is recommended over freezing or chemical fixation.

There are unlicensed point-of-care tests available. These are *not* recommended due to validity concerns, intermittent viral presence in tissues outside of the brain, and the public health risk of unreliable results. There are currently no reliable confirmatory antemortem diagnostic tests for rabies infection in animals.

### 17.8.3 Prevention and Control in Dogs and Cats

#### 17.8.3.1 Serology in Animals

Antibody titers are not a reliable substitute for vaccination due to unknown correlation with actual protection when the immune system responds to infection. Although rabies virus antibody levels rise as a result of vaccination or infection, other immunologic factors that determine virus progression or repression are not well understood. Vaccination and postexposure management decisions should not be based on rabies virus antibody titers in animals.

#### 17.8.3.2 Pre-exposure Vaccination

Vaccination is critical to rabies prevention in domestic animals. Local laws may dictate that parenteral rabies vaccination must be administered by or under the direct supervision of a veterinarian to ensure correct product storage and administration.

Full immunologic response to vaccination is considered complete by 28 days after the first injection. All animals should receive another vaccine 1 year later, unless using an approved 3 year product. Vaccination intervals should follow the manufacturer's label. Any animal overdue for vaccination should be vaccinated immediately and is then considered current and can follow the manufacturer's label for future vaccination intervals.

#### 17.8.3.3 Importation of Dogs from Rabies Endemic Countries

Dogs moved from countries with endemic canine rabies virus variant are a significant public health concern. Imported dogs should have a documented history of current rabies vaccination, and all appropriate public health authorities in the destination country or region should be notified.

#### 17.8.3.4 Postexposure Management of Dogs and Cats Exposed to Rabies

A rabies exposure is considered to be introduction of infected saliva or neural tissue into an open wound or mucous membrane. Wild carnivores, skunks, and bats that cannot be tested are considered to be a possible source of rabies exposure. Progression of rabies virus from initial exposure to development of clinical signs can take months; observation and quarantine of exposed dogs and cats are determined by vaccination status:

- Current on rabies vaccination: provide wound care and rabies booster vaccination. In-home quarantine for 45 days.
- Overdue for rabies booster vaccine with documentation of previous licensed vaccination: wound care, immediate vaccination, and 45 day in-home quarantine.
- No history of rabies vaccination: either immediate vaccination and 4-month quarantine in strict confinement or euthanasia.

#### 17.8.3.5 Management of Dogs and Cats Following a Bite to a Human

Rabies virus is present in the saliva of infected animals for only days before clinical signs are apparent, followed by death; observation and quarantine of potentially rabid animals is not impacted by vaccination status:

- All dogs and cats should be observed for 10 days following a bite to a human, regardless of vaccination history.
- Administering a rabies vaccine booster during this quarantine period is not recommended due to the risk of an adverse vaccine reaction that could appear similar to early signs of clinical rabies.
- Development of illness consistent with rabies should result in euthanasia and submission of the brain for diagnostic testing.

## 17.9 Enteric Diseases

### 17.9.1 Introduction

Enteric diseases primarily originate from the gastrointestinal tract of source animals and people, and the typical transmission route is fecal-oral [11–18]. These diseases are among the most frequently occurring zoonoses, and it is not uncommon for healthy animals and people to shed infectious pathogens without exhibiting any clinical signs (Table 17.3).

### 17.9.2 Important Prevention Strategies

Avoid stress and overcrowding of dogs and cats and provide routine veterinary preventive care including parasite control to dogs and cats. The feeding of raw diets should also be avoided.

Ensure that all staff and volunteers are informed about potential zoonotic risks and facilitate good

**Table 17.3** Selected enteric diseases of importance in transmission from dogs and/or cats to humans.

| Pathogen | Type | Notes |
|---|---|---|
| *Campylobacter jejuni*<br>*C. upsaliensis* | Bacteria | • Significant cause of human enteritis.<br>• Cats and dogs can be subclinical or have GI signs including vomiting, bloody diarrhea, and fever. |
| *Clostridium difficile* | Bacteria | • Considered a significant cause of enteritis, especially diarrhea, in humans, cats, and dogs.<br>• Interspecies transmission has not been proven.<br>• Zoonotic risk, as well as transmission from humans to pets, is suspected. |
| *Salmonella* spp. | Bacteria | • Not part of the normal intestinal flora of most dogs and cats.<br>• Ingesting contaminated food can cause fecal shedding for a week in dogs.<br>• Signs in dogs and cats range from subclinical-to-mild diarrhea to hemorrhagic gastroenteritis.<br>• Transmission to humans has been documented more frequently from cats than from dogs. |
| *Escherichia coli* | Bacteria | • Found in healthy animals and can cause diarrhea in dogs and cats and hemolytic uremia in dogs. |
| Dogs:<br>*Ancylostoma caninum,*<br>*A. braziliense*<br>*Unicinaria stenocephala*<br>Cats:<br>*A. tubaeforme,*<br>*A. braziliense*<br>*Unicinaria stenocephala* | Hookworms | • Dogs and cats ingest larvae from the environment or through vertical transmission.<br>• Can cause anemia and pneumonia in young animals.<br>• Prompt removal of feces, fecal testing, and routine deworming of dogs and cats, especially puppies and kittens, are important for prevention.<br>• Can cause cutaneous larval migrans in humans.<br>• Eggs are very difficult to remove from the environment. |
| *Baylisascaris procyonis* | Raccoon Roundworms | • Raccoons are the reservoir, but dogs can be infected, usually subclinically.<br>• Can cause severe neurologic, visceral, and ocular disease in humans due to larval migration.<br>• Eggs are very difficult to remove from the environment.<br>• Routine deworming of dogs is important for prevention. |
| Dogs:<br>*Toxocara canis*<br>*T. leonina*<br>Cats:<br>*T. cati* and *T. leonine* | Roundworms | • Dogs and cats ingest larvae from the environment or through vertical transmission.<br>• Prompt removal of feces, fecal testing, and routine deworming of dogs and cats, especially puppies and kittens, are important for prevention.<br>• Can cause visceral larval migrans in humans.<br>• Persists in the environment. |
| *Strongyloides stercoralis* | Threadworms | • Of greater potential zoonotic significance in dogs than in cats.<br>• Most infections in dogs and cats are subclinical and self-limiting.<br>• Genetic typing is now indicating that differences in strains between species infecting dogs and humans could make zoonotic potential less concerning; however, species and host adaption is known to occur. |
| *Echinococcus multilocularis*<br>*Echinococcus granulosus* | Tapeworms | • See disease profile section.<br>• Most infections in dogs and cats are subclinical.<br>• Routine deworming of dogs and cats with praziquantel every 3–4 weeks is recommended in endemic areas.<br>• Eggs shed in feces of infected dogs and cats are immediately infective to humans. |
| *Cryptosporidium* spp. | Protozoa | • Most infections in dogs and cats are subclinical.<br>• Significant zoonotic concern for immunocompromised people and animals. |
| *Giardia* spp. | Protozoa | • Common in dogs and cats but can be difficult to diagnose due to intermittent shedding.<br>• Test symptomatic animals with diarrhea.<br>• Prevention is prompt removal of feces and bathing of treated animals to remove fecal contaminants.<br>• Persists in the environment. |
| *Toxoplasma gondii* | Protozoa | • See disease profile section. |

hand hygiene (see Chapter 11). It is also prudent to take extra precautions to prevent exposure of people at high risk of clinical infection including individuals who are

- <5 years of age
- >65 years of age
- Pregnant
- Immunocompromised.

## 17.10 Vector-Borne Diseases

Dogs and cats are important sentinels of diseases transmitted by arthropod vectors; however, these diseases are not primarily zoonotic and are not described in detail here. Prevention methods for diseases transmitted by ticks and mosquitoes were outlined earlier in the chapter. Note that direct transmission potential from dogs and cats to humans is still under investigation for many of these diseases, and barrier precautions are strongly advised when handling animals and diagnostic samples with suspected infection. A selected list of these diseases is provided in Table 17.4 for further reference.

## 17.11 Diseases with Zoonotic Risk of Transmission from Dogs and Cats to Humans

This section is intended to provide basic key information on distribution, clinical signs, and specific prevention recommendations for selected zoonotic diseases of dogs and cats. It is not intended as an exhaustive list or as a guide for diagnosis or treatment; rather, it should allow for quick reference of zoonotic diseases that are relatively common, rare but highly significant, or of note in a particular geographic area.

**Table 17.4** Selected vector-borne diseases of dogs and cats that also infect humans.

| Flea-borne | Tick-borne | Sandfly-borne |
| --- | --- | --- |
| *Rickettsia felis* | *Borrelia burgdorferi* | *Leishmania infantum* |
| *Rickettsia typhi* | *Anaplasma phagocytophilum* | *L. chagasi* |
| | *Ehrlichia spp.* | |
| | *Rickettsia rickettsii* | |

Not included in this list are diseases that have a common environmental source but that are not directly transmitted from dogs and cats to people such as *Blastomyces dermatitidis* and screw-worm myiasis. Dogs and cats are important sentinels of environmental risk to humans for these diseases, but as they are not generally considered truly zoonotic, they have been omitted.

Diseases in this section are listed in three ways: in a summary table (Table 17.5), by geographic distribution (Table 17.6), and alphabetically with key details.

### 17.11.1 Alphabetical Disease Listing

#### 17.11.1.1 Anthrax

*Basic Information*
- *Caused by bacteria. Bacillus anthracis*
- *Arthropod vectors.* No
- Potential bioterrorism pathogen
- *Geographic distribution.* Worldwide, particularly in warm, damp environments [19–21].

*Risk Factors for Human Exposure from Dogs and Cats*
- Dogs and cats are rarely infected and are an uncommon source of human exposure.
- Veterinary personnel handling infected dogs and cats, performing necropsies, or processing diagnostic samples are at greatest risk.

*Clinical Manifestation in Humans*
- *Presentations based on exposure route.* Cutaneous, inhalation/pulmonary (severe), and gastrointestinal (rare)
- *Cutaneous is most common.* Skin ulceration resembling a spider bite followed by edema, lymphadenopathy, and flu-like illness.

*Clinical Manifestation in Dogs and Cats*
- *Oral exposure is most common.* Inhalation is rare.
- Fever, anorexia, lymphadenopathy, toxemia, shock, and hemorrhagic gastroenteritis.
- Cutaneous disease is not reported.

*Prevention*
- Wear gloves and institute barrier protection when working with dogs and cats with suspected history and clinical presentation.
- Use full barrier protection with a face shield when bathing exposed dogs and cats for decontamination.

Table 17.5 Diseases with zoonotic risk of transmission from dogs and cats to humans.

| Disease | Route | | | | | | Species | |
|---|---|---|---|---|---|---|---|---|
| | Contact | GI | Resp | Genital | Urine | Vector | Dog | Cat |
| Anthrax | X | | X | | | | X | X |
| Bartonellosis | X | | | | | X | X | X |
| *Bordetella bronchiseptica* | | | X | | | | X | Rare |
| *Brucella canis* | X | | | X | X | | X | |
| *Capnocytophaga* spp. | X | | | | | | X | X |
| *Cheyletiella* spp. Infection | X | | | | | | Rare | X |
| *Chlamydophila felis* | X | | | | | | | X |
| Cowpox | X | | | | | | | X |
| Glanders | X | | X | | | | X | X |
| Echinococcosis | X | X | | | | X | X | X |
| Hendra | X | | X | | | | Undocumented | Undocumented |
| Influenza | | | X | | | | X | X |
| Leptospirosis | | | | | X | | X | |
| Listeriosis | X | | | | | | X | X |
| Melioidosis | X | | X | | | | X | X |
| Nipah | X | | | | | | Undocumented | Undocumented |
| Plague | X | | X | | | X | rare | X |
| Rat bite fever | X | | | | | | rare | rare |
| Ringworm | X | | | | | | X | X |
| Rift Valley fever | X | | X | | | X | Rare | Rare |
| Sarcoptic mange | X | | | | | | X | rare |
| *Staphylococcus* spp. | X | | | | | | X | X |
| *Streptococcus* spp. | X | | X | | | | X | X |
| Toxoplasmosis | | X | | | | | | X |
| Tuberculosis | X | | X | | | | X | X |
| Tularemia | X | | X | | | X | | X |
| Q fever | | | | X | | rare | X | X |

- Anthrax is not susceptible to most routine disinfectants: use 1 : 10 bleach dilution with complete removal of organic material beforehand.
- Prevent dogs and cats from ingesting livestock carcasses particularly in endemic areas.
- A human vaccine is available with limited access to those with specific high risk of exposure.
- A vaccine for livestock is available.
- No vaccine exists for dogs and cats.

### 17.11.1.2 Bartonellosis

*Basic Information*

- *Caused by bacteria. Bartonella henselae*
- *Arthropod vectors.* Fleas and ticks (unconfirmed)
- *Geographic distribution.* Worldwide, with increased incidence in regions with high temperature and humidity [22–25].

**Table 17.6** Summary table of disease geographic distribution.

| Worldwide | North America |
|---|---|
| Anthrax | *Brucella canis* (South) |
| Bartonellosis | Leptospirosis |
| *Bordetella bronchiseptica* | Plague (West) |
| *Capnocytophaga* spp. | Rat bite fever |
| *Cheyletiella* spp. | Tuberculosis (sporadic) |
| *Chlamydophila felis* | Tularemia (West) |
| Dermatophytosis | |
| Echinococcosis | **Middle East** |
| Influenza | Glanders |
| Listeriosis | Melioidosis |
| Sarcoptic mange | Rift Valley fever |
| Sporotrichosis | Tuberculosis |
| *Staphylococcus* spp. | Tularemia |
| *Streptococcus* spp. | |
| Toxoplasmosis | **Asia** |
| Q fever | *Brucella canis* |
| | Glanders |
| **Central and South America** | Leptospirosis |
| *Brucella canis* | (Southeast) |
| Glanders | Melioidosis (primarily |
| Leptospirosis | Thailand, Malaysia, and |
| Melioidosis | Singapore) |
| Plague (South) | Nipah (primarily |
| Rat bite fever | Malaysia, Bangladesh, |
| Sporotrichosis | northern India, and the |
| (focal area in Brazil) | Philippines) |
| | Plague |
| **Europe** | Rat bite fever |
| *Brucella canis* (rare) | Tuberculosis |
| Cowpox (West and the United | Tularemia (Central) |
| Kingdom) | |
| Plague (East) | **Australia** |
| Rat bite fever | Hendra |
| Tuberculosis (sporadic) | Melioidosis |
| Tularemia (rare) | |
| | **New Zealand** |
| **Africa** | Tuberculosis (sporadic) |
| *Brucella canis* | |
| Glanders | |
| Melioidosis | |
| Plague | |
| Rift Valley fever | |
| Tuberculosis | |
| Tularemia (North) | |

## Risk Factors for Human Exposure from Dogs and Cats

- Most human cases occur due to a scratch from a cat.

- Cats under 2 years of age are at a higher risk of transmitting infection.
- *B. henselae* is of greatest zoonotic significance.

### Clinical Manifestation in Humans

- *Cat scratch disease.* Fever, enlarged lymph nodes, pustules
- *Complications.* Endocarditis, uveitis, neurological conditions
- *Increased risk with immunocompromise.* Bacillary angiomatosis with skin, bone, and organ lesions, and bacillary peliosis with lesions of the liver and spleen.

### Clinical Manifestation in Dogs and Cats

- *Dogs.* Rare. May be subclinical carriers or can present with clinical signs including fever, endocarditis, lymphadenitis, and epistaxis. Transmission from dogs to humans is rare.
- *Cats.* Reservoir species with a high prevalence of subclinical bacteremia:
  - Infection sources for cats are from fleas, ticks, or direct contact with infected blood through bite wounds, scratches, or transfusions.
  - Significant bacteremia occurs most commonly in cats under 2 years of age.
  - Transient, self-limiting fever occurs in some infected cats.
  - Antibiotic treatment is only indicated in the presence of clinical signs.

### Prevention

- Control flea vectors on dogs and cats (but avoid the use of permethrin pesticides on cats).
- People with immunocompromise should take extra handling precautions to avoid being scratched, particularly by young cats.
- Clean scratch wounds well and seek medical treatment as indicated.
- No vaccine is currently available for humans or for animals.
- Prophylactically, treating healthy animals or declawing cats are not recommended as prevention strategies.

### 17.11.1.3 Bordetella bronchiseptica

*Basic Information*

- *Caused by bacteria.* Bordetella bronchiseptica
- *Arthropod vectors.* None
- *Geographic distribution.* Worldwide [25–27].

*Risk Factors for Human Exposure from Dogs and Cats*

- Human infection is rare, but may occur following close contact with infected domestic species including dogs and, even more rarely, cats.
- Clinical illness in previously healthy adults and children has been reported, but primary risk factors in humans include immunocompromise, cystic fibrosis and chronic respiratory disease, and pregnancy.

*Clinical Manifestation in Humans*

- *Primary clinical sign.* Tracheobronchitis that may progress to respiratory complications, particularly in high-risk individuals.
- The causative agent of whooping cough, *Bordetella pertussis*, is closely related but distinct and not considered a zoonotic pathogen.

*Clinical Manifestation in Dogs and Cats*

- *Dogs.* Typical clinical signs include cough and nasal discharge that may progress to pneumonia. The bacteria can be found in the respiratory tract of asymptomatic dogs. Shedding can persist for weeks following infection.
- *Cats.* A primary differential for coughing cats. Respiratory signs range from mild fever, coughing, sneezing, ocular discharge, and lymphadenopathy to severe pneumonia, particularly in young kittens.

*Prevention*

- Wear gloves and institute barrier protection when handling dogs and cats with respiratory illness.
- No human vaccine is available. Cross protection from whooping cough vaccines has not been established.
- The vaccines for dogs and cats reduce, but do not eliminate clinical signs, shedding, and transmission potential.
- Susceptible to routine disinfectants. May persist in the environment for more than 10 days.

### 17.11.1.4 Brucella canis

*Basic Information*

- *Caused by bacteria.* Brucella canis
- *Arthropod vectors.* None

- *Geographic distribution.* Widespread in the southern United States, Central and South America, Asia, and parts of Africa. It has only sporadically been reported in Europe and in Canada [28–30].

*Risk Factors for Human Exposure from Dogs and Cats*

- Routes of human infection: mucous membranes, ingestion, open skin wounds, and needle-stick injuries.
- Transmission from dogs occurs through contact with mucous membranes of the canine reproductive tract, fomite transmission, and direct contact with body fluids including vaginal discharge, semen, fetal fluid, urine, saliva, blood, and feces.
- Occupational exposure is a key human risk factor: veterinary personnel, dog breeders, and others in close contact with breeding dogs.
- Cats have been very rarely documented to transmit *Brucella suis* to humans but have not been documented to transmit *B. canis*.

*Clinical Manifestation in Humans*

- Nonspecific flu-like illness, fever, sweats, and lymphadenopathy.
- *Complications (rare).* Waxing and waning fever, arthritis, chronic fatigue, neurologic signs, and endocarditis
- *Incubation period.* 2 weeks to 3 months.

*Clinical Manifestation in Dogs and Cats*

- *Dogs*
  - Females: abortion at 40–60 days of gestation.
  - Males: epididymitis, scrotal dermatitis, and scrotal necrosis.
  - May be asymptomatic.
  - Transmitted venereally and through ingesting placental material.
- *Cats.* Brucella spp. infection is not considered an important cause of reproductive disease in cats.

*Prevention*

- Wear gloves, institute barrier protection, and wash hands thoroughly when handling intact male, pregnant, or postpartum dogs, particularly when in contact with reproductive tract mucous membranes, aborted fetuses, birth fluids, and urine.
- The bacteria can survive for months in water, aborted fetuses, feces, equipment, and clothing.
- There is no vaccine for dogs or cats.
- *Brucella* spp. are susceptible to routine disinfectants.

#### 17.11.1.5 Capnocytophaga spp

*Basic Information*

- *Caused by bacteria.* *Capnocytophaga* spp., particularly *Capnocytophaga canimorsus*
- *Arthropod vectors.* None
- *Geographic distribution.* Worldwide [31, 32].

*Risk Factors for Human Exposure from Dogs and Cats*

- Dog bites are the most common route of exposure, followed by dog scratches, dog licks, and other contact with dogs and cats. This is a rare infection.
- Other important human risk factors:
  - Lacking a spleen (primary risk factor)
  - Liver disease
  - Alcoholism
  - Immunocompromise
  - Over 40 years of age.

*Clinical Manifestation in Humans*

- *Common symptoms.* Blisters around the bite wound, inflammation of bite wound, fever, gastrointestinal pain, diarrhea, vomiting, headache, mentation change, and muscle or joint pain
- *Complications.* Gangrene, endocarditis, meningitis, heart attack, kidney failure, and rapid fatality (case fatality rate may be as high as 30%)
- Infection during pregnancy can cause chorioamnionitis, sepsis, and low birth weight.

*Clinical Manifestation in Dogs and Cats*

- Present in the normal oral cavity of healthy dogs without causing disease.

*Prevention*

- Animal bite prevention.
- Seek medical care promptly for animal bites.
- Individuals without a spleen should take increased precautions to avoid animal bites, scratches, and licks.

#### 17.11.1.6 Cheyletiella spp

*Basic Information*

- *Caused by mite.* *Cheyletiella blakei* (cats) and *Cheyletiella yasguri* (dogs)
- *Other names.* Hair-clasping mite and walking dandruff mite
- *Geographic distribution.* Worldwide [33, 34].

*Risk Factors for Human Exposure from Dogs and Cats*

- Transmitted from cats and dogs to humans by close skin contact
- Transmission from cats is reported more frequently than from dogs.

*Clinical Manifestation in Humans*

- Mild, pruritic dermatitis with papules and erythema in areas that came in contact with an infected animal
- *Complications.* Vesicles, crusts, central necrosis, hives, and bullae.

*Clinical Manifestation in Dogs and Cats*

- Alopecia, dermatitis, and flaking; particularly distributed dorsally
- In cats, military dermatitis is frequently seen.

*Prevention*

- Wear gloves and institute barrier protection when handling dogs and cats with skin lesions.
- Infections in humans are generally self-limiting, but medical treatment should be sought based on severity and discomfort.

#### 17.11.1.7 Chlamydophila felis Infection

*Basic Information*

- *Caused by bacteria.* *Chlamydophila felis*
- *Arthropod vectors.* None
- *Geographic distribution.* Worldwide [35–37].

*Risk Factors for Human Exposure from Dogs and Cats*

- Direct contact with infected cats.

*Clinical Manifestation in Humans*

- Minimal evidence of significant zoonotic risk
- Case reports of keratoconjunctivitis. Association between *C. felis* and pneumonia in immunocompromised individuals has been reported, but causation is not proven.

*Clinical Manifestation in Dogs and Cats*

- *Dogs.* *C. felis* has been isolated from dogs with conjunctivitis but is considered primarily a feline pathogen.
- *Cats.* Highly host-adapted to cats:
  - Clinical signs are mostly seen in cats less than a year of age.
  - Severe conjunctivitis, chemosis, blepharospasm, pain, and ocular discharge.

– The primary ocular complication is conjunctival adhesion.
– A minority of infected kittens can have fever and inappetence.

*Prevention*

- Wear gloves and institute barrier protection when handling cats, particularly kittens, with conjunctivitis.
- Requires close contact for transmission.
- Very limited survival in the environment.
- The vaccine for cats is recommended in high-density environments, where *C. felis* has been documented in the population.

### 17.11.1.8 Cowpox

*Basic Information*

- *Caused by virus.* Cowpox virus
- *Arthropod vectors.* No
- *Geographic distribution.* The United Kingdom and Western Europe [38, 39].

*Risk Factors for Human Exposure from Dogs and Cats*

- Contact with cats is frequent route of human exposure in endemic areas.

*Clinical Manifestation in Humans*

- Lesions on the legs, arms, and face
- Complications: systemic disease resembling smallpox.

*Clinical Manifestation in Dogs and Cats*

- *Dogs.* Rare reports
- *Cats.* Cats are infected by rodents:
  – Slow-healing skin lesions of the face and paws: inflammation, crusting, pruritus, and ulceration with hard edges
  – Complications, seen most frequently in kittens, and when infected cats are treated with corticosteroids: secondary infections, conjunctivitis, pharyngeal or esophageal ulceration, pneumonia.

*Prevention*

- Wear gloves and institute barrier protection when handling cats with suspect history and clinical signs in endemic areas.
- Can survive in an environment under ideal conditions for months.

- Most disinfectants are effective; rubbing alcohol alone is not recommended.
- No vaccine.

### 17.11.1.9 Dermatophytosis (Ringworm)

*Basic Information*

- *Caused by fungi. Microsporum* spp. and *Trichophyton* spp. are of greatest zoonotic significance
- *Arthropod vectors.* None
- *Geographic distribution.* Worldwide [40–43].

*Risk Factors for Human Exposure from Dogs and Cats*

- Skin contact with animals through petting, grooming, restraint, and handling of bedding
- Young and advanced age, as well as immunocompromise increase risk of infection.

*Clinical Manifestation in Humans*

- Ringworm, also called *tinea.*
- Signs and symptoms: itchy, red, sometimes circular rash that can occur on any area of the body.
- Uncomplicated infections may respond to non-prescription anti-fungal topical treatment.
- Persistent or progressive infections and infections of the scalp require treatment by a healthcare provider.

*Clinical Manifestation in Dogs and Cats*

- *Dogs.* Alopecia, scaly patches, folliculitis, and furunculosis.
  – Most common cause is *Microsporum canis* followed by *Microsporum gypseum* and *Trichophyton mentagrophytes.*
- *Cats.* Focal alopecia, scaling, crusting, particularly of the face and extremities:
  – Clinical signs vary widely in cats and may be quite subtle.
  – Primary cause is *M. canis* followed rarely by *Trichophyton* spp.

*Diagnosis*

- Ultraviolet (Wood's) lamp
- Direct microscopic examination of fluorescing hairs
- Fungal culture (gold standard).

*Prevention*

- Always wash hands with soap and water after handling animals.

- Wear gloves and protective clothing when handling animals with any skin or hair-coat abnormalities and when touching bedding or upholstered surfaces in contact with those animals.
- Immunocompromised individuals, the young, and the elderly should take extra caution or avoid handling animals with skin abnormalities.
- Mechanical removal of spores from the environment through vacuuming nonporous surfaces and laundering bedding is critical. Upholstered surfaces are extremely difficult to decontaminate.
- Once surfaces are visibly clean of organic material, utilize a disinfectant effective against dermatophytes with 10 min of contact time. Options include the following:
  - Sodium hypochlorite (studies are now showing that a dilution of 1 : 32 is adequate)
  - Enilconazole (dilution of 1 : 100)
  - Accelerated hydrogen peroxide (dilution of 1 : 16)
  - 2% potassium peroxymonosulfate.

#### 17.11.1.10  Echinococcosis

*Basic Information*

- *Caused by tapeworm. Echinococcus multilocularis* and *Echinococcus granulosus* [44, 45].
- *Arthropod vectors.* Flies and beetles can be mechanical vectors.
- *Other disease names.* Hydatid disease.
- *Geographic distribution.*
  - *E. multilocularis.* Northern Hemisphere including Europe, north central Asia, and North America
  - *E. granulosus.* Worldwide with strain-specific geographic ranges.

*Risk Factors for Human Exposure from Dogs and Cats*

- Dogs and cats are definitive hosts and become infected when they consume cysts in the issues of intermediate hosts, which are typically herbivores. Ingested cysts mature into tapeworms in the intestine and shed eggs (proglottids) in the feces that are immediately infective for consumption by intermediate hosts.
- Humans can act as intermediate hosts. Within the intermediate host, ingested eggs become larvae, which move through the intestinal wall into the blood and are carried to the organs, particularly the liver and lungs, where they form cysts and await ingestion by a carnivore.

- Petting an infected or mechanically contaminated dog or cat is a source of transmission to humans. Other sources of human infection not caused by dogs and cats include consuming an infected definitive host, consuming contaminated food or water, and handling a contaminated wild animal carcass or contaminated soil containing eggs.

*Clinical Manifestation in Humans*

- *E. multilocularis.* Large, slowly progressive cyst tumors in the liver eventually causing epigastric pain, ascites, jaundice, and liver failure. Cysts can also spread to other organs including the spleen, brain, and lungs. Cysts can remain asymptomatic.
- *E. granulosus.* Slowly progressive cyst tumors that most commonly occur in the liver and lungs but can be found throughout the body including bones, muscles, eye, nervous system, and other organs. Clinical signs depend on the location of the cyst, and single cysts are more common than multiple cysts. Cysts can remain asymptomatic.
- *Incubation period.* Months to years.

*Clinical Manifestation in Dogs and Cats*

- As definitive hosts, dogs and cats are typically asymptomatic other than rare enteritis and diarrhea with exceptionally heavy parasite burdens.

*Prevention*

- Routinely deworm dogs and cats with praziquantel every 3–4 weeks in endemic areas.
- Discourage dogs and cats from consuming the viscera of suspected intermediate hosts in endemic areas.
- Prevent dogs and cats from accessing livestock pastures.
- Wear gloves and use strict hand hygiene when handling dog and cat feces.
- Extremely resistant to routine disinfectants but bleach may reduce surface contamination with eggs.
- Eggs are inactivated by heat and drying.
- There is no vaccine available for dogs and cats.

#### 17.11.1.11  Glanders

*Basic Information*

- *Caused by bacteria. Burkholderia mallei*
- *Arthropod vectors.* Flies can act as mechanical vectors
- *Other disease names.* Farcy, Malleus, Droes

- Potential agent of bioterrorism
- *Geographic distribution.* Endemic in parts of the Middle East, Asia, Africa, and Central and South America [46–48].

*Risk Factors for Human Exposure from Dogs and Cats*

- This is a rare zoonotic pathogen.
- Primarily a disease of horses, but dogs and cats can carry and transmit infection to humans.
- Transmitted to humans from the tissue and body fluid of infected animals.
- Entry routes are open wounds, ingestion, and inhalation of aerosolized particles.
- Also transmitted on fomites including equipment.

*Clinical Manifestation in Humans*

- *Four presentations.*
  - *Localized.* Nodules and ulcers of mucous membranes and skin.
  - *Disseminated.* Similar lesions to above as well as fever, headache, and lymphadenopathy
  - *Pulmonary.* Effusion and pneumonia.
  - *Septicemic.* Pustular rash, cellulitis, cyanosis, necrotizing wounds, and multi-organ failure.
- *Incubation period.* 1–14 days.

*Clinical Manifestation in Dogs and Cats*

- This is a rare disease in dogs, while cats are highly susceptible.
- Dogs and cats can present with one of four recognized presentations: nasal, pulmonary, cutaneous ("farcy"), and subclinical carrier.
- The clinical forms result in nodules and ulcerations of the respiratory tract and skin that results in symptoms such as purulent to hemorrhagic nasal discharge, lymphadenopathy, coughing, dyspnea, and diarrhea.

*Prevention*

- Wear gloves and institute strict barrier protection when working with dogs and cats with suspect history and signs
- Susceptible to routine disinfectants
- Inactivated by heat and sunlight but can survive weeks in moist environments
- There is no vaccine available.

#### 17.11.1.12 Hendra

*Basic Information*

- *Caused by virus.* Hendra virus
- *Arthropod vectors.* No

- *Geographic distribution.* Limited to parts of Australia inhabited by flying foxes (fruit bats) [49].

*Risk Factors for Human Exposure from Dogs and Cats*

- This is a very rare disease that originates in fruit bats.
- Although primarily a zoonotic disease of horses, dogs are thought to be at risk of infection based on a small number of case reports and are assumed to pose a transmission risk to humans.
- Transmission to humans could occur through direct contact with tissues or body fluids or through aerosolization of infectious material.
- Intranasal and oronasal infection routes are important in horses.
- Fomite transmission is also possible.

*Clinical Manifestation in Humans*

- Flu-like illness, multi-organ failure, and encephalitis
- Incubation period: 5–21 days.

*Clinical Manifestation in Dogs and Cats*

- *Dogs.* Limited case reports of natural infection with minimal nonspecific to absent clinical signs:
  - One dog had respiratory lesions on necropsy.
  - Virus was detected in blood and tissues on PCR.
  - Dogs were thought to be infected through close contact with infected horses.
- *Cats.* Experimentally infected cats experienced fever, dyspnea, and rapid death. No reports of natural infection.

*Prevention*

- Wear gloves and institute strict barrier protection when handling mucous membranes, open wounds, blood, fluid, and tissue samples of dogs and cats in endemic areas
- Susceptible to routine disinfectants
- Inactivated by heat and sunlight but can survive for days in the environment under cool damp conditions
- No vaccine available.

#### 17.11.1.13 Influenza

*Basic Information*

- *Caused by virus.* Influenza. Three primary species: A, B, and C:
  - *Influenza A viruses.* Widely distributed in birds and mammals with current primary host

adaptation of virus subtypes to birds, pigs, horses, dogs, and humans.
  – *Influenza B viruses.* Primarily found and circulated in human populations. Serologic evidence of natural infection, case reports of clinical illness, and experimental infection in other species are rare and sporadic.
  – *Influenza C viruses.* Same as for Influenza B.
- *Arthropod vectors.* None
- *Geographic distribution.* Worldwide [50–53].

*Risk Factors for Human Exposure from Dogs and Cats*

- There are two primary zoonotic concerns with dogs and cats at present:
  – The potential for transmission of avian influenza from dogs and cats to humans
  – Antigenic shift that would increase the transmission potential and pathogenicity of other influenza subtypes from dogs and cats to humans.
- Canine influenza is not currently considered to be zoonotic.
- Human infection with avian influenza originating from dog or cat exposure has not yet been confirmed but is presumed to be possible.
- Most viral replication occurs in the respiratory tract. Cross species transmission potential is greatest by aerosolization of respiratory secretions, close contact with tissues, or direct inoculation of mucous membranes or the eye.
- Primary risk factors for severe disease in humans with any type of influenza: young age, old age, young adult age (for some viral subtypes), chronic disease (lung, heart, renal, liver, and diabetes), immunocompromise, and pregnancy.

*Clinical Manifestation in Humans*

- Uncomplicated infections with human influenza viruses cause nonspecific illness with both respiratory and gastrointestinal signs possible. Complications include pneumonia and neurological syndromes.
- Infection with other types of influenza can cause a wide range of clinical presentations in humans ranging from conjunctivitis and mild-to-serious disease, mirroring human influenza, to acute respiratory distress syndrome, septic shock, and organ failure.

*Clinical Manifestation in Dogs and Cats*

- *Dogs.* Respiratory signs such as mild-to-severe lethargy, fever, and anorexia.

- *Cats.* Rapid progression of fever, lethargy, lower respiratory disease, conjunctivitis, and neurologic signs:
  – *Key risk factor.* Contact with birds, particularly consumption of bird meat, in an area where avian influenza is present
  – Cat-to-cat transmission of avian influenza has been documented.

*Prevention*

- Wear gloves and institute barrier protection when working with dogs and cats with suspect history and clinical signs. Consider saliva, respiratory secretions, urine, and feces as potentially infectious.
- Institute isolation protocols for housing.
- Avoid feeding undercooked poultry to dogs and cats.
- No avian influenza vaccine is available for dogs and cats. Subtype vaccines are not cross-protective.
- Susceptible to routine disinfectants.

### 17.11.1.14 Leptospirosis

*Basic Information*

- *Caused by bacteria. Leptospira* spp:
  – Classified into serovars that are adapted to mammalian maintenance hosts.
- *Arthropod vectors.* None
- *Geographic distribution.* Worldwide, although Central America, Southeast Asia, and parts of the United States have the highest incidence due to tropical and subtropical environmental conditions [54–57].

*Risk Factors for Human Exposure from Dogs and Cats*

- Transmission is direct through close contact with the urine or blood of dogs shedding spirochetes.
- Routes include open wounds and mucous membranes of the mouth, eye, nose, and throat.

*Clinical Manifestation in Humans*

- *Biphasic disease.*
  – *Acute (septicemic) phase.* Nonspecific flu-like illness, fever, myalgia, lymphadenopathy, and abdominal pain
  – *Immune phase.* Meningitis, icterus, kidney or liver failure, and hemorrhage.
- *Complications.* Uveitis, multi-organ failure, pulmonary hemorrhage, and edema.
- Most infections are asymptomatic or resolve after the acute phase.
- *Incubation period.* Typically 7–12 days.

## Clinical Manifestation in Dogs and Cats

- *Dogs.* Infections range from subclinical or mild and nonspecific to severe:
  - Classic presentations include renal or hepatic failure, uveitis, pulmonary hemorrhage, fever, and abortion.
  - Complications include acute renal failure, leptospiral pulmonary hemorrhage syndrome (LPHS), multi-organ hemorrhage, vasculitis, hepatitis, and cardiac damage.
  - Shedding in urine can continue for weeks to months, including with subclinical infection.
  - Risk factors are drinking from ponds or rivers, close proximity to rodents and other urban wildlife, ingesting sewage or raw meat.
- *Cats.* Infection is documented but rare and usually subclinical:
  - Interstitial nephritis with or without clinical polyuria and polydipsia is sometimes seen. Renal failure is a possible complication.
  - Healthy cats can shed bacteria in urine.

## Prevention

- Dogs with acute renal failure should be leptospirosis suspects. Wear gloves, institute barrier protection, wash hands thoroughly, and a use face shield when aerosolization of urine is possible.
- Avoid pressure-washing kennels of leptospirosis suspects, which can aerosolize urine.
- Take extra care to avoid needle-stick injuries when drawing or handling the blood of leptospirosis suspects.
- Vaccinate dogs at geographic and lifestyle risk of infection.
- Vaccines for humans have limited availability.
- Stable in soil for weeks to months.
- Susceptible to routine cleaning and disinfectants.

### 17.11.1.15  Listeriosis

## Basic Information

- *Caused by bacteria.* Listeria monocytogenes
- *Arthropod vectors.* No
- *Geographic distribution.* Worldwide [58].

## Risk Factors for Human Exposure from Dogs and Cats

- Although dogs and cats are a rare source of infection to humans, direct contact with infected animals through tissue handling and necropsies poses a risk.

- *Important risk factors.*
  - Occupation
  - Pregnancy
  - Young and advanced age
  - Immunocompromise.

## Clinical Manifestation in Humans

- Flu-like illness, conjunctivitis, miscarriage, premature birth, newborn septicemia, and meningitis
- Most common in veterinarians handling tissue of infected animals: rash, sometimes with fever, chills, and pain.

## Clinical Manifestation in Dogs and Cats

- *Dogs.* Septicemia, neurologic signs
- *Cats.* Lethargy, anorexia, abdominal pain, vomiting, diarrhea:
  - Complications are septicemia and encephalitis.

## Prevention

- Wear gloves and institute barrier protection when handling sick animals and their tissues and performing necropsies.
- Susceptible to routine disinfectants.
- There is no vaccine available.

### 17.11.1.16  Melioidosis

## Basic Information

- *Caused by bacteria.* Burkholderia pseudomallei.
- *Arthropod vectors.* Not recognized in field conditions.
- *Other disease names.* Whitmore disease and Pseudoglanders.
- *Geographic distribution.* Primarily Thailand, Malaysia, Singapore, and northern Australia. Rare reports throughout Asia, Central and South America, the Middle East, and parts of Africa [59, 60].

## Risk Factors for Human Exposure from Dogs and Cats

- This is a rare disease.
- Human exposure is primarily directly from the environment, but zoonotic transmission from dogs and cats is possible. Transmitted to humans from the tissue and body fluid of infected animals.
- Entry routes are open wounds, ingestion, and inhalation of aerosolized particles.

## Clinical Manifestation in Humans

- Acute localized infections, pulmonary disease, septicemia, organ abscesses, neurological syndromes.

- *Incubation period.* Typically 9–21 days with a range of days to years.

### Clinical Manifestation in Dogs and Cats

- *Dogs.*
  - *Acute.* Lymphadenitis, septicemia, fever, diarrhea, respiratory disease, and pneumonia.
  - *Chronic.* Any organ can be affected, anorexia, limb edema, and skin abscesses.
- *Cats.* Rare. Reports of jaundice, anemia, organ abscesses, and neurological disease.

### Prevention

- Wear gloves and institute strict barrier protection when working with dogs and cats with suspect history and signs.
- Susceptible to most routine disinfectants; however, 0.3% chlorhexidine and hand soap may not be adequate. Chlorination may not reliably clear it from water.
- Protect open wounds from contamination and clean thoroughly.
- Inactivated by heat and sunlight, but prolonged survival in moist environments such as soil.
- No vaccine.

#### 17.11.1.17 Nipah

### Basic Information

- *Caused by virus.* Nipah virus
- *Arthropod vectors.* No
- *Geographic distribution.* There have been documented cases in humans and domestic animals in Malaysia, Bangladesh, northern India, and the Philippines. It has also been detected in bats across Southeast Asia [61].

### Risk Factors for Human Exposure from Dogs and Cats

- Although primarily a zoonotic disease of bats and pigs, infections in dogs and cats have been confirmed. There is speculation but no confirmed evidence for potential dog-to-human transmission.
- This is a geographically isolated disease that originates in fruit bats (flying foxes).
- Transmission to humans could occur through direct contact with tissues or body fluids or through aerosolization of infectious material.

### Clinical Manifestation in Humans

- Flu-like illness, respiratory disease, and encephalitis.

- *Complications.* Septicemia, gastrointestinal hemorrhage, renal failure, and late-onset encephalitis months or years after initial infection.
- Infections may be subclinical.
- *Incubation period.* Typically 2–14 days.

### Clinical Manifestation in Dogs and Cats

- *Dogs.* Case report of fever, respiratory distress, conjunctivitis, and nasal discharge
- *Cats.* Experimentally infected cats experienced fever and severe respiratory disease:
  - During a naturally occurring outbreak, three cats with suspected infection were reportedly found dead with hemorrhage.

### Prevention

- Wear gloves and institute strict barrier protection when handling mucous membranes, open wounds, blood, fluid, and tissue samples of dogs and cats in endemic areas.
- Susceptible to routine disinfectants.
- Can survive from hours to days under ideal conditions in bat urine or fruit juices.
- No vaccine.

#### 17.11.1.18 Rat Bite Fever

### Basic Information

- *Caused by bacteria.* Streptobacillus moniliformis and *Spirillum minus* [62–65]
- *Arthropod vectors.* No
- *Geographic distribution.*
  - *S. moniliformis.* Primarily North America; rare reports in Central America, South America, and Europe
  - *S. minus.* Primarily Asia.

### Risk Factors for Human Exposure from Dogs and Cats

- Constitute part of the normal respiratory flora of rodents; primarily transmitted to humans by handling rodents, a bite or scratch from a rodent, or contaminated food or water (Haverhill fever).
- Rare case reports have attributed human infection to a dog source. In a small study, there was evidence of *S. moniliformis* in the oral flora of several dogs following close contact with wild rats.
- There is a case report of transmission of *Sp. minus* to a human through a cat bite.
- The infective dose and incubation with rat to dog or cat transmission are unknown.

- Dogs and cats are a suspected, but unconfirmed source of transmission to humans, particularly with close contact between a dog or cat and a rodent followed by the dog or cat biting a human.

*Clinical Manifestation in Humans*

- *S. moniliformis.*
  - Fever, chills, headache, rash on extremities, and vomiting
  - *Incubation period.* 3–10 days.
- *S. minus.*
  - Fever, ulceration at bite site, lymphadenopathy, and rash
  - *Incubation period.* 7–21 days.
- *Complications.* Endocarditis, myocarditis, meningitis, arthritis, abscessation, sepsis, pneumonia.

*Clinical Manifestation in Dogs and Cats*

- *Dogs.* Isolated case reports of abscessation, arthritis, endocarditis, pneumonia, and vomiting attributed to *S. moniliformis;* causation not proven
- *Cats.* No reports.

*Prevention*

- Clean bite wounds appropriately and seek medical care promptly.
- Wear gloves and institute barrier protection when handling dogs and cats following known contact with rodents, particularly regarding bites and licking.
- Wash hands thoroughly following animal and diagnostic sample handling.

### 17.11.1.19 Rift Valley Fever

*Basic Information*

- *Caused by virus.* Rift Valley fever virus
- *Arthropod vectors.* Mosquitoes
- *Geographic distribution.* the disease is endemic in southern and eastern Africa, and there have been sporadic reports in Egypt, the Middle East, and Madagascar [66].

*Risk Factors for Human Exposure from Dogs and Cats*

- Human exposure is primarily from occupational exposure to infected animal blood and tissues, but mosquitoes also transmit the disease in endemic areas.
- Exposure through aerosolization is also possible.

*Clinical Manifestation in Humans*

- Febrile flu-like illness, myalgia, headache, hepatomegaly.
- *Complications.* Renal failure, neurologic syndromes, ocular involvement, and hemorrhagic syndrome.
- Most infections are subclinical or self-limiting.
- *Incubation period.* 3–6 days.

*Clinical Manifestation in Dogs and Cats*

- *Dogs.* Neurologic signs and acute death in puppies younger than 2 weeks of age. Not reported in adult dogs other than possible reduction in fertility of adult females
- *Cats.* Neurologic signs and acute death in kittens younger than 3 weeks of age. Not reported in adult cats.

*Prevention*

- Wear gloves and institute strict barrier protection when working with dogs and cats, particularly neonatal puppies and kittens, with suspect history and signs in endemic areas.
- Utilize mosquito protection measures.
- Susceptible to most routine disinfectants.
- Can persist for days to months in tissues, and for an hour or more in the environment when aerosolized. Breaks down quickly in decomposing tissue.
- The vaccine for humans has limited availability.

### 17.11.1.20 Sporotrichosis

*Basic Information*

- *Caused by fungus. Sporothrix schenckii*
- *Arthropod vectors.* None
- *Geographic distribution.* Worldwide with a focal area of zoonotic transmission between cats and humans reported in Brazil, particularly in and around Rio de Janeiro [67–69].

*Risk Factors for Human Exposure from Dogs and Cats*

- This is a rare infection.
- Cat scratches and bites can be a source for human exposure. Immunocompromise is an important human risk factor.

*Clinical Manifestation in Humans*

- *Symptoms.* Initial painless, discolored nodule progressing to a nonhealing ulcer and possible additional nodules
- *Complications.* Spread of infection to bones, joints, or nervous system.

*Clinical Manifestation in Dogs and Cats*

- *Dogs.* Rare and generally mild:
  - Dermal and subcutaneous nodules of the head, nose, distal limbs, and thorax with possible ulceration and lymphatic involvement
- *Cats.* Highly susceptible:
  - Forms include cutaneous, cutaneolymphatic, and disseminated.
  - Nodules and ulcers are frequently seen on the tail-base, distal limbs, and nose and can occur in conjunction with lymphangitis, lymphadenitis, lethargy, fever, and respiratory signs.

*Prevention*

- Wear gloves and institute barrier protection when working with dogs and cats with skin lesions.
- Institute safe handling practices to decrease the risk of scratch injuries when examining and treating animals with suspected lesions.
- Thoroughly wash bite and scratch wounds and seek professional medical treatment.

### 17.11.1.21  Staphylococcus spp

*Basic Information*

- *Caused by bacteria.* Multiple species of concern including *Staphylococcus aureus, Staphylococcus haemolyticus,* and *Staphylococcus pseudintermedius*
- *Arthropod vectors.* None
- *Geographic distribution.* Worldwide [70–72].

*Risk Factors for Human Exposure from Dogs and Cats*

- Humans may become infected by handling, petting, restraining, or treating animals carrying the bacteria on skin or in wounds.
- Other important risk factors:
  - Immunocompromise
  - Densely populated conditions
  - Healthcare settings
  - Residential institutions
  - Compromised skin.

*Clinical Manifestation in Humans*

- Methicillin-resistant *S. aureus* (MRSA).
- Other related *Staph* species may acquire the methicillin-resistant gene such as Methicillin-resistant *S. pseudintermedius* (MRSP) and Methicillin-resistant *S. haemolyticus* (MRSH).
- Signs and symptoms: infected area of the skin that is red, swollen, painful, and warm with purulent exudate and a fever. Initial appearance may be a bump mistaken for a spider bite.
- Can progress to serious systemic infections.

*Clinical Manifestation in Dogs and Cats*

- Postoperative and wound infections presenting with redness, pain, swelling, and drainage.
- Persistent skin infections.
- More rarely occur as ear infections, urinary tract infections, or pneumonia.
- Bacterial colonization can occur without clinical signs.
- Therapeutic animals in healthcare settings may be at increased risk of both colonization and infection.

*Prevention*

- Wear gloves and institute barrier protection when working with dogs and cats with skin lesions and open wounds.
- Judicious use of systemic antibiotics is important in preventing development of resistant infections. Consider antibiotic susceptibility based on culture and sensitivity when available, for wounds and skin infections in dogs and cats that fail to heal or respond to routine antibiotics as expected.
- Utilize additional wound management strategies including topical antimicrobial treatment, drainage, and debridement as indicated to decrease sole reliance on systemic antibiotics in dogs and cats.
- Screening of healthy animals for bacterial colonization is not recommended.
- Thorough handwashing by all handlers between and after animal contact is critical.

### 17.11.1.22  Toxoplasmosis

*Basic Information*

- *Caused by protozoa. Toxoplasma gondii.*
- *Arthropod vectors.* Flies and cockroaches can be mechanical vectors.
- *Geographic distribution.* Worldwide, particularly in warm, humid climates [73–76].

*Risk Factors for Human Exposure from Dogs and Cats*

- Human exposure is primarily from ingesting raw or undercooked meat, but zoonotic transmission from cats is possible through contact with cat feces or occupational contact with cat blood and tissues.
- The zoonotic route of human infection is ingestion of material contaminated with oocysts.

- Human risk factors include pregnancy and immunocompromise.

### Clinical Manifestation in Humans

- Most human infections are subclinical.
- Clinical signs include flu-like illness, fever, lymphadenitis, and rash.
- Immunocompromise during infection can lead to encephalitis, nervous tissue abscessation, chorioretinitis, myocarditis, and pneumonia.
- Infection during pregnancy can cause congenital toxoplasmosis for the infant with a range of severity that can include the following:
  - Ocular pathology – Chorioretinitis, strabismus, and microphthalmia
  - Neurologic pathology – Hydrocephalus, cerebral calcification, and seizures
  - Systemic disease – fever, rash, pneumonia, and liver or spleen enlargement
  - Miscarriage or stillbirth.
- *Incubation period.* 5–20 days.

### Clinical Manifestation in Dogs and Cats

- The dog is not a definitive host, which means that infections are "dead-end" and do not lead to shedding of oocysts or infectious risk to other animals or humans.
  - Most infections are subclinical.
  - Puppies under 6 months and immunosuppressed dogs are at highest risk of clinical disease.
  - Signs can include encephalitis, myositis, hepatitis, pneumonia, myocarditis, lymphadenopathy, and ocular pathology.
  - Similar clinical presentation to canine distemper virus and *Neospora caninum.*
- Cats are the definitive hosts, which means that infections lead to shedding of oocysts, infectious risk to other animals and humans, and the lifelong potential for reactivation of infection.
  - Most infections are subclinical.
  - Kittens and immunosuppressed cats are most likely to have clinical disease including ocular disease (mostly commonly retinitis), fever, pneumonia, hepatitis, pancreatitis, and neurologic signs.

### Prevention

- Infectious oocysts shed in cat feces require 24 h to become infectious; therefore, removing fresh feces from the environment promptly reduces the risk of human exposure.
- Pregnant women should employ extra vigilance with barrier protection or avoid handling cat feces.
- Oocysts can remain infectious for months in warm, moist conditions.
- Oocysts are extremely resistant to almost all routine disinfectants. Very hot water and steam are most effective.
- Disposable litter pans are recommended for cats at risk of shedding.
- Avoid feeding raw or undercooked meat to cats.
- There is no vaccine available.

### 17.11.1.23   Tuberculosis

### Basic Information

- *Caused by bacteria. Mycobacterium* spp.
- *Arthropod vectors.* No
- *Geographic distribution.* Endemic in Africa, Asia, and the Middle East, while sporadic infections in the United States, the United Kingdom, and New Zealand still occurs [77–80].

### Risk Factors for Human Exposure from Dogs and Cats

- This is primarily a zoonotic disease of cattle (*Mycobacterium bovis*):
  - Contact with infected cats and dogs, particularly through bites and scratches, is a rare but possible source of infection for humans.
  - Inhalation of aerosolized pathogen and ingestion are also possible infection routes.
- Dogs and cats have natural resistance to *Mycobacterium tuberculosis*, the most common cause of tuberculosis in humans, but can rarely become infected and transmit infection to humans and other animals.
- Immunocompromise is a risk factor in humans.
- Dogs and cats may be at risk of acquiring infection from humans.

### Clinical Manifestation in Humans

- A wide range of symptoms can result from infection, most commonly including fever, night sweats, weight loss, cough, gastrointestinal pain.
- Cutaneous lesions are most likely to occur when the route of infection was through the skin.
- Subclinical infection is possible.

*Clinical Manifestation in Dogs and Cats*

- *Dogs.* Respiratory signs are classic, but most infections are subclinical or have mild, nonspecific signs.
- *Cats.* Digestive and respiratory signs are most common with *M. bovis*:
  - Other signs can include fever, lymphadenopathy, neurologic syndromes, liver and spleen enlargement, and ocular pathology.
  - Cutaneous signs including ulceration, nonhealing tracts, and nodules on the face, tail base, ventrum, and extremities are typically caused by the following three zoonotic mycobacteria species:
  *Mycobacterium microti.* Results from contact with small rodents
  *Mycobacterium lepraemurium* (feline leprosy). Results from contact with rodents or wound contamination from soil
  Nontuberculous mycobacteria results from wound contamination with soil.
- Risk factors for infection in both dogs and cats include consumption of raw milk and close contact with wildlife.

*Prevention*

- Wear gloves and institute barrier protection when handling sick dogs and cats with suspect history and clinical signs, particularly skin lesions.
- Rodent control can reduce exposure risk for dogs and cats.
- Prevent dogs and cats from ingesting raw milk.
- *Mycobacteria* spp. survive for months under cool, dark, damp conditions in the environment.
- Difficult to inactivate through disinfection; recommended disinfection is bleach (1 : 10 concentration) with at least 10 min contact time.

#### 17.11.1.24   Plague

*Basic Information*

- *Caused by bacteria. Yersinia pestis*
- *Arthropod vectors.* Fleas
- *Geographic distribution.* Semiarid climates of Asia, Africa, Eastern Europe, South America, and western North America [81–84].

*Risk Factors for Human Exposure from Dogs and Cats*

- Flea bites are the primary route of infection.
- Contact with the tissues and respiratory secretions of infected cats, and even more rarely dogs, is a less common but documented source of infection for humans.

*Clinical Manifestation in Humans*

- Depending on exposure route, there are three primary clinical presentations in humans. They are all frequently accompanied by fever:
  - *Bubonic.* Headache, chills, and swollen, and painful lymph nodes (buboes). Most likely to occur following a bite by an infected flea.
  - *Septicemic.* Chills, abdominal pain, shock, skin or organ hemorrhage, and superficial necrosis of the extremities. Exposure routes include flea bites, progression of the bubonic presentation, or direct contact with the tissue of an infected animal, such as a cat.
  - *Pneumonic.* Headache and acutely progressive pneumonia that can lead to shock and respiratory failure. Can result from other presentations or from the aerosolization of respiratory secretions from an infected person, cat, or other animal.
- *Incubation period.* 3–7 days.

*Clinical Manifestation in Dogs and Cats*

- *Dogs.* Typically subclinical or only a mild, transient fever. Clinical disease and transmission to humans are very rare but reported.
- *Cats.* Bubonic presentation is most common with necrotic stomatitis and abscessation of mandibular or sublingual lymph nodes. Septicemic and pneumonic presentations may occur. Overall mortality rate in cats is around 50%.

*Prevention*

- Wear gloves and institute barrier protection when handling sick cats, and their blood and tissue samples, in endemic areas. Consider plague as an uncommon differential for sick dogs in endemic areas.
- Utilize appropriate flea control methods for dogs and cats (do not apply products containing permethrin to cats).
- Prevent human exposure to fleas by using repellents on skin and clothing during outdoor activities and when in close contact with animals in endemic areas.
- A human vaccine has limited availability.

#### 17.11.1.25   Q Fever

*Basic Information*

- *Caused by bacteria. Coxiella burnetti*

- *Arthropod vectors.* Ticks (uncommon)
- *Geographic distribution.* Worldwide [85, 86].

*Risk Factors for Human Exposure from Dogs and Cats*

- Exposure to placenta and fetal fluids of cats and dogs, both healthy and postaborting
- Other key risk factors considered more important than dog and cat exposure:
  - Age > 46 years
  - Contact with ponds
  - Treatment of cattle, swine, and wildlife
  - Immunocompromise.

*Clinical Manifestation in Humans*

- Most infections are asymptomatic or mild and self-limiting.
- *Acute.* Flu-like illness, severe headache, pregnancy complications.
- *Chronic (uncommon).* Endocarditis, osteoarthritis, hepatitis, pregnancy complications. May develop months or years after initial infection.
- *Complications.* Pneumonia and hepatitis.
- *Incubation period.* Typically 2–3 weeks.

*Clinical Manifestation in Dogs and Cats*

- Infections are typically subclinical but may result in aborted pregnancy.
- Fever, anorexia, and lethargy are very rare.
- Source of infection may be tick bite, ingestion of infected carcasses, and aerosol exposure.
- For dogs, contact with sheep is considered an added risk factor.

*Prevention*

- Wear gloves, institute barrier protection, and wash hands thoroughly when handling dogs and cats during birthing and abortions.
- There is no vaccine for dogs and cats.
- The vaccine for humans has varying availability.
- The bacteria are very persistent in the environment and can survive for weeks to months.
- Resistant to routine cleaning, it is recommended to use 1 : 10 bleach solution for disinfection with a 10 min contact time.

#### 17.11.1.26 Sarcoptic Mange

*Basic Information*

- *Caused by mites. Sarcoptes scabiei*
- *Arthropod vectors.* No
- *Geographic distribution.* Worldwide [87–89].

*Risk Factors for Human Exposure from Dogs and Cats*

- Transmitted from dogs to humans by close skin contact.
- Cats are rarely infected but can be a transient source of human infection.

*Clinical Manifestation in Humans*

- Severe pruritus and dermatitis in areas that were in contact with the infected dog.

*Clinical Manifestation in Dogs and Cats*

- *Dogs.* Alopecia, hyperkeratosis, excoriation with serous exudate, and severe pruritus:
  - Typical distribution includes ear margins, flanks, ventrum, and lateral limbs.
- *Cats.* Rarely seen; isolated case reports of mild-to-moderate skin lesions similar to dogs but with less pruritus apparent.

*Prevention*

- Wear gloves and institute barrier protection when handling dogs and cats with skin lesions.
- Infections in humans are generally self-limiting, but medical treatment should be sought based on severity and discomfort.

#### 17.11.1.27 Streptococcus spp. Infection

*Basic Information*

- *Caused by bacteria. Streptococcus* spp.
- *Arthropod vectors.* None
- *Geographic distribution.* Worldwide [90–92].

*Risk Factors for Human Exposure from Dogs and Cats and Clinical Manifestations*

- There are three antigenic groups of *Strep* bacteria that pose a risk of transmission from dogs and cats to humans:
- Group A beta-hemolytic *Streptococcus* spp. (primarily *S. pyogenes*)
  - *Risk factors.* Zoonotic potential from dogs to humans is uncertain and considered to be very low with occasional suspected cases reported.
  - *Clinical manifestation in humans.* Pharyngitis ("strep throat"), skin infections, septicemia, and a wide range of severe systemic diseases including toxic shock syndrome. This is primarily a pathogen transmitted from human to human.

– *Clinical manifestation in dogs.* Subclinical and transient infection originating from close contact with humans.
– *Clinical manifestation in cats.* Not reported.

- Group C beta-hemolytic *Streptococcus* spp. (primarily *S. equi* subsp. *zooepidemicus*)
  – *Risk factors.* Horses are the primary zoonotic origin, but transmission from dogs and cats is thought to be possible through aerosolization of respiratory secretions, skin contact including bite wounds and fomites.
  – *Clinical manifestation in humans.* Respiratory disease, pneumonia, endocarditis, ocular inflammation, arthritis, meningitis, nephritis, septicemia, and toxic shock syndrome.
  – *Clinical manifestation in dogs.*
    Hemorrhagic pneumonia and septicemia.
    Clinical disease progression is similar to human toxic shock syndrome.
    Generally recognized as a copathogen but reported both as a primary cause of pneumonia and as a subclinical infection. Not considered to be a normal component of canine microflora.
    High population density is a risk factor.
  – *Clinical manifestation in cats.*
    Upper respiratory infection, purulent nasal discharge, cough, severe pneumonia, and meningoencephalitis
    High population density is a risk factor.

- Group G beta-hemolytic *Streptococcus* spp. (primarily *S. canis*)
  – *Risk factors.*
    Close contact with the skin or mucous membranes of a dog or cat, particularly through bite wounds
    Immunocompromise.
  – *Clinical manifestation in humans.* Soft tissue infection, septicemia, urinary tract infection, and osteomyelitis
  – *Clinical manifestation in dogs.*
    Can be normal inhabitants of the respiratory, intestinal, urinary, and genital tracts without clinical signs.
    Clinical manifestations can include pneumonia, abortion, septicemia, endocarditis, urinary tract infections, necrotizing fasciitis, hepatitis, and encephalitis.
    Young age is a significant risk factor. Consider as a primary differential in neonatal death.

– *Clinical manifestation in cats.* Same as in dogs with the addition of upper respiratory tract infection as a primary clinical sign.

*Prevention*

- Wear gloves and institute barrier protection when handling dogs and cats with respiratory illness.
- Clean bite wounds thoroughly and seek appropriate professional medical treatment.
- Recognize stress and overcrowding as population-level risk factors in animals.
- No vaccines are available.
- Susceptible to routine disinfectants.

### 17.11.1.28 Tularemia

*Basic Information*

- *Caused by bacteria. Francisella tularensis.*
- *Arthropod vectors.* Ticks, biting flies (especially deer flies in the western United States), mosquitoes (particularly in northern Europe). Other vectors including fleas, mites, and fruit flies can carry infection but have an unconfirmed role in transmission.
- *Geographic distribution.* Northern Hemisphere. The most virulent species, *F. tularensis* (Type A), is nearly exclusive to North America with rare reports in Europe. Other subspecies are found in Europe, Central Asia, the Middle East, and North Africa [93–95].

*Risk Factors for Human Exposure from Dogs and Cats*

- Contact with infected cats, particularly through bites and scratches, is a rare but possible source of infection for humans.

*Clinical Manifestation in Humans*

- Six clinical presentations occur in humans depending on inoculation site. All can cause fever. Those relevant to handling an infected cat are the following:
  – *Ulceroglandular (infection through skin or mucous membrane).* Ulcer at infection site, enlarged regional lymph nodes, nonspecific flu-like illness
  – *Glandular.* Same as above without an ulcer at the infection site
  – *Oculoglandular (infection through touching the eye).* Unilateral purulent conjunctivitis, regional enlarged lymph nodes; occasionally with

chemosis, conjunctival, or corneal ulceration; rarely with corneal perforation or iris prolapse
- *Pneumonic (typically from inhalation of infection but can be progression of other forms).* Cough, chest pain, and difficulty breathing. Most serious form
- *Typhoidal (can occur with any route of exposure).* Flu-like illness, rash, and pneumonia.
- *Complications.* Meningitis, endocarditis, osteomyelitis, kidney failure, hepatitis, and acute respiratory distress.

*Clinical Manifestation in Dogs and Cats*

- *Dogs.* Relatively resistant to infection. May have transient mild fever. Unlikely to be a direct source of transmission to humans

- *Cats.* Very susceptible to infection, particularly due to ingestion of infected wildlife. Lymphadenopathy, fever, and oropharyngeal ulceration
- Reportable disease in the United States. Culture and necropsy of suspected cases should be performed in designated facilities with elevated biosecurity.

*Prevention*

- Wear gloves and institute barrier protection when handling sick cats, and their blood and tissue samples, in endemic areas.
- Utilize arthropod vector control including effective repellents, long clothing, and prompt removal of ticks.
- A human vaccine exists, but availability is limited and varies by country.

# References

1 Wright, J.G., Jung, S., Holman, R.C. et al. (2008). Infection control practices and zoonotic disease risks among veterinarians in the United States. *Journal of the American Veterinary Medical Association* **232** (12): 1863–1872.

2 Buttke, D. Safe practices to avoid zoonotic diseases from wildlife: quick reference guide. National Park Service https://www.nps.gov/public_health/di/vb_ia.htm (accessed 2 August 2016).

3 National Association of State Public Health Veterinarians (2013). Compendium of measures to prevent disease associated with animals in public settings. *Journal of the American Veterinary Medical Association* **243** (9): 1270–1288.

4 Williams, C., Scheftel, J., Elchos, B. et al. (2015). Compendium of veterinary standard precautions for zoonotic disease prevention in veterinary personnel. National Association of state public health veterinarians: veterinary infection control committee. *Journal of the American Veterinary Medical Association* **247** (11): 1252–1277.

5 World Health Organization (2013). Animal bites. http://www.who.int/mediacentre/factsheets/fs373/en/ (accessed 2 August 2016).

6 National Guideline Clearinghouse: Agency for Healthcare Research and Quality (2013). Management of cat and dog bites. https://www.guideline.gov/summaries/summary/46428 (accessed 2 August 2016).

7 Presutti, R.J. (2001). Prevention and treatment of dog bites. *American Family Physician* **63** (8): 1567–1572.

8 World Health Organization (2016) Rabies. http://www.who.int/ith/vaccines/rabies/en/ (accessed 2 August 2016).

9 Brown, C.M., Slavinski, S., Ettestad, P. et al. (2016). Compendium of animal rabies prevention and control. *Journal of the American Medical Association* **248** (5): 505–517.

10 WHO Expert Consultation on Rabies (2013). Second Report: World Health Organization. *Tech. Rep. Ser. 982*, Geneva Switzerland.

11 Companion Animal Parasite Council (2016). Baslisascaris procyonis. http://www.capcvet.org/capc-recommendations/baylisascaris-procyonis-also-raccoon-roundworm/ (accessed 1 August 2016).

12 Companion Animal Parasite Council (2016). Cryptosporidium. https://www.capcvet.org/capc-recommendations/cryptosporidia/ (accessed 1 August 2016).

13 Companion Animal Parasite Council (2016). Cyclophyllidean tapeworms. https://www.capcvet.org/capc-recommendations/cyclophyllidean-tapeworms/ (accessed 1 August 2016).

14 Companion Animal Parasite Council (2016). Giardia. http://www.capcvet.org/capc-recommendations/giardia/ (accessed 1 August 2016).

15 Companion Animal Parasite Council (2016). Hookworms. http://www.capcvet.org/capc-recommendations/hookworms/ (accessed 1 August 2016).

16 Companion Animal Parasite Council (2016). Roundworms. http://www.capcvet.org/capc-recommendations/roundworms/ (accessed 1 August 2016).

17 Thamsborg, S.M., Ketzis, J., Horii, Y., and Matthews, J. (2016). *Strongyloides* spp. infections of veterinary importance. *Parasitology* **144** (3): 274–284.

18 Weese, J.S. (2011). Bacterial enteritis in dogs and cats: diagnosis, therapy, and zoonotic potential. *Veterinary Clinics of North America: Small Animal Practice* **41**: 287–309.

19 Centers for Disease Control and Prevention (2015). Anthrax. https://www.cdc.gov/anthrax/basics/index.html (accessed 2 August 2016).

20 Langston, C. (2005). Postexposure management and treatment of anthrax in dogs: executive councils of the American Academy of veterinary pharmacology and therapeutics and the American college of veterinary clinical pharmacology. *The American Association of Pharmaceutical Scientists Journal* **7** (2): E272–E273.

21 Weese, J.S., Peregrine, A.S., Anderson, M.E. et al. (2010). Bacterial diseases. In: Companion Animal Zoonoses, 1e (ed. J.S. Weese and M. Fulford), 110–114. Ames: Wiley-Blackwell.

22 Centers for Disease Control and Prevention (2015). Bartonella infection (cat scratch disease). http://www.cdc.gov/bartonella/index.html (accessed 3 August 2016).

23 Pennisi, M., Marsilio, F., Hartmann, K. et al. (2013). *Bartonella* species infection in cats: ABCD guidelines on prevention and management. *Journal of Feline Medicine and Surgery* **15** (7): 563–569.

24 Regier, Y., O'Rourke, F., and Kempf, V. (2016). *Bartonella* spp: a chance to establish one health concepts in veterinary and human medicine. *Parasites & Vectors* **16** (9): 261.

25 Egberink, H., Addie, D., Belak, S. et al. (2009). *Bordetella bronchiseptica* infection in cats. ABCD guidelines on prevention and management. *Journal of Feline Medicine and Surgery* **11** (7): 610–614.

26 Ford, R.B. (2012). Canine respiratory disease. In: Infectious Diseases of the Dog and Cat, 4e (ed. C.E. Greene), 55–65. St. Louis, MO: Elsevier.

27 Register, K.B., Sukumar, N., Palavecino, E.L. et al. (2012). *Bordetella bronchiseptica* in a pediatric cystic fibrosis patient: possible transmission from a household cat. *Zoonoses and Public Health* **59** (4): 246–250.

28 The Center for Food Security and Public Health (2012). Canine brucellosis: Brucella canis. http://www.cfsph.iastate.edu/Factsheets/pdfs/brucellosis_canis.pdf (accessed 2 August 2016).

29 Graham, E.M. and Taylor, D.J. (2012). Bacterial reproductive pathogens of cats and dogs. *Veterinary Clinics of North America: Small Animal Practice* **42** (3): 561–582.

30 Krueger, W.S., Lucero, N.E., Brower, A. et al. (2014). Evidence for unapparent *Brucella canis* infections among adults with occupational exposure to dogs. *Zoonoses and Public Health* **61** (7): 509–518.

31 Butler, T. (2015). *Capnocytophaga canimorsus*: an emerging cause of sepsis, meningitis, and post-splenectomy infection after dog bites. *European Journal of Clinical Microbiology and Infectious Diseases* **34** (7): 1271–1280.

32 Centers for Disease Control and Prevention (2016). Capnocytophaga. http://www.cdc.gov/capnocytophaga/index.html (accessed 3 August 2016).

33 The Center for Food Security and Public Health (2012). Ascariasis. http://www.cfsph.iastate.edu/Factsheets/pdfs/acariasis.pdf (accessed 3 August 2016).

34 Companion Animal Parasite Council (2013). Hairclasping mite. http://www.capcvet.org/capc-recommendations/hairclasping-mite (accessed 2 August 2016).

35 Browning, G.F. (2004). Is *Chlamydophila felis* a significant zoonotic pathogen? *Australian Veterinary Journal* **82**: 695–696.

36 Gruffydd-Jones, T., Addie, D., Belak, S. et al. (2009). *Chlamydophila felis* infection: ABCD guidelines on prevention and management. *Journal of Feline Medicine and Surgery* **11** (7): 605–609.

37 Pantchev, A., Sting, R., Bauerfeind, R. et al. (2010). Detection of all *Chlamydophila* and *Chlamydia*

*spp.* of veterinary interest using species-specific real-time PCR assays. *Comparative Immunology, Microbiology and Infectious Diseases* **10** (33): 473–484.

**38** Chomel, B.B. (2009). Emerging and re-emerging zoonoses of dogs and cats. *Animals* **4**: 434–445.

**39** Mostl, K., Addie, D., Belak, S. et al. (2013). Cowpox virus infection in cats: ABCD guidelines on prevention and management. *Journal of Feline Medicine and Surgery* **15** (7): 557–559.

**40** Moriello, K.A. and Newbury, S. (2009). Dermatophytosis. In: Infectious Disease Management in Animal Shelters, 1e (ed. L.A. Miller and K. Hurley), 243–273. Ames: Wiley-Blackwell.

**41** Moriello, K.A. (2015). Kennel disinfectants for *Microsporum canis* and *Trichophyton* sp. *Veterinary Medicine International* 853937.

**42** Centers for Disease Control and Prevention. (2015). Ringworm. http://www.cdc.gov/fungal/diseases/ringworm/index.html (accessed 2 August 2016).

**43** World Health Organization (2001). Ringworm (Tinea). http://www.who.int/water_sanitation_health/diseases/ringworm/en/ (accessed 1 August 2016).

**44** The Center for Food Security and Public Health (2011). Echinococcosis. http://www.cfsph.iastate.edu/Factsheets/pdfs/echinococcosis.pdf (accessed 2 August 2016).

**45** Companion Animal Parasite Council (2016). Intestinal parasites: Cyclophyllidean tapeworms. https://www.capcvet.org/capc-recommendations/cyclophyllidean-tapeworms/ (accessed 2 August 2016).

**46** Centers for Disease Control and Prevention (2015). Glanders. http://www.cdc.gov/glanders/index.html (accessed 3 August 2016).

**47** The Center for Food Security and Public Health (2015). Glanders. http://www.cfsph.iastate.edu/Factsheets/pdfs/glanders.pdf (accessed 3 August 2016).

**48** World Organisation for Animal Health (OIE). Glanders. http://www.oie.int/doc/ged/D13968.PDF (accessed 4 August 2016).

**49** The Center for Food Security and Public Health (2015). Hendra virus infection. http://www.cfsph.iastate.edu/Factsheets/pdfs/hendra.pdf (accessed 4 August 2016).

**50** Chomel, B.B. (2014). Emerging and re-emerging zoonoses of dogs and cats. *Animals* **4**: 434–445.

**51** The Center for Food Security and Public Health. (2014). Influenza. http://www.cfsph.iastate.edu/Factsheets/pdfs/influenza.pdf (accessed 5 August 2016).

**52** Munoz, O., De Nardi, M., van der Meulen, K. et al. (2016). Genetic adaptation of influenza a viruses in domestic animals and their potential role in interspecies transmission: a literature review. *EcoHealth* **13** (1): 171–198.

**53** Thiry, E., Addie, D., Belak, S. et al. (2009). H5N1 avian influenza in cats: ABCD guidelines on prevention and management. *Journal of Feline Medicine and Surgery* **11** (7): 615–618.

**54** Guerra, M.A. (2009). Leptospirosis. *Journal of the American Veterinary Medical Association* **234** (4): 472–478.

**55** Hartmann, K., Egberink, H., Pennisi, M.G. et al. (2013). *Leptospira* species infection in cats: ABCD guidelines on prevention and management. *Journal of Feline Medicine and Surgery* **15** (7): 576–581.

**56** The Center for Food Security and Public Health (2013). Leptospirosis. http://www.cfsph.iastate.edu/Factsheets/pdfs/leptospirosis.pdf (accessed 2 August 2016).

**57** Sykes, J.E., Hartmann, K., Lunn, K.F. et al. (2011). 2010 ACVIM small animal consensus statement on leptospirosis: diagnosis, epidemiology, treatment, and prevention. *Journal of Veterinary Internal Medicine* **25** (1): 1–13.

**58** The Center for Food Security and Public Health (2005). Listeriosis. http://www.cfsph.iastate.edu/Factsheets/pdfs/listeriosis.pdf (accessed 2 August 2016).

**59** Centers for Disease Control and Prevention (2012). Melioidosis. https://www.cdc.gov/melioidosis/index.html (accessed 2 August 2016).

**60** The Center for Food Security and Public Health (2016). Melioidosis. http://www.cfsph.iastate.edu/Factsheets/pdfs/melioidosis.pdf (accessed 1 August 2016).

**61** The Center for Food Security and Public Health (2016). Nipah. http://www.cfsph.iastate.edu/Factsheets/pdfs/nipah.pdf (accessed 2 August 2016).

**62** Elliott, S.P. (2007). Rat bite fever and *Streptobacillus moniliformis. Clinical Microbiology Reviews* **20** (1): 13–22.

**63** Centers for Disease Control and Prevention (2015). Rat-bite fever (RBF): information for health care workers. http://www.cdc.gov/rat-bite-fever/

health-care-workers/index.html (accessed 3 August 2016).

64 The Center for Food Security and Public Health (2013). Rat bite fever. http://www.cfsph.iastate. edu/Factsheets/pdfs/rat_bite_fever.pdf (accessed 1 August 2016).

65 Wouters, E.G., Ho, H.T., Lipman, L.J., and Gaastra, W. (2008). Dogs as vectors of *Streptobacillus moniliformis* infection? *Veterinary Microbiology* **128** (3–4): 419–422.

66 The Center for Food Security and Public Health (2015). Rift valley fever. http://www.cfsph.iastate. edu/Factsheets/pdfs/rift_valley_fever.pdf (accessed 2 August 2016).

67 Gremião, I.D.F., Menezes, R.C., Schubach, T.M. et al. (2014). Feline sporotrichosis: epidemiological and clinical aspects. *Medical Mycology* **53** (1): 15–21.

68 Pacheco Schubach, T.M., Caldas Menezes, R., and Wanke, B. (2012). Sporotrichosis. In: Infectious Diseases of the Dog and Cat, 4e (ed. C.E. Greene), 645–651. St. Louis, MO: Elsevier.

69 Centers for Disease Control and Prevention (2014). Sporotrichosis. http://www.cdc.gov/fungal/ diseases/sporotrichosis/index.html (accessed 1 August 2016).

70 Chomel, B.B. (2014). Emerging and re-emerging zoonoses of dogs and cats. *Animals* **4** (3): 434–445.

71 American Veterinary Medical Association (2009). Methicillin-resistant Staphylococcus aureus. https://www.avma.org/KB/Resources/Reference/ Pages/Methicillin-resistant-Staphylococcus-aureus. aspx (accessed 3 August 2016).

72 Centers for Disease Control and Prevention (2016). Methicillin-resistant Staphylococcus aureus (MRSA). http://www.cdc.gov/mrsa/index.html (accessed 2 August 2016).

73 Hartmann, K., Addie, D., Belak, S. et al. (2013). *Toxoplasma gondii* infection in cats: ABCD guidelines on prevention and management. *Journal of Feline Medicine and Surgery* **15** (9): 631–637.

74 Companion Animal Parasite Council (2014). Toxoplasma gondii. http://www.capcvet.org/capc-recommendations/toxoplasma (accessed 1 August 2016).

75 Centers for Disease Control and Prevention (2015). Toxoplasmosis. http://www.cdc.gov/ parasites/toxoplasmosis/ (accessed 2 August 2016).

76 Centers for Disease Control and Prevention (2005). Toxoplasmosis. http://www.cfsph.iastate. edu/Factsheets/pdfs/toxoplasmosis.pdf (accessed 1 August 2016).

77 The Center for Food Security and Public Health (2009). Bovine Tuberculosis. http://www.cfsph. iastate.edu/Factsheets/pdfs/bovine_tuberculosis. pdf (accessed 3 August 2016).

78 Lloret, A., Hartmann, K., Pennisi, M.G. et al. (2013). Mycobacterioses in cats: ABCD guidelines on prevention and management. *Journal of Feline Medicine and Surgery* **15**: 591–597.

79 Centers for Disease Control and Prevention (2012). Mycobacterium bovis (Bovine Tuberculosis) in humans. http://www.cdc.gov/tb/ publications/factsheets/general/mbovis.htm (accessed 2 August 2016).

80 Pesciaroli, M., Alvarez, J., Boniotti, M.B. et al. (2014). Tuberculosis in domestic animal species. *Research in Veterinary Science* **97**: S78–S85.

81 Pennisi, M.G., Egberink, H., Hartmann, K. et al. (2013). *Yersinia pestis* infection in cats: ABCD guidelines on prevention and management. *Journal of Feline Medicine and Surgery* **15**: 582–584.

82 Centers for Disease Control and Prevention (2015). Plague. https://www.cdc.gov/plague/index. html (accessed 1 August 2016).

83 World Health Organization (2014). Plague. http:// www.who.int/mediacentre/factsheets/fs267/en/ (accessed 2 August 2016).

84 Runfola, J.K., House, J., Miller, L. et al. (2015). Outbreak of human pneumonic plague with dog-to-human and possible human-to-human transmission – Colorado, June–July 2014. *MMWR. Morbidity and Mortality Weekly Report* **64**: 429–434.

85 Egberink, H., Addie, D., Belak, S. et al. (2013). Coxiellosis/Q fever in cats: ABCD guidelines on prevention and management. *Journal of Feline Medicine and Surgery* **15** (7): 573–575.

86 The Center for Food Security and Public Health (2007). Q Fever. http://www.cfsph.iastate.edu/ Factsheets/pdfs/q_fever.pdf (accessed 15 December 2017).

87 The Center for Food Security and Public Health (2012). Ascariasis. http://www.cfsph.iastate.edu/ Factsheets/pdfs/acariasis.pdf (accessed 15 December 2017).

**88** Malik, R., McKellar Stewart, K., Sousa, C.A. et al. (2006). Crusted scabies (sarcoptic mange) in four cats due to *Sarcoptes scabiei* infestation. *Journal of Feline Medicine and Surgery* **8** (5): 327–339.

**89** Companion Animal Parasite Council (2013). Sarcoptic Mite. http://www.capcvet.org/capc-recommendations/sarcoptic-mite (accessed 15 December 2017).

**90** Frymus, T., Addie, D.D., Boucraut-Baralon, C. et al. (2015). Streptococcal infections in cats: ABCD guidelines on prevention and management. *Journal of Feline Medicine and Surgery* **17**: 620–625.

**91** Lamm, C.G., Ferguson, A.C., Lehenbauer, T.W., and Love, B.C. (2010). Streptococcal infection in dogs: a retrospective study of 393 cases. *Veterinary Pathology* **47** (3): 387–395.

**92** The Center for Food Security and Public Health (2005). Streptococcus. http://www.cfsph.iastate.edu/Factsheets/pdfs/streptococcosis.pdf (accessed 2 August 2016).

**93** Fritz, C.L. (2009). Emerging tick-borne diseases. *Veterinary Clinics of North America: Small Animal Practice* **39**: 265–278.

**94** Centers for Disease Control and Prevention (2015). Tularemia. http://www.cdc.gov/tularemia/index.html (accessed 1 August 2016).

**95** The Center for Food Security and Public Health (2009). Tularemia. http://www.cfsph.iastate.edu/Factsheets/pdfs/tularemia.pdf (accessed 3 August 2016).

# 18

# Emergency Animal Sheltering

*Adam Parascandola*

*Humane Society International (Global Headquarters), 1255 23rd Street, NW, Suite 450, Washington, DC 20037, USA*

## 18.1 Introduction to Emergency Sheltering

The concept of emergency sheltering originated in the context of natural disasters when members of the public were offered shelter by organizations such as the Red Cross. While this provided for human health and safety, rarely were companion animals permitted in such emergency shelters due to public health and safety regulations [1]. As a result, many animal welfare organizations began to construct emergency shelters during times of crisis, which served as places of refuge for both owned pets and rescued animals. In 2009, Hurricane Katrina in New Orleans highlighted the fact that many citizens will refuse to evacuate disaster areas without their pets [2]. As a result, the Pets Evacuation and Transportation Standards (PETS) Act was enacted, which ensured that state and local emergency operational plans addressed the needs of citizens with pets prior to, during, and following a disaster [3, 4]. The field of emergency animal sheltering has since grown dramatically owing to both the increasing number of cruelty cases prosecuted and response to natural disasters.

## 18.2 What is an Emergency Animal Shelter?

Animal shelters are intended to provide refuge for animals that are abandoned, lost, or otherwise homeless until they can be reunited with their owners or rehomed into adoptive homes. Emergency shelters are a special type of shelter, designed to quickly house large numbers of animals requiring shelter during a crisis situation. Animals are temporarily sheltered until either returned to their owners, moved to more permanent facilities, adopted into new homes, or, if warranted, euthanized. Emergency shelters are then typically disassembled and supplies stored until the next crisis arises.

As these shelters are designed to provide safe and temporary housing of animals with potentially limited staff, enclosure sizes may be smaller than what is traditionally acceptable for long-term housing; enrichment provisions and medical resources may also be limited.

## 18.3 Making the Decision to Set Up an Emergency Shelter

The decision to set up an emergency shelter should not to be taken lightly as they are expensive and taxing for an organization. What may first be envisioned as a two-week temporary housing situation can drag on for months if disaster recovery takes longer than expected, or if the responding agency is not awarded immediate legal custody of the animals. Realistically, most local animal welfare groups lack the budget for operating an emergency shelter long-term. For organizations that anticipate the need for emergency sheltering (for example, they are located in disaster-prone areas), it can be helpful to amass supply caches that can be accessed during an emergency.

*Field Manual for Small Animal Medicine*, First Edition. Edited by Katherine Polak and Ann Therese Kommedal.
© 2018 John Wiley & Sons, Inc. Published 2018 by John Wiley & Sons, Inc.

## 18.4 Planning and Setting Up an Emergency Shelter

Emergency shelters are typically established in existing structures that are modified to provide safe and humane animal housing. Empty buildings, warehouses, airline hangers, commercial properties, and even farms/barns can serve as suitable locations for an emergency shelter if the property has the appropriate facilities.

When evaluating potential facilities, it is important to consider animal containment, particularly when sheltering cats due to their ability to escape. At a minimum, chain-link pens should be set up to enclose examination areas, and all cats must be transported in secure crates to prevent escapes.

Considerations when planning an emergency shelter include:

1) *Location:* Determine a suitable facility. See the Emergency Animal Sheltering Checklist (Appendix 18.A) to ensure that the chosen location provides for both animals and staff/volunteers. When choosing a location, consider properties that are secure, but allow easy access for people and vehicles. Ideally, the shelter should have no more than two entry and exit points to control people entering and leaving and prevent theft of animals or equipment.

---

**Textbox 18.1  Space considerations for animal housing**

The following are recommendations for animal housing:

a) *Dogs:* Provide 25–100 ft$^2$ (2.3–9.2 m$^2$) per dog. If small dogs are housed in wire cages, the lower end of the estimate can be used, whereas larger dogs kept in pens require the upper end of the estimate.
b) *Cats:* Provide 10–25 ft$^2$ (0.9–2.3 m$^2$) per cat when housed in cages.

Sample calculation:
*In a case requiring the temporary housing of 100 small dogs in wire cages, one would need a minimum of 2,500 ft$^2$ or 230 m$^2$, whereas 100 large dogs would require up to 10,000 ft$^2$ or 920 m$^2$. In the case of small dogs, cages could be stacked two high to maximize upon limited space.*

---

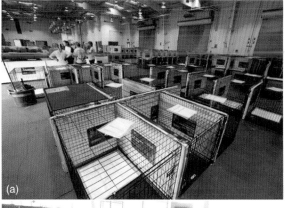
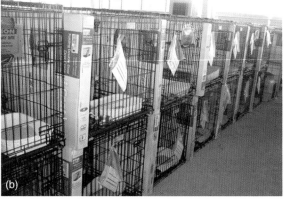

**Figure 18.1** (a) Temporary dog shelter in an airline hanger. (b) Temporary cat shelter. Cages are stacked two high with cardboard boxes in between, providing a physical barrier between cats. Copies of the intake examination form and treatment sheets are hung in a plastic cover on the front of each cage. Source: Courtesy of The HSUS.

2) *Space:* Assess space requirements, which will depend on the anticipated number and species of animals. Space requirements will vary depending on whether dogs or cats are being housed in wire or plastic crates versus larger pens. Wire and plastic crates can be stacked if needed (never stack more than two cages for dogs and three cages for cats). The stacking of crates is used when space is limited, as it requires less total square footage (Figure 18.1).

Chosen locations should also allow for the following separate areas:

- Animal housing/enclosures
- Wash station/decontamination
- Command center/record-keeping area
- Veterinary examination and treatment area
- Supply storage area.

3) *Utilities:* Assess what utilities are required. Running water or an accessible well is critical for performing cleaning and feeding activities. The facility should also have electricity and provide protection from the elements. Buildings must be well ventilated, ideally with several strong fans. In colder climates, if heat is not provided, then appropriate bedding and shelter will need to be provided for the animals to keep warm.

4) *Flooring:* Determine flooring needs. Epoxy flooring is ideal as it is easy to clean and maintain. Carpeting should be avoided as it is extremely difficult, if not impossible, to disinfect. If absolutely necessary, the entire floor can be lined with thick plastic sheeting. If dogs are housed in outdoor pens with dirt flooring, caution should be taken to prevent dogs from digging their way out.

5) *Trash disposal:* Ensure proper waste management to keep shelters sanitary and disease-free. There are two commonly used systems for waste management:
   a) Place a large dumpster on-site, which can then be emptied by a sanitation company.
   b) Implement a system for transporting trash in bags off-site to another trash collection site.

There may be times when an appropriate structure to house animals does not exist. With careful planning, alternate structures can be created, but one must consider supply availability. For example, temporary shelters can be constructed using tents and tarps. When constructing such a shelter however, drainage should be considered as rain can easily flood the shelter if care is not taken to find a spot where the rain can run-off, away from the shelter. It is also possible to build a lean-to, which is a simple structure constructed by adding rafters "leaning" against the side of a building and covered with a tarp. The ground must provide adequate drainage to prevent flooding. Dome-shaped livestock housing tents are handy to have on hand for use during an emergency. Such tents are sold both online and in various countries as greenhouse tents. When setting up an emergency shelter in a tent during hot weather, utilize fans and place the tent under existing shade to prevent overheating.

Another option, although less ideal, is to house animals in outdoor pens. When doing so, it is crucial that animals are provided adequately sized shelters/dog houses and that these houses either have a lip to prevent water from entering or are placed on wooden pallets off the ground. Adequate shade must also be provided.

Sheltering organizations may be tempted to group-house large numbers of dogs in outdoor fenced areas. To avoid fighting and potential disease transmission, animals should be kept either individually or in smaller groups, at least initially. Remember that during a natural disaster, owned animals should always be individually housed unless the owner has given permission to co-house them.

## 18.5  Shelter Layout

When creating a layout for an emergency shelter, consider the following points:

1) The emergency shelter must contain separate areas for general housing, isolation, owned animals, maternity ward, animal examination and treatment area, supply storage area, command center, food preparation, animal exercise area, and allow for the separation of species.

2) The shelter layout should facilitate animal and human flow-through. It should also minimize animal stress and overcrowding, and facilitate cleaning and feeding.

3) Animals can be housed individually or in pairs/small groups. As a general rule, animals that were previously housed together, either in a private home or hoarding situation, should be kept in the same housing area in the shelter. For individual housing, the animals should be housed in "family" pods of 15–20 enclosures per pod to facilitate care, cleaning, and minimize disease transmission. Pods can be separated from one another using cardboard dividers. Pods are essentially small groupings of animal enclosures that are self-contained. All cleaning supplies are assigned to specific pods (and not moved between pods), and animal care staff are assigned to clean by pod. Staff should use appropriate disease containment techniques including the changing of gloves, booties, etc. in between pods. This ensures that pathogens are not spread through fomites including cleaning supplies, clothing, etc. but rather stay contained within the pod (Figure 18.2).

4) Shelter animals are prone to stress. As such, the shelter layout must account for both the physical and behavioral needs of the animals.

**Textbox 18.2 Case study**

An adult dog rescued from a puppy mill was housed in a temporary shelter in the US in a 5′ × 5′ pen. The solid walls of his pen precluded him from seeing other dogs or any activity in the shelter. He refused to eat or engage with people, and lay huddled in the corner. In an effort to improve his behavioral well-being, he was moved to a pen with chain-link walls whereby he could visualize other dogs on either side of him. Within minutes, this once depressed dog was playing with the neighboring dogs, began eating, and approached and sniffed the hand of a caretaker. For this dog, interaction with other dogs played a key role in improving his behavioral and physical health.

Consider the following to minimize animal stress in a shelter environment:

- Walking a dog by other caged dogs can arouse the entire shelter population. Be sure to design exit walkways from the animal enclosures at strategic locations so that an animal can be walked without other animals seeing him. A walkway along the back of the kennels that is hidden from view using tarps hung along the backs of the enclosures can facilitate this.
- When receiving animals into a shelter, always house them in the farthest enclosures first (except for animals going to special housing areas) working your way closer to the loading point as kennels become occupied. This will prevent having to walk dogs past dogs already housed in enclosures, which helps minimize animal arousal and excitement.
- In shelters housing multiple species, designate separate entrances to the various species-specific areas to minimize foot traffic and animal stress. This is particularly important for cats who do not appreciate being transported past barking kennelled dogs.
- Pay attention to individual animal personalities. Some dogs benefit from having other dogs close by, while others become highly aroused and demonstrate signs of frustration. The shelter layout should ideally be flexible, allowing for the movement of enclosures depending on individual animal needs (Figure 18.3).

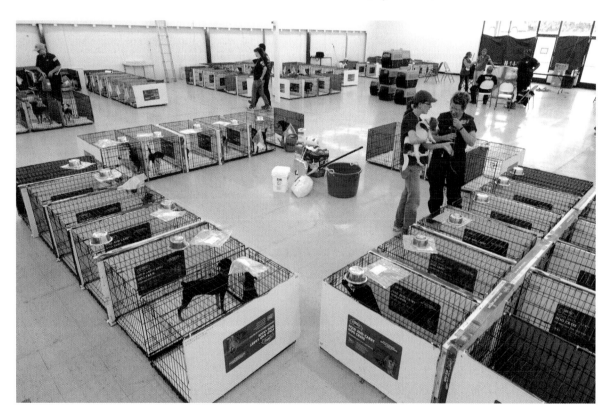

Figure 18.2 Aerial view of a temporary dog shelter using pods. Source: Courtesy of The HSUS.

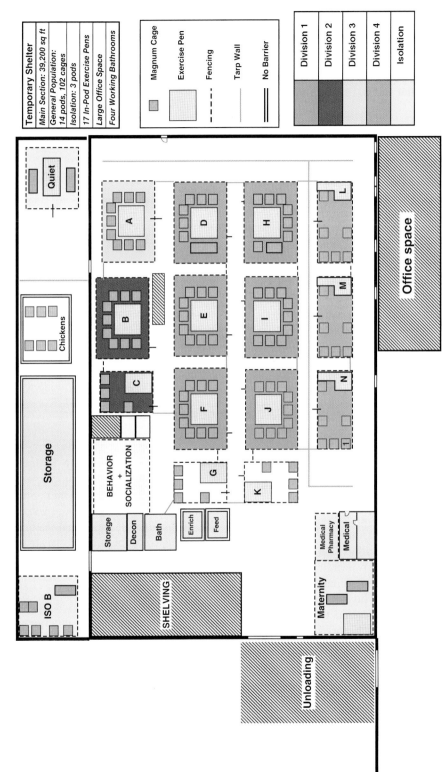

Figure 18.3 Sample layout for a basic emergency shelter. Source: Courtesy of Ehren Melius and the ASPCA.

## 18.6  Basic Supplies for an Emergency Shelter

The Shelter Equipment and Planning Checklist (Appendix 18.B) provides a sample temporary shelter supply list. Note that not all of the items will be available in every situation.

### 18.6.1  Animals Enclosures

Individual animal enclosures will typically consist of wire or plastic crates at least initially, but as resources allow, larger enclosures should be established to provide for better physical and behavioral health. Oftentimes, the larger the enclosure the more comfortable the animal is, allowing him or her to stretch out, stand up, and turn around. Feline enclosures must be large enough to allow for separate bedding and food areas, away from the litter box. All enclosures require adequate space for food and water bowls. Both dogs and cats benefit from having a safe hiding spot in their enclosures as well. This can be achieved by simply covering the back part of the cage to create a dark corner or by placing a smaller transport crate with the door removed inside the larger enclosure.

### 18.6.2  Food/Medication

Reliable suppliers are needed for procuring vital shelter supplies including food, medication, and cleaning supplies. In times of natural disasters, shelters should aim to have enough food on hand to last 7–10 days in case of delays in obtaining supplies. At a minimum, dry dog and cat food should be present if housing both species. Smaller dogs or puppies can eat adult dog food softened with warm water if needed; however, it is advisable to have canned food available for animals that are unable or refuse to eat dry food. The emergency shelter must have an appropriate location to store food to avoid spoilage. If food cannot be stored indoors, it will need to be placed on wooden pallets and under a tarp or tent. Whenever possible, food should be stored in a cool, dry place as even unopened canned food can spoil when stored improperly.

### 18.6.3  Bedding

If animals are housed on concrete or dirt, consider using shavings or straw to provide warmth and comfort. In cold weather, this type of bedding is crucial for safeguarding animals against hypothermia. If using shaving and straw however, beware of the potential for ophthalmic issues (corneal ulceration) particularly in dogs. For housing in wire or plastic crates, commercially available urine-absorbent liners are ideal to use as bedding. Blankets can also be used if they can be laundered. Another option is to use shredded newspaper for bedding and cat litter.

### 18.6.4  Miscellaneous Shelter Supplies

A variety of required items are needed to keep a temporary shelter operational (Appendix 18.B), and many of them may be available through donations. Large grocery stores or big box stores can be a great source for dog/cat food. Such stores may be willing to donate food and supplies once the product has reached its expiry date. However, it is important to ensure that the food has not spoiled. For this reason, open bags or cans of food that are donated should be discarded and not used. Similarly, any food showing signs of mold or discoloration should be discarded.

## 18.7  Emergency Shelter Staffing

Due to the sheer number of animals presenting to emergency shelters, most local and even national organizations will lack sufficient staff to properly manage all aspects of an emergency shelter. Staff from other animal welfare organizations and volunteers can be a valuable source of additional staffing. Adequate personnel and a clear organizational structure are crucial for ensuring humane animal care.

### 18.7.1  Staffing Requirements

Calculating staffing requirements for emergency shelters can be challenging as the numbers of animals requiring sheltering may be difficult to predict, or change by the day. However, there are general recommendations that can help determine the optimum number of staff required.

Key staffing positions within the shelter include:

- Incident Commander
- Shelter Manager
- Veterinary Medical Manager

---

**Textbox 18.3 Animal:staffing ratio**

The National Animal Control Association (NACA) in the United States and the Humane Society of the Unites States (HSUS) recommend allocating a minimum of 15 min per animal per day for basic feeding and cleaning activities in animal shelters [5, 6].

*Example:*
*A shelter houses 100 dogs in individual kennels. It opens at 8:00 a.m. and all animal cleaning and feeding tasks should be performed by 12:00 p.m. This gives staff 4 h to perform these duties.*

$$100 \; dogs \times 15 \, \text{min}/day = 1500 \, \text{min}$$
$$1500 \, \text{min}/60 \, \text{min}/h = 25 \, h$$
*25 h/4 h allowed to complete tasks = 6.25 staff members are required*
*To ensure adequate care, this shelter should employ at least 7 staff devoted solely to animal care.*

When animals are group housed, in the author's experience, one caretaker per 25–30 dogs or cats is required. This provides for basic feeding and cleaning – additional staff is required for administering medications, enrichment, etc.

---

- Logistics Manager
- Administrative Manager/Recordkeeper
- Volunteer Manager.

These positions should generally only be filled by staff members or trusted volunteers. Depending on the size and medical needs of the population, there may be a need for additional team leaders (divided by species or sections of the shelter), treatment staff to administer daily treatments, and specialized behavior staff. One person may fill multiple roles depending on the number of personnel available.

### 18.7.2 Utilize Volunteers

If the organization setting up the temporary shelter already has an active volunteer program, utilizing these volunteers as animal care staff in the shelter is easy to facilitate. While volunteers can be a tremendous help in a crisis situation, they must be managed appropriately.

#### 18.7.2.1 Determine Volunteer Recruitment Strategies

##### 18.7.2.1.1 Temporary Staffing
One quick recruitment strategy is to hire temporary labor from temporary labor agencies. These individuals may not be experienced in animal handling but can be taught the basics of cleaning and feeding. Many temporary labor staff employed at emergency shelters have gone on to later seek employment in the animal welfare field. Using temporary labor can be a real win–win to provide jobs for people in need and spark an interest and empathy for animals.

##### 18.7.2.1.2 Collaborating with Other Shelters
Collaborating with other local or regional animal shelters is an important way to bolster shelter staffing and animal care. However, the responsibilities and duties of each organization, as well as media and public relations issues should be made clear from the start. An incident command system (ICS) can facilitate a clear chain of command. It is always a good idea to have a memorandum of understanding (MOU) detailing specific responsibilities of partnering organizations in place to ensure transparency and accountability.

##### 18.7.2.1.3 Animal Care Professionals
Groomers, dog trainers, pet supply vendors, boarding facilities, veterinary hospitals, and veterinary schools can all be excellent sources for skilled volunteers or discounted services.

##### 18.7.2.1.4 Lay Person Volunteers
Local media outlets can successfully attract well-meaning individuals interested in assisting. As discussed earlier, volunteers can be an excellent source of labor if managed appropriately.

---

**Textbox 18.4 Tips for successful volunteer management**

- *Volunteers are not staff.* Volunteers can be reliable, but may have other obligations that limit their time to volunteer. Volunteers should not be given the same responsibilities as staff.
- *Set volunteers up for success.* Set clear expectations and guidelines for volunteers in writing and have them signed. It is important to ensure that all volunteers understand the rules of the shelter. New volunteers brought in to the emergency shelter should be partnered with more seasoned volunteers until they learn policies and procedures.
- *Communicate, Communicate, Communicate.* A volunteer briefing should be held twice daily.
  - In the morning, deliver an overview of the day, new volunteer introduction, and description of the day's activities.
  - Once the initial feeding and cleaning is finished, hold another briefing to discuss specific afternoon tasks. Set time aside (lunch is always a good time) for volunteers to ask questions regarding individual animals, the situation from which the animals came from (particularly useful in hoarding cases), etc.
- *Protect the organization.* When working with volunteers, a liability waiver must be signed by every volunteer. A confidentiality clause should be added to the waiver if the animals at the shelter are

involved in a legal case. Consult with a lawyer if needed to create these forms.
  - Emergent volunteers are volunteers who show up to help who were not already volunteers with the organization responsible for the shelter. These volunteers should receive an orientation explaining the emergency shelter objectives, rules, social media policy, etc. This is also a good time to have the volunteer waiver signed. Consider having the emergent volunteers fill out a short survey as to any specific skills they may have that might be useful in the shelter.
- *Scheduling.* Maintain a daily volunteer schedule. Volunteers should sign in and out of the shelter every day so that an accurate log is maintained of which volunteers were at the shelter when. Volunteers should be scheduled for specific shifts and should be expected to adhere to them unless they notify the shelter of a change in schedule.
- *When it's not working.* While volunteers can be a critical asset to any shelter, they must be managed appropriately. An initial orientation and explanation of policies and procedures should help set volunteers up for success. However, if there are continued problems with a volunteer, it is reasonable to ask him or her to leave.

---

## 18.8 Incident Command System

The ICS was designed for natural disaster response by rescue responders and is an excellent way to quickly create an organizational chart specific to the needs of a shelter [7]. An ICS is a must for emergency situations that bring together staff from different organizations, volunteers, veterinary partners, and the public. It is a system designed to create an organizational chart and ensure appropriate and timely communications for a specific response where multiple agencies are working together. It ensures an appropriate chain of command, which facilitates communication and prevents duplication of work. The ICS has been adapted by many animal welfare organizations to provide structure for a variety of situations ranging from natural or man-made disasters to mass spay/neuter surgical operations (Figure 18.4).

Positions typically included within an emergency sheltering ICS are as follows:

- *Incident Commander (IC):* Ultimately responsible for managing the entire operation. The IC makes high-altitude decisions; day-to-day operational decisions are left to others. The IC may also oversee Public Relations/Media, Finance, and Logistics; however, the Operations Chief should be his or her only direct report.
- *Operations Chief:* The vision and goals of the IC are put into practice by the Operations Chief.
- *Shelter Manager:* Responsible for the day-to-day care of the animals, including feeding, cleaning, and enrichment as well as volunteer management.
- *Veterinary Medical Manager:* Ensures the medical care of shelter animals, bringing medical conditions to the attention of the veterinarian, and ensuring medical care is outsourced when needed.

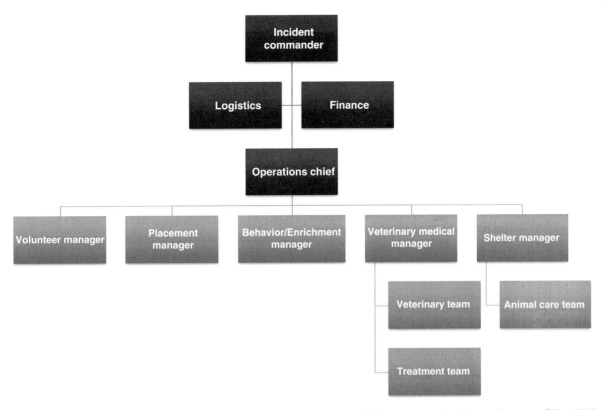

**Figure 18.4** Sample shelter incident command structure for an emergency sheltering operation. Source: Courtesy of The HSUS.

- *Volunteer Manager:* Ensures that volunteers are scheduled and tasked appropriately.
- *Enrichment/Behavior Manager:* Depending on the shelter and animals housed, there may be a need for a behavior or enrichment manager to assess individual animals and determine their enrichment needs. This staff member issues recommendations for behavioral enrichment, and the Shelter Manager then oversees the implementation of such activities.
- *Placement Manager:* Determines the placement of shelter animals following the cessation of sheltering activities, through transfer to other shelters or rescue groups, return-to-owner, or adoption.

All communications proceed upward through the chain of command. For example, an animal caretaker reports to their lead on the ICS chart (Shelter Manager) and that lead reports to the Operations Chief, who would then decide if the issue needed to be elevated to the IC. This method of organization ensures that all relevant parties are kept notified and reduces unnecessary communications.

## 18.9 Animal Intake

Once the emergency shelter is established and staffed, animal intake can begin. Intake procedures in an emergency shelter are critical for setting animals up for success. Intake protocols should be created well before the first animal comes through the doors. Intake protocols are frequently standardized by organizations and are used repeatedly for various sheltering situations, with minor changes made depending on the situation. Appendix 18.C is a sample intake protocol from an emergency shelter.

Although protocols should be tailored to the individual situation, there are general guidelines that can be followed.

### 18.9.1 Medical Evaluation and Vaccinations/Treatments

A veterinarian should be on-site to perform an initial intake examination on all animals. If a veterinarian is not available during intake, a veterinary technician or other trained personnel should screen the animals and arrangements should be made to have a veterinarian follow up as soon as possible. Based on the examination results, the appropriate housing decisions can be made for individual animals. Except for situations where owners have medical records for their pets, it should be assumed that incoming animals have had no prior vaccination and preventive care. All animals should be vaccinated immediately upon intake to the shelter. At a minimum, all dogs and cats should receive

- *Dogs:* Rabies vaccine, DHPP (or DHLPP) vaccine, and endo- and ectoparasite treatment.
- *Cats:* Rabies vaccine, FVRCP vaccine, and endo- and ectoparasite treatment. All cats should ideally be tested for FeLV and FIV, particularly if co-housed. Retroviral positive cats should not be co-housed with negative cats.

A thorough intake protocol will dictate what additional diagnostics and treatment are required. For example, organizations working in countries with a high incidence of canine parvovirus may decide to test all incoming animals with diarrhea or vomiting using a commercially available antigen test. Shelters working in areas with a high prevalence of canine influenza may choose to vaccinate all dogs on intake for this pathogen. Additional diagnostics such as heartworm and tick-borne disease point-of-care tests can also be performed at intake depending on available resources.

All shelters must have a microchip scanner available to scan animals upon entry in an attempt to reunite lost pets with their owners. All detected microchips should be documented in the patient's intake record and followed-up by calling the microchip company or searching an online database.

### 18.9.2 Animal Identification

Individual animals must be identified and tracked while at the shelter. Accurately identifying animals in the shelter is important for ensuring animal health,

proper housing, the legal protection of the sheltering group, and, during a legal case, is part of the evidence process.

#### 18.9.2.1 Individual Animal Numbering

Create a system for identifying animals by name or number. Numbering systems are advisable in situations involving large numbers of animals (>100). This system can simply be 1, 2, 3, etc. for situations involving a single species but slightly more complicated when multiple species are involved. If a shelter houses both cats and dogs, one may utilize C1, C2, etc. for cats and D1, D2, etc. for dogs. If there is more than one team processing animals at the time of intake, it may be necessary to assign colors (for example, a red and blue team) so the first dog completed by the red intake team (in a multispecies shelter) would be RD1 and the first dog completed by the blue intake team would be BD1. This helps avoid the duplication of numbers. Names can be given to the animals as well but numbers should be used as a consistent identifier.

#### 18.9.2.2 Physically Affixed Identification

The best way to physically identify animals is to affix a tab band or paper collar with the number of the animal written on it. These tend to fade and fall off over time and need to be replaced regularly. For shorter-term identification, write a number using a permanent marker on the inside of each ear. If the organization operating the emergency shelter has legal custody of the animals, microchip them. This can be done in conjunction with a collar or ID band since the microchip cannot be read without a scanner.

#### 18.9.2.3 Photographs

Photograph every animal during the intake process. The animal can be photographed next to a dry erase board or index card with the assigned animal number, date, and name of the event. Multiple views should be taken to capture all identifying marks to distinguish between animals that look similar (imagine a large-scale seizure involving hundreds of black cats!) (Figure 18.5).

#### 18.9.2.4 Mapping the Animals

Once the shelter is established, create a map (see Section 18.5) labeling all animal housing sections and

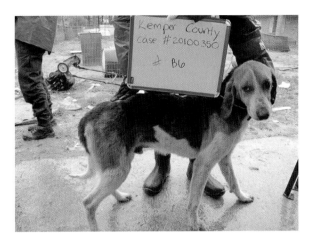

**Figure 18.5** Intake photograph of a dog confiscated from a hoarding site. Source: Courtesy of The HSUS.

enclosures. Each row, pod area, or section should be identified by a distinct letter or number. Within each section, number each enclosure. For example, if the first row of enclosures is row A, the first cage would be A1. Each row or section and each cage should be labeled with a number. This map can then be used by the Shelter Manager (or their appointee) to direct each animal upon intake to a specific enclosure. This person then notes the number of that enclosure on the master inventory log (Appendix 18.E) along with the animal identification information. This ensures an accurate and up-to-date record of all animal locations in the shelter.

### 18.9.2.5 Documentation and Paperwork

Operating an emergency shelter involves copious amounts of paperwork. It is absolutely essential that animals are identified appropriately, medical conditions and treatments are documented, and paperwork is stored and maintained properly. Many emergency shelters are designed to house animals confiscated after investigations of animal cruelty. Record-keeping is especially critical in such cases to help document the animal's condition upon entry and to protect the shelter from accusations regarding lapses in in-shelter care. During intake, there are several key forms that should be utilized (Appendices 18.C–18.F).

#### 18.9.2.5.1 *Intake Forms/Animal Medical Record*

During the initial intake examination, use a standardized intake form to record all vaccinations and medical treatments administered, and document specific medical information such as follow-up tests required, abnormalities noted, etc. (Appendix 18.C). This medical record serves as an additional backup form of identification. Ideally, this form is in duplicate or triplicate form, so one copy can be attached to the animal's enclosure and one copy kept at the vet station to be placed in a master binder located in the command center.

#### 18.9.2.5.2 *Treatment Forms*

Treatment forms are used to document individual animal medical treatments (Appendix 18.D). The veterinarian fills this form out during the initial intake examination and gives it to the person assigned to oversee medical care. These forms are then used to facilitate individual animal treatments which may include special diets, medications, and even medicated baths. If animals that are co-housed require separation during treatment or feeding, it should also be noted on this form.

#### 18.9.2.5.3 *Cage Cards*

Create an individualized cage card to accompany all animals at the shelter. The ideal cage card includes the following information:

- Photo of the animal
- Unique identifying number
- Date of entry
- Sex/sterilization status
- Disease status if known (FeLV, FIV, heartworm infection)
- Special dietary needs
- Other identifying information.

#### 18.9.2.5.4 *Master Inventory*

Record every animal on a master inventory log prior to being placed in an enclosure (Appendix 18.E). This inventory list records the identifying number and description of each animal, as well as the enclosure in which the animal will be housed in the shelter. This ensures an accurate animal inventory and that the right animal is in the appropriate kennel or cage. This list can be provided to animal care staff to facilitate treatments or to anyone else who might need to locate specific animals.

### 18.9.2.6 Sorting the Population

On intake, sort and house animals in appropriate areas depending on their health status, species, and behavioral or medical needs. At a minimum, animals exhibiting signs of infectious disease should be separated from healthy animals. Pregnant and nursing animals should also be housed in a quiet maternity area. A manager or appointee equipped with a shelter map should assist in assigning each animal to a specific cage or run following the intake examination.

### 18.9.2.7 Post-intake Cool-down Period

Intake to the emergency shelter can be very stressful for animals unfamiliar with the shelter environment. Provide animals time to adjust to this new environment. Following an initial intake examination, provide cats and dogs with 72 h to "cool down." During this period, provide food, water, and necessary medication, and keep enclosures clean. Minimize unnecessary animal interaction, such as intensive enrichment and socialization work. The exception to this are highly socialized dogs and cats craving attention or those that can be walked to go to the bathroom.

### 18.9.2.8 Animal Handling

Handle animals in such a way as to minimize animal stress and discomfort. In crisis situations, animals are often frightened and at high risk for escape. Some animals may have never been outside of a cage before and unaccustomed to handling; this is typical of dogs rescued from puppy mills and hoarding cases. Therefore, during intake processing, minimize the amount of animal handling. Very fearful or aggressive animals may require sedation. Alternatively, if the animal appears healthy, it is reasonable to let the animal acclimatize and attempt the examination the next day. Every effort should be made however to vaccinate animals as soon as or even before they enter the shelter.

When moving unsocialized animals around the shelter, use a transport crate. Allow the animal to enter the crate on his own so that he feels like it is a safe space, and then close the door. The animal can then easily be moved from one enclosure or area to another without handling. Always remember to remain calm, move slowly, and use a towel or blanket to cover the animal's head and eyes when needed during handling. For more information on humane handling, refer to Chapter 4.

## 18.10 Animal Care

The primary objective of any emergency shelter is to provide quality animal care. The majority of staff and volunteer time is therefore devoted to cleaning, feeding, and medical care. Documentation of these activities is crucial.

### 18.10.1 Daily Shelter Schedules

Dogs and cats are creatures of habit and benefit from consistent shelter schedules.

It is important to establish and publish consistent hours of operation:

- Hours the shelter is occupied by staff and volunteers
- Hours that donations can be dropped off (if being received at the shelter)
- Hours for public visitation (if owned animals are being held)
- Hours animals can be received or reclaimed (in situations of natural disaster). As there may not always be telephone access, it is especially important during natural disasters to make sure these hours are well advertised to the public.

When determining schedules, work around the shelter's designated feeding and cleaning times, as well as the hours designated as "quiet time" for any activities that involve the public entering the shelter's animal housing areas.

### 18.10.2 Cleaning Procedures

Detailed cleaning protocols are listed in Chapter 11. Special sanitation considerations specific to emergency shelters are included here. In general, cleaning should cause the least amount of disruption to the animal as possible. Keep in mind that during emergencies supplies may be limited and specialized cleaning products unavailable.

### 18.10.2.1 Products

When cleaning products are limited, household bleach is one of the most useful and readily available products for disinfecting animal bowls, toys, litter boxes, and even animal enclosures. Bleach must be diluted appropriately, however. As a general rule, a 1 : 32 (1 part bleach to 32 parts water) dilution is

---

**Textbox 18.5 Sample daily shelter schedule**

| Time | Activity |
|------|----------|
| 7:00–7:30 a.m. | • Unlock doors and perform a walk-through of all animal areas, ensuring all animals are safe and are not in critical need of attention |
| | • During the walk-through, double check that all areas are fully stocked with supplies |
| | • Ensure appropriate air flow, adjust the temperature if needed |
| | • Return to the command center to greet volunteers and staff, ensuring that they have signed in |
| 7:30–8:00 a.m. | • Morning staff/volunteer briefing |
| | • Feed and water all animals |
| 8:00–11:30 a.m. | • Clean kennels and enclosures |
| | • Collect and clean food and water bowls, toys, Kongs®, litter boxes, and other items that are in the animal enclosures that require cleaning |
| 11:30 a.m.–1:30 p.m. | • Provide quiet time for the animals to reduce animal stress. During this time, keep the lights low in animal housing areas and try to minimize human foot traffic and animal interaction as much as possible |
| | • Send staff and volunteers to lunch |
| 1:30–3:00 p.m. | • Provide enrichment as directed by the Shelter Manager |
| 3:30–6:00 p.m. | • Feed and top off water dishes |
| | • Assign volunteers to end-of-day duties including sweeping, mopping, and washing of any items not cleaned in the morning |

---

appropriate for routine disinfection. Allow a 10-min contact time prior to rinsing. Remember that bleach is inactivated by organic matter (i.e. blood, feces) and must be applied after the object requiring disinfection has been cleaned. Commercially available dish soap is often used as a detergent followed by bleach.

### 18.10.2.2 Spot Cleaning Versus Deep Cleaning

Most animals (especially cats and fearful dogs) only require their enclosures to be spot cleaned, rather than deep cleaned daily. This refers to simply removing dirty items, topping up food and water, and spot cleaning the dirty areas in the enclosures. This ensures minimal disturbance to the animals. Enclosures and all items in them must be thoroughly disinfected between animals however.

Deep cleaning of enclosures should be performed once weekly and more frequently if too soiled for spot cleaning. This involves removing the animal from the enclosure, removing any feces, urine and visible dirt, cleaning the surfaces with a detergent solution, followed by applying a bleach dilution or other disinfectant to all the surfaces of the enclosure, and allowing it to sit for at least 10 min before rinsing. If resources and space allows, having a second cage or enclosure for each animal to go into during cleaning is desirable, especially for cats, to reduce handling and stress. Volunteers can also walk the dogs during deep cleaning. For unsocialized animals, a carry crate can be placed inside the cage that the animal can enter. Once inside, the door can be shut and the crate removed during cleaning of the enclosure.

### 18.10.2.3   Triple-basin Cleaning Technique

To clean large numbers of bowls, litter boxes, Kong® toys, and other small, removable items, consider using the triple-basin cleaning technique. This technique involves three basins placed side by side. The first basin is filled with hot water and a detergent (i.e. dish soap), the second basin is filled with warm water, and the third basin is filled with cool water with the appropriate amount of bleach or other disinfectant.

The first step is to remove all organic material from the items requiring cleaning into a garbage can. Next, all items are scrubbed in the first basin using a sponge or brush, rinsed in the second basin, and dipped in the third basin for at least 45 s. The final step is to allow the items to air dry. The basins will need to be emptied and refilled periodically when the water becomes dirty.

## 18.10.3   Feeding

Ideally, animals should be fed twice daily except for very young or underweight animals who require more frequent feedings. A system must be in place to clearly identify enclosures of animals requiring additional feeding or a specialized diet. This can be marked on a standardized treatment sheet (Appendix 18.D). The person responsible for administering treatments should also oversee additional feedings. For the entire shelter population, feeding should be recorded on a daily care sheet (Appendix 18.F). Animals not eating should be clearly marked on this form. Water bowls should be kept filled and clean at all times. Watering cans can be used to easily top-up water bowls in wire cages when needed.

## 18.10.4   Treatments and Medical Care

Many animals presenting to emergency shelters require some type of medical care. It is advisable to assign one person, commonly referred to as the Veterinary Medical Manager, the responsibility of managing this task. The following are recommendations to assure adequate medical care in an emergency shelter.

### 18.10.4.1   Veterinary Oversight

A veterinarian must be involved in the emergency shelter, even if he or she is not able to visit daily. Veterinarians can perform the following tasks:

- Perform initial intake examinations
- Control in-shelter disease transmission
- Determine intake and treatment protocols
- Design isolation, quarantine, and treatment areas in the shelter
- Perform humane euthanasia when warranted
- Assist with supply ordering.

### 18.10.4.2   Treatment Sheets

Fill out treatment sheets during the initial intake examination and store in a master binder. The Veterinary Medical Manager is responsible for ensuring that the instructions on these sheets are carried out. Check off treatments when performed (Appendix 18.D).

### 18.10.4.3   Commonly Observed Disease Protocols

To ensure consistency of care, prepare standardized treatment protocols for commonly observed diseases. Such protocols should contain enough details to guide medical diagnostics, treatments, and housing recommendations based on testing results. Depending on the species and case, some commonly observed diseases requiring protocols include feline upper respiratory disease, dermatophytosis (ringworm), wounds, otitis externa, kennel cough, and canine parvovirus.

### 18.10.4.4   Emergency Contacts

Although most emergency shelters are equipped to handle basic medical treatments, emergencies are usually best treated off-site. For this reason, establish memorandums of understanding with local veterinary clinics to provide off-site care. Doing so also helps engage the local veterinary community during the emergency response.

## 18.11   Animal Enrichment

Enrichment is a critical tool in an emergency shelter to ensure the mental well-being of sheltered animals. Emergency shelters frequently house dogs and cats unaccustomed to kenneling, and long-term confinement frequently leads to boredom, anxiety, and mental deterioration, which can affect the overall health of the animals. Therefore, sheltered animals must be kept engaged and stimulated. Long-term sheltering also provides an opportunity to socialize

---

**Textbox 18.6 Simple enrichment tools for use in emergency shelters**

1) *Exercise pens.* Simple leash walking or time in an enrichment pen can be a fundamental component of an enrichment program. Pens can also be used to socialize shy dogs.

2) *Playgroups.* Dogs that enjoy interacting with other dogs can greatly benefit from regular exercise and play with other dogs. Such playgroups must be done carefully and with appropriate supervision.

3) *Auditory enrichment.* A radio playing soft music, talk radio, or a relaxation CD can have a calming effect on dogs. These can be played during quiet time in the kennel or throughout the day.

4) *Scent of the day.* Fill a spray bottle with water and 10–20 drops of an essential oil such as vanilla, almond, or lavender. Spray a new scent each day over dog beds, blankets, or kennel walls. When disease transmission is not an issue, some shelters will exchange unsoiled blankets from various kennels as a form of olfactory enrichment.

5) *Food dispensing toys.* Durable rubber Kong®-type toys can be stuffed with dog kibble, filled with peanut butter, and frozen to provide a long-lasting treat. If Kongs® are unavailable, frozen treats can be made by placing food or treats in chicken broth and freezing into cubes.

6) *"Busy boxes/buckets".* Use a cardboard box (leftover pizza containers are perfect) or bucket and fill it with a variety of scents (pizza boxes already come with great smells!), treats, kibble, etc. Either tape the box closed or stuff the items in the bucket tightly so it requires a significant effort to get them out.

7) *Blanket shredders.* Smear peanut butter, beef broth, or anything other edible item with a strong smell on the center of a towel, then tie a knot over it. Dogs will be kept busy as they attempt to shred their way to the area with the strongest smell.

8) *Touch time.* Have volunteers or staff enter the dog's enclosures, sit quietly, and pet the dog or cat for up to 10 min. Interaction should be done in a calm and quiet manner.

---

any undersocialized animals to increase their chances for adoption.

### 18.11.1 Canine Enrichment

Canine enrichment can consist of a variety of activities including physical exercise outside the enclosure to simple in-kennel treats and toys that can keep dogs mentally stimulated for hours.

Many items used in the shelter on a daily basis such as plastic bottles, paper towel rolls, and disposable staff lunch containers can be repurposed for animal enrichment. When using such items however, ensure animals are appropriately monitored to prevent the ingestion of non-consumable items such as plastic and towels.

#### 18.11.1.1 Shy/Unsocialized Dogs

Shy or fearful dogs may require special enrichment techniques to facilitate adjustment to the shelter environment. The following are a few suggestions specific to fearful dogs:

- *Read and Relax:* During Read and Relax, a volunteer (or staff member) sits in front of a dog's kennel (facing to the side and not directly towards the dog) and reads a book in a calm voice. This helps the dog acclimate to both the presence and voice of people. If the dog approaches the front of the enclosure, a treat can be dropped into the kennel to encourage further interaction.

- *Treating:* There are simple ways to use treats with shy dogs in their enclosures. Both techniques can be used to encourage certain behaviors.
  - Roll-by treating is performed when a container with treats is hung on each dog's enclosure. As staff and volunteers move around the shelter, they take treats from the container and drop them into the kennel. Dogs learn to correlate humans with positive events happening.
  - Sit and treat happens when volunteers or staff sit outside the dog's enclosure (much like in Read and Relax) and give treats to the dog. Be sure to not directly face the dog and from time to time turn your back to encourage the dog to come up behind and perform a stealthy sniff.

When socializing a dog, pay attention to the dog's behavior in order to determine when to progress to the next step. Every dog progresses at his or her own pace. The Dog Enrichment Cheat Sheet (Appendix 18.G) helps guide which activities are appropriate given the observed behavior.

### 18.11.2 Feline Enrichment

Cats are particularly prone to stress in the shelter environment. Simple environmental adjustments can dramatically affect a sheltered cat's quality of life.

- For social cats, touch can be an effective enrichment tool. Petting, brushing, and massaging cats can lower their stress levels. Additionally, interactive toys such as pipe cleaners and strings with fake mice on the end can be great tools for engaging cats. In fact, almost anything can be a great cat toy including a paper bag or wadded-up ball of tape. Most cats love anything that crinkles.
- For cat enclosures, creating hammocks (made of fabric with holes cut in the corners and tied to the edges of the enclosure) is a very simple way to make a nice bed and hiding spot for cats. For shy cats, a hiding crate inside the enclosure or a visual barrier consisting of a towel draped over the cage can help relieve stress. House cats in the quietest area of the shelter, away from barking dogs. Consider using Feliway® spray on blankets or towels.

## 18.12 Disposition and Release of Animals

Emergency shelters are designed to serve as temporary refuges for animals. Following cessation of the emergency or once animals are legally released to the organization operating the shelter, decisions must be made about animal disposition. There are four possibilities for animal disposition: return-to-owner, adoption/transfer, long-term sheltering, and euthanasia.

### 18.12.1 Return-to-owner

This occurs most commonly following natural disasters. Animals may have been sheltered during a crisis but are then reclaimed by the owners following cessation of the emergency. Lost pets may also be reunited with their owners. Any time an animal is reclaimed ensure that owners sign release paperwork. During the reclamation process, owners may be asked to present proof of ownership. Because many people may have lost all their belongings during a disaster, a lost pet report and description of the animal usually suffices.

### 18.12.2 Adoption/Transfer of Animals for Adoption

Whether an emergency shelter decides to host an adoption event themselves or transfer animals to existing sheltering facilities to adopt out will depend on a number of factors. Operating a successful adoption program requires a tremendous amount of resources. However, if the emergency shelter is operated by a permanent shelter, also referred to as a brick-and-mortar facility, this might be an appropriate option. Keep in mind that large numbers of animals in emergency shelters can overwhelm the adoption capacity of a local town and transferring to partner shelters in other areas can help maximize the chance of successful adoptions. Consider the following when deciding whether to transfer animals to other facilities or hold an adoption drive at the emergency shelter.

- *Returned adoptions:* How will adoption returns be handled? If adopters have an issue or cannot keep an animal, who will they turn to? An established brick-and-mortar shelter may already have these resources in place.
- *Media:* Media attention can help draw large crowds of potential adopters to an emergency shelter. If transferring animals to brick-and-mortar shelters, assure that media attention is generated at a local level as well.
- *Personnel/staffing:* Large-scale adoption events require a significant number of personnel. Does the emergency shelter have enough staff and volunteers to facilitate an event?

Regardless of the type of adoption event, ensure that copies of all paperwork from that animal's time at the emergency shelter accompany the animal, including both medical and behavioral notes.

### 18.12.3 Long-term Sheltering

Generally, long-term sheltering of animals is a last resort for those with medical or behavioral issues that preclude adoption. This includes cats that are FeLV- or FIV-positive or aggressive animals. An emergency shelter should not turn into long-term housing, and if animals require long-term housing, they should be transferred to a facility with the appropriate resources.

### 18.12.4 Euthanasia

While controversial, it is worth noting that euthanasia may be appropriate for animals without adoption options, with untreatable medical conditions, or whose suffering cannot be ameliorated. Every organization must assess their resources for long-term care and options for live release.

## 18.13 Breakdown and Deconstruction of the Shelter

Once animals have been moved out of the emergency shelter, all equipment and supplies must be cleaned, disassembled, and stored. The facility itself also needs to be cleaned and decontaminated.

### 18.13.1 Animal Care Supplies

Clean and disinfect all enclosures, bowls, enrichment items, blankets, and animal care supplies. Use the triple-basin method for non-laundry items as described in the cleaning section. For enclosures too large for the basin, wash, rinse, and then spray all surfaces with a 1:32 bleach solution or other appropriate disinfectant, and leave to dry. Items that cannot effectively be cleaned or decontaminated should be thrown away.

### 18.13.2 Facility

Specific cleaning and decontamination procedures will depend on the particular facility. In general, clean the walls and cement or tile flooring, and cover with a 1:10 bleach dilution or other appropriate disinfectant. For dirt or similar flooring, lime can be used to decontaminate the area. If the area is a barn or similar structure laced with shavings, remove the old shaving and line the floor with new shaving.

### 18.13.3 Supply Storage

Store any remaining shelter supplies in a manner that minimizes contamination and spoilage. Distribute food and other perishable items to other shelters and rescue groups in the area. Maintain a written inventory of all equipment and institute a system to sign the equipment in and out to prevent loss.

Once the shelter has been emptied, cleaned, and decontaminated, conduct a walk-through with the property owner to ensure any issues can be addressed immediately.

## 18.14 Utilizing Media Outlets

During times of crisis, the public often responds with overwhelming support and assistance. A community can quickly progress from a situation in which they have very few visible resources to being suddenly engulfed with public support. Knowing how to best harness this increased public attention can ensure the organization continues to have the resources to operate.

### 18.14.1 Traditional Media

Traditional media (newspaper, radio, television) can help increase awareness and support for an emergency sheltering operation. Media outlets will often provide their readers, viewers, or listeners with ways that they can help (often by providing the contact information for the organization operating the shelter). It is important to decide prior to starting media outreach who will be the primary contact for media, where to direct the public, and who will receive public enquiries. Instruct staff and volunteers not to talk to the media unless they go through this designated point of contact. This helps ensuring that all messaging is consistent. Traditional media can also put the crisis situation into context. For example, if the emergency shelter is for dogs rescued from dog meat farms, the media can help highlight the issues surrounding the dog meat trade. Doing so generates support for the shelter and increases community awareness of the overall issue.

### 18.14.2 Social Media

The rise of social media has been a game changer for organizations struggling with day-to-day and/or emergency operations. Social media provides a direct outlet to appeal to the public for help, as well as to keep the public up-to-date on shelter activities. During an emergency, shelters can ask for monetary donations, provide updates on specific animals or the overall situation, solicit for volunteers or in-kind donations, and during times of disaster, provide lost and found reports, and requests for rescue of specific animals. Enact policies for all staff and volunteers regarding social media postings. Once an organization is using social media, many people will try to initiate contact. Assign a point person to monitor and respond to public comments to maintain control of the messaging and outward communication.

### 18.14.3 Donations

The public's response to a crisis situation can be generous, and an organization can be easily overwhelmed by donated goods. When planning the emergency shelter, consider allocating an area for receiving donations. Assure clear messaging to provide a list of specific items needed and locations that these items can be dropped off. It is also recommended to investigate where donated items can be redirected locally should too many be received at the emergency shelter (local shelters and rescue groups or, in times of natural disaster, even a food bank for animal owners).

### 18.14.4 Volunteers

Use of media and social media is a great way to recruit volunteers but the response can be overwhelming. Designate a point-of-contact person to handle volunteer inquiries.

## Suggested Websites

Animal Sheltering Magazine and website – Publication and informational website of the Humane Society of the United States (www.animalsheltering.org).

ASPCA Professional – Website with webinars to provide tools and resources for all aspects of animal welfare work (www.aspcapro.org).

Global Wildlife Resources, Inc. – Website providing detailed techniques and equipment on most methods for capturing and handling street dogs (http://wildliferesources.com).

Guidelines for Standards of Care in Animal Shelters – Comprehensive guidelines to help sheltering operations meeting the physical, medical, and behavioral needs of sheltered animals (http://www.sheltervet.org).

# Appendix

## 18.A   Emergency Animal Sheltering Checklist.

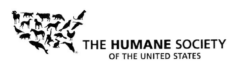

## Emergency Animal Sheltering Checklist

**PHYSICAL FACILITY:**

**Access from a main road**
- ☐ Hazard-free access
- ☐ Signage identifying the facility and its purpose
- ☐ Safety markings and signage
- ☐ Separate entry for rescue teams, etc.
- ☐ 24/7 access for staff and volunteers (*if shelter is in curfew area, obtain clearance*)
- ☐ Easy access for large trucks and supply vehicles to get in and out
- ☐ Minimal hazards for staff and volunteers, as well as for animals
- ☐ On or near a main evacuation route

**Parking area**
- ☐ Signage directing the public bringing animals in; emergent volunteers; in-kind donations; people looking for lost animals; etc.
- ☐ Safety–hazards mitigated and/or marked, etc.
- ☐ Poop area for dogs coming in, plastic bags, garbage cans
- ☐ Parking for response equipment: RVs, trailers, trucks, etc.
- ☐ Parking for the public
- ☐ Parking for staff & volunteers
- ☐ Able to accommodate 50' transport trailer and PetsMart Charities trailer
- ☐ Able to accommodate large numbers of vehicles to enter/exit easily and not obstruct parking areas or roads
- ☐ Solid surface for parking areas to avoid getting vehicles stuck in mud, sand, ice, or snow
- ☐ Security

**Facility entrance**
- ☐ Signage directing the public bringing animals in; emergent volunteers; in-kind donations; people looking for lost animals; etc
- ☐ Areas where people can wait with their animals and not have animal interaction, is this area protected from the elements?
- ☐ Safety–hazards mitigated and/or marked, etc.
- ☐ Security

## 18.A    Emergency Animal Sheltering Checklist. (*Continued*)

**Facility Design and Construction**

☐ Non-porous floors, easily disinfected
☐ Ventilation, heat/cooling
☐ Electricity (lighting)
☐ Plumbing

**Utilities and Services**

☐ Power
☐ Emergency lighting
☐ Water (municipal supply, delivered, etc.)
☐ Trash disposal service
☐ Telephone
☐ Internet access

**Floor Plan and Layout**

☐ Ability to separate animals by species and health status
☐ Logical flow for processing animals, people, and supplies/equipment
☐ Separate public and private areas
☐ Separate human and animal areas; allowing smooth flow of functions

**Animal Related Areas**

☐ Animal intake and registration
☐ Initial Assessment
☐ Isolation; Quarantine facility and procedures
☐ Triage, veterinary, and first aid
☐ Decontamination
☐ Small animal housing: Healthy dogs, Isolation dogs, Aggressive/Quarantine, Healthy cats, Isolation cats; Feral/Quarantine; Caged birds; Rabbits; Pocket pets; Reptiles; Ferrets; Other
☐ Large animal housing: Cows; Goats & sheep; Poultry; Ratites; Pigs (potbelly & hogs); Horses (separate stallions individually; pregnant mares & mares w/foals); Horse with unknown Coggins status
☐ Food preparation and storage, food sanitation (wash bowls, etc.)
☐ Cleaning station for cages
☐ Animal exercise and dog relief areas
☐ Animal visitation and reunion processing
☐ Grooming / bathing

**Security**

☐ Personnel
☐ Medications
☐ Equipment
☐ Personal effects

# 18.A Emergency Animal Sheltering Checklist. (*Continued*)

- [ ] Procedures-screening of volunteers and staff
- [ ] Human service areas
- [ ] Donations management security,
- [ ] Animal housing areas

**Human Service Areas -** Areas available and delineated:

- [ ] Bathroom/shower facilities
- [ ] Staff break area
- [ ] Volunteer intake/orientation
- [ ] Canteen area with food and drinks
- [ ] Quiet office area
- [ ] First aid station
- [ ] Housing
- [ ] Team information (bulletin boards) for staff and volunteers
- [ ] Public information

**PROCEDURES:**

**Animal intake**

- [ ] Accountability paperwork–personnel trained and supervised how to complete paperwork and secure identification to animals
- [ ] Waiting area for owners–seating, separation from other owners and animals
- [ ] Triage set up–identify infectious diseases, emergency situations, critical illness
- [ ] Decontamination area

**Keeping Track of the Animals**

- [ ] Identification
- [ ] Daily care schedule
- [ ] Lost & found
- [ ] Foster
- [ ] Adoptions
- [ ] Euthanasia
- [ ] Transfers to rescue (chain of custody)

**Intake Procedures**

- [ ] Written procedures
- [ ] Forms
- [ ] Identification photo–cameras, printers, etc.

**Special Policies and Protocols**

- [ ] Vaccines
- [ ] Spay/neuter
- [ ] Euthanasia
- [ ] Presence of endangered orprotected species

## 18.A   Emergency Animal Sheltering Checklist. (*Continued*)

**Initial Assessment**
- ☐ Animals assessed for pre-existing or potential medical problems; behavioral or temperament issues affecting care or handling (aggressive, fearful, high-stress, timid, feral, etc.)

**Identification Protocol and Supplies:**
- ☐ Jiffy tags; Hospital ID bands; Microchip
- ☐ Halter tags; Paint sticks; Shaver; Neck ID bands

**Daily Care Record**
- ☐ Keep track of Food; Water; Exercise; relief; Medication; Behavior changes; Any unusual observations

**Lost & Found Protocol**
- ☐ System of logging & cross referencing found and lost records
- ☐ System of notification of owners
- ☐ Photo books –Polaroid / digital photos
- ☐ Owner provides photos of lost pets
- ☐ Shelter takes photos of incoming animals
- ☐ Internet database of found animals in shelter

**Strategy for Special Need Animals**
- ☐ Special interest/fanciers clubs or groups to assist with special needs animals
- ☐ Pre-existing foster/rescue networks as primary source of off-site care
- ☐ Veterinary clinics and boarding kennels for overflow or animals with medical, behavioral or emotional needs

**Adoption**
- ☐ Holding period protocol and adoption guidelines established
- ☐ Transfers to rescue groups

**Animal Mental Health Issues**
- ☐ Recognition of and meeting emotional and environmental needs of animals

**Ongoing Procedures**
- ☐ Limit people in shelter
- ☐ Log when care provided
- ☐ No visitors except animals' owners during authorized visitation hours
- ☐ Monitors condition of animals–notify vet staff of problems

## 18.A  Emergency Animal Sheltering Checklist. (*Continued*)

### Worker Health Issues

- ☐ Vaccinations: Rabies; Tetanus; Hepatitis A and B; Influenza and others suggested
- ☐ Control of and protection from environmental hazards
- ☐ Use of "Universal Precautions" in dealing with animals and humans
- ☐ Protective clothing available and in proper use
- ☐ Mental health/stress management capability for staff and volunteers: peer-to-peer CISM; orientation, training, referral resources.

### SUPPLIES AND EQUIPMENT:

### Shelter Housing/Containment

- ☐ Appropriate physical environment
- ☐ Weather/season (can limit sheltering options)
- ☐ Temperatures match animal needs (warmer for reptiles & birds)
- ☐ Type of caging (crates, cages, portable fencing, aquariums, stables/corrals)
- ☐ Cold weather considerations including additional heat needs, check for frozen pipes, etc.

### Animal Care Supplies (excluding food and water–*see equipment/supply list*)

- ☐ Adequate containment capability (crates, cages, corrals, pens, etc.) for expected number and types of animals
- ☐ S/S dog bowls
- ☐ Collars, leashes, muzzles
- ☐ Animal Handling equipment: Control pole; Muzzles; Gloves (different types for different species); Traps; Nets, etc
- ☐ Cat litter/newspapers; litter pans, scoops, paper (disposable) food containers, water bowls
- ☐ Sanitation supplies: Plastic sheets; Paper towels; Cleaners/Disinfectants; garbage bags; Covered trash containers; poop bags; cleaning gloves; nitrile gloves for decontamination;
- ☐ Blankets, towels, sheets
- ☐ Card board, metal sheeting, etc. for cage separation

### Animal Food

- ☐ Protocols for food type; appropriate for species, age, and health of each animal
- ☐ Written feeding protocol and meal record for each animal
- ☐ Alternate or specialty foods
- ☐ Supplements
- ☐ Proper storage of food (covered containers)

## 18.A Emergency Animal Sheltering Checklist. (*Continued*)

**Water**

- [ ] Potable water for drinking (human and animal)
- [ ] Non-potable for cleaning (fire departments/National Guard may provide)
- [ ] Quantity sufficient for each type of animal and humans, appropriate to activity level & weather

**Basic Veterinary Care:**

- [ ] Basic first aid supplies; Thermometer; bandages, sponges; adhesive bandages; gauze roll; Vet wrap; splints; Gauze; Muzzles; Syringes/needles (assorted sizes); Stethoscope; medications; etc
- [ ] On-call or on-site veterinarians and/or veterinary technicians

**Human First Aid**

- [ ] First aid kit; Sterile gloves; Stethoscope; Thermometer; Waterless hand sanitizer;
- [ ] Eye wash; Saline, hydrogen peroxide
- [ ] Insect repellent and sunscreen
- [ ] Aspirin/Ibuprofen/acetaminophen, Benadryl, antibiotic ointment; and other over-the-counter medications
- [ ] Blankets and cots

**Food and Hydration for People**

- [ ] Adequate water and sports drinks;
- [ ] Snacks with protein and carbohydrates; appealing; single-serving packages
- [ ] Food sanitation; plates, cups, utensils, etc.

**Tools and Equipment**

- [ ] Fencing (pens & perimeter): chain link, portable panels, portable corrals, construction barricade, hog wire/field fence
- [ ] Tarps (for roofing & shade)
- [ ] Fans/heaters, Extension cords
- [ ] Locks
- [ ] Dumpster
- [ ] Generators
- [ ] Forklifts and pallet jacks if necessary for supply management

**Sanitation and Disposal Areas:**

- [ ] Decontamination
- [ ] Garbage
- [ ] Biohazard waste
- [ ] Haz-mat disposal
- [ ] Dead animal holding facility

## 18.A   Emergency Animal Sheltering Checklist. (*Continued*)

**ICS SECTIONS AND OFFICES:**

**Incident Management**

- ☐ Shelter staffed according to the ICS
- ☐ ICS chart posted
- ☐ Distinct facilities available and marked for Incident Command; Communications; Finance and Administration; Public Information Officer (PIO) and Media; Operations staging area; Transportation staging area; Resources Staging Area; Base Camp; Equipment and supply storage; etc.

**Volunteer Management**

- ☐ Reception desk or area–staffed –check-in/check-out procedures
- ☐ Orientation and training provided
- ☐ Daily briefings to include safety issues
- ☐ Information bulletin board
- ☐ Controlled area preventing access to animals until/if assigned
- ☐ Printed instructions/manual/etc for volunteers

**Donation Management**

- ☐ Signage saying what is needed
- ☐ Information on how to donate money
- ☐ Ability to store donated supplies properly
- ☐ Donations manager–acknowledgement, update wish list, etc.

Source: Courtesy of The HSUS

## 18.B  Shelter Equipment Planning Checklist.

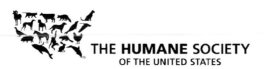

THE **HUMANE** SOCIETY
OF THE UNITED STATES

**SHELTER EQUIPMENT PLANNING CHECKLIST**

### *Minimal* Shelter Set-up Equipment Needs:

☐ 300-350 Wire Crates (Med-Large)
☐ 25-50 Airline Crates (Med & Large)
☐ 300-350 S/S bowls (Various sizes)
☐ 5000 3 to 5# capacity Dixie paper food trays
☐ 100 slip leads
☐ Soft muzzles (Med-Large sizes)
☐ 1000 ID bands (Large)
☐ 200-250 sheets of cardboard

### Office Supplies
☐ Pens
☐ Copy paper
☐ 1 Printer / Copier
☐ 1 dozen legal pads
☐ Permanent Markers
☐ Stapler
☐ Scissors
☐ File box w/folders
☐ Dry erase boards and markers

### Forms
☐ Animal Intake Forms (triplicate)
☐ Animal Care Sheets
☐ Volunteer Sign-In/Out Roster
☐ Volunteer Release of Liability
☐ Animal Release Forms
☐ Animal Health Assessment Forms

### Sheltering Tools and Supplies

☐ 100+ clip boards

☐ 300-500 shower hooks
☐ 3 rolls 55-gallon garbage bags
☐ Large garbage cans
☐ 20 buckets
☐ Duct tape (silver, lime, orange, pink)
☐ 1000 zip ties
☐ 500 gallon-size ziplock bags
☐ Paper towels
☐ Digital or Instant camera w/film
☐ 2 doz. Spray 32-oz. bottles
☐ 5 bottles Dawn
☐ 3 case Bleach
☐ Can opener
☐ Brooms and dust pans
☐ Minimum 6 folding tables
☐ Tool box
☐ 3 50' electrical cords
☐ 6 large tarps
☐ Garbage dumpster w/regular pick-up service
☐ 3 80-85 Gallon Poly (or carbon fiber) stock tanks for wash station
☐ 3-6 scrub brushes
☐ 6-1cup measuring cups
☐ Exam Gloves
☐ Exam Gowns
☐ Booties
☐ First Aid Kit
☐ Wire Cutter and Pliers for Tool Box
☐ Snaps for Kennel / Cage Crates
☐ Puppy Pads

Source: Courtesy of The HSUS

## 18.C   Canine Veterinary Intake Examination

**THE HUMANE SOCIETY**
OF THE UNITED STATES

Intake Number: _____

Deployment: _____

**VETERINARY INTAKE EXAM**     Location: _____

### ANIMAL PATIENT MEDICAL RECORD - DOG

Intake Exam Date: _____ Clinician(s): _____ Initials: _____

Breed: _____ Color: _____ Neuter:  Y / N (circle)   Gender:  M / F (circle)

Age / Birth: _____ est./Act. (circle)    Current Weight: _____ kg/lb. (circle)    est./act. (circle)

Ear Tag#: _____ Brand/Tattoo: _____ Already Chipped?  Y/N  Microchip: _____

**EXAM**

| T | Ears ☐ NSF ☐ F | Eyes ☐ NSF ☐ F | Nose ☐ NSF ☐ F | Mouth ☐ NSF ☐ F |
|---|---|---|---|---|
| P | Abdomen ☐ NSF ☐ F | Heart ☐ NSF ☐ F | Lungs ☐ NSF ☐ F | Hydration ☐ NSF ☐ F |
| R | MuscSkel ☐ NSF ☐ F | Neurol. ☐ NSF ☐ F | Dental Grade: NSF    1    2    3    4 | |

| Body Condition: | Emaciated (1) | Very Thin (2) | Thin (3) | Underweight (4) |
|---|---|---|---|---|
| | Ideal (5) | Overweight (6) | Heavy (7) | Obese (8) | Grossly Obese (9) |

**Medical Findings:** _____
_____
_____
_____
_____
_____

**Assessment/Plan:** _____
_____

**Vaccinations:**
☐  No Vaccination due to Age     ☐  No Vaccination due to Medical

| ☐ CBC/Chem ☐ UA ☐ Fecal <br> ☐ 4DX:   ☐ Neg. ☐ Pos. | Rabies: ☐ 1 Year   ☐ 3 Year <br> Date: _____ | (Label) |
|---|---|---|
| Dewormer: _____ <br> Dosage: _____ Date: _____ | Distemper:  ☐ DHPP  ☐ DHLPP <br> Date: _____ | (Label) |
| Ext.Parasite: ☐ Frontline ☐ Revolution <br> Date: _____ | Bordatella:   Date: _____ | (Label) |

## 18.D Animal Medical Treatment Form

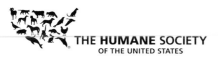

THE **HUMANE** SOCIETY
OF THE UNITED STATES

# ANIMAL TREATMENT

Animal I.D.#: _____ Cage Location: _____

Breed: _____ Color: _____ Sex: _____

Medication: _____ RX Veterinarian: _____

Reason for Medication: _____

Directions/Duration: _____

Recheck Date (if needed): _____

Special Instruction: _____

| DATE | AM | | MID AM | | MIDDAY | | PM | | NOTES |
|------|------|------|------|------|------|------|------|------|-------|
| | Time | Intl. | Time | Intl. | Time | Intl. | Time | Intl. | |
| | | | | | | | | | |
| | | | | | | | | | |
| | | | | | | | | | |
| | | | | | | | | | |
| | | | | | | | | | |
| | | | | | | | | | |
| | | | | | | | | | |
| | | | | | | | | | |
| | | | | | | | | | |
| | | | | | | | | | |
| | | | | | | | | | |
| | | | | | | | | | |
| | | | | | | | | | |
| | | | | | | | | | |
| | | | | | | | | | |
| | | | | | | | | | |
| | | | | | | | | | |
| | | | | | | | | | |
| | | | | | | | | | |
| | | | | | | | | | |
| | | | | | | | | | |
| | | | | | | | | | |

## 18.E    Master Intake Log

THE **HUMANE** SOCIETY
OF THE UNITED STATES

Page _____ of _____

Date: _____

Scribe:_____

# MASTER INTAKE

**Deployment / Case :** _____

| Animal ID | Breed | Color | Gender | Notes |
|-----------|-------|-------|--------|-------|
|           |       |       |        |       |
|           |       |       |        |       |
|           |       |       |        |       |
|           |       |       |        |       |
|           |       |       |        |       |
|           |       |       |        |       |
|           |       |       |        |       |
|           |       |       |        |       |
|           |       |       |        |       |
|           |       |       |        |       |
|           |       |       |        |       |
|           |       |       |        |       |
|           |       |       |        |       |
|           |       |       |        |       |
|           |       |       |        |       |
|           |       |       |        |       |
|           |       |       |        |       |
|           |       |       |        |       |
|           |       |       |        |       |
|           |       |       |        |       |
|           |       |       |        |       |
|           |       |       |        |       |
|           |       |       |        |       |
|           |       |       |        |       |
|           |       |       |        |       |
|           |       |       |        |       |

## 18.F   Daily Care Sheet

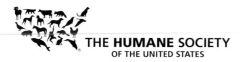
THE **HUMANE** SOCIETY
OF THE UNITED STATES

INTAKE NUMBER

# DAILY CARE SHEET

| ANIMAL DESCRIPTION |
|---|

**TYPE:**

☐ DOG   ☐ CAT   ☐ HORSE   ☐ OTHER _____

**CHARACTERISTICS:**

BREED:_____   GENDER: ☐ MALE  ☐ FEMALE COLORS: _____

**SPECIAL INSTRUCTIONS:** _____

_____

_____

_____

_____

| RECORDS (always date, time and initial) | | | | | | | |
|---|---|---|---|---|---|---|---|
| DATE | TIME | DIET / PORTION | FECES/URINE | EXERCISE | BEHAVIOR | COMMENTS | INT. |
| | AM : | / | ☐ F ☐ U | | | | |
| | MID : | / | ☐ F ☐ U | | | | |
| | PM : | / | ☐ F ☐ U | | | | |
| | AM : | / | ☐ F ☐ U | | | | |
| | MID : | / | ☐ F ☐ U | | | | |
| | PM : | / | ☐ F ☐ U | | | | |
| | AM : | / | ☐ F ☐ U | | | | |
| | MID : | / | ☐ F ☐ U | | | | |
| | PM : | / | ☐ F ☐ U | | | | |
| | AM : | / | ☐ F ☐ U | | | | |
| | MID : | / | ☐ F ☐ U | | | | |
| | PM : | / | ☐ F ☐ U | | | | |
| | AM : | / | ☐ F ☐ U | | | | |
| | MID : | / | ☐ F ☐ U | | | | |
| | PM : | / | ☐ F ☐ U | | | | |
| | AM : | / | ☐ F ☐ U | | | | |
| | MID : | / | ☐ F ☐ U | | | | |
| | PM : | / | ☐ F ☐ U | | | | |
| | AM : | / | ☐ F ☐ U | | | | |
| | MID : | / | ☐ F ☐ U | | | | |
| | PM : | / | ☐ F ☐ U | | | | |

## 18.G   Canine Enrichment Cheat Sheet

### Approved Enrichment for Dogs

| Behavior Plan | Body Language | Approved Enrichment | Be Aware Of |
|---|---|---|---|
| Tier 1:  Highly Adaptable | Loose, wiggly body language on all or most handlers' approach to kennel.  Accepts touch and general handling, may still be sensitive about touching certain areas<br>Accepts or is learning about leash<br>Normal stool and toileting habits<br>Eating regularly | -- In-Kennel human socialization<br>-- Experiment with touch, petting, and gentle physical play<br>-- Leash On/Leash Off<br>-- Hand Feeding<br>-- Read and Relax in kennel<br>-- Explore novel object approved by Shelter Manager | -- Stress signs during petting or Leash On/Leash Off<br>-- Reserved body language asking to increase distance or space<br>Review "Signals" handout<br>-- Notify Shelter Manager if rough mouthing, jumping, or taking food roughly during hand feeding |
| Tier 2:  Developing Social Skills | Shows inviting language on approach but may become aloof or stressed during cleaning routine.  May often shows stress signals.  May show stress at sight of leash<br>Occasional loose stool or diarrhea after stressful interactions | -- In-Kennel human socialization as long as not cowering, shaking<br>-- Hand Feeding<br>-- Quiet Sitting in kennel<br>-- Read and Relax out of kennel<br>-- Explore novel object approved by Shelter Manager<br>-- Experiment with touch if body language remains loose and dog solicits attention (5 Second Rule) | -- Different response to different handlers<br>-- Stress signs during inkennel enrichment<br>-- Behavior may change with sudden human movements/position changes.<br>-- Notify Shelter Manager if rough mouthing, jumping, or taking food roughly during hand feeding |
| Tier 3:  Stressed or Fearful | Obvious signs of fear or stress when human approaches.  May become rigid  or timid during cleaning routine | -- Observing regular routine<br>-- Have meals or snacks in Kongs<br>-- Quiet Sitting outside Kennel | These dogs will respond differently to different handlers |
| Caution | Growl or cower and shake on approach | -- Observing regular routine<br>-- Have meals or snacks in Kongs | Only Shelter Manager or Enrichment Lead should be in-kennel on for enrichment or necessary treatments |
| Puppy | Varying depending on socialization | -- Modified Puppy Rules of 12<br>-- Hand feeding<br>-- Supervised group play with siblings as approved by Shelter Manager | Signs that show puppy is scared or stressed.  Keep everything positive |

Remember: A dog's adaptability and stress throughout can change throughout the day and always "listen" to what a dog's body language is telling you.  At no time should any dog be given loud verbal or physical correction, or be encouraged to engage in rough mouthing.

## References

1 American Red Cross (ARC) (2002). Standards for Hurricane Evacuation Shelter Selection. Washington, DC: American Red Cross.

2 Brackenridge, S. and Zottarelli, L.K. (2015). Dimensions of the human–animal bond and evacuation decisions among pet owners during hurricane Ike. *Anthrozoös* **25** (2): 229–238.

3 GovTrack.us (2006). H.R. 3858-109th Pets Evacuation and Transportation Standards Act of 2006, legislation https://www.govtrack.us/congress/bills/109/hr3858 (accessed 12 December 2016).

4 Leonard, H.A. and Scammon, D.L. (2007). No pet left behind: accommodating pets in emergency planning. *Journal of Public Policy & Marketing* **26** (1): 49–53.

5 Mays, D. (2009). National Animal Care and Control Association Training Manual. Kansas City: National Animal Care and Control Association.

6 Humane Society of the United States (HSUS) (2010). General staffing recommendations for kennel caretaking. https://www.animalsheltering.org/ (accessed 15 December 2017).

7 FEMA (2017). Incident command system resources. https://www.fema.gov/incident-command-system-resources (accessed 22 January 2017).

# 19

# Program Monitoring and Evaluation

*Elly Hiby[1] and J.F. Reece[2]*

[1]International Companion Animal Management (ICAM) Coalition, Chaired by IFAW, International Headquarters, 290 Summer Street, Yarmouth Port, MA 02675, USA
[2]Help in Suffering, Maharani Farm, Durgapura, Jaipur 302018, Rajasthan, India

## 19.1　Introduction

Veterinary staff have a responsibility to record details about an animal's condition, treatment, and recovery in order to evaluate the impact of veterinary intervention on the individual. This evaluation should consider potential improvements to the veterinary intervention and selection of individual animals for intervention, in a way that maximizes benefit and minimizes costs to the individual. All staff and volunteers involved in an intervention also have a responsibility to consider how the intervention is impacting the wider population and contributing to the ultimate goals of the project.

This chapter introduces the principles of monitoring and evaluation, briefly describes indicators and methods available for monitoring, and provides a list of ideal data to collect for each animal presented to the clinic. A fuller discussion is available from the International Companion Animal Management Coalition's (ICAM) "Are we making a difference? A guide to monitoring and evaluating dog population management interventions" [1].

## 19.2　Responsibility to an Individual Animal's Welfare

Veterinary surgeons on admission to the profession in most countries swear an oath to uphold certain professional standards regarding animal welfare. In the United Kingdom, the oath places responsibility to animal welfare: "ABOVE ALL, my constant endeavor will be to ensure the health and welfare of animals committed to my care," and places the health and welfare of animals as the "first consideration" when attending to animals [2]. In India and the United States, veterinary surgeons promise to swear to "use my . . . skill for . . . the protection of animal health and welfare . . . and the prevention and relief of animal suffering" [3]. In Australia, veterinary surgeons swear "to practice veterinary science ethically and conscientiously for the benefit of animal welfare." In Iran, the oath is to "reduce the suffering of animal," in Canada, to "strive to promote animal health and welfare," and in Hungary, to "benefit the well-being of my patients."

It is clear that veterinary surgeons across the world must consider animal welfare as a very important, if not the most important, part of their professional life. The duty to consider animal welfare is imposed by professional regulators on all veterinary surgeons and, importantly, in all their professional dealings with all animals. Whether the animal is a pet, valuable farm animal, wildlife, or an unowned stray animal does not affect these responsibilities. All animals must receive a treatment that minimizes any potential suffering.

In order to ensure this, professional regulators usually require veterinary surgeons to continually improve their professional knowledge and competence (India and the United States for example) and to ensure clinical governance forms part of their professional activities [2]. Clinical governance involves monitoring and evaluating veterinary activity to ensure it meets the strict requirements to benefit patients. Clinical governance should reveal situations where resources (of any kind) are insufficient to allow the prevention and relief of suffering. In other words, monitoring and evaluation by veterinary surgeons is required to evaluate any clinical intervention to ensure it is not creating animal welfare problems. If resources are limited, effective interventions can still occur, but there comes a point where it is impossible to undertake the intervention without imposing negatively on the animals' welfare. When this occurs, it is the veterinary surgeon's responsibility to halt these professional activities until standards can be improved to an acceptable level.

## 19.3 Responsibility to the Wider Population

A person may choose to work or volunteer for a field project for many reasons, including the personal challenge of contributing in less than ideal circumstances and wanting to improve the welfare of individual animals that are struggling to cope in resource-limited environments. Many would also want to know that their personal resources, and the wider project finances, are making a significant impact on the problems experienced by both people and animals in the local community, including those not directly intervened upon by the veterinary team. This concept of a project contributing to change in wider problems is at the heart of monitoring and evaluation; but if this is the heart, the head of monitoring and evaluation is analyzing and interpreting the data collected in a way that allows evidence-based improvement of the project over time. By utilizing resource-efficient methods of monitoring and making time for evaluation to assess impact and learn where improvements are required, the investment in monitoring and evaluation should repay through greater project effectiveness and/or improved animal welfare.

Successful monitoring and evaluation requires an understanding of what changes, or *impacts*, the project hopes to contribute toward, for example, improved feral cat welfare, a reduction in rabies cases in both dogs and people or an improved perception of the roaming dog population. This goal setting may appear obvious, but projects can develop from the activity level, born out of a need to "do something," rather than a vision of project impact. Where project impacts have been defined, monitoring and evaluation requires *indicators*, which are the measurable signs that a change is happening. For example, an indicator of dog welfare could be the percentage of dogs brought into a clinic in an emaciated body condition; an indicator of public health could be the number of dog bites treated with postexposure prophylaxis for suspect rabies at the local hospital bite center. For each indicator, there needs to be an agreed *method of measurement* that can be followed repeatedly over time to collect data consistently for each indicator (Figure 19.1).

Veterinary staff and volunteers will almost inevitably be involved in collecting data and should be diligent in following the agreed methods of measurement including data recording. They may also be able to contribute to developing new monitoring and evaluation tools or taking part in evaluation events where the data collected through monitoring is analyzed and interpreted.

## 19.4 Methods of Measurement

Record-keeping for individual animals as they pass through the clinic environment is the method of measurement that veterinary staff and volunteers will most likely be involved in; this is tackled in more detail in Section 19.4.2 Clinic Records. Other common methods of measurement are covered in Section 19.4.1 Methods of Measurement Outside the Clinic.

### 19.4.1 Methods of Measurement Outside the Clinic

Most methods of measuring indicators of dog and cat populations outside the clinic environment can be categorized into three types:

1) Monitoring animals roaming on public property
2) Questionnaires of people who own and live among dogs and cats
3) Accessing secondary sources of information about animals or their effects, such as dog bite figures.

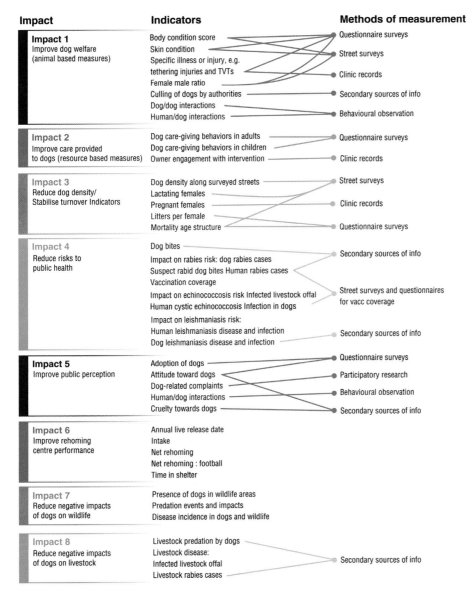

**Figure 19.1** Eight potential impacts of dog population management with associated indicators to reflect change in each impact over time and methods of measuring those indicators. Source: Reproduced with permission from ICAM (2015) [1]. Are we making a difference? A guide to monitoring and evaluating dog population management interventions.

Each category is briefly described here, and more details on practical implementation and examples of other methods are available in "Are we making a difference?" [1] for dogs and in "A generalized population monitoring program to inform the management of free-roaming cats" [4] for the monitoring of free-roaming cats.

**19.4.1.1 Monitoring Animals Roaming on Public Property**

Monitoring animals roaming on public property is most commonly achieved through street surveys. These involve visual identification of dogs and/or cats and recording their position along standard routes. The routes can be designed to cover a random selection of the project area, with or without stratification (splitting the project area into area types, such as urban and rural, and selecting routes within those types). Or they can focus on areas of particular concern regarding roaming animals, such as locations where complaints about roaming animals are most frequent. Additional information can be captured at the same time, including gender, age, signs of sterilization or vaccination (e.g. ear tips, tags, or collars), lactation, body condition, and skin condition. These street surveys are then repeated over time, along the same routes and using the same protocol to ensure a consistent search effort. Not every roaming animal will be observed on these surveys, but the assumption is that a consistent proportion will be seen over time and so the results will provide an indicator of how the wider population is changing in terms of density, composition, and welfare. To support this assumption, surveyors must not influence animal behavior, for example, through feeding while surveying. When signs of project intervention are also recorded, for example, ear tip removal for sterilized free-roaming cats or collars for vaccinated dogs, the survey will provide a measure of population coverage by the intervention. When staff or volunteers take part in these street surveys, they must record the protocol used in the case of a baseline survey and be diligent to follow the protocol used for previous surveys. This minimizes any potential error resulting in changes in observer, so that any changes over time are due to changes in the animal population and not to how the method was conducted. The protocol should include the survey start time for each route, the route itself, mode of transport, and definitions of attributes such as age, body condition, and skin condition.

### 19.4.1.2 Questionnaires

Questionnaires of people in the project area can be relatively time consuming to implement but can deliver a wide range of information about owned animals and people's perception about dogs, cats, or the project itself. The questionnaire can include questions about the number of animals owned, where they were sourced, and how there are cared for. It can also ask about people's experience of problems, such as asking if they have been bitten in the last year, or if they know of anyone in their community that abandoned an animal in the past year; providing a time frame allows for a comparison of responses between repeated questionnaires. They can also present positive and negative attitude statements and ask for people's agreement with these, such as "I like having dogs around on my street" and "I think stray cats should be collected and euthanized." As with street surveys, when questionnaires are repeated it is important to follow the same protocol, including the sampling frame used to select respondents, so that data can be compared across time. Staff and volunteers involved in questionnaires have to be aware that their interview style and question phrasing can influence how the interviewee responds, so the way questions are asked should be kept consistent over time.

### 19.4.1.3 Secondary Sources of Information

A final example of measuring indicators is using secondary sources of information. For dog and cat projects, this tends to involve asking government veterinary departments and hospitals for data, e.g. numbers of dog rabies cases and numbers of dog bites (e.g. Reece et al. [5] showed a decline in dog bites recorded by the local hospital over the time span of the Animal Birth Control project in Jaipur). Accessing secondary sources of information can be a resource-efficient method of measurement for the project, as the raw data collection has been done by someone else. However it has challenges, including securing regular access to the data, changes to the way the data has been recorded by the source, and data only being recorded in hard copy making data analysis laborious. Veterinary staff and volunteers may be able to help establish or maintain access to data, enter data from hard copy into an electronic database, or conduct data analysis and interpretation.

### 19.4.2 Clinic Records

Every animal that enters the clinic should have basic data recorded. At a minimum, this provides the necessary information to follow up on patient progress and review the veterinary intervention used. If there are clinical problems revealed by the monitoring process, the intervention must be changed. If the monitoring process shows no clinical problems, veterinary surgeons and managers can take comfort from this but need to regularly undertake evaluations to ensure high standards of individual care are maintained. Published literature detailing both best practice and acceptable rates of clinical problems are available for a range of clinical conditions and treatments (resources to search and assess relevant literature include PubMed, Google Scholar, and the RCVS Knowledge site – http://knowledge.rcvs.org.uk/home – this provides access to the journal Veterinary Evidence and links to other useful resources, such as the clinical audit toolkit).

This data may also be useful for assessing how the population in general is responding to the project. When using clinic data to assess changes in the wider population, the selection of animals for entry to the clinic needs to be considered, as these animals are likely a biased sample of the general population. This does not render the information useless, but it may make interpretations from the data relevant for only a specific subpopulation of animals. Potential changes

in which animals enter the clinic over time should also be considered, as changes in the clinic population's welfare may reflect changes in animal selection policy rather than changes in the wider population's welfare.

The following is a list of ideal data requirements for each individual animal (Table 19.1) [5,6].

## 19.5 Conclusions

Methods of monitoring require time and resources to implement that would otherwise be spent on project activities. However, monitoring the progress of a patient through the clinic is essential to ensure good patient care and refinement of veterinary

**Table 19.1** Recommended data collection points for individual animals in field clinics.

- Date of entry to clinic
- Identification of the animal – its name, any microchip or tattoo (potentially added while in the clinic), any temporary ID provided to track the animal as it is caught/received and passes through the clinic
- Gender – if female, include reproductive status (heat/pregnant/lactating)
- Sterilization status – intact or already sterilized
- Age
- Weight
- Description of the animal
- Whether the animal was brought to the clinic by an owner or caught on the street
  - If the animal is owned or has a caretaker – owner/caretaker name, address and contact details. Also include owner's description of why the animal was brought to the clinic.
  - If the animal was caught on the street – who caught the animal and a precise location of where it was caught. Preferably, the place of capture is recorded as a precise GPS location on a smart phone/device, so that the animal can be returned at the exact spot of capture, as returning to the wrong place can reduce the chance of survival.
- Whether this is first attendance or a repeat presentation – if a re-treatment this record should be linked to previous records for this same animal.
- Basic welfare measurements – body condition score, skin condition, presence of wounds
- Medical/surgical records
  - Medical history, if available
  - Results of clinical examination
  - Results of diagnostic tests, if conducted
  - Differential diagnosis list
  - Diagnosis
  - Treatment plan
  - Treatment conducted:
    ○ Which veterinarian/veterinary technician
    ○ All drugs – name, dose, route of administration, time of administration
    ○ Anesthetic record – minimally this must include the record of drugs (name, dose, route of administration, time of administration) and any irregularities or complications
    ○ Surgical record if the procedure involved anything other than a standard ovariohysterectomy or castration
    ○ If euthanized, for what reason
  - Recovery – include description of surgical site and results of pain assessment at every check
- Return date and how returned.

Source: Adapted from ICAM [1] and Loeffler [6].

procedures and patient selection. Regular evaluation also allows learning and improvement of project efficiency based on the data collected. Further, evidence of project impact can help to sustain project funding and lobby for project support and replication.

Volunteers and short-term staff can be well suited for supporting projects through monitoring activities. Where these volunteers and staff are engaged in monitoring themselves, they must be diligent to follow or create protocols to ensure data collection is as consistent as possible. Evaluation of data to capture evidence of project impact, and interpret where efficiencies can be made in the project, also takes time. There may be opportunities for volunteers and short-term staff to contribute to evaluation, bringing perspective of someone usually outside the project but also respecting the knowledge and perspective of those working long term within the project.

## References

1 ICAM Coalition (2015). Are we making a difference? A guide to monitoring and evaluating dog population management interventions. http://www.icam-coalition.org/downloads/ICAM_Guidance_Document.pdf (accessed 11 November 2016).

2 RVCS (2016). Code of professional conduct for veterinary surgeons and supporting guidance. http://www.rcvs.org.uk/advice-and-guidance/code-of-professional-conduct-for-veterinary-surgeons/pdf/ (accessed 2 March 2017).

3 AVMA (2016). Veterinarian's oath. https://www.avma.org/KB/Policies/Pages/veterinarians-oath.aspx (accessed 13 December 2017).

4 Boone, J. and Slater, M. (2014). A generalized population monitoring program to inform the management of free-roaming cats: report for ACC&D. http://www.acc-d.org/docs/default-source/think-tanks/frc-monitoring-revised-nov-2014.pdf?sfvrsn=2 (accessed 26 January 2017).

5 Reece, J.F., Chawla, S.K., and Hiby, A.R. (2013). Decline in human dog-bite cases during a street dog sterilisation programme in Jaipur, India. *The Veterinary Record* **172** (18): 473.

6 Loeffler, I.K. (2016). Field manual of veterinary standards for dog & cat surgical sterilization. http://www.fao.org/fileadmin/user_upload/animalwelfare/asset_upload_file726_61605.pdf (accessed 11 April 2017).

# 20

# Formulary

*Rachael Kreisler*

*Midwestern University, 5715 W. Utopia Rd., Glendale, AZ 85308, USA*

## 20.1 Introduction

This formulary is intended to serve as a readily available and practical source of drug information and reference charts for use in the field. Drugs were selected based on their frequency of use in limited-resourced environments, affordability, and potential to have the largest impact on animal welfare in field projects. The author recognizes that there are significant geographical differences in the availability of such drugs, and therefore, alternative drugs are suggested as appropriate substitutes. Legal and practical considerations, compounding recipes, and helpful reference charts are also included.

## 20.2 Legal and Practical Considerations in the United States

### 20.2.1 Veterinarian–Client–Patient Relationship (VCPR)

The delivery of effective and legal veterinary care is dependent on a veterinary–client–patient relationship (VCPR); this includes the dispensing of prescription drugs. Per the American Veterinary Medicine Association (AVMA), a VCPR exists when all the following conditions have been met: [1]

- The veterinarian has assumed the responsibility for making clinical judgments regarding the health of the patient and the client has agreed to follow the veterinarian's instructions.
- The veterinarian has sufficient knowledge of the patient to initiate at least a general or preliminary diagnosis of the medical condition of the patient. This means that the veterinarian is personally acquainted with the patient through a timely examination, or medically appropriate and timely visits by the veterinarian to the site where the patient is housed.
- The veterinarian is readily available for follow-up evaluation or has arranged for the following: veterinary emergency coverage and continuing care and treatment.
- The veterinarian provides oversight of treatment, compliance, and outcome.
- Patient records are maintained.

Per the AVMA, these conditions are not designed to define a VCPR for a herd. Some regulations, such as state practice acts, may have slightly different definitions for the VCPR.

### 20.2.2 Extra-Label Use of Drugs

Veterinarians working in the field often encounter difficulties acquiring the specific veterinary drugs they need or other challenges requiring extra-label drug use (ELDU). ELDU is the use of an approved drug in a manner that differs in *any* way from the drug's approved labeling. This includes use of a drug for a species or indication not on the label, or a different dose, frequency, or route of administration. Use of human drugs for animals is ELDU, and an approved human drug may be used for treatment in an extra-label manner even if an identical, approved animal drug exists [2]. Drug listings submitted to the Food and Drug Administration (FDA) may be looked up at https://dailymed.nlm.nih.gov/dailymed/. Trade names used internationally may be found at http://www.drugs.com/international/.

Per the Animal Medicinal Drug Use Clarification Act of 1994 (AMDUCA), extra-label use of approved animal or human drugs is legal in the United States if all the following conditions are met:

- The ELDU is by or on the lawful order of a veterinarian within the context of a valid VCPR.
- The health of an animal is threatened, suffering, or death may result from failure to treat.
- Use of the drug does not threaten public health.

ELDU for dogs and cats requires record keeping so that the FDA may evaluate risk to public health. Like all medical records, these should be legible, accurate, timely, accessible, and traceable to individual animals. The information should include the following:

- Name of the drug(s) and the active ingredient(s)
- Condition treated
- Species treated
- Dose administered
- Duration of treatment

Medical records must be kept for 2 years (potentially longer if required by State or Federal law) and be provided to the FDA upon request. Veterinarians are liable for problems that may arise from ELDU.

### 20.2.3 Over-the-Counter Drugs

Some drugs useful in veterinary medicine are available over-the-counter (OTC). These drugs may not be legally used by laypersons in an extra-label manner unless prescribed by a veterinarian.

### 20.2.4 Compounding

Compounding is the manipulation of approved drugs by a veterinarian or a pharmacist upon the prescription of a veterinarian to meet the needs of an individual patient. In the Unites States, compounding is regulated by both the federal (FDA) and state governments. The FDA regulates compounding via the Food, Drug and Cosmetic Act (FDCA) and Animal Medicinal Drug Use Clarification Act of 1994 (AMDUCA) available at https://www.fda.gov/AnimalVeterinary/GuidanceComplianceEnforcement/

ActsRulesRegulations/ucm085377.htm [3]. A summary of state regulations is provided by the AVMA at https://www.avma.org/Advocacy/StateAndLocal/Pages/compoundinglaws.aspx [4]. The compliance policy guide issued in July 2003 and previously used to guide compounding, "Section 608.400 Compounding of Drugs for Use in Animals," was withdrawn in May of 2015.

Note that there are very specific instructions and exclusions regarding food animals that are not addressed here.

The compounding source should be an FDA-approved substance and/or United States Pharmacopeia and The National Formulary (USP/NF) grade substance. Compounding from bulk drugs is illegal and not permitted. However, the FDA recognizes that there are circumstances where there is no drug available to treat a particular animal with a particular condition.

EDLU from the compounding of approved animal or human drugs is permitted if in compliance with state laws and the following conditions have been met:

- No approved animal or human drug is appropriate to treat the condition diagnosed as labeled with the available dosage form and concentration.
- Adequate procedures are followed to ensure the safety and effectiveness of the compounded product.
- The scale of the compounding operation is commensurate with the need for compounded products.

The veterinarian compounding or requesting compounding from a pharmacy is ultimately responsible for the compounded product and assumes liability for any adverse effects or efficacy failure. There is potential for additional liability if the client is not fully informed regarding the risk of the compounded substitute. In extreme cases, a veterinarian may be liable for veterinary malpractice or negligence in the case of treatment failure. Liability coverage may not cover this activity if there are exclusions for "gross negligence" or "intentional acts."

To reduce the risk for legal liability, provide full disclosure about the compounded drug, its risks, and why it is being prescribed and comply with all aspects of the federal ELDU regulations including record-keeping and labeling requirements. Clients should be informed that the compounded preparation has not been evaluated by the FDA for potency, purity, stability, efficacy, or safety, and client consent should be obtained. While a drug labeled for use in humans can be administered even if an animal-labeled drug for that species and medical condition exists, the risk of treatment failure and liability can be minimized by following this hierarchy:

- *First Choice.* An FDA-approved veterinary medication indicated for that species and marketed for that condition.
- *Second Choice.* An FDA-approved veterinary medication that might be indicated for another species.
- *Third Choice.* An FDA-approved human medication indicated for that condition.
- *Fourth Choice.* A compounded drug if there are no FDA-approved medications appropriate for the individual animal and condition.

If drugs are compounded by a compounding pharmacy, veterinarians should evaluate the integrity of the compounding pharmacy as well as the quality and consistency of the pharmaceuticals they produce. Check whether the pharmacy is certified by an independent body, such as the Pharmacy Compounding Accreditation Board (PCAB). PCAB-accredited pharmacies may be viewed by state at http://www.pcab.org/accredited-locations.html. Contact the state board of pharmacy to find out the status of the pharmacy within the state and assure that it is licensed to compound in that state. Use a compounding pharmacist that follows FDA Guidelines for Good Compounding Practices and has product liability insurance. Although drug manufacturers are required to carry product liability insurance, pharmacies are not.

### 20.2.5 Telemedicine

Field medicine is frequently episodic with limited ability for in-person follow-up patient care. Telemedicine, the remote diagnosis and treatment of patients by means of telecommunications technology, is an option for providing patient aftercare. The delivery of telemedicine is complicated by the fact that it is often regulated at the state level, if addressed at all.

Telemedicine for the purposes of follow-up care is likely to be permitted by most practice acts, as a valid VCPR has already been established. The AVMA Practice Advisory Panel recommends that telemedicine only be conducted within an existing VCPR, except for emergency situations before the patient being seen by a veterinarian. Per the AVMA model practice act, the basis for many state practice acts, a VCPR cannot be established solely by telephonic or other electronic means.

Telemedicine is a topic of concern, and the AVMA Practice Advisory Panel is actively working to guide the profession's responsible use of telemedicine. It is anticipated that resources from the AVMA regarding telemedicine will be aggregated at http://www.avma.org/telemedicine in the near future.

### 20.2.6 Transport of Controlled Substances Within the United States

The transport of controlled substances is legislated by the Controlled Substances Act [5]. The Veterinary Medicine Mobility Act of 2014 amended the Controlled Substances Act to allow veterinarians who are registered to manufacture or distribute controlled substances to transport and dispense controlled substances in the usual course of veterinary practice at a site other than the veterinarian's practice. The transporting and dispensing site must be in a state where the veterinarian is licensed to practice and must not be a principle place of business or professional practice. However, the veterinarian does not need to be registered with the Drug Enforcement Agency (DEA) in the state where the dispensing occurs as long as they are registered with the DEA in another state.

### 20.2.7 Transport of Controlled Substances From the United States Internationally for Medical Missions

Export of controlled substances requires registration with and authorization from the DEA unless the exportation is for a medical mission and a waiver is granted by the DEA [6]. The DEA-registered practitioner wishing to export controlled substances from the United States for a medical mission must request a waiver at least 30 days before the scheduled US departure date. The practitioner must also obtain import authorization from the Competent National Authority of the country of destination before submitting the waiver request. Waiver requests must contain all items on the Medical Mission Waiver Letter Checklist located at http://www.deadiversion.usdoj.gov/imp_exp/med_missions.htm and be submitted to the DEA via email or fax. Class I and II substances require more paperwork than those classified as Class III–V drugs.

## 20.3 Fluid Therapy in the Field

Fluid therapy is a mainstay treatment for many cats and dogs in the field for a variety of conditions including dehydration (loss of fluid from the interstitial space), hypovolemia (loss of fluid from the intravascular space), distributive shock, and intoxication where the agent is excreted via the kidneys [7]. This brief overview on fluid therapy is designed to provide the reader with a quick reference for fluid administration using isotonic crystalloids. See Chapter 15 for additional information on administering fluids to critical patients.

### 20.3.1 Initial Patient Assessment

Signs of dehydration are typically absent until dehydration is at least 5% of the patient's body weight. Loss of skin turgor or tenting is one of the first signs of dehydration. Gently pull the skin on the back of the neck and evaluate the length of time it requires to return to the patient's body. A prolonged or sluggish return is indicative of dehydration. Note that not all patients may exhibit all signs of dehydration and assessment may be complicated by age (particularly very young or very old patients), breed, or recent weight loss [8]. See Table 20.1 for clinical signs of dehydration.

### 20.3.2 Replacement Therapy

Depending on the severity of illness and disease process, fluids can be administered either subcutaneously (SQ) or intravenously (IV). The intravenous administration of fluids for replacement therapy is typically the preferred route of administration, but ongoing administration may be challenging under field conditions. Subcutaneous fluids are best used to prevent, not treat, losses. Some clinics may find it preferable to administer IV fluids as a bolus or via a fluid pump when staff are present and use SQ fluids to bridge gaps in time when staff are not available. Smaller volumes of fluid or use of

Table 20.1 Clinical assessment of dehydration.

| Dehydration | Percent | Clinical signs |
| --- | --- | --- |
| Mild | 5% | Minimal loss of skin turgor, semidry mucous membranes, eyes appear normal |
| Moderate | 8% | Moderate loss of skin turgor, dry mucous membranes, weak rapid pulses, enophthalmos |
| Severe | >10% | Severe loss of skin turgor, severe enophthalmos, tachycardia, extremely dry mucous membranes, weak/thready pulses, hypotension, altered level of consciousness |

a buretrol is preferred to reduce the chance of fluid overloading, particularly if a fluid pump is not available. A volume as small as 250 ml can potentially volume-overload a small patient.

### 20.3.3 IV Administration

For IV administration, replace the deficit over 12–24 h. Doses and frequency of monitoring should be adjusted for each animal and its condition, particularly in animals with cardiovascular, renal, or pulmonary abnormalities. All animals, but particularly cats, should be re-evaluated frequently to prevent over-hydration. Ideally, a new bag of fluids and line should be used for each patient when fluids are given IV.

### 20.3.4 SQ Administration

For SQ administration, the estimated volume should be administered and reassessed within 6 h. Generally, up to 10 ml/kg may be given in a single SQ injection site, with a maximum of approximately 200 ml per site. Excess pressure may cause leakage or discomfort, so it is advisable to give SQ fluids in multiple sites or more frequently if the total volume to be given exceeds these limits or excess pressure is noted [9]. In veterinary emergency rooms, there is evidence for mild bacterial colonization of fluids after moderate use, likely due to injection port contamination [10]. If fluid bags and administration sets are used with strict asepsis, even bags used frequently may remain sterile for a maximum of 30 days [11].

**Table 20.2** Evaluation and monitoring of hydration parameters based on available resources.

| Minimal resources | Moderate resources | Significant resources |
|---|---|---|
| Pulse rate and quality | Packed cell volume/total solids | Creatinine |
| Capillary refill time | Total protein | Electrolytes |
| Mucous membrane color | Urine-specific gravity | Serum lactate |
| Respiratory rate and effort | Blood pressure (Doppler or oscillometric) | Blood urea nitrogen |
| Lung sounds | Blood urea nitrogen (reagent strip) | Venous or arterial blood gas |
| Skin turgor | Oxygen saturation | |
| Blood pressure (pulse)[a] | Serum lactate (handheld point-of-care device) | |
| Urine output (estimated, weighing of preweighted pad[b] or free catch) | Urine output (catheter and closed system) | |
| Mental status | | |
| Temperature of extremities | | |

a) Pulse quality is also referred to as the "poor man's blood pressure monitor." A palpable femoral pulse indicates a systolic blood pressure of >60 mm Hg. A palpable dorsal metatarsal (pedal) pulse indicates a systolic blood pressure of >90 mm Hg. This is a simple tool for use in the field to assess response to fluid resuscitation during shock.
b) One gram to one milliliter urine, in absence of other contaminants.

Aseptic technique includes capping the ends of fluid lines when not in use.

### 20.3.5 Evaluation and Monitoring

Patients receiving fluids must be closely evaluated and monitored to ensure fluid administration is appropriate and effective. Assessment, evaluation, and monitoring can be performed even with minimal resources [8] (Table 20.2).

Practitioners must also be able to recognize signs of over-hydration when administering fluids (Table 20.3).

### 20.3.6 Calculating Fluid Volumes

#### 20.3.6.1 Correcting Dehydration

To estimate the amount of fluids required to correct dehydration, simply multiply the patient's body weight in kilograms by the estimated percent

**Table 20.3** Clinical signs of over-hydration.

| | |
|---|---|
| Serous nasal discharge | Subcutaneous edema |
| Ascites | Tachypnea/coughing |
| Restlessness | Vomiting/diarrhea |
| Pulmonary edema/pleural effusion | Increased respiratory effort |
| Chemosis/exophthalmos | |

dehydration [8] (Textbox 20.1). Ideally, dehydration deficits should be replaced over 12–24 h.

---

**Textbox 20.1 Calculating dehydration deficits**

Patient weight (kg) × % dehydration (as decimal) × 1000 = ml deficit

Source: Adapted from Davis et al. 2013 [8].

---

To determine the total amount of fluids required for ongoing administration, add the deficit with maintenance to arrive at the volume necessary to correct the patient's hydration. See Tables 20.7–20.10 for more quick reference on fluid rates for dogs and cats according to weight and conditions.

#### 20.3.6.2 Maintenance Fluids

Maintenance fluids is the amount of fluids estimated to be lost by a patient that is not eating or drinking but does not have abnormal losses such as vomiting or diarrhea. It is better to calculate the exact daily fluid volume for very small or very large animals, but the estimated rates provided here (Table 20.4) can be used as a guideline [8]. See Chapter 15 for additional information.

#### 20.3.6.3 Anesthetic Fluid Rates

The routine practice of administering patients undergoing anesthesia IV fluids at 10 ml/kg/h has fallen out

**Table 20.4** Calculating daily maintenance rates.

|  | Exact daily fluid volume (ml/day) | Estimated fluid rate (ml/kg/h) | Estimated daily fluid rate (ml/kg/day) |
|---|---|---|---|
| Feline | $80 \times \mathrm{kg}^{0.75}$ | 2–3 | 48–72 |
| Canine | $132 \times \mathrm{kg}^{0.75}$ | 2–6 | 48–144 |

Source: Adapted from Davis et al. 2013 [8].

**Table 20.5** Calculating surgical fluid rates.

|  | Exact surgery fluid volume (ml) | Estimated fluid rate (ml/kg/h) | Estimated total fluid volume (ml/kg) |
|---|---|---|---|
| Feline | $80 \times \mathrm{kg}^{0.75}$ + replacement | 3 | 3 |
| Canine | $132 \times \mathrm{kg}^{0.75}$ + replacement | 5 | 5 |

---

**Textbox 20.2 Sample fluid calculation**

A 30-kg mixed-breed dog presents to a field clinic after being rescued from a road traffic accident. On physical examination, the patient appears to be 5% dehydrated.

Calculate the dehydration deficit

30 kg body weight × 0.05 dehydration × 1000 = 1500 ml

Determine the maintenance fluid rate

$$132 \times 30\,\mathrm{kg}^{0.75} = 1692\,\mathrm{ml}/24\,\mathrm{h} = 71\,\mathrm{ml/h}$$

Replace the deficit over 12 h. 1500 ml deficit/12 h = 125 ml

Add this to the hourly maintenance fluid rate. 125 ml + 71 ml = 196 ml/h

Administer 196 ml/h fluids IV for the first 12 h, and then re-evaluate patient. If sufficiently hydrated, decrease to the maintenance rate of 71 ml/h.

Source: Adapted from Powell 2014 [7].

---

of favor due to the risk of fluid overload. Fluid rates in such patients is estimated to be maintenance plus necessary replacement at <10 ml/kg/h (Table 20.5). The fluid rate should be decreased to maintenance after the first hour, unless there are significant ongoing losses.

### 20.3.6.4 Diuresis Fluid Rate

Recommended fluid rates for diuresis are typically 2–2.5 times maintenance, as long as the patient's clinical status indicates that this rate is appropriate. IV therapy is recommended for 48–72 h, depending on the patient's condition [7].

### 20.3.6.5 Hypovolemia/Shock Fluid Volume

Historically, shock doses for veterinary patients consisted of 60–90 ml/kg for dogs and 60 ml/kg for cats. Most practitioners no longer advocate using the entire shock dose when attempting to stabilize patients in hypovolemic shock. Instead, if a patient presents in shock, give a shock bolus of one-fourth to one-third of the total shock volume (one complete blood volume) IV over 15–30 min, then reassess vital parameters for response to therapy (Table 20.6). An easy way to remember this is to add a zero to the weight of a dog in pounds and add a zero to the weight of a cat in kilograms [12].

Additional boluses can be given if perfusion abnormalities persist. If patient has not responded to 50–65% of the total shock volume, colloids or a transfusion are likely indicated [8].

**Table 20.6** Shock fluid volumes.

|  | Shock bolus (ml/kg) | Total shock volume (ml/kg) |
|---|---|---|
| Feline | 10–20 | 50–55 |
| Canine | 30 | 80–90 |

Table 20.7 Feline dehydration fluid replacement rates and volume.

| | Dehydration | | | | | | | | | | | | | | |
| --- | --- | --- | --- | --- | --- | --- | --- | --- | --- | --- | --- | --- | --- | --- | --- |
| | 5% | | | | | | 8% | | | | >10% | | | | |
| | Total water | SQ bolus | | | IV rate for 24 h | | Total water | | IV rate for 24 h | | Total water | | IV rate for 24 h | | |
| Patient body weight (kg) | Amount (ml) | Amount (ml) | Frequency, q (h) | ml/h | Drops/min for 15 drop/ml set | Drops/min for 60 drop/ml set | Amount (ml) | ml/h | Drops/min for 15 drop/ml set | Drops/min for 60 drop/ml set | Amount (ml) | ml/h | Drops/min for 15 drop/ml set | Drops/min for 60 drop/ml set |
| 1 | 130 | 130 | 24 | 5 | 1 | 5 | 160 | 7 | 2 | 7 | 180 | 8 | 2 | 8 |
| 2 | 235 | 235 | 24 | 10 | 2 | 10 | 295 | 12 | 3 | 12 | 335 | 14 | 3 | 14 |
| 3 | 332 | 332 | 24 | 14 | 3 | 14 | 422 | 18 | 4 | 18 | 482 | 20 | 5 | 20 |
| 4 | 426 | 426 | 24 | 18 | 4 | 18 | 546 | 23 | 6 | 23 | 626 | 26 | 7 | 26 |
| 5 | 517 | 259 | 12 | 22 | 5 | 22 | 667 | 28 | 7 | 28 | 767 | 32 | 8 | 32 |
| 6 | 607 | 303 | 12 | 25 | 6 | 25 | 787 | 33 | 8 | 33 | 907 | 38 | 9 | 38 |
| 7 | 694 | 347 | 12 | 29 | 7 | 29 | 904 | 38 | 9 | 38 | 1044 | 44 | 11 | 44 |
| 8 | 781 | 390 | 12 | 33 | 8 | 33 | 1021 | 43 | 11 | 43 | 1181 | 49 | 12 | 49 |
| 9 | 866 | 433 | 12 | 36 | 9 | 36 | 1136 | 47 | 12 | 47 | 1316 | 55 | 14 | 55 |
| 10 | 950 | 317 | 8 | 40 | 10 | 40 | 1250 | 52 | 13 | 52 | 1450 | 60 | 15 | 60 |

Table 20.8 Feline fluid rates and volume for maintenance, anesthesia, hypovolemia/shock, and diuresis.

| Patient body weight (kg) | Maintenance | | | | | | Anesthesia | | | | Hypovolemia/shock | | Diuresis | | | |
|---|---|---|---|---|---|---|---|---|---|---|---|---|---|---|---|---|
| | Total water | SQ bolus | | IV rate | | | Total water | IV rate for first hour | | | Total water | IV bolus | Total water | IV rate | | |
| | Amount per day (ml) | Amount (ml) | Frequency, q (h) | ml/h | Drops/min for 15 drop/ml set | Drops/min for 60 drop/ml set | Amount (ml) | ml/h | Drops/min for 15 drop/ml set | Drops/min for 60 drop/ml set | Amount of total blood volume (ml) | Amount (ml) | Amount per day (ml) | ml/h | Drops/min for 15 drop/ml set | Drops/min for 60 drop/ml set |
| 1 | 80 | 80 | q24h | 3 | 0.8 | 3 | 3 | 3 | 0.8 | 3 | 50 | 13 | 160 | 7 | 2 | 7 |
| 2 | 135 | 135 | q24h | 6 | 1.4 | 6 | 6 | 6 | 1.5 | 6 | 100 | 25 | 269 | 11 | 3 | 11 |
| 3 | 182 | 182 | q24h | 8 | 1.9 | 8 | 9 | 9 | 2 | 9 | 150 | 38 | 365 | 15 | 4 | 15 |
| 4 | 226 | 226 | q24h | 9 | 2.4 | 9 | 12 | 12 | 3 | 12 | 200 | 50 | 453 | 19 | 5 | 19 |
| 5 | 267 | 134 | q12h | 11 | 2.8 | 11 | 15 | 15 | 4 | 15 | 250 | 63 | 535 | 22 | 6 | 22 |
| 6 | 307 | 153 | q12h | 13 | 3.2 | 13 | 18 | 18 | 5 | 18 | 300 | 75 | 613 | 26 | 6 | 26 |
| 7 | 344 | 172 | q12h | 14 | 3.6 | 14 | 21 | 21 | 5 | 21 | 350 | 88 | 689 | 29 | 7 | 29 |
| 8 | 381 | 190 | q12h | 16 | 4.0 | 16 | 24 | 24 | 6 | 24 | 400 | 100 | 761 | 32 | 8 | 32 |
| 9 | 416 | 208 | q12h | 17 | 4.3 | 17 | 27 | 27 | 7 | 27 | 450 | 113 | 831 | 35 | 9 | 35 |
| 10 | 450 | 225 | q12h | 19 | 4.7 | 19 | 30 | 30 | 8 | 30 | 500 | 125 | 900 | 37 | 9 | 37 |

Table 20.9 Canine dehydration fluid replacement rates and volume.

| Patient body weight (kg) | Dehydration | | | | | | | | | | | | | |
|---|---|---|---|---|---|---|---|---|---|---|---|---|---|---|
| | 5% | | | | | | 8% | | | | >10% | | | |
| | Total water Amount (ml) | SQ bolus Amount (ml) | Frequency, q (h) | IV rate for 24 h ml/h | Drops/min for 15 drop/ml set | Drops/min for 60 drop/ml set | Total water Amount (ml) | IV rate for 24 h ml/h | Drops/min for 15 drop/ml set | Drops/min for 60 drop/ml set | Total water Amount (ml) | IV rate for 24 h ml/h | Drops/min for 15 drop/ml set | Drops/min for 60 drop/ml set |
| 1 | 182 | 182 | 24 | 8 | 2 | 8 | 212 | 9 | 2 | 9 | 232 | 10 | 2 | 10 |
| 2 | 322 | 161 | 12 | 13 | 3 | 13 | 382 | 16 | 4 | 16 | 422 | 18 | 4 | 18 |
| 3 | 451 | 225 | 12 | 19 | 5 | 19 | 541 | 23 | 6 | 23 | 601 | 25 | 6 | 25 |
| 4 | 573 | 287 | 12 | 24 | 6 | 24 | 693 | 29 | 7 | 29 | 773 | 32 | 8 | 32 |
| 5 | 691 | 346 | 12 | 29 | 7 | 29 | 841 | 35 | 9 | 35 | 941 | 39 | 10 | 39 |
| 6 | 806 | 403 | 12 | 34 | 8 | 34 | 986 | 41 | 10 | 41 | 1 106 | 46 | 12 | 46 |
| 7 | 918 | 459 | 12 | 38 | 10 | 38 | 1 128 | 47 | 12 | 47 | 1 268 | 53 | 13 | 53 |
| 9 | 1 136 | 379 | 8 | 47 | 12 | 47 | 1 406 | 59 | 15 | 59 | 1 586 | 66 | 17 | 66 |
| 10 | 1 242 | 414 | 8 | 52 | 13 | 52 | 1 542 | 64 | 16 | 64 | 1 742 | 73 | 18 | 73 |
| 12 | 1 451 | 484 | 8 | 60 | 15 | 60 | 1 811 | 75 | 19 | 75 | 2 051 | 85 | 21 | 85 |
| 14 | 1 655 | 552 | 8 | 69 | 17 | 69 | 2 075 | 86 | 22 | 86 | 2 355 | 98 | 25 | 98 |
| 16 | 1 856 | 464 | 6 | 77 | 19 | 77 | 2 336 | 97 | 24 | 97 | 2 656 | 111 | 28 | 111 |
| 18 | 2 054 | 513 | 6 | 86 | 21 | 86 | 2 594 | 108 | 27 | 108 | 2 954 | 123 | 31 | 123 |
| 20 | 2 248 | 562 | 6 | 94 | 23 | 94 | 2 848 | 119 | 30 | 119 | 3 248 | 135 | 34 | 135 |
| 25 | 2 726 | 454 | 4 | 114 | 28 | 114 | 3 476 | 145 | 36 | 145 | 3 976 | 166 | 41 | 166 |
| 30 | 3 192 | 532 | 4 | 133 | 33 | 133 | 4 092 | 171 | 43 | 171 | 4 692 | 196 | 49 | 196 |
| 35 | 3 649 | 608 | 4 | 152 | 38 | 152 | 4 699 | 196 | 49 | 196 | 5 399 | 225 | 56 | 225 |
| 40 | 4 100 | 683 | 4 | 171 | 43 | 171 | 5 300 | 221 | 55 | 221 | 6 100 | 254 | 64 | 254 |
| 45 | 4 543 | 757 | 4 | 189 | 47 | 189 | 5 893 | 246 | 61 | 246 | 6 793 | 283 | 71 | 283 |
| 50 | 4 982 | 830 | 4 | 208 | 52 | 208 | 6 482 | 270 | 68 | 270 | 7 482 | 312 | 78 | 312 |
| 60 | 5 846 | 974 | 4 | 244 | 61 | 244 | 7 646 | 319 | 80 | 319 | 8 846 | 369 | 92 | 369 |
| 70 | 6 694 | 558 | 2 | 279 | 70 | 279 | 8 794 | 366 | 92 | 366 | 10 194 | 425 | 106 | 425 |
| 80 | 7 531 | 628 | 2 | 314 | 78 | 314 | 9 931 | 414 | 103 | 414 | 11 531 | 480 | 120 | 480 |
| 90 | 8 357 | 696 | 2 | 348 | 87 | 348 | 11 057 | 461 | 115 | 461 | 12 857 | 536 | 134 | 536 |
| 100 | 9 174 | 765 | 2 | 382 | 96 | 382 | 12 174 | 507 | 127 | 507 | 14 174 | 591 | 148 | 591 |

Table 20.10 Canine fluid rates and volume for maintenance, anesthesia, hypovolemia/shock, and diuresis.

| Patient body weight (kg) | Maintenance | | | | | | Anesthesia | | | | Hypovolemia/shock | | Diuresis | | | |
|---|---|---|---|---|---|---|---|---|---|---|---|---|---|---|---|---|
| | Total water Amount (ml) | SQ bolus Amount (ml) | Frequency q (h) | IV rate ml/h | Drops/min for 15 drop/ml set | Drops/min for 60 drop/ml set | Total water Amount (ml) | IV rate for first hour ml/h | Drops/min for 15 drop/ml set | Drops/min for 60 drop/ml set | Total water Amount (ml) | IV bolus Amount (ml) | Total water Amount per day (ml) | IV rate ml/h | Drops/min for 15 drop/ml set | Drops/min for 60 drop/ml set |
| 1 | 132 | 132 | 24 | 6 | 1 | 6 | 3 | 3 | 1 | 3 | 80 | 20 | 264 | 11 | 3 | 11 |
| 2 | 222 | 222 | 24 | 9 | 2 | 9 | 6 | 6 | 2 | 6 | 160 | 40 | 444 | 18 | 5 | 18 |
| 3 | 301 | 301 | 24 | 13 | 3 | 13 | 9 | 9 | 2 | 9 | 240 | 60 | 602 | 25 | 6 | 25 |
| 4 | 373 | 373 | 24 | 16 | 4 | 16 | 12 | 12 | 3 | 12 | 320 | 80 | 747 | 31 | 8 | 31 |
| 5 | 441 | 441 | 24 | 18 | 5 | 18 | 15 | 15 | 4 | 15 | 400 | 100 | 883 | 37 | 9 | 37 |
| 6 | 506 | 506 | 24 | 21 | 5 | 21 | 18 | 18 | 5 | 18 | 480 | 120 | 1012 | 42 | 11 | 42 |
| 7 | 568 | 284 | 12 | 24 | 6 | 24 | 21 | 21 | 5 | 21 | 560 | 140 | 1136 | 47 | 12 | 47 |
| 9 | 686 | 343 | 12 | 29 | 7 | 29 | 27 | 27 | 7 | 27 | 720 | 180 | 1372 | 57 | 14 | 57 |
| 10 | 742 | 371 | 12 | 31 | 8 | 31 | 30 | 30 | 8 | 30 | 800 | 200 | 1485 | 62 | 15 | 62 |
| 12 | 851 | 426 | 12 | 35 | 9 | 35 | 36 | 36 | 9 | 36 | 960 | 240 | 1702 | 71 | 18 | 71 |
| 14 | 955 | 478 | 12 | 40 | 10 | 40 | 42 | 42 | 11 | 42 | 1120 | 280 | 1911 | 80 | 20 | 80 |
| 16 | 1056 | 528 | 12 | 44 | 11 | 44 | 48 | 48 | 12 | 48 | 1280 | 320 | 2112 | 88 | 22 | 88 |
| 18 | 1154 | 385 | 8 | 48 | 12 | 48 | 54 | 54 | 14 | 54 | 1440 | 360 | 2307 | 96 | 24 | 96 |
| 20 | 1248 | 416 | 8 | 52 | 13 | 52 | 60 | 60 | 15 | 60 | 1600 | 400 | 2497 | 104 | 26 | 104 |
| 25 | 1476 | 492 | 8 | 61 | 15 | 61 | 75 | 75 | 19 | 75 | 2000 | 500 | 2952 | 123 | 31 | 123 |
| 30 | 1692 | 564 | 8 | 71 | 18 | 71 | 90 | 90 | 23 | 90 | 2400 | 600 | 3384 | 141 | 35 | 141 |
| 35 | 1899 | 475 | 6 | 79 | 20 | 79 | 105 | 105 | 26 | 105 | 2800 | 700 | 3799 | 158 | 40 | 158 |
| 40 | 2100 | 525 | 6 | 87 | 22 | 87 | 120 | 120 | 30 | 120 | 3200 | 800 | 4199 | 175 | 44 | 175 |
| 45 | 2293 | 382 | 4 | 96 | 24 | 96 | 135 | 135 | 34 | 135 | 3600 | 900 | 4587 | 191 | 48 | 191 |
| 50 | 2482 | 414 | 4 | 103 | 26 | 103 | 150 | 150 | 38 | 150 | 4000 | 1000 | 4964 | 207 | 52 | 207 |
| 60 | 2846 | 474 | 4 | 119 | 30 | 119 | 180 | 180 | 45 | 180 | 4800 | 1200 | 5691 | 237 | 59 | 237 |
| 70 | 3194 | 532 | 4 | 133 | 33 | 133 | 210 | 210 | 53 | 210 | 5600 | 1400 | 6389 | 266 | 67 | 266 |
| 80 | 3531 | 294 | 2 | 147 | 37 | 147 | 240 | 240 | 60 | 240 | 6400 | 1600 | 7062 | 294 | 74 | 294 |
| 90 | 3857 | 321 | 2 | 161 | 40 | 161 | 270 | 270 | 68 | 270 | 7200 | 1800 | 7714 | 321 | 80 | 321 |
| 100 | 4174 | 348 | 2 | 174 | 43 | 174 | 300 | 300 | 75 | 300 | 8000 | 2000 | 8348 | 348 | 87 | 348 |

Table 20.11 Abbreviations used.

| Units | Administration route | Dosing | Other |
|---|---|---|---|
| kg = kilogram | PO = per os (oral) | q = every | Rx = prescription |
| g = gram | IM = intramuscular | h = hour | OTC = over-the-counter |
| mg = milligram | IV = intravenous | d = day | NSAID = nonsteroidal anti-inflammatory drug |
| ml = milliliter | IC = intracardiac | w = week | UTI = urinary tract infection |
| | SQ = subcutaneous | PRN = as needed | URI = upper respiratory infection |
| | SL = sublingual | | BSA = body surface area |
| | TM = transmucosal | | |

## 20.4 Formulary

The drugs included in this formulary are not an exhaustive list nor are all indications for use included. Selected drugs were chosen based on their frequency of use and/or overall usefulness in the field. Due to varying availability, drug shortages, and volatile pricing, drugs that may serve as potential substitutes for desired medications are included. Prescription and controlled drug status are per US laws and regulation; this may vary outside of the United States.

Suggested doses included here are derived from various sources including the manufacturer, veterinary textbooks, journal articles, symposium notes, and clinical experience. Table 20.11 summarizes commonly used abbreviations. The reader should understand that the doses listed in this formulary are a suggested guideline and are not the *only* dose that can be used (Table 20.12). The author assumes no responsibility for, and makes no guarantee, with respect to the results that may be obtained from the uses or doses listed. This formulary should not substitute professional veterinary judgment.

Table 20.12 Formulary.

| Generic name (Common trade names) | Type and field indications | Canine dose | Feline dose | Potential substitutes | Comments, cautions, and contraindications | Rx/controlled status and forms |
|---|---|---|---|---|---|---|
| Acepromazine (PromAce®) | *Phenothiazine* Sedation, antiemetic, urethral spasm | 0.055–0.22 mg/kg PO or 0.055–0.11 mg/kg IV, IM, or SQ (max 3 mg) | 0.055–0.22 mg/kg PO or 0.055–0.11 mg/kg IV, IM, or SQ (max 1 mg) | Gabapentin (cats) | Antiemetic properties. Current recommended doses are lower than on label; much less concern for dogs with ABCB1-1Δ (MDR1) mutations and boxer dogs at these doses. May disinhibit biting. May use atropine concurrently to help compensate for bradycardia. *Contraindications: Conditions exacerbated by hypotension* | Rx 10 mg/ml injection. 5, 10, 25 mg tablets |
| Acetylcysteine | *Antidote* Acetaminophen, xylitol, or phenol intoxication | 140–180 mg/kg IV or 280 mg/kg PO loading dose; 70 mg/kg PO or IV q6h for 7–17 treatments | 140–180 mg/kg IV or 280 mg/kg PO loading dose; 70 mg/kg PO or IV q6h for 7–17 treatments | | Increases glutathione levels to treat hepatotoxic conditions involving glutathione synthesis or oxidative stress. Poor oral absorption and unpalatable taste make IV dosing preferred to oral. May cause nausea and vomiting. Treatment of acetaminophen intoxication should be initiated within 8–10 h of exposure, while treatment of phenol intoxication should be initiated within 12–24 h of exposure. Methemoglobinemia due to acetaminophen intoxication may be monitored via blood smear, whereas xylitol intoxication may be monitored via blood glucose. *Caution: IV solution should be diluted to 5% (50 mg/ml) and given slowly over 15–20 min* | Rx human-labeled 200 mg/ml injection, 600 mg capsules OTC capsules (nutritional product) |

| Drug | Class / Indication | Dose (dog) | Dose (cat) | Alternative | Comments | Availability |
|---|---|---|---|---|---|---|
| Alcohol, ethyl | *Antidote* Ethylene glycol or methanol intoxication | 5.5 ml/kg of 20% ethanol q4h for six treatments then q6h for four treatments | 5 ml/kg of 20% ethanol q4h for six treatments then q6h for four treatments | Fomepizole | In cases of ethylene glycol ingestion, ideally start treatment within 1 h of ingestion; treatment must be started within 8 h to be efficacious. Solution can be made from ethanol or grain alcohol using the equation (% desired custom solution × final volume desired)/% stock solution = volume of stock solution. Add this volume of stock solution to final volume desired of diluent − volume of stock solution. The percent of alcohol is half of the proof. In this case, if using 190 proof alcohol to make 100 ml of a 20% solution, you would add 21 ml of alcohol to 79 ml of sterile saline. Ideally cold sterilize by passing through a 0.2 μm filter | OTC Various proof/percentages |
| Alfaxalone (Alfaxan®) | *Synthetic neuroactive steroid* Anesthetic agent, induction of anesthesia | 1–3 mg/kg IV slowly to effect | 2–5 mg/kg IV slowly to effect | Propofol, etomidate | Required dose depends on other drugs that may have been used for premedication. Little or no cardiovascular effects and less apnea as compared with propofol. May see agitation in recovery if used as sole agent, particularly cats. Can be used IM (2–4 mg/kg) in conjunction with midazolam (0.3 mg/kg) for critical patients that will not tolerate restraint for procedures of less than 5 min (due to volume, only practical for dogs <10 kg) | Rx (Schedule IV) 10 mg/ml injection |
| Amoxicillin | *Beta-lactam antibiotic* Skin infection, UTI | 11–15 mg/kg PO q8h for 7–14 days | 11–15 mg/kg PO q8h for 7–14 days | Amoxicillin–clavulanic acid, ampicillin | Susceptible to inactivation by beta-lactamases. Powder for oral suspension may be divided before reconstitution for more economical dosing of cats | Rx Various veterinary- and human-labeled tablets, capsules, and suspensions |

*(continued)*

**Table 20.12** (Continued)

| Generic name (Common trade names) | Type and field indications | Canine dose | Feline dose | Potential substitutes | Comments, cautions, and contraindications | Rx/controlled status and forms |
|---|---|---|---|---|---|---|
| Amoxicillin-Clavulanic acid (Clavamox®, Augmentin®) | *Beta-lactam antibiotic and beta-lactamase inhibitor* Skin infection, wounds, URI (cats) | 13.75 mg/kg PO q6–12h for 5–7 days (wounds), 21 days (superficial pyoderma), 28 days (deep pyoderma) | 62.5 mg/cat PO q6–12h for 5–7 days (wounds), 12.5 mg/kg PO q12h for 14 days (URI) | Amoxicillin, ampicillin, ampicillin sulbactam | Veterinary-labeled products are in the ratio of 4:1 amoxicillin and clavulanic acid and expressed as total of both compounds. Human-labeled products have various ratios and are expressed as the amount of amoxicillin only | Rx Various veterinary- and human-labeled tablets and oral suspension |
| Ampicillin (Polyflex®) | *Beta-lactam antibiotic* Wounds, sepsis | 20–40 mg/kg IV q6–8h (sepsis, typically used in conjunction with a fluoroquinolone), 10–20 mg/kg IV, IM, SQ, PO q6–8h | 20–40 mg/kg IV q6–8h (sepsis, typically used in conjunction with a fluoroquinolone), 10–20 mg/kg IV, IM, SQ, PO q6–8h | Amoxicillin, amoxicillin-clavulanic acid, ampicillin sulbactam | For oral dosing, amoxicillin preferred due to better absorption. Reconstituted trihydrate injection should be refrigerated and discarded after 3 months, reconstituted sodium injection within 1 h. Reconstituted oral suspension should be discarded after 14 days if refrigerated, 7 days if kept at room temperature | Rx Veterinary-labeled 10 and 25 g trihydrate injection, various human-labeled injection (sodium), capsules, and oral suspension |
| Ampicillin Sulbactam (Unasyn®) | *Beta-lactam antibiotic and beta-lactamase inhibitor* Wounds, sepsis | 15–30 mg/kg IV q6–8h (sepsis, typically used in conjunction with a fluoroquinolone), 10–20 mg/kg IV, IM q8h | 15–30 mg/kg IV q6–8h (sepsis, typically used in conjunction with a fluoroquinolone), 10–20 mg/kg IV, IM q8h | Amoxicillin, ampicillin, amoxicillin-clavulonic acid | | Rx Human-labeled 1.5 and 3 g injection |
| Apomorphine (Apokyn®) | *Centrally mediated emetic* Emesis in dogs | 0.03 mg/kg IV, 0.04 mg/kg IM, 0.08 mg/kg SC, 0.3 mg/kg topically into the conjunctival sac | Not effective | Hydrogen peroxide (dogs, dexmedetomidine or xylazine (cats)) | Emesis typically within 20–30 min. If emesis does not occur, do not administer repeat doses. If animal is symptomatic is likely too late for emesis and gastric lavage may be more appropriate. *Caution: Brachycephalic breeds. Contraindications: Intoxication with substances such as hydrocarbons or corrosive agents or patients that cannot protect airway* | Rx 10 mg/ml injection |

| Drug | Classification / Indication | Dose | Dose | Alternatives | Comments | Availability |
|---|---|---|---|---|---|---|
| Aspirin | *NSAID* Analgesic, antipyretic, anti-inflammatory | 10 mg/kg q12h | 10 mg/kg q48h | NSAIDs | Last resort substitute, veterinary-labeled products that are COX-2 selective strongly preferred. Do not use combination products that contain acetaminophen. *Caution: Cats. Contraindications: Bleeding disorders, concomitant steroid use, bleeding gastric ulcers, dehydration* | OTC Various human-labeled |
| Atipamezole (Antisedan®, Revazol®) | *Alpha-2 antagonist* Reversal of alpha-2 agonists, treatment of amitraz toxicity | 3.75 mg/m² IM (reversal of (dex)medetomidine), 0.05 mg/kg IM (treatment of amitraz toxicity) | 0.01 mg/kg IM (reversal of dexmedetomidine), 0.025–0.05 mg/kg IM (reversal of sedation when xylazine used for emesis) | Yohimbine | Volume of reversal same as the volume of dexmedetomidine. Rapid effect. Some concern for vascular collapse if given quickly IV; recommend IV only for CPR. Additional doses may be required for treatment of amitraz toxicity. Cats may become excitable and dogs dysphoric upon reversal | Rx 5 mg/ml injection |
| Atropine | *Anticholinergic* Adjunct to anesthesia or CPR, treatment of muscarinic signs associated with carbamate or organophosphate intoxication | 0.02 mg/kg IM or IV (preanesthetic), 0.04 mg/kg IV (CPR, bradycardia), 0.2 mg/kg (antidote) | 0.02 mg/kg IM or IV (preanesthetic), 0.04 mg/kg IV (CPR, bradycardia), 0.2 mg/kg (antidote) | Glycopyrrolate | Can test for organophosphate/carbamate poisoning by noting heart rate, then administering 0.02 mg/kg IV atropine. An increase in heart rate and dilation of pupils indicates that poisoning is unlikely. *Contraindication: Concurrent use of dexmedetomidine* | Rx 0.54 and 15 mg/ml veterinary-labeled injection. Various human-labeled concentrations for injection |
| Azithromycin (Zithromax®) | *Macrolide antibiotic* Susceptible infections | 5–10 mg/kg PO q24h for 5 days | 5–10 mg/kg PO q24h for 5 days | | Wide range of safety. Discard reconstituted oral suspension after 10 days. May divide powder for suspension into smaller course of treatment amounts before reconstitution. *Caution: Hepatic disease* | Rx 250, 500, and 600 mg tablets. 20 and 40 mg/ml powder for suspension in various amounts |
| Bacitracin (Neosporin®, Polysporin®) | *Topical antibiotic* wounds and minor burns | Apply to affected area q8h for up to 1 week | Apply to affected area q8h for up to 1 week | Mupirocin, silver sulfadiazine (SSD), nitrofurazone | Do not use around the eyes. May use veterinary-labeled ophthalmic ointment topically. *Caution: Rare anaphylactic shock in cats* | OTC Various human-labeled ointments, may be combined with polymyxin B and neomycin. Veterinary-labeled ophthalmic ointment |

(continued)

Table 20.12 (*Continued*)

| Generic name (Common trade names) | Type and field indications | Canine dose | Feline dose | Potential substitutes | Comments, cautions, and contraindications | Rx/controlled status and forms |
|---|---|---|---|---|---|---|
| Bismuth Subsalicylate (Pepto-Bismol®, Kaopectate®) | *Antacid and adsorbent* Antidiarrheal, gastroprotectant | 4.4–35 mg/kg PO q6–8h | 4.4–17.5 mg/kg, with caution | Sucralfate | May darken stool. *Extreme caution: Cats* | OTC Various veterinary and human-labeled paste, suspension, tablets, and caplets |
| Bupivacaine | *Amide* Local/topical anesthesia | 1.0 mg/kg (max 2 mg/kg) | 1.0 mg/kg (max 1.0 mg/kg) | Lidocaine (faster onset, shorter duration), mepivacaine (faster onset, shorter duration) | Time to onset 20–30 min, duration 3–5 h. Greater potential for toxicity as compared with lidocaine. May dilute with normal saline to reduce pain on injection in awake animals. *Contraindication: Do not give IV* | Rx 2.5, 5.0, 7.5 mg/ml injection |
| Buprenorphine (Buprenex®, Simbadol®) | *Partial mu agonist opioid* Analgesia, premedication for anesthesia | 0.01–0.04 mg/kg IM or IV | 0.01–0.04 mg/kg IM, IV, TM | | Higher doses lead to longer effects. IM route preferred in cats. May antagonize other mu-agonists like morphine, hydromorphone, fentanyl, oxymorphone. Relatively long onset to peak action, 30 min IV, 45–60 min IM. Available in a sustained release formula as buprenorphine SR with analgesia lasting 3 days | Rx (Schedule III) Veterinary-labeled 1.8 mg/ml (Simbadol). Human-labeled 0.3 mg/ml |
| Butorphanol (Dolorex®, Torbugesic® Torbutrol®) | *Mixed agonist (kappa)/antagonist (mu) opioid* Sedation, analgesia | 0.2–0.4 mg/kg IV, IM, SQ | 0.2 mg/kg IV < IM < SQ | Nalbuphine (not controlled) | Duration of action of 30–60 min (dogs), 1–3 h (cats). Usually used in conjunction with other anesthetic drugs. Better drugs for moderate-to-severe pain but may be useful as a bridge to opioid analgesics with a longer onset of action such as buprenorphine. Concentrations vary between products | Rx (Schedule IV) 0.5, 2, 10 mg/ml veterinary-labeled concentrations; 1, 2 mg/ml human-labeled concentrations |

| Drug | Class / Indication | Dose | Dose | Alternatives | Notes | Availability |
|---|---|---|---|---|---|---|
| Calcium gluconate, 10% | *Mineral* Puerperal hypocalcemia | 5–15 mg/kg/h elemental calcium slowly to effect | 5–15 mg/kg/h elemental calcium slowly to effect | Calcium chloride, 10% (27.2 mg/ml elemental calcium) | Calcium gluconate 10% contains 9.3 mg/ml elemental calcium. Doses must be calculated based on *elemental calcium*, which varies by formulation. Calcium gluconate preferred formulation as less irritating. Monitor heart rate during administration and stop infusion if an arrhythmia develops. Treat overdoses with normal saline diuresis and a loop diuretic such as furosemide | Rx and OTC Various veterinary-labeled and human-labeled products, some with additional additives such as phosphorus, potassium, or dextrose |
| Carprofen (Rimadyl®) | *NSAID* Analgesic, antipyretic, anti-inflammatory | 4.4 mg/kg SQ (injection) or PO (tablet) q24h 2 h before procedure, 4.4 mg/kg PO q24h PRN for up to 7 days | 4 mg/kg SQ once preoperatively at time of induction | Meloxicam, deracoxib, ketoprofen, tolfedine | *Contraindications: Bleeding disorders, concomitant steroid use, bleeding gastric ulcers, dehydration* | Rx Veterinary-labeled 25, 75, and 100 mg tablets and caplets, 50 mg/ml injection |
| Cefazolin | *1st generation cephalosporin* Surgical prophylaxis (Gram-positive bacteria) | 20–22 mg/kg IV, IM, SQ within 1 h of incision, then q1.5–2h until closure | 20–22 mg/kg IV, IM, SQ within 1 h of incision, then q1.5–2h until closure | Cefotaxime, cefovicin, cefpodoxime proxetil, ceftiofur, cephalexin | After reconstitution, use within 24 h at room temperature, 96 h refrigerated. May freeze for up to 12 weeks. IM injection may be painful. Give slowly over 3–5 min IV | Rx Various human-labeled powder for reconstitution and injection |
| Cefotaxime (Claforan®) | *3rd generation cephalosporin* Bacterial infections, septic peritonitis | 30–50 mg/kg IV, IM, SQ q8h | 30–50 mg/kg IV, IM, SQ q8h | Cefovicin, cefpodoxime proxetil, ceftiofur, cephalexin | Relatively wide spectrum of activity against both Gram-positive and Gram-negative bacteria | Rx Various human-labeled powder for reconstitution and injection |
| Cefovecin (Convenia®) | *Injectable long-acting cephalosporin* Staphylococcus skin infections, UTI, wounds, abscesses | 8 mg/kg SC once, may repeat q7d or q14d, max 2 injections | 8 mg/kg SQ once | Cefotaxime, cefpodoxime proxetil, ceftiofur, cephalexin | Opened bottle lasts 56 days. Therapeutic concentrations for 7–14 days, side effects may occur for up to 2 months post-injection. Local compounding pharmacies may sterilely split powder into smaller portions for reconstitution in smaller batches. Anecdotally, the product may be reconstituted, stored in sterile vials (such as vaccine diluent), and frozen, but this is counter to label | Rx 80 mg/ml injection |

*(continued)*

**Table 20.12** (*Continued*)

| Generic name (Common trade names) | Type and field indications | Canine dose | Feline dose | Potential substitutes | Comments, cautions, and contraindications | Rx/controlled status and forms |
|---|---|---|---|---|---|---|
| Cefpodoxime proxetil (Simplicef®) | *3rd generation cephalosporin* Skin infections | 5–10 mg/kg PO q24h for 5–7 days | 5–10 mg/kg PO q24h for 5–7 days | Cephalexin, cefovecin, cefotaxime, ceftiofur, cephalexin | Reconstituted oral suspension must be stored in refrigerator. Discard reconstituted oral suspension after 14 days | Rx 100 and 200 mg veterinary and human-labeled tablets. 50 and 100 mg/ml human-labeled suspension |
| Ceftiofur (Excenel®) | *3rd generation cephalosporin* Skin infections, UTI | 2.2 mg/kg SC q24 for 5–14 days | Unknown | Cephalexin, cefovecin, cefotaxime, cefpodoxime proxetil | Drug must be injected, not effective by mouth. Store at room temperature, shake before use. Not to be given IV due to risk for anaphylaxis | Rx 50 mg/ml veterinary-labeled suspension |
| Cephalexin (Cefalexin®) | *1st generation cephalosporin* Skin infections, UTI | 22–30 mg/kg PO q12h for 28 days | 22–30 mg/kg PO q12h for 28 days | Cefpodoxime Proxetil, cefovecin, cefotaxime, ceftiofur | Reconstituted oral suspension should be stored at room temperature and discarded after 2 weeks | Rx Various veterinary- and human-labeled tablets and oral suspension |
| Charcoal, activated (Toxiban®) | *Oral adsorbent* Intoxication | 1–4 g/kg PO | 1–4 g/kg PO | Kaolin/pectate (may have less significant adsorbent properties) | May give with sorbitol at initial dose to decrease GI transit time. Some formulations contain sorbitol (osmotic cathartic). Not helpful for ethanol, methanol, ethylene glycol, xylitol, heavy metals, or iron salts *Contraindications: Animals at risk for aspiration pneumonia* | OTC Various veterinary- and human-labeled formulations |
| Chlorhexidine scrub | *Topical antiseptic* Superficial pyoderma, wound irrigation | 0.05–0.1% dilution (wound irrigation), 2% dilution topical q2d for 1–3 weeks (superficial pyoderma) | 0.05–0.1% dilution (wound irrigation) | Benzoyl peroxide | Avoid contact with the eyes. Good residual effect, shorter duration of application than shampoo. Apply for 5 min, then rinse and dry. Successful treatment of superficial pyoderma may also require systemic antibiotics. Dose may be described as 1 cm diameter size application of scrub per 6 cm of lesional area. Equal efficacy with 2% chlorhexidine acetate and 2% chlorhexidine gluconate | OTC Large number of cleansers, shampoos, flushes, solutions, scrubs |

| Drug | Class / Use | Canine dose | Feline dose | Related drugs | Notes | Availability |
|---|---|---|---|---|---|---|
| Ciprofloxacin | *Fluoroquinolone antibiotic* | 20–25 mg/kg IV or 30 mg/kg PO q24h | 20–25 mg/kg IV or 30 mg/kg PO q24h | Enrofloxacin, orbifloxacin, ofloxacin | Bioavailability is variable and much lower than enrofloxacin, therefore should only be used if no approved fluoroquinolones are available. Ciprofloxacin may be the only economically viable fluoroquinolone for large dogs | Rx. Various human-labeled tablets, solution for injection |
| Clindamycin (Antirobe®) | *Lincosamide antibiotic* Wounds, abscesses, and osteomyelitis caused by *Staphylococcus* spp. dental infections, many anaerobic infections | 5.5–33 mg/kg PO q12h up to 28 days (wounds, abscesses), 11 mg/kg PO q24h for 21 days (pyoderma) | 11–33 mg/kg PO up to 14 days (wounds, abscesses, dental infections) | | Very good tissue penetration | Rx. Various veterinary- and human-labeled capsules, tablets, and solutions |
| Deracoxib (Deramaxx®) | *NSAID* Analgesic, antipyretic, anti-inflammatory | 3–4 mg/kg PO q24h PRN for up to 7 days | No feline dose | Carprofen, meloxicam, ketoprofen, firocoxib, tolfedine | *Contraindications: Bleeding disorders, concomitant steroid use, bleeding gastric ulcers, dehydration* | Rx. 25, 50, 75, 100 mg chewable tablets |
| Dexamethasone SP | *Glucocorticoid* Anti-inflammatory | 0.125–0.25 mg/kg IV, IM, PO (anti-inflammatory), 0.2–0.5 mg/kg IV once (Addisonian crisis) | 0.125–0.5 mg/kg IV, IM, PO | Prednisone or prednisolone (anti-inflammatory), epinephrine first-line treatment for anaphylaxis | No longer recommended for treatment of anaphylaxis, shock or CNS trauma. Most significant side effects come from continued use. Effects last 48 h. *Contraindications: Concurrent NSAID use, GI bleeding* | Rx. Various veterinary- and human-labeled tablets, solutions, and injection |
| Dexmedetomidine (Dexdomitor®, Sileo®) | *Alpha-2 agonist* Sedation, analgesia, emesis (cats) | 0.375 mg/m² IV or 0.5 mg/m² IM (sedation and analgesia), 0.125–0.375 mg/m² IM (preanesthesia), 0.01 mg/kg IV or 0.03 mg/kg IM (postoperative delirium) | 0.04 mg/kg IM (sedation, analgesia, preanesthesia), 0.007–0.01 mg/kg IM (emesis in cats), 0.01 mg/kg IV or 0.03 mg/kg IM (postoperative delirium) | Xylazine | Dosed based on BSA in dogs. Reversed with atipamezole. Safer than xylazine. Typically causes vomiting in cats when used as sole agent. Often used at lower doses in synergistic combination with other medications for sedation and anesthesia. Use of insulin syringes facilitates accurate dosing | Rx. 0.5 and 0.1 mg/ml injection, 0.1 mg/ml oromucosal gel |

(continued)

**Table 20.12** (Continued)

| Generic name (Common trade names) | Type and field indications | Canine dose | Feline dose | Potential substitutes | Comments, cautions, and contraindications | Rx/controlled status and forms |
|---|---|---|---|---|---|---|
| Dextrose 50% | *Glucose elevating agent* Hypoglycemia, xylitol intoxication | 0.25–0.5 g/kg IV | 0.25–0.5 g/kg IV | Corn syrup PO to effect in animals with the ability to swallow, gavage 5–10% dextrose solution 0.25–0.5 ml/100 g neonates (5 French soft red rubber) | Percent solution is g/100 ml; 50% means there is 50 g dextrose in 100 ml water. If given as bolus, concentration should be 25% or less and given quickly to avoid phlebitis upon injection. Use sterile water or saline as diluent. To calculate the amount of stock solution required to create a custom solution use the equation (% desired custom solution × final volume desired)/% stock solution = volume of stock solution. Add this volume of stock solution to final volume desired of diluent – volume of stock solution | OTC Injectable |
| Diazepam (Valium®) | *Benzodiazepine* Anticonvulsant, muscle relaxant, anesthetic agent | 0.5–1 mg/kg rectally up to three times in 24 h, but at least 10 min apart (anticonvulsant), 0.2 mg/kg to 0.4 mg/kg IV (anesthetic) | 0.5–1 mg/kg rectally up to three times in 24 h, but at least 10 min apart (anticonvulsant), 0.2 mg/kg to 0.4 mg/kg IV (anesthetic) | Methocarbamol, propofol (anticonvulsant), midazolam (anesthetic) | Usually combined with ketamine or an opioid for anesthesia. Reverse with flumazenil *Caution: Discomfort on IM injection, midazolam strongly preferred for this route* | Rx Various human-label tablets, oral solution, injectable, rectal gel |
| Diphenhydramine (Benadryl®) | *Antihistamine* preventive/adjunctive treatment for anaphylaxis | 2–4 mg/kg PO q12h (antihistamine), 1–2 mg/kg IM or PO once (before FNA) q12h (adjunct to anaphylaxis) | 0.5–2 mg/kg IM or PO q12h (adjunct to anaphylaxis) | Epinephrine first line treatment for anaphylaxis | May cause sedation. Give with or without food | Rx and OTC Various human-labeled tablets and capsules |
| Doxapram (Dopram-V®, Respiram®) | *Chemoreceptor stimulant* CNS/respiratory stimulant | 1.1–11 mg/kg IV (anesthesia), 1–5 mg/kg IV, SQ, SL (neonates) | 1.1–11 mg/kg IV (anesthesia), 1–5 mg/kg IV, SQ, SL (neonates) | Mechanical ventilation and oxygen support first-line therapy | Use in neonates is controversial | Rx Veterinary- and human-labeled 20 mg/ml injection |

| Drug | Indication | Dose | | Alternatives | Comments | Status | Formulations |
|---|---|---|---|---|---|---|---|
| Doxycycline | *Tetracycline antibiotic* URI, *Ehrlichia* spp., *Anaplasma* spp., rickettsial diseases, *Bordetella*, adjunctive heartworm, *Mycoplasma felis* | 10 mg/kg PO q24h for 10 days (*Bordetella*) 28 days (*Ehrlichia* spp., Lyme), 5 mg/kg PO q12h for 7 days (RMSF, *Bordetella*), 14 days (*Anaplasma* spp.), 10 mg/kg PO q12h for 30 days (adjunctive heartworm) | 10 mg/kg PO q24h for 14 days (*M. felis*) | Minocycline, tetracycline | Give with food to minimize side effects of vomiting, diarrhea, and anorexia. May compound to a liquid for safer dosing (see recipes). May have anti-inflammatory properties. *Caution: Must follow pilling of cats with liquid due to risk of esophageal stricture with dry pilling. May discolor permanent enamel when given to young animals* | Rx | Various human-labeled tablets, capsules, and powder |
| Electrolytes (Hydrolyte®) | *Minerals and electrolytes* Mild-to-moderate dehydration secondary to diarrhea or vomiting | ($0.07 \times$ kg body weight $\times 1000$) + ($48 \times$ kg body weight) | | Isotonic crystalloid fluids SQ or IV | Appropriate for patients with mild-to-moderate dehydration only. Animals may refuse to drink solution. Offer one-fourth to one-third total amount and replace as consumed over a 12-h period | OTC Veterinary-labeled packet. Various human-labeled packets and solutions | |
| Enrofloxacin (Baytril®) | *Fluoroquinolone* Susceptible infections | 5–20 mg/kg PO q24h up to 30 days. May start with one initial dose of 2.5 mg/kg IM before transitioning to oral | 5 mg/kg PO or IM q24h up to 30 days | Orbifloxacin, ofloxacin, ciprofloxacin | Give at least 2–3 days past resolution of clinical signs, up to a maximum of 30 days. 100 mg/ml formulation is not recommended for use in small animals *Caution: Young animals due to potential for articular cartilage abnormalities; potential for retinal degeneration in cats at higher doses. Not recommended as first-line empiric treatment or treatment of a herd due to concerns about resistance* | Rx | Veterinary-labeled 22.7, 68, 136 mg tablets. 22.7 mg/ml, 100 mg/ml injection |
| Epinephrine | *Alpha- and beta-adrenergic agonist* Anaphylaxis, cardiac resuscitation, topical hemostasis | 0.01 mg/kg IM repeated q5–15 min PRN (anaphylaxis), 0.01 mg/kg IV or 0.1 mg/kg IT (diluted 1:1 with saline or sterile water) q3–5 min (resuscitation) up to 0.3 mg, 0.005–0.02 mg/ml (topical hemostasis) | 0.01 mg/kg IM repeated q5–15 min PRN (anaphylaxis), 0.01 mg/kg IV or 0.1 mg/kg IT (diluted 1:1 with saline or sterile water) q3–5 min (resuscitation) up to 0.3 mg, 0.005–0.02 mg/ml (topical hemostasis) | | See Chapter 15 for CPR details For ease of dosing, can make a 1:10 000 solution from 1:1 000 by adding 1 ml epinephrine to 9 ml of normal saline, or use insulin syringe for smaller doses See recipes for topical hemostasis via vasoconstriction *Caution: Do not confuse concentrations* | Rx | Various vet and human-labeled injection 1 mg/ml (1:1 000), 0.1 mg/ml (1:10 000) |

(*continued*)

**Table 20.12** (Continued)

| Generic name (Common trade names) | Type and field indications | Canine dose | Feline dose | Potential substitutes | Comments, cautions, and contraindications | Rx/controlled status and forms |
|---|---|---|---|---|---|---|
| Famotidine (Pepcid®) | *H2 receptor antagonist* Acid reflux | 0.5–1.1 mg/kg PO q12–24h, 0.5 mg/kg IV (slowly), IM or SC q12–24h | 0.5–1.1 mg/kg PO q12–24h, 0.5 mg/kg IV (slowly), IM or SC q12–24h | Omeprazole | Tablets have bitter taste. Oral omeprazole may be superior to oral famotidine *Caution: Geriatric patients, patients with impaired renal or hepatic function. May see idiosyncratic intravascular hemolysis in cats* | Rx and OTC Human-labeled 10, 20, and 40 mg tablets, powder for oral suspension, 10 mg/ml injection |
| Fenbendazole (Panacur®, Safe-guard®) | *Benzimidazole* Parasiticide | 50 mg/kg PO q24h for 3 days (ascarids, hookworms, whipworms) to 5 days (*Giardia*) | 10 mg/kg PO q24h for 3 days (ascarids, hookworms), 50 mg/kg PO q24h for 5 days (*Giardia*) | | In dogs, fenbendazole (50 mg/kg q24h) in conjunction with metronidazole (25 mg/kg q12h) for 5 days may be more effective than fenbendazole alone for treating *Giardia* | OTC 22.2% granules (222 mg/g), 100 mg/ml suspension |
| Fipronil (Frontline®) | *Phenylpyrazole* Parasiticide | 6.7–15 mg/kg | 7.5–15 mg/kg | | Found in conjunction with IGR (s)-methoprene (Frontline Plus). EPA rather than FDA approved. Some generic products are said to contain an inadequate dose of fipronil and dosing should be adjusted | OTC Various veterinary-labeled single-application topical treatments and sprays |
| Firocoxib (Previcox®) | *NSAID* Analgesic, antipyretic, anti-inflammatory | 5 mg/kg PO q24h PRN (osteoarthritis) up to 3 days (postsurgical) | No data | Carprofen, robenacoxib, ketoprofen, meloxicam, tolfedine, deracoxib | Cannot be accurately dosed in dogs less than 5.7 kg. COX-2 selective. *Contraindications: Bleeding disorders, concomitant steroid use, bleeding gastric ulcers, dehydration* | Rx 57 mg, 227 mg chewable tablets |
| Fluconazole (Diflucan®) | *Triazole* Antifungal | 5 mg/kg PO q12h | 10 mg/kg PO q12h (susceptible systemic mycoses), 20 mg/kg PO q12h (severe infections) | Itraconazole, ketoconazole | Treatment is usually at least several months duration and should be continued for 1–3 months past clinical resolution | Rx Various human-labeled tablets and suspension |
| Flumazenil | *Benzodiazepine antagonist* Reverses sedation caused by benzodiazepines | 0.01 mg/kg IV repeat hourly if required | 0.01 mg/kg IV repeat hourly if required | | Routine use not advisable due to potential for side effects such as seizures | Rx Injectable |

| Drug | Classification / Indication | Dose | Dose | Related drugs | Notes |
|---|---|---|---|---|---|
| Fluralaner (Bravecto®) | *Insecticide, acaricide* Fleas, ticks, demodex mites, sarcoptic mites | 25 mg/kg PO q12w (chewable tablet), 25 mg/kg topical q12w (topical solution) | 40 mg/kg topical q12w | | Rx. Available as chewable tablets and topical spot-on in five different strengths for dogs weighing between 2 and 56 kg. Available as topical spot-on for cats weighing between 1.2 and 12.5 kg. Give tablets with food. After feeding onset of action is within 8 h for fleas and 12 h for ticks. Labeled for 12 weeks of control of fleas and ticks (Ixodes scapularis, Dermacentor variabilis, and Rhipicephalus sanguineus). Effective against Amblyomma americanum for 8 weeks. Not labeled for use in dogs weighing less than 2 kg or less than 6 months old. Not labeled for cats less than 1.2 kg or less than 6 months old. Wide range of safety. Reported single-use efficacy against demodex mites in dogs. |
| Furosemide (Lasix®) | *Loop diuretic* Pulmonary edema | 2.75–5.5 mg/kg IV or IM q12–24h (pulmonary edema), 1–4 mg/kg IV, IM, or SQ q1 – 2h until respiratory rate decreases (severe acute pulmonary edema) | 2.75 mg/kg IV or IM q12–24h (pulmonary edema), 4 mg/kg IV, IM, or SQ q1–2h until respiratory rate decreases (severe acute pulmonary edema) | | Rx. Various veterinary-labeled and human-labeled tablets, injections, and oral solutions. In the field, often used for accidental fluid-overload. *Contraindications: Anuria* |
| Gabapentin (Neurontin®) | *Anticonvulsant* Anxiolytic (cats), neuropathic pain | 10–20 mg/kg PO q8h (neuropathic pain) | 50–100 mg/cat PO 2–3h before stressor (anxiolytic) | Acepromazine, alprazolam | Rx. Various human-labeled capsules, tablets, oral solution. Cats may become mildly ataxic |
| Glycopyrrolate | *Anticholinergic* Adjunct to anesthesia, sinoatrial arrest, treatment of carbamate, or organophosphate intoxication | 0.011 mg/kg IV, IM, or SQ (adjunct to anesthesia), 0.01–0.02 mg/kg IV repeated as required (carbamate/organophosphate intoxication) | 0.011 mg/kg IV, IM, or SQ (adjunct to anesthesia), 0.01–0.02 mg/kg IV repeated as required (carbamate/organophosphate intoxication) | Atropine | Rx. 0.2 mg/ml injection. Various human-labeled injection, tablets, oral solution. Lasts longer (2–3h) than atropine, does not cross blood–brain barrier. Use as a preanesthetic adjunct is no longer routine, despite this being the FDA-approved indication. *Contraindication: Concurrent use of dexmedetomidine* |
| Griseofulvin | *Antifungal* Dermatophytosis | 50 mg/kg PO q24h (microsize), 5–10 mg/kg PO q24h (ultramicrosize) | 50 mg/kg PO q24h (microsize), 5–10 mg/kg PO q24h (ultramicrosize), with caution | Itraconazole, fluconazole, terbinafine, ketoconazole | Rx. Various human-labeled microsize (4 μm) and ultramicrosize (<1 μm) tablets, may have limited availability. Terbinafine and triazole antifungals preferred; typically used only if no alternatives due to potential for significant side effects (vomiting, diarrhea, anorexia, pancytopenia), particularly in cats. Bitter taste. Give with fatty foods or corn oil. Ultramicrosize form is absorbed 1.5 times as well. *Caution: Cats* |

(continued)

Table 20.12 (Continued)

| Generic name (Common trade names) | Type and field indications | Canine dose | Feline dose | Potential substitutes | Comments, cautions, and contraindications | Rx/controlled status and forms |
|---|---|---|---|---|---|---|
| Hydrogen peroxide 3% | *Chemical compound* Emesis | 1–2 ml/kg PO | Use in dogs only | Apomorphine (dogs), dexmedetomidine or xylazine (cats) | Repeat once after 10–15 min if no emesis *Caution: Max 45 ml/dog* | OTC |
| Hydromorphone (Dilaudid®) | *Mu-agonist opioid* Preanesthetic, analgesic | 0.1–0.4 mg/kg IM or IV | 0.05–0.2 mg/kg IM or IV | Morphine, oxymorphone | Lasts 4–6 h. Side effects include vomiting and bradycardia. Typically used in conjunction with other drugs in an induction protocol | Rx Various human-labeled injection concentrations, tablets, capsules |
| Imidacloprid (Advantage®, Seresto®) | *Neonicotinoid parasiticide* Fleas, chewing lice | 7.5–10 mg/kg topical q1m (topical), 1 q8m (collar) | 10 mg/kg topical q1m (topical), 1 q8m (collar) | | EPA rather than FDA approved. Found in conjunction with moxidectin (Advantage Multi), permethrin (Advantix), pyriproxyfen (Advantage II), permethrin and pyriproxyfen (Advantix II), flumethrin (Seresto collars). Seresto collars provide protection against fleas and ticks for 8 months. Low-cost program from manufacturer specifically for Native American communities | OTC Topical spot-on, shampoo, spray collar |
| Itraconazole (Sporanox®) | *Triazole* Antifungal | 5 mg/kg PO q24h (*Malassezia*), 5–10 mg/kg PO q24h (susceptible mycoses; duration varies with agent) | 5 mg/kg PO q24h for 21 days in conjunction with q2d lime sulfur dips (ringworm), 5–10 mg/kg PO q24h (susceptible mycoses; duration varies with agent) | Fluconazole, ketoconazole, terbinafine, griseofulvin (ringworm only) | Discontinue treatment or monitor biochemical parameters if patient becomes depressed or anorexic. Compounded versions not recommended | Rx 100 mg human-labeled capsules and tablets, 10 mg/ml oral solution |
| Ivermectin (Ivomec®) | *Macrocyclic lactone* Parasiticide | 0.05 mg/kg PO or SQ once (microfilaricide), 0.3 mg/kg PO or SQ q1w for 4 weeks (sarcoptic mange), 0.3 mg/kg PO q24 for 8 weeks past the first negative scraping (demodex mange), 0.3 mg/kg SQ (ear mites) | 0.02 mg/kg PO or SQ q24 for 8 weeks past the first negative scraping (demodex mange), 0.024 mg/kg PO (heartworm prevention and control of hookworms), 0.3 mg/kg SQ (ear mites) | | Found in combination with pyrantel in products for heartworm prevention and parasiticide. May see hypersensitivity like reaction when administered to dogs with large microfilaria burden. Starting at 0.1 mg/kg and increasing recommended to detect dogs sensitive to ivermectin for doses >1.1 mg/kg *Caution in dogs with ABCB1-1Δ (AKA MDR-1) mutation such as Collies* | Rx Various chewable tablets OTC 10 mg/ml (1%) injectable |

| Drug | Classification/Indication | Dose | Dose | Related drugs | Comments | Availability |
|---|---|---|---|---|---|---|
| Kaolin/Pectin | *Adsorbent, GI-mucosal protectant* Antidiarrheal (symptomatic) | 1–2 ml/kg (5.8 g kaolin/0.26 g pectin/fluid ounce) PO q2–6h | 1–2 ml/kg (5.8 g kaolin/0.26 g pectin/fluid ounce) PO q2–6h | Activated charcoal (antidiarrheal, adsorbent), sucralfate (GI-mucosal protectant) | May cause transient constipation. Changes consistency of feces, but does not appear to decrease fluid or electrolyte loss – not for management of severe diarrhea. May adsorb drugs administered at same time, separate doses by 2 h. Both veterinary- and human-labeled products available OTC, but be cautious of human-labeled products that contain bismuth salicylate, which may be toxic, particularly to cats | OTC 5.8 g kaolin/0.26 g pectin/fluid ounce suspension (veterinary-labeled), 90 g kaolin, 2 g pectin/30 ml human-labeled |
| Ketamine (Ketaset®, Ketaflo®) | *Dissociative anesthetic* General anesthesia | Not recommended for sole agent | 11 mg/kg IM (restraint), 22–33 mg/kg IM (anesthesia) | Tiletamine, thiopental | Typically used in conjunction with other drugs (diazepam, midazolam) to induce general anesthesia. Skeletal muscles do not relax, and corneas must be protected with lubricant | Rx (Schedule III) 100 mg/ml injectable (veterinary-labeled products), various concentrations human-labeled products |
| Ketoconazole (Nizoral®) | *Azole antifungal* Systemic mycoses, *Malassezia* dermatitis | 5–10 mg/kg PO q24h for 2–4 weeks (*Malassezia*) or q12–24h for 1 month past clinical signs (systemic mycoses) | 10 mg/kg q12–24h (only if no alternatives) | Fluconazole, itraconazole, terbinafine, griseofulvin (ringworm only) | Newer triazole agents are generally preferred as more effective and lesser potential for side effects. *Extreme caution: Cats* | Rx 200 mg tablets |
| Ketoprofen (Ketofen®) | *NSAID* Analgesic, antipyretic, anti-inflammatory | 2 mg/kg IM, IV or SQ once, may continue at 1 mg/kg q24h for 4 additional days | 2 mg/kg SQ once, may continue with 1 mg/kg PO tablets for up to 4 additional days | | May dilute with 0.9 NaCl at 1:10 ratio for easier dosing in cats. Not COX selective, may result in greater bleeding or GI side effects. *Contraindications: Bleeding disorders, concomitant steroid use, bleeding gastric ulcers, dehydration* | Rx 100 mg/ml injectable |
| Lidocaine (Xylocaine®) | *Local anesthetic* Local/topical anesthesia | 1–4 mg/kg SQ | 1–4 mg/kg SQ | Bupivacaine (slower onset, longer duration), mepivacaine. Similar onset, | Time to onset 5–10 min, duration 1–2 h. Also available as topical alone or in combination with prilocaine. May mix lidocaine with sodium bicarbonate in a ratio of 9:1 with double the | Rx 2% (20 mg/ml) injectable. Various concentrations of |

*(continued)*

Table 20.12 (Continued)

| Generic name (Common trade names) | Type and field indications | Canine dose | Feline dose | Potential substitutes | Comments, cautions, and contraindications | Rx/controlled status and forms |
|---|---|---|---|---|---|---|
| | | | | longer duration (2–3 h) | volume of sterile water to reduce sting in awake patients. *Caution: Cats – do not exceed maximum dose* | human-labeled injectable |
| Mannitol | *Osmotic diuretic* Diuresis, CNS trauma | 0.25–0.5 g/kg IV bolus over 10–20 min q4–6 (diuresis), 0.5 g/kg IV over 15–20 min q6h (CNS trauma) | 0.25–0.5 g/kg IV bolus over 10–20 min q4–6 (diuresis), 0.5 g/kg IV over 15–20 min q6h (CNS trauma) | | *Use with extreme caution in the field given limited ability to monitor electrolytes* | Rx Various human-labeled injection concentrations |
| Maropitant (Cerenia®) | *Neurokinin-1 (NK1) receptor antagonist* Antiemetic | 1 mg/kg SQ or IV or 2 mg/kg PO q24h up to 5 consecutive days | 1 mg/kg SQ or IV or PO q24h up to 5 consecutive days | Ondansetron, dolasetron, metoclopramide | To prevent vomiting (rather than treat), administer at least 2 h before stimulus. SQ injections sting, refrigerate to reduce discomfort or give IV. Protect remainder of sectioned pills from moisture and light by wrapping tightly. May reduce visceral pain | Rx 10 mg/ml vial, 16, 24, 60, and 160 mg in blister packs |
| Melarsomine (Immiticide®, Diroban™) | *Arsenic-based antiparasitic* Heartworm treatment | 2.5 mg/kg deep IM q24h twice, alternating sides | Toxic to cats | | Refer to Chapter 13 for heartworm treatment protocols *Caution: Low margin of safety* | Rx 50 mg/vial |
| Meloxicam (Metacam®, Loxicom®) | *NSAID* Analgesic, antipyretic, anti-inflammatory | 0.2 mg/kg PO, IV or SQ first dose, 0.1 mg/kg PO q24 subsequent PRN for up to 7 days | 0.3 mg/kg SQ once | Carprofen, robenacoxib, ketoprofen, tolfedine, firocoxib | Human-labeled tablets may be most cost-effective NSAID option for large dogs. *Caution: Repeated use of meloxicam in cats has been associated with acute renal failure and death. Contraindications: Bleeding disorders, concomitant steroid use, bleeding gastric ulcers, dehydration* | Rx 5 mg/ml injectable, 1.5 mg/ml oral suspension, 7.5 and 15 mg human-labeled tablets |

| Drug | Class/Indications | Dose | Dose | Related | Notes | Availability |
|---|---|---|---|---|---|---|
| Methocarbamol | *Muscle relaxant* Intoxications with muscle tremors | 55–200 mg/kg q6–8h titrated, max 330 mg/kg/day | 55–200 mg/kg q6–8h titrated, max 330 mg/kg/day | Diazepam, propofol | Appropriate for intoxications involving muscle tremors, including pyrethroids (some dog-only flea/tick preventatives), metaldehyde (snail bait), strychnine, CNS stimulants, and SSRIs. Side effects include CNS depression. *Caution: Renal disease with injectable (contains polyethylene glycol)* | Rx 500 and 750 mg tablets, 100 mg/ml injection |
| Metoclopramide (Reglan®) | *Antiemetic/ prokinetic* Secondary agalactia | 0.2–0.5 mg/kg q6–8h PO, SC or IM (antiemetic/prokinesis), 0.1–0.2 mg/kg SQ q12h (secondary agalactia) | 0.2–0.4 mg/kg SQ or PO q6 antiemetic/prokinesis) | Ondansetron, dolasetron, maropitant (antiemetic), cisapride (prokinetic) | May have changes in mentation or constipation as side effects. *Contraindications: Obstruction due to pro-kinesis* | Rx 5 and 10 mg tablets, 1 mg/ml oral syrup |
| Metronidazole (Flagyl®) | *Antibiotic* *Giardia*, enteritis/colitis | 10–15 mg/kg q12h for 5–10 days (enteritis/colitis), limit 65 mg/kg/day | 25 mg/kg PO q12h for 5 days (*Giardia*), 62.5 mg/cat PO q12h for 5 days (enteritis/colitis) | Fenbendazole (*Giardia*), tylosin, sulfasalazine (colitis) | Activity against other protozoal parasites. Bitter taste. Can compound liquid to aid in dispensing to cats. Neurologic signs with overdose or cumulative dose. As last resort substitute, 250 and 500 mg metronidazole tablets available OTC for use in fish tanks | Rx and OTC Various human-label tablets and capsules |
| Midazolam (Versed®) | *Benzodiazepine* Sedation | 0.1–0.3 mg/kg SQ, IM, IV in combination with other medication | 0.1–0.3 mg/kg SQ, IM, IV in combination with other medication | Diazepam | IV midazolam can be orally administered at a dose of 0.2–0.5 mg/kg | Rx (Schedule IV) 1 mg/ml, 5 mg/ml, oral solution |
| Milbemycin oxime (Interceptor®) | *Macrolide antiparasitic* Heartworm prophylaxis, roundworms, hookworms, whipworms | 0.5 mg/kg PO q30d | 2 mg/kg PO q30d | | Found in combination with lufenuron (Sentinel), praziquantel (Interceptor Plus), lufenuron/praziquantel (Sentinel Spectrum), spinosad (Trifexis) | Rx Chewables sold for dogs and cats, by weight |
| Minocycline | *Tetracycline antibiotic* *Bordetella*, *Ehrlichia* spp., *Anaplasma* spp., lyme | 10 mg/kg PO q12h | 5–12.5 mg/kg PO q12h | Doxycycline, tetracycline | May cause nausea and vomiting, give with food. May discolor deciduous teeth. *Caution: May lodge in the esophagus of cats and cause stricture, follow pilling with water* | Rx Various veterinary and human label tablets and capsules |

(continued)

**Table 20.12** (*Continued*)

| Generic name (Common trade names) | Type and field indications | Canine dose | Feline dose | Potential substitutes | Comments, cautions, and contraindications | Rx/controlled status and forms |
|---|---|---|---|---|---|---|
| Morphine | *Mu-opioid agonist* Moderate to severe pain, premedication protocols | 0.1–1.0 mg/kg SQ, IM, IV q3–6h | 0.05–0.5 mg/kg SQ, IM | Hydromorphone, methadone | Causes nausea and vomiting | Rx (Schedule II) Various human-label tablets, oral solution, injection |
| Mupirocin (Bactroban®) | *Topical antibacterial* Skin infection | Apply topically to affected areas q12–q24h until healed (max 30 days) | Apply topically to affected areas q12–q24h until healed (max 30 days) | Silver sufadiazine (SSD), nitrofurazone, bacitracin | | Rx Ointment |
| Nalbuphine (Nubain®) | *Kappa agonist, mu antagonist/ partial agonist opioid* Potentiate other anesthetic drugs, mild-to-moderate analgesia | 0.2–0.4 mg/kg IV, IM, SQ | 0.2 mg/kg IV, IM, SQ | Butorphanol | Potential substitute for butorphanol that is not a controlled substance. May have benefits in treatment of shock as it blocks the depressant effects of endogenous opioids and improves patient cardiovascular dynamics | Rx 10 and 20 mg/ml |
| Naloxone (Narcan®) | *Opiate antagonist* Opioid reversal | 0.01–0.04 mg/kg IV, IM, SQ | 0.01–0.04 mg/kg IV, IM, SQ | | Wide margin of safety | Rx 0.4 and 1 mg/ml human-labeled injection |
| Nitenpyram (Capstar®, Capguard®) | *Oral insecticide* Adult fleas, maggots | 0.8–5 mg/kg | 1–2.75 mg/kg | | Rapid acting (as quickly as 30 min) against adult fleas. Can be used safely with other flea control. May be given rectally to sedated animals, or crushed and applied to wound (maggots) *Contraindications: Animals under 2 pounds of weight or 4 weeks of age.* *Caution in animals younger than 8 weeks of age* | OTC 11.4 and 57 mg tablets |

| Drug | Class/Indication | Dose | Dose | Compatible drugs | Comments | Availability |
|---|---|---|---|---|---|---|
| Omeprazole (Prilosec®) | *Proton pump inhibitor* Acid reflux, esophagitis | 0.5–1.0 mg/kg PO q24h | 0.5–1.0 mg/kg PO q24h | Famotidine | May be more effective PO than famotidine. *Caution: Do not crush capsules or tablets* | Rx and OTC Human-labeled 10, 20, and 40 mg tablets and capsules, 2 mg/ml oral suspension |
| Ondansetron (Zofran®) | *5-HT3 receptor antagonist* Prevention of vomiting | 0.5–1 mg/kg PO or IV (give slowly over 2–15 min) q12h | 0.5 mg/kg IV or PO q12h | Maropitant, metoclopramide | IV doses may be best at low end, oral doses at high end of range. Can be given at same time (0.22 mg/kg) as dexmedetomidine to reduce dexmedetomidine-induced nausea in cats | Rx Various human-labeled tablets, oral solution, injection |
| Penicillin G procaine | *Beta-lactam antibiotic* Wounds, abscesses | 20 000–40 000 Units/kg SQ q24h | 20 000–40 000 Units/kg SQ q24h | Amoxicillin, ampicillin | Must be refrigerated. Do not give IV. Label syringes to ensure that it is not mistaken for propofol | Rx Various veterinary- and human-labeled forms |
| Pentobarbital sodium (Pentasol®, Fatal-Plus®, Socumb® Euthasol®) | *Barbiturate* Euthanasia | 85 mg/kg IV or IC (euthanasia), 250 mg/kg PO (heavy sedation before euthanasia) | 85 mg/kg IV or IC | Potassium chloride | IC administration only appropriate for animals at a surgical plane of anesthesia. See Chapter 12 for additional information on euthanasia protocols. *Caution: Toxic to wildlife, dispose of carcass appropriately to prevent scavenging* | Rx (Schedule II or III) Solution, powder (Pentasol, Fatal-Plus). Also formulated in conjunction with phenytoin sodium (Beuthanasia-D Special, Euthasol, SomnaSol), which moves from Schedule II to Schedule III |
| Permethrin | *Synthetic pyrethroid* Insecticide (adult), miticide, insect repellent | Refer to product label | Not safe for cats | | Permethrin intoxication of cats occurs between 2 and 24 h from exposure. Treat seizures/tremors with methocarbamol (preferentially) or diazepam. Bathe, maintain on fluids for 24–48 h *Contraindications: Cats or dogs that are in contact with cats* | OTC Various topical solutions, shampoos, and sprays, often in combination with other drugs |

*(continued)*

**Table 20.12** (Continued)

| Generic name (Common trade names) | Type and field indications | Canine dose | Feline dose | Potential substitutes | Comments, cautions, and contraindications | Rx/controlled status and forms |
|---|---|---|---|---|---|---|
| Ponazuril (Marquis paste®) | *Antiprotozoal* *Coccidia, Neospora, Toxoplasma* spp. | 55 mg/kg PO q24h | 55 mg/kg PO q24h | Toltrazuril, sulfadimethoxine | Must be diluted with 25 ml water or 12.5 ml water and 12.5 ml syrup before dosing of small animals (results in 75 ml of a 100 mg/ml oral suspension). Protect from light, shake thoroughly before dosing | Rx 4.5 oz. tubes |
| Potassium chloride | *Metal halide salt* Euthanasia alternative for anesthetized animals | 1–2 mmol/kg (74–148 mg/kg) IC or IV given to effect | 1–2 mmol/kg (74–148 mg/kg) IC or IV given to effect | Pentobarbital, propofol | Animals *must* be at surgical plane of anesthesia prior to administration. See Chapter 12 for more information. Minimal risk of relay toxicity (poisoning by eating a poisoned animal). Requires a large volume as compared with pentobarbital. Can make up to 360 mg/ml solution (saturation point temperature dependent) from OTC KCl powder or KCl (NOT NaCl) water softener crystals (see compounding recipes). Give as quickly as possible for best effect | Rx or OTC 2 mEq/ml (149 mg/ml, 4 mmol/ml), 4 mEq/ml (298 mg/ml), powder |
| Praziquantel (Droncit®) | *Anticestodal anthelmintic* Tapeworms | 2.5–5 mg/kg, maximum 170 mg | 2.5–5 mg/kg, maximum 34 mg | Epsiprantel, fenbendazole | Wide margin of safety. Labeled for cestodes, but extra-label dosing for schistosomes and trematodes | Rx 23 mg (feline), 34 mg (canine) tablets, 56.8 mg/ml injectable, many generics. Often found in combination with other dewormers for a broader spectrum of activity |
| Prednisone | *Corticosteroid* Anti-inflammatory | 0.5–2.0 mg/kg PO q12–24h | 0.5–2.0 mg/kg PO q24h or q12h | Dexamethasone | Prednisolone considered more effective for cats. *Caution: Must taper dose before stopping* | Rx 5 and 20 mg tablets, oral solution |

| Drug | Class / Indication | Dose | Dose | Alternatives | Notes | Availability |
|---|---|---|---|---|---|---|
| Proparacaine | *Topical ocular anesthetic* Diagnosing spastic entropion, removal of foreign bodies | 1–2 drops in affected eye | 1–2 drops in affected eye | | Onset of action around a minute, duration of action 5–10 min, can be repeated. For diagnostic/procedural use only | Rx |
| Propofol (PropoFlo®, PropoFlo 28®, Propovet®) | *Hypnotic anesthetic agent* Induction of anesthesia | 4–6 mg/kg IV, 1–4 mg/kg IV with premedication | 6–8 mg/kg IV, 1–4 mg/kg IV with premedication | Alfaxalone | Titrate dose against the response of the patient over 60–90 s. PropoFlo 28 has a shelf life of 28 days, whereas formulations without preservatives must be used within 6 h. Mild hypotension and transient apnea are common side effects. Expired bottles may be used as euthanasia alternative via respiratory arrest if no gross changes to solution (start with 10 mg/kg, titrated to affect). Delayed recovery in Sighthounds. *Caution: Hypoproteinemic animals Caution (PropoFlo 28): Cats (benzyl alcohol preservative)* | Rx (may be controlled in individual states) 10 mg vial |
| Pyrantel Pamoate (Nemex®, Strongid®) | *Pyrimidine anthelmintic* Removal of ascarids and hookworm | 10 mg/kg < 2.5 kg, 5 mg/kg ≥ 2.5 kg | 20 mg/kg | | Often found in combination with other dewormers for a broader spectrum of activity, including febantel and praziquantel (Drontal Plus), praziquantel (Drontal), ivermectin, and praziquantel (Heartgard) | Rx or OTC Various tablets and oral suspensions for small animal, large animal, and human |
| Robenacoxib (Onsior®) | *NSAID* Analgesia | 2 mg/kg PO, SQ, both for up to 3 days | 1 mg/kg PO q24h, 2 mg/kg SQ, both for up to 3 days | Meloxicam, carprofen, ketoprofen, tolfedine, firocoxib | Not evaluated in cats <4 months of age or <5.5 pounds. Can use injectable and oral forms interchangeably without need for washout. Selective COX-2 inhibition. *Contraindications: Bleeding disorders, concomitant steroid use, bleeding gastric ulcers, dehydration* | Rx 20 mg/ml inj., 6 mg tablet |

*(continued)*

Table 20.12 (*Continued*)

| Generic name (Common trade names) | Type and field indications | Canine dose | Feline dose | Potential substitutes | Comments, cautions, and contraindications | Rx/controlled status and forms |
|---|---|---|---|---|---|---|
| Selamectin (Revolution®) | *Macrocyclic lactone* Topical parasiticide. Prevention of fleas, heartworm, some ticks. Treatment of sarcoptic mange and ear mites. Treatment and control of roundworm and hookworm (cats) | 6 mg/kg topically every 30 days. For treatment of tick infestation, ear mites, and sarcoptic mange, additional dose 2–4 weeks after initial dose may be required | 6 mg/kg topically every 30 days. For treatment of tick infestation, ear mites and sarcoptic mange, additional dose 2–4 weeks after initial dose may be required | Fluralaner, imidacloprid, ivermectin | FDA approved and individually packaged doses may be combined and dosed via syringe | Rx 60 and 120 mg/ml |
| Silver nitrate | *Chemical coagulant* Superficial bleeding | Apply silver nitrate stick topically to superficial bleeding tissue | Apply silver nitrate stick topically to superficial bleeding tissue | Styptic powder | Do not use on eyes. Painless on intact skin but burning sensation on wounds (can prep with lidocaine). Apply only to area to be treated. Saline can be used to neutralize chemical reaction. Useful for stopping bleeding following ear tipping in cats | OTC Sticks |
| Silver Sulfadiazine (SSD) (Silvadene®) | *Topical antibacterial* Wounds and burns | Apply topically at a thickness of 1–2 mm on affected areas q24h or q12h until healed | Apply topically at a thickness of 1–2 mm on affected areas q24h or q12h until healed | Mupirocin, bacitracin, nitrofurazone | Wide spectrum of antimicrobial activity against both Gram-negative and Gram-positive bacteria. Also antimycotic. Dressings not normally required | Rx 50 and 400 g jar |
| Sucralfate (Carafate®, Antepsin®) | *GI-mucosal protectant* Treatment and prevention of esophagitis | 20–50 mg/kg PO q8h | 250 mg/cat PO q6–8h | | Give other oral drugs at least 2 h before sucralfate. Can be given when increased risk for reflux (surgery after a recent meal). May cause constipation | Rx 1 g tablets, 100 mg/ml suspension |
| Sulfadimethoxine (Albon®) | *Sulfonamide* Coccidia | 50–60 mg/kg PO q24h for 5–20 days | 50–60 mg/kg PO q24h for 5–20 days | Ponazuril, toltrazuril | An antibiotic most commonly used for treatment of coccidia (extra-label). Coccidiostatic rather than coccidiocidal, young animals may benefit from alternatives | Rx 50 mg/ml oral suspension, 125, 250, and 500 mg tablets |

| Drug | Class / Indication | Dose | Dose | Combined with / Alternatives | Comments | Availability |
|---|---|---|---|---|---|---|
| Terbinafine (Lamisil®) | *Antifungal* Dermatophytosis, *Malessezia* dermatitis | 20–40 mg/kg PO q24h with food until two consecutive negative DTMs | 20–40 mg/kg PO q24h with food until two consecutive negative DTMs | Fluconazole, itraconazole, ketoconazole, griseofulvin (ringworm only) | For dermatophytosis, best used in conjunction with twice per week topical lime sulfur. May pulse 2 weeks on, 2 weeks off. See Chapter 13 for more information on the treatment of dermatophytosis | Rx 125 and 187.5 mg granules, 250 mg tablets |
| Thiopental (Pentothal®) | *Thiobarbiturate* General anesthesia | 12–15 mg/kg IV, with 1/3 given rapidly, remainder to effect | 12–15 mg/kg IV, with 1/3 given rapidly, remainder to effect | Tiletamine, ketamine | Very short acting. *Caution: Use in animals with ASA status > 1, may cause apnea in cats* | Rx (Schedule III) No longer marketed in the United States |
| Tiletamine and zolazepam (Telazol®, Zoletil®) | *Dissociative/ muscle relaxant combination* Sedation/ anesthesia | 6–12 mg/kg IM | 9–12 mg/kg IM | Ketamine and diazepam | Often used in combination with an opioid and alpha-2 agonist. Dose adjusted for desired level of sedation/anesthesia. Minimal-to-moderate analgesia, depending on dose. Best to give as single dose rather than multiple smaller doses due to differential metabolism of constituents | Rx (Schedule III) Telazol and Zoletil 100®: 500 mg vial reconstituted to 100 mg/ml (50 mg tiletamine, 50 mg zolazepam). Zoletil 50® reconstitutes to 50 mg/ml |
| Toltrazuril 5% (Baycox®) | *Antiprotozoal* Coccidia, Neospora, Toxoplasma | 10–30 mg/kg PO once (can be repeated for 3 days) | 10–30 mg/kg PO once (can be repeated for 3 days) | Ponazuril, sulfadimethoxine | Available in several countries outside of the United States, potentially OTC. Ponazuril is an active metabolite of toltrazuril. Coccidiocidal rather than coccidiostatic. Wide range of safety. May cause drooling. Do not use 2.5% solution | Rx 5% solution |
| Tramadol | *Synthetic mu-receptor opiate agonist* Analgesia | 2–5 mg/kg, 10 mg/kg maximum PO q8–12h | No established dose | NSAIDs, other opiates | Tramadol injectable forms available in some countries. Avoid the human-labeled tramadol–acetaminophen combination tablets (Ultracet®), particularly in cats | Rx (Schedule IV) Various human-labeled tablets |
| Trazodone | *Antidepressant of the serotonin antagonist and reuptake inhibitor class* Anxiety | 20 mg/kg PO PRN (exam), 8–15 mg/kg PO q12h (post-op.) | Gabapentin preferred | Acepromazine, gabapentin | Can be used as a noncontrolled substance option for managing anxiety, particularly in shelter dogs. Some sedation, principally at higher doses. Cats experience some sedation, but not altered behavior. May facilitate post-surgical confinement | Rx Various human-labeled tablets |

*(continued)*

**Table 20.12** (Continued)

| Generic name (Common trade names) | Type and field indications | Canine dose | Feline dose | Potential substitutes | Comments, cautions, and contraindications | Rx/controlled status and forms |
|---|---|---|---|---|---|---|
| Trimethoprim/ Sulfonamide (Tribrissen®) | *Potentiated sulfonamide antimicrobial agent* Infection with sensitive organisms, uncomplicated UTI, toxoplasmosis | 30 mg/kg PO q24h for 7 days (sensitive organisms, UTI), 15 mg/kg PO q12h 7 days (severe infections, UTI), 15 mg/kg PO q12h 4 weeks (toxoplasmosis) | 30 mg/kg PO q24h (sensitive organisms), 15 mg/kg PO q12h 7 days (severe infections, UTI), 15 mg/kg PO q12h 4 weeks (toxoplasmosis) | | Combination of trimethoprim and sulfadiazine in the ratio of 1:5, dose is based on combined amount. Concerns about KCS in dogs when used for more than 7 days. *Caution: Dobermans, renal, or hepatic disease, urolithiasis, dogs with KCS* | Rx Human-labeled 480 and 960 mg tablets most common |
| Tylosin (Tylan®) | *Macrolide antibiotic* Colitis | 10–40 mg/kg PO q12h, 2–10 mg/kg IM q8–q24h PRN | 10–40 mg/kg PO q12h, 2–10 mg/kg IM q8–q24h PRN | Metronidazole, sulfasalazine | Used more for anti-inflammatory properties than antibiotic. Safer for long-term use than metronidazole. Bitter taste may require packaging in gelatin capsules for oral administration. Tylosin tartrate has better bioavailability than tylosin phosphate. Other concentrations exist, dose typically given in teaspoons. 1 tsp = 5 ml (pack powder into syringe to measure). Wide safety range | Rx 100 g tub, 50 mg/ml injection |
| Vincristine | *Mitotic inhibitor* Transmissible venereal tumor (TVT) | 0.025 mg/kg IV or 0.5 mg/m² BSA IV once per week until resolution (generally 3–6 weeks) | Not applicable | | Maximum dose 1 mg. Avoid extravasation | Rx 1 mg/ml |
| Vitamin B12 (Cyanocobalamin) | *Vitamin* Vitamin B12 deficiencies | 250–500 µg IM or SQ | 250–500 µg IM or SQ | | | Rx 1000 µg/ml |
| Vitamin K1 (Phytonadione) | *Vitamin* Anticoagulant rodenticide antidote | 2.2 mg/kg SQ initial, 1.1 mg/kg SQ or oral q12h | 2.2 mg/kg SQ initial, 1.1 mg/kg SQ or oral q12h | | Maintain 1.1 mg/kg SQ dose until active bleeding subsides. Duration of oral treatment is 1 week (warfarin) to 6 weeks (second generation) depending on rodenticide. Vitamin K2 or K3 is NOT an acceptable substitute. IV administration may cause a severe anaphylaxis-like reaction | Rx and OTC 10 mg/ml, 25 mg, and 50 mg capsules/tablets |

| | | | | | | |
|---|---|---|---|---|---|---|
| Xylazine (AnaSed®, Rompun®, Tranquived®) | *Alpha-2 agonist* Sedation, analgesia, emetic (cats) | 1 mg/kg IM or IV | 0.4 mg/kg (emesis) | (Dex) medetomidine | More likely to cause vomiting than medetomidine | Rx 20, 100, 200 mg/ ml injection |
| Yohimbine (Yobine®) | *Indolealkylamine alkaloid* Alpha-2 antagonist, amitraz toxicity, antiemesis | 0.1 mg/kg IV slowly (reversal and amitraz toxicity). 0.25–0.5 mg/kg SQ or IM q12h or q24h (antiemesis) | 1 mg/cat IV or IM | Atipamezole | Reverses analgesic effects of alpha-2 agonists as well as sedative effects. Approved in dogs only | Rx 2 mg/ml injection |
| Yunnan Baiyao | *Chinese herbal formula* Prevent perioperative bleeding | 250 mg <14 kg, 500 mg ≥14 kg PO q12h | No data | Aminocaproic acid | Formulations may vary. Capsules may be opened and topically applied to wounds | OTC 250 mg capsule |

## 20.5 Compounding Recipes

### 20.5.1 General Rules of Thumb

- If a drug is packaged in blister packs or with a moisture-proof barrier, it is probably subject to loss of stability and potency if mixed with aqueous vehicles [13].
- If the original packaging of a drug is in a light-protected or amber container, it is probably prone to inactivation by light.
- If an antibiotic is available in a powder that must be reconstituted in a vial or in an oral dispensing bottle before administration, it should not be mixed with other drugs.

### 20.5.2 Signs of Drug Instability

Altering drugs may alter the product's bioavailability or stability. It is important to monitor for signs of drug instability [13] (Table 20.13).

### 20.5.3 Beyond-Use Dating

The beyond-use date is the date after the compounded drug is not to be used. The following maximum beyond-use dates are suggested [13]:

- For solutions or nonaqueous liquids, should not be later than 25% of the time remaining until the product's expiration date.
- For water-containing formulations, should not be later than 14 days at cold temperatures.

- For all other formulations, not later than the intended duration of therapy or 30 days, whichever is earlier.

These suggested limits may be exceeded when there is supporting scientific data that applies to the specific compounded formulation.

### 20.5.4 Recipes

Evidence-based recipes are provided below for practitioner compounding by a licensed veterinarian. All liability for use lies with the practitioner. Some of these recipes may involve bulk ingredients. These should only be used under circumstances where Federal and State laws forbidding compounding from bulk substances do not apply, or when in compliance with regulatory guidelines for nonenforcement. See Section 20.2.4 for further information regarding compounding regulation and liability.

#### 20.5.4.1 Micro-dose of Dexmedetomidine
Indication: Management of postoperative delirium and differentiation from postoperative pain [14].

Compounding recipe and directions:
Dilute 0.1 ml of dexmedetomidine (500 µg/ml) with 0.9 ml of saline or sterile water to form a 50 µg/ml concentration of dexmedetomidine.
Dose:
0.1 ml per 5 kg IV
0.3 ml per 5 kg IM

Table 20.13 Signs of drug instability.

| Liquids | Solids |
| --- | --- |
| Color change (pink or yellow) | Odor (sulfur or vinegar odor) |
| Signs of microbial growth | Excessive powder or crumbling |
| Cloudiness, haziness, flocculence, or film | Cracks or chips in tablets |
| Separation of phases | Swelling of tablets or capsules |
| Precipitation, clumping, crystal formation | Sticking together of capsules or tablets |
| Droplets forming on inside of container | Tackiness of the covering of tablets or capsules |
| Gas or odor release | |
| Swelling of container | |

Comments:

Duration of effect is approximately 5–8 min. To differentiate delirium from painful recovery:

- If the patient returns to vocalization 3–5 min after micro-dose of dexmedetomidine is given, the patient is most likely painful.
- If the patient was exhibiting delirium, he will most likely remain calm and quiet after a micro-dose of dexmedetomidine.

### 20.5.4.2 Kitten/Puppy Milk Replacer

Indication: Emergency substitute or supplementation for neonates when commercial milk replacer is not available. Divide total amount into four to eight feedings [15].

Compounding recipe and directions:

- 250 ml whole cow's milk
- Three egg yolks
- One drop of oral multiple vitamin solution
- 15 ml corn oil
- Small pinch of salt

Blend uniformly and warm to 95–100 °F (35–38 °C). Refrigerate between uses.

Dose:

Week 1: 0.20 ml/g/day PO
Week 2: 0.22 ml/g/day PO
Week 3: 0.24 ml/g/day PO
Week 4: 0.26 ml/g/day PO

Comments:

Formula contains approximately 1 kcal/ml. Neonates' energy requirement is 20–26 kcal/100 g. Maximum comfortable stomach capacity is approximately 4 ml/100 g body weight.

### 20.5.4.3 Dakin's Solution 0.025%

Indication: Germicidal wound wash [16]
Compounding recipe and directions:

- 4.75 ml bleach (sodium hypochlorite solution 5.25%)
- 1/2 teaspoon of baking soda
- 995 ml sterile water

Place in sterile jar and protect from light.
Comments:

Discard unused portion after 48 h. Caution, solutions >0.5% retard wound healing. A 0.05% chlorhexidine solution (25 ml of 2% chlorhexidine in 975 ml of sterile saline or sterile water) or 0.1–1% povidone–iodine solution (10 ml of 10% povidone–iodine in 990 ml of sterile saline for 0.1% or 100 ml of 10% povidone–iodine to 900 ml of sterile saline for 1%) may be substituted if available.

A 0.025% solution of bleach (modified Dakin's solution) is effective against Gram-negative and Gram-positive bacteria, fungi, and viruses without being cytotoxic. At this concentration, it has also been found to promote quicker healing, have greater bactericidal effect, and was more cost effective than a 1% silver sulfadiazine (SSD) cream when managing partial thickness burns [17]. It does not debride, relieve edema, or have anti-inflammatory effects.

### 20.5.4.4 Three Percent Vinegar/Acetic Acid

Indication: Germicidal wound wash [18]
Compounding recipe and directions:

- 160 ml water
- 240 ml 5% white wine vinegar

Comments:

Vinegar/acetic acid controls infection and promotes healing by lowering the surface pH of wounds. A vinegar solution is an excellent therapeutic option if systemic antibiotics are unavailable or if antibiotic-resistant strains of bacteria exist within the wound. At appropriate concentrations, vinegar is effective against *Pseudomonas*, *Escherichia coli*, and *Enterococcus* spp. A 3% acetic acid solution is effective in eliminating *Pseudomonas aeruginosa* from superficial infection sites in human wounds and is also nontoxic [18].

The acidifying effect on the wound is short-lived, however. Flushes or bandage changes should be repeated ideally every 4 h, although success has also been seen with once daily use.

### 20.5.4.5 Normal Saline

Indication: Wound irrigation when supplies of commercial normal saline are unavailable or must be reserved for intravenous use [19].

Compounding recipe and directions:

- Eight teaspoons of table salt
- One gallon distilled water

Use and discard the remainder immediately, or refrigerate for up to 4 weeks. If no distilled water is available, you may boil filtered water and container for 5 min to make sterile.

Comments:

May be used SQ or IV only when used immediately and the benefit significantly outweighs the risk.

### 20.5.4.6 Oral Rehydration Solution

Indication: Mild-to-moderate dehydration caused by diarrhea or vomiting [20].

Compounding recipe and directions:

- 1/2 teaspoon table salt
- Six teaspoons of sugar
- 1 l clean drinking water or room temperature boiled water
- ± Salt substitute (KCl)

Dose:

$(0.07 \times kg$ body weight $\times 1000) + (48 \times kg$ body weight). Offer one-fourth to one-third total amount and replace as consumed over a 12-h period.

Comments:

Animals may refuse oral rehydration and require SQ or IV rehydration. Control nausea before offering oral rehydration solution.

### 20.5.4.7 Cefazolin Eye Drops

Indications: Gram-positive bacterial infection of the eye. May use in conjunction with a fluoroquinolone such as ofloxacin for broader coverage [21].

Dose:

Administer one drop in affected eye(s) q2h

Compounding recipe and directions:

Reconstitute a 1 g vial of cefazolin to 330 mg/ml. Aseptically remove the top of a new artificial tear drop bottle (15 ml) and with a sterile needle and syringe remove 2.4 ml. Add 2.4 ml of cefazolin to the bottle of artificial tears to create a final concentration of 50 mg/ml.

Comments:

Must be refrigerated. Stable for 42 days. Shake well before use.

### 20.5.4.8 Topical Ivermectin 1.1 mg/ml

Indication: Ear mites [22]

Compounding recipe and directions

1% injectable ivermectin, diluted 1:9 with propylene glycol

Dose:

Administer one drop (0.05 ml)/ear and massage ear base. For large dogs, administer two drops. Repeat in 2 weeks if needed.

Comments:

Exercise caution if rupture of the tympanic membrane (ear drum) is suspected.

### 20.5.4.9 Oral Ivermectin 1.1 mg/ml

Indication: Heartworm prevention and intestinal deworming [23]

Compounding recipe and directions:

- 1 ml 1% (10 mg/ml) ivermectin
- 5 ml water
- 4 ml propylene glycol

Creates a 1.1 mg/ml solution.

Dose:

0.05 mg/kg (0.05 ml/kg) PO for heartworm prevention. 0.2 mg/kg (0.18 ml/kg) PO for intestinal deworming.

### 20.5.4.10 Otitis Treatment

Note that cytology should be performed to guide selection of best empiric treatment. Often times, for mild otitis externa caused by cocci, ear cleaning products with antibacterial effect (chlorhexidine, Tris–EDTA, acetic acid, and isopropyl alcohol) alone are curative. An otoscopic exam should be performed to determine if the tympanic membrane is intact.

Several recipes are provided below for the treatment of otitis, depending on the cause (cocci, yeast, etc.)

#### 20.5.4.10.1 Otitis Recipe #1

Indication: Bacterial ear infections with rods present, moderate-to-severe otitis externa with the presence of bacteria [24,25]

Compounding recipe and directions:

- 13 ml of 100 mg/ml injectable enrofloxacin
  - 118 ml (4 oz) bottle of Tris–EDTA (ethylene-diaminetetraacetic acid) or T8
  - Tris–EDTA/keto or T8 Keto may be used if yeast present
  - Synotic, 1% hydrocortisone, or saline may be used if Tris–EDTA or T8 unavailable
- ±24 mg dexamethasone if severe inflammation

Dose:

Fill the ear canal q12h. Recheck cytology every 2 weeks and discontinue after two negative cytologies. At this time, switch to maintenance ear cleaning.

### 20.5.4.10.2  Otitis Recipe #2
Indications: Bacteria present and tympanic membrane is perforated [25]
Compounding recipe and directions:

- 1/2 of 22 g tube of mupirocin
- HB101 (hydrocortisone + Burow's solution)

Add the mupirocin to a 60-ml squeeze bottle and fill remainder of bottle with HB101. Mix thoroughly.
Dose:

Fill the ear canal q12h. Recheck cytology every 2 weeks, discontinue after two negative cytologies, and switch to maintenance ear cleaning.

Comments:

Mupirocin is safe in the middle ear.

### 20.5.4.10.3  Otitis Recipe #3
Indication: Yeast present [25]
Compounding recipe and directions:

- 30-ml bottle of miconazole lotion
- 3- to 5-ml fluocinolone acetonide 0.01% and dimethyl sulfoxide 60% (Synotic)

Remove 3–5 ml from miconazole bottle and add 3–5 ml of Synotic.
Dose:

Put 0.5–1 cc in each ear twice daily.

Comments:

Antibiotics should be avoided if no bacterial component.

### 20.5.4.10.4  Otitis Recipe #4
Indications: *Pseudomonas* spp. and/or perforated tympanic membrane [26]
Compounding recipe and directions:

- 1 g of SSD cream diluted 1:9 sterile water
  - May use HB101, Tris–EDTA, or Burrow's solution instead of sterile water

Dose:

0.5–1 ml/ear q12h

Comments:

Ears must be clean before use. Appears safe with ruptured tympanic membrane. Note that SSD cream comes in a water-soluble and -insoluble form – Silvadene is reported to work best for compounding. SSD powder can be obtained from compounding pharmacies to facilitate the compounding of a solution.

### 20.5.4.11  Ear Cleanser, 2.5% Acetic Acid
Indication: Ear cleaning [27,28,29]
Compounding recipe and directions:

- 1:2 5% white wine vinegar to water

Dose:

0.5–1 ml/ear q12–24h

Comments:

Best for healthy ears as the solution may be irritating to inflamed skin.

### 20.5.4.12  Doxycycline Suspension
Indication: Upper respiratory tract infections, tick borne disease [30]
Compounding recipe and directions:

- Ora-Sweet syrup
- Ora-Plus suspending vehicle
- 100 mg doxycycline tablets or capsules

Create a 50:50 mixture of Ora-Sweet syrup and Ora-Plus suspending vehicle for desired mixture volume. ((Patient weight × mg per unit of weight/desired final concentration × # of days) + 1 = desired mixture volume).

33.3 mg/ml: 1 100 mg crushed tablet or capsule per 3 ml mixture volume

50 mg/ml: 1 100 mg crushed tablet or capsule per 2 ml mixture volume

100 mg/ml: 1 100 mg crushed tablet or capsule per 1 ml mixture volume

200 mg/ml: 1 100 mg crushed tablet or capsule per 0.5 ml mixture volume

Comments:

The compounded doxycycline suspension is good for 7 days when stored in a light proof container. May use other suspension vehicles such as maple syrup, but the duration of efficacy of the compounded product is unknown.

### 20.5.4.13 Topical Hemostasis

#### 20.5.4.13.1 *Dilute Epinephrine*
Indication: Prevention of hematomas, hemostasis in absence of cautery [31]
Compounding recipe and directions:

- 1:1 000 epinephrine
- Sterile saline (ideally chilled)

1:200 000 dilution (5 mg/ml): 0.01 ml of 1:1 000 epinephrine in 2 ml of sterile saline
1:400 000 dilution (2.5 mg/ml): 0.01 ml of 1:1 000 epinephrine in 4 ml of sterile saline
Comments:

Recommended concentration for topical hemostasis is 1:200 000 or 1:400 000. Greater concentrations may cause cell necrosis. Splash on subcutaneous tissues to avoid complications such as scrotal hematoma. Maximum effect reached at between 4 and 5 min. May be added to appropriately diluted local anesthetic for a topical splash block with hemostatic powers.

#### 20.5.4.13.2 *Ear Tip Paste*
Indication: Hemostasis after ear tip
Compounding Recipe and Directions:

- 10 ml bupivacaine
- 0.05 ml epinephrine 1:1 000
- 0.25–1 teaspoon styptic powder

Mix bupivacaine and epinephrine and add resulting solution in 0.1 ml increments to a quantity of styptic powder sufficient for the needs of the day until a paste is formed. Discard paste at the end of the day. A

bupivacaine/epinephrine solution is likely stable in the refrigerator for up to 6 months [32].

### 20.5.4.14 "Miracle Mouthwash" Topical Pain Relief for Oral Cavity
Indication: oral ulceration [33]
Compounding Recipe and Directions:

- 5 ml lidocaine 0.5%
- 14.75 ml aluminum hydroxide suspension (Maalox)
- 0.25 ml diphenhydramine 12.5 mg/ml

Combine ingredients together
Dose:

dogs 2–5 ml, cats 2 ml; PRN up to q6h.

Comments:

Limit dosing to less than 2.5 ml/kg/day. Shake before use.

### 20.5.4.15 Euthanasia Alternatives
Indication: Euthanasia without access to barbiturates or approved potassium chloride injectable drug

#### 20.5.4.15.1 *Potassium Chloride (KCl)*
Compounding Recipe and Directions: [34–36]

- 6 g powdered KCl or water softener KCl crystals ground to a powder
- 20 ml water

One gram of powdered KCl is approximately 1 ml by volume. Mix to saturation. Warming the water before dissolving powder will allow for better dissolution. Ideally filter before use. Scale recipe as appropriate for anticipated use.
Dose:

To effect, IV or IC (preferred) as rapidly as possible. Dose will vary by health status of animal, but expect to administer around 0.3–0.5 ml/kg.

Comments:

Purchase as commercial powder, or water softener crystals may be blended in a heavy-duty blender. *Animal MUST be at surgical plane of anesthesia before administration*, and potassium chloride should only be used when barbiturates are unavailable.

### 20.5.4.15.2  Magnesium Sulfate (MgSO₄)

Compounding recipe and directions [35–38]:

- 60 g $MgSO_4$ (Epsom salt)
- 60 ml water

1.5 g of powdered $MgSO_4$ is approximately 1 ml by volume. Mix to saturation. Warming the water before dissolving powder will allow for better dissolution. Ideally filter before use. Scale the recipe as appropriate for anticipated use.

Dose:

To effect, IV or IC (preferred) as rapidly as possible. Dose will vary by health status of animal, but expect to administer around 1–2 ml/kg.

Comments:

Purchase as Epsom salts. Saturated solutions will be viscous. *Animal MUST be at a surgical plane of anesthesia*, and magnesium sulfate should only be used when barbiturates are unavailable.

## 20.6  Reference Charts

Empiric treatment is often required in the field when culture and sensitivity are unavailable (Tables 20.14–20.22). To ensure success, empiric treatment must target the most probable pathogen in the population from which the patient originates. Previous culture and sensitivity results or historic treatment successes and failures should be considered. Antibiotics listed here reflect pathogen probability derived from a wide range of veterinary practices, drugs commonly available in the field, and practices meant to minimize drug resistance. Doses and duration should be adjusted based on practitioner experience in a given population.

Due to concerns regarding antibiotic resistance, it is recommended to minimize the use of enrofloxacin, particularly in herd situations unless it is clearly indicated (such as rods visualized on ear cytology) and no alternatives exist. The Antimicrobial Reference Guide to Effective Treatment (TARGET) guide, available in print or freely accessible online format, is strongly recommended for further reference [45].

**Table 20.14** Blood collection tubes.

| Color | Content | Uses |
|---|---|---|
| Lavender/purple | EDTA anticoagulant | Hematology, Knott's heartworm, blood smear |
| Red | No active additives (but may contain other additives unless specifies "no additive") | Serum chemistries (wait at least 45 min before centrifuging blood), sterile urine/bodily fluid collection, Lee–White clotting time test[a]<br>Not a good choice for drug storage (use purpose bought sterile vials or emptied sterile water vials such as those provided with vaccines) |
| Red marble | Separation gel | Serum chemistries |
| Green | Heparin anticoagulant | Whole blood or plasma chemistries |
| Green marble | Heparin | Plasma separation |
| Gray | Diatomaceous earth, kaolin, celite, glass beads | Activated clotting time (ACT)[b] |
| Light blue | Citrate anticoagulant | Coagulation (PT, PTT, D-dimer, fibrinogen), DNA tests |

a) Lee–White clotting time[39]. Using gentle venipuncture technique, draw 0.5–1 ml of blood into a red top tube that has been heated to body temperature (suggest holding in armpit). Invert the tube every 30 s to observe for a clot. A Lee–White clotting time >10 min is likely to represent a coagulopathy in the intrinsic or common systems, such as seen with rodenticide toxicosis.

b) Activated coagulation time (ACT) [40,41]. Warm tube to body temperature (suggest holding in armpit). Use smooth venipuncture technique to avoid introducing tissue factor. Simultaneously draw the blood into the tube (mix well) and start a stop watch. Incubate for 1 min and then stop the stopwatch when the first formation of fibrin strands is seen. The reference values vary by substrate in humans and only MAX-ACT tubes have been validated in dogs and cats, with values >85 s considered abnormal. For other ACT tubes, the reference range is suggested to be <120 s for dogs and <100 s for cats. Note that factors must be markedly decreased to prolong the ACT.

**Table 20.15** Weights and measures equivalents and conversions.

| | Unit | SI unit equivalent |
|---|---|---|
| Length | Foot | 30.5 cm |
| | Yard | 91.4 cm |
| | Inch | 2.54 cm |
| Weight | Ounce | 28 g |
| | Pound | 0.45 kg |
| | Grain | 64.8 mg |
| | Ton | 907.2 kg |
| | Metric ton | 1000 kg |
| Volume | Teaspoon | 5 ml |
| | Tablespoon | 15 ml |
| | Ounce, liquid | 30 ml |
| | Pint | 473.2 ml |
| | Cup | 250 ml |
| | Quart | 946.4 ml |
| | Gallon | 3.8 L |

**Table 20.16** Temperature, pulse, and respiratory rate (TPR) reference ranges.

| | Dog | Cat |
|---|---|---|
| Temperature | 99.5–102.5 °F (37.5–39.2 °C) | 100–102.9 °F (37.8–39.4 °C) |
| Pulse (beats per minute) | 80–120 | 100–140 |
| Respiratory rate (breaths per minute) | 15–34 | 16–40 |

**Table 20.17** Hematologic reference ranges.

| | Units | Dog | Cat |
|---|---|---|---|
| PCV | % | 37.0–55.0 | 24.0–45.0 |
| Hemoglobin | g/dl | 12.0–18.0 | 8.0–15.0 |
| RBCs | $\times 10^6 \, \mu l^{-1}$ | 5.5–8.5 | 5.0–10.0 |
| Reticulocytes | % | 0–1.0 | 0–1.0 |
| Absolute reticulocyte count | $\times 10^3 \, \mu l^{-1}$ | <80 | <60 |
| MCV | fl | 60.6–77.0 | 39.0–55.0 |
| MCH | pg | 19.5–24.5 | 2.5–17.5 |
| MCHC | g/dl | 32.0–36.0 | 30.0–36.0 |
| Platelets[a] | $\times 10^3 \, \mu l^{-1}$ | 200–500 | 300–800 |
| MPV | fl | 5.4–9.2 | 12.1–15.1 |
| WBCs[b] | cells/μl | 6 000–17 000 | 5 500–19 500 |
| Neutrophils | % | 60–77 | 35–75 |
| Total protein | g/dl | 5.7–7.0 | 6.1–7.4 |

Source: Cowell et al. 2007 [42]. Reproduced with permission of Elsevier.

MCV, mean corpuscular volume; MCH, mean corpuscular hemoglobin; MCHC, mean corpuscular hemoglobin concentration.
a) 100× objective: average number of platelets in 10 monolayer fields × 15 000.
b) 10× objective: WBC estimate/μl = average number of WBCs in 10 fields × 150.

**Table 20.18** Temperature conversion.

| Fahrenheit | Celsius | Description |
|---|---|---|
| 32.0 | 0 | Freezing/melting point of water |
| 33.8 | 1 | |
| 35.6 | 2 | |
| 37.4 | 3 | |
| 39.2 | 4 | |
| 41.0 | 5 | |
| 42.8 | 6 | |
| 44.6 | 7 | |
| 46.4 | 8 | |
| 48.2 | 9 | |
| 50.0 | 10 | |
| 68.0 | 20 | |
| 69.8 | 21 | Room temperature |
| 86.0 | 30 | |
| 98.6 | 37 | |
| 101.0 | 38.8 | Typical rectal temperature |
| 104.0 | 40 | |
| 122.0 | 50 | |
| 140.0 | 60 | |
| 158.0 | 70 | |
| 176.0 | 80 | |
| 194.0 | 90 | |
| 212.0 | 100 | Boiling point of water |

$T_{(°F)} = T_{(°C)} \times 1.8 + 32.$
$T_{(°C)} = (T_{(°F)} - 32)/1.8.$

**Table 20.19** Urine volume and specific gravity.

| Species | Volume (ml/kg/day) | Specific gravity |
|---|---|---|
| Cat | 10–20 | 1.020–1.040 |
| Dog | 20–100 | 1.016–1.060 |

Source: Erickson et al. 2004 [43]. Reproduced with permission of John Wiley & Sons.

**Table 20.20** Body surface area (BSA).

| Weight | | BSA | Weight | | BSA |
|---|---|---|---|---|---|
| kg | lb | m$^2$ | kg | lb | m$^2$ |
| 0.5 | 1.1 | 0.06 | 26 | 57.2 | 0.88 |
| 1 | 2.2 | 0.1 | 27 | 59.4 | 0.9 |
| 2 | 4.4 | 0.15 | 28 | 61.6 | 0.92 |
| 3 | 6.6 | 0.2 | 29 | 63.8 | 0.94 |
| 4 | 8.8 | 0.25 | 30 | 66 | 0.96 |
| 5 | 11 | 0.29 | 31 | 68.2 | 0.99 |
| 6 | 13.2 | 0.33 | 32 | 70.4 | 1.01 |
| 7 | 15.4 | 0.36 | 33 | 72.6 | 1.03 |
| 8 | 17.6 | 0.4 | 34 | 74.7 | 1.05 |
| 9 | 19.8 | 0.43 | 35 | 77 | 1.07 |
| 10 | 22 | 0.46 | 36 | 79.2 | 1.09 |
| 11 | 24.2 | 0.49 | 37 | 81.4 | 1.11 |
| 12 | 26.4 | 0.52 | 38 | 83.6 | 1.13 |
| 13 | 28.6 | 0.55 | 39 | 85.8 | 1.15 |
| 14 | 30.8 | 0.58 | 40 | 88 | 1.17 |
| 15 | 33 | 0.6 | 41 | 90.2 | 1.19 |
| 16 | 35.2 | 0.63 | 42 | 92.4 | 1.21 |
| 17 | 37.4 | 0.66 | 43 | 94.6 | 1.23 |
| 18 | 39.6 | 0.69 | 44 | 96.8 | 1.25 |
| 19 | 41.8 | 0.71 | 45 | 99 | 1.26 |
| 20 | 44 | 0.74 | 46 | 101.2 | 1.28 |
| 21 | 46.2 | 0.76 | 47 | 103.4 | 1.3 |
| 22 | 48.4 | 0.78 | 48 | 105.6 | 1.32 |
| 23 | 50.6 | 0.81 | 49 | 107.8 | 1.34 |
| 24 | 52.8 | 0.83 | 50 | 110 | 1.36 |

Source: Adapted from Hill and Scott 2004 [44].

$BSA = 10 \times kg^{2/3}.$

**Table 20.21** Empiric antibiotic treatment of common medical conditions.

| Feline | Canine |
|---|---|
| *Pyoderma* | |
| Cefovecin 8 mg/kg once<br>Doxycycline 5 mg/kg q24h<br>Trimethoprim/sulfonamide 30 mg/kg q24h<br>Enrofloxacin 5 mg/kg q24h *(only if P. aeruginosa)* | Cefovecin 8 mg/kg once<br>Cephalexin 22 mg/kg q12h<br>Enrofloxacin 5 mg/kg q24h *(only if P. aeruginosa)* |
| *Urinary tract infection (UTI)* | |
| Cefazolin 15 mg/kg q12h<br>Cefovecin 8 mg/kg once<br>Trimethoprim/sulfonamide 30 mg/kg q24h<br>Enrofloxacin 5 mg/kg q24h *(only if P. aeruginosa)* | Cefovecin 8 mg/kg once<br>Cefpodoxime 5 mg/kg q24h<br>Ceftiofur 2.2 mg/kg q24h<br>Trimethoprim/sulfonamide 30 mg/kg q24h<br>Enrofloxacin 5 mg/kg q24h *(only if P. aeruginosa)* |
| *Upper respiratory infection (URI)* [a] | |
| Doxycycline 10 mg/kg q24h<br>Enrofloxacin 5 mg/kg q24h *(only if P. aeruginosa)* | Doxycycline 5 mg/kg q24h<br>Enrofloxacin 5 mg/kg q24h *(only if P. aeruginosa)* |
| *Soft tissue infection* | |
| Amoxicillin 11 mg/kg q12h<br>Amoxicillin-clavulanate 13.75 mg/kg q12h<br>Cefovecin 8 mg/kg once<br>Enrofloxacin 5 mg/kg q24h *(only if P. aeruginosa)* | Amoxicillin-clavulanate 13.75 mg/kg q12h<br>Cefovecin 8 mg/kg once *(not effective against P. aeruginosa or Enterococcus spp.)*<br>Enrofloxacin 5 mg/kg q24h |
| *Oral/gingival infection* | |
| Amoxicillin 11 mg/kg q12h<br>Amoxicillin-clavulanate 13.75 mg/kg q12h<br>Cefazolin 15 mg/kg q12h<br>Cefovecin 8 mg/kg once | Cefovecin 8 mg/kg once<br>Ceftiofur 2.2 mg/kg q24h<br>Cephalexin 22 mg/kg q12h *(poor efficacy against Enterococcus spp.)*<br>Clindamycin 5.5 mg/kg q12h *(not effective against Pasteurella multocida or E. coli)*<br>Enrofloxacin 5 mg/kg q24h |
| *Otitis (outer ear)* [b] | |
| Unusual; no established empiric treatment | Cefovecin 8 mg/kg once<br>Ceftiofur 2.2 mg/kg q24h<br>Enrofloxacin 10 mg/kg q24h *(middle/inner ear infections or if P. aeruginosa)* |
| *Osteomyelitis (bone)* | |
| Amoxicillin 11 mg/kg q12h<br>Amoxicillin-clavulanate 13.75 mg/kg q12h<br>Enrofloxacin 5 mg/kg q24h *(only if P. aeruginosa)* | Enrofloxacin 5 mg/kg q24h |

a) The Antimicrobial Guidelines Working Group of the International Society for Companion Animal Infectious Diseases recommends that antimicrobial treatment be considered only if fever, lethargy, or anorexia is present concurrently with mucopurulent discharge [46].

b) Physical exam findings that may indicate the presence of certain organisms in the absence of cytology [47]:
- Dark brown waxy or dry exudates: yeast (dogs), ear mites (cats)
- Creamy tan-colored moist exudates: gram + bacteria (*Staphylococcus* spp.)
- Purulent or mucoid exudates with a white, yellow, green, or black color: gram − bacteria (*Pseudomonas* spp.).

Table 20.22 Emergency drug doses.

| Indication | Drug | Concentration | Dose (IV) | Weight (kg) 2.5 / Weight (lb) 5 / ml | 5 / 10 / ml | 10 / 20 / ml | 15 / 30 / ml | 20 / 40 / ml | 25 / 50 / ml | 30 / 60 / ml | 35 / 70 / ml | 40 / 80 / ml | 45 / 90 / ml | 50 / 100 / ml |
|---|---|---|---|---|---|---|---|---|---|---|---|---|---|---|
| Cardiac arrest | Epinephrine low dose 1:1000 | 1 mg/ml | 0.01 mg/kg | 0.03 | 0.05 | 0.10 | 0.15 | 0.20 | 0.25 | 0.30 | 0.35 | 0.40 | 0.45 | 0.50 |
| | Epinephrine high dose 1:1000 | 1 mg/ml | 0.1 mg/kg | 0.25 | 0.50 | 1.00 | 1.50 | 2.00 | 2.50 | 3.00 | 3.50 | 4.00 | 4.50 | 5.00 |
| | Atropine | 0.5 mg/ml | 0.05 mg/kg | 0.25 | 0.50 | 1.00 | 1.50 | 2.00 | 2.50 | 3.00 | 3.50 | 4.00 | 4.50 | 5.00 |
| | Glycopyrrolate | 0.2 mg/ml | 0.01 mg/kg | 0.13 | 0.25 | 6.25 | 0.75 | 1.00 | 1.25 | 1.50 | 1.75 | 2.00 | 2.25 | 2.50 |
| | Vasopressin | 20 U/ml | 0.8 U/kg | 0.10 | 0.20 | 0.40 | 0.60 | 0.80 | 1.00 | 1.20 | 1.40 | 1.60 | 1.80 | 2.00 |
| Antiarrhythmia | Lidocaine (dog) | 20 mg/ml | 2 mg/kg | 0.25 | 0.50 | 1.00 | 1.50 | 2.00 | 2.50 | 3.00 | 3.50 | 4.00 | 4.50 | 5.00 |
| | Lidocaine (cat) | 20 mg/ml | 0.2 mg/kg | 0.03 | 0.05 | 0.10 | | | | | | | | |
| Reversal | Atipamezole | 5 mg/ml | 0.05 mg/kg | 0.03 | 0.05 | 0.10 | 0.15 | 0.20 | 0.25 | 0.30 | 0.35 | 0.40 | 0.45 | 0.50 |
| | Flumazenil | 0.1 mg/ml | 0.01 mg/kg | 0.25 | 0.50 | 1.00 | 1.50 | 2.00 | 2.50 | 3.00 | 3.50 | 4.00 | 4.50 | 5.00 |
| | Naloxone | 0.4 mg/ml | 0.04 mg/kg | 0.25 | 0.50 | 6.25 | 1.50 | 2.00 | 2.50 | 3.00 | 3.50 | 4.00 | 4.50 | 5.00 |

# References

1 AVMA. The veterinarian-client-patient relationship (VCPR) is the basis for interaction among veterinarians, their clients, and their patients and is critical to the health of your animal. https://www.avma.org/KB/Resources/Reference/Documents/VCPR_printable.pdf (accessed 12 December 2017).

2 eCFR. Code of federal regulations. http://www.ecfr.gov/ (accessed 12 December 2017).

3 US FDA (1994). Animal Medicinal Drug Use Clarification Act (AMDUCA) of 1994 (AMDUCA). https://www.fda.gov/AnimalVeterinary/GuidanceComplianceEnforcement/ActsRulesRegulations/ucm085377.htm (accessed 3 February 2017).

4 AVMA (2016). Administration and dispensing of compounded veterinary drugs. https://www.avma.org/Advocacy/StateAndLocal/Pages/compoundinglaws.aspx (accessed 13 January 2017).

5 FDA (1970). Controlled Substances Act. https://www.fda.gov/RegulatoryInformation/LawsEnforcedbyFDA/ucm148726.htm (accessed 10 February 2017).

6 DEA (2017). Import/export permit applications and declarations – medical missions. https://www.deadiversion.usdoj.gov/imp_exp/med_missions.htm (accessed 12 March 207).

7 Powell, L.L. (2014). Top five indications for fluid therapy. In: Veterinary Team Brief, 10–12. https://www.veterinaryteambrief.com/article/top-5-indications-fluid-therapy.

8 Davis, H., Jensen, T., Johnson, A. et al. (2013). 2013 AAHA/AAFP fluid therapy guidelines for dogs and cats. *Journal of the American Animal Hospital Association* **49**: 149–159.

9 Lee, J.A. Subcutaneous fluids: How much should you give to your veterinary patients? In: VetFolio.

10 Guillaumin, J., Olp, N., Magnusson, K. et al. (2013). Influence of hang time on bacterial colonization of intravenous bags in a veterinary emergency and critical care setting. *Journal of Veterinary Emergency and Critical Care* **23**: S6.

11 Matthews, K.A. and Taylor, D.K. (2011). Assessment of sterility in fluid bags maintained for chronic use. *Journal of the American Association for Laboratory Animal Science* **50** (5): 708–712.

12 Pachtinger, G.E. (2014). Hypovolemic shock. In: Clinician's Brief, 13–16.

13 Papich, M.G. (2005). Drug compounding for veterinary patients. *Journal of the American Association of Pharmaceutical Scientists* **7** (2): 281–287.

14 Ko, J.C., Knesl, O., Weil, A.B. et al. (2009). FAQs analgesia, sedation, and anesthesia. *Compendium on Continuing Education for the Practising Veterinarian* **31** (1): 1–16.

15 Lawler, D.F. (2008). Neonatal and pediatric care of the puppy and kitten. *Theriogenology* **70** (3): 384–392.

16 Heggers, J.P., Sazy, J.A., Stenberg, B.D. et al. (1991). Bactericidal and wound healing properties of sodium hypochlorite solutions: the 1991 Lindberg Award. *The Journal of Burn Care & Rehabilitation* **12** (5): 420–424.

17 Ahmed, N., Shahzad, M.N., Qureshi, K.H. et al. (2011). Effectiveness of 0.025% Dakin's solution versus 1% silver sulphadiazine for treatment of partial thickness burns. *Annals of Pakistan Institue of Medical Sciences* **7** (3): 127–132.

18 Nagoya, B.S., Deshmukh, S.R., Wadher, B.J., and Patil, S.B. (2008). Acetic acid treatment of pseudomonal wound infection. *European Journal of General Medicine* **5** (2): 104–106.

19 Fellows, J. and Crestodina, L. (2006). Home-prepared saline: a safe, cost-effective alternative for wound cleansing in home care. *Journal of Wound Ostomy & Continence Nursing* **33** (6): 606–609.

20 Suh, J.-S., Hahn, W.-H., and Cho, B.-S. (2010). Recent advances of oral rehydration therapy (ORT). *Electrolytes & Blood Pressure* **8** (2): 82.

21 How, T.H., Loo, W.Y., Yow, K.L. et al. (1998). Stability of cefazolin sodium eye drops. *Journal of Clinical Pharmacy and Therapeutics* **23** (1): 41–47.

22 Youssef, M., Sadaka, H., Eissa, M., and El-Ariny, A. (1995). Topical application of ivermectin for human ectoparasites. *American Journal of Tropical Medicine and Hygiene* **53** (6): 652–653.

23 Anderson, D.L. and Roberson, E.L. (1982). Activity of ivermectin against canine intestinal helminths. *American Journal of Veterinary Research* **43** (9): 1681–1683.

24 Petritz, O.A., Guzman, D.S., Wiebe, V.J., and Papich, M.G. (2013). Stability of three commonly compounded extemporaneous enrofloxacin suspensions for oral administration to exotic

animals. *Journal of the American Veterinary Association* **243** (1): 85–90.

25 Nuttall, T. (2016) Successful management of otitis externa. *Practice*, **38** (Suppl. 2), 17–21.

26 Griffin, C.E. (2007). Otitis topical and systemic. Proceedings of the SCIVAC Congress, Rimini, Italy, pp. 270–272.

27 Matousek, J.L., Campbell, K.L., Kakoma, I., and Schaeffer, D.J. (2003). The effects of four acidifying sprays, vinegar, and water on canine cutaneous pH levels. *Journal of the American Animal Hospital Association* **39** (1): 29–33.

28 Nuttall, T. and Cole, L.K. (2004). Ear cleaning: the UK and US perspective. *Veterinary Dermatology* **15** (2): 127–136.

29 Spohr, A., Schjoth, B., Wiinberg, B., et al. (2009). Antibiotic use guidelines for companion animal practice. http://www.fecava.org/sites/default/files/files/DSAVA_AntibioticGuidelines%20-%20v1-1_3 (1).pdf (accessed 12 December 2017).

30 Papich, M.G., Davidson, G.S., and Fortier, L.A. (2013). Doxycycline concentration over time after storage in a compounded veterinary preparation. *Journal of the American Veterinary Medical Association* **242** (12): 1674–1678.

31 Gessler, E.M., Hart, A.K., Dunlevy, T.M., and Greinwald, J.H. (2001). Optimal concentration of epinephrine for vasoconstriction in ear surgery. *Laryngoscope* **111** (10): 1687–1690.

32 Kjønniksen, I., Brustugun, J., Niemi, G. et al. (2000). Stability of an epidural analgesic solution containing adrenaline, bupivacaine and fentanyl. *Acta Anaesthesiologica Scandinavia* **44** (7): 864–867.

33 Dodd, M.J., Dibble, S.L., Miaskowski, C. et al. (2000). Randomized clinical trial of the effectiveness of 3 commonly used mouthwashes to treat chemotherapy-induced mucositis. *Oral Surgery, Oral Medicine, Oral Patholology, Oral Radiology* **90**: 39–47.

34 Harms, C.A., McLellan, W.A., Moore, M.J. et al. (2014). Low-residue euthanasia of stranded mysticetes. *Journal of Wildlife Diseases* **50** (1): 63–73.

35 WSPA (2007). Methods for the euthanasia of dogs and cats: comparison and recommendations. http://www.icam-coalition.org/downloads/Methods%20for%20the%20euthanasia%20of%20dogs%20and%20cats-%20English.pdf (accessed 12 December 2017).

36 AVMA (2013). AVMA Guidelines for the Euthanasia of Animals: 2013 Edition. https://www.avma.org/KB/Policies/Documents/euthanasia.pdf (accessed 3 March 2017).

37 Aranez, J.B., Caday, L.B., Avariez, J.B., and Caday, L.B. (1958). Magnesium sulphate euthanasia in dogs. *Journal of the American Veterinary Medical Association* **133** (4): 213–214.

38 Carding, T. (1977). Euthanasia of cats and dogs. *Animal Regulation Studies* **1**: 15–21.

39 Abrams-Ogg, A. (2011). Assessment & disorders of secondary hemostasis. Western Veterinary Conference, Las Vegas (20–24 February 2011).

40 David, M. (2009). Coagulation: guide to bleeding disorders. Wild West Veterinary Conference, Reno.

41 See, A.M., Swindells, K.L., Sharman, M.J. et al. (2009). Activated coagulation times in normal cats and dogs using MAX-ACT TM tubes. *Australian Veterinary Journal* **87** (7): 292–295.

42 Cowell, R.L., Tyler, R., Meinkoth, J., and DeNicola, D. (2007). Diagnostic Cytology and Hematology of the Dog and Cat, 4e. Mosby.

43 Erickson, H.H., Jesse, P.G., and Uemura, E.E. (2004). Dukes' Physiology of Domestic Animals. Cornell University Press.

44 Hill, R.C. and Scott, K.C. (2004). Energy requirements and body surface area of cats and dogs. *Journal of the American Veterinary Medical Association* **225** (5): 689–694.

45 Aucoin, D. (2007). Target: the Antimicrobial Reference Guide to Effective Treatment. North American Compendiums, Inc.

46 Weese, J.S., Blondeau, J.M., Boothe, D. et al. (2011). Antimicrobial use guidelines for treatment of urinary tract disease in dogs and cats: antimicrobial guidelines working group of the International Society for Companion Animal Infectious Diseases. *Veterinary Medicine International* 263768.

47 Gotthelf, L.N. (2016). Examination of the ear. *Clinician's Brief* 64–72.

# Index